TEXTBOOK OF
MEDICAL-SURGICAL NURSING

CONTRIBUTORS

Leonard S. Bushnell, M.D.

Departments: Anesthesia and Respiratory Therapy, Beth Israel Hospital and Harvard Medical School

Sharon Spaeth Bushnell, R.N.

Departments: Anesthesia and Respiratory Therapy and Nursing, Beth Israel Hospital, Boston

James F. Elam, Ph.D.

Clinical Biochemist, Pathology Department, Alexandria Hospital, Alexandria, Virginia

Robert J. Gill, M.D.

Associate Physician, Pennsylvania Hospital, Philadelphia, Pa.; Assistant Professor of Clinical Medicine, University of Pennsylvania, School of Medicine

Silvia Lange, R.N., M.N.

Psychiatric Nurse, Community Mental Health Services, Day Center, San Diego, California; formerly Assistant Professor and Director, Mental Health Program, Seattle University

Richard E. Palmer, M.D., F.A.C.P.

Pathologist, Alexandria Hospital, Alexandria, Virginia; Clinical Associate Professor, George Washington University Hospital School of Medicine, Washington, D.C.; formerly President, American Society of Clinical Pathologists

H. Millard Smith, M.D., Ph.D.

Formerly Director of Clinical Pharmacology, Schering Corporation; Associate Professor of Physiology, University of Arkansas; Associate Professor of Physiology, Loma Linda University

William D. Snively, Jr., M.D.

Clinical Professor, Department of Pediatrics, University of Alabama; formerly Vice-President; Medical Affairs, Mead Johnson & Company, Evansville, Indiana

Gerald H. Whipple, M.D.

Associate Professor of Medicine, University of California, Irvine

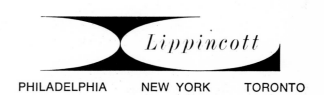

Lippincott

PHILADELPHIA   NEW YORK   TORONTO

TEXTBOOK OF

MEDICAL-SURGICAL NURSING

second edition

Lillian Sholtis Brunner

R.N., B.S., M.S., Consultant in Medical-Surgical Nursing at the School of Nursing, Hospital of the University of Pennsylvania and the Bryn Mawr Hospital School of Nursing; formerly Assistant Professor of Surgical Nursing, Yale University School of Nursing.

Charles Phillips Emerson, Jr.

A.B., M.D., Associate Professor of Medicine and Chief of Hematology Section, Department of Clinical Research, Boston University School of Medicine; Senior Visiting Physician and Director of Clinical Laboratories, Massachusetts Memorial Hospital, Boston University Medical Center; Hematology Consultant, U. S. Public Health Service.

L. Kraeer Ferguson

A.B., M.D., F.A.C.S., Late Professor of Surgery, School of Medicine and Graduate School of Medicine, University of Pennsylvania.

Doris Smith Suddarth

R.N., B.S.N.E., M.S.N., Consultant in Health Occupations, Job Corps Health Office, U. S. Department of Labor; formerly Coordinator of the Curriculum, Alexandria Hospital School of Nursing.

Preface

The practitioner of nursing in this decade will require ever increasing knowledge, understanding and overall sophistication in order to achieve professional standards of competence. The student of nursing must learn to observe and assess signs, symptoms, reactions and behavior, understand the pathophysiology underlying many disease conditions, and be able to apply principles from the biological, physical, social, behavioral and medical sciences in the care of medical and surgical patients. Involved are the processes of assessing patients, formulating nursing judgments and intervening on a rational basis. This textbook includes in-depth discussion of the clinical conditions and problems most frequently seen in nursing practice.

The first 5 units focus on the patient as a person and in relation to his problems, needs and care. The first unit assists in problem identification and observation skills, and in understanding the aging process. The completely new chapter *Illness as a Human Experience* explores common behavioral responses to illness. In Unit II, there is another new chapter, *The Internal Environment: Homeostatic Mechanisms and Pathophysiologic Processes*. This chapter presents a physiologic analysis of the causes of disease. Supportive and therapeutic modalities that are necessary in the care of all patients are presented in Unit III. The chapter on fluids and electrolytes, *Body Fluid Disturbances*, has been completely rewritten. The continuum of care of the surgical patient is described in Unit IV as preoperative, intraoperative and postoperative management. Principles of rehabilitation are in a separate unit. Throughout the book, the significance of the nurse's role in building the confidence of the patient is stressed because successful rehabilitation depends on this key factor.

Units 6 to 19 cover specific conditions of illness. Where pertinent, nutritional and pharmacologic aspects are included. For additional information the student is referred to appropriate textbooks. Teachers of nursing are free to adapt their own methods of subject presentation. The authors believe that therapeutic and nursing management cannot be separated, since each complements and is essential to the other. The nurse must understand the therapeutic regimen and its rationale in order to develop a personalized plan of care for each patient. Also inherent in planning care is the understanding of the emotional components of illness and the basic precepts of their management. Behavioral concepts are identified and given consideration as they relate to specific illnesses.

Because the practical and the theoretical sides of nursing are of equal importance, attention has been paid to "doing," knowing *why* and *how* to carry out specific nursing activities. The discussion of each has been made as complete as possible. This has been stressed because many of the activities which professional nurses usually performed are now being delegated to auxiliary personnel, and too often are performed less adeptly.

It is recommended that the student use this book on the patient unit in the development of nursing care plans and patient studies. The aims and objectives of medical and nursing management are set forth whenever possible so that the student will be assisted in the selection of realistic patient and nursing goals. The authors recommend that the student refer to the medical-surgical nursing textbook early in the first clinical assignment. As more complex experiences are presented, the textbook is designed to incorporate increasing depth.

Much thought and consideration were given to the acute and complex problems of patients in intensive care units. Specific entities are discussed in their appropriate chapters. Because research and experience indicate that a large percentage of patients in ICU need airway assistance and ventilation, a new chapter, *Respiratory Intensive Care Nursing*, is presented. This includes additional material on respiratory physiology, recognition of respiratory failure, and methods used in respiratory therapy. Another new chapter, *The Patient in the Cardiac Care Unit*, deals with this area of specialization. Principles of electrocardiography and the nursing management of patients requiring cardiac monitoring and cardiac pacing are emphasized. Because of the seriousness of these conditions and the necessity for immediate action, there is a series of guidelines for nursing in the cardiac care unit at the end of the chapter which summarize the principal management features for cardiac patients requiring specialized medical and nursing skills.

A new section on dental care is placed at the beginning of the chapter on upper gastrointestinal conditions. The chapter on burns has been completely redone; prevention and emergency therapy are stressed. The physiologic effects of burns, on local tissues as well as systemically, are explained in detail. The rationale for the various current therapies is also given.

Although not included in some contemporary nursing texts, much detail has been given in the area of dermatology, since patients with skin problems do seek the support of an understanding nurse. The authors also believe that communicable disease nursing takes on new meaning as nursing frontiers broaden to include world health problems, especially those of the peoples of developing nations. This section has been updated.

Emergency and disaster nursing requires a composite of knowledge and abilities that are gained in studying and caring for patients with a wide variety of conditions. This subject is covered in the latter part of the book, since the student must have competence in nursing practice to make the critical judgments so necessary for effective care of these patients.

Because of pressing space limitations, the most common laboratory tests and their clinical significance have been tabulated in the Appendix. However, diagnostic evaluation tests requiring significant nursing understanding and participation are discussed where applicable throughout the text. Nursing in the operating room is also found in the Appendix. The material has been made current and new illustrations are included to orient the nurse to this important clinical specialty.

Every chapter has been updated, and there have been particularly extensive revisions of the following:

Nursing in Conditions of the Nose and Throat
Patients with Medical and Surgical Conditions of the Chest
Patients with Vascular Disorders
Patients with Conditions of the Heart
Patients with Conditions of the Mouth, Neck and Esophagus
Patients with Disorders of the Liver and the Biliary Tract
Patients with Renal and Genitourinary Problems
Nursing the Patient with a Gynecologic Condition
Nursing in Endocrine and Metabolic Disorders
Patients with Problems of the Eye
Patients with Problems of the Ear and the Mastoid
Patients with Neurologic and Neurosurgical Problems
Patients with Musculoskeletal Conditions

In many clinical areas a specific vocabulary is necessary for understanding and communication, and this has been provided, with definitions.

Patients seek factual advice and simple answers to their questions concerning problems they anticipate after leaving the hospital. Patient education guidelines have been added to help the nurse know *what* to teach the patient. The medical and nursing management summaries that found such gratifying acceptance in the previous edition have been retained and new ones developed.

To further enhance the value of this volume, there is wide cross-referencing besides a complete index. The entries in the bibliography were carefully selected to ensure their being appropriate, up-to-date and authoritative. At the end of each chapter are listed agencies and materials for patient education. Many new illustrations have been added. Legends are designed to focus the attention of the student on key points in the illustrations.

Because the art is long, the subject matter vast and the value of human life immeasurable, the study of nursing is the task of a lifetime. We offer this volume in the hope that it will increase understanding and clinical expertise as the nurse engages in the most challenging and rewarding of tasks, that of caring for patients.

Acknowledgments

The authors are grateful to the many individuals listed below who have offered objective criticism and shared unselfishly their special knowledge.

For Medical Science:

Robert D. Dripps, Jr., M.D., Professor and Chairman
Dept. of Anesthesia, School of Medicine,
University of Pennsylvania

Ira Green, M.D.., F.A.C.A., Associate Radiologist,
Alexandria, Virginia

Inta A. Grots, M.D., Associate Professor of
Dermatology, Boston University School of Medicine

G. Khodadad, M.D., Assistant Professor of Neurological
Surgery, School of Medicine,
University of Pennsylvania

Philip Kimbel, M.D., Director, Pulmonary
Rehabilitation Project, Moss Rehabilitation Hospital,
Philadelphia, Pa.

Stephen Levin, M.D., Clinical Instructor in
Orthopedics, Howard University, Washington, D.C.

William R. McCabe, M.D., Associate Professor of
Medicine, Boston University School of Medicine

Cyril N. Luce, M.D., Associate Surgeon,
Wills Eye Hospital; Instructor, School of Medicine,
Temple University, Philadelphia, Pa.

Jesse Nicholson, M.D., Emeritus Professor of
Orthopedic Surgery, Graduate School of Medicine,
University of Pennsylvania

James Nixon, M.D., Assistant Professor of Orthopedic
Surgery, Graduate School of Medicine,
University of Pennsylvania

Richard Rhame, M.D., Assistant Clinical Professor of
Urology, George Washington University School of
Medicine, Washington, D.C.

For Nursing and Allied Health Specialties:

Special thanks to Jean DeVries, R.N., Operating Room
Supervisor, Alexandria Hospital, Alexandria,
Virginia, and Joan A. Safko, R.N., M.S.Ed.,
Assistant Director, School of Nursing, Hospital
of the University of Pennsylvania.

Gilbert Banenelli, Orthopedic Technician
Brenda Bare, R.N., Instructor in Nursing
Herman Brotman, Research Statistician
Loretta Call, R.N., Cardiac Nurse Clinician
Julita Gray, R.N., Educational Coordinator
Arleen Gordon, R.N., Project Nurse,
    Pulmonary Rehab. Project
Esther Lione, R.N., Operating Room Supervisor
Gerald E. Kay, Inhalation Therapist
Louise J. LaBorwit, Speech Pathologist
Marian Korczowski, M.S., Dietitian
Miriam Zumwalt, R.P.T. Rehabilitation Consultant

For Art Work:

Steven Gigliotti
Patricia Kenny
Lt. Col. Constance Ferebee, A.N.C.
John O'Connor, M.D.

For Research and Library Assistance:

Mrs. Evelyn F. Bowling, Bryn Mawr Hospital
Naomi Lanham, Alexandria Hospital
Laura Stewart, Fairfax Hospital
Lois Topping, Alexandria Hospital
Edith Blair, Alvin Barnes, and Howard Drew,
    all of the National Library of Medicine

For Editorial Assistance:

J. Stuart Freeman, Jr.
Margaret· Sommer
Carol Kerr
Vincent Gordon

Last, but far from least, for his guidance, determination, understanding . . . we are indeed grateful to David T. Miller, Editorial Manager, Nursing Department, J. B. Lippincott Company.

Contents

UNIT SIXTEEN: *Nursing in Conditions of the Nervous System*

UNIT SEVENTEEN: *Nursing in Musculoskeletal Conditions*

TEXTBOOK OF

MEDICAL-SURGICAL NURSING

CHAPTER 1

The Patient and His Problems

- *The Patient's Problems: His Troublesome Symptoms*
- *The Patient's Basic Needs*
- *Patient Assessment and Planning Patient Care*
- *The Team Approach to Patient Care*
- *Nursing Abilities*

Nursing is a service devoted to the prevention and the relief of physical suffering. Inherent in nursing is the control of disease, the care and rehabilitation of the sick and the promotion of health through teaching and counseling. The nurse, applying her technical knowledge, experience and skill, combats the physical disabilities of her patients, and through the contribution of her wisdom and insight, she assists them to overcome their emotional difficulties.

The central figure in and the principal object of these services is, of course, the patient. The patient comes to the hospital as an individual, a member of a family and a citizen of the community. He comes with a health problem and is laden, in addition, with a number of personal concerns that have been exaggerated and compounded by illness. Confronting him, perhaps, are problems that he feels are at once inescapable and insurmountable; problems that demand a solution but are incapable of solution; problems for which he feels solely responsible, which he is reluctant to share and refuses to delegate. He may be wholly absorbed in problems that are of minor consequence while dismissing others that truly are of paramount importance relative to his illness, which may bear, for example, on the prevention of complications or recurrences of his disease, or on the pursuit of his rehabilitation. As a potential source of frustration and anxiety

and as an impediment to recovery, these personal problems naturally are of concern to the nurse; and to help her patient to sort them out, reduce them to their essentials, place them in proper perspective and cope with them effectively is one of her important functions.

The nurse, by virtue of her proximity and accessibility to the patient, is in a position to discover and identify his problems, to establish his needs and to plan his care appropriately. And while directing her attention to the problems of immediate importance—the overt problems—she must be ever alert to sense the subtle, unexpressed needs of her patient, needs that may be influencing his behavior and may be producing, or at least modifying, his symptoms.

THE PATIENT'S PROBLEMS: HIS TROUBLESOME SYMPTOMS

From the standpoint of the symptomatic patient, the most important problem confronting him is his major symptom. If he is gasping for breath, his most pressing need is to be relieved of his respiratory distress. Dyspnea is his primary problem. The nurse must undertake to evaluate this symptom and alleviate it.

If she is to deal with this problem effectively she must understand correctly the pathologic physiology underlying her patient's dyspnea. Is it caused by pul-

TABLE 1-1. Deaths and death rates for 10 leading causes of death in specified age groups: 1965*

Rank	Age and Cause of Death	Number	Rate per 100,000 population in age group
	25-44 Years		
	ALL CAUSES	108,402	233.2
1.	All accidents	22,228	47.8
2.	Diseases of heart	20,852	44.9
3.	Cancer and other malignant neoplasms	18,980	40.8
4.	Suicide	6,785	14.6
5.	Homicide	5,037	10.8
6.	Cerebral hemorrhage and other vascular lesions affecting central nervous system ("stroke")	4,810	10.3
7.	Cirrhosis of liver	4,427	9.5
8.	Influenza and pneumonia, except pneumonia of newborn	2,708	5.8
9.	Diabetes mellitus	1,725	3.7
10.	Other diseases of circulatory system	1,688	3.6
	45-64 Years		
	ALL CAUSES	450,313	1,155.1
1.	Diseases of heart	176,474	452.7
2.	Cancer and other malignant neoplasms	108,207	277.6
3.	Cerebral hemorrhage and other vascular lesions affecting central nervous system ("stroke")	31,617	81.1
4.	All accidents	22,900	58.7
5.	Cirrhosis of liver	13,815	35.4
6.	Influenza and pneumonia, except pneumonia of newborn	8,973	23.0
7.	Diabetes mellitus	8,754	22.5
8.	Suicide	8,594	22.0
9.	Other bronchopulmonic diseases	7,627	19.6
10.	Other diseases of circulatory system	7,456	19.1
	65 Years and Over		
	ALL CAUSES	1,110,841	6,118.3
1.	Diseases of heart	512,707	2,823.9
2.	Cancer and other malignant neoplasms	163,657	901.4
3.	Cerebral hemorrhage and other vascular lesions affecting central nervous system ("stroke")	163,586	901.0
4.	Influenza and pneumonia, except pneumonia of newborn	38,795	213.7
5.	General arteriosclerosis	36,121	198.9
6.	All accidents	28,134	155.0
7.	Diabetes mellitus	22,308	122.9
8.	Other diseases of circulatory system	17,679	97.4
9.	Other bronchopulmonic diseases	16,593	91.4
10.	Other hypertensive disease	8,593	47.3

* From "Facts of Life and Death," Public Health Service, 1967.

monary congestion? by pneumonia? by pleurisy? or by asthma? Does the patient have respiratory obstruction? Should he be placed in an orthopneic position? or in low Fowler's position? or should he lie flat? Should he be receiving oxygen? Is he in need of tracheal suction? Is a tracheotomy likely to be required? Should a sedative be administered, or is sedative medication strictly contraindicated in this patient? Close scrutiny of an occasional patient might convince the nurse that his breathing, although abnormally rapid and deep, is not attended by discomfort and does not involve undue effort. In other words, this particular patient is not dyspneic but hyperpneic. Hyperpnea is a different symptom altogether, and the problems it entails are quite different from those of dyspnea. Is this a case of hysterical hyperventilation? or diabetic acidosis? or has this patient been poisoned? On the appropriate answers to these and to a host of other pertinent questions may hinge the correctness of diagnosis, the effectiveness of treatment and, in many instances, the very survival of such a patient.

Every step in the care of the patient represents a team effort, as will be discussed later; and a key member of the medical team that is charged with this responsibility is the professional nurse. Among the most important of her contributions to this joint effort are her clinical observations. To what extent these observations are significant, informative and helpful depends on how well she knows and understands symptoms. Confronted with one, she must be able to recognize it as a pathologic deviation from the normal. Moreover, she should be able to relate the abnormal manifestation to the particular organ system whence it is likely to have originated and accordingly which might be the site of disease. Details concerning the nature, the mechanism and the significance of specific symptoms and other nursing observations are discussed in later chapters of this text.

The nurse's knowledge of symptomatology, and of causative factors, treatment and prevention as well, should extend to all of the common medical and surgical conditions. Most of the serious illnesses she will encounter will represent various stages of the diseases listed in Table 1-1, specifying the leading causes of death in the United States.

THE PATIENT'S BASIC NEEDS

Common to all human beings are certain needs that are basic and demand satisfaction. Unfulfilled needs in this category are among the patient's most pressing problems. These differ in their urgency; as each is satisfied, a "higher" one emerges and takes precedence. Ranked in order of priority* they include the following: physiologic needs, safety needs, the need to belong, the need for recognition, esteem and affection, the need to create, the need for knowledge and comprehension; and aesthetic needs.

Physiologic Needs. These needs predominate in the motivation of human behavior and drive the mechanisms that maintain *homeostasis*—the constancy of the internal environment of an organism. It involves the regulation of respiratory, nutritive and excretory functions, as well as maintenance of the water content of tissues, adjustments of body temperature and the operation of numerous protective mechanisms. These needs are powerful; unless satisfied, they dominate the conscious mind. For example, if a patient is obliged to restrict his fluid intake for therapeutic reasons, thirst will absorb his thoughts. He may discuss nothing but drinking, complain incessantly of thirst and repeatedly question his nurse and physician as to when fluids will be forthcoming. During this period he is not likely to be too concerned about the aesthetic features of his environment. As soon as his thirst is quenched he becomes aware of other needs; now he may be disturbed by the absence of privacy.

* Maslow, A. H.: *Motivation and Personality*, New York, Harper, 1954.

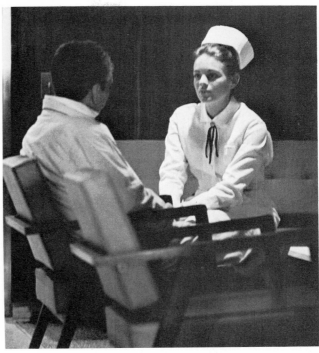

Courtesy of Peter Dechert.

FIG. 1-1. A basic emotional need is the need to communicate with others. Listening to the patient express his feelings helps him maintain his sense of security and self esteem.

Safety Needs. If the physiologic needs are satisfied, the concern for safety emerges. The normal adult is able to protect himself and usually does not feel endangered. He is relatively "safe" from death. His job is "safe." His insurance program and his savings account furnish a sense of economic security.

Illness naturally poses a threat. The sick person may be apprehensive in response to the many different persons with unfamiliar functions who enter his room. Diagnostic tests and therapeutic procedures may contribute to his fears. He wants to feel safe and secure. Although he may not express his feelings in these terms, he wants the health team to be aware of his insecurity. In order to help to protect the patient from danger the nurse must know the nature of his illness and be cognizant of its possible complications, so that she may be in a position to forestall the latter, if they are preventable, and to supply intelligent care if they should occur. The nurse's role in promoting the psychological safety of the patient is discussed in Chapter 3.

Need for Affection and Recognition. His physiologic and safety needs having been satisfied, the patient's need for affection will become apparent. Every individual, sick or well, desires the companionship and recognition of others. A sick person wants and needs his family or, in its absence, friends, or even just friendliness. The wise nurse is constantly aware of this need and of its importance in relation to her patient's morale. She will help the family members to feel that they have a definite contribution to make to his recovery. She will seek relevant information from them concerning his habits, his preferences and his antipathies, and will be guided by this information to whatever extent may be possible.

Man is by nature a social being, abhorring isolation. Illness removes him from his relatively convivial world and transplants him into a strange environment, an environment that is entirely unsought and unfamiliar, one in which he feels incompetent and alone. Previously an actively contributing member of society, he now must accept a position of dependency. This patient needs to preserve his self-esteem. He needs to be recognized as an individual, a distinct personality. The professional nurse, imbued with the concept of the individual worth and the dignity of man, sees to it that this need is fulfilled. She takes time to listen to her patient. To the extent that he desires it and opportunity permits it she joins him in conversation. She exhibits interest, not only in matters that concern her, but also in all matters that seem important to him—her attentiveness, thoughtfulness and kindliness conveying the conviction that he is held in esteem and affection, and that his needs and problems are recognized.

The Creative Impulses. His physiologic needs having been compensated, feeling secure, esteemed and wanted, the patient's creative impulses may now emerge. During the course of a short hospital stay this need is not likely to be frustrated. However, the patient with a protracted illness must be assured an opportunity to express himself creatively and to be, or at least feel, useful.

The Need to Know and to Understand. This need is a strong drive. The intelligent person seeks information, organizes it, analyzes it and searches for its meaning. In general, patients want to know what is in store for them, and they are thwarted by explanations that are too brief or vague. Many have studied and know a surprising amount concerning the bodily functions. However, while some of their information may be factual some of it is likely to be erroneous, and correction or clarification is usually necessary. Their instruction is the responsibility of the nurse, and the teaching of patients is one of the most responsible functions of her profession. To teach correctly and effectively the nurse must have a thorough knowledge of her subject, be skilled in communication and cognizant of the basic mechanisms of learning. Her explanations, while simple for the sake of comprehension, at the same time must be meaningful if they are to be accepted.

Much of her instruction will refer to specific tests or treatments that are in prospect, describing the technical steps that are involved, the sensations likely to be experienced and the after-effects to be anticipated, and specifying what the patient can do to facilitate the procedure, minimize his discomfort and reduce complications. Of course, when discussing anything with her patient the nurse must take into consideration his physical and emotional status, his intelligence, his experience as a patient and his awareness of the situation, as well as the urgency of his need to know and understand. She also must consider the possible implications of her intended remarks and guard with equal care against inaccuracies on her part and misunderstandings on the part of the patient.

Aesthetic Needs. These needs vary in importance from individual to individual, but for all patients the most salutary environment is one that is orderly and one in which there is beauty. The patient with acute aesthetic sensibilities will be distressed by unpleasant sights, sounds and odors, and intolerant of disarray. He may crave flowers, books or music, and when supplied, these amenities add immeasurably to his well being.

Concluding this discussion, it may be pointed out that most of the needs of the average individual, ill or well, can be satisfied only in part. Moreover, the nurse whose responsibility and privilege it is to help the patient meet his problems must recognize the fact that some problems can be neither eliminated nor solved. In relation to the patient with such a problem her role is to help him to make a mature, objective and compensatory adjustment to its continued existence or to its imperfect solution, if this solution is the best that can be achieved.

THE TEAM APPROACH TO PATIENT CARE

The professions devoted to healing constitute an organized team in which numerous and diverse arts, sciences and industries function in coordinated and mutually dependent roles. Those individuals and institutions engaged in the health professions serve in the greatest of all enterprises—the relief and the prevention of suffering, the improvement of human effectiveness, and the prolongation of life. Key personnel are the practicing nurses and the physicians who, for the furtherance of these objectives, have elected to accept responsibilities of the gravest sort. Few disciplines are as demanding. The labors of nursing and medicine are extremely taxing; many of their problems are not solved easily, but the rewards are correspondingly great. Opportunities for effective contributions never end, and the value of each successful accomplishment is immediately or eventually obvious.

The Health Team. Whether a particular project is designed to provide relief from intractable pain suffered by one individual or to protect an entire population from a variety of communicable diseases, its success depends on the contributions of innumerable practitioners, past as well as present, representing many areas of endeavor.

Those responsible for actually executing the mission of the entire vast medical organization are, however, members of the health team, or, more specifically, the professional nurses, the practicing physicians, the occupational therapists, the physical therapists, the nutritionists, the social workers, the practical nurses and the auxiliary employees. Through their teamwork the fruits of scientific investigation and the technical achievements are distributed. On them depend the successful accomplishments of the medical profession as a whole. Obviously, were it not for the endeavors and the accomplishments of these members, medical science could be classed as little more than an academic exercise, devoid of any acute sense of obligation or high responsibility—a sterile pursuit motivated by intellectual curiosity, perhaps, but certainly not by compassion.

The responsibility for patient care is a communal one, whether shared by many, as in hospital practice, or by few. The principal participants are the professional nurse and the physician; their roles are interdependent and mutually complementary, each bearing a well-defined portion of the responsibility. The physician evaluates each individual patient on the basis of the medical history, the course of the disease, the physical examination of the patient and a laboratory investigation. He then outlines the therapeutic program which he considers is indicated and performs whatever technical procedures may require his personal participation. The physician's decisions regarding treatment require implementation, of course, or they are worthless. Implementation, through the actual performance of the prescribed treatment, is one of the functions of nursing.

The Nursing Team. Team nursing, as the term implies, refers to the care of patients by an organized group of nursing personnel, rather than by an individual nurse. Nursing duties are apportioned among a team, the members of which represent various levels of training and competence, and which is so constituted as to provide optimum nursing care with maximum efficiency. Comprising the team are professional nurses, nursing students, and nursing assistants. To each of these individuals specific responsibilities are delegated that are in keeping with his or her educational background and experience.

The *team leader* is responsible for planning and evaluating the care of each patient. She delegates responsibilities and assigns specific duties to the personnel in her charge. She guides and supports the activities of every team member. The major decisions are hers.

The functions of the *professional nurse* are deter-

mined largely by the needs of the patient and the nature of his problems. She undertakes the care of patients whose conditions are complex, requiring judicious decisions, experienced teaching or advanced nursing skills. In addition, she assists the other team members in the care of their patients.

The *nursing student* participates to an extent commensurate with her education and in a manner that should prove of mutual benefit to her and to the patients whose care she is assigned.

The role of the *practical nurse* is dictated by her educational background, clinical experience and individual competence, and by the needs of the team. The nursing assistants perform the functions for which they are trained. Each member has a distinctive contribution to make to the patient's care and to the smooth functioning of the team.

The *team conference* serves as a "clearinghouse" for the exchange of information concerning each patient. Such a conference is scheduled daily, and usually is held as soon as possible after the completion of the major portion of the patient's care. The team leader inscribes pertinent notations on the nursing-care plan, revising the latter according to the suggestions offered and the solutions proposed at the conference. Thus, the patient benefits promptly and directly from the combined observations, the cumulative knowledge and the joint problem-solving ability of the several team members, all of whom are operating in concert to provide nursing care of the highest possible quality.

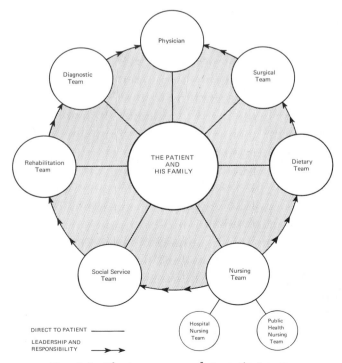

FIG. 1-2. The team approach to patient care.

PATIENT ASSESSMENT AND PLANNING PATIENT CARE

Patient Assessment

A patient comes to the hospital because he has a problem and needs help. This problem may be urgent, simple or complex. Nurses and other members of the health team are concerned with assisting the patient to gain a solution of his problem. The physician evaluates the patient, conducts the physical examination, orders laboratory and other investigative studies, initiates a therapeutic regimen and constantly evaluates the patient's response to treatment. The nurse, too, has a responsibility in developing a plan of nursing care for the patient. The nurse also constantly assesses the patient's symptoms, fluctuation of vital signs, the direction of his clinical course, reactions, attitudes and complaints. The nurse has the advantage of being where the action is, at the bedside of the patient.

Nursing assessment is an orderly process of determining the problems of a patient, utilizing all available data so that a nursing care plan can be formulated, implemented and evaluated. The first phase of assessment is gathering the facts about the patient. In studying all available data, one quite naturally begins with the health record or chart. What is the problem that caused the patient to seek help? A tentative diagnosis has usually been formulated by the physician upon the patient's admission to the hospital. It is absolutely essential to understand the pathophysiological processes underlying this diagnosis. "Therapeutic conversation" is no substitute for knowing the effects of altered physiology, rationale of treatment and potential complications. This knowledge helps the nurse to anticipate problems that may evolve and to formulate a nursing approach to their solution.

The Patient Interview. In addition to the information obtained from the chart, the *patient interview* is a method of gathering data. The interview is a dialogue between the patient and the nurse and is a very personal experience. Interviewing is an art that requires wisdom, judgment, tact and experience. It involves the sensitive direction of a conversation with a patient in order to obtain information about him. The

---

CHART 1-1. GUIDELINES FOR INTERVIEWING PATIENTS

Guiding Principle: At the beginning of the interview, focus on what is most troublesome to the patient—what are his symptoms or complaints.

What brought you to the hospital?
What is causing you the most discomfort?
When did the complaints appear?
Do you believe you are getting better or worse? (the directional trend: improvement or deterioration)
What do you think made you sick?
What do you do for yourself at home when you are sick?

What factors aggravate or help your condition?
Are you taking any medications?
Do you have any allergies? (food, drugs)
Do you have any elimination (bowel or urinary) problems?
What is your greatest concern?
Are you being informed about tests and treatment?

Guiding Principle: Learn about the patient's background and experience in order to determine his needs.*

Where is your home?
Do you have a family? (Who is caring for your children?)
What type of work do you do?

Has your illness interfered with your work?
What activities, hobbies and forms of recreation do you enjoy?

Guiding Principle: Ascertain what can be done to support the patient and help him make the best use of his resources.

What are your food preferences? Dislikes?
What are your sleeping habits?
  Regular retiring time?
    Do you like a night light?
Do you have any limitations of seeing? hearing? walking?
What personal preferences do you have?
  Sleep late?
  Hot water bottle for feet?
  Ice or tap water to drink?

Would it be helpful to have a family member or friend stay with you?
What annoys you the most about being in the hospital?
What do you miss the most in the hospital?
What could the nursing staff do that would be most helpful to you?

---

* Cultural and educational levels can be assessed throughout the interview. Clues to the patient's financial status are obtained from his belongings, room, data on the chart, etc.

nurse's approach to the patient will largely determine the amount and quality of information that she receives. To achieve a relationship of mutual trust and respect requires the ability to communicate a sincere interest in the patient. The patient should be made as comfortable as possible and privacy afforded for the interview. The principles involved in interviewing a patient are: (1) listening and questioning; (2) observing and interpreting; and (3) synthesizing and incorporating what is learned into a plan of care. To learn about a patient one must talk little and listen a lot. Listen to the patient with "hearing ears." What is he saying? Because an ill person is so suggestible, do not put words in his mouth. Let him tell his story in his own way. A person also communicates with gestures, posture, facial expression and other subtle forms of non-verbal behavior. Give him time, without interruptions, to tell why he is seeking help. Anxiety is present in almost every patient; it may be well concealed but it is there. Anticipate the patient's anxieties and try to relieve them during the conversation. All inquiries should be relevant. The patient has the right to expect something from each interview. He should especially be made to feel that he is being understood.

A guidesheet may help the beginning nurse formulate meaningful questions. Because patient interviewing is individualized, questioning cannot be a stereotyped procedure. The guidesheet is used only to help the nurse gain skill in this phase of nursing; in time, a special form should not be needed. The questions in the chart on p. 8 are offered as guidelines for interviewing, but the questions actually asked are determined by the reaction of the individual patient.

During the interview listen for patient clues. Throughout the interaction process the nurse is assessing the cultural and intellectual capacity of the patient. She listens to the theme of his conversation and gets the "feeling" of his emotional and mental state. Before leaving, ask the patient, "Is there anything else that you wish to tell me?" This encourages communication. As soon as possible a summary of the major features of the interview is written. The patient's major problems are identified and an impression of the nursing needs is recorded.

Observation. Observation of the patient is the most important phase of nursing assessment. Indeed, observation may be recognized as the unique function of the nurse. Because observation is so important and complex, a chapter has been devoted to this nursing function (see Chap. 2). This chapter requires careful study in order to help the nurse observe with "seeing" eyes and understand what is being observed. Significant observations that should be made with each clinical condition appear in the appropriate chapter in which the condition is discussed.

Planning Nursing Care. A *nursing care plan* is a plan of action which includes a résumé of the patient's problems, a description of the proposed nursing approach, and a continuous evaluation of the effectiveness of the nursing approach. Included in the plan is a statement of the patient goals and the nursing staff goals if this is necessary. These may be short term, intermediate or long term goals based on the patient's condition and needs. A nursing care plan has to be flexible because the patient's condition changes, his problems vary, his reactions shift and the unexpected can occur. Therefore, alternative nursing actions may also be identified. (A sample nursing care plan appears on p. 10.)

Who does the planning? Ideally, this is a group activity involving the nurse with other members of the nursing team, the patient and his family, and perhaps a resource person from the community health agency. In planning with other members of the nursing team, the nurse recognizes that each team member has a role that is supported and respected. Of course, the physician initiates the medical regimen and is a valuable resource person, counselor and teacher. After as much data as possible has been collected the team captain and the members discuss the problem, goals and possible methods of solution, i.e., their nursing management. If a nurse specialist is a member of the staff agency, she is consulted.

Because the plan revolves around a patient, he should have a part in it. The ultimate goal is to help the patient help himself. This means the patient is accepted as a worthy individual and his right to self-determination is respected. If the plan is oriented in terms of the patient's goals and capabilities, he has every right to express his feelings and voice his opinions about his care.

The patient is part of a family. The family members have needs that arise from the patient's illness. They may be included in the planning by questioning them about the patient's reactions and informing them about the nursing care plan and the expected results of treatment. The family may also make pertinent observations and offer effective suggestions.

The patient comes from the community. Community agencies have an interest in the patient and are involved in planning. This means that at least those nurses in administrative positions (supervisor, head nurse, team captain) know the community services that may be offered a patient following discharge from the hospital. These agencies can be informed of the goal to be reached and decisions made for the type of services that will be needed. Many communities have a directory listing all community resources available. These include public health and visiting nursing services, homemaking services, meals on wheels, welfare and recreational services, etc. A knowledge of these resources and the method of referral is of inestimable value in helping to cope with long term health needs.

Implementing the Plan of Care. *Implementation* refers to carrying out the proposed plan of care. It includes all the nursing activities that help the patient meet his needs and solve his problems. Some of these needs have already been discussed in this chapter (pp. 5-6). Those needs specific to certain conditions are discussed elsewhere in the book.

Included among nursing activities are hygienic care, promotion of physical and psychological comfort, support of respiratory and elimination functions, environmental management, promotion of a therapeutic relationship, and a host of therapeutic nursing abilities. The nurse utilizes judgment in the selection of nursing measures that are based on physiologic fact.

This knowledge of physiology must be constantly sought, integrated and applied. Consider this clinical example:

A patient with bronchiectasis is exhausted from repeated episodes of unproductive coughing. Traditionally the doctor would be notified and a medication for cough given. The more self-directing nurse, using nursing abilities based on an understanding of altered pathophysiology, will listen to the patient's lungs with a stethoscope, locate the area of congestion, position him for drainage and then sit him upright while he coughs up the mucus. Of course the physician is notified and his medical regimen for the patient is followed.

Utilizing nursing knowledge, the nurse with others of the team decides how each situation is to be

---

EXAMPLE OF NURSING CARE PLAN

Mr. Gerald Moorehouse, a 62-year-old bus driver, was admitted to the nursing unit via the emergency room. He had been experiencing shortness of breath for the past week. He was in obvious distress and had generalized edema. Ten years ago he had been hospitalized for three weeks with acute glomerulonephritis. The blood urea nitrogen level taken on admission was 120. His provisional diagnosis was listed as "uremia."

DIAGNOSIS: Uremia

IMMEDIATE GOALS:
1. To relieve dyspnea and reduce edema
2. To prevent complications

LONG RANGE GOALS:
1. To prevent further renal damage
2. To aid patient in accepting restrictions and in adjusting to limitations

PROBLEMS	NURSING APPROACH	EVALUATION	OUTCOME
Dyspnea	Maintain oxygen at 4 liters/min. via nasal cannula.	Minimal relief of dyspnea → patient mouth-breathing; cannula irritates nares.	Change cannula to mask → more response to O_2 therapy.
	Elevate head of bed at 60° angle.	Slides down in bed.	Apply foot board to bed.
	Administer Aminophylline Supp. 500 mg. q. 8 hr.	Unable to retain suppository.	Notify dr. → changed to Aminophylline 750 mg. IV 1000 ml 5% Dextrose in water/24 hrs. for 24 hrs.
	Restrict IV fluids to 1000 ml/24 hrs.	Difficult to regulate fluid flow to such a slow drip.	Apply minimeter to IV drip chamber.
Generalized edema, oliguria.	Administer diuretics on schedule.	Abdomen less distended. Feet, ankles, legs less edematous.	
	Prevent dependence of extremities.	Patient sits on side of bed for long intervals and walks to bathroom.	Explain necessity of bedrest and elevation of legs → more accepting of restrictions.

handled. The format for writing the care plan varies with each health agency. The Kardex or a loose leaf notebook is most commonly used. A problem in current nursing practice is failure to revise the nursing care plan. The patient is not static. His problems, needs, condition and reactions change. During the nursing conference more knowledge, understanding and insight may be gained. This data should be immediately written on the plan. At the end of each tour of duty additions or changes may be made. The nursing care plan facilitates communication between members of the team and acquaints them thoroughly with the patient. Information obtained from the physician and family may initiate a change in priorities and a shift in the method of nursing approach.

Evaluating the Plan of Care. How effective is the nursing management of the patient? Are his problems less troublesome? Are the goals being achieved? Is he responding to treatment? Continuing evaluation is necessary. *Evaluation* is a process of value determination in terms of specific objectives or criteria. All available and pertinent objective and subjective data about the patient are used. Evaluation cannot be done by feeling. To evaluate something one must find a set of criteria or standards to set up as the ideal

TABLE 1-2. Steps in patient assessment and nursing care planning

Gather the Facts
1. Study the health history and clinical record
2. Interview the patient
3. Observe the patient

Analyze the Facts
1. Evaluate the collected data
   (a) Review history, physical examination, clinical studies
   (b) Study information obtained from physician, patient, and family
   (c) Assess patient during entire clinical course
2. Rank problems in order of importance
   (a) Determine what problems have priority
   (b) Anticipate what problems may arise
3. Synthesize the data

Develop a Plan of Nursing Care
1. State the goals
2. Formulate the nursing approach that will help attain the goals
3. Communicate with the patient about his plan of care
4. Implement the plan
5. Keep the plan current and flexible to meet the patient's changing problems and needs
6. Evaluate the effectiveness of the nursing approach and the extent to which the goals are achieved
7. Determine what can be done to improve the care

PROBLEMS	NURSING APPROACH	EVALUATION	OUTCOME
Generalized edema (cont.)	Restrict oral fluids to 500 ml./24 hrs.; accurate intake and output record.	Requests extra fluid at night.	Reserve 100 ml. of allowed fluid, to be taken at night.
	Prevent pressure and irritation of edematous areas; turn, position, skin care.	Heels and ankles reddened and tender to touch.	Apply lamb's wool heel pads.
Mouth dry, lips cracked.	Frequent mouthwash; lemon and glycerin swabs to lips and tongue frequently.	Mouth less dry.	
Nausea and vomiting.	Administer Thorazine 25 mg. IM q. 6 hr. p.r.n.	Vomiting persists. Drowsiness.	Notify Dr. → Digoxin discontinued. Siderails; frequent observation.
Non-palatable diet.	Provide calm aesthetic atmosphere at mealtime; explain purpose of diet and importance of eating.	Requests foods not included on 25 gm. protein 500 mg. sodium diet.	Alert dietician to food preferences included on diet. Notify Dr. → salt substitute ordered.
Incontinent of urine at night.	Offer urinal at frequent intervals; clean, dry linen.	Anxious and embarrassed.	Reassure patient; urinal within close reach.
Elevated blood pressure.	Observe and record vital signs q. 2 hr.; observe for symptoms of cerebral irritability.	Anxious about frequent blood pressure reading.	Explain necessity of procedure.

that is to be achieved, so that a comparison can be made. While there are no specific criteria established for effective care, each health agency can set forth acceptable standards. There are well known standards of hygienic care. Nursing records, charts and care plans reflect whether there is an understanding of the patient's needs, and are a tool in the evaluation process. Evaluation of the patient's response to treatment is accomplished by knowing the expected response to the disease process and its treatment. This knowledge is basic for patient observation and evaluation.

The patient and his family are part of the evaluation program. Their comments, commendations and criticisms should be listened to and acted upon. While "good care" to them is not always based on scientific knowledge, the patient and his family understand intuitively if he is understood and his needs met. A dissatisfied patient (or family) reflect that the nursing care is ineffective.

It is not enough to evaluate the effectiveness of the nursing care. An important phase in evaluation is "What should be done to improve?" Other nursing measures may have to be substituted. A new nursing approach may be tried. There must be a continuous and thorough scrutiny of the patient; then changes are made, plans altered and a course of action initiated that will be most supportive to the patient.

NURSING ABILITIES

Promoting a Therapeutic Nurse-Patient Relationship

An understanding of one's self, what one means to the patient and what the patient means to the nurse is basic for satisfactory interaction. Very early in her contact with the patient, the nurse needs to know the effect of illness and hospitalization on the patient. C. R. Rogers, Professor of Psychology, University of Chicago, expressed his hypothesis of human relationships in this manner:

If I can create a relationship characterized on my part:
By a genuineness and transparency, in which I *am* my real feelings,
By a warm acceptance of and liking for the other person as a separate individual,
By a sensitive ability to see his world and himself as he sees them,
Then the other individual in the relationship:
Will experience and understand aspects of himself which previously he has repressed,
Will find himself becoming better integrated, better able to function effectively,
Will become more similar to the person he would like to be,
Will be more self-directing and self-confident,

Will become more of a person, more nearly unique, and more self-expressive,
Will be able to cope with the problems of life more adequately and more comfortably.[*]

Teaching the Patient

In current practice, the patient has a role in his own therapy. It is expected that the patient will purposefully participate in his own recovery, will focus his own energy and spirit on the goals of therapy.

The patient is informed of the therapeutic goals and his cooperation sought in attaining them. Here, too, the nurse needs facts to impart, judgment as to what and when to inform, and the proper accompanying attitude.

In the past one of the weaknesses with regard to the care of the patient has been in offering him the kind of assistance necessary to carry on when he leaves the hospital environment. Throughout this text a concerted effort has been made to emphasize this important aspect of care. At the end of the chapters on the clinical areas, a list of patient teaching aids are given; however, it must be understood that merely to hand a patient a list of instructions or a brochure is not enough. He must be prepared to absorb and practice that which he needs to know. The following guide is offered to assist in the nurse's instruction of patients.

A Guide to Teaching the Patient[†]

A. *Approaching the Learning Situation*
   1. Readiness for learning
      a. The need to learn exists, but does the patient recognize this need?
         (a) Is the patient ready physically?
         (b) Is he psychologically ready?
      b. Are there other problems more important to him at this time that take priority?
   2. Content
      a. What do I know or need to know about this patient and his disease or condition?
      b. How much does the patient already know and what more does he need to know? (Consult with physician.)
   3. Factors affecting the patient's learning ability
      a. How does his educational experiences or occupation affect or influence the learning process?
      b. What adaptations must be made because of his cultural or religious background?
      c. What economic factors should be considered?

[*] Rogers, C. R.: A counseling approach to human problems, Am. J. Nursing 56:997, 1956.

[†] In collaboration with Martha E. Warstler, formerly Dir. School of Nursing, Reid Memorial Hospital and School of Nursing, Richmond, Ind.

d. Will his illness affect his ability to learn?

e. Where would be the best place for the patient to learn? Is this place optimal?

B. *Selection of Teaching Methods*

1. To begin with, ascertain from the patient his understanding and needs regarding the problem.

2. Select materials and methods appropriate to the level of the particular patient.

    a. Discussion

    b. Demonstration and use of equipment

    c. Charts, pamphlets and other visual aids

    d. Return demonstration

    e. Consider modifications necessary for patient in order to perform effectively in his own environment with his own equipment. Suggest improvisations.

3. What other resources, such as dietitian, physical therapist and so forth, might be helpful?

4. Ascertain how much can be taught in a given period of time.

5. Provide time for questions and offer encouragement.

6. Learning is facilitated if the patient knows "why" he is doing something as well as "how" to do it.

C. *Evaluation and Referral*

1. Provide opportunity for the patient to practice and to ask questions.

2. If he has problems or questions when he is at home, provide him with the sources he can contact, e.g., visiting nurse association, his physician, the hospital clinic, community health agencies.

Communicating With Others

In order to communicate effectively with patients, the nurse needs to know how and when to listen, to recognize and evaluate patient's feelings, to communicate supportive attitudes, to ask and to answer questions, to manipulate conversation into desired channels and to recognize the high communication value of touch, manner, expression and attitude. The nurse will recognize that when an ill person moves from the routine activities of a busy world into the very different atmosphere of a hospital, in many instances he tends to exaggerate what he feels, sees and hears. Fears often are responsible for this change. By communicating effectively with the patient, the nurse assures that his understanding will be broader and his misconceptions and fears will be reduced.

BIBLIOGRAPHY

Books

Bonney, V., and Rothberg, J.: Nursing Diagnosis and Therapy— An Instrument for Evaluation and Measurement. New York, The League Exchange, National League for Nursing, 1963.

Henderson, V.: The Nature of Nursing. New York, Macmillan, 1966.

Little, D. E., and Carnevali, D. L.: Nursing Care Planning. Philadelphia, J. B. Lippincott, 1969.

National League for Nursing: Evaluation—The Whys and The Ways. New York, National League for Nursing, 1965.

————: Perspectives for Nursing. New York, National League for Nursing, 1965.

Skipper, J. K., and Leonard, R. C. (eds.): Social Interaction and Patient Care. Philadelphia, J. B. Lippincott, 1965.

Straub, K. M., and Parker, K. S. (eds.): Continuity of Patient Care: The Role of Nursing. Washington, D. C., Catholic University of America Press, 1966.

Wemsley, E.: Nursing Service Without Walls. New York, National League for Nursing, 1963.

Yura, H., and Walsh, M. (eds.): The Nursing Process, Washington, D. C., Catholic University of America Press, 1967.

Articles

Alman, B.: Patients participate in nursing care conferences. Amer. J. Nurs., 67:2331-2334, Nov., 1967.

Standards for organized nursing services, Amer. J. Nurs., 65:76-79, March, 1965.

Cooke, R. V.: Clinical diagnosis and clinical judgment. Ann. Int. Med., 68:239, 1968.

Enelow, A. J., et al.: The medical interview. Med. Times, 93: 1192-2000, 1965.

Goodall, J.: The difficult historian. Lancet, 1:776-799, 1967.

Hammond, K. R.: Clinical inference in nursing. II. A psychologist's viewpoint. Nurs. Res. 15:27-38, Winter, 1966.

Keller, N. S.: Care without coordination. Nurs. Forum, 6:280-323, 1967.

Kelly, K.: Clinical inference in nursing. I. A nurse's viewpoint. Nurs. Res., 15:23-26, Winter, 1966.

Ledley, R. S.: Computer aids to medical diagnosis. JAMA, 196: 933-943, 1966.

Lewis, L.: This I believe about the nursing process—key to care. Nurs. Outlook, 16:26-29, May, 1968.

Lineham, D. T.: What does the patient want to know? Amer. J. Nurs., 66:1066-1070, May, 1966.

Lipkin, M. et al.: The formulation of diagnosis and treatment. New Eng. J. Med., 275:1049-1052, 1966.

Little, D., and Carnevali, D.: Nursing care plans: let's be practical about them. Nurs. Forum, 6:61-76, 1967.

McCain, R. F.: Nursing by assessment—not intuition. Amer. J. Nurs., 65:82-84, April, 1965.

McPhetridge, L. M.: Nursing history: one means to personalize care. Amer. J. Nurs., 68:68-75, Jan., 1968.

Paltrow, K. G., et al.: The review of areas: a simple way to take a comprehensive medical history. J. Med. Education, 42:72, 1967.

Phaneuf, M.: The nursing audit method for the evaluation of patient care. Nurs. Outlook, 14:51-54, June, 1966.

Slack, W. V., et al.: Computer-based patient interviewing I. Postgraduate Med., 43:68-74, 1968. (Part II, 43:115-120, 1968.)

Tayrien, D., and Lipchak, A.: The single problem approach. Amer. J. Nurs., 67:2523-2527, Dec., 1967.

Yochelson, L.: Psychiatric principles in medical interviewing. Postgraduate Med., 42:80-86, 1967.

Team Nursing

Books

Kron, M.: Nursing Team Leadership. Philadelphia, W. B. Saunders, 1966.

Swansburg, R.: Team Nursing: A Programmed Learning Experience (Units 1, 2, 3, 4). New York, Putnam's Sons, 1968.

Articles

Dietrich, B. J., and Miller, D.: Nursing leadership—a theoretical framework. Nurs. Outlook, *14*:52-55, Aug., 1966.

Fosberg, G. C.: Teaching management skills in a team nursing setting. Nurs. Outlook, *15*:67-68, April, 1967.

Ingmire, A., and Blansfield, M.: A development program for the hospital team. Nurs. Forum, *6*:382-398, No. 4, 1967.

Lambertsen, E. C.: Defining the right roles helps assure the right team. Mod. Hospital, *109*:128, December, 1967.

———: Reorganize nursing to re-emphasize care. Mod. Hospital, *108*:68-71, Jan., 1967.

Logsdon, A.: Preparing for unexpected responsibilities. Nurs. Clin. N. Amer., *3*:143-152, March, 1968.

Mercadante, L. T.: Leadership development seminars. Nurs. Outlook, *13*:59-61, Sept., 1965.

Swansburg, R.: An experiment in team nursing (part I). Nurs. Outlook, *16*:45-47, Aug., 1968.

———: An experiment in team nursing (part II). Nurs. Outlook, *16*:42-43, Sept., 1968.

Walker, V., and Hawkins, J.: Management: A factor in clinical nursing. Nurs. Outlook, *13*:57-58, Feb., 1965.

CHAPTER 2

Observation of the Patient

- *Symptoms and Their Significance*
- *Detection and Recording of Physical Signs*

The initial step in the evaluation of any patient is the securing, by skillful questioning and careful listening, of a detailed historical account of all subjective symptoms that might conceivably pertain to his present illness. The second component of the clinical examination is the eliciting of physical signs, an exercise in trained observation involving a systematic and exhaustive search for any significant physical deviations from the normal. The history and the physical examination together furnish information containing clues of diagnostic value, and on the basis of this a provisional program of therapy is adopted.

The eliciting of symptoms and signs is not concluded with the first clinical examination, nor is it solely the prerogative of the examining physician. Symptoms which were forgotten by the patient may be recalled later and described to the nurse; symptoms may change or may disappear, and physical signs may become altered in their character under her observation. Entirely new symptoms and signs may come to her attention first. In view of her opportunities for clinical observation, which are exceptionally great, it is important that she familiarize herself with the character and the significance of the cardinal signs and symptoms, for as a competent reliable observer, her contributions to the diagnosis and the treatment of her patients can be of inestimable value.

SYMPTOMS AND THEIR SIGNIFICANCE

Early in her experience, the nurse should learn to draw a sharp distinction between the patient's *subjective symptoms,* such as his sensations of pain, numbness, dizziness or nausea, which he alone can reveal, and those objective evidences of disease called *physical signs,* which are visible, audible, can be smelled or felt by the examiner and can be elicited by means of a laboratory procedure or some technical diagnostic aid. Skin rashes, lymph node enlargements, abdominal masses and sounds from the heart and the lungs heard with the stethoscope are examples of physical signs; concerning these, the examiner, with little or no assistance from the patient, can form a judgment.

The eliciting and the reporting of symptoms are very definitely within the scope of nursing care. Indeed, of all members of the professional team, the nurse may be the only one to whom some of these data are completely and readily accessible. In order for her to perform her functions as clinical observer, it is essential that the patient's complaints be described fully and with care, evaluated with discrimination and recorded as nearly as possible in the patient's own words.

The Nurse's Role in Evaluating Symptoms

The nursing student quickly learns that a patient may have a serious disease and yet express but few complaints of a relatively minor character, or he may be altogether symptom free. This is the situation in several serious disorders during most of their clinical course and in many ultimately fatal diseases during their early, curable stages.

Some patients tend to be uncommunicative regarding their discomforts and disabilities; they must be "drawn out" and questioned with persistence and persuasiveness lest information of diagnostic value escape the examiner. In the majority of instances, however, this problem does not exist or is overcome readily, and overzealous questioning is not only unnecessary but also distinctly disadvantageous for the patient's morale. Patients with certain types of neuroses may express their anxiety predominantly in the form of multiple complaints, all of which would seem to imply serious disability but which merely represent an acute awareness of normal bodily sensations. Inasmuch as therapy in such cases often is designed to de-emphasize the importance of these symptoms and to distract the patient from his subjective discomforts, it behooves the nurse to desist from persistent questioning, which can serve only to reinforce the patient's psychogenic disability.

The following generalizations are often helpful in evaluating symptoms with respect to their importance and severity. If a patient exhibits abnormal lack of concern in connection with a disability that is obviously serious, or if he displays a high-spirited optimism that is unwarranted in circumstances that are obviously grave, he is apt to be relatively uncommunicative as regards his subjective discomforts and, if he discusses them at all, they may be minimized to a misleading extent. Conversely, if a patient describes a multiplicity of complaints for which there is relatively little or no confirmatory objective evidence in the form of physical signs or manifest incapacity, the observer must reserve judgment in attempting to grade the discomfort.

Finally, it should be observed that individuals with neurotic tendencies are quite as susceptible to organic disease as are individuals without neuroses, but they are in far greater danger of medical neglect because of the suspicious nature of their complaints, which may color the judgment of their family, associates and professional advisors.

The Nurse's Role in Reporting Symptoms

The nurse should become practiced in the description of symptoms, learning to specify their characteristics according to a definite pattern. The following attributes, if possible, should be elicited and reported in connection with each: total duration, time of onset or first occurrence, constancy since onset, character of onset, location and degree of severity. In describing pain, the presence or absence of "radiation," i.e., spread of the pain from its point of origin or greatest intensity, should be specified, and the pain itself should be described in terms as informative as the patient can supply, such as "knifelike," "dull," "boring," "pressurelike," "steady," "wavelike," "crampy," "spasmodic," etc.

The final interpretation of symptoms is, of course, the responsibility of the physician, the nurse's role in diagnosis being chiefly that of observer and recorder. It is an essential role, however, and one requiring knowledge that can be derived only from study, from judgment based on clinical experience and, above all, from keen interest in the problems of her patients.

DETECTION AND RECORDING OF PHYSICAL SIGNS

General Appearance

Certain features of the patient's appearance are invariably important in diagnosis and never should escape the attention of the nurse. These signs include, in addition to the quality of his physical development and the degree of nourishment, manifestations indicative of the patient's physical comfort and mental state, his facies, posture and, if ambulatory, his gait.

The observing nurse soon learns to judge the mental and emotional status of her patient. Is he comfortable? If not, what is the apparent source of his discomfort? Is he alert? Is he stuporous or comatose? Is he accurately oriented, aware of his present location and identity? Does he recognize his visitors and attendants? Does he know what hour of the day, what day of the week, what month and what year it is? Does he appear to have adequate insight into his situation? Is he unduly depressed and anxious or is he euphoric, experiencing an abnormal sense of well-being and prowess? Does he describe hallucinations (visual, auditory or tactile sensations not founded in reality) or delusions (gross misinterpretations of true perceptions)? Can he move all 4 extremities?

Evidence of mental aberrations should be detected and recognized speedily so that close observation, active therapy and, if necessary, protective measures can be instituted in time to forestall any unfortunate developments. Any suggestion that the patient is suffering from ideas of persecution or any sign of delirium should put the nurse on her guard at once. Abnormalities of mood, unusual behavior and defective orientation may be the result of drug toxicity, uremia, severe infection or a metabolic disorder, as well as of a primary psychosis. Whatever the cause of the mental disturbance, the consequences of neglect in reporting or failure to realize the true gravity of the situation may be serious.

Facies, Posture, Movements and Gait

Facies. The patient's facial color and expression should be noted carefully, for they often contribute greatly to the formulation of a correct diagnosis.

Anemia and Edema. Pallor is suggestive of anemia but is by no means diagnostic of that condition. A pale, puffy complexion may indicate the presence of edema, i.e., excessive accumulation of water in the subcutaneous tissues; therefore, it is encountered in nonanemic patients with nephritis and other disorders complicated by edema formation. In anemic individuals, pallor involves not only the skin but the lips and the conjunctivae as well. This is important, inasmuch as pallor of the skin, even in severely anemic individuals, may be obscured by skin pigmentation.

Cachexia. This is characterized by the appearance of marked wasting of the soft tissues of the face; the eyes are sunken and the cheek bones prominent. This type of facies is indicative of severe, long-standing malnutrition, due, for example, to a far-advanced neoplastic disease.

Dehydration. This condition likewise contributes the appearance of thinness, hollowness of cheeks and temples and sunken eyes, but in addition there are a lead-colored or grayish discoloration of the skin, a relaxation of the muscles about the mouth and the lips, the latter being parched and loosely apposed, and a dry, thick coating on the tongue. This, the "hippocratic facies," is observed in patients with advanced peritonitis, in which fluid is lost into the abdominal cavity, and in diarrheal diseases such as dysentery and cholera, in which voluminous and frequent liquid stools are responsible for rapid and severe dehydration.

Thyroid Disease. Often thyroid disease is suspected from the facial configuration and expression. The physiognomy of the patient with myxedema, which may be described as "moon face," with puffy lids and lack of expression, betrays his sluggish metabolism and retarded psychomotor activity. On the other hand, the patient with hyperthyroidism exhibits characteristically a staring expression suggesting "crystallized fear"; this is attributable to exophthalmos and to retraction of the eyelids, exposing the white sclerae, as well as to the smoothness of the forehead and the evident tension of all the facial muscles.

Liver Disease. The hepatic facies, encountered in patients with cirrhosis of the liver, may be recognized by the thinness of the face and the neck, the muddy, yellowish discoloration of the skin and the sclerae, the sunken eyes and the localized dilatations of small blood vessels arranged in spiderlike configurations ("spider angiomata") on the face and the neck.

Posture. The positions in which patients lie or sit and the bodily attitudes adopted when standing are of diagnostic importance.

Congestive Heart Failure. The patient with congestive heart failure, particularly when there is fluid accumulation in the chest or the abdomen, sits propped up in bed, breathing being easiest in that position. The greater the respiratory distress, the more erect the posture (*orthopnea*). He may lean forward and elevate his shoulders by bearing down with his hands on the bed or on the arms of a chair, thereby increasing to an even greater extent the capacity of his thorax.

Arthritis. Patients with acute arthritis of the spine, as a result of which each breath is painful, usually lie in such a fashion that the weight of the body keeps the inflamed costovertebral joints as motionless as possible, that is, in the supine position with the back hyperextended. Those with acute arthritis involving 1 or more peripheral joints hold the latter in the position of semi-flexion, which affords the greatest capacity to the synovial sac distended with fluid and reduces to a minimum the tension of the surrounding muscle groups.

Intra-abdominal Disease. When caused by an inflammatory process involving the peritoneum, abdominal pain is aggravated by pressure; therefore, persons with acute appendicitis, an infection of the gallbladder or peritonitis tend to lie supine with knees flexed in order to relax the abdominal muscles.

Movements. *Tremors.* These may be rhythmic or arrhythmic, their speed slow or rapid, and their quality coarse or fine. In patients with hyperthyroidism, the tremor may be so rapid and its excursion so small that it may not be apparent until the examiner places a sheet of paper on the back of the patient's extended hand. The "intention tremor" of multiple sclerosis appears only in the course of directed movements of the extremities; when the patient attempts to place a finger on a specific object or point, the excursion of the tremor increases in amplitude as the finger approaches its goal. Parkinson's disease often is accompanied by a tremor involving the hands; the presence of this tremor is quite unrelated to voluntary muscular activity. This type of tremor is repetitive and stereotyped in quality, and the movements suggest "pillrolling."

Peculiar to patients with impending liver coma is the so-called "liver flap," characterized by irregular bursts of rapid, arrhythmic movements of the wrist in flexion and extension, appearing as the patient attempts to hold his arm and hand in rigid extension. Comparable movements may be exhibited by the elbows and shoulder girdles, the protruded tongue and the retracted lips.

Tics. Tics are involuntary muscular contractions involving whole groups of muscles; they result in a coordinated, stereotyped movement of the head or an extremity or cause a facial contortion. They seem to be devoid of purpose and serve no useful function. Common varieties of tics include a sudden jerking or twisting of the head to one side (torticollis), the winking of an eye and particular types of facial grimaces. Although clearly involuntary, tics are replicas of perfectly natural, although perhaps unusual, voluntary movements and occasion no disability.

Chorea. Choreal movements are irregular, jerky, purposeless, involuntary and unpredictable muscular movements which may involve all extremities and the entire trunk as well. This sign occurs as a transient complication of acute rheumatic fever, when it is referred to as "Sydenham's chorea," and is displayed persistently in one specific degenerative disease of the nervous system designated as "Huntington's chorea."

Athetosis. This term is applied to involuntary, more or less constant, slow wormlike twistings and bendings of the fingers and alternate flexion and extension of wrists, arms and feet, with coarse, jerky choreal movements affecting the entire extremity. The appearance of athetosis signifies the presence of a serious organic disease of the brain.

Convulsions. Such movements may be described as spontaneous paroxysms of involuntary, purposeless muscular contractions. The implications of this sign, diagnostically and therapeutically, are invariably important. There are several possible causes to be considered, and, since the character of the convulsion is usually the most helpful diagnostic clue, an accurate description of the seizure is essential. The nurse must be prepared to take advantage of every opportunity that may present itself to serve as expert observer and witness in such patients. Her observations at the time of the convulsive seizure should enable her to report the following pertinent information: the duration of the episode; the character of the onset, including the presence and the character of antecedent and associated signs (for example, the appearance of pallor, flushing, changes in facial expression, mental confusion, instability of gait, irregularity of respirations and pulse); the portions of the body involved and the sequence in which they are involved; the position of the eyes and their movements, if any, during the episode; the onset of stupor or coma; the occurrence of involuntary micturition or defecation; and, finally, signs and symptoms displayed following the seizure.

Convulsions may be "tonic" or "clonic" in type, the former being characterized by generalized muscular rigidity and the latter by rhythmic but violent flexion-extension jerkings. Characteristic types of seizures are observed as the predominant manifestation of epilepsy, neoplastic, vascular and infectious diseases involving the brain, eclampsia, uremia, hypoglycemia, calcium deficiency, tetanus, toxic states attributable to certain drugs and conditions resulting in gross interference with the oxygen supply to the brain.

Gait. Disorders involving the nervous and the musculoskeletal systems may be quite apparent and their diagnoses suspected on the basis of the gait.

Limping Gait. A limp may be attributable to pain on walking, to inequality of length or strength of the legs or to the limitation of motion of one or more joints in the lower extremities. Patients with partial hemiplegia, with motor weakness affecting one leg and the corresponding arm, tend to drag the affected leg when walking, characteristically supporting the arm on the affected side stiffly and in a position of slight flexion. Patients with impaired position sense due, for example, to combined system disease or tabes dorsalis, characteristically walk with a slapping or flail-like gait, fixing their gaze on the ground, keeping their feet well apart and raising their legs high between steps.

Propulsive Gait. Patients with Parkinson's disease, or "paralysis agitans," typically walk with the so-called propulsive gait. Head and body forward, the patient trots toward his goal, the tempo of his gait progressively increasing until the objective is reached or until he is able to check his forward movement and resume at a slower pace.

Spastic Gait. The spastic gait, encountered in patients with multiple sclerosis and other disease affecting the central nervous system, may be described as a slow, stiff, choppy walk, obviously entailing considerable effort.

Other Abnormal Gaits. Other abnormal gaits characteristic of specific diseases include the *waddling* gait of patients with congenital dislocation of the hips; the slow, clumsy, *high-stepping* gait seen in patients with peripheral neuritis and related to the presence of numbness or acute pain affecting the feet; and the grossly irregular, reeling, *swinging* gait of the patient suffering from ataxia due to cerebellar disease. This last gait results from the patient's inability to place his feet in their intended location, a problem of faulty regulation of muscular movement rather than lack of position sense.

Body Temperature

The heat that maintains body temperature is generated as a result of biochemical reactions associated with metabolic activities constantly in progress throughout the body.

The constancy of the body temperature is explained by the activity of nerve centers located at the base of the brain. These centers control all of the physiologic mechanisms that are concerned with the control of heat production and heat loss, including the volume of blood flow through the skin and the respiratory mu-

FIG. 2-1. Course of normal body temperature, measured orally, for 24 hours.

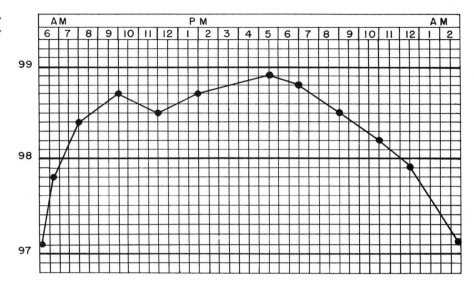

cosa and the phenomena of sweating, shivering and panting. The precision by which this regulation is accomplished is attested to by the fact that in normal individuals the body temperature rarely fluctuates beyond a range of 2° F., day or night, despite extreme variations of the surrounding temperature. A progressive accumulation of body heat, resulting in fever, normally is prevented by an increased volume and rate of blood flow in the skin and the subcutaneous tissues. This increased blood flow permits a greater volume of blood to be cooled in a given period of time as a result of radiation. Sweating increases the cooling effect of vaporization on the skin, and panting produces a similar result in the respiratory tract. These mechanisms effectively increase the rate of heat loss and protect against fatal overheating in hot weather and in the course of muscular exertion. Cooling of the body to subnormal temperatures in cold environments is prevented chiefly by two mechanisms. One of these constricts the peripheral blood vessels, decreasing the blood flow in the skin and the respiratory tract, and the other mechanism stimulates vigorous muscular exertion in the form of voluntary activity or involuntary shivering.

Normal Temperature Variations. The course of the normal body temperature is by no means constant, as is evident from the inspection of a 24-hour chart (Fig. 2-1). At 4 A.M. the temperature of normal individuals may be as low as 97.0° F.; between 9 and 10 A.M. it attains a peak of approximately 98.6° F. and then it declines to about 98.2° F. before the noonday meal. Afterward it rises slowly, reaching its maximum, between 98.7° and 98.9° F., during the early evening hours and thereafter falls slowly until 4 A.M. the following morning. The temperature charts characteristic of individuals working during the night, although similar in form, are quite different with respect to the timing of the fluctuations; the maximum peaks occur not during the late afternoon or the early evening hours but early in the morning.

The maximum degree of body temperature that is customarily regarded as normal is 99.0° F. Values in excess of 99.0° F. are considered indicative of fever, although individuals are encountered who habitually exhibit oral temperatures as high as 99.4° F. without other evidence of ill health. Normal variations in the lower temperature ranges are much greater; the lowest temperature recorded in most individuals is 97.0° F., but readings as low as 96.0° F. are not uncommon.

Hypothermia. Abnormal conditions responsible for an unusual reduction of body temperature are relatively few. Hypothermia is attributable either to a lessened production of body heat, as in hypothyroidism, or to excessive heat loss resulting from prolonged exposure to cold or from profuse sweating (diaphoresis). It is observed in circulatory failure due to severe blood loss (oligemic shock), in patients who have ingested large doses of antipyretic drugs such as aspirin and as a complication of diseases, which involve the temperature-regulating centers in the brain or the nerve pathways through which these exercise their physiologic functions.

Fever. An abnormal elevation of temperature is one of the most valuable of all clinical signs, not only because it occurs with great regularity in a large proportion of disease states, but also because of its specific characteristics in many types of disorders. By the same token, the absence of fever is equally important because of its usefulness in the exclusion of diagnostic possibilities.

Symptomatology of Fever. The onset of fever may be accompanied merely by a subjective sense of malaise, fatigue, loss of appetite, headache and generalized aches and pains of a mild degree. If, on the other hand, the onset is rapid and the elevation is of marked degree, the accompanying symptoms are correspondingly severe; the symptoms usually include the appearance of chills, severe malaise, occasionally nausea, vomiting and mental changes ranging from mild confusion to frank delirium or deep stupor. Convulsive seizures, rather than chills, may mark the onset of fever of this type, particularly in young children.

During an episode of chills, all of the mechanisms described as contributory to the production of fever are manifest, and all are operating at full capacity, which explains the speed with which the temperature peak is attained. The peripheral skin vessels become markedly constricted; as a result, the circulating blood is shunted away from the superficial tissues, and the heat-producing organs are cooled less efficiently. Moreover, because of the accompanying muscular contractions, which may be so vigorous as to shake the entire bed, the total heat production in the body is greatly increased.

The abatement of fever, or "defervescence," may occur very abruptly, within a few hours, or gradually over a period of many days. In the former instance, the temperature is said to fall by "crisis" and in the latter by "lysis." Symptomatic improvement occurs at a corresponding rate, preceded, in rapid defervescence, by the appearance of profuse sweating.

Interpretation of Fever. Fever most often denotes the presence of an active infection, and, when attended by chills, a bacterial infection is the probable diagnosis. Alternate possibilities include various neoplastic diseases, especially carcinoma of the kidney or the lung, and tumors of the lymphoma group; immune reactions of many types, including those which follow the administration of vaccines or prophylactic serums of animal origin; toxic reactions to certain drugs; and conditions in which the temperature-regulating centers are directly damaged by heat (heat stroke), trauma or a disease involving the central nervous system.

The nurse can be extremely helpful in the diagnosis of obscure fever, not only by routinely recording the vital signs, but also as a clinical observer. She must be constantly on the alert for novel and significant developments in her patients—for example, the onset of cough, headache, nausea, pain, mental changes or skin rash, and she should maintain the attitude that any unusual phenomenon deserves reporting.

Factitious Fever. Sooner or later in the course of her professional career, the nurse is very likely to become the victim of the deception of an emotionally disturbed patient who appears to be running a febrile course but whose "fever" is, in fact, spurious and fraudulent. These individuals, in order to attract attention, create concern and prolong their hospitalization, falsify their temperature charts by manipulating thermometers, warming them on adjacent light bulbs or cigarette lighters, or by applying friction, before they are retrieved and read by the nurse. A more sophisticated method involves the possession of 1 or more extra thermometers which can be manipulated at opportune times and substituted for those actually placed by the nurse. Most patients in this category have had some medical background, either as patients or hospital employees in the past.

The alert nurse is aware of the possibility of factitious fever, and is not likely to be deceived for long. Her suspicions will be aroused by the exhibition of fever by a patient solely when his temperature is recorded in her absence, i.e., when she is not in his immediate vicinity throughout the procedure, or by a patient's refusal to permit his temperature to be taken in her presence. (However, expert prestidigitators have been encountered with an uncanny ability to substitute thermometers undetected, under the very noses of suspicious doctors and nurses!) She will become suspicious on observing certain discrepancies in the patient's clinical chart, particularly the absence of the expected diurnal temperature variation and the lack of correlation between pulse rates and temperature readings.

In the event of suspicion, steps must be taken immediately to establish or exclude fraudulence. With no indication of distrust, she should place a thermometer in the patient's mouth or rectum in the usual manner and at the scheduled time, having first noted the serial number of that thermometer. While the temperature is registering, he should be observed no more, but less, closely than usual. If the instrument which she retrieves and reads bears a different serial number, the deception is unmasked; if it is the correct thermometer and records an elevation, it should be readjusted to a normal reading, replaced immediately in mouth or rectum and read again after 3 minutes, during which period the nurse will be standing by and observing closely.

If the serial numbers check and the reading is the same, the latter is obviously valid and has been so proved without embarrassment to patient or nurse. Otherwise, if the temperature proves to be normal or a thermometer substitution is discovered, the attending physician is to be notified at once, without preliminary comment to the patient. An elaborate, expensive and time-consuming investigation of F.U.O. (fever of unknown origin) is thus avoided.

Respiration

Aspects of breathing which are of clinical importance and which should be noted by the nurse as routine in all patients are its rate, rhythm and depth; the effort it involves and the discomfort it causes; the position which the patient adopts in order to breathe most comfortably; the sounds which accompany it and the presence or the absence of cyanosis.

Respiratory Rates. The normal rate of respiration in adults is from 16 to 20 per minute; in children, from 20 to 40, depending on age and size; and in infants, 40 or over. *Hyperpnea* and *polypnea* indicate a very rapid respiratory rate, and *oligopnea*, one that is abnormally slow; *apnea* signifies the temporary cessation of breathing.

Hyperpnea. A rapid respiratory rate is normal in children and young adults, occurring in response to exercise, painful stimuli or emotional distress. Although deep, hyperpnea requires no unusual effort, a feature distinguishing this type of respiration from dyspnea. Hyperpnea is as much a part of the fever syndrome as are the elevations of body temperature and pulse rate. The rate of respiration increases on the average about 5 per minute for each degree of temperature elevation, except in patients with pneumonia and infarcts of the lung which are accompanied by increases in the respiratory rate which are relatively much greater. Hyperpnea is also a common manifestation of hysteria; in some cases the rate approximates 50 to 60 per minute, and each breath is full, easy and painless. Inasmuch as hysterical hyperpnea is not stimulated by oxygen lack or carbon dioxide excess, as is hyperpnea due to exercise, it is often designated as "hyperventilation." The latter is not without effect on the physiologic state of the individual, for, as a result of "washing out" the carbon dioxide, the blood becomes abnormally alkaline, and the patient experiences spasmodic muscular contractions, as well as subjective numbness of the extremities, dizziness and faintness.

Oligopnea. Oligopnea (slow respiration) is most often attributable to toxic depression of the respiratory centers by opiates, particularly morphine and its derivatives.

Apnea. The temporary cessation of respiration is termed apnea. It is best exemplified in one of the respiratory arrhythmias termed *Cheyne-Stokes respiration.*

Cheyne-Stokes Respiration. This is a type of breathing characterized by periods of apnea, lasting from a few seconds to almost a minute, alternating with periods of similar length during which breathing is resumed (Fig. 2-2). Following periods of apnea the respiration is at first quiet and shallow; it then ac-quires a definite crescendo quality, with rate, depth and effort steadily increasing to peak intensity. After this it becomes progressively quieter and shallower until the return of apnea. This abnormality of respiration is frequently associated with increased intracranial pressure due, for example, to meningitis or cerebral tumor. It is exhibited also by patients with cerebral arteriosclerosis, who may exhibit Cheyne-Stokes breathing for periods lasting many months—usually, however, only when asleep or under the influence of sedative medication.

Respiratory Movements. When the predominant respiratory movement is confined to the ribs and the clavicles the term "costal breathing" is applied. This is in contrast to "abdominal breathing," which refers to respiration that is accomplished chiefly by the diaphragm as evidenced by the appearance of abdominal expansion and contraction, the excursion of which exceeds that of the chest movements. Normal breathing employs both types of movement, the costal component predominating in women, and the diaphragmatic in men. Excessive predominance of either, however, requires explanation.

Abdominal Respiration. This may be due to pleurisy or to acute arthritis of the costovertebral joints, motion of the chest being inhibited by pain. It also is found in patients with bilateral pleural effusion and extensive pneumonia. A long persistence of this respiratory abnormality suggests either fixation of the costovertebral joints due to chronic arthritis or bilateral paralysis of the intercostal muscles.

Costal Breathing. This may result from paralysis of the diaphragm or the abdominal musculature. It also may be related to the presence of fluid in the peritoneal cavity or to gaseous distention of the abdomen, which forces the diaphragm into an elevated position and restricts its normal excursion. Persistent limitation of both costal and diaphragmatic movements indicates that the lungs have lost their normal elasticity. In pulmonary emphysema, for example, the chest becomes immobilized in a position of inspiration, with the ribs and the clavicles elevated and the costal angle widened.

Asymmetric Respiration. Unilateral predominance of respiratory movements on the right or the left side,

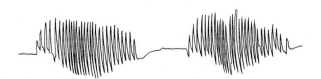

FIG. 2-2. Respiratory movements of a patient exhibiting Cheyne-Stokes breathing.

may be indicative of acute pleurisy, the respiratory movements on the affected side being limited by pain. It also may be attributable to scarring and contracture of one lung as a late complication of chronic tuberculosis.

Dyspnea. This implies labored breathing. The respiratory rate may be rapid or reduced, the rhythm regular or irregular, each breath shallow or deep. The important characteristic is its labored quality, unusual effort being entailed in each respiratory movement. There is active participation on the part of the accessory muscles of respiration, especially the sternocleidomastoid muscles in the neck, which visibly contract, lifting the clavicles with each inspiration, while the nostrils actively dilate. The dyspneic patient appears anxious; his pupils are dilated, his mouth is held open, his tongue and lips are dry, and the entire skin is moist and usually cyanotic. Severe dyspnea almost always is accompanied by *orthopnea,* the patient maintaining an erect position or leaning forward in order to breathe with optimum efficiency and comfort.

Dyspnea may result from the mechanical obstruction of the trachea, of a major bronchus or of numerous bronchioles within the lung tissue. It also may occur as a result of a reduction in the area of functioning respiratory surface within the lungs; this may be due to an infectious process, an invading tumor or fibrous scarring. Heart failure may cause the lung capillaries to become overdistended with blood and the alveoli, or air cells, to fill with edema fluid. A portion of the lung may be collapsed due to a fluid accumulation in the pleural cavity or the pericardial sac, or the lung may be compressed externally by air which has leaked into the mediastinal or pleural cavity.

Asthma. This is a type of breathing which is accompanied by an audible wheeze, which is more pronounced on expiration than on inspiration. It is due to partial obstruction of the small bronchi as a result of their spasm and edema, as in bronchial asthma. It may be attributable to the presence of fluid secretions within the bronchioles, which is the situation in asthmatic bronchitis and in congestive heart failure.

"Kussmaul Breathing." A classic finding in diabetic acidosis, this is characterized by a continuous dyspnea in which the respiratory movements are unusually deep, although not necessarily hurried. Considerable effort may be entailed, but there is little or no evidence of discomfort. Neither cyanosis nor orthopnea is associated with Kussmaul breathing, which distinguishes it from most other types of dyspnea. The cause of the disorder is abnormal acidity of the blood which provokes a persistent and excessive stimulation of the nerve centers controlling respiration.

Noisy Respiration. Stertorous breathing, or snoring, is produced by the vibration of the relaxed soft palate when an individual breathes simultaneously through nose and mouth and is observed commonly in association with stupor and deep, normal sleep. *Stridor,* the production of harsh, whistling noises, is attributable to partial obstruction of the larynx or the trachea by an infectious inflammatory disease by a foreign body or by spasm of the laryngeal muscles. Tracheal rales, responsible for the "death rattle" in terminal cases of pulmonary edema, are gurgling, bubbling sounds which are synchronous with respiration, indicating the presence of fluid in the major respiratory passages.

Arterial Pulse

The Pulse Examination. Each beat of a normally functioning heart propels approximately 100 ml. of blood into the arterial system and simultaneously initiates a fluid wave. This wave is propagated throughout the entire extent of this system and is palpable as a vibration called the "pulse," the rate and the character of which are highly informative as regards the state of the circulation. The pulse is examined by applying digital pressure over one of the large superficial arteries, preferably one which courses just beneath the skin and directly over bone and is surrounded by relatively little soft tissue. The temporal, the external maxillary (facial), the brachial and the femoral arteries fulfill these criteria, and circumstances occasionally require their selection, but the vessel that is most suitable for examination, and usually most readily accessible, is the radial artery at the wrist.

Normally, the pulse waves, when palpated from moment to moment, appear to be approximately equal in force and are separated by time intervals of equal length. In other words, the pulse is expected to be regular with respect to rate, rhythm and force, and any deviation from the normal in any of these qualities suggests the possibility of heart disease. However, as will become evident from the following discussions, abnormalities of the pulse occur in certain diseases other than cardiac, as well as in individuals who present no evidence of ill health.

Pulse Quality. The normal arterial pulsation, as observed by palpation, reaches its maximum intensity very rapidly and subsides more slowly. A small "dicrotic" impulse may be discerned as it subsides; this impulse is related to the closure of the aortic valve. If unduly pronounced, the term "dicrotic pulse" is applicable.

A forceful or "bounding pulse" suggests an increase in the magnitude of the pulse wave and a high "pulse pressure." This may be associated with a decrease in the diastolic arterial pressure, the systolic pressure remaining normal, or an increase in the systolic pressure while the diastolic is normal or low. Contrariwise, when the difference between systolic and diastolic pressures is unusually small (i.e., when the pulse pressure is low), the peripheral pulse is endowed with a feeble quality. A "thready pulse" is one that is not only feeble but also rapid. The "Corrigan" or "water hammer pulse" is one which strikes the palpating finger with a quick, sharp stroke. This abnormality in pulse quality, usually attributable to incompetence of the aortic valve (see p. 380), is elicited best by grasping the patient's wrist in the whole hand with the palmar surface of the fingers clasped firmly against the flexor surface of the patient's wrist and by elevating the wrist to a vertical position. A converse type of abnormality is the "slow pulse," one that is characterized by an unusually slow development of maximum force. It is encountered in patients with aortic stenosis, a condition in which, because of a reduction in the size of the aortic orifice, egress from the ventricles into the arterial system is impeded, blood being slowly squeezed with each contraction from the heart into the aorta.

Pulse Rates. The pulse rate is influenced by the degree of muscular activity. For example, that of a normal recumbent man may be approximately 66 beats per minute, slower when he sleeps, 70 while sitting or leaning and 80 while standing. During strenuous physical exercise, and for a short period thereafter, rates between 100 and 140 normally are attained, depending on the degree of exertion and the condition of the individual. Another influential factor is the emotional state; an increase in pulse rate occurs in response to anxiety, fear, displeasure, discomfort and accompanying excitement of any type.

Tachycardia, a rate greater than 100 per minute, may represent either a normal response to stimuli of the types mentioned or a manifestation of some disorder.

When the heart rate is consistently less than 50 beats per minute, the condition is described as *bradycardia.*

Abnormalities of pulse rate or irregularities of pulse rhythm are described in Chapter 19.

Pulse Deficit and Its Measurement. The pulse rate in untreated patients with atrial fibrillation is usually between 100 and 120 per minute. Its value, however, may not necessarily indicate the actual ventricular rate, for, unless the fibrillation is unusually slow, a certain proportion of the pulse waves do not possess sufficient force to be palpable at the wrist. There results, therefore, a "pulse deficit," which refers to the numerical difference between the ventricular and the peripheral pulse rates. The existence of a pulse deficit is important in establishing a diagnosis of atrial fibrillation and in differentiating this type of arrhythmia from others similarly characterized by pulse irregularities, such as premature beats, sinus arrhythmia and flutter with varying degrees of block. Moreover, the amount of deficit is one of the most valuable therapeutic guides in the treatment of patients with fibrillation.

The pulse deficit is determined by the simultaneous measurement of the rate of arterial pulsation, palpated at the wrist, and the rate of ventricular contraction, determined by direct auscultation of the heart with a stethoscope applied over the cardiac apex. (See p. 370.) Two individuals perform this maneuver, each making an independent count, one counting the radial pulsations and the other counting the audible heart beats, both counting from the same watch and both counts being started and completed simultaneousy. A full minute of counting is required as a minimum, and a 2-minute count is preferable for accurate measurements of pulse deficit.

Arterial Pressure

The force exerted by each systolic contraction of the left ventricle is normally sufficient to increase the pressure of the blood in the aorta and in all of the major arteries to a peak between 120 and 150 mm. of mercury (or between 5 and 7 feet of water). Venous pressure, by contrast, differs widely throughout the body, being greatest in the areas which are most dependent on their relation to the heart. The normal value, calculated with reference to the position of the right atrium, is approximately 7 mm. of mercury (or 4 inches of water).

The level of arterial pressure is determined by 2 factors: (1) the *cardiac output,* in other words, the rate with which blood is ejected from the heart into the aorta; and (2) the ease with which blood flows from the larger arteries through the smallest arterial branches, or the *degree of peripheral resistance* to blood flow. The magnitude of cardiac output depends on the speed and the force of ventricular contractions, as well as on the volume of blood filling the left ventricle before its contraction; the peripheral resistance is determined by the caliber of the arterioles.

The measurement of the arterial blood pressure is one of the most important aspects of the clinical examination. It, together with measurements of the pulse rate, the body temperature and the respiration, should be performed routinely as an integral part of every diagnostic investigation, for these pressure values supply vital information with respect to the efficiency of cardiac function and the status of the peripheral vascular system.

Systolic Pressure. This is defined as the peak level of arterial pressure that is attained during the cardiac cycle; it coincides with the crest of the pulse wave. This pressure, in a normal adult at rest, varies between 110 and 140 mm. of mercury; in normal children it lies between 95 and 110, and in infants between 75 and 90 mm. of mercury. It is precisely equal to the degree of arterial compression that is necessary and just sufficient to halt the flow of arterial blood completely and continuously. It is recorded at the level on the sphygmomanometer where the first sound is heard.

Diastolic Pressure. The diastolic pressure, normally between 70 and 85 mm. of mercury, is the lowest level of pressure in the cardiac cycle, occurring immediately following the subsidence of each ventricular contraction when the musculature of the heart is relaxed most completely. Its height depends, in part, on the elasticity of the arterial vessels—in other words, on the degree of compression exerted by their muscular walls as they contract from the state of stretch after each systolic wave. In part, its height also depends on the rapidity with which blood escapes from the arteries through the arterioles. It is recorded at the level where the sounds disappear.

Pulse Pressure. The difference between systolic and diastolic pressure is termed the pulse pressure; normally it is about ⅓ the value of the systolic arterial pressure. A "wide" pulse pressure, with a reduced diastolic and a normal or elevated systolic pressure, usually denotes the presence of a normal or increased cardiac output and a simultaneous reduction of peripheral arteriolar resistance; this is a situation observed in febrile states, in patients with hyperthyroidism and in normal individuals following exertion attributable both to a subnormal diastolic and an increased systolic pressure. It also is observed in certain types of heart disease affecting the aortic valve, failure of its effective closure in diastole permitting blood to flow back into the left ventricle from the aorta after each systolic contraction.

Errors in Sphygmomanometry. Transient elevations of blood pressure may be attributable solely to an increase in cardiac output caused by emotional stress or recent physical exertion. Failure to elicit audible sounds of any type may be due to malposition of the stethoscope or, in hypertensive patients, to failure of the examiner to elevate the cuff pressure high enough to exceed the systolic pressure.

Guidelines for Taking the Blood Pressure. The first step in determining the source of the difficulty is to palpate the radial pulse while simultaneously elevating the pressure cuff to the precise level at which the pulse is obliterated completely; this corresponds approximately with the systolic arterial pressure. If the latter is substantially above or below the range tested previously, the observer then proceeds by the auscultatory method, as indicated; otherwise the difficulty must be attributable to failure to locate the end piece of the stethoscope in correct relation to the brachial artery, assuming of course that the instrument itself is patent and functioning properly. This artery may have been obliterated as a result of disease or it may be located in an unusual position. In any event, it is necessary to establish the location of the brachial pulse by means of palpation and to repeat the determination with whatever modifications are indicated.

Erroneously high arterial blood pressure values are obtained in very obese individuals because of the excessive girth of the upper arm. Valid recordings under these circumstances require the use of an unusually broad cuff. Otherwise, the latter impinges unevenly, and the distribution of pressure is not as an even band but as a wedge. In this case, the manometric readings are recording certain components of pressure that are directed tangentially toward the shoulder and the elbow and are spreading the soft tissues rather than compressing the deeper structures of the arm.

Difficulty in determining the diastolic pressure may arise from the fact that the pulse occasionally remains audible throughout the entire reading range until the cuff pressure is reduced to zero. This situation emphasizes the importance of learning to recognize and interpret correctly the quality of sounds, for one must depend exclusively on one's ability to detect the point at which there is a disappearance of sound. Occasionally, as in aortic insufficiency, the sound never entirely disappears and then the diastolic is recorded as 2 numbers—the change of sound and zero, i.e., 160/40/0. Blood pressure is recorded as systolic over diastolic (i.e., 120/70).

The "auscultatory gap," a potential source of error in occasional patients with severe hypertension, is a phenomenon marked by the complete disappearance of sound between the systolic and the diastolic pressure levels. Thus, the systolic pressure may be estimated at a level of 260 mm. of mercury and, with gradual release of the cuff pressure, the sounds suddenly disappear at a reading of 220. Were the test abandoned at this point, it obviously would be interpreted as indicating an arterial pressure of 260/220. However, if the nurse is accustomed to continue auscultation until the cuff pressure has been completely released, she will note, in such cases, that sounds again become audible at a much lower level—for example, at 150—and disappear at 130 mm. of mercury, so that the arterial pressure should be recorded as 260/130.

Arterial Hypertension and Hypotension. Temporary elevations of blood pressure normally occur as a result of emotional excitement and muscular exertion, explainable on the base of an increased cardiac output and peripheral arteriolar resistance, for which the activities of the sympathetic nervous system and of the adrenal glands are responsible. Hyperactivity of the thyroid gland usually results in a more prolonged elevation of arterial pressure, which can be related to a marked increase in cardiac output. However, in most patients with chronic arterial hypertension the cardiac output is normal, and the abnormality is assumed to result from an increase in peripheral resistance due to sustained, generalized arteriolar vasoconstriction throughout the body, with consequences which are damaging to the kidneys, the heart and the brain.

Hypotension. The term "low blood pressure," as generally applied, has no precise significance. In many normal individuals the arterial pressure consistently ranges between 90 and 100 mm. of mercury.

On the other hand, transient acute hypotension is of great importance. It is a regular occurrence in some individuals upon arising suddenly from a reclining or sitting position ("postural hypotension") and may be accompanied by attacks of dizziness or even temporary loss of consciousness. This usually is attributable to marked loss of muscular "tone" in the lower extremities due to neurologic disease, prolonged bed rest or debility; for these muscles, instead of providing a firm support for the veins in the dependent areas or assisting them to empty in the direction of the thorax, permit them to dilate and retain an excessive volume of pooled blood. Acute hypotension also occurs in patients afflicted with carotid sinus sensitivity; nerve impulses originating in these centers produce sudden dilatation of the peripheral arterioles, with consequent loss of peripheral resistance to blood flow, or cause temporary heart block with transient cessation of cardiac output. Acute hypotension is also one of the most significant features of "shock," whether due to excessive blood loss or to "forward heart failure." Chronic hypotension is an important clinical sign of Addison's disease (see Chap. 31) and of severe cachexia, whether due to inadequate function of the pituitary gland, to prolonged infection or to severe malnutrition.

Venous Pressure

The pressure in the venous system is low in comparison with the arterial pressure, although it is quite sufficient to ensure the adequate return of blood to the right atrium. The venous pressure is elevated abnormally in patients with congestive heart failure due to myocardial or valvular disease, to compression of the heart by a scarred, inelastic pericardial membrane or by a fluid accumulation within the pericardial sac. A local increase in venous pressure in 1 portion of the body, i.e., in 1 or more extremities, is a common sequel of local venous obstruction due to mechanical causes or to incompetence of the venous valves. These structures greatly facilitate the return of venous blood to the thorax and to the right atrium by reducing the hydrostatic venous pressure in dependent portions of the body; moreover, they protect the capillary vessels in those regions from exposure to processes which would almost certainly exceed their tolerance. But for the valves in the femoral and the saphenous veins, for

example, the venous and the capillary pressure in the feet would approximate the diastolic arterial pressure (i.e., 40 inches of water or about 120 mm. of mercury, instead of 2 mm. of mercury) and fluid would escape rapidly through the capillary loops into the surrounding tissues.

A local increase in venous pressure, complicated by edema formation in the dependent areas, can result from venous varicosities with valvular destruction, from malignant tumors impinging on the femoral or the iliac veins or on the vena cava, from intraperitoneal fluid accumulation (ascites) compressing the vena cava and from inflammatory diseases of the veins resulting in thrombosis and the obliteration of these channels. Obstruction of a brachial or an axillary vein or of one of the great veins in the superior mediastinum into which they drain results in edema of a single upper extremity. Edema of the upper trunk, both upper extremities, the neck and the head, while the lower trunk and the limbs are edema-free, suggests obstruction of the superior vena cava.

A generalized increase in venous pressure usually is detected without difficulty upon routine inspection of the patient by observing neck vein distention when the patient is sitting or standing. Normally, in these positions, venous filling is not visible much above the clavicles. However, in cases of congestive heart failure, filling is generally seen at a much higher level, distention of the neck veins occasionally being apparent at the angle of the jaw. Another observation of similar significance is the observation of venous distention in the upper extremities when the latter are raised above the level of the chest.

SUMMARY OF NURSING ROLE

Because of her frequent and intimate contacts with the patient, the nurse is indispensable as an observer and a recorder of signs and symptoms. She has numerous opportunities daily to solicit information which is potentially of diagnostic value. The confidence of patients is readily established as they become acquainted with her in her role as their nurse. She must learn to be accurate and discriminating in her observations and must train herself to record them in complete and explicit terms for the physician.

BIBLIOGRAPHY

Books

Delp, M. H., and Manning, R. T.: Major's Physical Diagnosis. Philadelphia, W. B. Saunders, 1968.
Fuerst, E. V., and Wolff, L.: Fundamentals of Nursing. ed. 4. Philadelphia, J. B. Lippincott, 1969.
Hochstein, E., and Rubin, A. L.: Physical Diagnosis. New York, McGraw-Hill, 1964.

MacBryde, C. M. (ed.): Signs and Symptoms. ed. 4. Philadelphia, J. B. Lippincott, 1964.

McClain, M. E., and Gragg, S. H.: Scientific Principles in Nursing. ed. 5. St. Louis, C. V. Mosby, 1966.

Matheney, R. V., *et al.:* Fundamentals of Patient-Centered Nursing. St. Louis, C. V. Mosby, 1964.

Matousek, W. C.: Differential Diagnosis. Chicago, Year Book Medical Publishers, 1967.

Sjöstraand, T.: Clinical Physiology. Philadelphia, J. B. Lippincott, 1967.

Articles

Bean, M. A., *et al.:* Monitoring patients through electronics. Amer. J. Nurs., *63*:65-69, April, 1963.

Brown, C., Iannarella, F., Menchetti, G., and Tuman, M.: Body function monitoring. Nurs. Clin. N. Amer., *1*:569-576, Dec., 1966.

Carriker, D. B., and Rosenberg, M.: Automation—a facilitator of nursing practice. ANA Clinical Sessions, 83-89, 1966.

George, J. H.: Electronic monitoring. Amer. J. Nurs., *65*:68-71, Feb., 1965.

Hershey, M.: Automation in patient care, the legal perspective. Amer. J. Nurs., *67*:1039-1047, May, 1967.

Keezer, W. S.: The clinical thermometer. Amer. J. Nurs., *66*: 326-327, Feb., 1966.

Manning, R. T., *et al.:* Signs, symptoms and systematics. JAMA, *198*:1180-1184, 1966.

Nichols, G. A., and Verhonick, P. J.: Time and temperature. Amer. J. Nurs., *67*:2304-2306, Nov., 1967.

Perloff, J. K.: A modern view of an ancient art—feeling the pulse. GP, *33*:78-86, 1966.

Rosenberg, M., and Carriker, D.: Automating nurses' notes. Amer. J. Nurs., *66*:1021-1023, May, 1966.

Tarrant, B. J.: Automation: its effect on the patient, the nurse and the hospital. Amer. J. Nurs., *66*:2190-2199, Oct., 1966.

CHAPTER **3**

Illness as a Human Experience

- *Aspects of Communication*
- *Basic Emotional Needs*
- *Anxiety*
- *Body Image*
- *Stages in Adaptation to Illness*
- *Anger and Hostility*
- *Grief and Mourning*
- *Denial*
- *Psychosomatic Interactions*
- *Dying and Death*

ASPECTS OF COMMUNICATION

The experience of illness precipitates many stressful feelings and reactions, e.g., anxiety, anger, denial, shame, guilt, and uncertainty. The diagnostic tests, the medical treatment, the prognosis, the body changes, the reactions of family and friends, the experience of hospitalization, and the projected changes in life style—all take part in a person's adaptation to the new situation. Usually, a sick person is exceptionally sensitive and vulnerable. His whole life has been changed at least temporarily, and he often struggles with the resurgence of past experiences as he copes with the present reality and the anticipated future. The nurse is a central figure in the patient's immediate life. Through sensitive understanding and intelligent action she can provide many opportunities for the patient to maintain his basic security, self-esteem, and integrity.

The basic nurse-patient relationship takes into account the physician, the family, other patients, the rest of the health team and society at large. The relationship is established and maintained by the communication process—a complex, dynamic exchange of verbal and nonverbal messages. Communication is based on mutually intelligible symbols. To be understood, a person must have a knowledge of himself and his needs, be able to speak the language, be able to express himself clearly, and be familiar with the usual conventions of the situation. To understand others, he must be able to observe and evaluate behavior. To make oneself understandable and to understand others is vital to the establishment of relationships. The patient whose English is inept or who speaks a foreign langauge, or whose ability to express himself is markedly impaired through physical or psychological causes, poses a challenge to the nurse.

The process of communication may be considered to consist of 4 segments: (1) *I* (2) *am communicating something* (3) *to you* (4) *in this situation*. Breakdowns in communication can be pinpointed by identifying the segment in which the interference is taking place. The sender of the message, the *I*, is affected by such factors as age, sex, socioeconomic status, marital status, occupation, intelligence, physical condition (especially as related to the nervous system and the organs of communication), personality, and current emotional status. The message, *am communicating something*, consists of both verbal and nonverbal elements that may be complementary or incongruent. The patient who says, "Oh, I'm fine. Nothing is the matter," while restlessly moving about, wringing her hands and sighing frequently illustrates the latter.

The receiver of the communication, *to you*, is influenced by the same factors as the sender as regards behavior. The ability to hear or "read" a patient's behavior depends largely upon the ability to listen openly and sensitively. The presence of stereotypes, misconceptions, and her own anxiety may prevent the nurse from correctly identifying the message from a particular patient. The context of the communication, *in this situation,* refers to the sociocultural status of the patient, the context of illness, the social order of the hospital, and immediate environmental aspects. The importance of understanding the cultural background and the values of patients has gained recognition in all areas of nursing. When patients enter the hospital world, they may be overwhelmed and bewildered by the change in their status and role. The nurse plays a vital part in orienting patients to their new position. She also needs to acquaint them with the scope of her professional services. Many people do not know that the nurse is prepared and eager to help them with a wide variety of health needs. In addition to performing the traditional services related to physical needs, she offers help as a health teacher, a rehabilitation worker, a liaison between other professional services, and in some instances, a psychotherapeutic counselor.

A person in the first stages of adapting to illness, who is taking the defensive measure of denying his illness, does not seek or welcome accurate information about his condition or treatment. A nurse who attempts to do effective health teaching will find her efforts of little avail in such a case. The behavior of the patient, the questions he asks or avoids, and his reactions to the changes in his health status all give clues to his readiness and his needs. In turn, the patient is also very sensitive to the reactions of the medical and nursing staff. Very often patients seek to interpret nonverbal messages in regard to their prognosis, especially when it is not favorable. Patients are particularly aware of the commodity of time, and are often reluctant to ask for attention because the nurses are "too busy."

Developing skill in listening to and talking with patients is a continuous process that improves with experience. The nurse communicates with patients in order to identify their health needs, to clarify misconceptions, to help them verbalize their fears and reactions to their situations. Anxiety can be lessened or channeled through sharing it with another person. The nurse concerns herself with the impact of illness in the patient's life situation in order to arrive at a position where she can be helpful in sorting out the answers to his problems. She must be aware of the right of the patient to privacy about his life and recognize that the purpose of talking with him is to be of benefit to him.

The expressive function of the nurse has been identified as that of helping the patient maintain his motivational equilibrium. This consists of helping him to cope with the experience of illness and treatment by providing direct gratifications that reduce his tension level and help him to adapt to the process. The provision of physical comfort and support is combined with such interpersonal activities as explaining, reassuring, understanding, protecting, and simply being with the patient. When a patient is acutely ill, communication generally takes place on a primitive, chiefly nonverbal level. The nurse evaluates the ability of the patient to communicate and simplifies her verbal interaction with him. A touch, a soft but reassuring tone of voice, and the presence of the nurse may convey to the patient that he is not alone and that he is being cared for. When it is anticipated that a patient will have a direct interference with communication patterns as a result of treatment, it is a vital part of his care to set up a system of communication prior to that treatment. One patient reported: "The worse part about my laryngectomy was that I couldn't talk or tell anyone what I needed, but the magic slate helped."

An important part of the development of interpersonal and communication tools is the nurse's understanding of herself, her characteristic interpersonal needs, and her usual patterns of communication. As she becomes more aware of her own needs, she is better able to identify those of her patients and to know when her own perceptions and reactions are preventing her from accurately assessing the situation. This is particularly true when the patient's behavior is frustrating, puzzling, or otherwise upsetting to her personally. When a patient is hostile or demanding, the nurse must be able to evaluate her own responses so that she does not retaliate with anger or rejection. The situations that lead to feelings of helplessness and hopelessness must be talked about and shared so that the nurse can maintain her own equilibrium and give optimal nursing care to patients with incurable, repulsive, or terminal conditions. The nurse's awareness of her own need for approval and recognition plays an important part in her reaction to patient behavior and that of her coworkers, supervisors, and the medical staff. Nurses must come to grips with the vast amount of knowledge that is available and ever increasing. The many varieties of human personalities pose a constant challenge to find effective ways to help patients in the crisis situation of illness.

BASIC EMOTIONAL NEEDS

Everyone has the same basic emotional needs. These have been categorized by some authorities as love, trust, autonomy or self-control, self-esteem, identity and productivity. Another list includes the desire for recognition, for new experiences, for security, and for response—to give and receive personal appreciation, love and affection. Boiled down, the foregoing needs might be divided into 3 categories: (1) inclusion, (2) control and (3) affection. These are helpful guides in understanding the behavior of both patient and nurse as they relate to each other. The nonrealization of a need leads to undesirable consequences. The discrepancy between the need and its fulfillment results in feelings that are labeled *anxiety*.

The *need for inclusion* is defined behaviorally as the need to establish and maintain a satisfactory relation with people with respect to association and interaction. It refers to the establishment and maintenance of a feeling of mutual interest in others. In relation to the self-concept, the need for inclusion is the need to feel that the self is significant and worthwhile. Inclusion behavior refers to association between individuals and is indicated by such words as "associate," "interact," "belong," "join," and "communicate." Lack of inclusion is connoted by words such as "excluded," "ignored," "withdrawn," "aloof," or "isolated." The need to be included is shown by the desire to attract attention and interest. The "demanding" patient who frequently signals and monopolizes the staff with extensive conversation may simply be indicating strong needs for inclusion. The nurse who feels personally slighted when a patient ignores her attempts at polite conversation or treats her like a servant rather than a professional person may be demonstrating her own inclusion needs. The desire for prestige and status is a part of inclusion needs, and indicates a need for people to pay attention to a person, know who he is, and distinguish him from others. Identity is closely related to inclusion. One is known as a distinct individual, who therefore deserves attention paid to him. The height of inclusion is to be understood, which implies that someone is interested enough to seek and discover a person's particular characteristics, likes and dislikes.

When people enter a hospital situation, their first crises involve inclusion needs. Will the staff know who they are? Will they be treated like a person and not just another case—"Room 111" or "the new cardiac"? Many routines of hospital admission strip the patient of his outward signs of prestige and status. His clothes and belongings, even his dentures, may be taken away. He receives a uniform and often humiliating hospital gown. He may be bombarded by a series of questions relating to the most intimate details of his life. He is expected to join the patient "group" but may be given little explanation or few guidelines as to what to do. When it is necessary to place a patient in isolation, attention should be given to his inclusion needs—the nurse becomes a vital link in satisfying them. Other ways to help a patient with his inclusion needs include a thorough and considerate orientation to his physical surroundings. The nurse can inquire about any questions the patient has, what he expects from his treatment, and how he expects her to help him. She can give him some guidelines in terms of her professional responsibility—that she will be available to help him in a variety of ways—and that she will maintain her interest in him as an individual.

The patient who is withdrawn and avoids association with others may have unmet inclusion needs. He may not talk to his roommates or the nurse and may spend long periods sleeping or with the curtains pulled. A certain amount of regression and isolation is often a necessary part of adaptation to illness and recovery, but extremes over a period of time are significant. Underneath an apparent indifference to others may lie a basic anxiety in relation to people. The patient's worst fear may be that others will ignore him and show no interest in him, which he disguises with a lack of interest in others and a seeming independence. Feelings of worthlessness and inferiority may prevail or be heightened by illness and incapacitation, and may progress to the point where the motivation to live is lacking. Patients who feel abandoned and isolated from their families and friends, who believe that they are so changed now as to be unacceptable, or who feel rejected and ignored by the medical and nursing staff, may give up the struggle. On the other hand, such patients may get lifesaving reassurance and support from the nurse who continues to include them in the human race and communicates her recognition of their individuality and worth.

Excessive need for inclusion may be seen in the patient who is always demanding attention. Patients who demand "VIP" treatment, who ask for many little favors, or who brag about themselves all give clues to their inclusion needs. Part of the decision of where to place a patient is based on his need for inclusion. Will he do better in a room with three other people? How close to the nursing station should he be? Patients who are together for long periods of time, such as on an orthopedic ward or a facility for the treatment of tuberculosis, demonstrate a particularly wide variety of inclusion needs.

The second major need is *control*. This is the need to establish and maintain a satisfactory relation to others with regard to power, decision-making, and authority. It has to do with the feeling of mutual respect for the competence and responsibility of the self and others. Control needs are suggested by such words as "dominance," "influence," "boss," "rebellion," "submission," "leader," "noncooperation," and "follower." Control represents assumption of power over others and therefore over one's own future, while to *be* controlled means giving up responsibility for oneself.

When a person comes to a hospital, he struggles

with his need for control. In addition to the problems of inclusion, he may find other people making decisions for him that he would ordinarily make for himself—when to get up, what to eat, and when to go to the toilet. The rules of the hospital may take away his usual decision-making capacity. An extreme example of control behavior is the person who completely gives up or abdicates his own responsibility. He is a clinging, helpless patient who seeks direction from everyone as to what to do and how to do it. This reinforces his conviction that he is incompetent, unresponsible, and powerless. Behind these beliefs often lie anxiety, hostility, and a lack of trust in others as well as oneself. Helping the patient to assume early responsibility and decision-making for his own care are nursing actions that help to increase a sense of self-control and responsibility.

The other extreme in control behavior is reflected in actions of constant rebellion and domination. Although the patient's overt behavior may be that of a strong, competent, responsible person, his underlying feelings may be those of uncertainty in his own power. He takes every opportunity to disprove these fears and therefore has a great deal of difficulty in allowing necessary dependency such as bed rest or following "doctor's orders." Nurses also need to examine their own needs for power and control in relation to patients, coworkers, and physicians.

The third major need is that of *affection*. This represents the need to establish with another person a give-and-take relationship based on mutual liking. Affection is suggested by such words as "love," "like," "emotionally close," "personal," "friendship," "intimacy." Lack of affection is connoted by "hate," "dislike," and "emotionally distant." The need for affection is usually met by family members, spouses, and close friends. When a person is separated from these sources by illness or hospitalization, he may not have the need satisfied sufficiently. To be emotionally close to another generally results in confiding innermost anxieties, wishes, and feelings. In the hospital setting, the patient may turn to the nurse to share these things, especially if the family member is unavailable or too anxious to listen. One difference between a social and a professional relationship is that the former implies mutuality of need-satisfying, the latter, that the patient's needs are the focus without the nurse's burdening him with her own problems. However, the need for affection in both patient and nurse must be considered, particularly when the relationship continues over a period of time.

Aspects of inclusion, control, and affection behavior are overlapping and continuous. Inclusion is primarily related to the formation of a relationship, while control and affection are demonstrated within the relationship. Inclusion is related to feeling "in" or "out"; control, to "top" or "bottom"; and affection, to "remote" or "close." Generally, a person establishes an equilibrium between himself and other people in these 3 different areas. Sickness with hospitalization disturbs this equilibrium, giving rise to a wide variety of new stresses. The nurse-patient relationship is a dynamic, shifting experience in which the nurse uses her knowledge, understanding, and compassion to help the patient resolve personal conflicts in the most meaningful ways possible.

ANXIETY

Anxiety is a normal reaction to stress and threat. It is an emotional reaction to the perception of danger, real or imagined, that is experienced physiologically, psychologically, and behaviorally. Anxiety and fear are often used synonymously; however, fear generally refers to a specific threat, anxiety to a nonspecific one. A person experiencing anxiety may feel uneasy and apprehensive, having a vague sense of dread. Feelings of helplessness and inadequacy may be present along with a sense of alienation and insecurity. The intensity of these feelings may range from mild to severe enough to cause panic, and the intensity may be increased or diminished by interpersonal means.

Anxiety is caused by a threat to the functioning of the organism—either to physical survival or to the integrity of psychosocial self (self-image). Often, the threat affects both these areas: a person who is anxious because of acute pain may also be anxious in response to his feelings about his level of courage and dependency. Illness and hospitalization include the following anxiety-precipitating threats: general threat to life, health and body integrity; exposure and embarrassment; discomfort from pain, cold, fatigue, and changes in diet; deprivation of sexual satisfaction; restriction of movement; isolation; interruption or loss of one's means of livelihood; precipitation of a financial crisis; dislike, rejection or ridicule from others as the result of the condition; inconsistent and unpredictable behavior of the authority figures on whom one's welfare depends; frustration of goals and expectations; confusion and uncertainty about the present and the future; separation from family and friends.

Physiologic reactions to anxiety are primarily reactions of the autonomic nervous system and are defensive in nature. They include increased heart beat and respiration, shifts in blood pressure and temperature, relaxation of the smooth muscles in the bladder and bowel, cold, clammy skin, increased perspiration, dilated pupils and dry mouth. The bodily responses to mild anxiety initially promote learning and the ability to function, but as the reaction increases in severity, learning decreases, perception is reduced or distorted, and the ability to concentrate is greatly reduced. Nurses must be able to evaluate the level of anxiety in a patient so that they can be effective in reducing it, and thus help the patient cope with his immediate situation. An extremely anxious person is suffering and is very uncomfortable. He has difficulty giving or receiving information of any kind. As far as health matters are concerned, he learns little and magnifies or distorts what he hears.

Characteristic manifestations of anxiety reflect a person's individuality. They include withdrawal, muteness, hyperactivity, swearing, talking and joking excessively, striking out verbally or physically, phantasizing, complaining and crying. The specific means of coping with anxiety, whether successful or not, varies with individuals and with the situation. One disadvantage of enforced immobility and isolation is that a person used to active approaches in handling anxiety is prevented from his usual means and so must develop alternate channels.

Nursing intervention in anxiety includes 4 aspects:

1. Recognition by the nurse that the patient is anxious. She is aware of situations that can potentially precipitate anxiety and is alerted to physiologic, emotional, and behavioral clues.

2. The nurse verbally encourages the patient to recognize and express his feelings of anxiety.

3. If the source of the anxiety is external, such as poor orientation to the ward or disturbing noises and sights, the nurse may take steps to change these conditions or, if this is impossible, help the patient understand and cope with his reactions. By identifying the source of anxiety, the nurse can help the patient adapt more readily. She encourages the patient to share his immediate experience by open-ended statements such as "Tell me what happened" or "What was going on?" Patients often need help in describing their reactions and thoughts. To ask initially "Why are you anxious?" may or may not result in the information. The person may be too afraid or unsure to tell you, he may not know why he is anxious; or he may resent the inquisition.

4. The nurse helps the patient cope with what is now a specific threat. He may be helped to re-evaluate the situation and his reaction to it. Many times just the sharing of a feeling reduces its intensity. The nurse asks the patient what he usually does to handle anxious feelings and helps him to use similar or other means. The physical presence of the nurse may help, as well as the appropriate use of touch, physical care, and tones of voice.

The apprehension of patients recovering from surgery may be demonstrated by their anxiety as to whether the operation was a success and whether they will survive the bewildering, painful, often uncertain postoperative period. The expert physical nursing care given in the recovery room or intensive care unit must take into consideration the patient's fears resulting from isolation, the weird noises and equipment attached to all parts of the body, the blinking, beeping monitor signalling the body's functioning, and the periods of disorientation and loss of physical and emotional control. In this tense situation the nurse must be constantly aware of her own behavioral manifestations of anxiety, so that she does not communicate them to the patient.

Illness and its treatment are anxiety-precipitating. For many people, early conflicts are revived. There is often a great deal of uncertainty about the future. The nurse sometimes may be powerless to decrease the patient's anxiety at all, but she can avoid adding to it. For some patients, getting well and leaving the hospital is anxiety-producing. The nurse can be helpful to these people by encouraging them to mobilize their strengths and by encouraging decision-making and the reacquisition of responsibility.

Nursing in almost all areas is a profession that deals continually with anxiety. The intimate association with life, death, and all the stages in between arouse conscious and unconscious fears of her own vulnerability in the nurse. Recognition, achievement, and attention are all important to her; she must be able to say that she did all that was possible. There are emotional "high risk" situations in nursing, such as the intensive care unit and the emergency room, in which the nurse's understanding and management of her own anxiety as well as that of patients and their families is vital.

BODY IMAGE

The concept of body image is useful in understanding the many complex reactions of people to changes in their health status. Body image may be considered as the total, constantly changing and evolving perception of one's physical self as separate and distinct from all others. This perception is based on inner sensations and functionings as well as on information derived from the external environment. Society prescribes norms of physical appearance and behavior. The perception of body image operates on both a conscious and unconscious basis.

Integration of experiences regarding the use of the body takes place over a long period of time. The formative years of childhood are particularly significant in laying down the basic body image and its relation to the personality. While a child is being held, fondled, fed, played with and toilet-trained, he gradually accumulates related concepts pertaining to his ability to use his physical body, his degree of pride, and his sense of identity. Through sensory impressions, motility, and touch he experiences pleasure, pain, shame, failure or pride of accomplishment as he tests out his boundaries and abilities. As the small child becomes aware of his separation from others, he grows increasingly conscious of his own body, its relation to others, and his ability to control his muscles in the acts of locomotion, bowel and bladder retention and release, motor coordination and speech. During this period, he begins to master these abilities, which results in pride and self-esteem. If he is not able to do so because of loss of self-control or parental overcontrol, he may develop basic attitudes toward his body as being inadequate, worthless, and shameful. Illness, with enforced dependency and lack of body control, reactivates in persons of all ages many of these early conflicts and perceptions of body image. Feeling ashamed of a disfigurement or deformity stems from early attitudes toward smallness, weakness, and ugliness as compared to others. The prominent sociocultural values on youth, physical attractiveness, health, and wholeness are incorporated early and reinforced throughout life.

Threats to the body image, and therefore to self-esteem, are recognizable in many nursing situations. Feelings of shame, inadequacy, and guilt may precipitate, depending on the patient's definition of the situation. Violation of modesty and invasion of privacy causes anxiety and embarrassment. Exposure of the body during physical examinations and such treatments as enemas and catheterizations may be upsetting, even though expected as part of the therapeutic regimen. The disturbance in usual elimination processes and the need for using a bedpan or talking about bowel and bladder habits threatens self-esteem. This is a major problem for people requiring surgery that produces such drastic changes as a colostomy or ileostomy. Major changes in the body image are brought about by amputation of any part, or surgery of the face, hands, and reproductive organs—areas particularly related to identity and self-esteem. Other parts of the body may have unconscious symbolic meaning to a person, and so he may react in an unexpected way to relatively minor, external changes. Besides the sudden changes in body structure and functioning that occur through accident or surgical intervention, subtle changes occur in progressive diseases such as arthritis, obesity, and multiple sclerosis. Even normal changes in the body pose a problem of altering the body image, such as in puberty and pregnancy. During adolescence there is a sensitive, often painful awareness of the body with its many changes. Complexion, weight, and development of primary and secondary sexual characteristics are intricately linked to feelings of worth and sexual desirability.

Changes in the body image may result from the side effects of medication that cause development of a moon face, changes in the secondary sex characteristics, and growth of facial hair. The reaction of the body to radiation treatment may further threaten the body image, as may changes in skin color:

> A man who was dying developed a marked jaundice. When the nursing student commented, "My, you're yellow," he became very upset. "No, no, I'm not!" he insisted. Communication stopped at this point. Later, in conference, the students explored the possible meanings of his remarks. Was it complete denial of his actual condition? Was he aware he was dying and his skin condition confirmed this? Or did he interpret the comment to mean he was "yellow"—cowardly?

Changes in medical technology require that nurses meet the challenge of new and different approaches to helping people. A person with chronic kidney damage extends his body image to include the "artificial kidney." Organ transplants are another development that raises questions about body image. What does it mean to a person to have another person's heart beating in his chest? What would it be like to have parts of your own body live on after you are clinically dead?

The first step in understanding the concept of body image is to become more aware of one's own attitude toward health, illness, mutilation, disfigurement, and changes in body functioning. Anxiety, revulsion, disgust, and pity are often automatic responses to abnormal body appearance and functioning. But to help patients who have these conditions, nurses must come to grips with their own feelings. A patient has a right to expect that nurses will be knowledgeable about his condition, will be impartial toward it, will be willing to help him, and will be concerned about him. A patient often uses the nurse's reactions as a test of whether he is still a worthwhile person in spite of his altered appearance or functioning.

The nurse needs to learn about the possible meanings and adjustments that alteration in the body image will cause the individual patient. Both the patient and his family should be considered, because ideally the adjustment that takes place is mutual. Careful interviewing helps to determine the proper approach, based on the strengths and needs of the patient and the family. A person who denies that he is anxious, frightened, angry, or even concerned is often protecting himself from facing the reality of the situation. This may be the only way for him to cope at this particular time, but it may delay necessary shifts in his body image. In formulating the nursing care plan for a particular patient, include the ability of the family to help the patient cope with changes, his orientation to reality, the specific problems in coping and his methods of coping, and the nursing care. The nurse needs to determine how she can help support the family and the steps she will take in response to the patient's positive moves. She can anticipate grief, mourning, and anger as reactions to changes in body appearance and functioning. The need for hope and steps toward full rehabilitation must be supported.

Even after the patient has begun to alter his body image and feels worthwhile and accepted in the hospital setting, he is faced with adjusting to society. Many conditions of altered appearance and functioning are stigmatizing. Because of their close proximity to illness, nurses may lose sight of the fact that to be disfigured or incapacitated still carries a negative connotation and means rejection by most of the population. Any such stigma implies that the person is not quite human—that he is a disabled person, rather than a person having a specific disability. The tendency to stereotype denies the person's individuality. A person with an obvious physical disability has a major problem in handling tensions in interpersonal situations. He may be subject to curiosity and stares. He may be asked invasive questions about his condition or treated as if he were completely helpless.

> A woman who had been blind for some time was admitted to the hospital for flu. She was roused by an aide to eat and as she sat up, she was jabbed in the face by a teaspoon full of food. "What's this?" she asked, and was told that because she was blind, the doctor had said that she had to be fed. The patient replied indignantly, "After all, madam, I do know where my own mouth is," and proceeded to demonstrate.

If the condition is not readily visible, learning to exercise information control may be helpful in decreasing stigma. For instance, a prosthesis for a mastectomy serves to suppress general knowledge about such radical surgery. Talking about one's health status, body functioning, and difficulties in adjustment are appropriate with health personnel and close family and friends. With other people, excessive dwelling on these topics may lead to ostracism and rejection.

A person making necessary adjustments to alterations in his body is often faced with physical and social insecurity. A physically normal person has a general idea of how high the bus steps are and is able to read from a menu. However, the person with a physical impairment may have to make constant and vigilant adaptations to his physical world. The person who uses a wheelchair must find a restroom large enough for him to maneuver in; one with diabetes must calculate his allowed intake at a cocktail party; a man with crutches may find a revolving door almost impossible to manage. Energy, ingenuity, and persistence are necessary to adapt. Sometimes an individual limits his living space and activities in order to provide more predictable situations. Although this arrangement may be safer, it also limits a person's full participation in life. Nurses can help patients increase their ability to anticipate and cope with problems in the physical world, and to find social and vocational settings in which they can function to the fullest capacity.

Reactions of others toward a disabled person and his condition are ambiguous and conflicting. Acceptance and rejection, sympathy and pity, trust and fear, curiosity and revulsion, valuation and devaluation face him in countless interpersonal situations. He is often unsure of where he stands, particularly with strangers. He is also often unsure of himself, because the process of adaptation and self-acceptance is a shifting one.

STAGES IN ADAPTATION TO ILLNESS

The transition from health to illness is a complex and highly individualized experience. The 2 main tasks to be faced by anyone with a developing condition are: (1) to modify his body image, the concept of himself and his relation to people and work; and (2) to readjust to the realistic limitations and adaptations of the condition. These 2 tasks begin to take place within a setting in which the person is being treated for his physical disturbance. In the cycle of health and illness, most people go through 3 stages: (1) the transition from health to illness, (2) the period of "accepted" illness, and (3) convalescence. The length of time and quality of experience an individual has in these stages vary with his personality, the specific disorder, and the changes made in his life.

The development of symptoms usually is accompanied by unpleasant sensations, loss of vigor and stamina, and a decrease in ability to function. Certain symptoms such as chest pain, indigestion or headache may increase in frequency and intensity. Anxiety is often present, which the person handles with his usual coping devices. To ward off the prospect of sickness, one person may plunge into activity, keeping late hours with extra work and social activities. Another may become passive and withdrawn, hoping that the vague symptoms will go away. A person may put off going to the doctor for fear of the diagnosis, which may be particularly threatening if a familiar disease such as cancer is suspected. Anxiety, guilt, shame and denial are prominent during this initial period. If the symptoms persist, the person may be impelled to seek medical attention. He may have marked ambivalent feelings toward examination and diagnostic tests, of which cancelled or missed appointments are often indices. Some patients go from doctor to doctor, hoping to find out "what is really the matter" or seeking evidence that a previous diagnosis was inaccurate.

If a person experiences a serious injury or a sudden catastrophe such as a heart attack or a cerebral vascular accident, he is instantly shifted from health to illness. His immediate concern is that help will not arrive in time, or that the strangers he is suddenly so dependent upon are not competent. If he is unconscious, his family may experience similar fears. This apprehension may be expressed through excessive demands, refusal to cooperate or accept the proposed treatment, and suspicion of the motives and methods of those trying to help. To reduce anxiety and prevent panic, it is helpful to obtain information about close relatives and to contact the person's own physician, if possible. Calm explanation of the necessary procedures and technical skill will convey to the patient that he is being cared for adequately.

When a patient is experiencing shock, disbelief, and denial of his condition, the nurse can help by being available to listen to him. In a noncritical way, she does not support the denial, but does allow the patient to cope with his situation in this way at the present time. She establishes herself as a helpful professional person who wants to understand the patient and his current dilemma. She orients him to his immediate environment and makes herself available to answer his questions.

The second stage is a shift to the period of accepted illness. The patient recognizes and admits that he is sick and in need of help from others, specifically from the medical and nursing staff. Temporarily, he withdraws interest and concern from his usual adult responsibilities and applies himself to the task of getting well. He becomes preoccupied with himself, his symptoms and treatment. Interest in current events and even concern about family and friends may be quite limited. The patient becomes egocentric, with increased dependency and increased somatic concerns. His behavior is often described as regressed, in that earlier forms of acting, feeling, and participating with others occurs. A certain amount of regression is considered necessary so that the person can allow himself bedrest, regulation in his eating, and just letting his body heal. People who normally resist being dependent may find being in a situation in which dependency is expected and permitted very difficult. They may be so frightened that they continue to deny their condition in part or refuse to follow prescribed treatment. They push themselves beyond their physical limits and leave treatment before it is indicated. Other dependency problems evolve when a person receives so much gratification from this state that he attempts to continue it indefinitely; the term "hospitalitis" refers to this situation.

Nursing students are often concerned that the patient will become too dependent on them. There must be a realistic evaluation of the stage of illness, the patient's needs for dependency, and his need for a trusting, caring person. Nurses who care for the same patients over a long period of time should evaluate their own needs for dependency and for having people dependent on them. Patients must be helped to move through the stages of illness, and nurses can help them to do so.

During the stage of accepted illness, the patient may express anger, guilt and resentment. He may be very critical of his care and medical management, attacking the very people on whom he so depends. In such a case, the most helpful nursing approach is to view this reaction as the patient's way of dealing with his situation and to try to understand how he feels. The nurse should encourage the patient to express his feelings, without passing judgment, moralizing, or arguing. She assumes responsibility for his care, but should be alert to individual differences and provide opportunities for him to make decisions and assume responsibility whenever indicated. As the patient becomes more assured of the nurse's availability, interest, and competence, he is less anxious and more willing to relinquish his dependence on her. During this period, the patient may be experiencing an acute sense of loss, of which the clinical picture is often depression with sadness, hopelessness, and anger. He may be mourning the loss of his state of health and vigor, the loss of a body part or function, or the changes in his job or family. He may be mourning his own death in advance.

The third stage in adaptation is called the convalescent period or the period of restitution. The return of health and physical strength often precedes the patient's feeling and acting "well." Just as a lag usually occurs in the initial stage between the appearance of physical symptoms and the emotional acceptance of illness, a reverse lag occurs at the other end. Getting well implies giving up a dependent, regressed, egocentric position and resuming adult responsibilities and normal relations with others. This stage has been compared to the period of adolescence, in which the individual must leave the protective world in which responsibilities were minimal and satisfaction of his own needs the prime concern. Although some people are reluctant to give up the patient role, most are motivated toward health but are afraid or hesitant to try out new skills. This is particularly true if the illness and treatment requires major changes in work and family relations. The nurse can help the patient in this stage by assuming a role analogous to that of an adequate parent of a teenager. The nurse gradually relaxes protection and offers guidance, advice and encouragement to progress. She quietly retires to the sidelines, ready to reassure the patient but encouraging him to experiment with new skills; she steps in only when gross errors in judgment occur. The patient senses the confidence of the nurse and is reassured by it, especially when ideal or perfect results are not expected.

During this stage the nurse can stimulate the patient

to renew his interest in the world, to communicate better with his family, and to make plans for the future. For example, for patients with radical surgery such as colostomy or laryngectomy, groups of people with similar conditions have formed clubs in the community. These club members may be called upon to talk to the patient both pre- and postoperatively, in order to convey hope and to give realistic, firsthand information on coping with their common disability. At first, the patient may be overwhelmed by anxiety or grief and be unable to use this service to his full advantage. As he recovers, he may be reminded and encouraged to avail himself of their help. It is important, however, to keep in mind individual differences, since some people prefer not to affiliate themselves with a group of this type. The connotation of being "different," of having a stigmatizing condition, may be too painful to accept.

The stages of transition from health to illness and back to health are most clearly defined when a person has an acute, discrete condition that responds favorably to treatment. A similar series of steps takes place in adapting to a chronic condition, as identified by Crate. She described the stages as disbelief, developing awareness, reorganization, resolution and identity changes. In a successful adaptation to a chronic illness, the person can comfortably or resignedly regard himself as having a specific condition. He acknowledges and copes with the necessary changes in his life imposed by the condition. Although he may have gone through periods of despair, anger, and self-depreciation, he is able to regard himself as a worthwhile person who happens to be dependent. The nurse needs to be aware of the changes in feelings during the adaptation, to recognize deviations from the usual patterns, and to help the patient move forward through the process. Adaptation to chronic illness is a lengthy and continuous process. The extent of adaptation required depends on the type of illness, the degree of disability, and the patient's unique personality. Some chronic illnesses are relatively stable with little changes; others have acute remissions and slow degeneration; others are terminal. Throughout, the nurse is in a position to provide skilled nursing care along with compassion, concern, and intelligent approaches to help guide the patient and his family in their struggles.

ANGER AND HOSTILITY

In addition to anxiety, expressions of anger are common in nursing situations. Conflict and frustration often precipitate aggression, a complex reaction of feelings and behavior that varies in intensity, duration and expression. Words such as "irritated," "sullen," "unfriendly," "hostile," "assertive," "belligerent," "defiant," "uncooperative," "resentful," "enraged," "furi-ous" and "indignant" describe differences in aggressiveness. Anger, the general term for this emotion, is one way of handling anxiety, particularly in response to real or perceived threat, insult or injury. To be a patient means to be sick, helpless, controlled by others, and assaulted—however therapeutically—by needles, catheters, enemas and surgical procedures. To be told to wait for medication angers many patients who are in pain. Being awakened in the middle of the night to cough and take deep breaths taxes anyone's patience. Hospital rules such as lights out and restrictions on visitors may precipitate feelings of anger. When a patient is new to the hospital or clinic, he is often uncertain and anxious about his diagnosis, treatment, and prognosis; as a defense he may flare out at the nurse or withdraw in sullen noncommunicativeness. Expressions of anger may decrease markedly as the element of the unknown is reduced and the patient becomes more familiar with his surroundings, the personnel, and the treatment program. On the other hand, anger may increase if the threat grows and the patient's needs are not met adequately.

A person who has been angry, unhappy, and chronically dissatisfied with himself and others brings this behavior with him to the clinical setting. He may be argumentative, demanding, unappreciative, sarcastic and unwilling to go along with nursing care. Extreme over-friendliness, ingratiation, and refusal to make any decision concerning one's care are opposite but nonetheless valid expressions of aggression. Occasionally, a patient is aggressive to the point of violence—throwing his dinner tray, shouting, cursing, doing or threatening to do physical harm. Nonverbal expressions of anger—glaring eyes, clenched fist, a sneer—can be nearly as eloquent.

Anger hinders progress. The usual social response to anger is to counterattack, withdraw, or avoid the situation. Generally, a nurse's initial response to an angry patient is to treat the situation much as she would in social circumstances. Many times this is not appropriate from the therapeutic standpoint. The professional nursing responsibility is to try to help this person even with and in spite of his anger. The nurse does this by first recognizing her own responses to angry behavior. It is not unusual for a nurse to experience feelings of irritation and annoyance in reaction to expressions of a patient's anger. She may be frightened, embarrassed and hurt. When a patient lashes out at her verbally, she may feel inadequate and guilty even if she has acted appropriately. She may feel helpless or immobilized to the extent that she dreads caring for the patient and begins to avoid him whenever possible. This kind of behavior may heighten the patient's frustration by leaving him isolated, helpless, and unable to depend on the nursing staff to meet his physical and emotional needs. Thus a vicious circle is established.

Aggressive behavior that is ascribable to a toxic condition is acceptable; the patient can be excused because he was delirious or "not in his right mind." The continuously hostile patient who is fully conscious and in control is much harder to understand and deal with. The expression of anger in the clinical situation may reflect the person's best manner of coping with threats that surround him. Anger may be an attempt to relieve feelings of helplessness and dependency. In other situations, anger may indicate part of the grief process or emergence from apathy and depression. A patient's anger may vanish when someone helps him to identify what is frustrating or threatening him and to take steps toward successfully dealing with the threat.

It is not unusual for people to displace feelings of anger—that is, to express them toward someone or something other than the original frustrator. When one believes oneself to be in a vulnerable position, it may not be safe to express dissatisfaction and anger directly. Therefore, one takes it out on somebody less likely to retaliate or less vitally important to one's emotional and physical well-being. A patient may be very angry with his physician but is afraid to complain for fear he will receive less attention. Instead, he bawls out the nurse and later insists that she contact his doctor. Or, the nurse and the doctor may have a covert misunderstanding; she finds herself snapping at the aides and being irritable with the patients. Generally, direct expressions of anger are not socially acceptable, and outbursts may be followed by guilt, shame and profuse apologies. Moreover, there exist cultural and socioeconomic differences in the expression of anger, and the nurse may find herself bewildered, insulted, and overwhelmed by behavior considered normal and expected by another individual.

Therapeutic responses to angry patients are based on the attempt to understand the person and his situation. The nurse is aware of her own reaction to him and attempts to help him sort out the issues involved. She enables the patient to maintain his dignity, pride and self-esteem. She sets limits on his behavior so that he does not hurt himself or others, and helps him to find more appropriate means to express his feelings. Although she may feel angry or frightened in reaction to the behavior, she uses her feelings for further problem-solving rather than giving way to retaliation or withdrawal. Helpful questions in arriving at a nursing care plan for patients who are angry and hostile include the following: When does the patient get angry and how does he show it? Does his anger interfere with his receiving the care he needs? Why does his behavior bother me? How do I react? Does he get angry with other people too? Is there someone who

does get along with him? What does that person do that is different? Does the patient's hostility serve a useful purpose? How much of this behavior reflects his usual way of reacting to people? How much is he willing to change? What realistic goals shall we work toward? Are there any other resources—doctor, family, psychiatric nursing consultant, psychiatrist, occupational therapist, or other patients—that we could call in? If the patient stops expressing anger, will he develop more destructive patterns?

Learning to work therapeutically with angry, hostile patients is a challenging and rewarding part of nursing. Patients who disguise temporary fear and shame with anger appreciate the nurse who stands by them in the crisis without condemnation, rejection, or retaliation. Patients who have made a lifelong adjustment by means of hostile attack are also grateful, although they may never express it directly, to the nurse who refuses to be alienated and who uses herself to understand and care for him.

GRIEF AND MOURNING

Grief is a complex of emotional responses to the anticipated or actual loss of someone or something valued. The loss may be that of a relative or friend, a part of the body, a job, health or life. Feelings of anxiety, helplessness, hopelessness, guilt, anger, remorse, sadness, and loneliness are part of grief. Mourning refers to the processes that follow the loss and ultimately result in overcoming the grief. There are many cultural factors in the specific way in which grief and mourning take place, from the extremes of stoic acceptance to elaborate and ritualistic weeping, keening and public display.

The intensity of grief and mourning depends on the significance and extent of the loss to the person. It is generally greater if the loss, especially through death, comes suddenly. If the survivor had been particularly dependent upon the deceased person, or if in any way he had been responsible for the death, grief is intensified. A person who is very sensitive to separation as a result of early separations may be deeply affected. Ambivalence (mixed feelings) is present in all significant relationships. If the ambivalence is marked, grief may be particularly intense, partly because the object of one's hostility is no longer present. Guilt and irrational ideas about the causation of the death may prevent a person from facing himself and mourning effectively.

The stages of mourning are similar to the stages of adaptation to illness—shock and disbelief, awareness, and restitution. Upon recognition of a loss, people often experience a sinking feeling, tightness in the throat, loss of appetite, fatigue, tension and acute anxiety. The sensorium is altered, with a feeling of unreality and distance from people. There is a preoccupation with the deceased or lost object and a state of readiness for its return. Feelings of guilt may be present, and there may take place a soul searching for things that could have been done differently. The grieving person's relationships with other people lack warmth and are characterized by irritation and the desire not to be bothered. He is likely to slow up activities, neglect personal care, and be restlessly, purposelessly active. He may develop symptoms similar to those of the deceased one. Sometimes the shock of the loss is intellectually accepted and the person goes through the motions of making arrangements and caring for others. His emotional reaction is cut off in his attempt to protect himself from the pain of the loss.

In the stage of developing awareness, the person experiences pain, anguish, emptiness and acute sadness. Crying or the desire to cry is common and often elicits support from others. Many people cannot allow themselves to cry in public and need privacy to handle their grief.

In the stage of restitution, the physical reality of the loss is emphasized. In the case of death, the funeral makes this fact unavoidable. In the case of an amputation, the sight of the stump and beginning to use a prosthesis underline the reality. The mourner begins a long process of coping with the absence of the loved person or object. There may be repetitive talk about the person or object that is often idealized, so that only pleasant memories are reinforced. Gradually, this assists in emotional detachment. As dependence on the lost object decreases, the person begins to develop new interests and invests his energy in other people. He is able to remember the relationship more realistically, with its good and bad aspects, and can talk about it without an emotional dependence on the memory of the relationship.

Nursing intervention to help patients handle their feelings with the experience of grief and mourning includes anticipating reactions to loss, supporting the patient's usual coping mechanisms, and allowing the patient to express feelings when he wishes. The nurse should provide privacy and availability when needed. When a body part or function is lost, the nurse designs her nursing care and manipulates the environment to prevent additional loss of self-esteem. In order to maintain resources and give complete care, she includes the family in the plan of care. Her presence and willingness to participate in the painful experiences that precipitate grief help to prevent feelings of total abandonment. By being aware of the usual patterns of grief and mourning, she is able to recognize maladaptive patterns and help evaluate the need for other types of therapeutic intervention, such as psychotherapy.

DENIAL

It has been mentioned that a common response to a shift in health status is denial. When symptoms of illness threaten a person, he may avoid facing his fear of them by unconsciously denying their existence or their significance. Denial is an ego-defense mechanism that protects the person from recognizing painful and disturbing aspects of reality. As long as a person can maintain the denial, it serves to diminish anxiety. However, the reality of increased symptom formation may force a person to abandon the denial.

Denial may possibly underlie the behavior of patients who do not follow treatment regimens and who miss appointments or transfer to another doctor. Inappropriate cheerfulness or lack of concern about symptoms of the illness may indicate denial. If anxiety, depression and anger are not expressed in situations where they could be expected, the patient may be protecting himself by denial. The ignoring of certain aspects of reality may indicate denial, as in the case of a coronary patient who experiences substernal pain and attributes it to indigestion. Obese patients who explain their trouble as "glandular" and deviate from their reducing diets also demonstrate this behavior. Denial may prevent a person from seeking help or it may interfere with his treatment program. However, it is also a means of maintaining psychological equilibrium. When the stress and anxiety decrease, so does the need for denial. Denial mechanisms may be operating in members of the patient's family as they try to protect themselves from recognizing the severity of the condition. Even when the possibility of imminent death is discussed, the family may deny that this is possible and act (or fail to act) accordingly.

In dealing with denial of illness as a nursing problem, the nurse assesses the extent to which the denial is harmful and in which ways it is beneficial. On this basis, she makes the necessary nursing judgments and intervenes accordingly. Generally, the defense of denial is not challenged directly, because such an action tends to reinforce the denial or leaves the person without adequate ego protection. On the other hand, the nurse does not support or encourage the denial. She makes herself available so that when the patient can relinquish his denial, she can help him cope with the onset of reality. Sometimes a person appears to use denial defenses, although he is consciously acting in such a manner in order to protect the feelings of his family. This may happen when the patient is aware that he will die soon but perceives that his family would be more comfortable if he continues the mutual deception. If the nurse conveys her interest in and concern for this patient, he may choose to talk about his feelings with her, thus lessening his isolation.

Denial is a coping mechanism that nurses use to

handle their own painful feelings about illness, radical surgery and death. A nurse may find this defense necessary to continue functioning in some areas over a long period of time. If she can talk about her feelings with other nurses and develop more realistic ways to deal with the stresses, she may be better equipped to help patients cope with their use of denial.

A patient faced with a leg amputation encountered negative reactions from some of the nurses who entered her room with sad faces or forced smiles. After the operation they were unable to look at the empty spot in the bed and retreated from direct care of the stump. The patient praised the nurse who had explored with her the facets of the operation and what it would be like. The nurse had described the prostheses available along with other rehabilitative services. Not requiring the patient to be cheerful or pleased with the situation, she gave excellent nursing care that included insistence on exercises and crutch-walking regardless of the patient's initial reluctance.

In this example, a nurse who had come to grips with her feelings and reactions toward disability was able to offer the patient her knowledge, experience and compassion. Partly because of their own need for denial, the other nurses made it even harder for the patient to cope with the reality of the situation.

PSYCHOSOMATIC INTERACTIONS

Knowledge about the relationship between emotions and physical reactions is increasing. This is a highly complex and little-understood matter that mass media has simplified to the point where the terms "psychosomatic," "neurotic," "imaginary," "faking," "malingering," "psychogenic," and "somatopsychic" are used loosely with much confusion.

Anxiety is experienced as both an emotional reaction and as a physiologic reaction that may affect the total organism. Many people seek treatment for symptoms that are due directly to chronic, continued anxiety. The anxiety may represent a reaction to reality factors in the present, such as a job or a marriage, or to long-standing conflicts over sexuality, dependency, aggression and other factors.

Anxiety reactions in which the symptoms center around one organ system are described in the nomenclature as psychophysiologic reactions having autonomic and visceral responses (e.g., "psychophysiologic reaction, cardiovascular," if the symptoms are predominately cardiac in nature). Any organ system can be affected. When actual structural changes do occur, the condition is described as a psychosomatic illness that has resulted from a combination of emotional and physiologic factors. Common conditions that are generally considered to involve psychosomatic factors are: peptic ulcer, chronic ulcerative colitis, hyperthyroidism, bronchial asthma, essential hypertension and neurodermatitis. The frequency and severity of these illnesses point to the need for greater understanding of the relationship between mind and body.

Another manifestation of underlying emotional conflict that expresses itself in physical symptoms is hypochondriasis. A hypochondriacal patient may be totally absorbed in his body and its functioning, and presents endless complaints and reports. Generally, a person uses this means to adapt to his environment in an attempt to meet long-standing dependency needs. The nurse must evaluate her own reactions to such a patient's complaints and demands. The usual reaction is frustration and anger toward one who seems to be capitalizing on minor complaints. The hardworking nurse often resents someone who seems to avoid adult responsibility so easily. To express this anger directly to the patient is generally not very helpful, since he is struggling to maintain some kind of equilibrium. Not to recognize the anger in herself could result in the nurse's avoiding the patient and not caring for his realistic needs. If she goes overboard and attempts to meet all his unsatisfied dependency needs, she soon finds that the patient is insatiable—a bottomless pit. Finding a reasonable middle ground is a challenge in working with these patients. Very little is known about successful nursing approaches to hypochondriacal patients. Excessive preoccupation with one's body, accompanied by unusual ideation, may be a sign of more severe emotional disorders, such as psychotic depression or schizophrenia. Through proper assessment of needs and evaluation of behavior, the nurse may help plan for more appropriate treatment.

Another group of physical reactions that have an emotional basis are conversion reactions. Conversion is an ego defense mechanism in which anxiety is eliminated or reduced by the production of a physical symptom. This symptom is often directly related to the emotional conflict; the hand that would strike out is paralyzed; the eyes that would look at the forbidden become blind. However, in most instances the conflict and the symbolic meaning of the symptom are complex, disguised, and difficult to unravel. These patients come into a medical-surgical setting for differential diagnosis. A conversion reaction may possibly develop after an organic illness has occurred, which tends to prolong the secondary gains of dependency and security.

Generally, the symptoms of conversion reactions simulate disturbances in the voluntary nervous system or in the organs of the special senses. Disturbances of sensation and motion are the most common. Sensation changes include anesthesia, paresthesia, and pain. Loss of hearing and sight are much more common than loss of the other special senses. Disturbances of motion include paralysis, usually of the limbs or speech mechanism, and uncontrolled movements such as tics and nonorganic convulsions. If the symptom is diagnosed as a conversion reaction, the treatment is generally best directed by a psychiatrist. The nurse can help greatly by accurately observing the patient's behavior, including his reaction to other people. She must keep in mind that symptom formation in a person with a conversion reaction occurs on an unconscious level—the patient is not faking, nor are his symptoms imaginary. This is his way of coping with situations at the present time; with professional help he may be able to find more adequate ways to do so.

Disturbances in orientation occur frequently in patients on medical-surgical services. Acute brain syndrome, which may be a reaction to anesthesia, infection, surgical or metabolic disturbances, overdose of drugs or alcohol, or assault to the brain as in head injury, often produces delirium. *Delirium* is a state of altered consciousness or awareness manifested by disorientation and confusion. It is induced by interference with the metabolic processes of the brain and is generally acute in onset and reversible. The first signs are restlessness, anxiety, and suspicion, which quickly mount to agitation, excitement, and confusion. The patient often begins to hallucinate and experience delusions. These distortions of reality are extremely frightening, and the desperate behavior of the person experiencing them necessitates skilled nursing action. Patients recovering from cardiac surgery, in particular, often become delirious. It is necessary to reduce the terror and extreme anxiety of these patients not only for emotional reasons, but also to prevent overloading the body with more stress.

Nursing care for a delirious patient includes continual reorientation, a calm voice, and adequate lighting through the night. If possible, the same nurses should attend the patient much of the time, since they repeatedly demonstrate by familiar words and action that he is safe and cared for. It often helps to tell the patient that you know he is very frightened, but that the things he is experiencing are a reaction to his illness that will go away. Hallucinations caused by organic processes are often vivid and threatening. Along with visual hallucinations, the patient may experience tactile hallucinations in which he feels he is being touched or bugs are crawling on him.

Acute brain syndrome is treated by alleviating the causative agents, and the nurse must be aware that proper hydration, nutrition, and medication are directed toward this end. Restraints may be necessary to keep the patient in bed, but they may also frighten and irritate him. The nurse must be aware of his distortion of reality and poor judgment to protect him from injuring himself or others. Patients have walked out of unprotected windows while delirious.

Following an episode of delirium, a person may experience anxiety and shame over his behavior when not in full control. He may fear that he has acted inappropriately, hurt someone, or said vulgar or obscene things. He may be afraid of having told confidences and secrets about himself. If the patient gives evidence of such concern, the nurse can encourage him to talk about his fears and then reassure him that his behavior was understandable in the situation and that she will not betray his confidence. This is a potentially shameful situation in which the rights, dignity, and privacy of the patient must be protected.

Chronic brain syndrome may result from damage to brain tissue sustained by the causes of acute brain syndrome, or from long-term infections such as syphilis, heavy mental intoxication, circulatory disturbances such as cerebral arteriosclerosis, convulsive disorders, disturbances of growth, metabolism or nutrition, intracranial neoplasm, prenatal factors, and diseases of unknown etiology such as multiple sclerosis. The behavior common to people with these conditions is described as *dementia,* and it represents chronic, irreversible brain damage with deterioration of intellectual capacities due to structural changes. Both delirium and dementia are characterized by loss of abilities—defects in memory, orientation (of time, place, and person), and in judgment. Depending on the premorbid personality, chronic brain syndrome may result in secondary symptomatology. In planning nursing care and long-term treatment, the individual's strengths must be evaluated along with his limitations. Environmental manipulation and simplification may help him to live his life to the fullest.

DYING AND DEATH

In order to give maximal help to the dying patient and his family, nurses need to examine their own feelings about death and to understand better the reactions of other people toward death. Each person dies in his individual style, just as he lives in his own style. One of the major problems in understanding death is that, in our culture, it is a taboo topic. The sight of death is a strange and foreign experience to most people, even more so now that many people die in hospitals and nursing homes rather than in their own homes. Many nursing students come into contact with death for the first time in their medical-surgical clinical experience.

For most people, even the thought of death is frightening, and when one is in robust health, it seems almost impossible. Regardless of one's religious beliefs, it is difficult to imagine oneself as no longer existing in the world. Nurses are deeply committed to life and health. The dying patient, through no fault of his own, is in direct opposition to that commitment. Sometimes the medical and nursing staff react to a dying patient as if their failure of skill or care is responsible for the impending death. It helps to realize that, although nothing can be done to reverse the ultimate process, the dying person can be helped in his last human contacts. Hospital policies, cultural attitudes, family fears, and the personal reactions of the nursing staff may result in a dying person's being left alone to struggle with his fears, loneliness and abandonment. It is not uncommon on many wards to move the terminal patient to another room, often by himself. Although the dying patient's physical care may be adequately maintained, staff are reluctant to answer his bell and often relief staff or students are assigned to his care. Verbal communication may decrease markedly and is rarely future-oriented. Use of professional terms may serve to protect the nurse, as does social chitchat. Premature mourning on the part of the patient, family and staff may begin long before the patient actually becomes moribund.

People face death in many ways. To ward off emotional recognition, many use denial and isolation. Others may be openly anxious and frightened, and some are relieved. These reactions are present in the families as well as in the patient. The complexity of family relationships is highlighted when the problem of death is encountered. The nurse must be aware that the family as well as the patient must cope as best they can. Love, responsibility, guilt, hate, despair, respect, and resentment may all take part in their reaction to the dying person. Some patients and families want to talk about their experience; some want to make definite plans; others are too threatened to allow themselves to realize what is going on. The defense mechanism of denial is commonly used in dealing with impending death. Denial can serve to protect the person from painful realization—reality is distorted or ignored as he maintains hope. The reality of life is that no one knows just when he or another person will die. When a patient asks, "Am I going to die?" he rarely wants a "yes" or "no" answer. He may be expressing his fears, his concern about abandonment and isolation, his anger or relief in leaving life behind, his problems with his family, his fear of dependency and pain during the final stages, and his terror of the unknown. He may want to exert his rights without medication so that his senses are clear as long as possible; another may want the end to be as comfortable as possible.

It is generally accepted that it is the physician's responsibility to decide what information to give the patient about his diagnosis and prognosis. It is important that the doctor and the nurse share information that will help the doctor determine what is most helpful to the patient. The nurse, through her observations and interactions, can help assess the patient's and his family's understanding of the disease and their intellectual and emotional patterns, including their coping abilities. She is then more sensitive to verbal and nonverbal cues of the patient and his family and can determine how she can help them most in this time of great need. An understanding of the mechanisms of denial and grief guides her actions.

Although an underlying principle in all areas of nursing is that the person is an individual who should be treated with respect and dignity, studies have shown that the social value placed upon a person determines how he is treated when dying. Such factors as age, color, socioeconomic status, attractiveness, and former accomplishments greatly affect a patient's treatment, and results in different degrees of abandonment, isolation and loneliness while dying. Many times, the nurse caring for the dying patient becomes his most important link with life. She can not only make him as physically comfortable as possible, but also is in a privileged position to help him and his family with one of the most difficult and painful parts of life—leaving it. She stays with him to the end and tries to comfort the family left behind.

Although she develops defenses against the full impact of repeated deaths, a nurse who completely "stops caring" when patients die temporarily loses her ability to be completely helpful. It is an emotional strain to nurse people who are dying. Nurses assigned to areas in which death frequently occurs must be able to share their feelings and reactions with each other. It is also helpful that these nurses be shifted periodically to other wards in which the recovery rate is high, in order to recharge their hope.

BIBLIOGRAPHY

Books

Carlson, C., *et al.*: Behavioral Concepts and Nursing Intervention. Philadelphia, J. B. Lippincott, 1970.

Garrett, J. F. (ed.): Psychological Aspects of Physical Disability. Washington, D.C., Federal Security Agency, Office of Vocational Rehabilitation, 1952.

Goldin, P. and Russell, B.: Therapeutic communication, Amer. J. Nurs. 69:1928-1930, Sept., 1969.

Haley, J.: Strategies of Psychotherapy. New York, Grune and Stratton, 1963.

Hofling, C., Leininger, M., and Bregg, E.: Basic Psychiatric Concepts in Nursing. ed. 2. Philadelphia, J. B. Lippincott, 1967.

Schutz, W.: Joy: Expanding Human Awareness. New York, Grove Press, 1967.

Skipper, J. K., and Leonard, R. C. (eds.): Social Interaction and Patient Care. Philadelphia, J. B. Lippincott, 1965.

Wright, B.: Physical Disability—A Psychological Approach. New York, Harper and Brothers, 1960.

Articles

Basic Systems, Inc.: Anxiety: recognition and intervention. Programmed instruction. Amer. J. Nurs., 65:129-152, Sept., 1965.

Crate, M. A.: Nursing functions in adaptation to chronic illness. Amer. J. Nurs., 65:72-76, Oct., 1965.

Educational Design, Inc.: Understanding hostility. Programmed instruction. Amer. J. Nurs., 67:2131-2150, Oct., 1967.

Rehabilitation—prologue to the future. Proceedings of the California Nurses' Association Fall Institute, Nov., 1968, San Diego. Mimeo.

CHAPTER 4

The Aging Patient

- *Factors Modifying Illness*
- *Socioeconomic and Health Problems of the Aging*
- *The Nurse and the Elderly Patient*
- *Significant Characteristics of the Older Patient*
- *Surgery of the Elderly Patient*
- *Convalescence*
- *Long-Term Illness*

FACTORS MODIFYING ILLNESS

A medical problem almost never is found to be a simple product of a patient plus an illness. Other factors modify the character of the medical problem and frequently influence the conduct of both medical and nursing care. These aspects may have no direct relation to the disease itself but originate in the patient's environment or his general status. Situational elements in this category may include: the patient's age; the duration of his illness and its prognosis; his position in the family and community; his economic status and his financial responsibilities; the character of his family and its attitude toward him and his illness; stress-producing factors of all types; medico-legal complications, as in compensation cases; the climate and the weather.

There are many factors of comparable importance, but the significance of these is relatively restricted; they are discussed in conjunction with the disorders in which they are particularly influential. Of those cited above, 3, with therapeutic implications of peculiar importance, are now to be examined: the age of the patient, the chronicity of disease and the gravity of prognosis.

The aging process begins with conception and ends with death. The treatment of very young and of elderly patients often is complicated by problems that relate strictly to age—problems warranting a degree of specialization of medical and nursing practice in the respective fields of pediatrics, ephebiatrics and geriatrics. The sources of divergence between the problems of childhood and old age are multiple, principally related to differences in their susceptibilities, their responses to specific etiologic factors and their recuperative powers. Moreover, the psychological aspects of their individual situations are markedly different as regards both the psychogenic factors that are involved and the nature of the psychological responses characterizing their age group.

Pediatrics

This field of medicine and nursing is not included here, because this textbook is concerned primarily with the adult. The student is directed to pediatric textbooks and references.

Ephebiatrics

Adolescence marks a phase of rapid body growth, the stage of sexual maturation and a period of emotional turbulence. From the standpoint of nursing care, the most important feature distinguishing this age group is a psychological attribute, the effect of which is to impose a firm communication barrier between the adolescent and the adult. Neither child nor adult, the

TABLE 4-1. The older population: Discharges from short-stay hospitals—number per 1,000 persons, average length of stay, and percent surgically treated, by age and selected characteristics, July 1963-June 1965

Characteristic	Discharges per 1,000 persons			Average length (days) of hospital stay			Percent of discharges surgically treated		
	65+	65-74	75+	65+	65-74	75+	65+	65-74	75+
Both sexes	186.3	181.3	195.6	12.7	12.6	12.7	34.9	37.0	31.2
Male	190.5	182.4	206.3	12.9	13.1	12.5	37.5	40.0	33.1
Female	183.0	180.4	187.7	12.4	12.2	12.8	32.7	34.6	29.6
Family income									
Under $3,000	178.5	175.7	182.5	12.7	12.4	13.1	33.6	33.8	33.4
$3,000-3,999	214.6	210.6	224.0	11.0	11.1	10.6	34.0	35.8	29.1
$4,000-6,999	184.4	174.0	209.5	13.0	12.5	13.9	36.2	40.6	27.3
$7,000-9,999	185.8	185.3	184.2	12.4	12.3	12.7	34.5	32.9	38.6
$10,000+	203.6	187.9	239.6	14.0	14.6	12.8	41.6	50.3	26.5
Living arrangement									
Living alone	182.3	183.0	181.4	13.6	14.6	12.4	34.8	38.5	29.6
Living with nonrelatives	232.0	213.1	254.0	19.7	21.5	17.8	36.5	38.7	35.9
Living with relatives—married .	181.8	177.1	196.2	11.5	11.0	12.9	37.8	38.6	35.7
Living with relatives—other ...	194.5	190.1	198.9	13.1	14.3	11.9	28.0	29.8	26.4
Geographic region									
Northeast	167.1	170.9	159.7	15.4	15.5	15.2	40.0	42.4	34.9
North Central	177.4	183.2	167.2	12.1	11.3	13.9	35.2	36.3	33.2
South	214.0	187.6	263.1	11.5	11.6	11.3	29.3	30.4	27.7
West	184.5	183.7	185.9	11.9	12.6	10.6	38.3	42.1	31.4
Residence									
Inside Metropolitan Area	165.2	163.6	168.3	13.8	13.8	13.8	39.6	40.2	38.6
Outside Metropolitan Area									
Nonfarm	224.7	216.8	237.7	11.7	11.5	12.1	29.1	32.8	23.5
Farm	176.0	166.9	192.1	9.0	9.7	7.8	33.3	36.1	28.8

Source: Basic data—Public Health Service. Administration on Aging, Social and Rehabilitation Service, DEPARTMENT OF HEALTH, EDUCATION, & WELFARE, May 1968.

teenager is in an anomalous position. Vigorously rejecting the trappings of childhood, a status recently departed and now abhorred, he now strives in every way to establish himself as an adult, a tormenting aspiration with no prospect of materializing in the immediate future. Considerably inadequate in his own estimation and by his own standards of adulthood, he is constantly on guard against the likelihood of slight and humiliation at the hands of disparaging, patronizing adults who fail to identify him as another adult. Blanket protection against this threat is sought by adopting a defensive, i.e., hostile, attitude toward adults in general. There are all degrees of hostility and many ways in which it is reflected. Normally it expresses itself in the form of diffidence in the company of, and avoidance of close association with, older individuals. Exchanges of confidence are limited strictly to his contemporaries who, of course, share his basic attitudes and are "on his side."

This reluctance to confide in adults has a very definite influence on the doctor-nurse-patient relationship and therefore on the diagnosis, the treatment and the nursing care of the sick adolescent. Emotional disturbances are frequent and profound at this age, commonly overlying and distorting the clinical features of organic disease and occasionally engendering serious psychological aberrations. Problems of this type, demanding the closest rapport between patient, doctor and nurse for their solution, are especially difficult in this age group, owing to the natural obstacle in communications. Removal of the obstacle is a prerequisite to effective medical and nursing care. The patient will be induced to remove it, lower his guard and yield his confidence under one condition only, namely, that he be accepted by his seniors in the status of an adult. The nurse, as the principal observer and active therapist in immediate contact with the hospitalized adolescent, must not fail to take steps for the achievement and the maintenance of good rapport with her young patient. By a convincing display of personal interest in matters of interest to the patient and personal respect for him as an adult, the goal is accomplished.

Some hospitals now admit teen-age patients to a "Teen-Age" floor which is apart from pediatric and adult units. Snack bars, telephones, visiting hours and so forth are provided and geared to their interests.

Geriatrics

. . . Nobody grows old by merely living a number of years. People grow old only by deserting their ideals. . . . You are as young as your self-confidence, as old as your fear, as young as your hope, as old as your despair. In the central place of every heart, there is a recording chamber; so long as it receives messages of beauty, hope, cheer and courage, so long are you young. When the wires are all down and your heart is covered with the snows of pessimism and the ice of cynicism, then, and then only, are you grown old . . .

GENERAL DOUGLAS MACARTHUR

Much attention is being focused on how to age gracefully and on how to be healthier, happier and more active in later years. Geriatrics, i.e., care of the aged, has come to deserve specific emphasis in the nursing curriculum. This specialty has as its prime concern the health and the well-being of a large and an important segment of the patient population, and it deals with problems of therapy and rehabilitation that are inherently and uniquely complex.

Profile of the Aged American. There are 20 million people in the United States over the age of 65. They comprise 10 per cent of the total population. Each day 3,900 persons celebrate their 65th birthday, but approximately 3,080 of those who are over 65 die. Therefore, at the end of each day the aged population is increased by approximately 820 people. In the course of a year this is a net increase of 100,000. Also, there are more than a million persons over 85.

Such a large aged population is a new phenomenon and has a tremendous impact on nursing. Of our aged patients, there are more older women than older men —about 11 million to 8 million. Most of the older women are widows while most of the older men are husbands. Half of this group did not go beyond elementary school and 17 per cent of older people are functionally illiterate. At the other end of the scale, approximately 5 per cent are college graduates. These factors have an influence on earning capacity, understanding, attitudes and perhaps health knowledge and care. Contrary to popular belief, only 4 per cent of older persons live in institutions. Approximately 70 per cent live in a family setting while the remaining 26 per cent live alone or with nonrelatives. Table 4-1 gives some statistics on the older population.

The aging population is a changing group. To understand older people requires an understanding of their backgrounds. Those working with them need to identify them as individuals with experience and achievements who have coped with major social, economic and technological developments, and who have made (and are still making) worthy contributions to society.

SOCIOECONOMIC AND HEALTH PROBLEMS OF THE AGING

As a result of the scientific and sociologic advances that have occurred during the past century, man's life expectancy has increased remarkably. The older age group now comprises a relatively substantial segment of the population. Moreover, it is expected that this segment will continue to expand at an accelerated pace for many decades to come. The impact of its growth has been felt in many areas of our social and economic situation, including the fields of medicine and nursing.

Socioeconomic Factors

Current population trends, marked by an increasing accumulation of older members, must be followed by major adjustments in our socioeconomic planning. Individual attitude patterns must be reoriented on a similar scale. Youth must be educated to its inevitable responsibilities for the aged and educated to the concept of living cooperatively and effectively with the aged.

Social Isolation of the Aged. Among the aged person's greatest sorrows and trials is the death of his spouse, other family members and friends, until sometimes he is virtually alone. Although personal losses through death are inevitable, it is wise to develop avocational interests early in life. Such creative interests have therapeutic value and meet emotional needs.

Income. Level of income affects the quality of living as well as health. According to a governmental study, almost one-third of the aged live below the poverty line. In spite of higher Social Security benefits and general prosperity, persons over 65 remain the most poverty-stricken group in the nation. Aged people cannot work as regularly and they earn less than younger people when they do work. Usually aged couples or older individuals living alone must live on half the money income available to a younger couple or a single person. Older consumers spend proportionately more of their incomes on food, housing, household operations and medical care than do their younger counterparts. Medical care costs are a large item in the budget of the elderly. They spend an average of $50 per year on medicines. Since three-quarters of the older population have chronic health problems, they may well spend double this amount.

Housing. A place to live is a basic human need. There is a growing trend toward provision of housing especially designed for older Americans. It is desirable that older people live independently as long as pos-

TABLE 4-2. Summary of recent major legislation for older people*

Subject Area	Name of Act	Public Law No.	Summary of Provisions
General	Older Americans Act of 1965	89-73	Authorized a 5-year program of grants to the States for community planning, services, and training in the field of aging. Established an operating agency, the Administration on Aging, to provide national focus on aging and the aged. The agency supports research, demonstration, and training in the field of aging through grant programs, serves as a clearinghouse of information on problems of aging and the aged, and studies ways to make more effective the use of new and existing resources in the creation of programs for the elderly.
	Older Americans Act of 1967	90-42	Provides for extension of program through 1972.
Health	Social Security Amendments of 1965	89-97	*Medicare:* Established comprehensive national health insurance programs for the aged designed to help meet the costs of a wide range of health services.
			Medical Assistance Program: Established a more effective Kerr-Mills medical program for the aged and extended its more liberal provisions to the elderly on old-age assistance and other categories of recipients of assistance. Also removed prohibition on Federal sharing in assistance payments for the elderly in tuberculosis and mental hospitals if, among other things, Federal funds are used to assure that better care results for the patients in these institutions.
	Vocational Rehabilitation Amendments of 1968	90-391	Extends authorization of grants to the States for rehabilitation services and broadens the scope of services available for the handicapped, including individuals disadvantaged by reason of either advanced age, or other conditions which constitute a barrier to employment.
Mental Health	1965 Amendment to the Community Mental Health Center Act	89-105	Authorized Federal matching payments toward the costs of staff in community mental health centers during their first 51 months of operation.
Heart Disease, Cancer and Stroke	Regional Medical Center Act	89-239	Authorized funds for the establishment of programs for prevention, detection, and treatment of heart disease, cancer, stroke, and related diseases. Also authorized a 3-year program of Federal grants totaling $340 million for setting up regional cooperative arrangements among medical schools, research institutions, and hospitals for research, training, and demonstration of patient care to make available to patients the latest advances in the diagnosis and treatment of these diseases and to improve the manpower and facilities available.
Income Maintenance	Social Security Amendments of 1965	89-97	Increased across-the-board monthly social security cash benefits by 7 per cent; increased amount which beneficiaries may earn before the provisions for withholding benefits begin to apply; lowered age for widows to retire with reduced benefits to 60; liberalized eligibility requirements for disability benefits so that anyone with a disability lasting 12 months or one expected to result in death may receive them; liberalized or authorized benefit payments for dependents including improvements in benefits for remarried widows or widowers and divorced women.
	Social Security Amendments of 1967	90-248	Provides an across-the-board increase of 13 per cent to all beneficiaries; liberalizes retirement test to allow a beneficiary to earn $1680 a year.
	Civil Service Retirement Act of 1965	89-205	Increased by 11 per cent all annuities with a commencing date prior to October 1, 1965, and by 6 per cent all with a commencing date after October 1, 1965. Also revised the method of determining cost-of-living increases in computing subsequent benefits.
	Amendments to the Railroad Retirement Act	89-212	Increased railroad retirement benefits to reflect changes in social security cash benefit increases. Also eliminated the dual benefit restrictions which previously reduced railroad retirement annuities of spouses of retired railroad employees by the amount of certain types of social security benefits received by them.

*Adapted from *AGING*, February 1967.

TABLE 4-2. Summary of recent major legislation for older people (continued)

Subject Area	Name of Act	Public Law No.	Summary of Provisions
Housing	Housing and Urban Development Act of 1965 (*Aging*, September 1965, p. 3)	89-117	*Rent Supplement Program:* Authorized the Federal Government to enter into contracts with nonprofit, cooperative, or limited-dividend sponsors of housing, under which elderly or other eligible tenants would pay only 25 per cent of their income toward rent and the Government would pay the difference between that amount and established fair market rents. *Expansion of Public Housing:* Increased the authorization for annual contributions to provide for an estimated 60,000 additional public housing units for each of the next 4 years. On the basis of recent experience, it may be expected that as much as half of the new public housing authorized will be devoted to housing for the low-income elderly. *Direct Loan Program:* Placed a ceiling of 3 per cent on the interest rate on direct loans to nonprofit sponsors of housing for the elderly. In addition, the amount authorized for this program was increased. *Home Rehabilitation Grants:* Authorized the use of urban renewal grant funds for grants to owner-occupants of homes in urban renewal areas to enable them to make repairs required by codes or urban renewal standards. Grants up to $1,500 are available for repairs depending upon the incomes of the owner-occupants. *Neighborhood Facilities:* Established a program of grants to local public bodies and agencies to finance projects for neighborhood facilities, including senior citizens centers, to low-income persons (*Aging*, April 1966, p. 7).
Education	Higher Education Act of 1965	89-329	Established grants to strengthen the educational resources of higher education institutions to aid them in providing community services programs for adults and to assist in solving community problems (*Aging*, October 1966, p. 14).
Poverty	1965 Amendment to the Economic Opportunity Act of 1964	89-253	Added a new section entitled "Programs for the Elderly Poor," which stated that, whenever feasible, the special problems of the elderly poor shall be considered in the development, conduct, and administration of programs under the Economic Opportunity Act.
	Economic Opportunity Amendments of 1966	89-794	Provided that the Office of Economic Opportunity shall carry out studies and investigations to develop programs providing employment opportunities, public service opportunities, and education for the elderly poor. Older people can petition for representation on community action boards if they do not believe they are adequately represented. In addition, the Office of Economic Opportunity was directed to appoint an Assistant Director whose concern are the problems of the older poor.
Employment	Fair Labor Standards Amendments of 1966	89-601	Directed the Secretary of Labor to submit to the Congress in January 1967 specific legislative recommendations for implementing the conclusions and recommendations contained in the Labor Department's report on age discrimination in employment.
	Age Discrimination in Employment Act of 1967	90-202	Prohibits age discrimination against workers between 40 and 65 years old; authorizes an education and research program to reduce the barriers to employment for older workers.
Library Services	Amendments to the Library Services Construction Act	89-511	Makes available to the States funds for the establishment or improvement of library services to the physically handicapped, including the blind or visually handicapped.

SENIOR CITIZEN'S CHARTER*

Rights of Senior Citizens: Each of our Senior Citizens, regardless of race, color or creed, is entitled to:

1. The right to be useful.
2. The right to obtain employment, based on merit.
3. The right to freedom from want in old age.
4. The right to a fair share of the community's recreational, educational, and medical resources.
5. The right to obtain decent housing suited to needs of later years.
6. The right to the moral and financial support of one's family so far as is consistent with the best interest of the family.
7. The right to live independently, as one chooses.
8. The right to live and to die with dignity.
9. The right of access to all knowledge as available on how to improve the later years of life.

Obligations of the Aging: The aging, by availing themselves of educational opportunities, should endeavor to assume the following obligations to the best of their ability:

1. The obligation of each citizen to prepare himself to become and resolve to remain active, alert, capable, self-supporting and useful so long as health and circumstances permit and to plan for ultimate retirement.
2. The obligation to learn and to apply sound principles of physical and mental health.
3. The obligation to seek and to develop potential avenues of service in the years after retirement.
4. The obligation to make available the benefits of his experience and knowledge.
5. The obligation to endeavor to make himself adaptable to the changes added years will bring.
6. The obligation to attempt to maintain such relationships with family, neighbors and friends as will make him a respected and valued counsellor throughout his later years.

*From the 1961 White House Conference on Aging

sible. Housing requirements of the elderly differ, and it is difficult for them to adapt to a changing environment. Younger retirees usually do not need any modifications in their dwellings. Those in their 70's may require additional safety measures such as grab bars in strategic places, nonslip flooring and single-level living quarters. The very aged may need facilities offering group dining and nursing and medical services. The Federal Government has special housing programs for older citizens. Of those living in substandard housing, over 80 per cent have annual incomes under $3000. Before the Housing and Urban Development Act, many elderly were paying 35 to 50 per cent of their monthly funds for shelter. The Housing Assistance Administration of the Department of Housing and Urban Development is providing housing units for the older segment of the population. The buildings are planned and designed to avoid accidents, easy to maintain, modest in size and within walking distance of varied facilities. The Rent Supplement Program allows poverty-stricken elderly to live in decent housing by providing them with rent supplements. This is of special interest to public health nurses as well as health workers who are engaged in helping the aged solve their problems.

Employment. Our society is youth-oriented, by which emphasis is placed on the development of the potential of the young. We need also to utilize the potential of the older individual. His physiological capacity should be considered rather than his chronological age. Studies show that the older person learns as easily as the younger, although he requires more time to solve certain problems. His accumulated knowledge and skills have value. He should remain gainfully employed as long as possible. Working at a job keeps the individual in the mainstream of life and helps maintain his dignity and self-esteem. The Age Discrimination in Employment Act of 1967 prohibits discrimination in employment against workers between 40 and 65 years old and authorizes a research program to reduce the barriers to employment for older workers.

Federal Programs for the Aged. Concern for the aged has been manifested through programs of the Federal Government. The Senate Special Committee on Aging attempts to gain information about older Americans and send this data to appropriate legislative committees. As an outgrowth of the historic White House Conference on Aging in 1961, the programs of Medicare, Medicaid and the Older Americans Act were enacted into law in 1965. This Conference also produced the Senior Citizen's Charter, which appears above. Other legislation which has been enacted includes low-income housing for the elderly (1964), tax benefits on medicine and drug expenses and on the sale of residences (1964), increase in Social Security benefits (1967), and prohibition of job discrimination because of age (1967). The Social and Rehabilitation Services has been created within the U. S. Department of Health, Education and Welfare. The Administration on Aging is a part of this agency and is responsible for services to older people.

Table 4-2 is a summary of legislation recently passed that is specifically helpful to older people.

Physiology of Aging

The process of aging starts before birth and varies with each individual. Hereditary and environmental factors influence longevity. Intensive and systematic study of aging, both experimental and clinical, is developing and expanding. Certain facts have become apparent. Aging occurs on all levels of bodily function: cellular, organic and systemic. Grossly speaking, loss of cells and loss of physiologic reserve make up the dominant processes. Given a sedentary occupation and a routine familiar task, the difference in performance between those aged 30 and those aged 60 is difficult to demonstrate. However from 35 to 80 years, the ability to do maximum work for short periods of time falls almost 60 per cent; the maximum breathing capacity, 57 per cent. However the basal metabolic rate is reduced on the average only by 10 per cent and the cardiac output at rest by 30 per cent.

Metabolic processes also change; the glucose tolerance curve tends toward that of the diabetic and the same dose of insulin in a younger person will reduce his blood sugar more rapidly. (If normal standards were applied to the aged, 50 per cent of this population would be classified as diabetic.)

Part of these changes are reflected in loss of tissues. The brain, kidneys and muscles decrease in weight. The number of nerve fibers in the nerve trunk decreases 27 per cent in advanced age.

Thus, aging is associated with loss of cellular and functional (physiological) reserve. The aging body lacks reserve power. It can function adequately at rest or during short periods of moderate activity, but when external stresses such as trauma or infection are exerted, there are little or no reserve capacities. Breakdown of bodily function can follow. The aging individual has to cope with these physiological changes within himself. In general, adjustment is made by reducing the level of activity.

Health Problems of the Aged

The aged, because of their lowered resistance, are more vulnerable to disease. Seventy-five per cent of those over 65 are affected by one or more chronic diseases. The major disorders of old age are heart disease, malignancy and diseases of the central nervous system. Coronary heart disease is the most frequently seen heart condition. Cancer of the alimentary tract, especially of the colon, is common. In fact, cancer is so frequently seen that those who live past 88 years will often have one or more cancers.

Many of the disabilities that are particularly associated with old age develop as a result of degenerative vascular disease, namely, arteriosclerosis. Multiple occlusions of the arteries in the cerebral cortex are responsible for the mental deterioration of the "senile" patient; because of these occlusions he can no longer integrate his thoughts or observations, he loses the ability to recall recent events, becomes increasingly irritable and exhibits signs which in many respects seem to represent a childhood reversion. The individual caring for the patient of advanced years must take cognizance of this difficult complication, namely, mental disability due to cerebral degeneration. The professional approach should be guided accordingly. Firmness in opposition to the expressed desires of the patient is often necessary; invariably, however, this should be accompanied by a display of reassurance and friendly understanding in order to preserve his sense of security. The elderly patient is always most fearful of becoming incapacitated and dependent without protection.

Disorders of motor and sensory function are common in elderly individuals. These are manifested in the form of muscular weakness, spasticity, tremors and various types of sensory disturbances. Loss of pain perception can be responsible for dangerous accidents —burn injuries, for example, through prolonged exposure to heat which is not perceived. In this regard, an extra blanket is safer than a hot-water bottle. Damaging falls may be caused by loss of position sense, related to a difficulty in maintaining equilibrium and to an uncertainty of gait, and it may be impossible to perform any act requiring precise muscular control. A cerebral hemorrhage, or the sudden occlusion of a large arteriosclerotic artery in the brain, if not immediately fatal, may seriously disable the patient, sometimes rendering him permanently unable to perform any serviceable motion of his extremities and completely incapable of caring for himself in any way. In other instances the degree of incapacity may be less, perhaps involving but one extremity and only to a partial degree.

However, regardless of the exact character of ·the neurologic disability, the medical management of these patients is a very real responsibility and, considering the details of protective care alone, may be a difficult problem.

Occlusive vascular disease involving the lower extremities, another complication of arteriosclerosis, is responsible for "intermittent claudication," that is, pain in the legs on walking, and may even provide the basis for gangrene, necessitating amputation of one or both extremities.

Arteriosclerosis is equally prone to involve the coronary arteries of the heart and those supplying the kidneys. Therefore, the elderly patient is unusually subject to cardiac disorders which may limit seriously his capacity for physical exertion, as well as to impairment of his kidney function with the ultimate prospect of chronic uremia. Gastrointestinal disturbances commonly occur in the older age groups because of a reduction of the blood supply to the gastrointestinal tract, arteriosclerotic changes or neoplastic disease involving that organ system. Gastrointestinal disturbances create problems in dietetic management and symptomatic therapy.

Softening of the bones due to their demineralization (senile osteoporosis) must be regarded as a possible hazard in any elderly individual, rendering him abnormally susceptible to major fractures. The joints are very often affected by degenerative ("hypertrophic") arthritis, causing pain and limiting the motion of the back and of the weight-bearing joints of the legs.

There are a variety of disorders that occur with increasing frequency with advancing age: pulmonary emphysema with fibrosis and impairment of respiratory function; atrophic and ulcerative lesions affecting the skin and the mucous membranes; and, in the male, enlargement of the prostate gland with urinary obstruction. Descriptions of these and of other degenerative disorders are included in the appropriate sections of this text.

Falls are the major cause of fatal accidents to the elderly. Older people are the victims of falls due to failing eyesight, diminishing muscular strength and coordination and osteoporosis.

THE NURSE AND THE ELDERLY PATIENT

Is the nursing care that the older person needs any different from that given to a younger person? Essentially it is not different, but it has more depth—more is required of the nurse. The elderly individual not only has multiple medical problems but psychological and socioeconomic problems, too. Aging certainly is a psychological stress. The greatest stresses to the aged are in the form of loss of resources: physical, social and economic.

Patient Assessment

To understand the patient in his totality, the nurse seeks information to develop a nursing care plan. One of the best ways of gathering data is through conversation with the patient. The objective is to answer the question: "What are the assets and liabilities of this patient?" In addition to knowing the medical problem(s) of the patient, the following is offered as a guide in assessment:

Physiological:
  How much physical capacity does he possess?
  How much muscle strength and coordination does he have?
  How well does he see and hear?
  What are his usual eating, sleeping and activity patterns?
  What will the patient have to do to regain/maintain functioning ability?
Socioeconomic:
  What is his family structure?
  How well does he relate to his family?
  Who are his social contacts?
  Is he economically self-sufficient?
  How much independence does he possess?
  Does he participate in any phase of community life?
Psychological:
  What does he identify as his major concerns and problems?
  What are his attitudes toward aging?
  What are his attitudes toward himself? Does he feel needed? Useful?
  What psychological defenses does he use?
  What are his interests and hobbies?

All of these factors affect the patient's reaction to his illness and hospitalization. The more the nurse knows about the patient the more effective is her care. The aged person's problems are more marked and his flexibility for solving them is less. The nurse may be the only one to whom he can turn for help in identifying, facing and solving his problems.

Psychological Considerations. The pursuit of happiness does not necessarily mean resting in a warm climate, fishing and being free of problems. In fact, the Committee on Aging of the American Medical Association feels that "the key to positive health lies in struggle rather than avoidance of the stress of living." If all challenges are removed from the older person, he will have no problems to confront him. But problem-solving motivates all human activity. It is a mistake to keep the aged in a problem-free environment. To do this is to literally "kill with kindness."

In order for the elderly to make successful adjustments to old age, it is necessary for them to accept their own aging as a *natural process*. The individual must cope with the physiologic changes within himself as well as adapt to external social changes. Studies suggest that the individual's basic personality determines the way he adjusts to aging. His capabilities, modes of adjustment and satisfactions are the sum total of his earlier experiences. The nurse is dealing with an individual who has been confronted with many of life's developmental crises and has creditable inner

SUMMARY OF THE PRINCIPLES UNDERLYING NURSING MANAGEMENT OF THE ELDERLY

1. Nursing care must be individualized, taking into consideration the patient's past experiences, needs and individual goals.
2. The patient should be an active participant in his own plan of care.
   A. Consult him for his preferences.
   B. Ask his opinions.
   C. Encourage him to make choices and decisions.
   D. Support him during his anxieties and feelings of inadequacy.
   E. Urge him to remain active.
3. Nursing activities should be done *with* the patient rather than *for* him.
4. Necessary modifications and compromises imposed by the physiological limits of aging must be made in the medical and nursing management of the patient.
5. Realistic and attainable goals, understood by the aged patient, should be set to help him gain a sense of accomplishment and purpose.
6. The elderly should be kept in the mainstream of life to prevent mental deterioration.
7. The nursing approach must communicate to the patient that he has value as an individual and status as a family member and member of society.

---

resources of courage and durability. Older persons respond to suggestions. Remind the patient that he has been successful in the past, and that each period of life also has its unique problems, benefits and gratifications. Accept him just as he is, and assure him that there are caring persons who will help when needed. The demonstration of respect and friendship will do much to enhance his self-esteem and mobilize his own resources to help himself.

The elderly fear loneliness and dying. As soon as the patient enters the hospital, references and plans should be made concerning his leaving the hospital. This dispels much of the ever present fear of invalidism, dependency, and death. *All nursing activities are directed toward restoration of the ability for self-care.* An elderly person seems to want physical contact. The use of the sense of touch, taking his hand during explanations or touching his shoulder, gives him a feeling that he is cared for. Many of the elderly have lost all their social contacts, and the nurse may be his only "caring" person.

On greeting the newly admitted patient the nurse should make him feel welcome and at home. If his condition permits, he should be introduced to nearby patients. At this early meeting, the nurse can observe any incapacities such as difficulty in hearing, tremor of an extremity, a stiff joint and so forth. In elderly patients more than in patients of the younger age group, a sudden change from accustomed surroundings to the impersonal routine of a hospital produces a feeling of insecurity and emotional disturbance. The understanding nurse can do much to help the patient over this hump of transition between home and institution. If he can be placed near another patient with whom he can talk, it will help him to adjust to the hospital environment.

Sometimes the transition to a new environment may bring on temporary states of anxiety, confusion and disorientation. Senile behavior may be exhibited without physiological cause. The patient may be misjudged as being senile when in reality he is fearful, depressed and has a feeling of hopeless inadequacy. When symptoms and behavior of senility occur, such as confusion, incontinence, etc., act on the assumption that they are temporary. The nursing approach should be a positive one, conveying the idea that the problem can be altered. The following nursing actions have proved to be beneficial:

> Call the person by name each time a contact is made.
> Show the patient the nurse's name tag.
> Keep the patient oriented to time and place. (A calendar with easily seen numbers and a clock should be within vision.)
> Schedule his daily activities and adhere to the schedule to promote his security.
> Learn of former interests and talk about them.
> Keep on a night light during the night.

The successful nurse early recognizes differences in older people. Some may be old and decrepit physically but are alert mentally and fresh in spirit. Very readily one may detect an inherent sense of humor, a philosophical frame of mind or a thwarted and depressed personality. Often the patient's temperament will direct his course of progress. Keen observation of these manifestations will present a challenge to the nurse as she develops a plan of care for her geriatric patient.

A fixed routine may provide a sense of security for some elderly persons. To know that a certain activity takes place at a certain time provides a schedule which allows him to anticipate and to do a certain amount of his own planning. The nurse can strengthen his further belief that he matters when she remembers his desires and idiosyncrasies even when they seem trivial. Having very little ice in the water pitcher may account for an adequate or an inadequate intake of fluids. These little things are significant aspects of individualized patient care.

During the period of diagnostic study or preoperative build-up, diversional aids such as visits, radio, television, newspapers, letters and gifts are significant. The older person has less tendency to live in the past if his present is filled with interesting activities.

Before procedures or examinations are done they should be described to the older patient in order to eliminate fears and tensions. Most of these individuals object to being hurried; therefore, sufficient time should be planned in preparation for a treatment. Every effort should be made to establish the confidence of the older patient in those individuals responsible for his care.

SIGNIFICANT CHARACTERISTICS OF THE OLDER PATIENT

Environmental and Physical Needs

One of the most disturbing *environmental factors* to the older patient is noise. Therefore, every attempt should be made to control unpleasant sounds such as dropping metal objects on a hard floor, handling dishes carelessly in the kitchen, banging elevator doors and so forth.

In general, the older patient does not like very much fresh air; therefore, indirect means of ventilation must be utilized. It is difficult to alter the *sleeping habits* of an individual; hence, any adjustment that can be made in the patient's behalf is desirable. Frequently, one has a patient who takes naps during the day and then complains of inability to sleep at night. In most instances, day napping should be discouraged in favor of a good night's sleep.

The nurse should employ whatever nursing measures that seem to be indicated to overcome insomnia, using every effort to make the patient comfortable, but reserving the use of soporific medications for such times as specific indications may exist, and then only as a final resort. Drugs pose a greater hazard to the elderly than to the younger patient because of a slowing in the rate at which the aged metabolize and excrete drugs. Drug administration on a routine basis should be governed by an attitude of conservatism and circumspection on the part of the nurse.

The aging process and the inelasticity of the *skin* predispose the elderly to decubiti. The older patient

is often content to lie in bed without moving. He must be encouraged to move and to get out of bed as frequently as is permissible. Mineral oil, lanolin creams or baby oil can be used on dry skin; alcohol should not be used, since it causes drying of the cutaneous tissues. Some authorities say that bathing once or twice a week is sufficient, since frequent bathing removes the natural oil from the skin. It is exceedingly important that adequate attention be given to the removal of soapy water from the skin after each bath. The danger of residual soap and consequent lysis of the skin is greatest between the toes and the fingers and in areas where there are folds. The feet especially become dry. It is well to remember that before cutting nails, the feet should be soaked in warm water. Nails should be cleansed and trimmed with care in order to prevent infection as well as injury to the patient. Corns and calluses and tough toe nails may require the care of a podiatrist. Shower or bathtub bathing using water of moderate temperature is preferred to the bed bath. The hair and the scalp should be inspected regularly and given whatever attention the nurse may find necessary. The nurse should anticipate that the geriatric patient needs help to prevent accidents. Safety measures should be utilized. The patient often experiences stiffness and pain when he begin to move or change his position. Because neuromuscular control as well as sensory function may be impaired, the aged bone structures are injured easily.

Further, *visual impairment* may predispose the patient to accidents. Side rails in the bathroom should be available, and all rooms should be well lighted. The older patient's bed is equipped with side rails to remind him to remain in bed at night. They are useful to hold onto when raising oneself to the sitting position and when turning over in bed.

The nurse who takes care of the older patient should know of any *hearing impairment*. Perhaps only one ear is involved, or he may not hear certain ranges of sound; whatever the difficulty, simple gestures and signals by the nurse may be understood clearly. Most patients who have diminished hearing are reluctant to call attention to it; therefore, it is up to the nurse to take the initiative in discovering this or any other handicap.

Many of our older patients have lost a number of their own *teeth* or possess remnants of them. Those who have dentures occasionally present difficulties with poorly fitting sets. This can be serious, inasmuch as constant irritation from a jagged tooth or an ill-fitting denture can lead to cancer of the mouth. Dentures should be cleaned at least twice daily; when they are not being worn a receptacle should be available for them. Frequently, the mouth is the most neglected part of the body. The nurse should encourage and help the patient in carrying out good mouth hygiene. By a careful evaluation of the condition of the mouth, the nurse is able to meet the patient's nutritional needs better, to request dental attention if necessary and to prevent postoperative pulmonary and systemic infections.

Nutritional Needs

Diet for the elderly patient demands consideration. Persons in this age group are especially prone to develop faulty dietary habits. Many depend to an undesirable extent on foods that are prepared with the least effort and which, in the individual's opinion, can be purchased most economically. Therefore, the proportions of carbohydrates in their diet may be excessively high, as in the "tea-toast" regimen, and their protein consumption far below the minimum requirements. Surveys show that calcium, ascorbic acid and riboflavin are the nutrients most lacking in the diets of the aged.

Interest in food may be very slight; social and environmental factors which usually operate to stimulate the appetite may be altogether lacking. Physiological changes also produce this loss of interest. Years of poor eating contribute to old age frailty. There is a diminished loss of taste buds (up to 50 per cent) in many of the elderly, along with the diminished ability to smell. Therefore, the selection of food items and the character of the environment are important to consider.

Merely because the patient is old, it does not necessarily follow that his food must be soft and bland. Reduced activity may have diminished the appetite, in which event it is especially important that the food be served attractively and be as palatable as possible. Orders for special diets may be furnished by the physician, if indicated; otherwise, food should be selected for the elderly patient on the same basis as for any other patient. An adequate, well-balanced regimen should be planned and presented. The nurse should have checked the condition of the mouth and the teeth in advance to be certain that the patient can chew. If the patient is unable to feed himself, arrangements should be made for his feeding, which should be accomplished in a leisurely manner. Unfamiliar foods or methods of cooking should be avoided when feeding the elderly.

The foregoing discussion refers primarily to the problem of undernutrition in the aged. Less of a problem from the standpoint of numerical incidence but even more serious in individual cases, and equally deserving of consideration, is the problem of overnutrition. The majority of persons who have been constantly overnourished for many years retain with tenacity until death their habit of overeating and their

obesity. An overweight patient with a disorder of locomotion due, for example, to hemiplegia, a fractured femur or arthritis affecting the weight-bearing joints, poses a vastly more difficult problem in treatment, rehabilitation or restoration than does an individual who is not burdened with excess poundage. Standing may prove impossible and a state of self-sufficiency unattainable because of obesity complicating a disorder of locomotion which otherwise would not have been incapacitating. In a patient with an acute pulmonary infection or congestive heart failure the effect of obesity may be lethal.

Weight reduction, when it can be achieved, invariably accelerates the rehabilitation of such patients. Its accomplishment, however, is no more simple than in younger individuals. In a large proportion of cases the attempt is doomed to failure or is rewarded by no more than limited success. Efforts to revise an eating habit of several decades' standing are apt to provoke extreme emotional distress or to meet flat rebellion, and therefore should be undertaken with circumspection and a proper sense of values.

Elimination Problems

The aged tend to be very concerned about bowel elimination. A bedside commode is easier to use and is more acceptable than a bed pan. Bowel incontinence positively can be reduced through *systematic* habit training. (See page 175.) Indwelling catheters should not be used to treat urinary incontinence; evidence shows that catheterization is a means of introducing organisms into the urinary tract. The cause of urinary incontinence should be determined. If no pathological problem can be found, fear, social withdrawal and loneliness may be factors. Experience in long term care facilities has shown that systematic bladder and bowel training programs, combined with exercises, ambulation and social activities, can produce significant decreases in the frequency of incontinence.

Exercise

Inactivity is a serious threat to the aged. Lack of muscle use causes atrophy of muscles and deterioration of the body. *Activity* is the key in the prevention of premature aging.

Exercise maintains a good muscular tone throughout the body, including the heart. Good muscle tone is necessary for proper circulation. Exercise aids in relaxation and helps restore the sense of equanimity. It exerts a favorable effect on digestion. And of special importance to the elderly, exercise has a retarding effect on the evolution of atherosclerosis.

(The President's Council on Physical Fitness and Sports and The Administration on Aging has published an exercise program for older Americans titled "The

Fitness Challenge in Later Years."* In it are graded exercise programs that give a balanced workout, utilizing all major muscle groups.)

The Patient's Family

Another aspect of geriatric nursing involves the family of the elderly patient. It may be the responsibility of the nurse to educate and orient its members to various aspects of the social situation and to give instruction concerning responsibility or the immediate and follow-up care of the elderly relative. The family's cooperation should be enlisted as early as possible in the therapeutic planning in order to assure satisfactory convalescent care and maximum protection for the patient against possible complications and further recurrences of his disease.

The Elderly Person and Accidents

Accidents constitute a major, but insufficiently emphasized, cause of death and disability among the aged. Although persons of 65 and over comprise only 10 per cent of our population, they experience a far greater share of fatal accidents. The National Safety Council figures show that this age group accounts for:

> 26% of all accidental deaths
> 10% of all bed disability injuries
> 13% of all hospitalized accident patients
> 11% of the costs of accidents

Mersdorf, National Safety Council specialist, stresses that persons above 65 usually are less able or less willing (1) to perceive danger, because of failing sensory abilities; (2) to organize and interpret warning signals rapidly, because of slowing mental abilities; (3) to move in a rapid and coordinated manner, because of muscular and skeletal impairment; and (4) to compensate for physical impairment, because they do not wish to burden others or even to admit that they are growing older.

The home is where most of the accidents involving older persons take place. Falling is the greatest single cause; the staircase is the most dangerous place. Here are some suggestions to help older persons to avoid accidents: (1) all stairs should have handrails; (2) grab bars should be next to the bathtub, the shower and the toilet; (3) shoes should fit, and the laces must be tied securely; loose slippers are a hazard; (4) belongings and whatever an older person uses should be stored at a level that is between the hip and the eyes, in order to avoid climbing or bending; and (5) older pedestrians, who are prone to think that they have the right of way on streets and highways must be reminded to take precaution, since their hearing and

vision often are impaired, and the conditions listed by Mersdorf above often are present.

(See also "Accidents" in Chapt. 6—Prevention of Disease (includ. Accidents) pp. 69-74.)

SURGERY OF THE ELDERLY PATIENT†

Preoperative Nursing and Medical Management

Due to advances in evaluation techniques and surgical procedures, older patients tolerate elective surgery very well. The principle to be kept in mind during preoperative evaluation, surgery and postoperative care is that the aged patient has *less functional reserve* (the ability of an organ to return to normal after a disturbance in its equilibrium). The special requirements of an aged surgical patient are (1) skillful preoperative evaluation and treatment; (2) experienced and careful anesthesia and surgery; and (3) meticulous and competent postoperative management. The hazards of surgery for the aged are proportional to the number and severity of coexisting diseases.

Psychological Aspects. Confidence will be strengthened if the geriatric patient fully realizes that the contemplated operation is less hazardous than the disease it is expected to remedy. Years of living have a tendency to broaden his ability to adjust to crises. He accepts adjustments more easily; this is particularly advantageous when he is given an anesthetic, for usually he has a smooth induction, maintenance and recovery. On the other hand, one must not assume that he is unconcerned. His attachment to life may be as real as the younger individual's, because in old age one is more conscious of the shortness of the remaining years. The patient may require repeated explanation and reassurance. The objective is to secure his *active* cooperation; if this is to be achieved, a kindly, considerate approach is basic.

Preoperative Preparation. A careful preoperative evaluation is done to determine the patient's ability to adapt to operative stress and to correct, as far as possible, existing defects.

Preparation for surgery demands a meticulous evaluation of the cardiovascular, respiratory and urinary systems as well as the nutritional status of the older patient. Although he may be admitted for a specific problem, it is usual for him to have several other difficulties. Ideally, all deficiencies should be eliminated before he goes to the operating room; practically, some compromises are necessary.

The Heart. In the presence of atherosclerosis, the heart, brain and kidneys are very sensitive to the further reduction of perfusion and oxygenation that anesthesia may produce. Since most elderly patients have some degree of arteriosclerosis, an electrocardiogram is

---

*Administration on Aging, Publication No. 802, May, 1968.

† Review also Chapter 9, pp. 99-157.

done preoperatively to demonstrate evidences of hypertrophy, conduction abnormalities and cardiac abnormalities. Cardiac arrhythmias can be controlled and congestive heart failure improved, but other manifestations of arteriosclerosis are altered very little by preoperative treatment. Coronary artery disease is considered the most serious heart disease for this aged group; its presence increases the operative risk. If the patient is in congestive heart failure, digitalization, diuretics, sodium restriction and bed rest are indicated before surgery is done. As with other patients, tranquilizing drugs, reserpine or other sympatholytic agents preferably are discontinued 10 days preoperatively. (Under stress, these agents may produce alterations of cardiovascular responses.)

The Peripheral Vascular System. Varying degrees of arterial insufficiency and tissue ischemia are present in the aged. The peripheral pulses should be evaluated (and marked) preoperatively. A nursing responsibility is to see that the patient avoids positions that permit venous stasis or pressure on the blood vessels. Instruct the patient to avoid crossing his legs while sitting. The head and foot of the bed must not be elevated at the same time as this position encourages venous stagnation in the pelvic veins. Elastic stockings, worn throughout the hospital stay, help keep venous blood in the deeper circulation. Sitting in a chair with the feet hanging down should be discouraged. Ambulate the patient as much as possible.

RESPIRATORY SYSTEM. The lungs of the elderly may be impaired by fibrosis and emphysema, thus rendering them less efficient in oxygenating the blood. Diminished respiratory activity may be caused by atelectasis, distention and metabolic acidosis. Preoperative assessment includes chest roentgenograms, pulmonary function studies and arterial blood gas and pH values when indicated. Positive pressure breathing, bronchodilator aerosols and antibiotic preparations (for patients with bronchitis, emphysema) may improve the respiratory reserve.

Fluids and Electrolytes. Electrolyte and water deficits should be restored before surgery is undertaken. Many elderly have a reduction of blood volume from chronic bleeding. During transfusion of the elderly the central venous pressure should be monitored (see p. 364). The urinary output also serves as a guide in the correction of dehydration states.

Urinary Tract. Urinary disturbances and disorders of renal function are common in old people. Between the ages of 50 to 80, the average urea clearance declines 50 per cent. In the male, urethral stricture and urethritis, prostatic hypertrophy, prostatitis and cystitis are frequently observed genitourinary lesions. Urine tests, serum electrolyte evaluations and roentgenograms of the G.U. system may be done preoperatively.

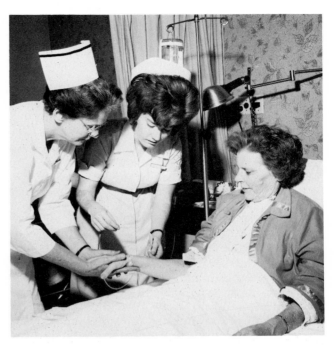

FIG. 4-1. Correct positioning for older patient receiving an intravenous infusion. The head and shoulders should be elevated. Utilizing a hand vein permits greater mobility for the patient. (Courtesy of Loma Linda University School of Nursing)

Preoperative Medication. Drug sensitivity usually is increased in elderly individuals, so that dosages are generally smaller. Preoperative medication is given earlier in the aged because of delayed absorption. In those individuals who have cerebral arteriosclerosis, barbiturates and scopolamine are likely to cause excitement; therefore, paraldehyde, chloral hydrate or tincture of opium may be preferable. Some physicians do not prescribe morphine for the older person. When it is given, the respiratory rate must be observed carefully. If sedatives are given, often one third to one half the usual adult amount is prescribed.

Enemas may be ordered the evening before rather than the morning of surgery because of the inclination of the rectum to retain fluid for several hours.

Position on Operating Table. In the operating room the older patient should be handled gently with no unnecessary exposure. One must have utmost patience in positioning him, since he cannot relax and allow others to move him as desired. Often his joints and muscles are painful when moved. His final position should be relaxed and as comfortable as possible. Extremes in positioning are to be avoided since they hinder circulation.

Anesthesia. Practically all the anesthetic agents used in the younger patient can be used in those past 65.

Intravenous Thiopental has been used as a very satisfactory induction anesthetic. Complicated gas machines may be frightening; consequently, the prick of a needle may be more tolerable than a face mask. Most experienced anesthesiologists prefer to give a mixture of cyclopropane and oxygen by the endotracheal method. This, combined with drugs as needed for relaxation, has the advantage that there is complete control of the anesthesia at all times. The gas concentration can be varied as needed, and adequate oxygenation can be maintained at all times.

Spinal anesthesia also may be used for geriatric patients. It must be remembered that even though their blood vessels may be quite inelastic, they may have a profound drop in pressure. If the blood pressure drop is sudden and prolonged it may lead to circulatory insufficiency. This in turn may cause thrombosis, followed by embolism, infarction and anoxemia. To maintain blood pressure at a normal level is of utmost importance in these individuals.

Going to the other extreme, it is well to remember that sudden increases in blood pressure from excessive or over-rapid infusions may cause pulmonary edema.

Postoperative Management

The immediate postoperative care is the same as that for any patient, but additional support is given to any impaired function of the cardiovascular, pulmonary and renal systems. The older person can chill more easily, and the possibility of shock is greater. Keeping him warm and turning him from side to side after he regains consciousness are essential. His position should be changed frequently not only for his comfort, since he often complains of aches when lying in one position, but also to avoid pulmonary and circulatory complications.

Prevention of Complications

Ever bearing in mind the patient's lesser margin of reserve, complications should be prevented rather than treated. Postoperative complications lead to other complications, and the aged cannot tolerate prolonged periods of stress. The most frequent respiratory complication of the aged is pneumonia. Decreased lung expansion, weakness, relative fixity of the rib cage and drug depression of cough reflexes contribute to its occurrence. Frequent turning, early ambulation, use of small doses of analgesia, removal of tracheobronchial secretions and breathing exercises are preventive measures. Yawning is an effective way to prevent or correct atelectasis. Taking a deep breath and holding it as long as possible helps clear the respiratory tract. If the tracheobronchial tree cannot be cleared, a tracheostomy may be necessary.

Shock. Shock causes death more frequently among those over 60 than among younger patients. The aged individual cannot tolerate a reduction of blood volume or hypotension for even a short period of time. The aged heart and blood vessels do not constrict as readily. Also the patient with sclerotic and narrowed arteries who develops hypotension from shock has a serious reduction in the perfusion of coronary or cerebral vessels. Therefore, the blood pressure must be maintained as closely as possible to the patient's normal blood pressure. The urinary output, an indication of adequacy of blood volume and perfusion, should be between 15 to 25 ml. per hour.

Hydration. Hydration and replacement of electrolyte losses postoperatively are the same as for any surgical patient (see p. 148). After the first few postoperative hours, the patient's head and back should be raised while he is receiving parenteral infusions. This reduces the pressure in the pulmonary circuit that can lead to pulmonary edema. The aging heart and circulatory system cannot stand overloading; infusions and transfusions are given slowly. If there is any question, central venous pressure monitoring will reveal circulatory overloading. It is desirable to use a vein in the hand for infusions so that the patient can be turned and moved readily.

As soon as they can be tolerated, oral fluids should be encouraged for many known reasons. Occasionally, the older patient will not take liquids because the nurse has used too much ice, and he may not be used to that. One older man did not drink fluids because the nurse always filled his glass full; the prospect of drinking a glass full of water overwhelmed him. When another nurse poured a quarter of a glassful at a time, he drank it willingly. This incident illustrates the fact that each individual is a person in his own right. Many older persons have set ways which may seem unusual to the nurse, but the sooner such a quirk is recognized, the more successful the nurse will be in her total care of that patient.

Usually the older patient needs to be encouraged to drink enough fluids. An output of one liter or more indicates that his intake is sufficient for his needs. Obviously, the recording of intake and output is important.

Postoperative Distention. Most often, postoperative distention is due to retention of swallowed air in the intestinal tract. This can be avoided by aspiration of the air from the stomach through a suction tube introduced through the nose and the esophagus into the gastric lumen. Suction may be provided in many ways, and in many cases is maintained until peristalsis is recovered, usually on the second or third day.

In older people, the sluggish peristalsis in the colon

frequently results in incomplete evacuation and therefore retention of fecal material in the sigmoid colon and the rectum. The absorption of fluid produces a hard fecal mass which is irritating to the intestine and often produces frequent small stools, a sort of pseudo-diarrhea. Digital examination reveals a hard mass of fecal material in the rectum. When the mass is broken up by the finger and by enemas, the symptoms are relieved.

Management of Postoperative Pain. Postoperative pain relief may be achieved with fairly small amounts of narcotic drugs. Codeine has proved to be effective. The side effects of narcotics, depressed ventilation and diminished circulation, are dangerous. Enough drug should be given to reduce the pain but not enough to make it difficult for the patient to perform his exercises. If the patient experiences a slight to moderate degree of discomfort, he will move about in bed and be more active. This is a much more desirable state than that of being in a prolonged stuporous condition from oversedation. A certain degree of relaxation can also be achieved with reassurance.

Exercise and Ambulation. Activity in as well as out of bed is essential to recovery. Bed exercises include turning from side to side, flexing and extending the legs and the arms, deep breathing and deliberate coughing. In getting out of bed, the patient should turn to his operated side and bend his knees up. As he swings his feet over the side of the bed, the nurse can assist him to a sitting position. Sitting positions that promote venous stasis in the lower extremities are to be avoided. *Ambulation means that the patient walks, not sits in a chair.*

Patients with pre-existing cardiovascular and pulmonary conditions should be watched carefully, because overexertion may cause a breakdown of these functions. The period out of bed can be gradually increased. The stability of the vital signs is a measure of the patient's reaction to exercise and ambulation activities.

CONVALESCENCE, REHABILITATION AND RECREATION

Convalescence may be difficult because strength is regained slowly. Above all, the elder one needs a great deal of patience. He has a tendency to fret about his limitations. Some authorities advocate that one day be allowed for each decade of one's age for convalescence from acute illness. Patients often find this difficult to accept.

Every attempt should be made to maintain an interest in people or things. Diversional and recreational therapies are of invaluable help for the aged and deserve a generous part of the patient's time. All phases of the rehabilitative program must be within the realm of possibility. The older person must be encouraged to do things for himself in order to become self-sufficient. The nurse must refrain from becoming overly motherly in this respect.

Appearance

A great morale booster is to look well; to look well implies that one feels well. The older person may be neglectful of his appearance; hence, a bit of encouragement by the nurse may direct his attention to "how he looks" rather than "how he feels." An attractive hair-do brightens a woman's spirit; this may be done by simple brushing and combing, setting a wave or braiding long hair. A cleverly placed ribbon, flower or small ornament in the hair may bring compliments from those who come in contact with the elderly woman. Both men and women enjoy a new garment or a bit of color on their person. Even conservative men seem to like bright-colored pajamas. A small flower on the lapel of a man's bathrobe will brighten his spirits. A shave and a haircut do for a man what lipstick does for most women. Almost everyone finds the fragrance of certain dusting powders and colognes refreshing. This has special appeal if it is a scent that is in keeping with the individual's personality. Surely the nurse will be able to find some one thing that will help immeasurably to cheer her older patient.

Physical Activity

The goal of rehabilitation of the elderly patient is to re-establish his ability for self-care and, if possible, to improve his ambulatory capacity. An exercise program in accordance with the patient's exercise tolerance is necessary to achieve this goal.

Walking activities should be encouraged as soon as the patient is able. Instruction in the proper use of aids, such as a walker, crutches or a cane, must be given to the patient. He should be taught why it is important to maintain proper body posture, and how to do it.

The dangers of prolonged bed rest, even prolonged sitting, are numerous and should be avoided even when the patient objects to a change. The rocking chair is more helpful than a straight or an overstuffed chair. The rocking chair is an inexpensive, easily obtainable therapeutic device that enables all but the most feeble to exercise with dignity at any time. Use of the calf and forearm muscles encourages venous return and increases cardiac output. Pulmonary ventilation is increased and hypostatic pulmonary congestion is discouraged. From the psychological point of view, rocking is socially acceptable; in such a chair, one can participate in home activities and be an integral part of the family.

Learning

Mental as well as physical activity is the nucleus of successful rehabilitation. It must be emphasized that old people can learn; the learning process is not limited to the young. Hence, the older person can learn to care for himself and can learn absorbing and interesting hobbies. It is for the nurse and all other members of the health team to teach and direct this potential learner. Instructions must be clear and complete. They must be repeated frequently enough to allow the patient to grasp them. He should be aware of the reasons for doing prescribed activities; many times the patient misinterprets such activities as measures to release the nurse from her many duties rather than accepting them as a means essential for his recovery (see also Chap. 10, pp. 170-177).

Recreation

In the words of Piersol and Bortz, "The society which fosters research to save human life cannot escape responsibility for the life thus extended. It is for science not only to add years to life, but more important, to add life to the years."

Recreation is more than just having fun; it is fundamental to physical and mental well-being. No matter how old or disabled one becomes, the desire for the dignity that comes only through purposeful activity is never lost.

Rusk* states that some surveys have shown that among older people who participate actively in Golden Age Clubs, day centers and similar programs, there are 50 per cent fewer visits to physicians' offices and clinics, 50 per cent fewer general hospital admissions and 800 per cent fewer psychiatric breakdowns than among persons of the same age not participating in active recreation programs.

As soon as the patient is capable of participating in any type of group activity or is willing to undertake some project on an individual basis, such should be planned. The nurse can enlist the help of others, such as occupational therapists, volunteer aides and members of the family, in the organizing of activities designed to occupy the patient's time pleasantly, maintain his enthusiasm and keep him in possession of his faculties and aware of his own personal worth. If a project is successful in this respect, one of the most important goals in the therapeutic process will have been accomplished.

No plan for rehabilitation will be successful unless it is continued beyond the walls of the hospital. Con-

*Rusk, H. A.: Recreation for the aged, The New York Times, p. 62, July 9, 1961.

tinuity of care can be planned with the visiting nurse programs and other community agencies as well as the patient's own family. In many instances, the geriatric patient does not have a family to whom he can return. Real adjustments may have to be made. The smoother the transfer, the more graceful will be the resumption of normal living for the elderly.

LONG-TERM ILLNESS

The duration of an illness, depending on its course, its nature and the degree of disability, deserves serious consideration in the planning and the conduct of medical and nursing care. Such planning should be done by the nurse in collaboration with the physician and other coworkers, in order that she may be informed adequately and advised properly concerning her responsibility for the instruction and the rehabilitation of the patient and the re-education of his family.

In most cases, the adaptation of the patient to prolonged disability is accomplished without apparent difficulty. More important, however, is the quality of the patient's ultimate readjustment to normal life following his recovery from organic disorders. The risk of chronic psychological invalidism never can be discounted, and its consequences are far from benign. At best, convalescence may be prolonged unduly, creating unnecessary hardships for the patient's family. At worst, the patient may be unwilling to assume the responsibilities he should accept and of which he is physically capable, obstinately resisting the loss of his passive and protected status. In either case, without capable instruction in the significance of the patient's attitudes and reactions, the family may be quite defenseless. The fostering of invalidism, which is frequently the unintended result of the family's attitude, seriously compounds the difficulties of rehabilitation and should be discouraged by those who are in a position to advise.

The treatment and the prevention of psychiatric disability in patients with chronic disease is essentially a problem of appropriate psychotherapy. The patient should be diverted continuously, by means of every available device, from his personal problems and discouraged from indulging in morbid self-absorption. Facilities should be made accessible for his intellectual stimulation, artistic satisfaction or productive accomplishment of any type that seems to be desirable and potentially effective. Occupational therapy, expertly conducted, should be incorporated into the program of treatment at the earliest opportunity and continued throughout convalescence. The requirements of individual patients are highly variable, but whatever the problems involved or therapeutic methods employed, the individuals responsible for their management must be acutely aware of the psychological complications that threaten, must be alert to any untoward developments of this character and, most important, must be sufficiently impressed by their own responsibilities in its prevention.

BIBLIOGRAPHY

Books:

Cowdry, E. V. (ed.): The Care of the Geriatric Patient. St. Louis, C. V. Mosby, 1968.

Freeman, J. T.: Clinical Features of the Older Patient, Springfield, Ill., Charles C Thomas, 1965.

Kastenbaum, R. (ed.): New Thoughts on Old Age. New York, Springer, 1964.

Kemp, R. C.: A New Look at Geriatrics, London, Pittman, 1965.

Mitty, W. F.: Surgery in the Aged. Springfield, Ill., Thomas, 1966.

Moss, B. B.: Caring for the Aged, New York, Doubleday, 1966.

Newton, K., and Anderson, H. C.: Geriatric Nursing. St. Louis, C. V. Mosby, 1966.

Powers, J. H. (ed.): Surgery of the Aged and Debilitated Patient. Philadelphia, W. B. Saunders, 1968.

Reynolds, F. W., and Barsam, P. C.: Adult Health. New York, Macmillan, 1967.

Rudd, T. N.: The Nursing of the Elderly Sick. London, Faber and Faber, 1966.

Schwartz, D., et al: The Elderly Ambulatory Patient. New York, Macmillan, 1964.

Williams, R. H., et al.: Processes of Aging. Vols. 1 and 2. New York, Atherton Press, 1963.

Articles:

Amburgey, P. I.: Environmental aids for the aged patient. Amer. J. Nurs., 66:2017-2018, Sept., 1966.

American Medical Association, Committee on Aging: Report on conference on aging and long-term care. October, 1964.

Armbruster, R. J. (ed.): A long look at aging. Johns Hopkins Mag., 13-17, Spring, 1968.

Beck, L. C., and Stangle, E. K.: Geriatric rehabilitation. Geriatrics, 23:118-126, July, 1968.

Brink, M. F., et al.: Current concepts in geriatric nutrition. Geriatrics 23:113-120, March, 1968.

Brotman, H. B.: A profile of the older American. Administration on Aging Publication No. 228. Address before the Conference on Consumer Problems of Older People, New York City, Oct., 1967.

Brown, M., et al.: Nursing care of the aged. An annotated bibliography for nurses. U.S. Public Health Service Publication No. 1603, January, 1967.

Busse, E. W.: Geriatrics today. Amer. J. of Psychiatry, 123:1226-1233, April, 1967.

Cohen, S.: Improve emotional health of the elderly. Geriatric Nurs., 2:39-41, March-April, 1966.

Davis, R. W.: Psychological aspects of geriatric nursing. Amer. J. Nurs., 68:802-804, April, 1968.

Fendell, N.: Foster grandparents join the rehabilitation team. J. Rehabilitation, 33:22-23, May-June, 1967.

Fromm, E.: The psychological problems of aging. Geriatric Nurs., 3:14-21, April, 1967.

Gilliam, M. L.: Assessing the patient. Geriatric Nurs., 3:12-14, June, 1967.

Goldfarb, A.: Psychiatry in geriatrics. Med. Clin. N. Amer., 51: 1515-1527, November, 1967.

Gramlich, E. P.: Recognition and management of grief in elderly patients. Geriatrics 23:87-92, July, 1968.

Hecht, A.: Meeting the needs of the geriatric individual. Geriatric Nurs., 3:21-33, Oct., 1967.

Hulicka, I. M.: Fostering self respect in aged patients. Amer. J. Nurs., 64:84-89, March, 1964.

Hurvitz, M.: Emotional problems of aging patients. Postgrad. Med., 42:115-119, August, 1967.

Kistner, R. L.: Management of severe leg ischemia in the elderly patient. Geriatrics 23:93-96, July, 1968.

Kobrynski, B.: Rehabilitation of the elderly patient. J. Amer. Geriatrics Soc., 14:400-406, April, 1966.

Lamb, D.: Nurse-geriatric patient relationship in a stress situation, phases in human development: relevance in nursing, No. 16. Amer. Nurses Assoc., 1962, pp. 30-38.

McGinity, P. J., and Stotsky, B. A.: The patient in the nursing home. Nurs. Forum, 6:238-261, Summer, 1967.

Miller, A., and Miller, M. E.: Psychiatry of the aging. Applied Therapeutics 9:266-271, March, 1967.

Neely, E., et al.: Problems of aged persons taking medications at home. Nurs. Res., 17:52-55, Jan.-Feb., 1968.

Novick, L. J.: Understanding makes the difference. Canadian Nurse, 62:21-25, January, 1966.

Peck, A.: Psychotherapy of the aged. J. Amer. Geriatrics Soc., 14: 748-753, July, 1966.

Perry, J. F.: Surgery in the aged. Postgrad. Med., 41:414-417, April, 1967.

Sax, S.: The goals of gerontology. Gerontologist, 7:153-160, Sept., 1967.

Schwartz, D.: Problems of self-care and travel among elderly ambulatory patients. Amer. J. Nurs., 66:2678-2681, Dec., 1966.

Warner, B. A.: The processes of aging. Nurs. Clin. N. Amer., 1: 407-415, Sept., 1966.

Wolff, K.: The emotional rehabilitation of the geriatric patient. J. Amer. Geriatric Soc., 14:75-79, January, 1966.

PATIENT EDUCATION

Periodicals:

Aging. U.S. Dept. of Health, Education and Welfare (monthly)
Supt. of Documents
Washington, D.C. 20402 ($2.00 per yr.)

Adding Life To Years (monthly)
University of Iowa
26 Byington Road
Iowa City, Iowa 52240 ($1.00 per yr.)

Current Literature on Aging (quarterly)
National Council on the Aging
315 Park Avenue, South
New York, New York 10010 ($2.25 per yr.)

Geriatric Focus (semi-monthly)
Knoll Pharmaceutical Co.
Orange, New Jersey (free)

Geriatric Nursing (monthly)
Miller Publishing Co.
2501 Wayzata Boulevard
Minneapolis, Minnesota 55440 ($10.00 per yr.)

Harvest Years (monthly)
    Harvest Years Publishing Co.
    104 East 40th Street
    New York, New York 07050 ($4.50 per yr.)
Journal of the American Geriatrics Society (monthly)
    American Geriatrics Society
    10 Columbus Circle
    New York, New York 10019
Journal of Gerontology (quarterly)
    Gerontological Society
    660 South Euclid Avenue
    St. Louis, Missouri 63310 ($26.00 per yr.)
More Life for Your Years (monthly)
    American Medical Association
    535 North Dearborn Street
    Chicago, Illinois 60610 (free)
Senior Citizens News (monthly)
    National Council of Senior Citizens
    1627 K Street, N.W.
    Washington, D.C. 20006 ($3.00 per yr.)

Pamphlets:

U.S. Government Printing Office
    Supt. of Documents
    Washington, D.C. 20402
        Public Health Service Publication No. 993
        Mental Disorders of the Aging
U.S. Dept. of Health, Education and Welfare
    U.S. Government Printing Office
    Supt. of Documents
    Washington, D.C. 20402
        Administration on Aging Publications:
            Aging—Fact and Fancy. (AoA No. 224)
            Are You Planning on Living the Rest of Your Life? (AoA No. 803)
            Consumer Guide for Older People. (AoA No. 801)
            Employment and Volunteer Opportunities for Older People. (A 4-page fact sheet.)
            Meeting the Needs of Older People at the Community Level. (AoA No. 223)
            Part-Time Employment for Older People. (AoA No. 225)
            Protective Services for the Aged. (AoA No. 226)
            The Fitness Challenge in the Later Years. (AoA No. 802)
            You, the Law and Retirement. (AoA No. 800)
U.S. Office of Economic Opportunity
    Washington, D.C. 20506
        Resources for the Aging: An Action Handbook.
Public Health Affairs
    381 Park Avenue South
    New York, New York 10016
        Stern, E. M.: A Full Life After 65. (F1347)
        Ogg, E.: When Parents Grow Old. (F1208)
        Osborne, E.: When You Lose a Loved One. (F1269)
        Alexander, R. S. and Podair, S.: Medicaid: The People's Health Plan. (F1422)

American Medical Association
    Dept. of Health Services
    535 North Dearborn Street
    Chicago, Illinois 60610
        A New Concept of Aging
        Education of Children for the New Era of Aging
        Health Aspects of Aging
        Health Promotion for Adults
        How the Older Person Can Get the Most Out of Living
        Retirement: A Medical Philosophy and Approach
National Safety Council
    425 North Michigan Avenue
    Chicago, Illinois 60611
        Accidents to the Elderly
        Forget Things? Here's How to Avoid Accidents.
        Poor Sight? Here's How to Avoid Accidents.
        Tire Easily? Here's How to Avoid Accidents.

AGENCIES

Governmental:

Administration on Aging
Department of Health, Education and Welfare
Washington, D.C. 20201

Project SCORE (Service Corps of Retired Business Executives)
Small Business Administration
Department of Labor
Washington, D.C. 20212

VISTA
Office of Economic Opportunity
Washington, D.C. 20506

Voluntary:

American Association of Retired Persons
DuPont Circle Building
Washington, D.C. 20036

American Medical Association
Committee on Aging
535 North Dearborn Street
Chicago, Illinois 60610

National Council on Aging
315 Park Avenue South
New York, New York 10010

National Council of Senior Citizens, Inc.
1627 K Street, N.W.
Washington, D.C. 20006

The Gerontological Society
660 South Euclid Avenue
St. Louis, Missouri 63310

CHAPTER **5**

The Internal Environment: Homeostatic Mechanisms and Pathophysiologic Processes
A Physiologic Analysis

- *A Physiologic Definition of Disease*
- *Mechanisms for Maintaining A Stable Internal Environment*
- *Brief Survey of Other Mechanisms of Disease*
- *General and Local Defenses Against Disease*
- *Representative Pathophysiologic Processes*

INTRODUCTION

The great French physiologist, Claude Bernard, laid down a major biological principle when he wrote: "The condition for a free life is the constancy of the internal environment." By "internal environment" is meant the fluid bathing the cells of the body, as contrasted with the external environment that surrounds man as a whole organism. As long as this fluid, a water solution of gases, ions, and nutrients, is relatively constant in composition and temperature, the cell can carry on its functions, despite the fact that man as a whole lives in an external environment hostile to the existence of the cell. Because the cell is protected, man is not confined like the amoeba to a pond sufficiently rich in oxygen and nutrients, but is free to move in his external world to the extent that his inventive ingenuity permits. In short, the range and variety of activities and choices available to man depend upon both the functional integrity of the cell and the stability of the internal environment.

A PHYSIOLOGIC DEFINITION OF DISEASE

For the purposes of this chapter, disease is defined as any process or event that promotes a change in the internal environment resulting in loss of cell function, thus limiting man's freedom to act in the external world. To the nurse, disease is displayed as a changing state or shifting pattern of patient response that is the result of disease processes on one hand and bodily defenses and therapeutic responses on the other. Disease described in the context of physiology or pathophysiology is most useful to the nurse at the bedside as she attempts to answer two questions: what is the current status of the patient, and what is the response of the patient to therapy?

The physiologic definition given above is used for two reasons: (1) many serious illnesses provoke and evoke change in the internal environment; and (2) most therapy is directed toward the restoration of a normal internal environment. Moreover, such a viewpoint facilitates an analysis of the seriousness of a disease or the rate of recovery from it. For instance, the patient with advanced emphysema who is cyanotic, acidotic, fighting for every breath and able to climb only a few stairs without rest has his freedom of choice severely restricted because his oxidative energy supply for cell function is limited. Furthermore, the hydrogen ions produced by oxidative metabolism are not neutralized fast enough to avoid change in the blood pH, and respiratory acidosis results. Since the structure of most body proteins are pH-dependent, such a change in pH results in a change of structures and cell functions, especially of the cell wall. This patient is se-

TABLE 5-1. Composition* of serum, intercellular fluid, cerebrospinal fluid and intracellular fluid of muscle cells

	Serum	Intercellular Fluid	Cerebrospinal Fluid	Intracellular† Fluid
Na	138	140	141	10
K	4	4	3	150
Ca	7	7	2.5	—
Mg	—	—		40
Cl	102	114	127	15–20
HCO₃	26	29	18	10
PO₄, SO₄	3	3	1.5	150
Protein	15	—	—	40

*mEq./L. These substances are frequently reported in terms of mg./100 ml.
†Skeletal muscle.
Note: Only ions are considered, including the ionic equivalency of protein, which is a charged molecule at bodily pH values.

TABLE 5-2.* The kidney as a homeostatic organ

Substance	Amount Filtered per 24 hours	Amount Excreted per 24 hours	Per Cent Reabsorbed
Water	170 L.	1.5 L.	99%
Glucose	170 gm.	0 gm.	100%
Sodium	560 gm.	5 gm.	99%
Potassium	29 gm.	2.7 gm.	90%
Urea	51 gm.	30.0 gm.	60%
Ammonia†	—	1.0 mg.	0%

*The examples given are typical of a healthy man at rest and do not show the range possible in disease, exercise, or water excess or deprivation.
†Secreted after formation by the renal tubules.

riously ill because his internal environment is altered.

The chronic smoker with mild to moderate bronchitis and bronchoconstriction is not ill while carrying on sedentary activity, but if he must run to the bus stop, the reduction in ventilatory function would force a slackened pace. This means that his freedom of choice of action is restricted, and therefore he would be considered not healthy. A patient who has had a coronary occlusion is confined to bed lest the output of the heart be insufficient to maintain adequate transport of gases in the blood, or to maintain adequate blood pressure. Recovery is associated with increasing activity (freedom of choice) without breathlessness, fatigue, or unusually rapid or erratic heart rate.

Mental disease is not discussed because the pathogenesis is largely unknown, although evidence points to biochemical changes at the cellular level as one basis for such disease.

MECHANISMS FOR MAINTAINING A STABLE INTERNAL ENVIRONMENT

The bodily state associated with a stable internal environment is called *homeostasis*. The machinery and method for obtaining homeostasis is discussed next.

The *internal environment* is the intracellular or interstitial fluid bathing each cell, a water solution of inorganic salts and organic substances filtered from the plasma through the capillary wall. Its composition is similar to that of plasma without protein. However, the interstitial fluid of the brain (cerebrospinal fluid) is produced by active cellular processes and differs somewhat from interstitial fluid derived from blood plasma (Table 5-1).

Although the composition of the internal environment may vary locally from tissue to tissue because of differences in cellular activity and metabolism, its average composition is relatively constant, a consequence of the free exchange of substances back and forth between blood and interstitial fluid. Blood, in turn, is continuously being "mixed," through the process of collection and redistribution in the blood vessels of the body and lungs. This relative constancy of composition is the result of a *dynamic* type of equilibrium, the stability achieved by continuous small reciprocal exchanges of chemical substances between cell, interstitial fluid and blood. This situation is analogous to two equally skilled and powerful wrestlers who have brought one another to a standstill, equilibrium being achieved by continuous small and opposing shifts in muscular activity.

Various exchanges take place between the external and internal environments: respiratory gases, foodstuffs, water and heat. These exchanges are effected by the lungs, kidneys, gastrointestinal tract and skin, and the activity of these organs varies to compensate for cell activity ranging from rest to extreme exercise. The circulatory system acts as the middleman between the variable organ and the stable fluid. For instance, carbon dioxide, one end product of energy production in the cell, when dissolved in water forms a weak acid capable of changing the internal environment as it diffuses out of the cell and into the bloodstream. However, the CO_2 is buffered by the acid-neutralizing capacity of the blood and is transported to the lungs for elimination into an external environment that is low in CO_2 content.

Even more dramatic is the role of the kidney, which filters the blood and removes certain substances by tubular secretion. It then returns most of the filtered chemicals to the blood and eliminates excess or unwanted substances by way of the urine.

Table 5-2 illustrates the overall activity of the kidney; several consequences of renal function are apparent. About 170 L. of kidney filtrate are formed per 24 hours by the recirculation of about 3 L. of plasma through the kidney, thus providing for a continuous adjustment of the composition of the blood. Some substances important to cell function (such as glucose) are almost totally reabsorbed, while other substances are produced or eaten in excess of need (e.g., potassium) are excreted sufficiently to avoid accumulation. Thus, the kidney is capable of a wide variety and range of activities. A small change in renal function results in a major deviation in the internal environment, or departure from homeostasis. Were the kidney to excrete 10 per cent instead of 1 per cent of the filtrate water, a man would spend much of his time simply drinking and eliminating water. (Diabetes insipidus, produced by a deficiency of antidiuretic hormone of the anterior pituitary, is such a disease state.)

The other organs of homeostasis have analogous abilities and the capacity for wide changes in function to provide for continuous adjustment in the composition of the blood. Diseases of the organs of homeostasis (heart, lungs, kidney, liver, gastrointestinal tract, skin) are serious because the internal environment changes, and as a consequence cellular activity in general is altered, diminished or halted. For this reason, then, examination of blood to determine the status of the interstitial fluid and examination of the heart, lungs, liver, and kidney to determine the status of the organs of homeostasis constitute the crux of all diagnostic procedures and allow an estimate of prognosis.

Approximately 70 per cent of the lungs, kidney, liver or heart muscle can be surgically removed or damaged before homeostasis during bodily rest is altered. The enormous *physiologic reserve* of function allows a wide range of variation in total bodily activity, ranging from sleep to Olympic competition.

Though the end-function of the organs of homeostasis is to keep the internal environment constant, they act on molecules and use energy sources that are not reused or recycled, but that enter and leave the body in a one-way flow pattern termed *open-ended*. For example, in the adult, each day about 2000 ml. of water, about 2500 kilocalories of energy in the form of food, and varying quantities of oxygen and various ions enter the body and leave as water containing various molecules in solution, or heat, or CO_2, etc. This flow of materials and energy through the body is necessary for two reasons: (1) the molecular structure of the cell is continuously degraded, removed and replaced; and (2) the cells manufacture new substances such as fat, glycogen, or hormones, or perform such energy-consuming mechanical functions as shortening

and lengthening of muscles. From day to day adult man appears to be the same, but this apparent stability or steady state actually is dynamic. The molecules of his body are being exchanged for identical molecules at a variable but continuous rate. If a wall contained a million bricks, and if each day 100 original bricks were removed from various parts of the wall and replaced, in 10,000 days the entire wall would have been entirely replaced. Yet on any one day the wall functioned as a wall and with little apparent change. Entirely analogous is the situation of the body cellular structure. For this reason the patient is analyzed for "balance" or intake-output of water, minerals and energy because alteration of the flow of energy or materials means a loss of the steady state. Disease frequently causes an unsteady state with gradual but inexorable loss of cell integrity and a change in homeostasis. Vomiting, gastrointestinal obstruction, diarrhea or pneumonia cause a decreased input or increased output of material and energy. For this reason therapy often is directed toward maintaining the open-ended steady state: intravenous fluids with glucose and salts, diuretics, oxygen and so forth. Any analysis of disease must include an estimate of the disruption of the open-ended steady state, since in many cases cellular or organ malfunction that is trivial in terms of cellular integrity, such as viral enteritis, may be rapidly fatal in an infant because of water and salt loss.

The function of the organs of homeostasis is regulated by means of hormones and/or the activity of the nervous system. Insulin and the regulation of blood sugar via the liver; parathyroid hormone and the regulation of blood calcium and phosphorous via the kidney; neural control of the respiratory muscles regulating the rate and depth of respiration and thus of gas exchange; neural control of the rate and force of cardiac contraction—all are examples of *regulation of homeostasis*. Obviously, deficiency or excessive action of hormones, or of the nervous system, must result in disease. A blow on the head may cause sufficient neuronal injury to cause muscular paralysis so that respiratory muscles may not contract, so that the victim is unable by himself to supply the needs of his open-ended energy system.

The regulating organ receives continuous information about the results of regulation by way of the nervous system or the blood stream, a situation termed *feedback*. The feedback then alters the function of the regulator, enhancing or diminishing its activity. For instance, the level of sugar in the blood flowing through the pancreas determines the amount of insulin released from the islet cells of the pancreas. After a meal the blood sugar rises because of the intestinal absorption of glucose. Insulin then is released to enhance absorption of glucose into the body cells and to promote the formation of glycogen in the liver, thus correcting the postprandial rise in blood glucose.

During exercise when glucose is metabolized and tends to leave the blood, insulin secretion is reduced, glycogen storage is reduced, and epinephrine is released to aid the breakdown of glycogen to glucose in the liver by a process called glycogenolysis, with release from the liver to the blood stream. Meanwhile the mean blood glucose level remains relatively unchanged because production and use are balanced.

Feedback is called *positive* if the substance regulated enhances the action of the regulator, and *negative* if it decreases the action of the regulator. An example of negative feedback is ingestion of excess water which reduces the release of antidiuretic hormone from the anterior pituitary, and less renal tubular absorption of water occurs until the excess water is voided as urine.

Disease may be a consequence of abnormal regulation of homeostasis. Examples are diabetes insipidus due to deficiency of anti-diuretic hormone; paroxysmal atrial tachycardia following excess sympathetic nervous system stimulation; and renal edema due to excessive aldosterone, a hormone of the adrenal cortex which decreases the loss of sodium by way of the kidney.

Finally, the role of *compensation* must be discussed. The organs of homeostasis or their regulators are capable of a wide range of activity. Witness the range of the volume of air breathed: 0.3 to 150 L/min; or of the heart rate: 40-150 beats/min.; or urinary volume and concentration. These organs can increase their activity in the presence of disease processes which continuously tend to change the internal environment. Consider now an example.

The thyroid hormone controls the rate of energy metabolism, as generally measured by oxygen consumption or heat exchange, through an iodine-containing hormone, thyroxine, produced by its cells. If the food is deficient in iodine the continuous loss of iodine to the open-ended system is halted by means of a compensatory enlargement or hypertrophy of the thyroid cells which capture with great efficiency all iodine from the food or previously released hormone. The enlarged thyroid is called a goiter, and what is termed a disease is actually compensation to provide for homeostasis. The enlargement is due to the release of thyroid-stimulating hormone (TSH) from the anterior pituitary, a consequence of decreased circulating thyroid hormone (positive feedback).

Disease also follows loss of compensation. Rising from a sitting or lying position suddenly reduces the venous return to the heart because about 1 liter of blood is temporarily pooled in the legs. A fall in blood pressure is avoided by a compensatory increase in heart output. Ordinarily, however, the adjustment is

rapid, the change in heart rate is small and the blood pressure is steady. After squatting for a few minutes and then rapidly standing, even the young may experience transient dizziness because of the decreased cardiac output, loss of blood pressure, and decreased perfusion of the brain. The dizziness occurs because some brain cells have no energy reserve, and hence adequate blood pressure and flow to the brain to provide oxygen and glucose homeostasis are of the utmost importance. In the treatment of hypertension, drugs which block or diminish the activity of the sympathetic nervous system, such as reserpine or guanethidine, interfere with the vascular and cardiac compensation to change in posture, and orthostatic hypotension follows. Getting out of a chair becomes a study in slow motion and a search for support to reduce the dizziness and its consequences.

To summarize briefly, homeostasis in an open-ended system results from the varying activities of organs of homeostasis regulated by hormonal, humoral, and neural mechanisms often via a positive or negative feedback, circulation being the common mediator. The equilibrium achieved is a dynamic steady-state. Disease results when any of these interacting and interrelated organs and phenomena are altered by (1) a change in the organ cells themselves by infection, trauma, degeneration, (2) a change in formation, release or action of the regulators or (3) over- or undercompensatory action of the organs for changes elsewhere.

BRIEF SURVEY OF OTHER MECHANISMS OF DISEASE

Developmental defects are not an uncommon cause of disease. Overt anatomic defects such as imperforate anus or cardiac abnormalities make homeostasis impossible or else attainable only by restricted activity. Other defects, more subtle in expression, are molecular or cellular in scope, and are often a result of genetic abnormality. Examples are clotting defects such as hemophilia; anemia in sickle-cell disease; and enzyme defects such as phenylketonuria.

Common and important are diseases associated with the development of antibodies to abnormal proteins in the body—the allergic and auto-immune diseases. One of the allergic diseases, asthma, produces readily demonstrable changes in homeostasis. Because of constriction of bronchial muscle, resistance to air flow is increased, ventilation of the lungs is decreased, and exchange of respiratory gases is altered. Carbon dioxide accumulates, oxygen supply is insufficient and respiratory acidosis, anoxemia and reduced reserves for energy from oxidative sources result. By marked muscular effort the severe asthmatic may obtain sufficient oxygen to support life under conditions of reduced activity while the kidney excretes acid to compensate for the acidosis.

Diseases of metabolism and the endocrine glands may best be considered in their relationship to homeostasis. Abnormalities of growth or of the sex hormones do not usually alter homeostasis, or else alterations are confined to specific tissues not vital to survival. Metabolic diseases involving blood vessels, such as atherosclerosis, are most serious when the blood vessels of the organs of homeostasis are involved.

Deficiency of calories, protein, or other essential nutrient elements is a common cause of human misery and a serious one because man exists in an openended system. Many diseases cause malnutrition: diarrhea, malabsorption syndromes, intestinal obstruction; but poverty, ignorance, poor habits, and faulty dentition or ill-fitting teeth are more often the causes. In the United States, obesity caused by calorie excess is the most common nutritional defect. Although not usually classed as a disease, obesity is associated with an increased incidence of heart and arterial disease and a shorter life span. In fact, most acute illnesses are laid on a foundation of chronic disease either fully compensated by physiological means or ignored until the acute episode.

Altered regulation of cell growth and reproduction is also an important cause of disease and in this class may be placed growths, benign or malignant, of any tissue. Generally, in these instances, death comes from malnutrition or interference with the organs or regulators of homeostasis. Diseases of striated muscles, the skeleton, the sense organs, the motor control of skeletal muscles and the skin (save for sweating and heat regulation) may not disturb homeostatic mechanisms, but may change our relation to the external environment. Since the bulk of man's thought and activity is directed to the external environment, such diseases are serious tragedies. The victim of stroke may linger on for years, his mechanism for homeostasis intact; yet he is restricted in choice and freedom because still-living muscle cells are not stimulated and coordinated to permit purposeful movement.

Infection, parasitic infestation, trauma and poisoning come from without. There are bodily defenses for these: white cells, blood clotting, fibrous tissue repair, vomiting. Generally, cause and effect can be traced in these instances.

Finally to be mentioned but not discussed is the interaction between the mind and the body. Anxiety, depression and neurotic behavior with attendant physical symptoms are the major contributors to the discomfort of modern man, though life is not threatened **and** homeostasis generally is secure. Pain, though not a disease, may seriously influence behavior and restrict activity, thus providing a disease-like state.

GENERAL AND LOCAL DEFENSES AGAINST DISEASE

Cell injury due to any cause generally produces to a greater or lesser degree a local response typified by capillary dilatation with increased capillary wall permeability and, if sufficiently severe, the migration of white blood cells to the area: neutrophils to bacteria, eosinophils in allergy, and lymphocytes in chronic irritation conditions. If cell damage leads to cell death, compensatory hypertrophy, or hyperplasia, of remaining cells or fibrous tissue replacement may occur.

The blood vessel response is often, for convenience, termed the triple response: following cell injury dilatation of small vessels occurs due to (1) locally produced chemical substances or (2) neuronal influences and (3) local edema. The effects are typical of those found after a local injection of histamine and are reproduced similarly after mechanical injury, infection, and heat or chemical injury. The classical and cardinal signs are redness, swelling (edema), pain and loss of function. Pain may be due to the action of histamine or simple peptides split from tissue protein by enzymes called kinins. In chronic inflammation or irritation, the vascular component may be minimal, lymphocytes and monocytes migrate to the area and fibrosis may be prominent.

In addition to the local response there may be general responses and these stem from two sources: the hormonal system of the adrenal cortex and anterior pituitary gland, and the sympathetic nervous system.

In response to injury and to what is termed stress, the cortex of the adrenal gland, through the stimulus of a hormone released from the anterior pituitary called adrenocorticotrophic hormone (ACTH) releases another hormone called cortisol. Cortisol mobilizes some bodily resources such as glucose by promoting the conversion of protein to glucose by a process called gluconeogenesis and inhibits others, especially the local response to tissue injury and to antigen-antibody reactions. These latter so-called allergic reactions are modified or suppressed and at the same time body defenses against foreign protein are diminished. This property of the adrenocortical hormones is used to delay rejection of organ transplants.

Walter Cannon pointed out the role of the sympathetic nervous system in protecting the body against external events threatening to homeostasis, especially hunger, cold, trauma and sudden environmental change. In addition, some of the same responses occur in states of fear and rage.

Nerves from the sympathetic nervous system are distributed throughout the body; and in addition a hormone, epinephrine, whose actions mimic those of sympathetic nerve stimulation, can be released from the adrenal medulla by a variety of stimuli.

Cold, anoxia, low blood sugar and severe cutaneous pain, among many other stimuli, can provoke sympathetic responses. These are: (1) activation of a liver enzyme, phosphorylase, to promote glycogenolysis; (2) increase in rate and strength of contraction of the heart to maintain blood pressure; (3) constriction of blood vessels of skin, to reduce heat loss and reduce skin hemorrhage; (4) increased clotting ability of the blood; (5) dilatation of skeletal muscle arterioles and constriction of splanchnic vessels, to redistribute blood; (6) inhibition of the intestinal wall muscle, and (7) dilatation of bronchial muscle to provide easier air flow. All the above protect against external hazards. In addition, fatigue is postponed and energy sources are mobilized. Thus, the sympathetic nervous system is a defense system against external threat and can be considered a general homeostatic mechanism.

SUMMARY

Disease is a dynamic, ever-changing expression of the balance between cell damage or abnormal cell activity and the body defense mechanisms or compensations. It becomes serious when a major organ of homeostasis is extensively damaged or when it is functioning maximally. Once the internal environment is substantially altered, then all cells are damaged or die. Death is generally defined as cessation of the activity of the heart and lungs, the principal organs of homeostasis. More recently, the absence of cerebral function as measured by the electroencephalogram is now considered an indication of death, and so a regulator of homeostasis is included in the definition of death.

REPRESENTATIVE PATHO-PHYSIOLOGIC PROCESSES

The aim of the rest of this chapter is to present pathogeneses of several diseases as examples of the principles discussed. Flow diagrams indicate major events in the development of disease and for clarity are divided into *antecedent* events that may be considered the prime cause of disease, and *action* events that show the interrelation of disease and bodily response. In the latter case, cause and effect are displayed for the major facets of the disease. Regretably, arrows and words but dimly portray the shifts in the patient's condition, moment by moment or day by day in acute illness; or week by week in chronic illness. The influence of normal or abnormal physiological cycles, of social adjustments between patient and hospital personnel or family, of unknown or expressed anxiety and concern, of the patient's total life experience on the development and course of disease, is well recognized by the health team. However, these variables cannot be placed into a flow diagram. Yet, they may be major factors governing the course of the disease.

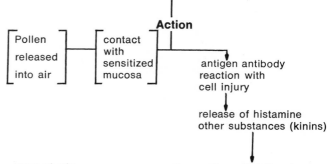

PATHOPHYSIOLOGY OF POLLINOSIS
(Flow Diagram I)

Antecedents

Inherited tendency to abnormal immune response (atopy)
Entry of antigen protein substance (pollen)

Formation of circulating protein antibodies (globulins) by immune cells (probably lymphocytes) that not only *immunize* but *sensitize* (skin-sensitizing antibodies or reagin)

Attachment of "skin sensitizing" antibodies to nasal mucosa

Action

Pollen released into air — contact with sensitized mucosa — antigen antibody reaction with cell injury

release of histamine other substances (kinins)

sympathetic nervous system activity diminishes these responses

1. capillary dilatation (congestion)
2. tissue fluid transudation (nasal discharge, sneezing)
3. stimulation of mucous production
4. stimulation of naked nerve endings ——▶ itching

Addenda

Repeated antigen challenge leads to desensitization (mechanisms unknown)

Four diseases are discussed and the major characteristics of each are pointed out. Pollinosis (seasonal allergic rhinitis due to pollens) is associated with an abnormal defense mechanism, that of defense against foreign protein. Sickle cell anemia is an example of the effect of a genetic defect, in this case of the formation of hemoglobin. The disease is caused by a small change in the structure of a molecule. Addison's disease, caused by decreased function of the adrenal cortex, is an example of loss of regulation of a part of the internal environment, principally sodium and water, and carbohydrate metabolism.

Left-sided heart failure shows the effect of abnormal function of an organ of homeostasis.

Seasonal Allergic Rhinitis Due to Pollens (Pollinosis) (Flow Diagram I)

Typically, allergies are characterized by a marked cellular response to trivial challenge and represent an exaggerated immune reaction. The protein structure of the body is, in part, unique to the organism and is a product of genetic inheritance. Invasion by a foreign protein, called an antigen (through bacteria, blood transfusion, gastrointestinal absorption of protein), provokes the formation of a body protein called an antibody which is able to combine with the antigen and render it incapable of injuring cells. The antibodies may circulate in the blood stream as globulins or be fixed in the tissues. Moreover, the bodily ability to provide antibodies is rather long term and easily invoked. Use of vaccines against common infectious diseases in a deliberate introduction of foreign protein is designed to stimulate antibody formation. Following vaccination against tetanus, the effective levels of antibody may be available for years, and the concentration or titer is readily increased by a so-called booster dose.

In seasonal allergic rhinitis, for some unknown reasons, tissue antibodies are found in the nose and eyes which not only react with very small doses of some specific pollen but also sensitize the cell. As a result cell injury occurs, indicated by copious secretions, edema of the mucosa, sneezing because of the secretions and local itching. When the offending pollen is blown away, the allergic condition ceases.

The cause of cell stimulation is due in part to release of histamine and other as yet poorly-identified substances. Therapy takes four major lines:

1. desensitization by repeated injections of the offending pollens in low concentration
2. administration of antihistamine; that is, substances protecting cells against the effects of histamine
3. removal of offending pollens (by air conditioning)
4. suppression of the immune response by means of corticosteroids

Sickle Cell Anemia (Flow Diagram II)

Sickle cell anemia is the result of the physical deformity of red cells following altered aggregation of hemoglobin molecules within the cell. The complex protein molecule, referred to as S hemoglobin, differs from normal hemoglobin by the introduction of a single amino acid, valine, instead of glutamic acid. The cause of this chronic inherited defect is a fault in the desoxyribonucleic acid of the gene controlling production of the abnormal S hemoglobin in the bone marrow. Since the sickle cell is resistant to invasion by the parasite of malaria, this latter disease may promote the survival of the genetic trait by natural selection.

In the capillaries serving actively metabolizing cells, the normal reduction in oxygen type and the production of acids such as carbonic and lactic acids cause the S hemoglobin to aggregate, and the coin-shaped red cell is distorted into a sickle-shape. The abnormal cells do not readily slip and squeeze through the

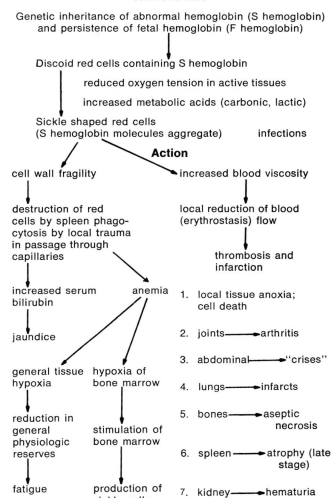

PATHOPHYSIOLOGY OF SICKLE CELL ANEMIA
(Flow Diagram II)
Antecedents

Genetic inheritance of abnormal hemoglobin (S hemoglobin) and persistence of fetal hemoglobin (F hemoglobin)

Discoid red cells containing S hemoglobin

reduced oxygen tension in active tissues

increased metabolic acids (carbonic, lactic)

Sickle shaped red cells
(S hemoglobin molecules aggregate)   infections

Action

cell wall fragility   increased blood viscosity

destruction of red cells by spleen phagocytosis by local trauma in passage through capillaries

local reduction of blood (erythrostasis) flow

thrombosis and infarction

increased serum bilirubin   anemia

jaundice

general tissue hypoxia   hypoxia of bone marrow

reduction in general physiologic reserves   stimulation of bone marrow

fatigue   production of sickle cells

1. local tissue anoxia; cell death
2. joints——►arthritis
3. abdominal——►"crises"
4. lungs——►infarcts
5. bones——►aseptic necrosis
6. spleen——►atrophy (late stage)
7. kidney——►hematuria

Compensation

1. Decreased oxygen is the stimulus for red cell production in the bone marrow which produces red cells sufficient to correct the anemia and attendant hypoxia. This is an example of positive feedback. The compensation produces further pathology in the bone vessels.
2. The greater the amount of F hemoglobin in the cells the less the sickling effect.
3. Local vessel dilatation following tissue injury and an inflammatory reaction are present. The white cells and other sources of proteolytic enzymes remove dead cells; fibrous tissue replacement occurs.

capillaries and a logjam of red cells causes local stases of blood flow with attendant cell damage due to hypoxia and altered local internal environment. In the general circulation, the red cells generally maintain the normal anatomic shape.

PATHOPHYSIOLOGY OF ADRENAL CORTICAL INSUFFICIENCY
(Addison's Disease)
(Flow Diagram III)

Antecedents

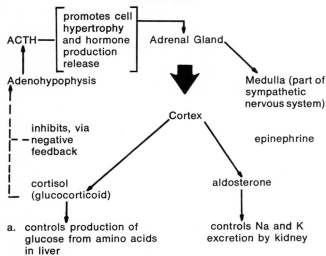

a. controls production of glucose from amino acids in liver
b. suppresses immune responses
c. suppresses lymphocyte formation and circulation
d. suppresses eosinophil circulation

Action

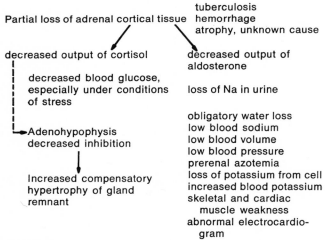

Compensation

1. hypertrophy of gland remnant by adenohypophysis via release of ACTH
2. salt "craving," a desire of unknown mechanism leads to intake of salt

Note: Hyperpigmentation occurs in Addison's Disease but the mechanism is not understood. Enhanced activity of a melanocyte stimulating hormone of the neurohypophysis has been advanced as an explanation.

The severity of the disease depends on the number of abnormal cells and local tissue factors governing blood flow at the arteriole-capillary-venule level. Ordinarily the course of the disease is chronic with exacerbations associated with infection or other disease. Though not life-threatening, sickle cell anemia does restrict the freedom of its victim to participate in a wide range of life's activities.

Adrenal Cortical Insufficiency (Addison's Disease (Flow Diagram III)

Certain disease states can cause the partial loss of adrenal cortical tissue. This loss leads to major changes in the internal environment because the hormone aldosterone, which normally controls the absorption of sodium by the kidney, is suppressed. Sodium is excreted in increased amounts. Sodium is the chief ion of the extracellular fluid from the standpoint of total concentration and of its key position in regulation of water volume and thus blood volume. Since the ionic concentrations of the internal environment must be kept relatively stable, retention of sodium ion by the kidney is always associated with water retention, with expansion of the fluid volume; and to a greater or lesser degree, sodium loss is usually associated with water loss, contraction of the fluid volume, and thus dehydration. Where sodium goes, water usually follows.

Loss of sodium and water is associated with decreased blood perfusion of the kidney and an increase of blood urea nitrogen, so-called prerenal azotemia.

The functional integrity of the cell wall in part depends upon the concentration of the sodium and potassium ions on the inside (high potassium) and outside (high sodium) of the cell. An important consequence of this asymmetrical distribution of ions is the creation of an ion-battery with excess positive electrical charge on the outer surface and a corresponding excess negative charge on the inside. Migration of these ions across the cell surface follows cell stimulation, and charged-particle migration causes an electric current which serves to initiate biochemical activities of the cell such as contraction of muscle protein and release of enzymes. The electrocardiogram is a graphic registration of the complex electrical fluctuations passing over heart muscle as the excited cell membranes allow small reversible migrations of sodium and potassium ions into and out of the cell. In Addison's disease, sodium loss causes the loss of potassium from the cell into the extracellular fluid. The increased potassium concentration in the extracellular fluid produced during exacerbations of the disease cause an abnormal electrocardiogram. A further consequence of the sodium and potassium shifts is muscle weakness, both skeletal and cardiac.

The adrenal cortex produces a second hormone, cortisol, as was noted earlier. Cortisol and its metabolites control the formation of glucose from amino acids in the liver, a process called gluconeogenesis. By this metabolic mechanism, glucose can be formed from non-carbohydrate stores and during periods of stress or starvation glucose homeostasis can be maintained. Because Addison's disease curtails cortisol production, the patient tends to have a low blood sugar and does not tolerate fasting.

Lymphocytosis occurs because the normal suppressive action of cortisol is absent or diminished. Because enhanced adrenal cortical activity is part of the bodily response to stress of any type, such as cold, heat, starvation, infection and injury, the Addisonian does not tolerate stress and major illness may rapidly become lethal. As in all endocrine disorders, the clinical picture varies with the degree of hormonal deficit.

Compensation is achieved by hypertrophy of the remaining cells of the adrenal cortex through the stimulus of the release of adrenocorticotropin hormone (ACTH) of the adenohypophysis released now from the inhibition of normally circulating levels of cortisol. Salt "hunger" leads to an appetite for salt which relieves the most serious aspect of this disease. Replacement therapy provides cure in the same sense that insulin provides a cure for diabetes mellitus.

Chronic Heart Failure Due to Mitral Stenosis (Flow Diagram IV)

Ordinarily, failure of the muscle of each heart chamber to pump out the incoming blood is a slowly developing process, though sudden demands on the heart may lead to acute failure. All organs, and in particular those of homeostasis, depend upon adequate blood flow for cell function, and by their cell function change or normalize the concentration of selected substances in the blood. Therefore, partial loss of the pumping action of the heart can lead to rapid and dangerous alterations of the internal environment. Symptoms rise from every organ and tissue. Left-sided failure is usually a way-station in course of total right and left heart failure.

Because in left-sided failure, blood cannot readily flow from the left atrium to the left ventricle, the lung serves as a reservoir for blood and pulmonary edema follows. Dyspnea, first on exertion and then as a paroxysmal nocturnal event, is the most important symptom. Hypoxemia is the consequence, and all tissues may function only to the limit allowed by reduced oxygen pressure. Poor perfusion of the myocardium by way of the coronary arteries leads to a still less efficient pump.

Because renal blood flow and pressure are reduced, sodium retention occurs, with retention of water as a

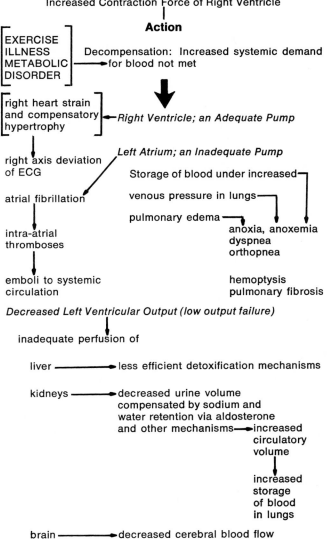

PATHOPHYSIOLOGY OF LEFT SIDED HEART FAILURE
(Flow Diagram IV)
Antecedents

MITRAL STENOSIS FOLLOWING RHEUMATIC FEVER

Decreased Input of Blood to Left Ventricle

Decreased Left Ventricular Output

Diminished Perfusion of Systems Organs

INTERIM COMPENSATION: Hypertrophy of Atrial Muscle with Increased Atrial Output, Increased Contraction Force of Right Ventricle

Action

[EXERCISE ILLNESS METABOLIC DISORDER] → Decompensation: Increased systemic demand for blood not met

[right heart strain and compensatory hypertrophy] ← *Right Ventricle; an Adequate Pump*

right axis deviation of ECG

Left Atrium; an Inadequate Pump

Storage of blood under increased

atrial fibrillation

venous pressure in lungs

pulmonary edema

anoxia, anoxemia
dyspnea
orthopnea

intra-atrial thromboses

emboli to systemic circulation

hemoptysis
pulmonary fibrosis

Decreased Left Ventricular Output (low output failure)

inadequate perfusion of

liver ——→ less efficient detoxification mechanisms

kidneys ——→ decreased urine volume compensated by sodium and water retention via aldosterone and other mechanisms ——→ increased circulatory volume

increased storage of blood in lungs

brain ——→ decreased cerebral blood flow cerebral edema, anoxia Cheyne-Stokes Respiration fatigue, personality change

skin ——→ compensation by vasoconstriction

consequence, leading to an expansion of blood and interstitial fluid volume. This increased circulating fluid is likewise stored in the lung and another vicious cycle is set up. In this case renal compensation for reduced cardiac output adds to the diseased state.

Cardiac compensatory activity also occurs. Stretch of the chamber wall by the blood left behind after a contraction of a chamber, combined with the normal incoming flow, results in a more forceful contraction of the atrium and a greater flow of blood past the narrowed valve orifice of mitral stenosis. Since no valves exist in the great pulmonary veins, the enhanced filling and contraction pressure is transmitted back to the lungs. Normally the pulmonary arterial and venous pressures are too low to cause filtration of water through the capillary to the alveoli. However, with enhanced venous pressures, edema fluid further accumulates and dyspnea follows. As the pulmonary venous pressure rises, the right ventricle must contract more forcibly to provide for a forward flow of blood. If the right ventricle fails then right heart failure with enhanced central venous pressure, generalized edema, liver and gastrointestinal congestion occurs.

An abnormal rhythm, artial fibrillation, frequently occurs and the atrium ceases to act as a pump at all. Stasis of flow of blood in the atrium may be sufficient to allow blood clotting, thrombus formation, and ultimately an embolus.

Although cardiac muscle and renal compensation may provide temporary improvement, the only effective compensation is a reduction in tissue activity, and this must necessarily be of skeletal muscle. Rest, reduced muscle activity, is essential to a mode of living making the fewest demands on the heart. An upright position to permit drainage of edema fluid to the lowest parts of the lung and body will relieve the dyspnea.

BIBLIOGRAPHY

Cannon, W. B.: Bodily Changes in Pain, Hunger, Fear, and Rage, ed. 2. N.Y., D. Appleton-Century Co., 1929.

Schoenheimer, R.: The Dynamic State of Body Constituents. Cambridge, Harvard Univ. Press, 1942.

Selye, H.: The general adaptation syndrome and diseases of adaptation. J. Clin. Endocrinology, 6:117, 1946.

Sodeman, W. A., and Sodeman, W. A. Jr.: Pathophysiologic Physiology, ed. 4. Philadelphia, W. B. Saunders, 1967.

CHAPTER **6**

Prevention of Disease and Accidents

- *Accomplishments and Challenges*
- *The Nurse's Role in Disease Prevention*
- *Environmental Health*
- *Accident Prevention*

ACCOMPLISHMENTS AND CHALLENGES

Since the turn of the century the mortality rate throughout the world has declined steadily and the average life span has increased, largely due to the successful control of many infectious diseases. Improvements in nutrition likewise have contributed significantly to the well-being of populations everywhere. Our environment unquestionably has become safer and more healthful. However, new problems arise constantly. For example, traumatic accidents have become a major cause of death between the ages of 1 and 34 years. Accidents, including poisoning, are the first largest cause of death in American children; cancer is the second.

As the average life span has increased, there has been a corresponding increase in the prevalence of chronic diseases. Cardiovascular disease and cancer now are responsible for over 70 per cent of the deaths in the United States. Ten per cent of this country's population are afflicted with chronic disease of one type or another. The resultant drain on individual economic and community resources is tremendous. Some of the worst health problems are found in the inner city areas of our metropolitan complexes, close to the larger medical centers. The Federal government is now sponsoring neighborhood medical centers in these areas to take medical care to the needy.

More than 50 per cent of the hospital beds in this country are occupied by patients with mental illness, and an estimated 6 per cent of the total population currently are in need of psychiatric care.

Public health problems confront us as a result of rapid industrial expansion and the development of large and overcrowded urban centers. The pollution of water, air and food by industrial waste products and the threat of damaging radiation from artificial sources are problems of great magnitude and long-range importance.

Hunger and malnutrition remain great problems even in the affluent United States. Ten thousand children die *daily* of malnutrition throughout the world.

During the past several decades medical research has advanced our knowledge at a fantastic pace. Among the most brilliant accomplishments have been those in the field of preventive medicine. But between the acquisition and the application of medical knowledge there may be unfortunate time lags. For example, although rheumatic fever is largely preventable by the prompt and vigorous treatment of streptococcal pharyngitis, nevertheless rheumatic fever and rheumatic heart disease still are responsible for more than 20,000 deaths in this country each year. Immunizations have reduced death rates from infectious diseases dramatically but neonatal mortality remains high in this country.

Glaucoma and diabetes remain the leading causes of blindness, solely because these diseases, although readily detectable even in their early stages if detection is sought, have escaped detection too often and too long, and the benefits of early treatment have been missed. Were all individuals over the age of 40 to undergo regularly a competent health examination, much human misery might be avoided. Executive health examinations sponsored by many business firms for their presumably healthy employees reveal that over 50 per cent of these people have abnormalities in need of medical attention.

THE NURSE'S ROLE IN DISEASE PREVENTION

Powerful ammunition for the battle against disease has been provided through the contributions of many basic sciences, including epidemiology, immunology, nutrition, sociology, psychology and biochemistry. However, the effectiveness of these weapons depends not only on their general availability but also on a wide knowledge of their application. *Education of the public, therefore, may be counted as the most important single aspect of this defense program.* This, of course, must be done in an intelligent fashion to avoid fright and panic.

Early in the nurse's professional career the significance of disease prevention becomes apparent and she becomes aware of her responsibilities in relation to its accomplishment. Throughout the period of her basic course she is instructed in the close relationships existing between individual health and group health, between health and economics, health and the physical environment, health and group immunization, standards of nutrition, sanitation and a host of other factors that mutually affect the public health.

There is a relationship between the status of an individual in his community and his attitude toward health practices. Patients in the lower socioeconomic groups are inclined to disregard their symptoms unless these prevent them from working or unless emergencies arise. These persons usually do not seek treatment early. Social scientists have observed that the behavior of an individual in relation to his health conforms to that which he considers acceptable to, and prevalent in, his social group. Moreover, it depends upon the importance that he and his family attach to health. Other factors that may have a bearing on attitude and behavior in this regard include the intellectual and the educational level, the age, the race and the sex of the patient.

In order to teach her patient effectively, the public health nurse must familiarize herself with the patient's concepts and system of values pertaining to illness and health. It may be her mission to convince him that he is not invulnerable, that he probably is susceptible and might well acquire a given disease, and that the preventive measures she is advocating are both safe and effective.

The instruction of patients and their families in the principles of health and disease prevention can be among the most valuable contributions of the nurse. If her instructions are to be realistic, she must evaluate her patients correctly with respect to their intelligence, physical capacity and handicaps—factors that determine the degree of responsibility they can accept for the protection of their own health and the extent to which this responsibility must be consigned to their families or to social agencies in their communities.

ENVIRONMENTAL HEALTH

In addition to health teaching, the nurse has numerous other functions in relation to preventive medicine. She must be cognizant of the environmental factors that pertain to each of the illnesses with which she deals—factors such as housing and sanitation, which, if defective, predispose the onset, progression, recurrence and spread of the illnesses. Such factors obviously are of importance, not only to the patient and his family, but also to the community as a whole. Modern medicine is not enough to eliminate illness and promote good health. Recent studies among the Indians of the southwestern United States reveal that infant and child mortality and morbidity and adult illness remain too high despite the introduction of modern medical facilities and physicians. Changes in mode of life, sanitation and diet need to be made before significant health improvements can occur.

In every home she visits, the nurse is a potential "case finder." People frequently voice their complaints and describe their symptoms to her. They may mention casually a problem that to them seems minor, but that the nurse recognizes as a potential clue to disease. She finds many opportunities to convince reluctant sufferers to report to a physician or clinic for medical attention that they have avoided.

Through direct referrals, the hospital nurse is able to assure continuity of patient care between the hospital and the community health and welfare agencies. The public health nurse represents the long arms of the hospital and the clinic. Not only is she familiar with the principles and the practice of preventive medicine, but she also knows the agencies, official and voluntary, whose services are available to the patient.

As agents of public health services, nurses are active in schools, industries, recreation centers and homes, serving as skilled observers, professional advisers, ad-

TABLE 6-1. Accidental deaths classified according to the international list of causes of death

Type of Accident or Manner of Injury	1966*	1965	Change 1965 to 1966
All Accidental Deaths	**113,563**	**108,004**	+ 5.1%
Motor-vehicle accident	53,041	49,163	+ 7.9
Railway accident (except collision with m.v.)	1,027	962	+ 6.8
Streetcar accident (except collision with train or m.v.)	9	4	+125.0
Other road transport accident (except collision with train or m.v.)	283	315	− 10.2
Water transport accident	1,630	1,493	+ 9.2
Aircraft accident	1,510	1,529	− 1.2
Poisoning by solid and liquid substances	2,283	2,110	+ 8.2
Poisoning by gases and vapors	1,648	1,526	+ 8.0
Falls	20,066	19,984	+ 0.4
Blow from falling or projected object or missile	1,459	1,493	− 2.3
Non-transport vehicle accident	115	85	+ 35.3
Machinery	2,070	2,054	+ 0.8
Cutting and piercing instruments	137	136	+ 0.7
Electric current	1,025	1,071	− 4.3
Explosion of pressure vessel	48	51	− 5.9
Fire and explosion of combustible material	8,084	7,347	+ 10.0
Hot substance, corrosive liquid, and steam	408	418	− 2.4
Radiation	1	2	− 50.0
Firearms	2,558	2,344	+ 9.1
Inhalation and ingestion of food	1,464	1,507	− 2.9
Inhalation and ingestion of other object	367	329	+ 11.6
Foreign body entering other orifice	1,131	1,138	− 0.6
Mechanical suffocation	1,263	1,340	− 5.7
Lack of care of infants	16	9	+ 77.8
Bites and stings of venomous animals and insects	48	54	− 11.1
Other animal accident	131	126	+ 4.0
Drowning	5,687	5,485	+ 3.7
High and low air pressure	11	6	+ 83.3
Excessive heat and insolation	531	106	+400.9
Excessive cold	365	298	+ 22.5
Hunger, thirst, and exposure	180	197	− 8.6
Cataclysm	155	431	− 64.0
Lightning	110	149	− 26.2
Accident in non-therapeutic medical and surgical procedures	123	168	− 26.8
Accident in therapeutic medical and surgical procedures	1,087	1,200	− 9.4
Late effect of accident (death more than a year after accident)	933	881	+ 5.9
Other and unspecified	2,559	2,493	+ 2.6

Source: National Center for Health Statistics.   *Latest official figures available.

ministrators of prescribed therapy. The improvements in health and living conditions in every department of community life in which they serve bear witness to their far-reaching accomplishments and professional influence.

Air Pollution—A Health Hazard

Authorities agree that the relation of air pollution to health is one of the most complex epidemiological problems. Only in the past decade have investigators turned their attention to the effects of certain combinations of environmental conditions. As air stagnation, fog, and the concentration of air pollutants have increased, so have the morbidity and mortality rates of elderly persons with cardiopulmonary disease.

Goldsmith* has made a useful classification of air pollutants according to their major physiologic effects on humans or animals. For example, one group of pollutants comprises those irritants that adversely affect the air-exposed membranous surfaces of the respiratory tract or the eye. These include sulfur dioxide, chlorine, formaldehyde and sulfuric acid. Irritants having a more chronic or delayed effect (as on the alveolar tissues of the lung) include nitrogen dioxide or ozone. Nitrogen dioxide results from crop fermentation in silos; its effect is observed in farmers and is known as "silo-filler's" disease. Other pollutants stimulate the formation of antibodies in the host, whose response is expressed as an allergic reaction. "Hay fever" is a common example of this effect. Still another group of pollutants are the so-called toxicants, which affect the body in various ways. Carbon monoxide blocks

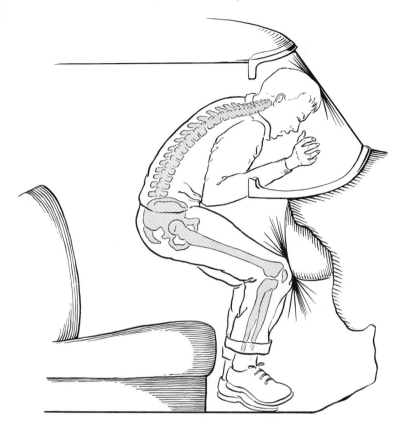

Fig. 6-1. Diagrammatic drawing to show the mechanism of injury for a front seat passenger when a car strikes an obstructing object. The head hits the windshield, and the knee strikes the dashboard; forces may be dissipated anywhere from the 1st cervical to the 5th lumbar vertebra.

the essential enzyme activity of the body. Lead seeks out bone and may affect the blood-forming areas. Chlorinated hydrocarbons are fat-seekers. Airborne insecticide and airborne lead are also potential hazards.

In summary, there is evidence that air pollutants above certain concentration levels have an adverse effect on health, particularly of older persons and all persons having cardiopulmonary disease. The nurse has two responsibilities in this broadening area of public health, concern. As a health teacher, she can emphasize the precautions to be taken and the reasons for them in order to reduce the exposure of susceptible individuals. The nurse can emphasize those aspects of preventive medicine that can reduce the incidence of cardiopulmonary disease, such as education of the public in the adverse effects of cigarette smoking. As a citizen, the nurse can support actively any efforts including legislation that is designed to reduce air pollution.

ACCIDENT PREVENTION

Industrial, vehicular and home accidents occur with such frequency that they now represent the nation's major peril to health and productivity. In both military and civilian populations, accidents are responsible for more deaths and lost working days than any single dis-

ease. For persons from 1 to 34 years of age, accidents are the first cause of death; for those from 35 to 44, they rank second only to heart disease.

The nurse learns, practices and teaches safety principles; she has a unique opportunity to participate in safety programs and to teach accident prevention. Posters, pamphlets and films are available from insurance companies and the National Safety Council.* Helpful aids in patient teaching are safety-instruction cards available from the National Safety Council.

The Traffic Accident Problem

Motor vehicle accidents head the list of causes of accidental death, as may be seen in Table 6-1.

Through automobile accidents, a life is lost every 15 minutes, and an injury occurs every 30 seconds. Furthermore, about 10 per cent of such injuries result in permanent disability. With an annual toll of over 55,000 traffic deaths, there is in addition well over a million disabling injuries.

The National Safety Council lists drinking, lack of alertness and fatigue to be important causes of motor

* *Accident Facts* also is published annually by the National Safety Council. This is a detailed analysis of the various types of accidents (425 N. Michigan Ave., Chicago, Ill. 60611).

vehicle accidents and excessive speed as the most common driver violation.* On our high speed highways this often involves several cars and many persons. Almost any type of injury may occur.

The Nature of Injuries. When the car stops suddenly, the occupants continue in motion, and they are killed by blows received when they are flung against the car interior, or they are killed by objects outside the car. One of the most common and most disabling injuries is the so-called *whiplash* (Fig. 6-1). This has been defined as the damage sustained by neck structures when the body, in propulsion, comes to a sudden stop, or when the body is suddenly propelled forward, and the head is thrust forcibly forward and/or backward, and/or to either side. The parts which may be damaged are the cervical vertebrae, the intervertebral disks and the odontoid process. Emotional and psychological disturbances frequently ensue later on.

The impact of a person against the interior of the automobile is responsible for many serious injuries. The dashboard with its various protuberances accounts for about 40 per cent of injuries, sometimes causing macerations of the liver and resultant hemorrhage, rib fractures, rupture of the spleen, and rupture or laceration of the kidneys. Blows received by the body against the windshield account for another 30 per cent of injuries, which most often consist of extensive lacerations of tissue with possible fractures of the sternum, the ribs, the zygoma, the maxillary sinus, or the frontal bone. Steering-wheel injuries, representing about 10 per cent of the total, most commonly involve a crushing blow to the thorax, with possible fractures of the sternum or the ribs and trauma to the heart and the lungs.

Safety Devices and Safety Suggestions. On the basis of studies, various safety devices have been suggested. As a member of the health team, the nurse can lend active support to all safety programs and legislation which have to do with (1) education of persons in accident and injury protection, (2) construction of safety features in automobiles, especially seat and shoulder belts, padding, collapsible steering wheels, and shatterproof glass, (3) adequate standards for driver licensure, (4) improved state inspections of all cars, and (5) adequate supervision of mechanics to do their job properly.

Another area of significance to the nurse and her patient is the danger of drugs to an automobile driver. Many highway deaths follow the use of drugs and alcohol taken by the driver either before or during driving. The average person cannot be expected to

know what drugs bring on lassitude or slow his reflexes and interfere with his judgment. The physician should advise him but even he cannot know fully what effect a drug will have on any given individual. Often someone in extreme pain or discomfort must drive and the physician has to decide what medication to give. For example, a dental extraction is performed with an intravenous anesthetic that wears off quickly, but some effects from it can linger up to 48 hours. The patient, therefore, usually is incapable of exerting his best judgment and will not regain his full reflex activity for one or two days. It is also possible that a tense person may find driving easier after taking small doses of a tranquilizer; however, many barbiturates induce hypnotic effects up to 14 hours.

Fatigue remains one of the most dangerous elements in driving, and too many people try to fight it with "pep" pills. Antidepressant and antispasmodic drugs also have a potent effect on the nervous system. A drug may be all right for a careful driver, but it would further impair the judgment of a driver used to taking risks.

Care of Injuries from Automobile Accidents. (See Chap. 38) The care of the injured from automobile accidents does not differ from the care of the injured from other civilian accidents except for the recognition of the frequency of cerebral and neck injuries, which demand caution in moving and positioning.

Home Accidents

Falls account for about half the accidents sustained in the home. Poor lighting, loose carpeting, misplaced toys and inadequate bases of support used in reaching articles placed on high shelves are the chief causes of falls. Home hobbies and repair jobs done by the novice who disregards safety rules contribute to the toll of injuries sustained at home. Fires, burns and poisons are other causes. Inasmuch as mothers, young children and elderly persons are at home most of the time, they are the principal victims, and it is to this group that educational efforts emphasizing safety and preventive measurse must be directed. Continued emphasis by radio, television, newspapers and magazines will help in reaching these persons.

Miscellaneous Accidents

Accidents will be reduced and lives will be saved when continued emphasis is placed on education of the public regarding hazards and risks, stressing the need for "built-in" safety features, and initiating legislation where indicated. The following are some areas in which much has been done but much remains to be done (the student will be able to add many more to this list):

Glass patio doors: It is estimated that 60,000 Ameri-

* Other causes of automobile accidents are hidden factors that often are never detected. These have to do with mechanical failures and not enough safety devices built into the car itself.

cans each year walk through such doors without opening them. Safety glass rather than thick plate glass would eliminate serious lacerations sustained by these people.

Shatterproof eyeglass lenses: The National Council for the Prevention of Blindness makes the informal estimate that less than 5 per cent of children's eyeglasses are made with non-shattering lenses.

Gasoline-powered lawn mowers: These machines injure more Americans (a minimum of 100,000) than any other mechanical device except the automobile. These injuries are mostly lacerations and amputations of the fingers and toes of the operators. Rotary mowers can eject a rock, nail, or piece of wire with the muzzle velocity of a shotgun. Manufacturers are still working on a safe rotary lawnmower.

Ski safety bindings: Although progress has been made in reducing the number of spiral fractures of the tibia, more ankle fractures (which take longer to heal) are occurring.

Football helmet face guards: These have reduced the incidence of broken noses but increased that of broken necks.

Boating accidents: Boating mishaps seem to be most prevalent not among novices, but among those with more than 100 hours of boating experience. Overloading boats, improper seating of passengers, using unseaworthy craft, sailing recklessly and not having life-saving equipment are the chief causes of accidents.

Golfing accidents: Approximately 20,000 disabling accidents occur annually on golf courses. These are caused by being hit with a golf ball or by a partner's club. In addition, reckless driving of golf carts by drunken golfers account for close to 10 per cent of all golfing injuries.

Cycling accidents: The incidence of pedal and motor cycling accidents continues to rise. Violation of safety rules are the major factor in cycling deaths. In many states, legislation has been passed to require the wearing of crash helmets by motor cyclists.

Aspirin-poisoning: Youngsters taking overdoses of aspirin have encouraged improvements in medicine-bottle caps.

Accidents involving hospitalized patients: Dangers in the hospital environment, dangers intrinsic in the patient population, plus oversights on the part of attending personnel, account for most accidents in the hospital. The medical-legal implications are great. Every hospital must have a constantly running safety program and stress preventive measures. (The student is referred to the Fundamentals of Nursing course for further information.)

See also:

Accidents caused by fire, Chap. 29.

Disaster and first aid, Chap. 38.

Accident prevention for the elderly, p. 52.

BIBLIOGRAPHY

Ashenburg, N. J.: Effects of air pollution. Nurs. Outlook, *16:* 22-25, Feb. 1968.

Crocke, W. M. and Meyer, K. K.: Splenic rupture due to improper placement of automobile seat belt. J.A.M.A. *183:*693, 1963.

Dasmann, R. F.: An environment fit for people. Public Affairs Pamphlet 421, 1968.

Goldsmith, J. R., *et al.*: Air pollution and health. Amer. Rev. Resp. Dis. 93:302-312, Feb., 1966.

Heimann, H.: Status of air pollution: health research, 1966. Arch. Environ. Health 1:488-503, Mar., 1967.

Middleton, J. T., Emik, L. O. and Taylor, O. C.: Air quality criteria and standards for agriculture. Jour. Air Pollution Control Assoc., *15*, No. 10 October, 1965.

National Tuberculosis and Respiratory Diseases Assoc.: Air Pollution—The Facts.

Rosenow, J. H. and Watkins, R. W.: How many traffic deaths are caused by mistreatment and mis-design? Mod. Med., 35:32-62, 1967.

Stone, E.: Accidents involving hospitalized patients. Hosp. Med., 4:54-60, June, 1968.

Westaby, J. R., Jones, H. M., Bubb, N. B. and Ryan, M.: Integrating accident prevention in total patient care. Nurs. Outlook, *11:*600-603, Aug., 1963.

PATIENT EDUCATION

Superintendent of Documents

U.S. Government Printing Office

Washington, D.C. 20402

    The Fundamentals of Accident Prevention

    (U.S. Dept. of Labor Bulletin No. 247)

    Maintenance and Safety

    (U.S. Dept. of Labor Bulletin No. 246)

National Safety Council

    425 N. Michigan Avenue

    Chicago, Illinois 60611

A variety of pamphlets and illustrative material. Listing of materials is available.

CHAPTER **7**

Body Fluid Disturbances

- *Gains and Losses*
- *Basic Imbalances*
- *Therapy*
- *Methods of Administration*
- *Complications of Therapy*

INTRODUCTION

Recent discoveries concerning body fluid and its role in the human body have brought about an increasing awareness of the importance of maintaining fluid balance in hospitalized patients. Body fluid disturbances represent the common denominator of a host of illnesses, and every seriously ill patient is a candidate for one or more of them. Even patients who have only moderate or mild illnesses can develop them, and their very lives depend upon how their medical attendants solve the problems posed by these disturbances. Therefore, it is important that those in the nursing and allied professions have a working knowledge of body fluid for the intelligent management of patients with diseases listed in the diagnostic nomenclature.

Body fluid is made up chiefly of water and certain dissolved substances called *electrolytes*. When placed in water, electrolytes (sometimes referred to as salts or minerals) develop tiny electrical charges. Those electrolytes that develop positive charges are called *cations* and include such substances as sodium (Na), potassium (K), calcium (Ca), and magnesium (Mg). Electrolytes that develop negative charges are called *anions*. These include chloride (Cl), bicarbonate (HCO₃), sulfate (SO₄), phospate (PO₄) proteinate, carbonic acid (H₂CO₃), and other organic acids. The term ion includes both cation and anion. (Fig. 7-1.)

The body fluid is divided into 2 major compartments —the cellular fluid and the extracellular fluid. The cellular fluid accounts for approximately ¾ of the total body fluid and represents the fluid contained within the body cells. The extracellular fluid, which comprises ¼ of the total body fluid, surrounds the cells. Approximately ¼ of the extracellular fluid exists as plasma and ¾ as interstitial fluid. (Fig. 7-2.)

The body cells feed themselves and excrete wastes by constantly exchanging materials with their environment, the extracellular fluid. These exchanges are continuous and of tremendous magnitude. This activity of the cells affects the composition of the extracellular fluid; the effects of this activity would be catastrophic were it not for the chemical regulatory activities carried out by the body homeostatic mechanisms, which keep the volume and chemical composition of the extracellular fluid within the limits of normal. (Fig. 7-3.)

In addition to keeping the cells healthy, the extracellular fluid has another important duty: it supplies the secretions and excretions, such as saliva, gastric juice, intestinal juice, bile, pancreatic juice, nasal secretions, perspiration, urine, and feces, with water and electrolytes. Just as the cellular and extracellular fluid each has its own characteristic chemical composition, so does each secretion or excretion exhibit a composi-

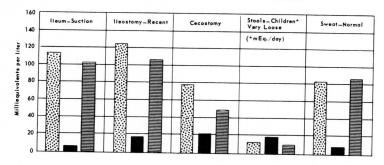

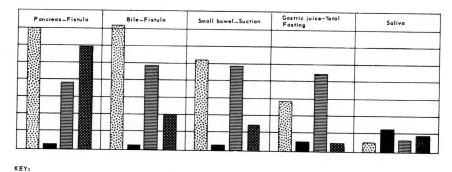

ELECTROLYTE COMPOSITION OF VARIOUS BODY SECRETIONS OR EXCRETIONS

FIG. 7-1. Electrolyte composition of various body secretions or excretions. (Metheny and Snively: Nurses' Handbook of Fluid Balance, Phila., J. B. Lippincott Co.)

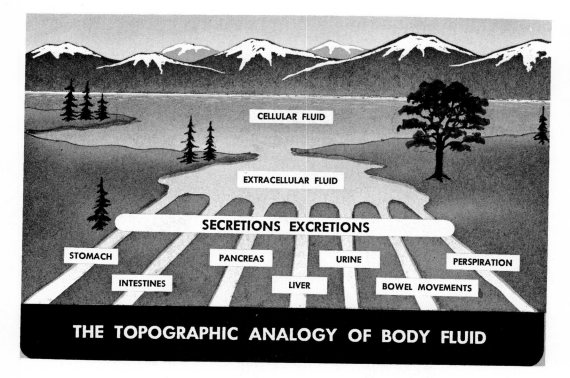

FIG. 7-2. The topographic analogy of body fluid. (Metheny and Snively: Nurses' Handbook of Fluid Balance, Phila., J. B. Lippincott Co.)

Fig. 7-3. A diagram illustrating the 3 main compartments of the body separated from each other by definite anatomic barriers, i.e., the capillary and the cell walls. The inner sphere is the intracellular space containing the fluid inside the cells of muscles, liver, etc., separated from the rest of the body by cell membrane. The outer space represents circulating blood. In the space between is the interstitial (or intracellular) fluid. The barrier between the blood and the interstitial fluid is the wall of the blood capillary membrane. (Adapted from Elman, Robert: Fluid balance from the nurse's point of view, Am. J. Nurs. *49*:222)

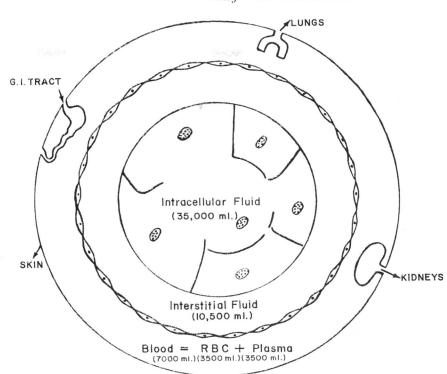

tion that is relatively constant during health but which may deviate widely from normal during disease. When the secretions and excretions are depleted, they deplete the extracellular fluid, which, in turn, depletes the cellular fluid. The time that it takes a depleted secretion or excretion to affect the extracellular fluid and the time that it takes the depleted extracellular fluid to affect the cellular fluid vary widely and depend, in general, upon the magnitude and rapidity of the depletion.

In order to understand, diagnose, and treat body fluid disturbances, we must have a simple, accurate unit of measure for the electrolytes of the body fluid. Since we are interested in their *activity*, we must have

Fig. 7-4. Fluid balance and imbalance in an individual. (*Left*) Normal fluid balance. (1) Water taken in as such. (2) Water lost by vaporization from the lungs and the skin (insensible loss). (3) Water lost in urine. The small amount normally lost in the feces is not indicated. The amount lost as sensible perspiration is highly variable and is not indicated. Daily intake and output are equal. (*Right*) Output exceeds intake. (1) Water lost by vomiting. None is taken in either as such or in food. The only source is the water of oxidation pro-

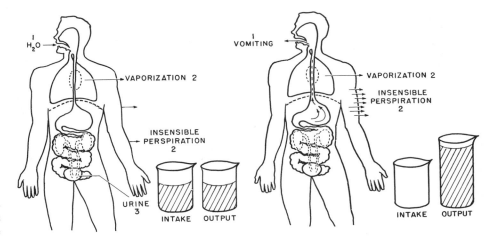

duced in the cells as the body tissues are consumed. (2) Water lost by vaporization. The insensible loss from the skin is increased, due to the elevation of the body temperature or to hot weather. Little or no urine is formed. The variable loss by sensible perspiration is not shown.

a unit that expresses chemical activity, or *chemical combining power* (the power of cations to unite with anions to form molecules). For this purpose, we use the milliequivalent (mEq.), which is equivalent to the activity of 1 milligram of hydrogen.

GAINS AND LOSSES

Water and electrolytes are gained and lost from the body in various ways. We gain water alone by drinking distilled water and through the oxidation of foodstuffs and body tissues. Water and electrolytes are gained when we drink well water, softened water, mineral water, or most city water and when we eat food. Hospitalized patients are often given water and electrolytes by way of nasogastric tube, intravenous needle, or rectal tube.

The body loses water and electrolytes normally through the lungs in breathing, from the eyes in tears, through the skin in perspiration, through the kidneys in urine, and in normal bowel movements. (Fig. 7-4.) Water alone is lost through the skin in insensible perspiration, which continues night and day. In illness or injury, additional losses can occur through burn or wound exudate, hemorrhage, vomiting, and diarrhea. Excessive water and electrolytes can also be lost through rapid breathing, the use of a gastric or intestinal suction tube, enterostomy, colostomy, or cecostomy. They are lost as a result of surgical operations (such as drainage from the biliary tract), in draining abscesses, or by way of paracentesis. (Fig. 7-5.) Fluids surrounding the brain and spinal cord can be lost when there is an abnormal opening to the exterior.

Sometimes fluids are lost within the body itself when abnormal closed collections of fluid occur, because these fluids are just as unavailable to the body economy as if they were outside the body.

The general state of fluid balance in the healthy adult can readily be assessed by comparing the volume of fluid ingested by mouth with the volume of urine. Since it is abnormal differences between gains and losses of water and electrolytes that cause body fluid imbalances, accurate intake-output records aid the physician in assessing the state of fluid balance in the hospitalized patient. (Fig. 7-6.)

BASIC IMBALANCES

Sixteen basic imbalances can occur that involve changes in volume of extracellular fluid, changes in composition of major electrolytes of extracellular fluid, and changes in position of water and electrolytes of the extracellular fluid. Imbalances can exist alone, in combination with one or more additional imbalances, or intimately associated with other disease states. Obviously, it is necessary to understand each of the basic 16 imbalances singly if one is to understand the combinations.

Changes in Volume of Extracellular Fluid

Extracellular Fluid Volume Deficit. Extracellular fluid volume deficit represents a deficit of water and electrolytes in roughly the same proportions as they occur in the extracellular fluid. This imbalance is sometimes called fluid deficit, hypovolemia, or dehydration (an incorrect term, since dehydration is the loss of

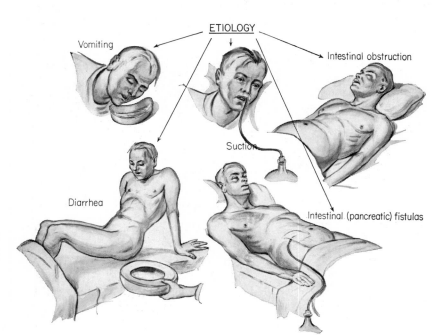

FIG. 7-5. The more common causes of primary salt depletion. (Thorek, P.: Illustrated Preoperative and Postoperative Care, Philadelphia, Lippincott)

water alone). The patient with extracellular fluid volume deficit usually has a history that includes one or more of the following: decreased water intake, vomiting, diarrhea, a systemic infection, fistulous drainage, or intestinal obstruction. The symptoms of this imbalance include dry skin and mucous membranes, longitudinal wrinkles or furrows of the tongue, oliguria or anuria, acute weight loss (in excess of 5 per cent in the child or adult, 10 per cent in the infant), lassitude, and a drop in body temperature. The laboratory findings reveal an increase in the red blood cell count, packed cell volume, and hemoglobin.

Extracellular Fluid Volume Excess. This imbalance represents an excess in the volume of the extracellular fluid caused by an incease in both water and electrolytes in roughly the same proportions as they exist in extracellular fluid. Other names frequently used in describing this imbalance are fluid volume excess and overhydration (an incorrect term, since overhydration represents an excess of water alone). The history of the patient with extracellular fluid volume excess may show that he has been given excessive quantities of an isotonic solution of sodium chloride intravenously. Volume excess also may be caused by congestive heart failure, excessive ingestion of sodium chloride or of electrolyte mixtures, administration of adrenal cortical hormones (especially for long periods), hyperaldosteronism, or renal disease. Symptoms exhibited in this imbalance include puffy eyelids, shortness of breath, edema, edema of tissues at surgical operation, moist rales in lungs, and acute weight gain, which can be in excess of 5 per cent. A decrease is shown in the red blood cell count, packed cell volume, and hemoglobin.

Changes in Properties of Extracellular Fluid

Sodium Deficit of Extracellular Fluid. Sodium deficit of extracellular fluid is caused either by decreased intake or increased output of sodium, or by increased intake or decreased output of water. Other names used to describe this imbalance include electrolyte concentration deficit, *hyponatremia*, low sodium syndrome, and hypotonic dehydration. Sodium deficit is often associated with heat exhaustion and a sodium-losing kidney. In the history of sodium deficit, we find that there has been excessive sweating plus drinking of plain water, gastrointestinal suction plus drinking of plain water, administration of repeated water enemas, administration of a potent diuretic, parenteral infusion of an electrolyte-free solution, or inhalation of fresh water (as occurs in fresh water drowning).

Symptoms of sodium deficit include apprehension (sometimes a bizarre, indefinable feeling of impending doom), abdominal cramps, convulsions, oliguria or anuria. In a severe deficit, hypotension, rapid thready pulse, cold clammy skin, and cynanosis can occur. Also, fingerprinting over the sternum may be observed. Laboratory findings reveal a plasma chloride below 98 mEq./L., a plasma sodium below 137 mEq./L., and the specific gravity of urine below 1.010.

Sodium Excess of Extracellular Fluid. In the history of the patient with sodium excess of the extracellular fluid, often called *hypernatremia*, hypertonic

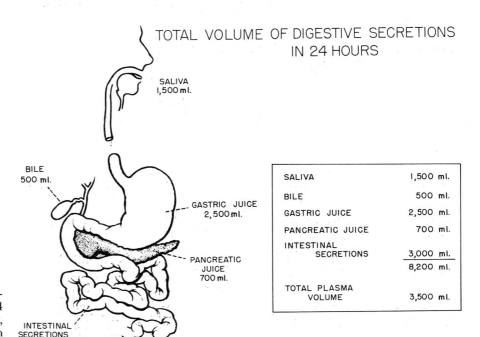

FIG. 7-6. Total volume of digestive secretions produced in 24 hours. (Adapted from Bowen, Arthur: Intravenous alimentation in surgical patients, Mod. Med.)

TOTAL VOLUME OF DIGESTIVE SECRETIONS
IN 24 HOURS

SALIVA
1,500 ml.

BILE
500 ml.

GASTRIC JUICE
2,500 ml.

PANCREATIC
JUICE
700 ml.

INTESTINAL
SECRETIONS
3,000 ml.

SALIVA	1,500 ml.
BILE	500 ml.
GASTRIC JUICE	2,500 ml.
PANCREATIC JUICE	700 ml.
INTESTINAL SECRETIONS	3,000 ml.
	8,200 ml.
TOTAL PLASMA VOLUME	3,500 ml.

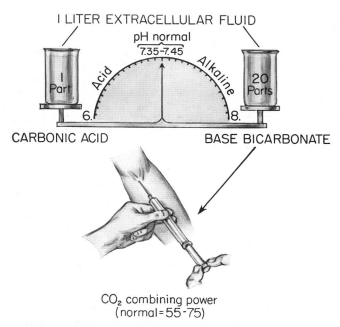

I LITER EXTRACELLULAR FLUID

pH normal
7.35-7.45

Acid   Alkaline

1 Part   20 Parts

6.   8.

CARBONIC ACID   BASE BICARBONATE

CO_2 combining power
(normal = 55-75)

FIG. 7-7. Normal acid-base balance is in a pH range between 7.35 and 7.45. If the pH drops below 7.35 acidosis (acidemia) results; if the pH is above 7.45, alkalosis (alkalemia) is present. In each liter of extracellular fluid there is approximately 1 part of carbonic acid to 20 parts of base bicarbonate. (Thorek, P.: Illustrated Preoperative and Postoperative Care, Philadelphia, Lippincott)

dehydration, salt excess, or oversalting, one may find decreased water intake, an excessive ingestion of sodium chloride, or perhaps a tracheobronchitis in which the rapid breathing and high fever have caused the loss of great amounts of water by way of the lungs. Sodium excess also may be brought on by profuse watery diarrhea or the inhalation of salt water (as in salt water drowning). The physician may also find this imbalance in the unconscious patient, who does not drink liquids.

The symptoms of sodium excess include dry, sticky mucous membranes, a flushed skin, intense thirst, oliguria or anuria, elevated temperature, a rough and dry tongue. The laboratory findings indicate a plasma sodium above 147 mEq./L., plasma chloride above 106 mEq./L., and the specific gravity of the urine above 1.030.

Potassium Deficit of Extracellular Fluid. Potassium deficit, sometimes known as *hypokalemia*, is often associated with a potassium-losing kidney. Potassium deficit is most frequently observed following the use of a potent diuretic—particularly a thiazide-type diuretic—or when there has been vomiting, ulcerative colitis, or diarrhea. The condition is encouraged by

the parenteral administration of a solution not containing potassium, by the loss of potassium through fistulas of the small intestine or colon, by the metabolic changes that occur in diabetic acidosis, or in a burn after the fifth day. It also occurs when there has been no potassium ingested for several days.

The symptoms of potassium deficit in the early stages are nonspecific. The patient has malaise, or is "just not feeling well." As the deficit develops, symptoms relating to the muscular system appear. In the *skeletal muscles,* there is generalized weakness and decreased to absent reflexes; the muscles are flabby, like half-filled water bottles, and the patient lies flat like a cadaver, not rounded. Symptoms of the *heart muscle* include weak pulse, faint heart sounds, heart block, and falling blood pressure. In the *gastrointestinal tract,* there is anorexia, vomiting, gaseous distention of the intestines, and paralytic ileus. Symptoms involving the *respiratory muscles* include shallow respirations. In addition to the above symptoms, thirst may be present. Laboratory findings reveal a plasma potassium below 4 mEq./L. The chloride is often below 98 mEq./L. The electrocardiograph shows evidence of potassium deficit.

Potassium Excess of Extracellular Fluid. Potassium excess of extracellular fluid is sometimes known as *hyperkalemia.* In the history, the physician usually finds burns or crushing injuries, kidney disease, excessive infusion of potassium solutions, or adrenal insufficiency. Potassium excess sometimes results from oliguria or anuria or because of kidney damage caused by mercuric bichloride poisoning.

The symptoms of mild potassium excess are irritability, nausea, intestinal colic, and diarrhea. If the excess becomes severe, the patient displays weakness and flaccid paralysis. There may be difficulty in phonation and respiration. Oliguria occurs and progresses to anuria. Finally, cardiac arrhythmia followed by standstill terminates the situation. Laboratory findings indicate a plasma potassium above 5.6 mEq./L. Renal function tests show severe renal impairment in most cases. The electrocardiograph shows a high T wave and a depressed ST segment.

Calcium Deficit of Extracellular Fluid. Calcium deficit, also called *hypocalcemia,* is often associated with calcium deficiency leg cramps. The history usually reveals sprue, hypoactive parathyroid glands, excessive ingestion of citrated blood, massive subcutaneous injections, generalized peritonitis, or surgical removal of parathyroid glands.

Symptoms include tingling of the ends of the fingers, tetany, abdominal cramps, muscle cramps, carpopedal spasms, and convulsions. The Sulkowitch test on urine reveals no precipitation, and the plasma calcium is usually below 4.5 mEq./L. The electrocardiograph and the X-ray are both helpful in diagnosing calcium deficit.

Calcium Excess of Extracellular Fluid. Calcium excess, or *hypercalcemia*, is often associated with pathologic fracture. It may be caused by tumor of the parathyroid glands, excessive administration of vitamin D for the treatment of arthritis, overactivity of parathyroid glands, or multiple myeloma. Symptoms of this imbalance include hypotonicity of the muscles, kidney stones, flank pain, deep bone pain, and bone cavities. The Sulkowitch test on urine reveals heavy precipitation, and the plasma calcium is characteristically above 5.8 mEq./L. Electrocardiograph and X-ray are helpful in making the diagnosis.

Protein Deficit of Extracellular Fluid. Repeated or chronic loss of whole blood often results in protein deficit, sometimes known as hypoproteinemia or protein malnutrition. Protein deficiency can also result from decreased food intake, drainage from wounds or decubitus ulcers, or as the aftermath of a severe burn, severe trauma, or fracture.

The symptoms of protein deficit include ready fatigue, pallor, soft, flabby muscles, and emotional depression. The patient also has decreased resistance to infection and exhibits chronic weight loss. The laboratory findings may sometimes (but not always) show a plasma albumin below 4.0 gm./100 ml.; the packed cell volume, hemoglobin, and red blood cell count are decreased. However, this decrease is not significant if the iron stores of the patient are inadequate, as he may be suffering from iron deficiency anemia rather than protein deficit. Closely related clinical states of protein deficit are kwashiorkor, pluri-carencial syndrome, and hypoproteinosis.

Magnesium Deficit. Magnesium deficit, or *hypomagnesemia*, is not common and is easily mistaken for potassium deficit. The patient usually has a history of chronic alcoholism, vomiting, or diarrhea. Gastrointestinal absorption may be impaired because of disease of the small intestine or because of surgical removal of portions of the intestine. Magnesium deficit may occur with enterostomy drainage or after prolonged parenteral administration of magnesium-free solutions. Symptoms include tremor, hyperactive deep reflexes, positive Chvostek sign, and convulsions. Confusion (even hallucinations), elevated blood pressure, and tachycardia may occur. There is a positive therapeutic response to magnesium therapy. Plasma magnesium is below 1.4 mEq./L.

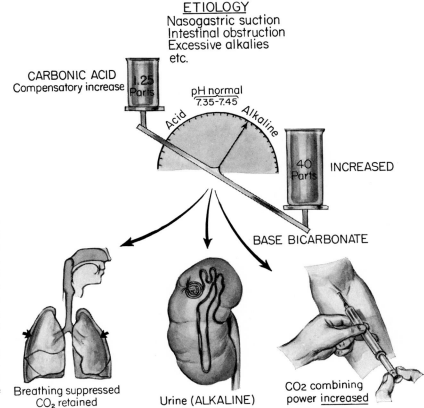

Fig. 7-8. Metabolic alkalosis (base bicarbonate excess). In this condition the base bicarbonates are increased, and the pH is increased. The normal acid-base ratio of 1 to 20 is now changed to 1.25 to 40. The lungs attempt to compensate by withholding carbonic acid (CO_2); hence the breathing is suppressed. A compensatory increase in carbonic acid may result. The kidneys attempt to compensate by retaining hydrogen ions and excreting bicarbonate ions; the urine becomes alkaline. The CO_2 combining power is increased. (Thorek, P.: Illustrated Preoperative and Postoperative Care, Philadelphia, Lippincott)

Acid-Base Disturbances

Deficits or excesses of base bicarbonate or of carbonic acid are usually called the acid-base imbalances. These imbalances occur as a result of abnormalities in the hydrogen ion concentration of the extracellular fluid. Although hydrogen is present in extracellular fluid in very tiny quantities, it is extremely important from the standpoint of health. When its concentration lies within certain narrow limits, the extracellular fluid is chemically and physiologically neutral. (Fig. 7-7.) When the concentration of hydrogen increases (pH decreases), the extracellular fluid becomes acid and the patient is said to have *acidosis*. When the concentration of hydrogen ion decreases (pH increases), the reaction of the extracellular fluid becomes alkaline or basic, and the patient is in *alkalosis*. (Fig. 7-8.)

Carbonic acid is formed in the extracellular fluid when carbon dioxide unites with water. When the cations sodium, potassium, calcium, and magnesium unite with the anion bicarbonate, they form an extracellular fluid complex, which Snively and Sweeney have designated as base bicarbonate. It is the ratio of carbonic acid to the base bicarbonate of the extracellular fluid that determines the concentration of hydrogen ions. As long as there is 1 mEq. of carbonic acid for each 20 mEq. of base bicarbonate in the extracellular fluid, the hydrogen ion concentration lies within normal limits.

Any condition that increases the carbonic acid or decreases the base bicarbonate causes acidosis. (Fig. 7-9.) Any condition that increases base bicarbonate or decreases carbonic acid causes alkalosis. The balance can be tipped by two types of disturbances—metabolic (systemic) and respiratory. Metabolic disturbances affect the base bicarbonate, and respiratory disturbances affect the carbonic acid.

Primary Base Bicarbonate Deficit of Extracellular Fluid. A primary deficit in the base bicarbonate concentration of the extracellular fluid is usually called *metabolic acidosis*. It also may be known as *acidemia*. This imbalance is often associated with diabetic ketosis and renal acidosis. It is caused by any clinical event that decreases the amount of base bicarbonate, such as decreased food intake, diabetic acidosis, systemic infection, the parenteral infusion of isotonic solution of sodium chloride, a ketogenic diet, renal insufficiency, or salicylate intoxication after the initial stages.

Symptoms of metabolic acidosis are stupor, deep, rapid breathing of Kussmaul type, shortness of breath

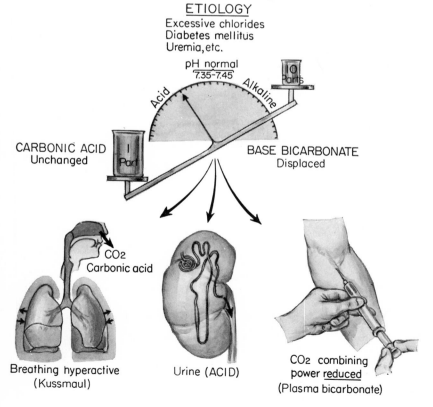

ETIOLOGY
Excessive chlorides
Diabetes mellitus
Uremia, etc.

pH normal
7.35-7.45

Acid   Alkaline

10 Parts

CARBONIC ACID
Unchanged

1 Part

BASE BICARBONATE
Displaced

CO_2
Carbonic acid

Breathing hyperactive
(Kussmaul)

Urine (ACID)

CO_2 combining
power reduced
(Plasma bicarbonate)

Fig. 7-9. Metabolic acidosis (base bicarbonate deficit). In this condition chlorides, organic acids and ketone bodies *displace* the base bicarbonate, and the pH of the extracellular fluid drops below 7.35. The lungs attempt to compensate by hyperactive breathing, thus blowing off excess carbonic acid (CO_2). The kidneys attempt to compensate by excreting hydrogen ions (acid) and conserving base bicarbonate. The CO_2 combining power is reduced. Although this illustration shows the carbonic acid unchanged, it may actually be lowered by hyperactive breathing. (Thorek, P.: Illustrated Preoperative and Postoperative Care, Philadelphia, Lippincott)

on exertion, weakness, and, if the imbalance is severe, unconsciousness. Laboratory findings show a urine pH below 6.0, plasma bicarbonate below 25 mEq./L. in adults and below 20 mEq./L. in children, and a plasma pH below 7.35.

Primary Base Bicarbonate Excess of Extracellular Fluid. A primary excess of base bicarbonate concentration, commonly called metabolic alkalosis or alkalemia, can be caused by any clinical event that weights the base bicarbonate side of the balance. It can result from the loss of a chloride-rich secretion, such as gastric juice. Metabolic alkalosis occurs following excessive ingestion of sodium bicarbonate or other alkalis, after vomiting, following the infusion of a potassium-free solution, when the taking of a potent diuretic for a long period has caused potassium deficit, following gastrointestinal suction, and with the administration of adrenal cortical hormones.

The symptoms of metabolic alkalosis include hypertonicity of the muscles, tetany, and depressed respiration. Laboratory findings include a urine pH of 7.0, plasma bicarbonate above 29 mEq./L. in adults and above 25 mEq./L. in children, a plasma pH above 7.45, and a plasma potassium below 4 mEq./L. The chloride is below 98 mEq./L. if the alkalosis is hypochloremic.

Primary Carbonic Acid Deficit of Extracellular Fluid. Any condition that results in an increased rate and depth of breathing with the resultant blowing off of carbon dioxide will bring on carbonic acid deficit, also known as respiratory alkalosis or alkalemia. This condition is seen with oxygen lack, with fever, in hysteria, with anxiety, with intentional overbreathing, following extreme emotion, and early in salicylate intoxication. The symptoms include tetany, convulsions, and unconsciousness. Laboratory findings include a urine pH above 7.0, plasma bicarbonate below 25 mEq./L. in adults and below 20 mEq./L. in children, and a plasma pH above 7.45.

Primary Carbonic Acid Excess of Extracellular Fluid. Primary carbonic acid excess, usually known as respiratory acidosis or acidemia, is brought on by any condition that impairs the exhalation of carbon dioxide by depressing breathing, such as pneumonia, emphysema, occlusion of the breathing passages, morphine poisoning, barbiturate poisoning, and asthma. It can also occur as a result of breathing excessive carbon dioxide. Symptoms of respiratory acidosis include disorientation, respiratory embarrassment, coma, and weakness. Laboratory findings reveal a urine pH below 6.0, a plasma bicarbonate above 29 mEq./L. in adults and above 25 mEq./L. in children, and a plasma pH below 7.35.

Position Changes of Water and Electrolytes of Extracellular Fluid

Plasma-to-Interstitial Fluid Shift. A shift of water and electrolytes from plasma to interstitial fluid is often seen on the first or second day of a severe burn or following a massive crushing injury, perforated peptic ulcer, or severe trauma. It may occur with intestinal obstruction or following the acute occlusion of a major artery. The symptoms of the shift are the same as those of shock—pallor, low blood pressure, tachycardia, weak to absent pulse, weakness, cold extremities, and unconsciousness. The red blood cell count, packed cell volume, and hemoglobin are increased since they are in a lesser volume of extracellular fluid. This shift is sometimes called *hypovolemia* and is closely related to shock and edema.

Interstitial Fluid-to-Plasma Shift. This shift may occur in a severe burn after the third day, in which case it is often called remobilization of edema fluid. The shift is also sometimes known as *hypervolemia*. It may occur after the loss of whole blood, as the aftermath of a fracture, or following the excessive infusion of large molecular solutions, such as plasma or dextran. Symptoms of this shift include pallor, weakness, air hunger, bounding pulse, engorgement of peripheral veins, and moist rales in the lungs. Cardiac dilatation and ventricular failure may occur. Because there is a volume increase in the plasma portion of the extracellular fluid, the red blood cell count, packed cell volume, and hemoglobin are decreased.

THERAPY

The physician keeps 3 goals in mind in his day-to-day planning of treatment for the patient with an actual or potential body fluid disturbance:

(1) Repairing pre-existing deficits of water and electrolytes;

(2) Providing water and electrolytes to meet the maintenance needs of the patient;

(3) Replacing water and electrolytes being lost through such routes as vomiting, diarrhea, tubular drainage, wound or burn drainage, diuresis, and so forth.

There are many different methods for achieving these goals, but rather than describe them all, we will present one simple method that has worked well in practice and that will give the nurse a basic understanding of the principles involved in fluid therapy. This method was developed by Butler and his co-workers at the Massachusetts General Hospital and has been used with great success in many parts of the world.

Because various types of solutions, particularly those containing potassium, can be hazardous if renal function is not adequate, the first step in fluid therapy is to determine the status of the kidneys. If any of the following criteria exists, a therapeutic test for functional renal depression is carried out: specific gravity of the urine above 1.030; less than 3 voidings in 24 hours; no urine in the bladder; massive acute loss of extracellular fluid, such as is seen in fulminating infantile diarrhea.

In any of these cases, a special solution, frequently called an initial hydrating solution or a pump-priming solution, is administered. Such a solution often provides sodium, 51 mEq./L., chloride, 51 mEq./L., and glucose, 5 gm./L. It actually represents a solution containing one part of isotonic solution of sodium chloride in 5 per cent glucose in water. The solution is administered at the rate of 8 ml./square m. of body surface/minute for 45 minutes. If the urinary suppression is due to volume deficit, the therapeutic test will re-establish urinary flow. If the kidneys begin to function, the initial hydrating solution is discontinued, and therapy is started with other appropriate solutions. If urinary flow is not restored, the rate of infusion is reduced to 2 ml./square m. body surface/minute and continued for another hour. If urination has not occurred at the end of this period, the physician assumes he is dealing with renal impairment and focuses his attention on the renal problem.

Administering Fluid Therapy

After the patient's kidneys have been shown to be functional, the physician can proceed to repair pre-existing deficits and to provide water and electrolytes for maintenance. To accomplish these goals, he may use a single solution of the type devised by Butler.

The patient's maintenance requirements can be met by the administration of 1,500 ml. of a Butler-type solution* per square meter of body surface per day.

* The solution of the type devised by Butler is formulated so that when one uses it to meet the patient's fluid volume requirement, it supplies electrolytes in quantities balanced between the minimal needs and maximal tolerances of the patient. Hence, it is sometimes called a *balanced solution,* as by Snively and Sweeney. The Butler-type solution is hypotonic, being only ⅓ to ½ as concentrated as plasma. Therefore, it provides free water to form urine and to carry out metabolic functions. It provides both cellular and extracellular electrolytes. It contains 5 or 10 per cent carbohydrate to reduce tissue destruction, counteract ketosis, and spare protein. What the Butler-type solution really does is to use the body homeostatic mechanisms that select the electrolytes that are required and reject those not needed. When used properly, it has a great margin of safety.

Current names applied by various pharmaceutical companies to their Butler solutions are as follows: Cutter Laboratories—Electrolyte No. 2, Electrolyte No. 48, Electrolyte No. 75, Polysal M; Baxter Laboratories—Electrolyte No. 2, Electrolyte No. 48, Electrolyte No. 75; McGaw—Electrolyte No. 2, Isolyte P; Amsco Hospital Liquids—Electrolyte B, Electrolyte F, Electrolyte D; Abbott Laboratories—Ionosol B, Ionosol MB, Ionosol T; Don Baxter, Inc.—Electrolyte No. 75.

If the patient has a moderate pre-existing deficit, this deficit can be corrected and the maintenance needs met by giving 2,400 ml./square m. body surface/day. If the patient has a severe pre-existing deficit, then one can correct the deficit and provide maintenance by giving 3,000 ml./square m. body surface/day.

The Butler-type solution is administered intravenously, by mouth, or by nasogastric tube, but not subcutaneously. In giving the solution intravenously, the usual rate of administration is 3 ml./square m. body surface/minute.

For correcting continuing abnormal losses, as in vomiting or severe diarrhea, replacement solutions with a composition resembling the body fluid being lost are employed. For example, if the patient loses gastric juice, a gastric replacement solution is administered intravenously. The rate of administration for replacement solutions is usually 3 ml./square m. body surface/minute. This simple plan of therapy can be used for treating body fluid disturbances that occur as a result of differences between intake and output, such as the following:

    (a) fluid volume deficit of extracellular fluid
    (b) sodium excess of extracellular fluid
    (c) potassium deficit of extracellular fluid
    (d) base bicarbonate deficit of extracellular fluid
    (e) base bicarbonate excess of extracellular fluid
    (f) carbonic acid deficit of extracellular fluid
    (g) carbonic acid excess of extracellular fluid

Several important imbalances require therapy specifically tailored to the imbalance.

Fluid Volume Excess of Extracellular Fluid

The object of therapy in this imbalance is to reduce the extracellular fluid volume to normal without altering the electrolyte concentration of the fluid. It may be necessary to withhold all liquids for a time.

Sodium Deficit of Extracellular Fluid

In treating sodium deficit, sodium chloride is provided in such concentration as to restore the sodium level of the extracellular fluid to normal without causing a fluid volume excess. If the extracellular fluid volume is normal or excessive, the imbalance is corrected by administering a 3 or 5 per cent solution of sodium chloride. If there is an extracellular fluid volume deficit, the physician administers an isotonic solution of sodium chloride.

Potassium Excess of Extracellular Fluid

The uncomplicated potassium excess with functional kidneys can be treated by avoiding additional potassium, either orally or parenterally. If the kidneys are impaired, however, several methods of removing excessive potassium from the extracellular fluid can be used.

FIG. 7-10. Sites of election for the insertion of intravenous needles for the parenteral administration of fluids or blood transfusion. Preferably, injections are made into the distal portion of the extremity, at the points indicated by dots, rather than in the anterior cubital fossa (e.g., at point x), to avoid the necessity for immobilizing the elbow and the risk of the needle's becoming dislodged during the injection.

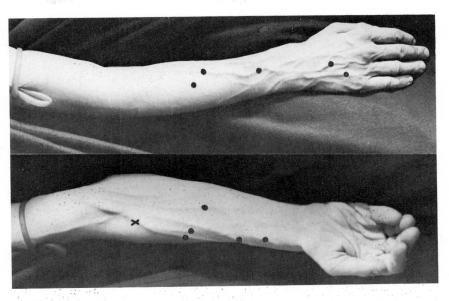

These methods include carefully measured replacement therapy, supplying fats and carbohydrates but no protein materials; administration of insulin and dextrose; administration of carbonic anhydrase inhibitors; the use of ion exchange resins; use of peritoneal dialysis; or employment of the artificial kidney.

Calcium Deficit of Extracellular Fluid

In acute calcium deficit, a 10 per cent solution of calcium gluconate should be administered intravenously. This is particularly important if tetany or convulsions have occurred.

Calcium Excess of Extracellular Fluid

Treatment of calcium excess should be directed at correcting the underlying condition. If other imbalances are also being treated, only calcium-free solutions should be used.

Protein Deficit of Extracellular Fluid

Protein deficit is corrected by the administration of high-protein foods or supplements, or by the administration of amino acids with provision of generous quantities of calories in the form of dextrose or alcohol or both. All three expedients may be required.

Plasma-to-Interstitial Fluid Shift

This shift can be restricted by relieving the condition causing it and by the application of a binder for localized shifts. Plasma volume can be maintained or restored by the parenteral administration of plasma dextran or a plasma-like electrolyte solution.

Interstitial Fluid-to-Plasma Shift

When remobilization of edema fluid causes this shift, the physician may employ phlebotomy, or he may apply tourniquets. If the shift results from internal or external loss of whole blood, blood transfusions should be given.

Whole Blood Deficit

Whole blood should be given to repair this deficit. Red cells should be given alone if the extracellular fluid volume is excessive.

Solutions Available

Solutions used from hospital to hospital vary greatly, and the nurse should become familiar with those used in the hospital where she is employed. She can do this by talking with physicians and by reading the literature provided by the hospital's pharmaceutical supplier.

METHODS OF ADMINISTRATION

Because the nurse plays a major role in the administration of parenteral fluids, it is imperative that she understand the basic principles of safe fluid administration.

Intravenous Route

An excellent route for the quick administration of water and electrolytes and other nutrients is through the veins, or intravenously. (Fig. 7-10.) Fluids administered intravenously pass directly into the extracellular fluid, and the body homeostatic mechanisms act rapidly to prevent the infusion from producing abnormal changes in volume or electrolyte concentration of extracellular fluid. When nutrients are needed in a hurry, the intravenous route is essential. Provided due care is exercised, relatively large volumes of fluids can be administered by this route.

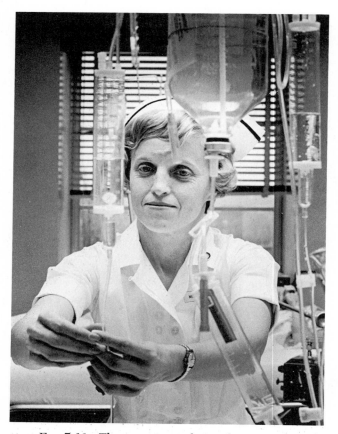

Fig. 7-11. The nurse is regulating the rate and volume of intravenous fluid administration. The use of a calibrated burette chamber enables her to infuse a specified volume of fluid per hour. When this volume is delivered, a flutter-valve closes and stops infusion. This system is helpful for administration of intravenous medications and for precise control of fluid intake. (National Institutes of Health)

The veins in and around the cubital fossa (antecubital, basilic, and cephalic veins) are the most common sites for venipuncture because they are large and easily accessible. They can accommodate large needles, large volumes of fluids, and all but the most irritating intravenous solutions. Other commonly used veins includes veins in the forearm (basilic and cephalic veins), veins in the radial area of the wrist, veins in the hand (metacarpal and dorsal venous plexus), femoral and saphenous veins in the thigh, veins in the foot (dorsal venous plexus, medial and lateral marginal veins), and scalp veins in infants and in the aged.

The selection of a vein depends upon a number of factors, including availability of sites (depends upon condition of veins), size of needle to be used, type of fluids to be infused, volume, rate, and length of infusion, degree of mobility desired, and the skill of the operator.

Fluids are introduced into the vein through a metal needle, a plastic needle, a plastic catheter threaded through a metal needle, or a plastic catheter introduced by means of a cut-down (minor surgical procedure performed only by a doctor). Metal needles are usually used for short-term infusions. The size of the needle to be used depends upon the vein and the type of solution. Nineteen- or 20-gauge, 1 or 1½ inch needles are the most commonly used; an 18-gauge needle is indicated for blood administration. (The smaller the gauge number, the larger the internal diameter of the needle.)

For therapy lasting longer than 12 hours, plastic needles or catheters are used because they allow the patient more freedom of movement than does a metal needle. A cut-down, which involves insertion of a catheter through a slit in the vein, is used when veins are hard to find and long-term fluid therapy is anticipated. Obese patients, infants, or those in or near shock frequently require cut-downs.

Before venipuncture, it is necessary to distend the vein. This can usually be accomplished by applying a tourniquet. The tourniquet should be applied lightly and should restrict only outflow. Sometimes it may be necessary to distend the vein by other methods, such as by placing the part in a dependent position for several minutes or by warming the entire extremity by applying warm towels, by immersion in warm water, or by the use of an electric hair dryer or an electric blanket.

If a large gauge needle is to be used, its insertion may be preceded by a small injection of 1 per cent procaine. This should only be done by order of the physician, and the patient should be questioned about a possible allergy to procaine before the injection is given. If the site chosen for venipuncture is hairy, the area should be shaved to eliminate some of the discomfort associated with the removal of adhesive tape after the infusion. The injection site should be wiped with alcohol before insertion of the needle. Sometimes the area is cleaned with pHisoHex or other detergents prior to the use of alcohol.

The bevel of the needle should be facing upward during insertion in most cases. However, when introducing a large needle into a small vein, it may be necessary for the bevel to face downward to prevent the needle from piercing the posterior wall of the vein when the tourniquet is removed. The needle should pierce the skin to one side of and about ½ to 1 inch below the point where the needle will enter the vein. The needle should enter the skin at a 45° angle; after the skin is pierced, the angle is decreased. The free hand is used to palpate the vein while the needle is being introduced. After the needle enters the vein, one should proceed very slowly with the insertion of the needle. It is threaded into the lumen approximately ½ to ¾ of an inch. The tourniquet is released. Frequently, a thin stream of blood is seen in the tubing when the needle enters the vein. To ascertain that the needle is in the vein, the infusion bottle may be lowered below the injection site; the negative pressure forces blood into the tubing.

Next, in order to anchor the needle comfortably and safely, a cotton ball or small gauze pad should be placed under the hub of the needle and fixed in place with adhesive tape. Another strip of tape should be placed over the needle to help hold it steady. A loop should be made in the tubing and taped in place to allow some slack and to minimize pull on the needle when the patient moves.

When the needle is secured in place, the fluid is then started and the proper flow rate established. Since the rate of most intravenous infusions slows 25 to 50 per cent during the first 3 to 5 minutes, it is best to start with a rate slightly above that of the desired rate. (Fig. 7-11.)

If swelling occurs, it is an indication that the needle is not in the vein and that the fluid is entering the subcutaneous area. The infusion should be stopped immediately and started in another vein.

If a plastic needle is used, it should not be used near a joint because flexion could obstruct the flow or cause the needle to break.

Hypodermoclysis

Hypodermoclysis, the administration of a solution subcutaneously, presents many problems and is not nearly as desirable as the intravenous route. Infections are common with hypodermoclysis. Some fluids, such as electrolyte-free solutions, hypertonic solutions, alcohol, amino acids, fat emulsions, and solutions that differ significantly from body pH (as gastric replacement solutions), are contraindicated for hypodermoclysis, and orders for their use should be questioned. The subcutaneous administration of a 5 per cent dextrose in water solution draws electrolytes from the surrounding tissues and from the plasma. The decreased plasma volume can cause hypotension and even shock. If the patient has a pre-existing sodium deficit, he may die.

Fluids generally considered safe for subcutaneous administration include hypotonic saline (0.9 per cent), half-isotonic saline (0.45 per cent) with 2½ per cent dextrose, Ringer's solution, half-strength Ringer's solution with 2½ per cent dextrose, lactated Ringer's solution, half-strength lactated Ringer's solution with 2½

per cent dextrose, and Darrow's solution. These solutions closely resemble the electrolyte content and tonicity of extracellular fluid and, therefore, can be absorbed in most cases.

Since subcutaneous infusions are easier to start than are intravenous injections, hypodermoclysis is often used for obese patients, infants, and the aged. Suitable sites for injection include the subcutaneous tissues in the lateral aspect of the thigh or abdomen. Two needles are usually used, and the fluid is injected into 2 sites at once. The rate of infusion depends upon how well the fluid is absorbed from the injection site. When the fluid is absorbed well, 250 to 500 ml. can be given at one site in 1 hour to an adult. An enzyme, Wydase, may be injected into the tissues at the injection site to hasten absorption. Unless the flow rate is adjusted carefully, a large amount of swelling can develop. A small sterile gauze pad should be placed under the needle hub and another should cover the injection site. When the needles are removed, a light sterile dressing should be applied since edematous injection sites are quite susceptible to infections.

COMPLICATIONS OF THERAPY

Complications sometimes occurring with intravenous injections include pyrogenic reactions, local infiltration, circulatory overload, thrombophlebitis, and air embolism. Patients receiving intravenous infusions should be observed often so that complications may be detected early.

Pyrogenic Reactions

Pyrogens, foreign proteins that can cause a febrile reaction, are sometimes present in the infusion solution or in the administration setup. The symptoms of a pyrogenic reaction usually begin about 30 minutes after the start of the infusion and include an abrupt temperature elevation (from 100° to 106° F., or 37.8° to 41.1° C.) accompanied by severe chills, backache, headache, general malaise, nausea and vomiting. Vascular collapse with hypotension and cyanosis may occur if the reaction is severe. The severity of the reaction depends upon the amount of pyrogens infused, the rate of flow, and the patient's susceptibility. If symptoms of pyrogenic reactions occur, the infusion should be stopped at once and the physician notified. Also, the nurse should check the patient's vital signs. The solution should be saved so that it can be cultured if necessary.

Commercially prepared solutions and administration sets are pyrogen-free, but contaminants can enter these solutions after the seal is broken. Solutions not used immediately after the seal is broken should be discarded. A solution should also be discarded if there is any evidence of cloudiness in a normally clear solution. A contaminated needle as the source of a pyrogenic reaction is easily overlooked. Any hypodermic needle that is to be reused must be properly cleaned and sterilized. The only safe alternative is to use new disposable needles exclusively. Special care must be taken when adding medications to the infusion fluid to avoid introducing organisms into the solution.

Local Infiltration

The dislodging of a needle and the local infiltration of solution into the subcutaneous tissues is fairly common, especially when a small, thin-walled vein is used and the patient is active. Edema at the site of injection, failure to get blood return into the tubing when the bottle is lowered below the needle, discomfort in the area of injection (the degree of discomfort depends on the type of solution), and a significant decrease in the rate of infusion or a complete stop in the flow of the fluid are indications of infiltration.

Some solutions, such as hypertonic carbohydrate solutions, solutions with a pH varying greatly from that of the body (such as protein hydrolysates, sixth molar sodium lactate, or ammonium chloride), and potassium solutions, often cause great pain if they infiltrate the subcutaneous tissues. The local irritation may cause tissue slough, especially when norepinephrine (Levophed) is the offending solution. When infiltration is apparent, the infusion should be immediately discontinued.

Circulatory Overload

Administration of excessive intravenous fluids may overload the circulatory system and cause increased venous pressure, venous distention, increased blood pressure, coughing, shortness of breath, increased respiratory rate, and pulmonary edema with severe dyspnea and cyanosis. Patients with cardiac decompensation are particularly prone to circulatory overload. If the patient displays signs of circulatory overload, the infusion should be stopped and the physician notified immediately. The patient can be raised to a sitting position to aid breathing.

Thrombophlebitis

Thrombophlebitis is a condition associated with clot formation in an inflamed vein. Some degree of venous irritation occurs with all intravenous infusions, but it is usually of significance only in infusions kept going in the same site for longer than 12 hours. Thrombophlebitis is indicated by pain along the course of the vein and redness and edema at the injection site. If the condition is severe, systemic reactions to the infection may occur (tachycardia, fever, and general malaise).

Irritating solutions, such as alcohol, can help cause thrombophlebitis. Hypertonic solutions are often associated with venous irritation; carbohydrate solutions in excess of 10 per cent almost always produce this reaction. Solutions with an alkaline or acid pH are more frequently associated with thrombophlebitis than are solutions that approximate body pH.

When thrombophlebitis is detected, the infusion should be stopped. The physician may change the order for the infusion to prevent more veins from being irritated and consequently unavailable. The infusion is best started in another site to allow the damaged vein to heal. Cold compresses usually are applied to the thrombophlebitic site. Later, warm, moist compresses can be employed to relieve discomfort and to promote healing.

Air Embolism

Even though air embolism occurs most often when blood is given under pressure, the danger of it occurring is present in all intravenous infusions. Small amounts of air are not always harmful; but in some patients, as little as 10 ml. may be fatal.

The nurse should take these measures to prevent the occurrence of air embolism:

(1) Discontinue an infusion *before* the bottle and tubing are completely emptied to prevent air from the bottle from entering the vein. The patient may be asked to notify the nurse when the infusion is about to run out. A tape can be placed on the side of the infusion flask to show the level at which the patient should notify the nurse.

(2) The needle and any other attachments should be tightly fitted to the infusion tubing.

(3) The first bottle to empty in a Y-type set (parallel hookup) should be completely clamped off so that air will not be drawn from the empty bottle into the vein.

(4) Instructions for use of blood pumping apparatus should be carefully followed when blood or any other fluid is given under pressure.

(5) The extremity receiving the infusion should not be elevated above the level of the heart since this results in venous collapse and negative venous pressure. Negative pressure in the vein receiving the infusion draws in large amounts of air if there are any defects in the apparatus.

(6) The clamp used to regulate fluid flow rate should be kept at a low level—preferably no higher than the level of the heart, certainly no higher than 4 to 11 cm. above the heart. Venous pressure normally causes a column of water to rise 4 to 11 cm. above the

level of the heart. If the flow regulating clamp is placed above this height, a negative pressure will result in the tubing below. The negative pressure can be great enough to draw in sizable amounts of air if there are any defects in the apparatus.

(7) Permitting the infusion tubing to drop below the level of the extremity may help prevent air from entering the vein if the infusion flask empties unobserved.

Air embolism is manifested by sudden vascular collapse, with symptoms of cyanosis, hypotension, weak rapid pulse, venous pressure rise, and loss of consciousness.

If an air embolism occurs, some physicians place the patient on his left side with his head down, on the theory that this allows the air to rise into the right atrium and permits some blood to empty from the right ventricle into the left side of the heart. Oxygen should be administered.

Speed Shock

Speed shock, a systemic reaction, may occur as a result of too rapid administration of solutions containing drugs. The drug floods the bloodstream, and toxic concentrations are supplied to organs that have a rich blood supply, such as the heart and the brain. Syncope and shock may occur. The nurse should check the flow rate often and reduce it if untoward symptoms (which vary with the offending drug) develop.

BIBLIOGRAPHY

Adriani, J.: Venipuncture. Amer. J. Nurs., *62*:66-70, March, 1962.

Collentine, G.: How to calculate fluids for burned patients. Amer. J. Nurs., *62*:77-79, March, 1962.

Crouch, M., and Gibson, S.: Blood therapy. Amer. J. Nurs. *62*: 71-76, March, 1962.

Drummond, E., and Anderson, M.: Gastrointestinal suction. Amer. J. Nurs., *63*:109-113, Dec., 1963.

Goldberger, E.: A Primer of Water, Electrolyte, and Acid-Base Syndromes. ed. 3. Philadelphia, Lea & Febiger, 1965.

Metheny, N., and Snively, W.: Nurses' Handbook of Fluid Balance. Philadelphia, J. B. Lippincott, 1967.

Snively, W.: The body's response to burning. GP, *20*:132-144, Sept., 1959.

————: Potassium salts and intestinal ulcer. J.A.M.A., *195*:977, 1966.

————: Toward a better understanding of body fluid disturbances. Nurs. Forum, *3*:1-17, Jan., 1964.

Snively, W., and Sweeney, M.: Fluid Balance Handbook for Practitioners. Springfield, Ill., Charles C. Thomas, 1956.

Snively, W., and Westerman, R.: Serum potassium determination. J.A.M.A., *197*:151, 1966.

Snively, W., Montenegro, J., and Dick, R.: Quick method for estimating body surface area. J.A.M.A., *197*:208-209, 1966.

Soffer, A.: Potassium Therapy. Springfield, Ill., Charles C. Thomas, 1968.

Weisberg, H.: Water, Electrolyte and Acid-Base Balance. ed. 2. Baltimore, Williams & Wilkins, 1962.

Westerman, R., and Snively, W.: Potassium deficit: clinical aspects. GP, *33*:85-93, June, 1966.

Wohl, M., and Goodhart, R.: Modern Nutrition in Health and Disease. ed. 3. Philadelphia, Lea & Febiger, 1964.

CHAPTER **8**

Blood Transfusion

- *The Nurse in the Donor Clinic*
- *Blood Groups and Blood Compatibility*
- *Transfusion Therapy*
- *Transfusion Complications*
- *Summary of the Problems of the Transfusion Recipient*

THE NURSE IN THE DONOR CLINIC

With the passage of time, nurses have been required to undertake an ever-increasing measure of responsibility in connection with transfusion therapy, including the taking of blood from donors and the conducting of donor clinics. The problems relative to blood procurement of most immediate concern are the selection and care of donors, the technical aspects of venisection and the possible complications of this procedure. Nursing responsibilities include the screening of potential donors on the basis of medical history and physical qualifications; the maintenance of sterile supplies and all other equipment and materials used in conjunction with donor phlebotomy; the training and the supervision of auxiliary workers assigned to the donor clinic; the performance of phlebotomy; the precise, unequivocal identification of donor blood and pilot samples, and the appropriate disposition of these donor units and test samples. The nurse is a key figure in public relations, the competence with which she performs her tasks in the donor clinic coloring the reputation not only of this unit but also of the entire hospital.

Donor Interviewing

Every prospective donor must be interviewed and examined before he donates blood, both for his own protection and that of the recipient. Only those persons are eligible to donate who appear to be in good health, are asymptomatic and are free of the following:

(1) Viral hepatitis, currently or at any time in the past, or a history of household contact within 6 months with a hepatitis patient (because of the possibility that this individual may have acquired the infection and, despite the absence of symptoms or signs, may be harboring the virus);

(2) A history of receiving within 6 months a blood transfusion or an injection of any fraction or product of human blood other than serum albumin or gamma globulin (all others being potential sources of hepatitis virus);

(3) A history, recent or remote, of any other infectious disease likewise transmissible by transfusion, such as syphilis or malaria;

(4) A history, or the stigmata, of acute or chronic alcoholism (because of its debilitating effects on the donor) or of narcotic addiction (because of the high hepatitis carrier rate among addicts);

(5) A skin infection of any type, in any location (because of the likelihood that the bacterial flora covering the entire skin surface including the venipuncture site will be abnormally dense, and contamination of the phlebotomy needle difficult to avoid);

(6) Symptoms of active respiratory or skin allergy (asthma or urticaria), or a history of drug allergy

within 6 months (because of the possibility that the corresponding hypersensitivity may be transferred to the recipient);

(7) The pregnant state, or a history of pregnancy within 6 months (because of the nutritional demands imposed thereby on the mother);

(8) A history of oral surgery including dental extraction within a 72-hour period (because of the frequency with which such procedures are attended and followed by bacteremia).

The standard routine for the screening of blood donors also involves measurements of the body weight, the oral temperature, the pulse rate, the arterial pressure and the hemoglobin level. Donors are expected to meet the following minimal requirements:

(1) The body weight should exceed 110 pounds for a standard 450 ml. donation. Donors weighing less than 110 pounds may be bled proportionately less.

(2) The oral temperature should not exceed 37.5°C (99.6°F).

(3) The pulse rate should be between 60 and 120 beats per minute.

(4) The systolic arterial pressure should be between 100 and 200 mm. Hg., and the diastolic, between 50 and 100 mm. Hg.

(5) The hemoglobin level in the case of a female should exceed 12.5 gm./100 ml.; in the case of a male, 13.5 gm./100 ml.

Individuals over 60 years of age generally are disqualified unless phlebotomy has been authorized, specifically and in writing, by the donor's physician. A person who is engaged in a hazardous occupation, e.g., an airplane pilot or high-rise construction worker, is not acceptable as a donor if he expects to work within a 12-hour period following his donation.

Phlebotomy

The technic of venisection may be described briefly as follows: The donor, having just received a full glass of water to assist the rapid restoration of his blood volume, is placed in a comfortable position, head resting on the same horizontal plane as the trunk. A blood pressure cuff is applied to the upper arm and inflated to a level between the diastolic and systolic pressure, e.g., approximately 100 mm. Hg, in order to distend and locate the antecubital vessels. After a vein has been selected the cuff is deflated and the skin overlying the puncture site is cleansed. Before venisection, the labeling of the donor-blood bottle and the tubes that are to receive the lab specimens is completed. Even if these labels have already been subjected to a routine check, they should be scrutinized once more with the utmost care, for it is quite clear that clerical errors, particularly those involving the placement of labels, are the most frequent cause of serious transfusion accidents. Numerous fatalities having been attributable to misdirection or faulty identification of donor blood.

Following reinflation of the cuff to the original pressure, venipuncture is performed, and the blood is allowed to flow until the volume of blood collected is sufficient. The volume of blood drawn from the donor should not exceed 450 ml. The donor tube is doubly clamped and cut. Its proximal end is permanently sealed; the distal end is then unclamped in order to fill 1 or 2 "pilot" tubes, after which the pressure cuff is deflated and the needle withdrawn.

The donor should be required to rest for a minimal period of 5 minutes and then adjust himself to the sitting posture. After the wound has been examined carefully for residual bleeding, a pressure dressing is applied to the arm, and the donor is permitted to regain his feet unless there is evidence of unusual weakness or faintness, in which event a longer rest is prescribed. Whatever his appearance, it is important that the donor remain in the near vicinity and under observation for a period of at least 20 minutes after leaving the table. During this interval he should drink a glass of liquid refreshment, one that is neither very hot nor very cold; permission to smoke, however, should be refused until he is considered for release.

Complications of Blood Donation

Local damage at the site of venipuncture occasionally occurs in blood donors. This may produce subcutaneous bleeding or inflammatory lesions, the former developing while the patient is still under observation and the latter many hours afterward. Continuous bleeding, although conceivably due to a blood disorder accompanied by a failure of the normal clotting mechanism, is usually due to laceration of the vein owing to some technical difficulty associated with the venipuncture or the withdrawal of the needle. Excessive probing within the subcutaneous tissue while searching for the lumen of the vein or through-and-through perforations of the vein often are responsible for damage adequate to explain the occurrence of both external and subcutaneous hemorrhage with subsequent hematoma production. A technical error that invariably results in bleeding of this type is failure to release the cuff pressure prior to the withdrawal of the needle. However, if the venipuncture has been performed carefully and correctly and a pressure dressing has been applied securely no earlier than 5 minutes following the bleeding, and if the arm has been extended in an upright position, hemorrhage is rarely encountered.

Fainting in blood donors is a fairly common occurrence for which there are many possible causes. Emotional factors play a decided role in the genesis of this phenomenon, as is evident from the contagious element apparent when several donors are bled in a common room. The observing of such an attack by individuals who are about to be, or just have been bled, often precipitates a similar response in other donors. The fasting state, if prolonged, is likewise a predisposing factor in the production of faints. Because of this correlation, most blood bank regulations that formerly forbade the ingestion of food within 6 or 8 hours now have been revised in the opposite direction; donors are requested to have a light meal within 4 or 6 hours prior to venisection, and at all events to drink a full tumbler of some fluid, e.g., water, milk or fruit juice, immediately before giving blood.

Attacks of fainting usually occur at the conclusion of the procedure, immediately after resumption of the upright posture or shortly thereafter, because this position aggravates the severity of hypotension that reflects the loss of blood volume. The warning signal to look for in all donors during the bleeding and afterward is the development of pallor. On the appearance of this sign, the donor should be obliged to lie down, or, if this cannot be arranged at once, he should sit with his head lowered between and below the level of the knees. This posture, and the reclining position with the feet on the bed and the knees flexed, improves the cerebral arterial circulation and tends to forestall fainting as well as to revive persons who have fainted. A donor who has fainted or feels faint should be kept under observation for a period of at least 30 minutes lest the phenomenon recur under less favorable circumstances.

Anginal pain, that is, pain located in the anterior chest in the region of the sternum or over the heart, is precipitated occasionally in donors afflicted with unsuspected coronary heart disease. The development of any symptom of this sort is always an occasion for serious concern because of its implication of a possible recent acute coronary thrombosis. Convulsions, the most dramatic sequel to venisection, may be precipitated in epileptic individuals, including those with a latent susceptibility to seizures. Angina pectoris and epilepsy are discussed elsewhere in this text (Chaps. 19 and 34).

Inflammation of the tissues in the area of venipuncture may result from the introduction of bacteria into the soft tissues owing to faulty technique in cleansing and sterilizing of the skin or in protecting the needle from contamination prior to its use. Sterile inflammatory processes that develop within a few hours following the procedure usually are due to procaine sensitivity.

BLOOD GROUPS AND BLOOD GROUP COMPATIBILITY

(The reader is referred to textbooks on anatomy, physiology, chemistry and microbiology.)

TRANSFUSION THERAPY

Clinical Uses of Blood and Blood Components

Traditionally, the term "transfusion" is taken to mean the therapeutic administration of whole donor blood. Even now, whole blood, while not the agent of choice for optimal therapy in most cases, is the material selected for the majority of transfusion recipients, for reasons of expediency. More often than not, however, transfusion requirements are more specific and can be met more efficiently, effectively and economically by appropriate blood fractions rather than by whole blood. All of the blood components in the following discussion are now widely available through the Regional Blood Centers of the American Red Cross and other community blood programs. Moreover, techniques for the preparation of most of these components are well within the competence and means of most hospital blood bank laboratories.

At least 7 blood derivatives are available that, selected and administered appropriately, will meet the needs of most prospective transfusion recipients as effectively as or more effectively than whole blood. These include packed red cells, platelet-rich plasma and platelet concentrates, whole plasma (liquid stored, fresh, or freshly frozen), plasma cryoprecipitate, human albumin, and desiccated human fibrinogen. Each of these types of transfusion, the indications and the rationale, are summarized below.

Whole Blood. This material is the logical choice for the treatment of acute hemorrhage and hypovolemic shock, actual or potential. If restoration of the patient's blood volume requires more than 5 units of donor blood within the space of a few hours, any additional transfusions should employ fresh blood, i.e., blood stored less than 24 hours (and therefore a source of labile as well as stable clotting factors). If the patient has become thrombocytopenic, he should receive blood that has been collected within a period of 4 hours (therefore a source of platelets as well as plasma clotting factors.)

Fresh whole blood collected within 24 hours should be specified for (1) all exchange transfusions, (2) postoperative transfusions following extracorporeal circulation with stored blood, and (3) recipients of massive transfusion therapy, as specified previously.

Fresh whole blood collected within 4 hours is indicated for the treatment of patients with certain specific hemorrhagic disorders who are bleeding actively, or who are anemic as a result of recent activity or recent bleeding. The hemorrhagic disorders in question are hemophilia A (factor VIII deficiency), factor V deficiency complicating severe liver disease or coumarin therapy, and severe thrombocytopenia.

Packed Red Cells. This form of transfusion is preferred for patients with severe anemia but with relatively normal blood volumes, especially if the anemia demands prompt correction because of its severity, if other antianemic therapy is likely to prove ineffective, or if major surgery is an imminent prospect. In contrast to whole blood, red cell concentrates contain a minimum of plasma colloids and sodium; thus, when they are transfused, they produce less expansion of the plasma volume and impose less risk of circulatory overload.

Platelet Transfusions. Platelets are given to patients with dangerous degrees of thrombocytopenia in order to control or prevent bleeding. The quantity of platelets needed to elevate the recipient's platelet count from a hemorrhagic to a safe level, e.g., from 5,000 to 50,000, represents the harvest from at least 4 to 6 units of donor blood and perhaps more, depending on the presence or absence of active bleeding or other factors that tend to consume platelets. Viable platelets may be supplied in the form of fresh blood (if the intent is to replace red cells as well), or as platelet-rich plasma (PRP), containing 80 to 90 per cent of the original platelets. However, to eliminate the risk of circulatory overload, inherent in the use of either PRP or whole blood, it is customary to prepare from the platelet-rich plasma a platelet concentrate (PC), reducing the volume to approximately 10 ml. per unit, while retaining nearly all of the original platelets in a viable state. The harvesting of donor platelets usually entails a double phlebotomy, i.e., the collection at one sitting of 2 units from each donor followed by the immediate return of the red cells. This entire procedure involving phlebotomy, centrifugation, supernatant separation and reinfusion is carried out simply, safely and speedily in a closed system comprised of multiple interconnected plastic bags. Confronted by the increasing incidence of thrombocytopenia, commensurate with the increasingly widespread use of myelotoxic drugs in cancer chemotherapy, many hospital blood banks throughout the country are adding to their agenda the collection, processing and transfusion of platelets.

Whole Plasma. The prime indication for plasma transfusions is the treatment of clotting defects, since all of the plasma factors can be supplied rapidly and effectively by this means without overexpanding the patient's blood volume. Plasma that has been separated from stored blood, or that has been stored in the liquid state after separation, contains the stable clotting factors VII, IX, X and XI, but lacks factor VIII, the antihemophilic factor, and factor V, one of the accelerators of prothrombin conversion. Freshly frozen plasma (FFP), i.e., plasma which has been separated immediately from freshly donated blood, then promptly frozen, contains all factors, including V and VIII. The latter, moreover, retain their activity for at least 12 months when stored at −30° C. Once thawed, however, FFP must be used immediately.

As a plasma expander in cases of hypovolemia, or as an exogenous source of plasma albumin for patients with hypoalbuminemia, whole plasma has been largely supplanted by pure preparations of serum albumin and other plasma fractions that are comprised largely of albumin.

Antihemophilic Cryoprecipitate. A material rich in factor VIII and exceedingly effective in the treatment of hemophilia can easily be prepared by freezing plasma that has been separated promptly from freshly donated blood. A precipitate forms that contains approximately 70 per cent of the original antihemophilic activity and, volume for volume, is about 20 to 30 times as potent as whole plasma. The material may be removed and stored separately at −30° C. pending its use. Once thawed it must be used immediately.

Human Serum Albumin (Cohn Fraction V) and Other Albumin Preparations. Plasma albumin comprises 50 to 60 per cent of the protein and therefore accounts for most of the oncotic pressure of the plasma. By the same token it is the chief determinant of plasma volume. This material, which is highly purified, and other fractions less pure, which contain most of the albumin, are used most logically and effectively to expand the blood volume of patients in hypovolemic shock and to elevate the level of circulating albumin in patients with hypoalbuminemia. These preparations, in contrast to all other fractions of human blood, cellular or soluble, are subjected to heating at 60° C. for 10 hours, and therefore can be certified unequivocally as free of all viral contaminants, including the hepatitis virus. Whereas the risk of hepatitis transmission is an important consideration in connection with every other type of transfusion therapy (gamma globulin excepted), no such complication has ever been known to attend the use of albumin.

Human Fibrinogen (Cohn Fraction I). This material is specifically indicated in cases of congenital and acquired hypofibrinogenemia complicated by active bleeding. Prior to its use the material, desiccated and packaged in 1- and 2-gm. vials, is reconstituted with sterile water and the final concentration adjusted to 1 per cent. This fraction has been responsible for transmitting hepatitis with a frequency exceeding that associated with any other blood component, probably for the following reasons: (1) each unit has been derived from a sizable donor pool; (2) factor I cannot be subjected to heat sterilization; and (3) the sequence of biochemical steps that lead to the separation of fibrinogen appear to favor the sequestration and concentration of virus in this particular fraction. Whatever the explanation for this high infectivity rate, this risk must be balanced very carefully with the clinical indications whenever fibrinogen therapy is contemplated.

Transfusion Technique

Methods of injecting blood are similar in most respects to those employed in other types of parenteral therapy. However, there are certain technical considerations of importance that apply specifically to blood transfusion and relate in part to the handling of the material before its injection. For example, blood never should be allowed to remain uncooled for any appreciable length of time (more than 2 hours) following its collection from the donor or its removal from the storage refrigerator, if rapid deterioration of the red cells is to be avoided.

Blood should be administered by a closed-system technique, using a glass transfusion bottle that is vented through a protected airway tube or a plastic system composed of a collapsible bag with attachments for phlebotomy and transfusion.

When blood is administered from the bottle or bag in which it was collected, a filter must be introduced into the connecting tubing to remove small clots before the blood enters the vein. The same precautions as for the giving of fluid by intravenous infusion must be observed. The nurse should observe and record the time at which the blood is given and the amount, any rise in temperature, rise in pulse, difficulty in respiration, nausea and vomiting.

Role of the Nurse. *The first step in the performance of every transfusion is to check the labels identifying the donor blood and to confirm the identity of the patient who is to receive it!*

The insertion of the intravenous needle and the arrangement of the recipient set, although classically the responsibility of the attending physician, is also quite properly and often necessarily within the capacity of the professional nurse. Judgment in the selection of a suitable vein and skill in the use of intravenous needles are usually acquired very readily, provided that the original technical instruction was correct and opportunities for practical experience have been sufficiently frequent. The importance of these techniques, formerly considered entirely outside the province of nursing care, stems from the fact that parenteral therapy has increased in usage to such an astounding degree that most hospitals, unless staffed with resident physicians, would find it impossible to conduct treatment of this sort on an adequate scale without the participation of competent nursing personnel. Moreover, even when professional medical assistance is amply available, there is often a tendency to schedule parenteral injections, including transfusion therapy, in a manner that is something less than ideal, large infusions being administered at infrequent intervals, whereas smaller injections, given regularly and more frequently, might be preferred on physiologic grounds. Finally, assuming that all such treatments could be performed by the attending physicians and scheduled in a manner that is always optimal from the patient's standpoint, the necessity for readjustment of the injection set is still an unavoidable problem. This function can be fulfilled best by a competent nurse who is close at hand in a position to recognize and remedy the situation at once.

Patients receiving whole blood or red cell transfusions should be attended closely for at least 10 minutes after the start of the infusion, and the rate of injection during this period should not exceed 20 drops per minute. Thereafter, if no untoward reaction is apparent, and unless rapidity of injection is undesirable for other reasons, the rate may be increased. It is important that the flow be continuous. If it ceases, corrective measures should be undertaken by the nurse, if able to do so; otherwise, the physician must be notified immediately. Most important, the nurse must be prompt to note the appearance of any unfavorable response on the part of the recipient that might signify the development of a transfusion complication.

TRANSFUSION COMPLICATIONS

Transfusion therapy, whether conducted with whole blood, red cells or plasma, entails a number of calculated risks, because some of its potential complications cannot be prevented with absolute certainty, and some are sufficiently dangerous to merit serious consideration whenever treatment of this type is contemplated.

Circulatory Overloading

Pulmonary congestion may occur, whatever the nature of the transfusate, if the volume of injected material is excessive in relation to the patient's cardiac reserve. This is an unusual complication in recipients who have sustained a blood loss sufficient to precipitate shock, unless therapy is conducted very carelessly, but it is far from uncommon in individuals whose blood volume is normal or excessive at the start. Precautions for the prevention of pulmonary edema are particularly important in elderly patients, especially those suffering from cardiovascular disease. Pulmonary congestion is suggested by the development of cyanosis and dyspnea. Later, if the injection is continued, pulmonary edema is precipitated, heralded by stertorous breathing, persistent coughing and the production of frothy sputum.

Treatment demands that the transfusion be stopped immediately. The patient is placed in an orthopneic position, tourniquets are applied on the extremities in rotation, and, unless there is obvious and prompt improvement, venisection is employed without delay as the surest method of relieving this dangerous situation.

Transmission of Infection

Infections of many types can be transmitted from a blood donor to a transfusion recipient if there are bacteria, viruses or parasites in the donor blood at the time of the venisection. Of these, the most important to consider are syphilis, hepatitis and malaria. Syphilitic infection by transfusion is a relatively uncommon accident because of the precautions usually enforced in the screening of prospective donors and the serologic tests that are required before donor blood is released for transfusion. Malaria is a more frequent complication, since exclusion of this disease in donors, particularly of those types of malaria characterized by prolonged symptom-free intervals, is very difficult.

Virus hepatitis, of all transfusion risks, at present is recognized to be one of the most important. There are two distinct varieties of hepatitis, one called "epidemic hepatitis" and the other, "homologous serum jaundice." The incubation period characteristic of the epidemic type is 3 to 4 weeks; of homologous serum jaundice, 2 to 6 months. The risk is multiplied with successive transfusions on the basis of statistical probabilities, because it is estimated that one or the other of these viruses is present in the circulating blood of one out of every 300 to 600 individuals. The highest incidence of these diseases is in recipients of plasma prepared from large pools of donor blood (See Chap. 23).

Allergic and Pyrogenic Reactions

Allergic reactions in the form of urticaria (hives) or, far less commonly, asthmatic breathing may appear in the course of transfusion. In an effort to avoid this type of complication, allergic individuals generally are disqualified as blood donors, owing to the possibility that their blood may contain antibodies capable of reacting with protein materials (allergens) in the recipient's circulating blood. Nevertheless, hives may be anticipated in approximately 3 per cent of the cases. Allergic manifestations are most successfully treated by means of epinephrine, 0.5 ml. of a 1:1,000 solution being injected subcutaneously or, if respiratory difficulty is severe, 0.25 to 0.5 ml. intravenously. The oral administration of one of the antihistaminic agents, such as Benadryl or Pyribenzamine, is usually quite as effective, although relief may not follow for a period of 10 to 20 minutes.

Pyrogenic reactions due to bacterial contaminants are quite as common, if not more so, in transfusion recipients as in patients receiving fluids of the crystalloid type. These reactions are characterized by the sudden onset of chills and fever 40 to 60 minutes following the start of a pyrogenic infusion or, in this case, transfusion. Headache, nausea and vomiting may accompany the fever at its height. The total duration of the reaction may be as brief as 20 minutes or as prolonged as 8 hours. Treatment consists in discontinuing the transfusion, supplying extra blankets, as needed, and reducing discomfort by administering analgesics. The salicylates usually are effective in such cases; intramuscular Demerol (25 to 50 mg.) may be indicated in some instances, when symptoms are severe and oral medication is not tolerated.

Some of these febrile, nonhemolytic transfusion reactions have been attributed to the presence of "leukoagglutinins" (white blood cell antibodies) in the blood of the recipient, implying the development of an immunity against foreign leukocyte antigens introduced in the course of earlier transfusions. Preliminary processing of the donor blood by removal of the buffy coat after centrifuging has been recommended as a means of rendering it nonpyrogenic for such individuals. The usual explanation, however, implicates the familiar airborne bacterial contaminants that likewise are responsible for the "intravenous chills" described on page 87. The pyrogenic reactions that result from the use of improperly prepared transfusion sets are not always brief and harmless; at best they are unpleasant in the extreme; for very ill patients they can be fatal. From this standpoint, commercial disposable transfusion sets are incomparably superior to reusable equipment of any type yet devised, and their exclusive use is highly recommended.

Incompatible Transfusions

Most dangerous of all transfusion complications is the hemolytic reaction following the injection of red cells that are agglutinated by the plasma of the recipient. Transfusions that cause this complication are those in which donor blood contains the A or B antigen, when this particular antigen is lacking in the recipient. This type of reaction may also follow the injection of a red cell antigen other than A or B, provided the recipient lacks it and has been sensitized to it as a result of previous transfusion or pregnancy.*

An example of an ABO incompatibility would be the use of a group A donor for a group O recipient. The second type of situation would be exemplified by the

---

* Such antigens are numerous and include, among others, those belonging to the Rh, the Kell, Kidd, Duffy and MNS blood group systems.

use of an Rh-positive donor for an Rh-negative recipient.

An incompatibility that involves one of the major (ABO) blood groups almost always precipitates an immediate reaction in an unanesthetized patient, symptoms usually developing before the injection has been in progress for 10 minutes. The recipient may complain first of chilliness, headache and backache or abdominal distress and then exhibits a shaking chill followed by a high fever. There may be a precipitous fall in arterial blood pressure, accompanied by clinical evidences of profound vascular collapse.

When symptoms of this sort appear, or, indeed, if there is *any* untoward manifestation in the course of a transfusion, this is the signal for halting the procedure immediately, recognizing that, whereas incompatible blood given in amounts of less than 100 ml. rarely causes death, such blood in amounts exceeding 300 or 400 ml. is lethal in a substantial proportion of patients. The promptness with which symptoms of incompatibility usually develop, namely, within 10 minutes, regardless of the precise volume of material injected, is the basis for insisting on the constant attendance of transfused patients for the first 10 minutes at least and on slowness of injection during the initial period. Patients receiving incompatible blood while under general anesthesia unfortunately may provide no overt evidence of incompatibility, except perhaps an inexplicable drop in arterial blood pressure, and the risk of blood transfusion under these circumstances, without an effective alarm system, is multiplied greatly.

The sequence of events that follow the initial clinical response in patients receiving large volumes of incompatible blood is usually as follows: the patient may void a small volume of urine, dark-red or wine-red in color, and thereafter excrete little or no urine for several days. During this period he may look and feel quite well, but if, by the end of the second week, there has been no spontaneous diuresis, the manifestations of uremia supervene. The patient becomes obviously ill, progressively more so each day, complaining of nausea, vomiting, general malaise, weakness, abdominal pain and diarrhea. Finally, after a few days of increasing lethargy and deepening stupor, death may be anticipated. A fatal outcome is by no means the rule, however, for in a considerable proportion of patients, after a period of oliguria lasting 2 weeks or more, there develops a brisk diuresis followed by rapid and complete recovery. In the mildest cases the only obvious indication of a transfusion accident may be transient hemoglobinuria unaccompanied by untoward symptoms of any sort, the subsequent clinical course being completely uneventful. Transfusion reactions attributable to an Rh incompatibility are generally of the milder variety, chills, fever and transient hemoglobin-

uria perhaps comprising the entire symptomatology, but with each succeeding transfusion of Rh-incompatible blood the severity of these reactions increases until they are entirely those characteristic of a major blood group incompatibility.

Hemolytic transfusion reactions that are entirely asymptomatic occasionally are observed following transfusions of "universal donor" blood; the donor red cells are completely unaffected, but the red cells of the patient sustain damage caused by the incompatible agglutinins contained in the donor plasma. This is particularly apt to occur when patients belonging to groups A, B or AB receive group O blood containing anti-A and anti-B agglutinins in high concentration. Hemoglobinemia and hemoglobinuria do not often occur as complications of such transfusions, or, if they do develop, they are of very brief duration and completely without residual impairment of kidney function. Patients belonging to groups A, B or AB who repeatedly receive large volumes of incompatible plasma over a period of several days may exhibit a mild degree of icterus because of the excessive destruction of their own red cells, but other than the appearance of jaundice and signs of progressive anemia, there is little evidence to indicate a hemolytic reaction. Such hemolysis is nonetheless undesirable, obviously, and can be avoided by neutralizing the incompatible agglutinins before they are injected into the patient. This is accomplished by adding purified blood group A and B substances to the plasma or group O blood prior to transfusion.

Responsibilities of the Nurse

If the nurse suspects that a transfusion reaction may be developing, the injection of blood must be stopped abruptly, and the physician responsible for the patient should be summoned immediately. During the interim the nurse prepares to carry out certain procedures indicated in all patients in which an obvious or suspected reaction has occurred or is in progress.

1. The transfusion set is disconnected, and the needle either is withdrawn or is connected to an intravenous set for the slow administration of sodium chloride or another crystalloid solution, if it is desirable to keep this particular needle in place and patent for the purpose of securing blood specimens or for continued therapy.

2. *Do not empty the contents of the blood bottle or set!* This equipment should be sent at once, intact and with all labels attached, together with an explanatory note, to the laboratory responsible for the blood grouping and compatibility tests for an immediate repetition of these tests.

3. Secure a test tube containing about 0.5 ml. of sodium citrate solution (approx. 3 per cent concentra-

SUMMARY OF THE PROBLEMS OF THE TRANSFUSION RECIPIENT

Transfusion Complications

Nursing Implications

1. *Circulatory Overloading*

   If the volume of the blood exceeds the cardiac output, the following symptoms of pulmonary congestion may occur:
   a. dyspnea
   b. cough
   c. frothy sputum

   Stop the transfusion immediately.
   Known cardiac patients and elderly patients should receive blood at a slower rate.
   Place the patient upright with his feet and legs in a dependent position.
   Apply rotating tourniquets if indicated.

2. *Transmission of Disease*

   The virus of hepatitis and malarial parasites may be transmitted from donor to recipient via infected blood.
   There is no known laboratory test to exclude these diseases in the donor.

   A careful history should be taken of every donor.

3. *Febrile (Pyrogenic) Reactions*

   These may be due to bacterial proteins in needles, blood, bottles, etc., or possibly to the presence of leuko-agglutinins in the recipient's blood.
   Symptoms: (may occur after blood is discontinued)
   a. sudden chilling and fever
   b. headache
   c. nausea and vomiting

   Stop the transfusion immediately.
   Take the temperature one-half hour after the chill and as indicated thereafter.

4. *Bacterial Contamination*

   Bacteria may gain access to the blood and multiply.
   Symptoms:
   a. severe fever and chills
   b. nausea and vomiting
   c. persistent shock-like state

   Stop the blood immediately. Send the remainder of the blood to the laboratory.
   Call the physician immediately.
   Use rigid asepsis with transfusion equipment.

5. *Allergic Reactions*

   Allergic individuals should not donate blood because their blood may contain antibodies capable of reacting with allergens in the recipient's blood.
   Symptoms:
   a. hives
   b. laryngeal edema
   c. asthmatic wheezing

   Stop the transfusion.
   The individual who has had a previous allergic reaction to blood may be given an antihistamine before subsequent transfusions.
   Prepare epinephrine if respiratory distress is severe.
   Watch for indications of laryngeal edema.
   Antihistamine drugs may be given orally.

6. *Hemolytic Reactions*

   Hemolysis follows when incompatible red cells are injected into the patient's circulating blood.

   Symptoms:
   a. chilliness
   b. feeling of head fullness
   c. oppressive feeling in the chest
   d. sharp pain in lumbar area
   e. flushing of face
   f. distention of neck veins
   g. fall of blood pressure
   h. vascular depression

   Positively identify patient and blood before transfusion is started.
   Stay with the patient during the first 10 minutes that he is receiving the transfusion.
   Administer blood at 20 drops per minute during this period.
   Stop the transfusion immediately if the symptoms occur.
   Call the physician at once.
   Give mannitol as indicated.
   Encourage fluid intake for next few hours.
   Measure and save all urine voided. Keep accurate intake and output record.
   Send blood and transfusion equipment to the laboratory for immediate repetition of typing and crossmatching.

tion) for the collection of a blood sample required for the exclusion of hemoglobinemia (the presence of free hemoglobin in the plasma is indicative of a hemolytic reaction).

4. Arrange that this collection be made as soon as possible. Use a 5-ml. or 10-ml. syringe rinsed with sterile sodium chloride or sodium citrate solution; this sample should be obtained with the utmost care and should be sent at once to a laboratory for immediate separation of the plasma and inspection of the latter for the presence or absence of free hemoglobin.

5. Arrangements are made in detail for a sampling of the next voided specimen of urine; this, as soon as it is secured, is likewise sent to the laboratory for hemoglobin tests.

If a hemolytic reaction is diagnosed on the basis of these examinations, an intravenous infusion of mannitol is given (approximately 100 gm. in 20 per cent concentration). After 1 liter of fluid is received, however, unless the patient is also suffering from dehydration or blood loss, no further parenteral treatment is indicated until the renal function can be estimated. Thus, one must foresee the possibility that practically no urine may be secreted for many days, and, if death occurs during this period, it is far more likely to result from excessive fluid therapy than from kidney failure alone. If complete anuria or severe oliguria does develop, oral feeding is halted; all nutrient and hydration therapy is supplied in the form of intravenous solutions, the selection of which must depend on the particular requirements of the individual patient. On no account must the total volume each day be allowed to exceed by a margin of more than 1 liter the amount of urine secreted within the preceding 24-hour period in extremely hot weather, or 500 ml. when the room temperature is moderate and perspiration is minimal.

The nursing staff must be fully aware of its responsibilities in relation to the measurements of fluid volumes received and excreted and of the necessity for complete and accurate recording of this information, vitally required for the control of water balance and the conduct of parenteral therapy in these patients. Precision in this regard is an absolute necessity, for as long as anuria persists the patient's life is balanced perilously between two threats: dehydration and gross electrolyte imbalance on the one hand and, on the other, overhydration resulting in pulmonary edema— in other words, therapeutic drowning. Either of these disasters may easily destroy life while there may yet be time for the spontaneous recovery of kidney function and the patient's own salvation.

BIBLIOGRAPHY

Foster, M. A.: Teaching blood groups and reactions. Nurs. Outlook, *14*:49-50, Feb., 1966.

Gurski, B. M.: Rationale of nursing care for patients with blood dyscrasias. Nurs. Clin. N. Amer., *1*:23-30, March, 1966.

Moore, F. D.: Blood transfusions: rates, routes and hazards. Nurs. Clin. N. Amer., *1*:285-294, June, 1966.

Seal, A. L.: The nurse's responsibility in anticoagulant therapy. Nurs. Clin. N. Amer., *1*:325-331, June, 1966.

Strumia, M. M., and Strumia, P. V.: Blood substitutes. Hosp. Med. 3:36, July, 1967.

The Preoperative Patient

- *Surgery in the Past*
- *Surgery at Present*
- *The Nurse and the Surgical Patient*
- *Preoperative Patient Care*
- *The Patient's Family*

SURGERY IN THE PAST

Surgery was performed long before the dawn of civilization with the aid of a sharpened flint. Neolithic skulls with trephined holes show evidence of bony repair and prove that patients did survive major operations. Surgery developed remarkably in ancient India; a clear-cut and logical classification of surgical operations is given in the famous writing, the Samhita. It is recorded also that women who helped with the sick had to have clean hands and nails cut short. In Greece (400 B.C.), Hippocrates knew and described surgical conditions varying from a clubfoot to a fracture of the vertebra. Prostheses, such as false limbs and dentures, were made for patients. Plastic operations were performed, and bladder stones were removed. Surgery advanced more rapidly than medicine, probably because its results were more dramatic. Surgical nursing as such is not mentioned in these early histories, but it must have existed.

One of the many stories in the New Testament at the beginning of the Christian era is:

And he went to him, and bound up his wounds, pouring in oil and wine, and set him on his own beast, and brought him to an inn, and took care of him.   LUKE 10:34

The good Samaritan gave nursing care. He found a man who had been beaten cruelly by thieves. After he had cared for his wounds, the Samaritan took his patient to an inn and continued to care for him. One realizes that the emphasis of his care was on the person with the wound and not the wound alone.

There were no remarkable developments in surgery or in nursing for many centuries after the beginning of the Christian era. Through these years there is reference to two groups of nurses: those associated with some religious group and those who nursed for hire. Little mention is made of nurses who cared specifically for surgical patients. At the time of Lister's introduction of carbolic acid as an antiseptic in the 19th century, one is made aware that nurses assisted in the operating room. About this time the seeds of present-day nursing were planted by Florence Nightingale as she cared for the wounded soldiers in the Crimean War. In particular, she emphasized the significance of good hygiene, and she was a strong advocate of planned instruction for nurses.

Up to the 19th century, tradition had a strong influence and a restricting effect on progress. The general practitioner treated all ills. There were few who limited their practice to surgery and almost none who limited their field to specialized types of surgery. However, following the industrial revolution, tradition relaxed, and the more highly skilled tasks necessary to operate machinery introduced specialization. A parallel in the medical field was the rise of the specialist. If a person had difficulty with his ear, he went to an ear specialist. Our emphasis today is not on the ear as such but on the person who has an ear problem. And so, in surgical nursing, our concern is not the appendectomy but the patient who has undergone surgery for appendicitis.

SURGERY AT PRESENT

The greatest progress in the care of the surgical patient has taken place since the beginning of the present century. An increasing knowledge of disease as a result of research has permitted the development of many diagnostic aids. Some of these depend upon roentgenograms, laboratory procedures such as chemi-

cal, bacteriologic, and pathologic determinations, as well as monitoring devices and computer aids. The result is that the diagnosis of disease is made with more exactness and certainty than was possible from the simple clinical examinations of previous days. It became apparent that the fluids, electrolytes and nutritional condition of the patient were important factors in the outcome of a surgical procedure.

In the operating room, the surgeon has been aided by progressive improvement in instruments, equipment and conveniences in construction. Improvement in the understanding and the practice of asepsis and various technical procedures enables surgeons to perform operations that would not have been possible before. Not the least of these improvements has been the

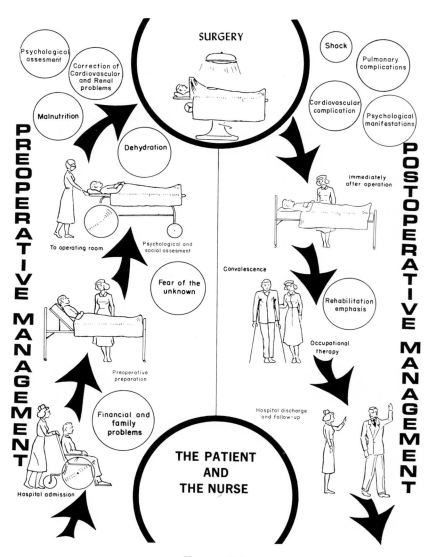

FIGURE 9-1.

development of the anesthesiologist, and with him have come many advances in the technique of the administration of anesthesia because of a better understanding of pharmacodynamics and physiologic function of the body. These advances have made it possible to deal surgically with lesions in the chest, the brain, the heart and the great vessels, and with extensive malignancies in many parts of the body—something unheard of before.

One of the most striking developments has been the result of research in the control of infection. The discovery of the sulfonamides and the production of more effective and less toxic drugs were followed by the advent of the antibiotics, so that many infections that led previously to surgery now can be treated conservatively. These drugs may be used to prevent infections after operations and to treat such infections should they arise, thus reducing greatly the operative hazard.

Many new fields of therapy have opened for the surgical patient. To mention them all would be impossible, but the therapeutic use of radiant energy, such as radium, x-rays and radioactive materials, may be used as an example.

A final advance in the care of the surgical patient is the change in attitude of all those who have a part in his care. It is recognized that the care of the surgical lesion is only a part of the care of the patient as a person: the important thing is to rehabilitate the patient and to return him to his home a healthy, happy, contributing member of society. This concept has many aspects. It may be concerned with the psychosomatic cause of the surgical disease, such as the influence of mental stress and overfatigue upon the production of peptic ulcer, or it may deal with the development of a mental attitude toward the acceptance of a colostomy or an amputation. In this rehabilitation, the patient and even his family frequently require training and instruction. Realizing that the best rehabilitation is a return to activities at an early date, the patient is gotten out of bed as soon as possible after the operation. Experience and study has proved that wounds heal well, that complications are decreased and that the general metabolism and the morale of the patient are improved by early ambulation. Prosthetic appliances that permit a more normal life for patients who have deformities have helped a great deal. Along with these important contributions to the rehabilitation of patients has come an increasing interest in the prevention of disease. Periodic health examinations, cancer detection clinics and industrial and public health education are playing an increasingly important part in the prevention of disease and the early detection of what would lead to serious surgical lesions if neglected.

THE NURSE AND THE SURGICAL PATIENT

With this improvement in the care of the surgical patient has come a change in the attitude, the functions and the responsibilities of the nurse. By being a vital member of the health team, the nurse is aware of her ability to assist the potential surgical patient even before his hospital admission. A neighbor, friend or relative is grateful for her answers to his questions about the surgical experience he will soon have. Concerns often arise after leaving the physician's office that are disturbing if unanswered. If the nurse disseminates information verbally or with instructional pamphlets, emotional concerns can be lessened. Often the nurse who is in close contact with the patient is able to relate pertinent information to the surgeon that may affect the patient's total care plan. The nurse also is expected to assess patient needs, develop a plan of care, and evaluate and modify this plan in line with the patient's progress.

PREOPERATIVE PATIENT CARE

Psychological Preparation (See also Chapter 3)

Any kind of surgical procedure always is preceded by some type of emotional reaction in a patient, whether it is obvious or not. From the psychological point of view, the student learns that a mind that is not at peace influences directly the proper functioning of the body. Fear of the unknown, of death, of anesthesia or of cancer may or may not be apparent immediately, but other fears may be more intangible and overt—those, for example, regarding the possible loss of a job, the need to support a family or the possibility of permanent incapacity. Not infrequently one sees a sick body that has resulted wholly from emotional insecurity, such as is evident many times in patients with a stomach ulcer or an inflamed, ulcerating colon. Emotional upsets are more apparent in illness. Consequently, the nurse who learns this early in her career will be more tolerant and understanding. Unfortunately, not all adults are mature persons. They may be adult physically but not emotionally.

Fear is expressed in different ways by different individuals. For example, fear may be expressed indirectly by the young woman who asks a lot of questions, many of them repeated even though the answers were given previously. For another person, the reaction may be withdrawal, such as deliberate avoidance of communication by concentrating on a book. Still another individual may talk incessantly about trivialities. Often such behavior ends abruptly as the patient turns to the nurse and says, "I guess you can tell I am a bit nervous about my operation." The need to keep the outlet of communication open is never greater than at this time. To belittle the patient's fears by saying, "Oh, there's nothing to be afraid of," immediately closes the door and causes the patient to lapse into his own less effective means of coping with his fears.

An essential part of the preoperative phase of patient care is the diagnostic study. The nurse should understand the purpose of each test and help to keep the patient informed. Too many times, a patient feels that he is being treated as a "guinea pig." There need be no such reaction if the nurse assumes her full role.

Bird* acknowledges the psychological contribution of comfort and reassurance but emphasizes that even more important is the need to

> *keep open the patient's lines of communication* to see that he is properly informed of everything he should know, that he does not receive misinformation, and that he himself can communicate freely with his surgeon and his relatives, thus allowing him to make his own requests and to ask his own questions. Other lines to be kept open are those between the relatives and the surgeon, between the nurse and the surgeon, and between all other working personnel.

Communication lines break down because of the number of persons who come in contact with the patient, the strangeness of the surgical floor (strange apparatus, a seemingly new language, increased tempo of activity) and the patient's own fears and anxieties. Such breakdowns in satisfactory interrelations leave the patient upset, bewildered and even unable to follow simple directions. Often in the course of conversation, something which was mentioned by a nurse or a physician becomes exaggerated out of all proportion to its importance. For example, because of a filled schedule, an operation had to be postponed. The patient was told that "something had come up." As he thought about this remark, the patient began to worry that something concerning himself was unsatisfactory; therefore, his condition must be deteriorating.

Let us examine the causes of fear that a preoperative patient may experience.

Fear of anesthesia was justified years ago, when little was known of the control and the effect of anesthetic agents. But with refined methods, tested drugs and skilled anesthesiologists, the hazards are minimized. The ease with which a patient accepts an anesthetic today is attributed to the adequate physical and mental preparation that he receives. The price of poor preparation is a difficult period of induction, followed by an unpleasant emergence from the anesthetic agent. The nurse in her daily association with

her patient can do much to dispel false conceptions and misinformation. In instances in which the anesthesiologist visits the patient the day before surgery, real confidence is established, and the patient accepts the anesthetic more gracefully.

Often the fear of the anesthetic is secondary to the *fear of pain or of death.* Will I feel the knife? What if the anesthesia wears off? The patient needs reassurance that the anesthesiologist will be in constant attendance to take care of these problems. Some surgeons will not operate on a patient who is convinced that he will die. This is a real fear, and it cannot be dismissed lightly. Good rapport between patient and nurse, together with tact on the nurse's part, may bring him to a realization that his fear is magnified. It will help him greatly if those responsible for his care build up his confidence.

The *fear of the unknown* is the worst of all. Part of this fear stems from a belief on the patient's part that he is not being told "everything" about his diagnosis or illness. Therefore, the more understanding one has of the probabilities for the future, the better is the adjustment. The nurse can do much to allay the anxieties of her patient and induce a certain peace of mind. A patient frequently expresses fears and misgivings to the nurse but hides them from the surgeon. In such circumstances the nurse should communicate these evidences of anxiety privately to the surgeon.

The *fear of destruction of body image* occurs more frequently than it did a few years ago because surgery in many instances has become more radical. Then too, there is greater emphasis today on youth, the body beautiful, and more revealing clothing as verified by magazine and television advertising. Consequently, any encroachment on the body that may be necessary by surgery is viewed with distress by many individuals.

Fear of separation from former activities, family and friends may compound the concerns and anxieties of the preoperative patient.

The average person has many *worries* when he is well, but he has more when he is ill. He may have financial problems, family responsibilities and employment obligations; in addition to these, he may fear a poor prognosis or the probability of a handicap in the future. These problems can be investigated by the nurse. If the difficulty is of such a nature that a medical social worker can give assistance, the aid of such a person should be enlisted. If the worry stems from fear of what the prognosis is likely to be, the physician should be informed.

When some of these fears have been expressed, brought to light and examined in their proper perspective, it is possible and even essential to get the patient to reveal what the operation means to him. Have him express his thoughts with regard to the importance and

---

* Bird, Brian: Psychological aspects of preoperative and postoperative care. Amer. J. Nurs. 55:685, 1955.

the meaning of this surgery for the immediate future and the more distant future. This is usually done by the surgeon, but, in the event that questions remain, the nurse may be in a position to elicit these from the patient. The importance of adequate lines of communication between surgeon and nurse must be emphasized here as they work together to prepare their patient for surgery.

The significance of *spiritual therapy* must not be forgotten. Regardless of the religious affiliation of the patient, the nurse must recognize that faith in a Higher Power can be as therapeutic as medication. Every attempt must be made to help the patient achieve the fullest spiritual help that he requests. This may be accomplished by participating in prayer, by reading passages from the Scriptures or by calling a

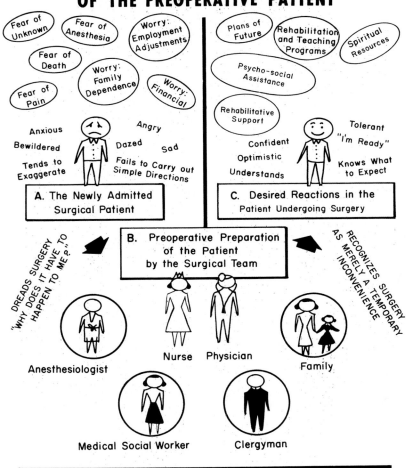

PSYCHOLOGICAL PREPARATION OF THE PREOPERATIVE PATIENT

FIGURE 9-2.

clergyman. Faith has great sustaining power; the beliefs of each individual patient should be respected and supported.

The interval of time preparatory to surgery may become very extended. *Recreational and diversional activities,* such as reading, listening to the radio, watching television, handcrafts, games and so forth, are useful. The nurse can arrange for individuals with similar interests to meet. Many times patients can help one another.

Perhaps the most valuable facility at the disposal of the nurse is her ability to *listen* to the patient. By engaging in conversation and using the principles of tactful interviewing, the nurse can acquire invaluable bits of information. An unhurried, understanding and kind nurse invites confidence on the part of her patient.

Lastly, every patient should be treated as an individual who has fears and hopes quite apart from the fears and hopes of the next person. To understand and help one patient may require a completely different approach from that used on another.* (See Fig. 9-2.)

Operative Permit

Before the surgeon has the right to operate, it is necessary to obtain a voluntary and informed consent from the patient. Such written permission, witnessed by the physician, nurse or other authorized person, protects the patient against unsanctioned surgery and protects the surgeon and the hospital against claims of an unauthorized operation. Prior to signing his permit, the patient should be told in clear and simple terms, using diagrams or models if necessary, what the surgeon proposes. This is usually done by the surgeon. The patient also ought to be informed by the surgeon of possible complications, disfigurement, disability, and removal of parts as well as what to expect in the early and late postoperative periods. Permission should be repeated for each operation, for each procedure in which it is necessary to enter a body cavity (cystoscopy, paracentesis, etc.) and when general anesthesia is given as for a closed reduction of a fracture.

The patient may sign his own permit for operation if he is of age and mentally capable. If he is a minor, unconscious, or irresponsible, permission must be obtained from a responsible family member. In an emergency, it may be necessary for the surgeon to operate as a life-saving measure without a permit. However, every effort should be made to contact the patient's

---

* A practice that is of inestimable value to the preoperative patient who has problems is the nursing conference in which members of the nursing team and members of associated disciplines participate. On occasion the patient may be a member of the conference and receive guidance and assistance.

family. In such a situation, consent by telephone, telegram or letter is acceptable.

The operative permit is placed in a prominent place on the patient's chart and accompanies the patient to the operating room.

Early Assessment and Physical Preparation of the Surgical Patient

Physical Evaluation and Diagnostic Tests

Before treatment is initiated, the patient is given a physical examination. The physician and the nurse must respect his feelings and his sense of modesty. In bathing the patient, the nurse may note significant physical findings, such as a rash, decubitus ulcer and so forth, that may be contributory. These preliminary administrations are ideal times for the patient to get acquainted with those who will be caring for him and provide the opportunity for him to ask questions.

There may be many diagnostic tests, such as blood counts, roentgenographic studies, gastric analyses, tissue biopsies and stool and urine examinations. In all these tests the nurse plays an important part. She is in a position to help her patient understand the need for diagnostic studies. She is aware that it is important to collect specimens and to describe them accurately in her charting.

Effect of the Aging Process

It is important for the nurse to remember that in the older person, reactions to injury are less pronounced and slower in appearing. The aged do not stand dehydration at all well. Their long established diabetes, anemia, obesity, hypoproteinemia and so forth must be considered. Certain drugs are dangerous because they are poorly tolerated. Scopolamine, morphia and the barbiturates are likely to cause confusion and disorientation, even excitement and apprehension. Some drugs have a cumulative effect. Sleeping and eating habits and the use of alcohol and laxatives, as well as the nightly "sleeping" medicine, must not be dismissed as unimportant (see pp. 52-55).

Fluid, Electrolyte and Nutritional Condition

Common conditions that adversely affect a surgical risk may be dehydration and malnutrition. Perhaps the patient has been vomiting or losing fluids in some other way; this results in a disturbed fluid and electrolyte balance. Parenteral fluids prescribed to meet the deficiency will be ordered. In such a situation it is important to keep a good record of total intake and output. Malnutrition may be alleviated by high caloric diets with adequate vitamins and proteins. Vitamin C and protein are significant in tissue repair and in increasing resistance to infection. The diet may be supplemented with these essentials. In marked protein deficiency, it may be necessary for the patient to have transfusions of whole blood or blood plasma; protein hydrolysates may be given intravenously. Dental caries and poor mouth hygiene may contribute to general debilitation and should be corrected. (Also see Chaps. 7 and 21.)

Obesity

If time permits, physicians will insist that a prescribed and systematic program of weight reduction be undertaken so that the surgical risk is lessened. Obesity increases the seriousness of complications to a great extent. During surgery, fatty tissues are not highly resistant to infection; the surgeon faces increased technical and mechanical problems, and therefore dehiscence and wound infections are more common. These patients are difficult to nurse because of their weight; they breathe poorly when lying on their side and so are subject to hypoventilation and postoperative pulmonary complications, distention and phlebitis. In addition, cardiovascular, endocrine, hepatic and biliary diseases are more common in obese patients. It has been estimated that for each 30 pounds of excess weight, about 25 additional miles of blood vessels are needed. The increased demands on the heart are obvious.

Presence of other Disease Conditions

Cardiovascular Disease. Since the margin of safety is less when a patient exhibits signs of cardiovascular disease, more than usual diligence during all phases of management are required. Depending upon the severity of symptoms, surgery may be deferred until maximal benefits have been obtained from medical treatment. At times, surgical treatment can be modified to meet the likely tolerance of the patient. For example, an obese patient with acute obstructive cholecystitis may also have diabetes and coronary artery disease. Simple gallbladder drainage with removal of calculi may be done rather than a more complete operation.

Of particular significance in the patient with cardiovascular disease is the necessity to avoid sudden changes of position, prolonged immobilization, hypotension or hypoxia, and overloading the body with fluids or blood.

Diabetes. In uncontrolled diabetes, the chief life-threatening hazard is that of hypoglycemia, which may develop during anesthesia or postoperatively. It results from inadequate carbohydrates or insulin overdosage. Other hazards which threaten but occur less rapidly are acidosis and glycosuria. In general, the surgical risk of the patient with controlled diabetes is not greater than the nondiabetic. (Also see p. 693.)

Upper Respiratory and Pulmonary Disease. It is necessary to maintain adequate ventilation during all phases of surgical treatment; therefore, elective surgery is usually contraindicated when the patient has a respiratory infection. Chronic disease of the air passages or lungs also increase the danger of postoperative pulmonary complications. Patients with emphysema or bronchiectasis are treated with aerosol medications and postural drainage for several days before surgery.

Renal Disease. Surgery is contraindicated when a patient has acute nephritis, acute renal insufficiency with oliguria or anuria, or other acute renal problems unless it is a life-saving measure or when surgery is necessary to improve urinary function as in a prostatectomy.

Alcoholism. The acutely intoxicated person is susceptible to injury. If surgery is required, local or regional block anesthesia is used for minor surgery; for more extensive injury, surgery is postponed if possible. Otherwise, the stomach must be intubated and aspirated before general anesthesia is administered to ensure against vomiting and aspiration.

The person with a history of chronic alcoholism often suffers from malnutrition and other systemic problems; therefore, the surgical risk is increased.

Prior Drug Therapy. Increasing attention is being paid to the history of drug usage by the patient. Potent medications have an effect on physiological functions; interaction of such drugs with anesthetic agents have caused serious problems such as arterial hypotension and circulatory collapse or depression.

How significant these drugs are is determined by the anesthesiologist by considering the length of time they were used by the patient, his condition and the nature of the proposed surgery. Those drugs that are particularly of concern are:

Adrenal steroids—It is not advisable to discontinue corticosteroids before surgery.

Diuretics—In particular, the thiazide drugs may cause excess respiratory depression during anesthesia; this is produced by an electrolyte imbalance.

Phenothiazines—These may increase hypotensive action of anesthetics.

Antidepressants—In particular, monoamine oxidase (MAO) inhibitors increase hypotensive effects of anesthetics.

Antibiotics—For example, neomycin, streptomycin, kanamycin, polymyxin A and B and viomycin. When combined with a curariform muscle relaxant, nerve transmission is interrupted and apnea due to respiratory paralysis may result.

General Preoperative Nursing Care

To summarize, the preparation and the care of the patient before operation are guided by an understanding of him as a unique, multifaceted individual. *Our*

TABLE 9-1. Classification of physical status for anesthesia prior to surgery

Classification	Description	Example
I. Good	No organic disease, no systemic disturbance	Uncomplicated hernias, fractures
II. Fair	Moderate systemic disturbance	Mild cardiac (I and II), mild diabetes
III. Poor	Severe systemic disturbance	Poorly controlled diabetes, pulmonary complications, moderate cardiac (III)
IV. Serious	Systemic disease threatening life	Severe renal disease, severe cardiac disease (IV), decompensation
V. Emergency, Good	Patients in Groups I and II with a complication needing treatment	Hemorrhage, open chest wound, perforated viscus, severe respiratory embarrassment
VI. Emergency, Poor	Patients in Groups III and IV with a complication needing immediate surgery	Hemorrhage, open chest wound, perforated viscus, severe respiratory embarrassment
VII. Special	Moribund patients	

From: American Society of Anesthesiology, Inc.: Codes for the Collection and Tabulation of Data Relating to Anesthesia, Inhalation Therapy and Therapeutic and Diagnostic Blocks.

objective is known; that is, to get the patient into the best possible condition for surgery. The means of achieving that goal are determined by the needs of the individual patient.

Surgeons and hospitals differ greatly in the detail of preparation for operation, but the general principle remains the same: to make the patient as clean as possible, externally and internally, and to cause the least possible amount of physical and mental exhaustion in doing so. The reasons for preoperative procedures are obvious. All sources of infection must be eliminated, hence the scrupulous cleanliness of the operative site. The intestines and the bladder must be empty to prevent their contents from being discharged involuntarily while the patient is under the influence of the anesthetic and to preclude an accidental incision in them, as sometimes occurs in an abdominal operation when these organs are distended. This is true particularly of the bladder and is the chief reason why it must be empty before a patient is sent to the operating room for a laparotomy.

Any preparation of the patient before operation should be carried out in the most efficient and capable way. Never approach a patient with an air of indecision: to do so causes him to lose confidence at once, and lost confidence is not regained easily. Determine exactly what procedures are to be performed and proceed with them in a systematic manner. If the treatment seems to be at all alarming to the patient, explain to him what you are about to do. Always work quietly, thoroughly and neatly; bustle, confusion and noise harass the patient.

During this period of preparation, from the time of admission to the actual operation, one of the most important responsibilities of the nurse is very close observation of the patient. Any sneezing, sniffling and coughing must be reported to the attending surgeon at once. Failure to do so may lead to postoperative pulmonary complications in the patient.

Hygienic Measures

The patient should have a warm bath the night before operation. A shampoo several days before operation is advisable, unless the condition of the patient does not warrant it. The teeth should be brushed thoroughly twice a day and the mouth rinsed with a mild antiseptic solution at least 3 times a day.

Nutrition

When the operation is scheduled for the morning, the meal the evening before may be an ordinary light diet. Water may, and should be, given freely up to 4 hours before operation. In dehydrated patients, and especially in older ones, fluids often are encouraged by mouth before operation. In addition, and especially in patients to whom fluids cannot be given by mouth, they are administered by vein. If the operation is scheduled to take place after noon and is not to be upon any part of the gastrointestinal tract, the patient may be given a soft diet for breakfast.

Starvation, exhaustion, prolonged loss of fluids from fistulous tracts or vomiting results in loss of calories, vitamins and proteins (hypoproteinemia). The preparation of such patients for operation demands the use of transfusions of blood, plasma or amino acid preparations. The particular vitamins needed may be added as indicated. (See Chapter 7.)

Enema

A warm cleansing enema may be given the evening before operation, and may be repeated if ineffectual. Unless the condition of the patient presents some contraindication, the commode, and not the bedpan, should be used in evacuating the enema.

Preoperative Skin Preparation

The aim of preoperative skin care is to render the skin as free as possible of microorganisms without damage to its physical and physiological integrity.

Where there is time, such as in surgery of a nonemergency nature, the physician may suggest that the patient use a soap containing hexachlorophene to cleanse the skin area for several days before surgery in order to help to reduce the number of skin organisms. After the bath, the area in the region of the operative field is cleansed particularly by the use of warm water and soap. The patient is told about the shaving procedure, placed in a comfortable position, and not exposed unduly. Any adhesive or grease may be removed readily with a sponge moistened in benzene or ether, if the odor is not objectionable to the patient. All hair must be shaved from the area to be operated upon (it is embarrassing to have a surgeon call for a razor after the patient is placed on the operating table). Be very sure to have a sharp razor and to shave thoroughly a liberal area including and surrounding the operative site to aid in reducing sources of contamination. Scratches should be avoided, and any skin eruptions must be reported because they are potential sites of infection.

In most hospitals, a male nurse or nursing assistant takes care of male patients. Skin shaving may be done by a special "prep" team, by the nurse assigned to the patient or by a member of the operating room team. Disposable "prep" trays are available which ensure individualized equipment.

Some surgeons require nothing further in the way of local preparation than thorough shaving and cleansing of the part until the patient reaches the operating room.

Certain factors need to be recognized in attempting to render the operative site as clean as possible for the proposed surgery:

(1) Human skin by nature harbors bacterial flora, both transients and residents; some of these are pathogens.

(2) Skin cannot be sterilized without destroying skin cells.

(3) No existing antiseptic produces instant skin disinfection.

(4) The practice of applying antiseptics on the skin (on the patient division) and covering the area with sterile dressings and towels until incision time is worthless.

(5) Effectiveness of the bactericidal agent against bacteria is hastened when gauze friction is used to apply the antiseptic.

Depilatory Cream.* Chemical compounds (creams to remove hair) have been perfected sufficiently to make them safe for preparing the skin of the surgical patient. Long hairs may be cut before applying the cream as an economy measure, since less cream would be required; however, cutting hair in the operating room area must be done very cautiously to eliminate loose-flying hair, which would be a source of contamination.

The depilatory cream usually comes in a collapsible metal tube and is expressed on the body surface. The cream is spread to a smooth layer of about ½ inch in depth over the entire operative site by a wooden tongue blade or a gloved hand. After the cream has been allowed to remain on the skin for 10 minutes, it is scraped off gently with the tongue blade or multiple moistened gauze sponges. When all cream and hair have been removed, the skin is then washed with soap and water and patted dry.

There are several advantages to using a depilatory cream for preoperative skin preparation. A clean, smooth and intact skin is produced. Scrapes, abrasions, cuts and poor hair removal are eliminated. It is more comfortable for the patient since he is less apprehensive and often finds this method relaxing. There is even the possibility of the patient preparing himself in selected operative procedures. Depilatory creams are more effective and safer for use on uncooperative or agitated patients. This method is no more expensive than other methods. A disadvantage is that a few patients have had some transient skin reactions involving rectal and scrotal areas.

Operative Fields

Cranial Operations. Obtain specific instructions from the surgeon as to the extent of shaving that is necessary.

Thyroid and Neck Operations. Shave the anterior neck from under the chin to the nipple line. The area should be shaved back to the hair line and to meet the bed line when the patient is lying supine.

* Ginsberg, F., Brunner, L. S. and Cantlin, V.: A Manual of Operating Room Technology. p. 134. Philadelphia, J. B. Lippincott, 1966.

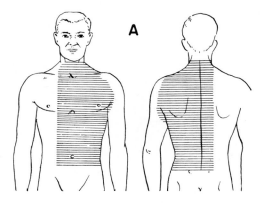

FIG. 9-3A. Area of preparation for operation on the thorax.

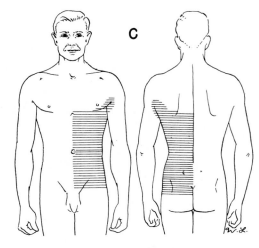

FIG. 9-3C. Area to be prepared for nephrectomy. Note that the preparation should be on both the anterior and the posterior sides of the trunk.

Operations upon the Chest. Shave the affected side from the spine posteriorly to beyond the mid-line anteriorly, and from the clavicle to the umbilicus. See Fig. 9-3A.

Breast Amputation. Shave the axilla on the affected side. Skin preparation should extend from above the clavicle to the umbilicus, from beyond the mid-line anteriorly to beyond the mid-line posteriorly. Particular care should be taken in cleansing the folds underneath the breast. See Fig. 9-3B.

Nephrectomy. Note that the preparation should be on both the anterior and the posterior sides of the trunk. See Fig. 9-3C.

Operations upon the Abdomen. Shave from the nipple line in males and from below the breast in females to, and including, the pubic area. Laterally, shaving should extend to the anterior axillary line. Particular care should be taken in cleansing the umbilicus and the inguinal creases. See Fig. 9-3D.

Inguinal Hernia. Shave the lower abdomen from the umbilicus downward, including the suprapubic area and about 6 inches of the upper thigh on the af-

fected side. Particular attention should be paid to cleansing the groin.

Operations on the Lower Bowel and the Rectum. Shave the entire abdomen as for any abdominal operation and prepare the perineum as for any anal operation. See Fig. 9-3E.

Anal Operations. Shave the area for a distance of about 10 inches from the anus. A suprapubic preparation is not necessary in male patients, but a partial perineal shave should be carried out in female patients. See Fig. 9-3E.

Amputations. The area should be shaved and the skin cleansed for a distance of about 12 inches above and below the proposed site of amputation. It is important for the nurse to know where the amputation is

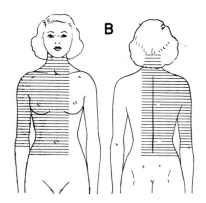

FIG. 9-3B. Preparation for amputation of breast.

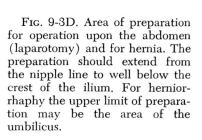

FIG. 9-3D. Area of preparation for operation upon the abdomen (laparotomy) and for hernia. The preparation should extend from the nipple line to well below the crest of the ilium. For herniorrhaphy the upper limit of preparation may be the area of the umbilicus.

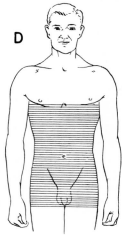

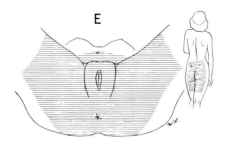

Fig. 9-3E. Area to be prepared for operations on the perineum. These areas should be shaved completely for all gynecologic operations, operations around the anus and for such combined operations as an abdominoperineal resection of the rectum.

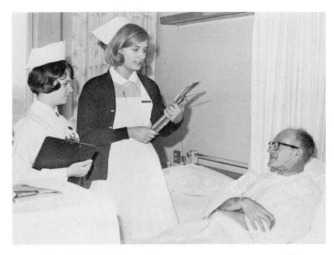

Fig. 9-4. Mr. J. is seeking answers to some troubling questions regarding his surgery which is scheduled for the next day. (Hospital of the University of Pennsylvania)

to be performed. Thus, in gangrene of the foot, the amputation often is through the thigh, and it is necessary, therefore, to prepare the thigh.

Skin Grafts. Shave both anterior thighs or the area from which a graft is to be taken. Request instructions. In many hospitals the preparation of the operative field is done by aids or technicians from the operating room staff.

Operations upon the Spine. Shave and prepare the skin for an area of 12 inches above and below the site of operation. Ask the surgeon for instructions.

When the nurse is not sure above the area to be prepared, she always should ask for instructions.

Instruction of the Preoperative Patient. The value of preoperative instruction to the patient about to have surgery has been recognized and is now substantiated by several studies. However, each patient is taught as an individual; he has certain anxieties, needs, and hopes. His background of relevant information is usually very different from that of the next patient. Once these differences are recognized and particular needs are assessed, a program of instruction can be planned. It is implemented at the proper time. If he is taught essential information several days before he needs it, it will not be remembered. If he is instructed too close to the time of surgery, he may not be in prime learning condition because of the effect of the preanesthetic medication. When offered at a time when the patient is most receptive and can participate in the learning process, instruction will be most useful to him at the time he needs the information.

Effective preoperative patient instruction has many advantages: (1) recuperation is more rapid; (2) drugs are used less frequently and in lower concentration; (3) fewer complications occur; and (4) hospitalization is shortened.

Deep Breathing and Coughing. The nurse first demonstrates to the patient how to take a deep breath slowly and how to exhale slowly. The patient is then asked to do it and is told to take deep breaths after the operation without being reminded by the nurse. He should know that he might be uncomfortable when taking deep breaths or coughing but that medication will be given to alleviate the discomfort. An effective bit of advice is to tell him that deep breathing and coughing may prevent the complication of pneumonia.

Maintain proper body position and utilize proper body mechanics. Before abdominal surgery, the patient is shown how to turn from side to side assuming the Sims' lateral position. This is encouraged every second hour for the first 24 hours postoperatively and is done to stimulate circulation, maintain muscle tone and prevent respiratory and circulatory complications. Rather than be assisted, the patient is encouraged to move himself.

Leg Exercises. Flexing the legs is done to lessen abdominal "gas" pain, facilitate moving from side to side, and adjust more easily to sitting, standing and walking. The patient is shown how to move his foot in a circle, and how to flex his leg slowly but often.

Medications and Control of Pain. The patient is told he will receive a preanesthetic medication and that it will help him to relax and perhaps to feel sleepy. He might notice that he may become thirsty. Postoperatively, he can expect medications to keep him comfortable but not to prevent him from regaining activity and maintaining an adequate air exchange.

Visiting Information and Spiritual Resources. The patient is placed at greater ease when he knows when

Patient: Date:

Division:

	Remarks	Yes	No
PATIENT PREPARATION			
1. Operative area prepared			
2. Operative area inspected by head nurse or supervisor (not necessary if done by "Prep" team)			
3. Oral hygiene given			
Dentures removed			
Dentures present			
Capped teeth present			
"Removable bridgework" removed			
4. Hair prepared—covered if necessary			
Hairpins removed			
5. Jewelry			
Removed			
Ring tied or taped on			
Other (medal, etc.) present			
6. Voided, catheterized, or indwelling catheter			
Amount			
Time			
7. Medications			
Those given in past 8 hrs. recorded			
Preanesthetic medication given			
Time a.m. p.m.			
8. Side rails applied after giving preanesthetic medication			
9. Identification wristlet applied			
10. Colored nail polish removed (from at least 2 fingers)			
CHART PREPARATION			
1. Operative permit signed and on chart			
2. Morning T.P.R. recorded			
3. Morning B.P. recorded			
4. Laboratory blood studies on chart			
5. Laboratory urine studies on chart			
6. Doctor's Order sheet on chart			

Fig. 9-5. Preoperative check list which is attached to the patient's chart and is checked immediately before the patient is taken to the operating room.

TABLE 9-2. Categories of contemplated surgery based on urgency

Classification	Indication for Surgery	Examples
I. Emergency—Requires immediate attention	Without delay	Extensive burns Major bone fractures Fractured skull Gunshot wounds Stab wounds Bladder or intestinal obstruction Severe bleeding Serious eye injuries
II. Urgent—Requires prompt attention	Within 24-48 hrs.	Acute gallbladder infection Kidney or ureteral stones Bleeding hemorrhoids or uterine tumors Cancer
III. Required—Requires operation	Plan hospital admission within a few weeks or months	Eye cataracts Thyroid operations Tonsillectomy Gallbladder problems without acute inflammation Prostatic hypertrophy without bladder obstruction Spinal fusion Bone deformities
IV. Elective—Should be operated on	Failure to have surgery is not catastrophic	Repair of scars Simple hernia Vaginal repair Superficial cysts
V. Optional—The decision rests with the patient	Personal preference	Cosmetic surgery

to expect his family or friends. It helps him to know that his family will be kept informed regarding the acute phases of his surgical experience. He appreciates information regarding the availability of a spiritual adviser of his preference.

Oxygen, Drainage Tubes and/or Special Equipment. If he knows beforehand that he will be on assisted breathing, have drainage tubes or be attached to special equipment, the patient is more likely to accept these accoutrements postoperatively without too much concern.

Immediate Preoperative Preparation

The patient is summoned to the operating room about 20 minutes before the anesthesia is to be started. Previous to this the nurse clothes the patient in the regulation short gown, leaving it untied and open in the back. Occasionally, long leggings are added. Further, for a woman, long hair is plaited in two braids, all hairpins are removed, and the head and the hair are covered entirely with a cap. The mouth must be inspected and all dentures or plates, chewing gum and so forth removed. Jewelry should not be worn to the operating room; even wedding rings should be taken off. If a patient has any real objection to the removal of a ring, a narrow tape may be tied to the ring and then fastened securely around the patient's wrist. All articles of value, including dentures, should

be labeled clearly with the patient's name and left in charge of the head nurse.

All patients (except those with urologic problems) should void immediately before being sent to the operating room. Unless the patient is in a weakened condition, the use of the commode or the bathroom rather than the bedpan should be urged. The bladder must be empty, but catheterization should not be resorted to except in an emergency. The amount of urine voided should be measured and recorded with the time of voiding on the preoperative check slip or the anesthesia chart.

Preanesthetic Medication

The administration of any anesthetic (general, spinal, regional or local) is facilitated greatly by the use of preanesthetic medication. Such medication is ordered to meet the needs of the particular patient. The drugs used most commonly are (1) the opiates—morphine and meperidine (Demerol), (2) the barbiturates—pentobarbital (Nembutal) and secobarbital (Seconal Sodium) and (3) the belladonna derivatives—atropine and scopolamine.

Opiates and barbiturates tend to allay the anxiety and the apprehension of the patient. They also reduce the metabolic rate and, by so doing, permit the induction of surgical anesthesia with smaller quantities of anesthetic agents. The belladonna derivatives reduce the amount of secretions in the mouth and the respiratory tract and help thereby to maintain a clear airway. They tend also to obtund certain harmful reflexes that may occur during operation on the chest and the abdomen.

These drugs should be given from 45 to 75 minutes before anesthesia is begun. Therefore, it is most important that the nurse give this medication precisely at the time it is ordered, otherwise its effect will have worn off or—what happens more often—it will not have begun to act when anesthesia is started.

Very frequently operations are delayed or schedules changed, and it becomes impossible to order medication for a given time. In these situations the preoperative medication is ordered "on call from operating room." Although this is far from ideal, and should be avoided whenever possible, the nurse can help by having the medication ready to give and by administering it as soon as the patient is called for. It usually takes 15 to 20 minutes to get a patient ready for the operating room. If the nurse gives the medication before she attends to the other details of preparing the patient, she will have allowed the patient at least partial benefit of the preoperative medication and will have contributed to a smoother and more pleasant anesthetic and operative course. A last-minute check concludes the preparation (Fig. 9-5).

*Transportation to the Operating Room**

The patient is transferred to the operating room in bed or on a previously prepared stretcher. This should be made as comfortable as possible and must be made up with a sufficient number of blankets to ensure against chilling from draughty corridors. A small pillow at the head usually is acceptable. The top covers of the stretcher should be long enough to tuck in at both the patient's feet and shoulders. The nurse always should remain with the patient until relieved by one of the anesthesiologists. The chart should be given to the anesthesiologist or a nurse; it never should be left with the patient.

THE PATIENT'S FAMILY

Most hospitals have a special waiting-room for the family of the patient who is having surgery. This room may be equipped with comfortable chairs, television, telephones and facilities for light refreshment. Volunteers may remain with the family, serve them coffee, boost their morale, and even keep them informed of the patient's progress. After surgery, the surgeon may meet the family here, join them for coffee and report his findings.

---

* *Film:* Transporting the Patient for Surgery (16 mm. color, sound, 18 min.) available from ANA-NLN Film Library, 13 E. 37th St., New York, N.Y.

The family never should judge the seriousness of an operation by the length of time the patient is in the operating room. He may be in surgery much longer than the actual operating time for several reasons:

(1) It is customary to send for the patient some time in advance of the actual operating time.

(2) Anesthesiologists often make additional preparations that may take from ½ to 1 hour.

(3) Occasionally, the surgeon takes longer than he expected with the preceding case, hence delaying the time of beginning the next operation.

(4) After surgery, the patient may be kept on the operating floor or recovery room to ensure satisfactory emergence from the anesthetic.

Those waiting for the postoperative patient should be told what to expect when the patient arrives, such as a blood transfusion, suction bottles, nasal tube, airway, oxygen tent, tracheostomy tube and so forth. A point needing emphasis is the situation in which it appears that the prognosis of the patient is more negative than positive. Even when the odds appear against the patient, it is not within the prerogative of the nurse to relay this information to the family.

BIBLIOGRAPHY

Aasterud, M.: Explanation to the patient. *In* Skipper, J. K., and Leonard, R. C.: Social Interaction and Patient Care. pp. 82-87. Philadelphia, J. B. Lippincott, 1965.

American College of Surgeons, Committee on Pre- and Postoperative Care: Manual of Preoperative and Postoperative Care. Philadelphia, W. B. Saunders, 1968.

Carnevali, D. L.: Preoperative anxiety. Amer. J. Nurs., *66*:1536-1538, July, 1966.

Dripps, R. D., Eckenhoff, J. E. and Vandam, L. D.: Chap. 1, Preanesthetic Care, Chap. 2, Effect of prior drug therapy upon the course of anesthesia, from Introduction to Anesthesia, 3rd ed., Philadelphia, W. B. Saunders, 1967.

Dumas, R. G., Anderson, B. J. and Leonard, R. C.: The importance of the expressive function in preoperative preparation. *In* Skipper, J. K. and Leonard, R. C.: Social Interaction and Patient Care. pp. 16-29. Philadelphia, J. B. Lippincott, 1965.

Dumas, R. G. and Leonard, R. C.: The effect of nursing on the incidence of vomiting. Nurs. Res. *12*:12, Winter, 1963.

Field, P. B.: Recordings ease fear of surgery. Hosp. Topics, *46*: 69-71, Sept., 1968.

Gregg, D.: Reassurance. *In* Skipper, J. K. and Leonard, R. C.: Social Interaction and Patient Care. pp. 127-136. Philadelphia, J. B. Lippincott, 1965.

Healy, K. M.: Does preoperative instruction make a difference? Amer. J. Nurs. *68*:62-67, Jan., 1968.

Lynch, J. D., Struck, R. M., and Wermers, D. F.: Anxiety and anxiety reduction in surgical patients. AORN Jour., *6*:58-60, July, 1967.

Magill, K. A.: How one patient handled fear. Amer. J. Nurs., *67*: 1248-1249, June, 1967.

Rosenberg, J.: Hazards of presurgical drug therapy. AORN Jour., *5*:89-91, June, 1967.

Weiler, Sr. M. C.: Postoperative patients evaluate preoperative instruction. Amer. J. Nurs. *68*:1465-1467, July, 1968.

Intraoperative Care

- *Reception and Greeting of the Patient*
- *The Anesthesiologist and the Patient*
- *Types of Anesthesiology*
- *Induced Hypothermia*
- *Artificial Hypotension During Operation*
- *Malignant Hyperthermia During Anesthesia*
- *Position on the Operating Table*

RECEPTION AND GREETING OF THE PATIENT

It is important that someone be with the preoperative patient at all times. Even though he has had preoperative medication, appears to be dozing and seems to be secure on the stretcher with a strap in place, he should not be left alone. It is desirable to have the patient brought directly to the anesthesia room, where he is greeted by name and made to feel that he is in safe hands. If no other waiting area is available, often he has to wait a few minutes in the corridor. Wherever he must wait before preparations for the administration of anesthesia are made, certain conditions should prevail. The area must be quiet for maximal effectiveness of the preoperative medication. He should not have to hear undesirable sounds from other patients or conversations which might be misinterpreted, exaggerated or out of range for accurate perception.

Patients occasionally assume an attitude of disinterest toward the equipment in an operating room; however, most people exhibit considerable curiosity. Some operating rooms are equipped with soft-playing piped music that is conducive to quiet relaxation.

It is assumed that preoperative preparation has covered quite a span of time before the patient comes to the operating room. However, many times the waiting patient with his eyes closed is reviewing some personal thoughts; then, a question or concern about some one thing may occur to him. Its value may even become overly exaggerated. Someone in attendance should be available to answer or attempt to find the answer to his query.

Skill in communication is accomplished not only verbally but also by facial expression, manner and a reassuring touch or warm grasp of the hand. Without a doubt it is important for the patient to have the security of someone nearby who is familiar, such as the nurse who helped to prepare him before coming to the operating floor, the nurse who greeted him in surgery and told him she would stay with him during his operation and be with him in the recovery room or the anesthesiologist who visited with him the day before and discussed his anesthetic agent and its induction.

Attention to physical needs will add greatly to his comfort. Keep the patient out of drafts, add a blanket if he is cold or remove a cover if he is too warm. Respect his modesty at all times and avoid unnecessary exposure. Knee straps should be applied loosely to prevent circulatory impairment. If there is any need to discuss somthing that the patient should not hear, this should be done well out of hearing range of the patient; even if he appears to be asleep, he may be acutely aware of all sounds.

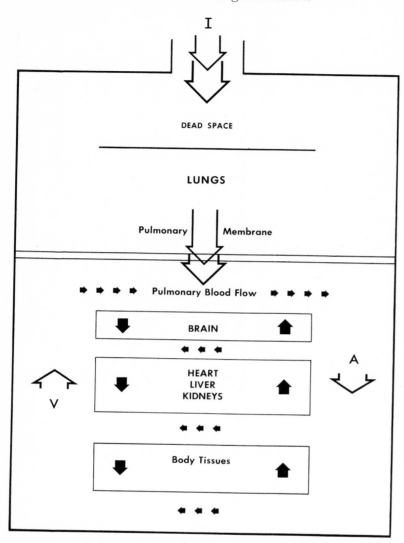

I

DEAD SPACE

LUNGS

Pulmonary   Membrane

Pulmonary Blood Flow

BRAIN

HEART
LIVER
KIDNEYS

A

V

Body Tissues

Fig. 9-6. Diagram illustrating some of the physiologic and physical factors underlying the uptake of inhalational anesthetics by the body. An anesthetic gas is given by mask at the mouth which, when carried to the brain by the circulating blood, will give rise to anesthesia. First, the anesthetic is breathed and mixed with the functional residual air of the lungs. Failure of the anesthetic in the tracheobronchial passages to come into contact with the pulmonary membrane is shown by the dead space area. The arrow pointing across the pulmonary membrane represents diffusion of the anesthetic gas across the membrane and solution of the anesthetic in the circulating pulmonary blood. The subsequent distribution of the anesthetic in the blood to the body is shown by the directional arrows. On the arterial side of the circulation, the tension of the anesthetic reaching the organs and the tissues is the same for all. The mass of the brain is pictured as being smallest, yet the volume of the blood flow to it is large. The body tissues, with the greatest mass, have the least blood flow. Diffusion of the anesthetic gas into and out of the organs and tissues according to the prevailing pressure gradient is shown by arrows. Finally, recirculation of the anesthetic to the lungs is shown on the venous side of the circulation. On the venous side, the tension of anesthetic gas is an average of the tensions of the anesthetic returned from the organs and the tissues. (Modified after Haggard, Journal of Biochemistry) (Dripps, R. D., Eckenhoff, J. E., and Vandam, L. D.: Introduction to Anesthesia, ed. 2, p. 60, Philadelphia, Saunders)

THE ANESTHESIOLOGIST AND THE PATIENT

The surgical patient usually is interested in and even concerned about the types of anesthesia that he is to receive. He has heard friends or relatives discuss the subject on the basis of personal experience or hearsay, and not infrequently he has formed definite opinions as to the merits or the demerits of the various methods in vogue. Therefore, it is helpful for the anesthesiologist to visit the patient in his own room before operation, introduce himself and point out that he has come for the purpose of allaying the fears that he knows exist in the minds of so many people. Choice of anesthetic agent is discussed and the patient has an opportunity to disclose any idiosyncracies as well as types of medications he is currently taking that may affect this choice (see p. 105). During this important visit, the anesthesiologist determines the condition of the patient's lungs, pre-existing pulmonary infections and extent of cigarette smoking. Of course, he is also concerned about the patient's general physical condition because this also may have an effect on the management of anesthesia. This preoperative contact builds up confidence and enables the patient to recognize a familiar face as he is being wheeled onto the operating floor. Uncertainty and anxiety are relieved, in part at least, and a much smoother course can be anticipated.

Today, with the increasing technical demands placed on the surgeon, it is of the utmost importance that he be freed of the responsibility of watching the patient's anesthetic progress while he is operating. The anesthesiologist, especially trained in the art and the science of anesthesiology, has acquired these functions. To him, after consultation with the surgeon, can be delegated the choice of anesthesia, the technical problems relating to the administration of the anesthetic agent and the supervision of the patient's condition during the operation. Such a "sharing" of responsibility obviously benefits the patient.

Such supervision and observation include not only attention to the blood pressure, the pulse and respiration but also, in many instances, the permanent recording of the patient's electrocardiogram, electroencephalogram, tidal volume, blood oxygen saturation, blood pH, pulmonary gas concentrations and body temperature. By meticulous attention to the cause-and-effect relationship of vital changes during operation, the anesthesiologist has contributed greatly to the development of devices with which to ventilate the patient's lungs or to circulate and aerate his blood, should his physiologic mechanisms become incapable of performing these functions.

In the anesthetizing room the patient is transferred to the operating table, and a last-minute check of his condition is made, blood pressure, pulse and respiratory rates in particular being noted. Then the anesthetic previously selected is administered. When all is in readiness for the beginning of the operation, the patient is wheeled into the operating room.

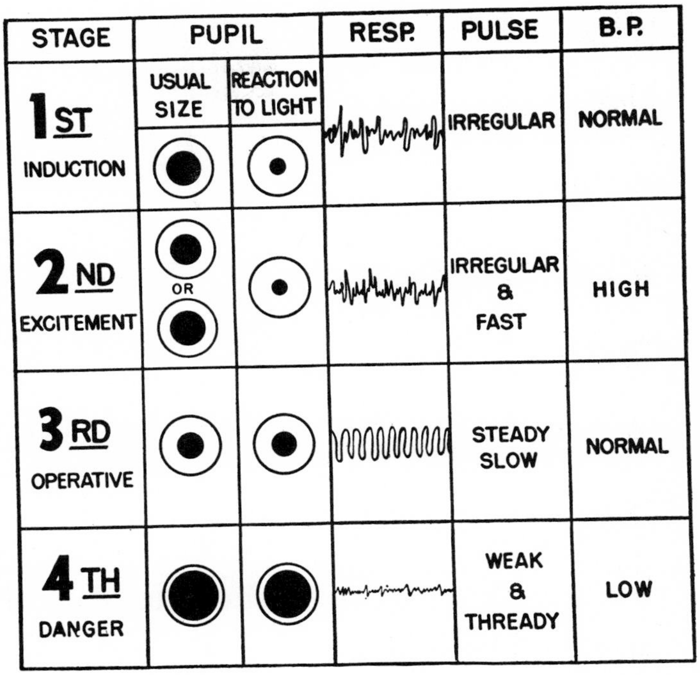

TYPES OF ANESTHESIA

Anesthetics have been divided into two classes according to whether they suspend the sensations (1) of the whole body (general anesthetics) or (2) of parts of the body (local, regional or spinal anesthetics). General anesthesia can be obtained by inhalation, intravenous or rectal techniques.

Inhalation Anesthesia

Liquids producing anesthesia by inhalation of their vapor: ethyl ether, halothane, divinyl ether, trichlorethylene, ethyl chloride, chloroform.

Gases also administered by inhalation, usually in combination with oxygen: nitrous oxide, ethylene and cyclopropane.

These substances, when inhaled, enter the blood through the pulmonary capillaries and, when in sufficient concentration, act on the cerebral centers in such a manner as to produce loss of consciousness and of sensation. When the administration of the anesthetic has been discontinued, the vapor or gas is eliminated by way of the lungs in respiration.

Physiologic and Physical Factors

General anesthetics produce anesthesia because they are delivered to the brain at high partial pressure. Relatively high amounts of anesthetic must be given during induction and the early maintenance phases because of recirculation of the anesthetic and its deposi-

STAGE	PUPIL		RESP.	PULSE	B.P.
	USUAL SIZE	REACTION TO LIGHT			
1ST INDUCTION	⬤	•		IRREGULAR	NORMAL
2ND EXCITEMENT	⬤ OR ⬤	•		IRREGULAR & FAST	HIGH
3RD OPERATIVE	•	•		STEADY SLOW	NORMAL
4TH DANGER	⬤	⬤		WEAK & THREADY	LOW

Fig. 9-7. Stages of anesthesia. (U.S. Army Manual, TM 8-230, Medical and Surgical Technicians)

tion in body tissues. As these depots become saturated, smaller amounts of the anesthetic agent are required to maintain anesthesia, since equilibrium or near equilibrium has been achieved between the brain, the blood and the other tissues. The relationship between the various parts of the body as it influences the course of anesthesia may be seen in Fig. 9-6.

On viewing this diagram, it becomes apparent that anything that influences peripheral blood flow, such as lean tissues or a condition of shock, may cause only small amounts of anesthetic to be required. Conversely, when peripheral blood flow is unusually high, as it is in the muscularly active or the apprehensive patient, the brain receives a smaller quantity of anesthetic which, in turn, means that induction is slower and that larger than usual quantities of anesthetic will be required.

Stages of Anesthesia

Anesthesia generally is described as having 4 stages, each of which presents a definite group of symptoms (Fig. 9-7).

Stage of Beginning Anesthesia

As the patient breathes in the anesthetic vapor, a feeling of warmth steals over his body, dizziness is experienced, and he seems to be detached from the world. He experiences a ringing, roaring or buzzing in his ears, and then, though still conscious, he is aware that he is unable to move his extremities voluntarily. During this stage noises are greatly exaggerated; even low voices or minor sounds appear distressingly loud and unreal. For this reason, unnecessary noise or motion must be prevented at all costs while anesthesia is being started.

Stage of Excitement

This stage—characterized variously by struggling, shouting, talking, singing, laughing or even crying—frequently may be avoided by judicious suggestion before anesthesia is begun and by its even and slow administration. The pupils of the eyes are dilated but contract if exposed to light, the pulse rate is rapid, and respiration is irregular.

Because of the uncontrolled movements of the patient during this stage, the anesthesiologist always should be attended by a nurse and an attendant, who should be ready to apply restraining straps if occasion demands. The patient should not be touched except for purposes of restraint, and in no circumstances should there be any palpation of the operative site.

Stage of Surgical Anesthesia

The stage of surgical anesthesia is reached by continued administration of the vapor or gas. The patient is then entirely unconscious, lying quietly on the table. The pupils are small, but they retain their contractile power on exposure to light. Respiration is regular, the pulse rate is about normal and of good volume, and the skin is pink or slightly flushed. By proper administration of the anesthetic this stage may be maintained for hours.

Stage of Danger

This stage is reached when too much anesthesia has been given and when the patient has not been observed carefully. The respiration becomes shallow, the pulse weak and thready; the pupils become widely dilated and no longer contract when exposed to light. Cyanosis develops gradually, and, unless prompt action is taken, death follows rapidly. If this stage should develop, the anesthetic is discontinued immediately, and artificial respiration is given. Stimulants may be administered.

During the administration of an anesthetic, there is, of course, no sharp division between the various stages. The patient passes gradually from one stage to another, and it is only by close observation of the signs exhibited by the patient that an anesthesiologist can have complete control of the situation. The condition of the pupils, the blood pressure and the respiratory and the cardiac rates are probably the most reliable guides to the patient's condition. The anesthesiologist should focus his attention entirely on the patient and not be diverted by an interest in the details of the operation or by other activities of the room.

The administration of an anesthetic is attended by other physiologic activities that have not been mentioned. Some anesthetics, especially ether, produce a hypersecretion of mucus and saliva. This may be eliminated largely by the preoperative administration of atropine. Vomiting occurs not infrequently, especially when the patient comes to the operating room with a full stomach. The head should be turned sharply to the side, if gagging occurs, and a basin provided to collect the vomitus. The head of the table should be lowered to permit material to flow out of the mouth by gravity. Suction apparatus always should be available.

During the anesthesia, the temperature may fall. Because of this, every precaution should be taken against chilling the patient. A warm bed and blankets always should be provided. Sugar metabolism is much reduced, with the result that acidosis may develop.

In addition to the dangers of the anesthetic itself, the anesthesiologist must guard against asphyxia. This may be due to foreign bodies in the mouth, spasm of the vocal cords, falling back of the tongue or aspiration of vomitus, saliva or blood.

Methods of Administration

Open-Drop Method

Sometimes this method is used for the anesthetics that are liquid. The fluid is dropped slowly on 8 layers of gauze held over the patient's nose and mouth. The patient inhales the vapor that evaporates from the gauze. Care must be taken to prevent a drop of the anesthetic from entering the eye. If this occurs, the eye should be irrigated immediately with saline solution and followed by a drop of sterile liquid petroleum.

Vapor or Gas Administration with Mask

Liquid anesthetics may also be given by causing the patient to breathe air or oxygen containing the vapor arising from the liquid. Ether, especially, is used in this manner, frequently in combination with the gas anesthetics. The vapor is conducted to the patient by a tube and a mask.

The gases (nitrous oxide, ethylene, cyclopropane and oxygen) are contained in tanks under pressure and are allowed to escape at the proper rate through valves opening into a mixing chamber and then usually into a large rubber bag. The bag is connected by a flexible tube to a mask, which is put over the patient's face. A reservoir containing ether often is attached to the mechanism so that, by turning a valve, a regulated amount of ether vapor may be given with the gas if this is desired.

Intrapharyngeal Anesthesia

Many operations upon the mouth and the lower part of the face will not permit the use of the ordinary inhaler. After anesthesia has been induced in such a patient, it is possible to continue its administration by the introduction of ether by the vapor method, through small rubber tube that leads into the pharynx by way of the nostril.

Endotracheal Anesthesia

The endotracheal technique consists of introducing a soft rubber or other variety of tube directly into the trachea, either by exposing the larynx with a laryngo-scope or by passing it "blindly." It may be inserted either through the nose or the mouth (Fig. 9-8).

This technique has many advantages, but the most important is the most obvious—the patient has a clear airway. There is no danger of respiratory obstruction, either from the falling back of the tongue against the posterior pharyngeal wall (swallowing the tongue) or from spasm of the vocal cords. The endotracheal method has its greatest use in chest surgery, in which the thorax is open and the patient must depend upon the anesthesiologist to assist him in breathing or take over breathing for him completely by rhythmic com-pression of the breathing bag. But many other types of operation have been made possible or made safer by this technique: for example, neurosurgical, dental, plastic and nose and throat procedures, in which the anesthesiologist does not have immediate access to the patient's face, or in any procedure on a patient in whom, because of obesity or anatomic abnormality, the airway may become compromised.

Another important advantage of endotracheal intu-bation is that it provides a convenient method of aspirating secretions, blood or other foreign material from the trachea and the bronchi. This is not only important in anesthesia, but it is invaluable in the nursing care of very ill patients.

Often the advantages overshadow some disadvan-tages. Care must be taken in inserting the tube to prevent injury to the lips, the tongue and the teeth. Other complications must be prevented, during intuba-tion, such as increased resistance to breathing, obstruc-tion or dislodgment of the tube, and coughing by the patient. Other complications may develop after re-moval of the tracheal tube: (1) laryngospasm, which may occur in the lightly anesthetized patient and can be treated by the administration of 100 per cent oxygen; (2) tracheal collapse; (3) edema or infection of the larynx or the trachea; (4) hoarseness; and (5) sore throat.

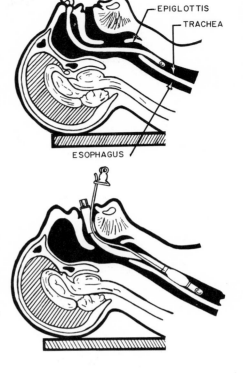

FIG. 9-8. En-dotracheal anes-thesia. (*Top*) Magill tube in proper position, intranasal intu-bation being used. Note metal elbow at proxi-mal end of tube. This adaptor is used to keep the tube from enter-ing the nose be-yond reach of extubation. It can be used also to attach to an-esthetic equip-ment. (*Bottom*) Oral intubation. The tube in po-sition with the cuff inflated. (Surgical Equip-ment)

Drugs Used for General Anesthesia

Inhalation Volatile Liquid Anesthetics

Ethyl ether generally is considered the best and the safest of the general anesthetics. It is a clear, volatile, inflammable fluid. It may be given by any of the methods mentioned.

ADVANTAGES. It produces anesthesia with relaxation admirably suited for surgical operations.

It is not highly toxic, and it has a wide margin of safety between the dosage required for anesthesia and the toxic dose. The signs of a toxic dosage usually appear in sufficient time to allow for resuscitation of the patient and to avoid a fatal outcome.

No accurate statistics are available, but various authors give mortality figures at from 1 death in 16,000 to 1 in 30,000.

In emergencies, ether may be given by unskilled persons under the guidance of the surgeon.

DISADVANTAGES. Ether vapor, especially in high concentration, irritates the respiratory mucous mem-brane. Its administration may be followed by increased secretions of the respiratory tract and by nausea and vomiting in the postoperative period. In the presence of respiratory diseases it is advisable to avoid ether whenever possible. The period of induction and of "coming out" is longer than for most of the other anes-thetics (Table 9-3, p. 119).

Halothane (Fluothane); Methoxyflurane (Penthrane). In recent years, great emphasis has been directed toward obtaining a non-explosive, potent general anesthetic that does not possess the toxicity of a drug such as chloroform. Two such drugs are now available—halothane and methoxyflurane. Both are clear, sweet-smelling liquids. Anesthesia is produced by inhalation of the vapor. They are both less volatile than ether and many times more potent. Evidence indicates they are even more potent than chloroform. Their main advantage is that they are neither explosive nor inflammable in therapeutic ranges even when mixed with oxygen. Induction with halothane is extremely rapid, with methoxyflurane considerably slower. Muscular relaxation is excellent with methoxyflurane, fair with halothane. To obtain good muscular relaxation with halothane, concentrations must be used that may severely depress circulation and/or respiration. Overdosage with these drugs is quite easy. They should be administered by special vaporizers that permit careful regulation of the inspired vapor concentration. In inexperienced hands, these drugs may be extremely dangerous. They do not possess the same margin of safety as ethyl ether.

Divinyl ether (Vinethene) is a clear, colorless volatile liquid. When given by the slow-drop method on gauze over the nostrils, it produces a rapid and a not unpleasant anesthesia from which the patient recovers rapidly with little or no nausea or vomiting. It is useful for short anesthesia. Kidney damage and liver damage may follow its use, particularly if it is given for operations of long duration.

Trichlorethylene (Trilene) is a weak anesthetic agent. It is useful to supplement nitrous oxide anesthesia and to provide pain relief without unconsciousness in obstetrics, urology and dentistry.

DISADVANTAGES. It may produce very rapid respiratory rates. It should not be used in a system containing soda lime.

Ethyl chloride at ordinary room temperature is a gas. Usually it is dispensed under compression from a glass tube with a tiny hole in one end. The spray tends to freeze tissues and render them less sensitive to a surgical incision.

As a general anesthetic it is rapid in its action and is administered by inhalation. It is used occasionally for short anesthesia and as a preliminary to ether. The cardiac depressant action of the drug makes it dangerous for general use.

* The Division of Simplified Practices of the National Bureau of Standards, Washington, D.C. has recommended the following color markings for the tanks containing these particular gases:

Inhalation Gaseous Anesthetics*

Oxygen	green
Carbon dioxide	gray
Nitrous oxide	light blue
Cyclopropane	orange
Helium	brown
Ethylene	red
Carbon dioxide & oxygen	gray and green
Helium & oxygen	brown and green

Nitrous Oxide. This general anesthetic causes the least disturbance of bodily function if it is given with a concentration of oxygen not less than that of air (21 per cent).

Advantages. The onset and the emergence from anesthesia are rapid and usually uneventful. Therefore, it is useful for short procedures on outpatients. It has a fairly pleasant smell. It is nonexplosive and can be used with the electrocautery.

Disadvantages. Nitrous oxide is a weak anesthetic. Its lack of potency can be overcome by adequate preanesthetic medication or by supplementation with an anesthetic vapor, such as ether, or an intravenous barbiturate or narcotic. Without these, if nitrous oxide alone is being used for induction, it may be necessary to reduce the oxygen to 10 per cent or less. This is dangerous in certain individuals, such as those suffering from heart disease or anemia.

Ethylene is a colorless, highly inflammable gas possessing a characteristic sweetish odor that reminds one somewhat of burnt matches. It is like nitrous oxide but has a more unpleasant odor and is explosive.

Advantages. Rapid induction of anesthesia and rapid recovery. No irritation of the respiratory mucous membrane.

Disadvantages. It has an odor that is offensive to some. Oozing from wounds seems to be increased, and the clotting time is prolonged.

Cyclopropane is much more potent than nitrous oxide or ethylene and can produce anesthesia in concentrations of 15 to 20 per cent. The remainder of the anesthetic mixture will consist of oxygen and nitrogen; therefore, the patient usually has a more than adequate supply of oxygen available at all times. Cyclopropane is relatively nonirritating. It is a powerful depressant to breathing. Occasionally, marked disorders of the heart rate and rhythm occur during cyclopropane anesthesia. These increase with respiratory depression and deepening of anesthesia (Table 9-4).

Explosibility

All the inhalation anesthetics discussed, with the exception of nitrous oxide, halothane and methoxyflurane, form explosive mixtures with air or oxygen. Therefore, they should be avoided if possible when the

TABLE 9-3. Volatile liquids as agents of general anesthesia

Agent	Administration	Advantages	Disadvantages	Implications
1. *Ethyl ether*	Open-drop; inhalation	Excellent relaxant Wide margin of safety Inexpensive Relatively non-toxic Used for all types of surgery	Slow induction: 10 minutes Long recovery; not eliminated for approximately 8 hours Irritating to skin, eyes, and kidneys May cause acidosis Causes nausea and vomiting Flammable and explosive	*Protect skin with lubricant.* *Instill sterile oil in eyes.* *Expect nausea and vomiting—turn head to side to prevent aspiration of vomitus.* *Practice safeguards in view of flammability.*
2. *Vinyl ether (Vinethene)*	Open-drop; inhalation	Induction very rapid Little postoperative vomiting Good for short procedures	Small margin of safety because of rapidity with which it acts May cause liver or kidney damage Increases salivation Flammable and explosive	*Protect skin and eyes to prevent irritation.* *Employ safeguards because of flammability.*
3. *Halothane (Fluothane)*	Inhalation; special vaporizer	Not explosive or inflammable Induction rapid and smooth Useful in almost every type of surgery Low incidence of postoperative nausea and vomiting	Expensive Requires skillful administration to prevent overdosage Has caused liver damage in a few cases May produce hypotension (low blood pressure) Requires special vaporizer for administration	*In addition to observing pulse and respiration postoperatively, it is important that blood pressure be determined frequently.*
4. *Methoxyflurane (Penthrane)*	Inhalation; special vaporizer	Nonflammable Nonexplosive Seldom causes postoperative nausea and vomiting Analgesic action continues several hours after surgery Excellent muscle relaxation	Requires skillful administration	*Prolonged postoperative depressant action calls for careful observation by recovery room personnel.*

electrocautery and the electric desiccator are to be used. In addition, the spark of static electricity may set off an explosion. For this reason, woolen blankets should not be used to cover the patient on the operating table, nor should nylon uniforms be permitted near the gas machine or the anesthetized patient. Finally, no one should touch the patient in the vicinity of the breathing mask lest a spark be generated and cause an explosion. The hazard of explosion is present always, but such unfortunate accidents are extremely rare if common sense is exercised.

Muscle Relaxants

Using muscle relaxants, it is possible to give a lighter degree of anesthesia by using a less potent anesthetic agent at a reduced dosage. Purified curare was the first widely used muscle relaxant; tubocurarine was isolated as the active principle. Since then, succinyl choline has been introduced to supplant the original drugs. It acts more rapidly than curare. The full effect of a dose occurs in 60 to 90 seconds after administration and persists for 1 to 2 minutes. The return to normal occurs in about 3 to 5 minutes. Because of its

TABLE 9-4. Gases as agents of general anesthesia

Agent	Administration	Advantages	Disadvantages	Implications
1. *Nitrous oxide* (N_2O)	Inhalation (closed method)	Induction and recovery rapid Nonflammable Nonexplosive Useful with oxygen for short procedures Useful with other agents for all types of surgery	Poor relaxant Weak anesthetic May produce hypoxia	*Most useful in conjunction with other agents.*
2. *Cyclopropane* (C_3H_6)	Inhalation (closed method)	Good relaxant Useful in all types of surgery Low toxicity	Explosive Expensive Powerful depressant; therefore should be administered skillfully Occasionally produces disturbances in heart rhythm May cause bronchospasm	*Employ precautions against explosions. Because cyclopropane may be followed by hypotension, it is important to observe blood pressure postoperatively.*

fast action and rapid elimination, the drug is repeated each time that relaxation is needed. Serious depression of respiration may occur if the dose that is given is too great; therefore, careful observation of the volume of breathing is of particular importance.

Intravenous Barbiturate Anesthesia

General anesthesia also can be produced by the intravenous injection of various substances. An extremely short-acting barbiturate, thiopental (pentothal sodium) is the anesthetic in most common use today for this purpose. This substance leads to unconsciousness within 30 seconds. The onset of anesthesia is pleasant; there is none of the buzzing, the roaring or the dizziness known to follow the administration of an inhalation anesthetic. For this reason induction of anesthesia with an intravenous agent is the favorite of patients who have experienced various methods. The duration of action is brief, and the patient awakens with little nausea or vomiting. Thiopental frequently is given in addition to other anesthetic agents. It is especially useful to relieve the anxiety of the patient with spinal anesthesia.

Thiopental is a powerful depressant of breathing, and its chief danger lies in this characteristic. It should be administered only by skilled anesthesiologists and only when some method of giving oxygen is available immediately should trouble arise. Sneezing, coughing and choking sometimes are noted.

Intravenous anesthesia has the advantage of being nonexplosive, of requiring little equipment and of being so easy to take. The low incidence of postoperative nausea and vomiting makes the method useful in eye surgery, in which retching endangers vision in the operated eye. It is useful for short procedures, but is used less often for abdominal surgery. It is not indicated for children, who have small veins and who are more susceptible to respiratory obstruction. The reasons in both instances are apparent.

TABLE 9-5. Intravenous barbiturate as an agent of general anesthesia

Agent	Administration	Advantages	Disadvantages	Implications
Thiopental (Pentothal Sodium)	Intravenous injection	Rapid induction Nonexplosive Requires little equipment Low incidence of postoperative nausea and vomiting	Powerful depressant of breathing Poor relaxant Sometimes produces coughing and choking Not useful for children because of small veins	*Requires intelligent and close observation because of potency and rapidity of drug action.*

Spinal Anesthesia

It must never be forgotten that the patient under spinal, regional or local anesthesia is awake and aware of his surroundings. Careless conversation, unnecessary noise, unpleasant odors—all are noticed by the patient on the operating table and reflect discredit on the operating room staff. Quiet must be insisted upon. The diagnosis must not be made aloud if the patient is not to be made aware of it at once.

Anesthesia of the lower extremities, the abdomen and even of the chest may be induced by the introduction of anesthetic drugs into the subarachnoid space (Fig. 9-9). A spinal puncture is made with sterile precautions, and the drug is injected in solution through the needle. As soon as the injection has been made, the patient is placed on his back. As a rule, the head and the shoulders are lowered, depending on the height of anesthesia desired. In a few minutes anesthesia and paralysis appear, first of the toes and the perineum and then gradually of the legs and the abdomen. The drugs generally used are procaine, Pontocaine and Nupercaine.

ADVANTAGES. It is administered easily, is inexpensive, and requires a minimum of equipment. The anesthesia produced usually is rapid in onset, and there is excellent muscular relaxation. The patient may remain awake, if that is desirable. It is a relatively safe anesthesia in experienced hands. Mortality figures compare favorably with those of the safer general anesthetics.

DISADVANTAGES. Soon after the administration of the drug there may be a marked fall in blood pressure, caused by a paralysis of the vasomotor nerves. This phenomenon is noted most often when the anesthesia ascends to the upper abdomen and the chest. The preoperative administration of drugs such as ephedrine or methoxamine may be used to prevent the marked decrease in blood pressure. The inhalation of oxygen, the intravenous administration of blood, plasma or saline and the injection of stimulant drugs such as ephedrine, methoxamine, or phenylephrine, are measures of value once the blood pressure has fallen. Nausea, vomiting and pain not infrequently occur during surgery under spinal anesthesia. As a rule, this is due to traction on various structures, particularly those within the abdominal cavity. These reactions may be avoided by the simultaneous intravenous administration of a weak solution of thiopenthal.

When the anesthetic drug reaches the upper thoracic and cervical cord in high concentration, a temporary, partial or complete respiratory paralysis may occur. This complication is treated by maintaining artificial respiration until the effects of the drug on the respiratory nerves have worn off.

Such postoperative complications as headache, paral-

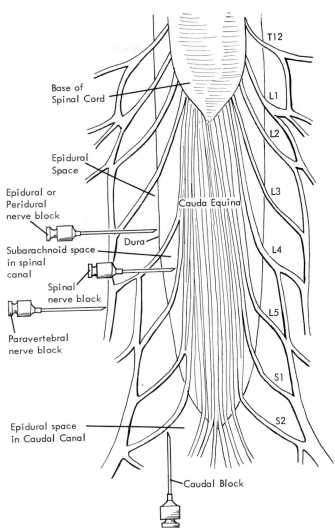

FIG. 9-9. Sites of injection for spinal anesthesia, showing position of needle for spinal and epidural types. Letters indicate vertebral level of injection.

ysis or meningitis may occur. Several factors are involved in the incidence of headache: the size of the spinal needle used, the leakage of fluid from the subarachnoid space through the puncture site, the activity of the patient and the degree of the patient's hydration. Any measure that can increase the cerebrospinal pressure is helpful in relieving headache. These include keeping the patient flat and quiet, applying a tight abdominal binder and injecting fluid into the subarachnoid space.

Nursing Care After Spinal Anesthesia

In addition to taking the blood pressure, the nurse should observe these patients closely and make notes

TABLE 9-6. Spinal anesthesia

Agents	Advantages of Spinal Anesthesia (Includes All Agents)	Disadvantages of Spinal Anesthesia (Includes All Agents)
Procaine (Novocaine) Tetracaine (Pontocaine) Dibucaine (Nupercaine)	Easily administered by a physician Inexpensive Minimum of equipment required Rapid onset Excellent muscular relaxation	Blood pressure may fall rapidly unless watched carefully and treated with such drugs as ephedrine, etc. If the spinal anesthesia ascends to the chest, there may be respiratory difficulties. Occasionally, postoperative complications occur, such as headache, paralysis or meningitis.

as to the time of return of motion and sensation in the legs and the toes. When there is complete return of sensation in the toes (appreciation of pin-prick) the patient may be considered to have recovered from the effects of the spinal drug.

"Serial" or Continuous Spinal

The tip of a plastic catheter may be left in the subarachnoid space during operation. Thus, more anesthetic may be injected as needed. Greater controllability of dosage is afforded by this technique, however, there is greater potential for postanesthetic sequelae.

Epidural or Peridural Anesthesia

This anesthesia is obtained by the injection of a local anesthetic into the spinal canal in the space surrounding the dura mater (Fig. 9-9). Interest in this approach has increased probably because of a desire to find a method of spinal anesthesia without the undesirable neurologic sequelae, notably headache, that occasionally result from the subarachnoid injection.

The advantages of epidural anesthesia appear to be the absence of neurologic complications and less disturbance of blood pressure. One disadvantage lies in the greater technical problem of introducing the anesthetic into the epidural rather than the subarachnoid space. Another is that the level of anesthesia is less controllable.

Regional Anesthesia

Regional anesthesia is that branch of local anesthesia in which, by an injection into or around the nerves, the area supplied by these nerve trunks is anesthetized. Motor fibers are the largest and have the thickest myelin sheath. Sympathetic fibers are the smallest and have a minimal covering. Sensory fibers are intermediary. Thus a local anesthetic blocks the motor nerves least readily and the sympathetic nerves most readily. An anesthetic cannot be regarded as having "worn off" until after all 3 systems (motor, sensory and autonomic) are no longer affected by the anesthetic. There are many types of this anesthesia, depending upon the various nerve groups that are injected.

Brachial Plexus Block

This produces anesthesia of the arm.

Paravertebral Anesthesia

This produces anesthesia of the spinal nerves supplying the abdominal wall and the viscera.

Transsacral (Caudal) Block

This produces anesthesia of the perineum and, occasionally, the lower abdomen.

An addition to obstetric anesthesia has been adaptation of caudal block analogous to the change from a single-injection spinal to serial spinal. This adaptation is called *continuous* or *serial caudal*. A malleable needle or a nylon ureteral catheter is inserted into the caudal canal. This is allowed to remain in place and is attached by a tube to a reservoir of anesthetic solution. When the woman in labor complains of pain, an injection is made, and subsequent injections are given as indicated. These may be continued for 20 to 30 hours. The patient is conscious during the entire labor, and the fetus is spared the depression caused by drugs given to relieve maternal distress. The mechanism of labor is changed somewhat by this method. The second stage is longer, and operative deliveries are more frequent.

The method is not entirely without harm. Infections have occurred at the site of the injection. The level of anesthesia may become too high, and respiratory and circulatory difficulties may follow. With a drop in blood pressure the fetus may be endangered. Convulsions can occur, and the nurse should report at once any marked restlessness, anxiety, tremor or twitching.

Local Infiltration Anesthesia

Infiltration anesthesia is the injection of a solution containing the local anesthesia into the tissues through which the incision is to pass. Often it is combined with a local regional block by injection of the nerves immediately supplying that area. Local anesthesia is popular for several reasons:

(1) It is simple to use, economical and nonexplosive. The amount of required equipment is minimal. Postoperative care is lessened.

(2) Undesirable effects of general anesthesia are avoided.

(3) It is ideal for use in short and superficial operations.

In operations upon the abdominal viscera, complete anesthesia is not obtained by infiltration or local block of the anterior abdominal wall, because the viscera are supplied by nerves that have not been affected by the anesthetic. For this reason, a separate injection must be made into the region of the splanchnic nerves, which supply the abdominal organs, except those of the pelvis. This injection may be made from the back (posterior-splanchnic anesthesia), or anteriorly, after opening the abdomen.

Local anesthesia is administered often in combination with epinephrine [0.3 to 0.6 ml. to the ounce (30 ml.)]. Epinephrine has the property of causing a local constriction of the blood vessels, which in turn prevents rapid absorption of the anesthetic drug and so prolongs its local action.

Contraindications for Local Anesthesia

Local anesthesia is the anesthesia of choice in every operation in which it can be used. However, it is contraindicated in surgical operations upon highly nervous, apprehensive patients. The emotional trauma experienced by these individuals under local anesthesia may be more harmful than that following a general anesthetic. A patient who begs to be put to sleep rarely does well under local anesthesia.

For some kinds of operations, local anesthesia is impractical because of the number of injections and the amount of anesthetic required, as for example, a radical mastectomy.

Technique of Local Anesthesia

The technique for the introduction of local infiltration requires few extraordinary materials. For the ordinary case the following are all that are needed:

1. Flask of sterile ½ per cent procaine solution.
2. Sterile beaker or medicine glass.
3. Sterile syringes and needles to fit.
4. Sterile sponges.

The skin is prepared as for an operation and, with a small-gauge needle, a little of the anesthetic is injected into the skin layers. This produces a blanching or wheal. The anesthetic then is carried ahead of the needle in the skin until an area as long as the proposed incision is anesthetized. A larger, longer needle then is used to infiltrate the deeper tissues with the anesthetic. The action of the drug is almost immediate, so that the operation may begin as soon as the injection is finished. The anesthesia lasts from ½ to 1 hour.

Drugs Used for Local Anesthesia

Cocaine

Cocaine is a white crystalline powder that is soluble readily in water. It was the first local anesthetic introduced and it is still used to some extent today. The high incidence of toxic reactions if injected and the liability to addiction has caused this medication to be less favored than the newer synthetic compounds.

Uses. It is used in 4 to 10 per cent solutions for anesthesia of the eye or of the mucous surface of the nose, the mouth and the urethra. It is used topically only; never injected.

Cocaine is a vasoconstrictor and tends to limit its own absorption.

DISADVANTAGES. It is highly poisonous, 1 gr. being regarded as the maximal dose for subcutaneous injections. Even this dose may produce acute toxic symptoms if rapidly absorbed or injected into a vein. The cause of the poisoning is the action of the drug on the centers of the medulla, causing respiratory failure and cardiac depression. The first symptom is a feeling of faintness. Nausea and vomiting occur, the pulse rate increases, and respiratory failure follows. In the event of cocaine poisoning with respiratory paralysis, life may be saved if artificial respiration is practiced until the effect of the drug wears off.

Prolonged sterilization by heat decomposes the drug.

Procaine (Novocaine)

Procaine is the least toxic of the local anesthetics. It is used in ½ and 1 per cent solutions, and as much as 2 gm. may be injected without toxic effects. It has supplanted cocaine for general use. Although its effects as an anesthetic are not quite as marked as those of cocaine, its lack of toxicity recommends its use.

ADVANTAGES. It may be sterilized by heat. It is very slightly toxic. Its anesthetic effects are sufficiently potent for all ordinary requirements.

Tetracaine (Pontocaine)

This local anesthetic agent has a toxicity from 3 to 5 times that of cocaine; however, it is used in much smaller doses. The chief use of tetracaine is for spinal anesthesia; the advantage being that it can give up to 2 hours of anesthesia.

Lidocaine (Xylocaine)

Lidocaine has achieved wide usage because of the rapid onset of action, the freedom from local irritative effect, and the longer duration of action as compared

TABLE 9-7. Local anesthetic agents

Agent	Administration and Action	Advantages	Disadvantages	Implications
1. Cocaine (white crystalline powder readily soluble in water)	*Only* used *topically* Produces temporary paralysis of sensory nerve fibers Pulse elevated Respiration elevated	Rapid Patient is awake and can cooperate	Possible idiosyncrasy (susceptibility) Possible addiction Cocaine Reaction 1. Exhilaration Excited Talkative Flushed face Muscular twitchings Rapid pulse 2. Shock Pallor Cyanosis Dilated pupils Apprehension Dyspnea Chills *Treatment:* Stop drug Oxygen Artificial respiration	*Never to be injected because of high toxicity* *Watch patient for reaction* *If reaction, stay with patient and reassure him* *Assist physician*
2. Procaine (Novocaine)	Solution, ½, 1, or 2% Subcut., I.M., I.V. or spinal	Low toxicity Inexpensive	Some idiosyncrasy (possibly skin flushing, increased pulse)	*Usually given with epinephrine, causing vasoconstriction, thereby slowing absorption and prolonging nerve-deadening effect*
3. Lidocaine (Xylocaine) and mepivacaine (Carbocaine)	Topical or injection	Rapid Longer duration of action (compared with procaine) Free from local irritative effect	Occasional idiosyncrasy Tends to spread from injection site	*Useful topically for cystoscopy* *Injected for use in dental work and surgery*

with procaine. Apparently, it has a tendency to spread from the site of injection. Lidocaine frequently is used intravenously to treat ventricular arrhythmias such as premature ventricular contractions and ventricular tachycardia. It may be given intravenously to depress the cough reflex; this permits patients to tolerate endotracheal tubes and oral airways at lighter planes of anesthesia.

Mepivacaine (Carbocaine)

Mepivacaine is most similar to lidocaine. It is found to act equally fast but to increase the duration of anesthesia by approximately 20 per cent. Tissue irritation appears to be minimal.

Prilocaine (Citanest)

This has a less toxic effect on the central nervous system but longer action than lidocaine. Disadvantages are the possibility of producing methemoglobin and cyanosis in some patients.

INDUCED HYPOTHERMIA

Deliberate cooling of the body (hypothermia) can be used as an adjunct to anesthesia in cardiac and neurosurgical operations, in which the reduction of tissue metabolism by cooling exerts a protective effect.

Induced hypothermia is a technique that is used to reduce the body temperature of the patient to below the normal (about 28° to 30° C. or 82° to 86° F.) in order to decrease the rate of metabolism. An individual who has been severely injured and is receiving an insufficient amount of blood flow to the tissues has a better chance of survival with the use of hypothermia because the body tissues and organs require less blood when the body temperature is kept at a subnormal level. That is, the oxygen uptake is reduced in linear fashion by the lowering of the body temperature.

Induction

The simplest way of reducing the body temperature is by the application of partially-filled ice bags* molded over the body and the extremities; however, specially devised blankets with coils for either heating or cooling by means of circulating water may be used. When the desired temperature is reached, some of the bags may be removed. A flexible electric thermometer provides an available temperature reading.

The nurse has special responsibilities when hypothermia is used for therapeutic purposes. These include: acute awareness of slight changes in the patient's blood pressure, pulse, respiration and level of consciousness which should be checked and recorded every 15 minutes. Thus, cardiac irregularities or respiratory difficulties can be detected early and treated. Other dangers of prolonged hypothermia are: cardiac arrest, edema, disturbance of fluid balance, and fat necrosis. During hypothermia, an indwelling catheter is usually in place in the bladder and a venisection is performed. An accurate recording of both the intake and the output is necessary.

Induced hypothermia may be used for the duration of an operation or it may be prolonged for 3 to 5 days, depending on the objective. For prolonged treatment, care of the eyes, the mouth and the skin are important. Maintenance of proper body alignment is essential and the patient should be turned to alternate sides every 2 hours.

Rewarming

Ice bags are removed and the patient is allowed to rewarm at his own rate. At this time, hot water bottles are contraindicated because of the danger of burning the skin. Following the return to a normal body temperature, the patient continues to have his vital signs checked periodically and a gradual return to a normal diet is planned. Problems that require special observation may include: an increased bleeding tendency, gastric distention, skin changes resulting from exposure to cold.

ARTIFICIAL HYPOTENSION DURING OPERATION

Another new development is that of producing *deliberate hypotension.* This is accomplished by spinal or intravenous injection of drugs that affect the sympathetic ganglia. Halothane is the anesthetic agent commonly used. This is supplemented with other means to lower blood pressure, such as a head-up position, positive pressure applied to the airway and administration of a ganglionic blocking drug such as pentolinium (Anolysen). The resultant hypotension reduces bleeding at the operative site, thereby allowing for more rapid surgery. Such a technique has been successful in brain surgery, radical neck dissection and radical pelvic surgery.

MALIGNANT HYPERTHERMIA DURING ANESTHESIA

Instances of severe hyperthermia have been reported recently, occurring during general anesthesia at which time the temperature may reach over $43.3°C$ ($110°F$). The mortality rate is about 75 per cent. Reasons for this phenomenon are unknown. However, careful monitoring can prevent its progression. Measures to combat the temperature rise include such treatments as ice packs, infusion of iced saline solution, administration of high concentrations of oxygen, and sodium bicarbonate to combat metabolic acidosis.

POSITION ON OPERATING TABLE

The position in which the patient is placed on the operating table depends upon the operation to be performed as well as the physical condition of the patient. Factors to consider:

(1) The patient should be in as comfortable a position as possible, whether asleep or awake.

(2) The operative area must be adequately exposed.

(3) Circulation should not be obstructed by an awkward position or undue pressure on a part (Fig. 9-10).

(4) There should be no interference with the patient's respiration as a result of pressure of the arms on the chest or from constriction of a gown about the neck or the chest.

(5) Nerves must be protected from undue pressure. Improper positions of arms, hands, legs or feet may cause serious injury or paralysis. Shoulder braces must be well padded to prevent irreparable nerve injury, especially when the Trendelenburg position is necessary.

(6) Concern for the patient as an individual must be practiced, particularly with the very thin, the elderly or the obese.

Dorsal Recumbent Position. The usual position is flat on the back, with the arms at the side on the table, palms down (Fig. 9-10). This position is used for most abdominal operations, except for those upon the gallbladder and the pelvis, and for other operations as described below (Fig. 9-10).

Trendelenburg Position. This position usually is employed for operations on the lower abdomen and the pelvis to obtain good exposure by displacing the intestines into the upper abdomen. In this position the

---

* Graves notes that 2 sizes of bags are most desirable. One that measures 36 x 12 inches is ideal for molding over the arms and the legs. The other measuring 12 x 12 inches is used to cover the chest and the abdomen.

head and the body are lowered, so that the plane of the body meets the horizontal at an angle. The knees are flexed by "breaking" the table, and the patient is held in position by padded shoulder braces (Fig. 9-10).

Lithotomy Position. This is the position in which, with the patient on his back and under the influence of an anesthetic, the legs and the thighs are flexed to right angles. The position is maintained by placing the feet in stirrups. Nearly all perineal, rectal and vaginal operations require this posture (Fig. 9-10).

For kidney operations, the patient is placed on his well side in Sims's position with an air pillow 5 or 6 inches thick under the loin, or he is placed on a table with a kidney or back lift (Fig. 9-10).

For chest and abdominothoracic operations, the position varies with the operation to be performed. The surgeon and the anesthesiologist place the patient on the operating table in the proper position.

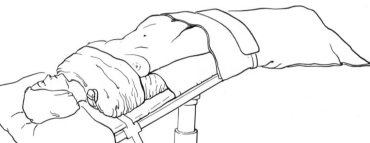

(*Left*) Patient in position on the operating table as prepared for a laparotomy. Note the strap above the knees and the arm holder in use.

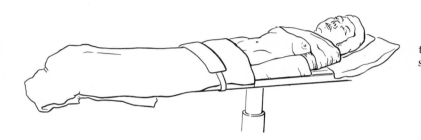

(*Right*) Patient in Trendelenburg position on operating table. Note padded shoulder braces in place.

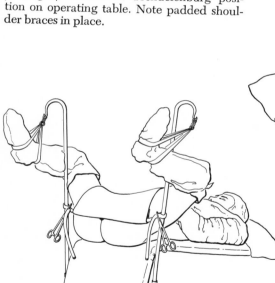

(*Left*) Patient in lithotomy position. Note that the hips extend over the edge of the table.

(*Right*) Patient on operating table for kidney operation, lying on his well side. Table is broken to spread apart space between the lower ribs and the pelvis. The upper leg is extended; the lower leg is flexed at the knee and the hip joints; a pillow is placed between the legs. Note the sandbag, which helps to support patient's chest.

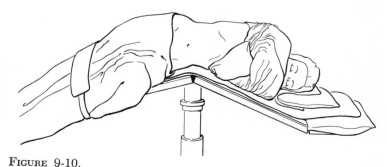

FIGURE 9-10.

Operations on the neck, as for goiter, are performed with the patient on his back, the neck extended somewhat by a pillow beneath the shoulders.

Operations on the skull and the brain demand special positions and apparatus, usually adjusted by the surgeon in charge. Restraining straps are applied after the anesthetic is begun.

BIBLIOGRAPHY

Alexander, E. L., Burley, W., Ellison, D., and Valleri, R.: Care of the Patient in Surgery. St. Louis, C. V. Mosby, 1967.

Carnes, M. A.: Postanesthetic complications. Nurs. Forum, *4*:46-55, 1965.

Clark, R. B.: The case for spinal anesthesia. Amer. J. Nurs., *67*:291-297, Feb., 1967.

Collins, V. J.: Positioning the patient for surgery. AORN J., *4*:55-66, Nov.-Dec., 1966.

Crawford, E. W.: Changing patterns in anesthesia and nursing problems. AORN J., *4*:88-91, March-April, 1966.

Dripps, R. D., Eckenhoff, J. E. and Vandam, L. D.: Introduction to Anesthesia. ed. 3. Philadelphia, W. B. Saunders, 1967.

Greisheimer, E. M.: The physiological effects of anesthesia. Amer. J. Nurs., *49*:337-343, 1949.

Hardy, J. D.: Emergencies in the intraoperative and immediate postoperative periods. *In* Randall: Manual of Preoperative and Postoperative Care. Philadelphia, W. B. Saunders, 1968.

Hickey, M. C.: Hypothermia. Amer. J. Nurs., *65*:116-122, Jan., 1965.

National Fire Protection Association: Tentative Standard for Inhalation Therapy. No. 56B-T, NFPA (60 Batterymarch St., Boston, Mass. 02110). 1966.

Rosenberg, J.: Hazards of presurgical drug therapy. AORN J., *5*:90-93, June, 1967.

Sr. M. Antonita: Pharmacology—a vital role in surgery. AORN J., *3*:59-70, May-June, 1965.

Stubbs, D. H.: Anesthesiology—what nurses should know about it. AORN J., *4*:75-81, 1966.

Tantum, K. R. and Dripps, R. D.: The scope and challenge of modern anesthesia. Nurs. Cl. N. Amer., *3*:591-600, Dec., 1968.

Zeppernick, R. G.: New trends in anesthesia. Nurs. Forum, *4*:41-45, 1965.

SECTION C, CHAPTER **9**

The Postoperative Patient

- *Recovery Room*
- *Removing Patient from Operating Table*
- *Principles of Immediate Postoperative Nursing Care*
- *Needs of the Patient Returning to Complete Consciousness*
- *Body Alignment and Good Body Mechanics*
- *Early Postoperative Ambulation*
- *Postoperative Fluid and Nutritional Needs*
- *Care of the Wound*
- *Charts and Nurses' Records*
- *Postoperative Discomforts and Complaints*
- *Postoperative Complications*

The prime objective of postoperative nursing care is to assist the patient in his return to normal function as quickly, safely and comfortably as possible.

Considerable effort should be expended on *anticipation* and *prevention*, if possible, of difficulties in the postoperative period. The nursing care of the patient after operation is second in importance only to the operation itself.

RECOVERY ROOM

The recovery room is a unit on the same floor as or near the operating rooms, where there is a concentration of (1) nurses who are especially prepared in caring for the immediate postoperative patient, (2) anesthesiologists and surgeons, (3) special equipment, medications and replacement fluids and (4) patients who are under anesthesia or are recovering from it. With this setting, the newly operated patient is given the best care available by those best qualified to give it.

The room should be quiet, neat and clean; unnecessary equipment should be removed. Many units are equipped with shelf space running the length of the wall, thus eliminating the use of inefficient small mobile tables. Other features of this room might be: (1) walls and ceiling painted in soft pleasing colors, (2) indirect lighting, (3) soundproof ceiling and (4) equipment that controls or eliminates noise, e.g., syn-

thetic emesis basins, rubber bumpers on beds and tables and so forth, as well as isolated quarters (glass encased) for noisy patients. These seemingly luxurious features may be added at little extra cost, yet psychologically they are of real value to the patient.

Equipment includes every type of breathing aid: oxygen, laryngoscopes, tracheotomy sets, bronchial instruments, catheters, mechanical ventilators and suction equipment; another necessity is equipment for meeting circulatory needs, such as blood pressure apparatus, parenteral equipment, universal donor blood, plasma expanders, intravenous trays and cut-down trays, cardiac arrest equipment, defibrillator, venous catheters and tourniquets. Surgical dressing materials, narcotics and emergency drugs should be available also. Monitoring devices provide an accurate and instant appraisal of the patient's condition.

The recovery bed should be one that affords easy access to the patient, is safe, easily movable, can assume Trendelenburg and reverse Trendelenburg position easily and possesses features that facilitate care, such as available receptacles for intravenous poles, side guards, wheel brakes and chart storage rack.

The temperature of the room should be about 68° F. to 70° F. during the day and about 60° F. at night. There should be an abundance of fresh air but no draughts.

A patient remains in this unit until he has reacted from the anesthetic agent, that is, has a stable blood pressure, good air passage and a reasonable degree of consciousness.

Many hospitals have set up an intensive care unit to which are admitted all patients requiring special care. These include those who have recovered from anesthesia but who demand intensive care, patients from other areas of the hospital who require special care, e.g., those with cardiac problems, hemiplegia, gastrointestinal bleeding, burns, and others in critical condition. The equipment is similar to that described for the recovery room, and the nursing staff is specially skilled in the care of critically ill patients.

REMOVING PATIENT FROM OPERATING TABLE

The removal of the patient from the operating table to the bed or the stretcher should be done with the least possible delay and exposure. Exposure of the perspiring patient predisposes to pulmonary complications and postoperative shock. The site of the operation should be kept in mind every time a newly operated patient is moved. Many wounds are closed under considerable tension, and every effort should be made not to place any further strain on the sutures. Thus, in patients in whom a thyroidectomy has been performed, the head should not be allowed to hyperextend; in breast amputations, the arm of the operated side should be held close to the body; in nephrectomy, the patient should not be allowed to lie on the affected side; and so on.

Attention has been called to the problem of serious arterial hypotension that may occur when a patient is moved from a lithotomy position to a horizontal position, from lateral to supine, from prone to supine and even from movement of the anesthetized patient to the stretcher; it must be done slowly and carefully.

As soon as the patient is placed on the stretcher or bed, he is covered with lightweight blankets that have been arranged previously on the stretcher. The wet and soiled gown and socks should be removed, a dry gown applied, and the bedding tucked in along the sides as well as at the bottom. On the stretcher the patient is held with straps above the knees and the elbows. The straps serve the double purpose of securing the blankets and of restraining the patient should he pass through a stage of excitement as he recovers from the anesthetic. Siderails should be raised to the position affording protection.

PRINCIPLES OF IMMEDIATE POSTOPERATIVE NURSING CARE

Transfer of the postoperative patient from surgery to the recovery room is the responsibility of the anesthesiologist, with some member of the special care unit in attendance. If a nurse has been assigned to a particular patient, she would assist also. The nurse needs to know what operation was performed, any untoward problem that has occurred in the operating room that may have a bearing on postoperative care, and what pathology was encountered (if a malignancy, whether the patient or his family know). She needs to know the patient's present condition, complications that might develop and special symptoms to watch for. She should be provided with immediate postoperative orders in writing. In most hospitals a physician remains in the unit while the nurse checks (1) the patient's blood pressure, pulse and respirations and (2) his airway, tubing, drains, catheters, infusions and other supportive aids as may have been instituted in the operating room.

The chief immediate postoperative hazards are those of shock and anoxemia due to respiratory difficulties. Shock can be avoided largely by the timely administration of intravenous fluids and blood and by appropriate drugs. The *respiratory difficulties* may be treated as they arise, or better, the patient can be treated so that they do not arise. These disturbances are confined almost entirely to those patients who are under prolonged or deep anesthesia. Patients given local anesthesia, nitrous oxide or ethylene usually are "awake" a few minutes after leaving the operating room. However, those patients having prolonged anesthesia usually are completely unconscious, with all muscles relaxed. This relaxation extends to the muscles of the pharynx; therefore, when the patient lies on his back the lower jaw and the tongue fall backward, and the air passages close more or less completely (Fig. 9-11).

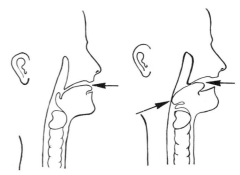

Fig. 9-11. Respiratory obstruction. (*Left*) With the tone of muscles normal, the tongue is in its usual position. (*Right*) With the muscles relaxed, the chin drops back, and the tongue comes in contact with the posterior wall of the pharynx, thereby shutting off the respiratory passages. (Greisheimer, Esther: The physiological effects of anesthesia, Am. J. Nursing 49:338)

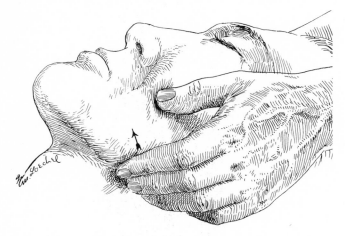

Fig. 9-12. Position of hand to hold the jaw forward after inhalation of anesthesia. Note that the fingers are placed behind the angle of the jaw, and the direction of the arrow shows the direction of pressure being exerted on the jaw. As the jaw is pushed forward the tongue is brought forward so as to keep an open airway. This is important, especially after operation under general anesthesia in children, for instance, in tonsillectomy.

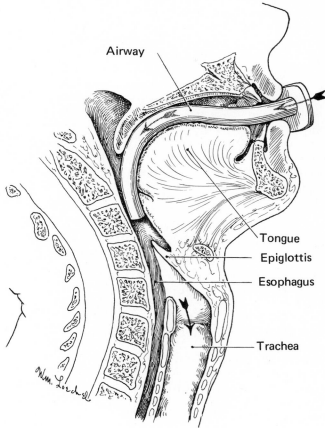

Fig. 9-13. Diagrammatic view to show methods by which an airway prevents respiratory difficulty after anesthesia. The airway passes over the base of the tongue and delivers air into the pharynx in the region of the epiglottis. Patients are often brought from the operating room with an airway in place. This should remain in place until the patient recovers sufficiently to breathe normally. Usually, as the patient regains consciousness, the airway causes irritation; then it should be removed.

The patient gives evidence of this difficulty in breathing by choking, noisy and irregular respirations, and in a short time a blue duskiness (cyanosis) of the skin appears. The treatment of this complication is to push forward on the angle of the lower jaw as if to push the lower teeth in front of the upper (Fig. 9-12). This maneuver pulls the tongue forward and opens the air passages. At times it may be necessary to grasp the tongue between gauze and pull it forward for a time. This prevents the respiratory obstruction, and the maneuver should be continued when necessary until the patient has regained reflex functions sufficiently to carry on normal respiration.

Often the anesthesiologist leaves a hard rubber or plastic "airway" in the mouth or a rubber nasal catheter in the nose. By both devices a patent airway is maintained. Such a device should not be removed until the patient expresses a desire to have it removed (Fig. 9-13).

Not infrequently the respiratory difficulty is produced by an excessive secretion of mucus. Turning the head to the side allows the collected fluid to escape from the side of the mouth. If vomiting occurs, the head should be turned sharply to the side and the vomitus collected in the emesis basin. The face should be wiped with gauze or paper wipes.

A very important point for the nurse to remember is that the only sure way of knowing whether a patient is breathing or not is to place the palm of her hand over the nose and the mouth of the patient in order to feel the exhaled breath. Movements of the thorax and the diaphragm do not necessarily mean that a patient is breathing. Mucus or vomitus obstructing the pharynx or the trachea should be aspirated with a nasal catheter introduced into the nasopharynx or the oropharynx. In most recovery rooms, wall suction or suction machines are available for this purpose. The introduction of the catheter into the nasopharynx or the oropharynx is not dangerous, and the catheter can be introduced safely a distance of 6 to 8 inches if secretions are obtained at this level. Oxygen may be given by mask, tent or intranasally. (See Chapt. 15.)

Nursing Activities During Recovery from Anesthesia

A nurse should be in constant attendance while the patient is recovering from anesthesia. *Never leave a patient alone, even for an instant.* The following are her chief responsibilities:

1. **Maintain a patent airway** (discussed in section immediately preceding this).

2. **Carry out any "stat" orders immediately.** This usually refers to drug or oxygen therapy.

3. **Turn the patient's head to the side when he vomits.** Wipe the lips and the mouth with paper wipes or gauze. Note the amount and the nature of the vomitus and record. Frequent aspiration of the nasopharynx and the oropharynx may be indicated. A clean rubber or plastic catheter is essential for this, and a basin of water for cleansing the suction tip. Caution is necessary in suctioning the throats of patients who have had tonsillectomies, since irritation of the operative area may cause bleeding or added discomfort. Moisten the lips to relieve thirst.

4. **Observe the patient and monitors for signs of respiratory obstruction, shock and hemorrhage.** The chief guides are the appearance of the patient, the pulse, the respiration and the temperature. The pulse and the respiration should be noted at frequent intervals for the first 2 hours, and every ½ hour for the next 2 hours. Thereafter they may be taken less frequently if they remain stable. The blood pressure is taken as often as ordered. A temperature of over 37.7° C. (100° F.) or under 36.1° C. (97° F.), respirations of over 30 or under 16 and a systolic blood pressure of under 90 are usually considered reportable at once. However, the patient's preoperative or base-line blood pressure should be known in order to make effective postoperative comparisons. Make notes on the general condition of the patient—for example, his color, good or cyanotic; skin, cold and clammy, warm and moist; excessive mucus in the throat and in the nostrils.

5. **Place patient in proper position.** Until the patient regains consciousness, the bed is kept flat. Unless contraindicated, the unconscious patient is positioned on his side with a pillow at his back and with his chin extended to minimize aspiratory danger. His knees are flexed to reduce strain on abdominal sutures.

6. **Promote comfort and maintain safety; keep the patient as quiet and as comfortable as possible.** When he is coming out of the anesthesia he may be restless. If it is at all possible, he should not be restrained, but he must be protected from injuring himself. Usually an infusion is running. If the arm is splinted, the needle will not be dislodged. However, the patient can pull the needle out with his free hand. Patients who have had hyoscine (scopolamine) or Amytal before operation should be watched closely for several hours after they have recovered from the effects of the anesthesia. Not infrequently, these drugs cause a type of delirium. Patients have been known to get out of bed and do other injurious things while under their influence. When the patient is fully conscious, deep breathing and turning every hour are necessary to prevent atelectasis or other pulmonary complications.

7. **Attach any drainage apparatus** when drainage is to be collected in a bottle—for example, from cholecystostomy or choledochostomy tubes, catheters, enterostomy drains and chest tubes. In case of underwater drainage tubes, such as those used after thoracotomy, clamps should be available to clamp the tube in order to prevent air from entering the chest if the bottle is accidentally broken or the apparatus disconnected.

8. **Begin postoperative treatment** as ordered—for example, attach nasogastric tube to suction-drainage apparatus.

9. **Inspect dressings** from time to time to detect signs of undue hemorrhage or abnormal drainage. Reinforce dressings, if necessary, making note of time of application on nurse's record.

10. **Report any alarming or peculiar signs or symptoms** to the surgeon at once. This includes any mental phenomena or uneasiness on the part of the patient. A patient's statements concerning his condition never should be disregarded entirely.

11. **Keep an intelligent and accurate record.** The volume and the character of the intake and the output must be charted conscientiously.

The Patient's Postoperative Symptoms

Often the inexperienced nurse is at a loss to differentiate between important and unimportant symptoms; and, in fact, the experienced nurse sometimes may be puzzled as to whether or not to notify the surgeon of a certain change in condition. The safest plan always is to call for advice when in doubt. However, in order to be able to decide intelligently, there are a few general rules that may be of some assistance. Of course, any severe symptom always is important. Any apparently slight symptom that tends to recur repeatedly or to increase in severity should be regarded as significant— for example, hiccups may or may not be of importance, depending on the duration. A symptom seemingly may be of no consequence in itself but when associated with other definite changes may foretell danger; for example, a repeated sigh means nothing, but, when accompanied by great restlessness, increasing pallor, rising pulse rate and so forth, it becomes one of the clinical signs of dangerous hemorrhage. Any progressive and steady change for the worse in the general condition of the patient, even with no outstanding symptoms evident, is of the gravest importance. And, as has been mentioned already, the patient's complaints and statements never should be passed over without investigation.

If the physician in charge of the patient is to be notified for any reason, be sure to have all necessary information literally at your fingertips before going to the telephone. Know the latest temperature, the pulse, the respiration and blood pressure readings, and always take the patient's chart and the nurse's record with you to the telephone, in order to refer to them should occasion arise. Learn to state the patient's condition concisely and accurately, and be prepared to answer all questions intelligently.

NEEDS OF THE PATIENT RETURNING TO COMPLETE CONSCIOUSNESS

As the patient returns to consciousness, he usually expresses concern about the outcome of the operation, his family, and his awareness of discomfort. Brief but appropriate information can be given to him. When his condition permits, a close member of his family may see him for a few moments. Thus, the family is reassured, and the patient feels more secure.

Hypodermic injections of morphine, Dilaudid, Demerol or Methadon often are ordered for pain and restlessness. Such an order usually is written "p.r.n." (Latin for "pro re nata"—as required by circumstances) for a certain number of doses. The time of administration frequently is left to the judgment of the nurse, but she should realize that pain in the first 24 hours after an operation requires relief by narcotics, and these drugs should not be withdrawn when the patient is in pain. There is seldom any method of relieving pain in the operative region, but the following suggestions may be useful in assuaging general discomfort temporarily and rendering the hypodermic medication more effectual when finally it is given:

1. Change position. Give added support with pillows. A small pillow in the hollow of the back is comforting.

2. Encourage deep breathing. A most important point in the care of the patient after the anesthesia is to prevent pulmonary complications. This is another significant reason why the *radical alteration in the position* of the patient is important. He is able to expand his lungs better when this is done. Patients are *encouraged to cough* in an effort to clear the respiratory passages of secretions. A third method of causing gas exchange in the lung is to encourage the patient to *take deep breaths.* This may be done by the use of a blow bottle. This is merely a gallon bottle half-filled with water. A length of tubing with a mouthpiece is attached to the bottle and the patient is asked to "blow bubbles" for 5 minutes in every hour. Unless the patient is told why it is important for him to do this

simple procedure, the nurse may not get his cooperation. Another method of stimulating deep respirations is by the use of carbon dioxide inhalations. This may be carried out by using a face mask attached to a gas tank or simply by instructing the patient to blow in and out of a paper bag. In a fourth method the patient should be shown how to take a deep breath, hold it a second and then give a hard cough as he starts to expel the air. On the second or the third exercise of this kind, he will often expectorate suddenly a viscid mass of mucus and clear his lungs.

3. Wash the face and the hands. Cold cloths applied to the forehead often are soothing.

4. Give a mouthwash. At the same time wipe the lips with a cool gauze sponge when water by mouth is not permitted.

5. Rub the back with lotion or alcohol. The extremities may be stroked very lightly with alcohol. *They never should be rubbed vigorously.* To do so may dislodge a thrombus and result in embolism and death.

6. If permissible give water in small quantities when nausea ceases. If small amounts are retained by the patient, the quantity given at one time may be increased gradually. Water is best either hot or cold; otherwise, it is likely to cause nausea. There are times when a large glass of water will do a patient no harm, even when he is nauseated, but this never should be given without the proper authority. Patients usually ask for cracked ice, and usually it does no harm in small amounts. If orders are that the patient is to have nothing by mouth, cracked ice wrapped in a piece of gauze is refreshing and soothing to the lips.

7. Remove blankets. If the patient has been put between blankets, they should be removed on complete recovery from the anesthesia—when the temperature, the pulse and the respirations are within normal limits, or they may be removed promptly but carefully when they are the cause of excessive perspiration. Recovery beds should be made in such a manner that the patient is left between sheets when these extra blankets are withdrawn. Cool sheets usually are a most gratifying change and often very soothing. However, care must be taken that the change is not too abrupt: if the patient complains of excessive heat, remove the under blanket first and the upper blanket a little later. In warm weather too many blankets cause marked perspiration and the consequent loss of a large amount of fluid. Therefore, it is advisable as a rule not to use blankets on the recovery bed during warm periods in the summer months. Remember that patients who have been anesthetized are susceptible to chills and draughts. Remember, also, that the obese patient perspires profusely and so loses fluid and salt much more rapidly than the patient who is of normal weight.

8. **Elimination.** URINATION. The length of time a patient may be permitted to go without voiding after operation varies considerably with the type of operation performed. Following gynecologic and abdominal operations patient catheterization may be required at the end of 8 or 10 hours (sometimes sooner), and in others it may be put off for 16 to 18 hours. Generally speaking, every effort must be made to avoid the use of catheter. Exhaust all known methods to aid the patient in voiding—let water run, apply heat and so forth. Never give a patient a cold bedpan. When a patient complains of not being able to use the bedpan, some surgeons permit the use of the commode rather than resort to catheterization. Of course, this applies only to suitable cases. Male patients sometimes are permitted to sit up or stand beside the bed, but this should not be allowed unless an orderly is in attendance to prevent any accidents from falling or fainting. All urine, whether voided or catheterized, must be measured and the amount noted on the nurse's record. A separate intake and output chart (p. 139) should be kept on all aged and all very ill patients. (See also p. 153, Urinary Retention.)

Defecation. Each defecation should be recorded. If the bowels do not move spontaneously every other day, a cleansing enema usually is given. As a rule, cathartics are not given to postoperative patients, especially if the operation has been on the abdomen.

9. **Psychological support.** Almost all postoperative surgical patients have need for psychological support during the immediate postoperative period. The questions posed by an awakening patient often indicate his deep feelings and thoughts. Perhaps he shows concern about the operation and the findings or about his future—whatever his expression, the nurse should be in a position to answer his query reassuringly without going into a discussion of details. The immediate postoperative period is not the time for discussion of operative findings or prognosis. On the other hand, these questions ought not to be dismissed lightly, for they may offer clues that suggest the method to select in directing future treatment and rehabilitation. The function of the recovery room nurse cannot be limited to bedside procedures, safety measures and the relief of pain; an understanding regarding the significance of psychological support is also important. If the nurse has never seen the patient before, a definite handicap is immediately presented. The nurse who knows the patient and accompanies him through the immediate preoperative and operative experiences is in a unique position to offer valuable support. In the absence of such continuous care by one nurse, pertinent nurses' notes on the chart help the recovery room nurse to recognize the particular needs of each individual patient.

BODY ALIGNMENT AND GOOD BODY MECHANICS

(Also see: Rehabilitation, Chapter 10, p. 161.) Poor posture for the surgical patient can result in the development of complications with subsequent delay in convalescence. These include pulmonary complications resulting from inadequate chest expansion, improper drainage from body cavities, contractures, decubiti, circulatory impairment and urinary and gastrointestinal difficulties.

The principles of proper body alignment and good body mechanics are an essential part of good surgical nursing. These apply to the nurse as well as to her patient.

Dorsal Position

The patient lies on his back without elevation of the head. In most cases this is the position in which the patient is placed immediately after operation. The head usually is turned to one side to facilitate easy evacuation of vomitus and to prevent its aspiration into the lungs. Bed covers should not restrict the movement of the toes and the feet of the patient.

This position is maintained until the patient has recovered from the effects of the anesthetic and has regained sufficient reflex activity to swallow, cough and so forth. This position may be employed to advantage many times when the necessity for drainage does not demand the Fowler position. It is believed that when the patient is flat in bed, respiration often is more free and turning is easier, advantages that are important in the prevention of respiratory complications.

Sims' or Lateral Position

The patient lies on either side with the upper arm forward. The under leg lies slightly flexed, the upper leg is flexed at the thigh and the knee. The head is supported on a pillow, and a second pillow is placed longitudinally under the flexed knee. This position is used when it is desirable to have the patient change position frequently, to aid in the drainage of cavities, as of the chest, the abdomen and so forth, and to prevent postoperative pulmonary, respiratory and circulatory complications.

Fowler Position

Of all the positions ordered for a patient, perhaps the most common, as well as the most difficult to maintain, is the Fowler. The difficulty in most instances lies in trying to make the patient fit the bed rather than having the bed conform to the needs of the patient. The patient's trunk is raised to form an angle of from 60° to 70° with the horizontal. This is a comfortable sitting position. Patients with abdominal drainage usually are put in Fowler position as soon as they have recovered consciousness, but great caution must be observed in raising the bed. It is not an unusual occurrence for a patient to feel faint after the raising of the head of the bed, and for this reason a close watch must be kept on the pulse rate and the color. If the patient complains of any dizziness, the bed must be lowered at once. However, if the condition of the patient is good, the head of the bed may be raised within 1 or 2 hours.

The nurse must determine whether or not the patient is in correct position and comfortable. Often very short people are most uncomfortable in the ordinary hospital bed and must be supported by pillows. It is advisable to place a support against the feet to prevent slipping down in bed, to prevent footdrop and to make the patient feel more secure.

When the Fowler position is ordered for a patient, it is the nurse's responsibility to see that this position is maintained at all times. It is not sufficient to arrange the patient in a faultless manner: he must remain so. No matter how correctly placed or how well supported by pillows the patient is, he will slip down in the course of time and frequent lifting up in bed and readjustment of the pillows will be necessary. Another significant reason for maintaining good body posture is that it affords better functioning of all organs, including those of respiration.

Jackknife or Semi-Fowler Position

This position is one used to relieve tension following the repair of inguinal or abdominal hernia. It is produced by raising the head of the patient from 10 to 12 inches and flexing the knees.

The Patient's Comfort and Changes of Position

Hampered by dressings, splints or drainage apparatus, the patient very frequently is quite unable to shift his position. Lying constantly in the same position may be the cause of pressure sores or hypostatic pneumonia, to mention only two of the more serious resulting complications. Turning a pillow from one side to another presents a cooler side as it touches the patient. Proper support for the arms and the hands offers a measure of comfort. A foot support encourages the patient to stretch his foot muscles and spread his toes, which is a relaxing maneuver. The helpless patient must be turned from side to side at least every 2 hours, and he should have his position changed as soon as he becomes uncomfortable.

When a patient is unable to turn himself, it may be necessary for the nurse to have 1 or 2 assistants. The number of persons needed depends on whether the patient must be moved in one unit or not and on his height and weight. At all times, the nurse should practice good body mechanics herself. Often back strain can be prevented if, instead of bending at the waist, the nurse can lift her patient with her back erect. bending at the knees and the hips.

EARLY POSTOPERATIVE AMBULATION

Almost all types of surgical patients are allowed and encouraged to be out of bed within 24 to 48 hours after operation. The advantages of early ambulation are seen in a reduction of postoperative complications. Atelectasis and hypostatic pneumonia are relatively infrequent when the patient is ambulatory. Ambulation increases respiratory exchange and aids in preventing stasis of bronchial secretions within the lung. Postoperative distention is almost absent, due to the increased tone of the gastrointestinal tract and the abdominal wall. Therefore, frequent enemata are unnecessary. Thrombophlebitis or phlebothrombosis are less frequent because ambulation increases the rate of circulation in the extremities, thereby preventing stasis of venous blood. Clinical as well as experimental evidence shows that the rate of healing in abdominal wounds is more rapid by early ambulation, and the occurrence of postoperative evisceration has been no greater than formerly: in some series of cases actually it has been less when the patient was allowed to be out of bed soon after operation. Statistics indicate that pain is decreased, as shown by the number of hypodermics required. Comparative records also indicate that the pulse rate and the temperature return to normal sooner when the patient attempts to regain his normal preoperative activity as quickly as possible.

Re-establishing a normal physiology includes a resumption of a full diet. Normal intestinal function returns in 2 or 3 days. This is indicated by the appearance of peristaltic sounds and the passage of gas. After this time the diet may be increased rapidly. In a few instances, a more adequate diet may be given earlier (usually, patients with operations on the extremities, following thyroidectomy, etc.). Finally, there are the further advantages to the patient of a shorter stay in the hospital, with the consequent lower expense.

Early ambulation should not be overdone. The condition of the patient must be the deciding factor. The very ill and feeble aged patient must be given every consideration. First of all, he must be placed almost upright in bed until all suggestion of dizziness has passed. This position can be obtained by raising the head of the bed. Then, he may be placed completely upright and turned so that his legs hang over the edge of the bed. After this preparation, he may be helped to stand beside his bed. When he has become accommodated to the upright position, he may take a few steps to a chair or around the bed. The nurse should be at his side to give support, both physical and moral.

Care must be taken not to tire the patient, and the extent of the first few periods of ambulation should vary with the type of operation and the physical condition and the age of the patient.

Convalescent Bed Exercises

When early ambulation is not feasible due to circumstances already mentioned, *convalescent bed exercises* may accomplish to some extent the same desirable results. General exercises should begin as soon after operation as possible—preferably within the first 24 hours—and they should be done under supervision to ensure their adequacy. These exercises are done to prevent the development of contractures and other deformities as well as to permit the patient the fullest return of his functions:

(1) Deep breathing exercises for complete lung expansion

(2) Arm exercises through full range of motion, with specific attention to abduction and external rotation of shoulder

(3) Hand and finger exercises

(4) Foot exercises to prevent foot drop and toe deformities and to aid in maintaining good circulation

(5) Exercises to prepare the patient for ambulation activities

(6) Abdominal and gluteal contraction exercises.

POSTOPERATIVE FLUID AND NUTRITIONAL NEEDS

Patients have nutritional and fluid needs even greater after operation than before it. Although these requirements may be supplied fairly well by the intravenous administration of amino acids, glucose, saline and blood (see pp. 85-87), this method of feeding a patient is much less efficient than giving food by mouth.

In many instances, even though a major operation has been performed, there is no reason why a normal diet cannot be given. Thus, after a thyroidectomy, a breast amputation, a lung resection or a herniorrhaphy, the patient may receive a full diet if he desires it. The patient should be encouraged to eat normally, because many patients are afraid to eat. By eating a normal diet, many of the unpleasant "gas pains" and enemas can be avoided. However, food should not be forced on the unwilling patient. The desire of the patient for food is one of the best indications of a normal recovery.

Usually liquids are desired first by the patient after operation. They also are tolerated by him. Water, fruit juices and tea with lemon and sugar may be given in increasing amounts if vomiting does not occur. Fluids administered should be cool, not ice cold or tepid. The fluids supply relatively few calories. If fluids are tolerated well, gelatin, junket, custard and cornstarch pudding may be added gradually; even buttered toast, milk and creamed soups. As soon as the patient tolerates liquids well, solid food may be given.

CARE OF THE WOUND
Careful Asepsis

The most important requisite for the successful care of wounds is careful asepsis. Bacteria are excluded from wounds during the period of operation to the full extent of the facilities for sterility in the operating room. Organisms that enter the wound usually are destroyed by the natural powers of resistance of the body. Accidental wounds are potentially infected wounds. Therefore, the surgeon is concerned with the removal of as much of the infection as possible and with the protection of the wound from further invasion by bacteria.

Wound Classification

Wounds are classified as (1) incised, (2) contused, (3) lacerated or (4) puncture, according to the manner in which they were made.

Incised wounds are those made by a clean cut with a sharp instrument. They are made by the surgeon in every operation.

Contused wounds are made by blunt force and are characterized by considerable injury of the soft parts, hemorrhage and swelling.

Lacerated wounds are those with jagged, irregular edges, such as would be made by glass, barbed wire and so forth.

Puncture wounds have small openings in the skin, such as those made by a bullet, a knifestab and the like.

Clean wounds (those made aseptically) usually are closed by sutures after all bleeding points have been ligated carefully. All other wounds are potentially infected and cannot be closed until every effort has been made to remove all devitalized tissue and infection. Therefore, a formal operation is performed for the purpose of cutting out the infected and devitalized tissue. This operation is called *débridement*. Often it is well to insert a small drain before suturing the wound to prevent the collection of blood and lymph, which would retard healing if it were allowed to remain.

Physiology of Wound Healing

Healing by First Intention (Primary Union). Wounds made aseptically and with a minimum of tissue destruction heal with very little tissue reaction "by first intention" (Fig. 9-14).

Healing by Second Intention (Granulation). In patients in which pus formation (suppuration) has oc-

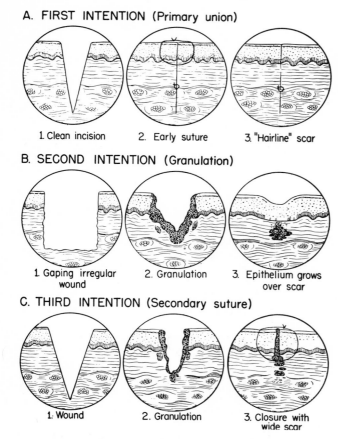

A. FIRST INTENTION (Primary union)

1. Clean incision   2. Early suture   3. "Hairline" scar

B. SECOND INTENTION (Granulation)

1. Gaping irregular wound   2. Granulation   3. Epithelium grows over scar

C. THIRD INTENTION (Secondary suture)

1. Wound   2. Granulation   3. Closure with wide scar

Fig. 9-14. Chronologic course of wound healing by first, second and third intention. In the final stage of second-intention healing it is to be noted that the underside of the epithelium is smooth and not serrated as normally. In the healing by second intention, the important role of contraction, which occurs in the patient in 3 dimensions and in the illustrations in 2, (B-2 and B-3), is shown. Contraction also plays a role in third-intention healing (C-2 and C-3). In C-3 an early phase is shown. Later the granulation tissue will be incorporated as a wide fibrous scar. (Rhoads et al.: Surgery: Principles and Practice, ed. 4, Philadelphia, J. B. Lippincott, 1970.)

curred, the process of repair is less simple and delayed longer. When an abscess is incised, it collapses partly, but the dead and the dying cells forming its walls are still being thrown out into the cavity. For this reason rubber tubes, rubber tissue or gauze packing often is inserted into the abscess pocket to allow the pus to escape easily. Gradually the necrotic material disintegrates and escapes, and the abscess cavity fills with a red, soft, insensitive tissue that bleeds very easily. It is composed of minute thin-walled capillaries, growing off from the parent vessels, each bud surrounded by cells that later form connective tissue. These buds, called granulations, enlarge until they fill the area of

the tissue destroyed. The cells surrounding the capillaries change their round shape; they become long and thin, intertwining with each other to form a *scar* or *cicatrix*. Healing is complete when skin cells (epithelium) grow over these granulations. This method of repair is called *healing by granulation,* and it takes place whenever pus is formed or when loss of tissue has occurred for any reason.

Healing by Third Intention (Secondary Suture). If a deep wound has either not been sutured early or breaks down and then is resutured later, two apposing granulation surfaces are brought together. This results in a deeper and wider scar.

Factors Affecting Wound Healing

In healthy tissue a wound heals at its normal optimal rate. There is no way in which this rate can be accelerated. In less healthy tissue certain aids can be introduced to assist the reparative process. This is brought about by providing an adequate nutritional level in the individual through proper diet. Protein elements and vitamin C are examples of essential needs. Whole blood may be given, since it is necessary to maintain the red blood cell count as near normal as possible; the wounds of anemic patients are known to heal less well than normally. Edema also interferes with the healing process. Tissues heal more readily in the younger patient; hence, age is a factor.

The Purpose of Dressings

A dressing is applied to a wound for one or more reasons: (1) to absorb drainage, (2) for splinting or immobilization of the wound, (3) to protect the wound from mechanical injury, (4) to promote hemostasis, as in a pressure dressing, (5) to prevent contamination from feces, vomitus and urine, and (6) for the mental and physical comfort of the patient.

On occasion, some surgeons prefer to eliminate dressings, either shortly after surgery or within the immediate postoperative period, wherever possible or feasible. On clean, dry incisions, when the initial dressing (applied in the operating room) is removed, usually it is not replaced. Generally, initial dressings on clean, dry incisions are left in place until the sutures are removed, and if a dressing is replaced at all, its purpose is more an esthetic than a necessary one.

In the absence of dressings, a wound heals with fibrin. The apparent advantages of no dressings are that it: (1) eliminates the conditions necessary for growth of organisms (warmth, moisture and darkness), (2) allows for better observation and early detection of wound difficulties, (3) facilitates bathing, (4) tends to minimize the operative procedure, (5) avoids adhesive tape reaction, (6) appears to be more comfortable for the patient and facilitates his activity and (7) is economical.

Substitute materials, such as sprayed plastic dressings, are being used, and they seem to provide satisfactory service for clean and dry incisions. This dressing usually lasts from 5 to 7 days. Depending upon the product, it either peels off or a dissolvent is used. On clean, dry wounds it seems superfluous to be concerned with the ability of the dressing to absorb secretions, since there are practically no secretions to be absorbed. Texture, comfort and perhaps screening ability against microorganisms (although this latter is a doubtful prerequisite) can be given more emphasis than power of absorption in such dressings. In spite of the advantages and the disadvantages mentioned above, most surgeons prefer to apply a dressing at the time of operation and a second dressing between 4 and 5 days later, after the removal of sutures. These dressings are purely protective from a mechanical point of view, and they give the patient a sense of security which is not present if wounds are treated without dressings.

Surgical Dressing Technique

The prerequisite to flawless surgical dressing technique is for surgeons and nurses to agree on a standard. Thereafter, it becomes a matter of repeated teaching and supervision to ensure that such handling of dressings actually is carried out.

Because of the dangers of contamination and spread of infection, the most desirable and safe technique is to use a sterile dressing pack for each patient. With this technique, a surgical dressing cart may be used as a stock table to hold the individually wrapped sterile supplies, including individual flasks of antiseptic solution.

Nursing Responsibility

The surgical nurse should be available to assist the physician in the changing of dressings for several reasons:

(1) The "team" working together assures the patient of expert care.

(2) The nurse, as a witness to the dressing, is better informed concerning her patient and therefore can give him more intelligent care.

(3) The nurse can obtain additional sterile materials as needed and can ensure proper disposal of contaminated articles.

(4) While all initial postoperative dressings are done properly only by the surgeon, subsequent applications may be done by the nurse.

(5) The condition of surgical dressings should be noted on the patient's chart as carefully as any medication or treatment, and pertinent observations should be recorded by the nurse.

Dressing Procedure

Preparation of the Patient. The patient should be told that the surgeon is going to change the dressing, and that it is a simple procedure associated with little discomfort. *Dressings should not be done at mealtime.* If the patient is in an open unit, the curtains should be drawn to ensure his privacy. When the dressing has a foul odor or the patient is unusually squeamish, it is better to wheel his bed to the treatment room, away from other patients. He should not be exposed unduly; his sense of modesty should be respected. At no time should the incision be referred to as a "scar." Psychologically, some patients react to scar as ugly or undesirable.

Stitches (black silk, nylon, or fine wire) or metal skin clips used to approximate the skin edges are of no value after the sixth or the seventh day. The nurse should be prepared for the first dressing at that time.

Removal of Adhesive. The adhesive should be removed by pulling it parallel with the skin surface and not at right angles (Fig. 9-15). Nonirritating solvents are available that come in aerosol containers and aid in removing adhesive tapes painlessly and quickly.

The old dressing and the pledgets used to clean the wound are removed by means of an unsterile forceps and deposited in a waterproof bag for easy closing and disposal by burning. Such dressings are never touched by ungloved hands because of the danger of transmitting pathogenic organisms. After instruments are used in the changing of dressings, they are placed in a receptacle such as an emesis basin and not placed on surfaces where contamination of clean areas is possible.

A Simple Dressing. To carry out aseptic technique, the nurse must know how to handle the transfer forceps correctly. (See p. 996.) For the routine dressing, an individual sterile pack usually contains scissors, forceps, hemostat and grooved director as well as cotton balls, dressings and perhaps a solution container. When the tray has been properly opened (see p. 998), the surgeon, using a forceps, grasps a cotton ball and holds it over the emesis basin as the nurse pours a small quantity of the desired antiseptic. After cleansing the wound and the surrounding skin with an antiseptic, the stitches are removed, and the nurse provides

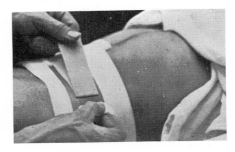

Fig. 9-15. Removing adhesive strips.

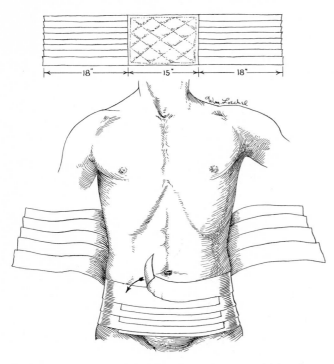

FIG. 9-16. Scultetus binder. Dimensions of binder and method of sewing are shown, also the method of application of binder. The tails should overlap from below upward, and the binder should fit snugly.

adhesive strips for the new dressing. A surgical tape is available for patients who are allergic to the rubber base in the usual adhesive tape. This 3M brand Micropore surgical tape is porous in structure and permits ventilation and prevents maceration. Tension sutures are allowed to remain in place for a longer period of time in some instances.

If there is any doubt concerning the sterility of an instrument or a dressing, it should be considered unsterile. In no circumstance should the nurse touch soiled dressings with her hands.

The Dressing of Draining Wounds. It may be necessary to dress draining wounds as soon as 24 hours after operation. Nothing causes a patient more unnecessary discomfort than a dressing saturated with drainage fluids. It dries on the edges and becomes stiff and scratchy, and the odor frequently is very offensive if not actually nauseating. The nurse may relieve such a situation by changing the outer layers of the dressing at frequent intervals between dressings.

When it is necessary to dress the wound daily, either adhesive with tapes or a laced dressing is more convenient than simple adhesive strips. These should not be applied to tightly that the dressings beneath are unable to retain drainage. A scultetus binder also makes an effective, convenient dressing (Fig. 9-16).

When the edges of the wound gape and the gauze has become adherent to the tissues, the patient may be spared considerable pain by moistening the dressings with peroxide of hydrogen. For this purpose a syringe and a basin containing the solution must be provided. As the surgeon applies the peroxide, the nurse should hold a waste pan to prevent the solution from soiling the bed.

When *drainage tubes* are being shortened, the nurse should have a sterile safety pin ready to insert in the new tube end. If the tubes are removed, the surgeon frequently inserts a piece of rubber tissue or packing to prevent too early a closing of the drainage tract. These materials should be at hand and ready for use.

The drainage from an infected wound frequently proves to be irritating to the surrounding skin. Often this situation may be avoided by the use of a protecting ointment or dressing. Petrolatum gauze, nitrofurazine (Furacin roll), and zinc oxide ointments are favorite preparations. When the discharge from the wound contains the digestive enzymes, as in pancreatic or intestinal fistulae, ileostomy and cecostomy wounds, more active measures to protect the skin must be taken. In some cases, the enzyme-containing secretion may be aspirated by constant suction (see Hemovac, below). In others, the skin surrounding the wound may be protected by such adhering ointments as zinc oxide ointment containing aluminum filings or by a creamy paste mixture of aluminum hydroxide gel and kaolin (Protogel, Wyeth), which is both soothing to the skin and a neutralizer of the enzymes in the secretions. These must be applied to an absolutely dry skin surface.

When a drainage tube is attached to drainage tubing and a bottle, it is necessary to check the tubing frequently for kinking, coiling and looping that would restrict the flow of drainage.

HEMOVAC SUCTION. Suction has been used in the past to evacuate blood and discharge underneath skin flaps. A commonly used and effective means of accomplishing such evacuation at present is the Snyder Hemovac. The principle involved in the Hemovac is the use of gentle, constant suction to effect drainage of serosanguineous fluid and collapse the skin flaps against the underlying tissue. The Snyder Hemovac is a sterile portable suction apparatus (Fig. 9-17) equipped with small multiple, perforated, inert polyethylene tubes. Such tubes are inserted in the drainage areas in the operating room and the wound is completely closed. An electric suction machine may be connected to the device or it may operate as an independent unit, depending upon the nature of the suction required and whether drip irrigation is to be used.

Hemovac suction has several advantages over conventional wound suctioning. It is silent, saves space and is disposable. It is light in weight and permits ambulation for the patient.

The Completion of a Dressing. Dressings are held in place by adhesive or Scotch tape. There are available many types and widths of adhesive tapes. The usual white adhesive tape is frequently used in locations on the extremities or when seepage of secretions is a factor; waterproofed adhesive is available. A transparent adhesive without cloth backing also is available. Some patients who are sensitive to the adhesive material may be better treated by the use of hypoallergic tape.

The correct way to apply tape is to place the tape at the center of the dressing and then press the tape down on both sides, applying tension evenly away from the midline. Unfortunately, the wrong method of applying tape is more common—fixing one end of the tape to the skin and then pulling it tight over the dressing, often wrinkling and pulling the skin in the process. The resulting continuous and forceful traction produces a shearing effect, causing the epidermal layer to slip sideways and become prematurely separated from the deeper dermal layers.

A commercial silicone aerosol is available that can be sprayed over the adhesive used to hold dressings in place; the silicone waterproofs the dressing so the patient can bathe or swim, and isolates the area from contamination. The spray is odorless, colorless, nonstaining, noninflammatory, heat stable and also nonallergenic.

Elastoplast (elastic adhesive bandage) is preferable for holding dressings in place over mobile areas, such as the neck or the extremities, or where pressure is required. When the dressing is completed, the soiled dressings are wrapped in a waterproof bag and deposited in the large covered utility can to await its removal to the incinerator.

CHARTS AND NURSES' RECORDS

To keep a record of all observations and treatments bearing on patient care is an essential nursing function. Accuracy and neatness in the matter of charts and records usually indicate thorough nursing with keen observation and attention to detail. For this reason, the record should be kept up to date. Such a nurse's report is worth more than one in which the whole record for the day is written in 5 minutes before the nurse reports to her successor.

In general, printing rather than script is preferable because usually it is more legible. Statements should be concise, pertinent and brief. The recording of the reactions of a patient to a treatment may be more important for his future therapy than the treatment itself. Hence, significant conversation, facial expressions, and general behavior of an individual ought to be charted. Cultural practices of the patient that reflect past experiences and indicate future tendencies may affect future treatment; therefore, these should be recorded

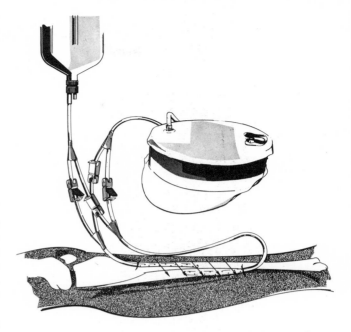

FIG. 9-17. The Snyder Hemovac apparatus can be used as suction alone or interchangeably with an irrigation set-up as this illustration depicts. The directional flow control permits the nurse to open or close the proper clamps so that irrigation or suction can be carried out as ordered. (Courtesy: Zimmer)

by the nurse. This will be of value not only to the physician but also to the next nurse coming to care for this patient.

The nurse prepares the important temperature chart that shows fluctuations in the vital signs of the patient. All medications and treatments should be recorded with the time of administration. The effects produced and/or the results noted must be recorded. For example, in recording the results of an enema, the kind, the amount of solution given and the effectiveness are desired. Merely to chart "Eff." or "Not eff." is not sufficient. By effectiveness is meant, what type of return (color and consistency as well as amount)? Was there much flatus? How did the patient feel during and after the enema?

At the end of each tour of duty, a brief summary is recorded. This may be merely fluid intake and output or it may be more extensive. A 24-hour résumé is more nearly complete and should include the condition of the patient, the medications and the treatments given during that time, the intake and the output and so forth.

Complete fluid intake and output charts are essential on some patients. The nurse must remember that the fluid intake includes all fluids given to the patient by any method during the 24-hour period. This includes liquid foods as well as water taken by mouth and all fluids given parenterally as well as fluids used for irrigating gastrointestinal suction tubes. Fluid output consists of all measurable fluids given off by the patient in 24 hours. This includes urine voided, vomitus and drainage. These fluids are recorded in milliliters and are totaled at periods of 12 and 24 hours.

In many hospitals it is required that each nurse sign or initial that portion of the nurse's record that represents the time she was responsible for the patient's care. When the patient is discharged, the nurse is responsible for seeing that the complete chart is in order and that the ward clerk sends it to the record room. This completes her responsibility.

POSTOPERATIVE DISCOMFORTS AND COMPLAINTS

By knowing that the patient may experience some discomforts postoperatively, the nurse is alerted to recognize their early manifestations and then proceed to alleviate them as best she can. This section should help the nurse to achieve these objectives.

Pain

Pain is among the earliest postoperative symptoms. It can be expected as soon as the patient returns to consciousness. Determination of the presence of pain is made by verbal means (asking the patient how he feels) and through nonverbal means (observation of behavioral evidence of distress). The major components of pain are (1) perception of the stimulus, (2) conduction of the sensation to the central nervous system, and (3) the patient's reaction to the pain. Postoperative pain may originate from the body surface, muscle, tendon, bone, peritoneum or viscera. During the first 24 hours the pain is considered to be due to the cutting, the retracting and the suturing incidental to the operation, and for this discomfort morphine or a similar narcotic should be given as ordered.

Assessment of the Nature of Pain

From studies, it has been determined that in general, only one-third of all postoperative patients have significant pain, one-third have moderate pain relieved by infrequent doses of narcotics, and one-third do not have significant discomfort. The time of maximal pain is between 12 and 36 hours postoperatively and usually disappears by 48 hours. When the patient complains of pain, the nurse should find its location, whether it is intermittent or constant, and whether it is dull, sharp or colicky in character. She should ascertain whether there is any constant radiation of the pain—whether it is down the legs; whether it is in the back; whether it occurs on taking a breath; or whether

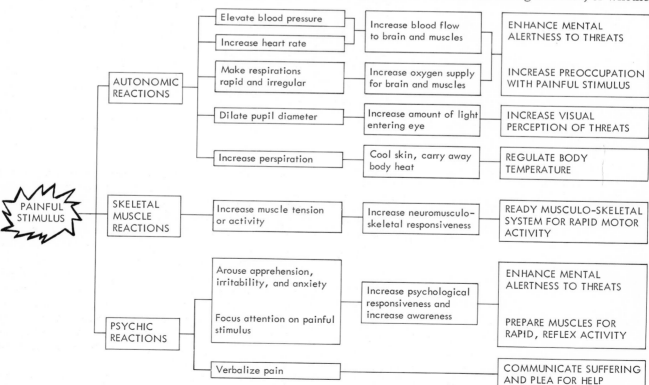

Fig. 9-18A. Biologic purposes of reactions to pain. (Amer. J. Nurs., Pain. *66*:1085-1108, May, 1966.)

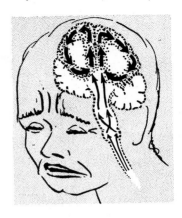
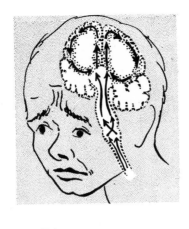
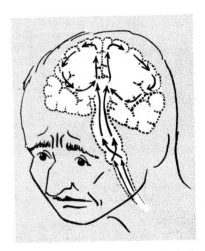

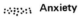 Anxiety   Pain

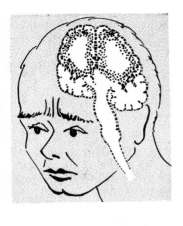
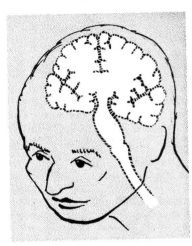
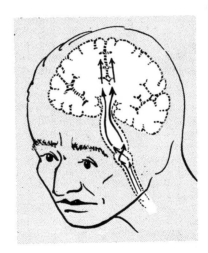

FIG. 9-18B. Reaction of two patients to a painful stimulus of the same intensity. Thicker arrows indicate greater intensity of pain. Notice that individuals react differently to the same pain. (Amer. J. Nurs., Pain. *66:* 1085-1108, May, 1966.)

it is worse at night than during the day. These facts should be noted on the nurse's record and communicated to the surgeon and/or anesthesiologist, because with this information he may be able to diagnose the cause more accurately and prescribe for its relief. In the recovery unit, a more accurate evaluation of the patient's condition can be made because of monitoring devices and the anesthesiologist's assessment of the effect of anesthetic agents and medications given during surgery.

Operation. Some operative procedures are followed by a greater or a lesser demand for analgesics than others. For example, the pain in abdominal and thoracic operations may be aggravated by vomiting, coughing and respiratory movements. It is the responsibility of the nurse to use discriminating judgment in evaluat-

ing the patient's need for narcotics. She can initiate mobilization and activities related to the prevention of complications, and introduce efforts to relieve distress by means other than the use of narcotics.

Type of Anesthetic Agent. The residual effects of anesthetic agents depend upon their solubility in blood and tissues and their excretion. Those with slow excretion rates are methoxyflurane, diethyl ether and trichloroethylene (soluble agents). Following the use of these, the depression of the central nervous system and analgesia may continue for hours postoperatively. On the other hand, insoluble agents, such as cyclopropane or nitrous oxide, produce rapid recovery but may be accompanied by restlessness and delirium.

Psychological Factors. Postoperative pain does not differ from other types of pain in perception and conduction, but the reaction of the patient to the stimulus is as varied and complex as his personality. *The psychological conditioning of an individual is considered the most important factor in the postoperative response to pain.* A neurotic patient with a small wound may complain much more than a phlegmatic individual after an extensive operation. Not only does the mental state of the patient affect the amount of pain he experiences, but there seems to be an actual difference in the amount of pain experienced by individuals of the same type.

Age. Pain seems to be experienced less keenly in old age than in youth and middle age. However, those elderly individuals who display a fear of death may show a markedly low tolerance of pain.

Sex. There is no documented proof that females tolerate pain better than males.

Management and Treatment of the Patient with Pain

Medication for pain is not given until the patient complains. Careful observation assists in the determination of the nature and amount of narcotic required. The ideal balance desired is to provide adequate pain relief and prevent the development of complications. With too much sedation, there is a tendency toward diminished ventilation, retention of airway secretions, pneumonia, atelectasis and depression of the cardiovascular and central nervous systems.

Although pain in the first 24 hours usually is due to the operative procedures, the nurse never should omit a thorough inspection of the wound and the dressings for causes of discomfort. Pins from dressings or drainage tubes may be sticking into the patient, or the bandage may be too tight. Pain occurring after operations on bones or joints in which splints or a cast has been applied demands immediate attention. Pressure points occur very frequently because of insufficient padding or because the bandages have been applied too firmly. These difficulties may be overcome easily if they are found early, but if the danger sign, pain, is disregarded, the patient may go without treatment until pressure causes necrosis of skin or tendons or paralysis of nerves. The pain in these patients may be very short-lived, but it never should be neglected for a single moment.

Abdominal distention is a common cause of pain, and often relief may be given by the insertion of a rectal tube or by the use of a small enema.

Drugs should be used in conjunction with other forms of treatment rather than instead of them. Morphine is the most effective, and it should not be withheld if the indications for its use arise. Morphine raises the patient's pain perception threshold, reduces fear and anxiety and produces sleep. The morphine habit rarely develops in a patient to whom it is given for actual pain. However, as soon as possible it may be replaced by codeine, acetylsalicylic acid, Empirin compound, or Darvon compound. A low or unstable blood pressure would be a warning sign to question the use of morphine because it may cause the patient to go into shock.

Synthetic analgesics are available that are more desirable than morphine for some patients. Examples are meperidine hydrochloride (Demerol), levorphanol tartrate (Levo-Dromoran), methadone hydrochloride (Dolophine, Adanon), phenazocine hydrobromide (Prinadol). Nalorphine hydrochloride (Nalline) is an effective synthetic narcotic antagonist.

Certain patients come to depend on their "hypodermic," especially at night, and complain of pain and discomfort that obviously are not as severe as they represent them to be. In such patients a hypodermic of sterile saline solution may act as a placebo. This procedure never should be resorted to without the knowledge and the written consent of the surgeon.

THE PATIENT IN PAIN

Principles of Nursing Management

1. Evaluate the quality, intensity and duration of the pain.
   A. Determine the time sequence of the pain.
   B. Ascertain if the pain is related to an activity (eating, moving, etc.).
   C. Ask the patient to localize the site of pain.
2. Note the patient's behavior and reaction to pain.
   A. Observe for evidences of disparity between pain intensity and patient's physical appearance.
   B. Note the circumstances under which pain occurs.
   C. Listen and record the patient's descriptions of his pain sensations.
3. Attempt to determine what the pain signifies to the patient.
   A. Accept the behavior of the patient.
   B. Develop a supportive relationship with the patient.
   C. Observe and listen for evidences of fear and anxiety.
   D. Listen with empathy and patience to complaints.
   E. Develop a therapeutic relationship with the patient.
4. Prevent the occurrence of pain.
   A. Relieve any evidences of pressure.
   B. Ascertain if the patient has a full bladder.
   C. Use measures to relieve intestinal distention.
   D. Encourage the patient to turn and move frequently.
   E. Maintain the patient in correct physiological positions.
5. Promote the general comfort of the patient.
   A. Handle the patient carefully and gently.
   B. Ensure general body warmth and relaxation.
   C. Relieve hunger and thirst.
   D. Relieve sensations of itching and burning.
   E. Promote a therapeutic environment (temperature, ventilation, visitors).
   F. Massage the patient's back.
   G. Offer diversional activities.

6. Support the patient during painful diagnostic procedures and treatment.
   A. Give a clear and adequate explanation to the patient.
   B. Enlist the patient's cooperation during the procedure.
   C. Teach the patient how to cope with his pain (deep breaths, immobilize parts).
   D. Observe for untoward physical reactions.
   E. Keep the patient informed of the progress of the examination or procedure.
   F. Praise the patient for his participation.
   G. Make the patient comfortable after a painful ordeal.
7. Relieve localized pain.
   A. Elevate edematous or painful extremities.
   B. Handle painful parts with care.
   C. Apply heat, cold and counterirritants as indicated.
   D. Encourage patient to participate in prescribed exercise program.
8. Administer agents to relieve pain when indicated.
   A. Use specific drugs for the relief of nausea and vomiting.
   B. Give ataractic agents to relieve anxiety.
   C. Apply local anesthetics as indicated.
   D. Give soporifics to induce sleep.
   E. Administer muscle-relaxant drugs and antispasmodics.
   F. Give analgesic drugs for more intense pain.
   G. Evaluate patient for signs of hypersensitivity, respiratory depression and toxic effects.

Vomiting

Nausea and vomiting may occur postoperatively particularly if the patient received ether as an anesthetic agent. Other causes may be the accumulation of fluid in the stomach or taking food or fluid before peristalsis returns. During anesthesia, inadequate ventilation increases the incidence of vomiting; also, inflation of the stomach contributes to this discomfort in the patient. Psychological factors often play a role; if the patient expects to vomit postoperatively, he usually will. Helpful preoperative instruction would minimize the likelihood of vomiting occurring after surgery.

Years ago vomiting was a common and expected postoperative occurrence; with other anesthetic agents and antiemetic drugs, it now is less common. When vomiting is likely because of the nature of surgery, a nasogastric tube is passed beforehand and functions throughout the operative procedure and immediately postoperatively. Otherwise, simple symptomatic therapy is usually all that is required. Many authorities believe that most antiemetic drugs (usually derivatives of phenothiazine) promote more undesirable effects, such as hypotension and respiratory depression, than beneficial ones. If a medication is required, short-acting barbiturates are often prescribed.

There are three types of postoperative vomiting, according to duration: (1) vomiting when coming out of the anesthetic, (2) vomiting that is continuous through the first day and night and (3) vomiting that is excessive or prolonged.

When Coming Out of the Anesthetic

The vomiting that occurs as the patient is coming out of the anesthetic relieves the stomach merely of mucus and saliva swallowed during the anesthetic period. This type of vomiting also may occur occasionally after operations done under local anesthesia. Its duration is short (from 2 to 8 hours at most), and it requires no special treatment beyond the washing out of the mouth and the withholding of fluids for a few hours.

When Continuous Through the First Day and Night

Vomiting that continues for the first day and night may be due to one of several causes:

Effects of the Anesthesia. These may persist so that a few patients may be nauseated and vomit long after they have regained consciousness.

Paralysis of Intestinal Activity. Frequently, there is considerable injury to the abdominal organs during an operation, with resultant paralysis of intestinal activity for a period longer than usual. Such patients have what in effect is a sterile peritonitis: fluids from the upper intestinal canal do not move onward; they dam back and are vomited. Nasal catheter drainage of the stomach for a time is the most effective treatment.

Idiosyncrasy to Medication. The patient may be affected in an unusual way by morphine or other medication if he vomits soon after the administration of the drug. An experienced nurse will recognize this idiosyncrasy and will report her observations to the surgeon and ask for instructions.

When Excessive and Prolonged

The causes of vomiting that continues without much remission for 3 to 7 days, retarding the patient's recovery or even threatening his life, usually are serious and are discussed separately. Such conditions may be enumerated as follows:

(1) Intestinal obstruction
(2) Acute dilatation of stomach
(3) Uremia or kidney insufficiency
(4) Hemorrhage in operations upon stomach
(5) Peritonitis

At times, even without any apparent marked organic cause, vomiting continues longer than usual. Such patients usually are highly nervous, apprehensive individuals, and it frequently taxes the ingenuity of both physician and nurse to the utmost to keep anything in their stomachs. In these patients, charged water, ginger ale or other effervescent drinks may be tried after evacuation of the stomach with nasogastric suction. The following medications give prompt relief:

phenothiazine antiemetics — thiethylperazine maleate (Torecan), or prochlorperazine maleate (Compazine); Nonphenothiazine antiemetics — trimethobenzamide (Tigan), cyclizine (Marezine), or meclizine (Bonine).

Restlessness

Discomfort. Restlessness is a postoperative symptom that should not be passed over lightly. The most common cause probably is the general discomfort following an operation, especially pain in the back, headache and thirst. This discomfort may be relieved largely by a gentle massage with lotion or alcohol, followed by a dose of acetylsalicylic acid (aspirin), which may be repeated if necessary.

Tight Drainage-soaked Bandages. Often these cause enough discomfort to make a patient restless and ill at ease. Fresh dressings usually improve the patient's spirits and make him more comfortable.

Retention of Urine. This occurs not infrequently after operation and may be the sole cause of restlessness.

Severe Toxemia. This condition frequently produces a very restless patient. For such a patient little can be done until the toxins have been eliminated from the blood. He is quieted best by adequate doses of morphine.

Flatulence and Hiccup. Flatulence and hiccup may be causes of restlessness. Their recognition and their treatment will be discussed later (pp. 145 and 154).

Hemorrhage. Probably the most serious cause of restlessness is hemorrhage. This is discussed on page 149.

Sleeplessness

Frequently, sleeplessness is associated with restlessness in patients after operation. However, there are many patients who simply cannot sleep. When this situation continues for 2 or 3 days, it is of concern to the surgeon. It is in such a situation that a competent nurse is most valuable. She must recognize that a patient taken suddenly from an active life and put to bed in strange surroundings may have cause for inability to sleep. The prolonged rest and periods of sleep secured during the daytime leave him wide awake at a time when in ordinary circumstances he would be asleep. Often, hospital noises prevent a patient from sleeping.

Treatment

The nurse should help to reduce noise to a minimum, provide diversion for her patient and cut the daytime naps short, so that at night he is ready to welcome a "good sound sleep." At bedtime she may give a gentle massage, particularly on the back and the neck, ventilate the room thoroughly and dim the lights. If these ordinary measures do not promote sleep, further causes of insomnia must be looked for. Many patients are used to some form of food before going to bed. Frequently these patients go to sleep after they have been given (their condition permitting) a cup of warm milk or cocoa and crackers or other food that is easily assimilated.

Worry and anxiety keep many patients awake. If it is possible to ascertain the cause of their worry, attempts can be made to relieve it. Perhaps it concerns their surgery, length of convalescence, readjustment to a new way of life—whatever it may be and however deep the worry, there is always a bright side of the picture. An understanding nurse can help such an individual. Spiritual comfort can provide an inner peace.

Medications. To this type of patient, bromides or barbiturates may be given with benefit. They should be given cautiously and in doses just sufficient to produce the desired effect. Demerol is a useful analgesic.

Thirst

Thirst is a troublesome symptom after many general anesthetics, and even after some cases of local anesthesia. It is due in large measure to the dryness of the mouth and the pharynx, caused by the inhibition of mucous secretion after the usual preoperative injection of atropine. Many patients operated on under local anesthesia complain of thirst during the operation. In addition, there is a considerable loss of body fluids due to perspiration, increased mucous secretion in the lungs and more or less loss of blood, so that the factor of fluid imbalance also enters into the cause. To combat the loss of fluids, solutions are given into the vein for the first few hours after operation. Even though an adequate amount of fluid is taken by this method, often it does not relieve the thirst.

The sticky, dry mouth demands fluids, and fluids may be given to most patients as soon as the postoperative nausea and vomiting have passed. Sips of water or hot tea with lemon juice serve to dissolve the mucus better than cold water. Small pieces of ice given to the patient may be very much enjoyed, and the amount of fluid given by this method is so small relatively that it is permitted even in patients in whom fluids are withheld by mouth. As soon as the patient can take water by mouth in sufficient quantities, the parenteral administration should be discontinued.

When operations have been performed on the mouth, the esophagus and the stomach, and about the duodenum, water usually is withheld for about 24 hours—often longer. Mouthwashes containing some weak alkali to dissolve the mucus are the best. A solution of equal parts of boric acid 4 per cent and glycerin also may be used. It seems to leave the mouth "wet" and allays thirst somewhat. A damp gauze cloth laid over the mouth tends to moisten the air breathed and is gratifying to many patients. Hard candies, chewing gum, even paraffin wax, may be chewed. This stimulates the flow of saliva and tends to keep the mouth moist.

Abdominal Distention

Distention of the abdomen after operation is very common. The trauma to the abdominal contents by operation produces a loss of normal peristalsis for 24 to 48 hours, depending on the type and the extent of the operation. Even though nothing is given by mouth, swallowed air and gastrointestinal secretions enter the stomach and the intestines and if not propelled by peristaltic activity, they collect in the intestinal coils to produce distention. Most often the gas collects in the colon; hence, a rectal tube or a small enema may be expected to give relief. After major abdominal surgery, distention may be avoided by frequent turning and movement by the patient and by the prophylactic use of a gastric or an intestinal tube. By this means the air that is swallowed (swallowed air provides most of the gas that produces distention) may be aspirated from the stomach and the upper intestine.

Certain patients swallow air as a part of anxiety reaction. If these characteristics can be recognized, the gastric suction tube may be used for a longer time than usual, until full peristaltic activity (passage of flatus) is resumed.

Bladder Distention. A distended bladder frequently is the cause of a distention of the lower abdomen. This is discussed on page 153.

Constipation and Diarrhea

The care of the bowels after operation is a responsibility shared alike by surgeon and nurse. The nurse, who is with the patient constantly, must be prepared to give accurate reports as to the number and the character of the stools, the effectiveness of enemas and so forth.

Constipation

The causes of constipation after operation may be innocent or serious. The irritation and the trauma to the bowel at the time of the operation may inhibit intestinal movement for several days, but usually peristaltic function returns after the third day, following early ambulation, perhaps a simple enema and an increase in diet. Local inflammation, peritonitis or abscess may cause constipation, in this instance treatment of the causal condition is indicated. Constipation has been mentioned as being a constant symptom of intestinal obstruction.

It must be borne in mind also, that many people, especially thin females and older people, are constipated habitually, and often give a history of having taken some form of laxative drug every day for years. These patients should be allowed to return to their former bowel habits as soon as possible after operation—at least until they have recovered from their operation. Liquid petrolatum (paraffin oil) or enemas usually are effective in evacuating the lower bowel, and cathartic drugs never should be given except on the physician's order.

Fecal Impaction. An avoidable cause of postoperative constipation is fecal impaction. This complication is a result of neglect and never should be permitted to occur. Early ambulation and regard for proper fluids and diet can prevent this problem in the majority of patients. Those affected usually are individuals past middle age, weakened somewhat by operation, whose bowel movements have been small in amount for several days. Enemas appear to be fairly effective, but distention usually continues and the patient has both general abdominal and local discomfort. He often states that he feels that the bowel wants to move but that movement gives no relief. Diarrhea may occur and persist, due to irritation of the upper rectum and the sigmoid by dammed-up fecal material. The diagnosis is made easily by inserting the gloved finger into the rectum. A hard fecal mass that fills the rectum can be palpated.

TREATMENT. The treatment of the condition is to remove the impaction. Enemas of 6 oz. of liquid petrolatum (oil enema) often are effective in softening the mass and helping its discharge. The harder masses may not be moved by this treatment. In these patients, the impaction may be broken up with the gloved finger, or by injecting from 1 to 2 oz. of hydrogen peroxide into the rectum. The foaming action of the drug tends to break up the fecal masses, which then may be evacuated.

Diarrhea

After operations diarrhea is rare. The patient may have 5 to 10 liquid stools of small amount a day. This should be reported at once. Fecal impaction has been mentioned as the most frequent cause of this complication in the aged.

Local irritation, such as a pelvic abscess, is the most frequent cause of diarrhea after operations in which a peritonitis was found. The gloved finger will find a tender mass bulging into the rectum. Surgical drainage usually is required, although at times these abscesses rupture spontaneously and drain into the rectum. Diarrhea due to a pelvic abscess is usually "spurious" in type—that is, not a true diarrhea but simply the expulsion of small amounts of liquid from the rectum. It is associated often with *tenesmus* (straining). The patient also may have painful urination.

POSTOPERATIVE COMPLICATIONS

The danger from a surgical problem is not only the risk of the operative procedure; there is also the very definite hazard of postoperative complications that may prolong the convalescence or even be an important contributing cause in an unsuccessful operative result. The nurse plays an important part in the prevention of these complications and in their early treatment should they arise. The signs and symptoms of the more common postoperative complications are discussed below. In each instance the most improved methods of prevention and the usual treatment are emphasized.

It should be borne in mind constantly that attention must be paid to the patient as an individual as well as to his particular surgical condition.

Circulatory Problems

Shock

One of the most serious postoperative complications is shock. It was, for a time, the cause of many operative fatalities. However, adequate attention in recent years to preoperative fluid balance and surgical prep-

aration, together with the intelligent use of whole blood and blood substitutes during and after operation, has prevented this complication to a large extent.

There are many causes of shock, and in almost all instances it is due to a combination of two or more factors. These factors may be of 5 main types. The first type is due to blood loss or *hematogenic* shock. Often there is more blood loss at operation than is realized. The handling of body tissues may cause local trauma and loss of blood and plasma from the circulation, thereby creating a decrease in the circulating blood volume. Shock due to vasodilatation and reflex inhibition of the heart brought about by an insult to the nervous system is *neurogenic* shock. When shock results from cardiac failure or an interference with heart function as in a myocardial infarction, coronary thrombosis or cardiac tamponade, it is referred to as *cardiogenic* shock. *Vasogenic* shock refers to diffuse vasodilatation. In this condition, the dilated vessels provide a sluggish system in which blood is circulating poorly and is not as available to the vital centers. Consequently, it pools in the small vessels and viscera. This type of shock may occur in anaphylaxis. *Toxic* or *bacteremic* shock is rather ill-defined and not well

MECHANISMS OF SHOCK*

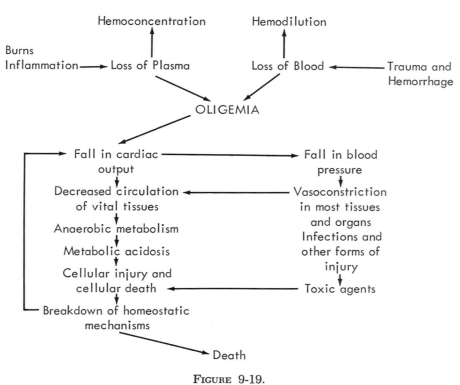

FIGURE 9-19.

* Simeone, F. A.: The nature and treatment of shock, Amer. J. Nurs., 66:1289, 1966.

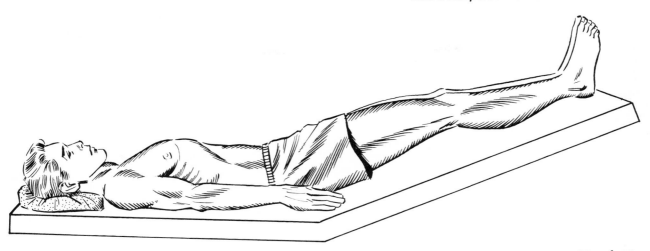

Fig. 9-20. Proper positioning of the patient who shows signs of shock is to elevate the lower extremities about 20° keeping the knees straight, trunk horizontal and head slightly elevated.

understood. It is characterized by a change in the capillary endothelium that permits loss of blood and plasma through the capillary walls into the surrounding tissues. This is thought to be caused by a toxic factor that enters the blood-stream from infection. Some authorities add a sixth category, *psychic shock,* to include shock resulting from extreme pain, deep fear or sudden emotionally disturbing information. The patient with a real fear of surgery or anesthesia would not be operated upon because of the shock potential.

Signs and Symptoms of Shock. No matter what the cause, the symptoms of shock are due to a breakdown of the vascular system and an insufficiency of the circulation. The result then is a patient who appears nervous and apprehensive but later is apathetic and in whom all sensations are markedly dulled. The skin is cold and moist, the lips are somewhat cyanotic, the pulse is rapid and thready, the respiration is rapid and shallow, and the temperature is subnormal. The blood pressure begins to fall.

Effects of Shock

Continued shock and its associated low blood pressure result in undesirable body changes. One of these is anoxia. *Anoxia,* a lack of oxygen in the body tissues, may be the result of *anoxemia,* decreased oxygen content in the blood. Oxygen, which combines with hemoglobin for transportation throughout the body, may be insufficient to provide the tissues with their normal requirements. Some of the more specialized tissues— the brain, the spinal cord and the kidneys—undergo degenerative changes rapidly when they are not supplied with adequate oxygen. These changes in the brain may be manifested by a permanent lack of nervous control of the vascular system and vascular

collapse, paralysis of one or more parts of the body, or by *hyperpyrexia.* The last is an excessive fever, sometimes as high as 42.2° or 42.8°C. (108° or 109°F.), that presages usually a fatal outcome and is the result of changes in the hypothalamic area. Later symptoms may include loss of memory and psychogenic alterations. When the kidney is deprived of oxygen for a sufficient period of time, kidney depression or failure may occur. Kidney depression, *oliguria,* is manifested by a decreased kidney secretion and urinary output. Kidney failure or *anuria* is evidenced by a lack of urinary secretion. Thrombosis with subsequent emboli also may occur throughout the body due to stasis of blood resulting from decreased circulation (see p. 150).

Depending upon the cause, shock can develop slowly or rapidly. The nurse, therefore, is on the alert for beginning signs enumerated on above. Note the following:

(1) If the signs result from external hemorrhage, this must be controlled immediately.

(2) Cyanosis indicates the need for oxygen.

(3) Place the patient on his back in shock position (see Fig. 9-20).

(4) Call the physician.

(5) Comfort and reassure the patient.

(6) Have oxygen available.

(7) The following articles must be ready for immediate use: sphygmomanometer and a stethoscope, fluid therapy equipment (transfusion or infusion), emergency drug tray, urine collecting equipment, vital sign and fluid records.

Where electronic equipment is available, data such as blood pressure, heart rate and output, circulation time, respirations, temperature, and urine flow are transmitted directly from body sensors into a computer. If data values go above or below predetermined settings, the equipment sounds an alarm.

Choice of treatment depends upon precipitating factors: nature of any disease process, if any; age of patient; cardiac, vascular, renal and respiratory reserve; and length of time the patient has been in shock.

Medical and Nursing Management of Patients in Shock

1. Prevention. The best treatment for shock is prophylaxis. This consists of adequate preparation of the patient, mental as well as physical, and anticipation of any complication that may arise during or after operation. The proper type of anesthesia should be chosen after careful consideration of the patient and his disease. Blood and plasma should be available if indicated. Blood loss should be accurately measured or intelligently estimated. In the operating room, a fairly reliable method is to weigh a dry sponge and then weigh the blood soaked sponge; the difference is the amount of fluid loss. If the amount exceeds 500 ml. replacement is usually indicated. Obviously, the individual patient and the particular circumstances must be considered in determining replacement therapy. An older, malnourished person requires this more readily than a healthy blood donor.

Operative trauma should be kept at a minimum. After operation, factors that may promote shock are to be prevented. Pain is controlled by making the patient as comfortable as possible and by using narcotics judiciously. Exposure should be avoided. In the recovery room the patient can be watched and cared for by nurses trained especially in the recovery of patients from anesthesia. In addition, a quiet room is advantageous in the immediate postoperative period in reducing mental trauma. Any moving of the patient is done gently. He is placed in the dorsal recumbent position to facilitate circulation. Lightweight, unheated covers prevent vasodilatation. Monitoring of vital signs is continued until the patient's recovery indicates that shock is unlikely.

2. Restoration of Blood Volume. This, of course, is the most important goal to be achieved in the treatment of shock. However, if the depressed circulation cannot be restored immediately, one must protect the vital centers of the brain. Irreversible changes may take place in a short period of time if the volume of the circulating blood is inadequate. The lower extremities are elevated to an angle of about 45°, keeping the knees straight; the trunk is horizontal with perhaps a slight lowering of the chest in relation to the abdomen and the head level with the chest or slightly elevated. In addition, some surgeons apply elastic bandages to the extremities, bandaging toward the trunk. By this procedure the available blood may be kept in a smaller circulating area, thus raising the blood pressure.

The quickest method of supplying an adequate amount of circulating blood is by transfusion. The deficit in circulating blood volume (hypovolemia) is best replaced in kind; for example, for hemorrhage, whole blood; for fluid loss in burns, plasma and electrolytes; for loss due to excessive vomiting or diarrhea, specific electrolytes. When blood is not available, a blood substitute, such as plasma or plasma volume expanders (Dextran), should be employed. Solutions of the electrolytes, glucose and saline solutions, should be used as blood substitutes only when blood or plasma is not available, and then only until one or the other can be obtained (see also Chapters 7 and 8).

Continuance of infusion or transfusion is determined by central venous pressure (C.V.P.) readings; at a normal level of 10 to 12 cm. there is no value to administering fluid. If the central venous pressure is below 10, fluids are continued but if pressure is at 15 or above, fluids are sometimes tapped by phlebotomy to prevent possible cardiac failure.

3. Oxygen. As patients in shock have some anoxemia, increasing the available oxygen to the blood may be beneficial. Done to improve oxygenation of vital organs and tissues, thereby decreasing the work of the heart, oxygen may be most easily administered by mask, intranasal catheter or through a clean airway (tracheostomy, intubation or respirator). If available, 100 per cent oxygen should be given to maximize the oxygen-carrying capacity of the circulating blood.

4. Relief of Pain. Pain should be relieved as far as possible by the intelligent use of narcotics. However, when the circulation is depressed, as it is in shock, the effect of morphine or other narcotics is delayed. Therefore, one must avoid overloading the patient with drugs that may accumulate during shock and become overwhelming when the circulation has been restored to normal. Other measures are used sometimes to alleviate pain. One of the most useful is procaine block of the peripheral nerves. This is satisfactory especially after operations on the chest, where relief can be obtained by intercostal nerve blocks.

5. Pharmacologic Agents. Certain drugs may cause a temporary rise in blood pressure. These drugs act by constricting the vessels in the peripheral circulation or by stimulating the brain centers, but they have a transient effect, and sometimes the effects are more harmful than beneficial. These drugs include 1-norepinephrine (Levophed) and metaraminol (Aramine, Pressoral, Pressonex) and are derivatives of the catecholamines. There are many who do not accept this form of therapy because of difficulty in regulating dosage and the risk of increased vasoconstriction. Experiments continue in the evaluation of those drugs that block the action of vasoconstricting nerve impulses or drugs. Such adrenergic-blocking agents are phenoxybenzamine (Dibenzyline) and phentolamine (Regitine). Patients on these medications must receive adequate transfusions to the degree of normovolemia or even hypervolemia so that fluid is available for the enlarged vascular space produced by the drug. Should this not be done, a rapid hypotension may be produced followed by circulatory collapse. All vasopressor drugs must be withdrawn gradually, for an abrupt discontinuance can produce a sudden hypotensive effect. They should be used with caution and the patient must be observed constantly by the nurse. Vital signs and cardiovascular assessment is continued until stability is apparent.

Adequate blood flow to tissues usually corrects any possibility of metabolic acidosis. However, if this becomes a problem, a buffer may have to be added to the circulating blood. Sodium carbonate given intravenously in an isotonic solution may be given slowly and with careful calculation as to amount based on the patient's weight and the acid-base evaluation. THAM (Trisbuffer) is a drug that provides a free base to neutralize acidosis but without the addition of sodium. It is an effective diuretic.

6. Urinary Output. In most forms of shock, oliguria is present. It is usually corrected in early shock by the restoration of blood volume to normal. However, in shock that occurs in toxic states or late in severe burns, oliguria may progress to anuria. Decreased urine output may be due to oligemia and dehydration or to renal tubular necrosis. Accurate recording of all fluid intake and output assists in determining the nature of the fluid balance in the body and its effect on the kidneys. Most patients have an indwelling catheter that may be attached to a urinometer to monitor urine outflow. The recording of time and amount of voiding is important even after the blood pressure has returned to normal. Amounts of 25 ml. or less voided in a 2-hour period is significant to call to the physician's attention. An osmotic diuretic such a mannitol may be effective in maintaining a diuresis when anuria has occurred.

7. Recovery and Convalescence. When signs and symptoms of shock are noticed and treatment is initiated promptly, the recovery is rapid. The longer the symptoms last before the problem is corrected, the more guarded is the prognosis and death may follow. This is why the prompt and intelligent recognition of early manifestations of shock by the nurse is important. By her initiating corrective measures and reporting to the physician, the patient can recover. As vital signs stabilize, therapeutic measures are slowly withdrawn but observation and monitoring are continued. A period for convalescence is required for the body to

recover fully. During this interval, the patient is observed for latent problems related to kidney function or thrombus formation.

Hemorrhage

Classification. Hemorrhage is classified as (1) *primary*, when it occurs at the time of the operation; (2) *intermediary*, when it occurs within the first few hours after an operation, due to a return of blood pressure to its normal level and a consequent washing out of the insecure clots from untied vessels; and (3) *secondary*, when it occurs some time after the operation, due to the slipping of a ligature because of infection, insecure tying or erosion of a vessel by a drainage tube.

A further classification frequently is made according to the kind of vessel that is bleeding. *Capillary* hemorrhage is characterized by a slow general ooze; *venous* hemorrhage bubbles out quickly and is dark in color; *arterial* hemorrhage is bright in color and appears in spurts with each heartbeat.

When the hemorrhage is on the surface and can be seen, it is spoken of as *evident;* when it cannot be seen, as in the peritoneal cavity, it is spoken of as *concealed.*

Symptoms. Hemorrhage presents a more or less well-defined syndrome, depending on the amount of blood lost and the rapidity of its escape. The patient is apprehensive, restless and moves continually; he is thirsty; and the skin is cold, moist and pale. The pulse rate increases, the temperature falls, respirations are rapid and deep, often of the gasping type spoken of as "air hunger." As the hemorrhage progresses, cardiac output decreases, arterial and venous blood pressure and the hemoglobin of the blood fall rapidly, the lips and the conjunctiva become pallid, spots appear before the eyes, a ringing is heard in the ears, and the patient grows weaker but remains conscious until near death. An interesting compensatory reaction of the human to blood loss or blood transfusion up to 500 ml. is that there generally is no change in cardiac output after 15 minutes. However, if greater volume changes occur, there is persistent change. For example, if a decrease in volume is great enough, hypovolemic shock occurs; if the increase in volume is great enough, pulmonary edema takes place. During World War II studies demonstrated that mild shock was usually associated with blood loss of 15 to 20 per cent, moderate shock, with 20 to 35 per cent, and severe shock with a loss greater than 45 per cent of the circulating blood volume.

The nurse must notify the surgeon immediately and carry out emergency measures until he arrives.

Management

Often the effects of hemorrhage after an operation are masked by those due to the anesthetic and to

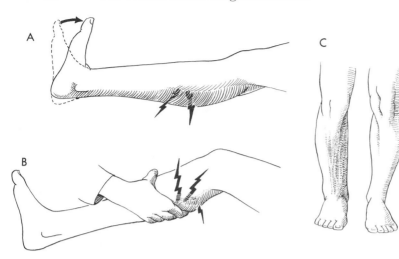

Fig. 9-21. Nursing assessment of signs and symptoms of phlebothrombosis. Signs of phlebothrombosis of the calf muscle veins. A, Homans' sign, pain in the calf on dorsiflexion of the foot with the leg in extension. B, tenderness of the calf muscles on gentle compression. C, slight swelling about the ankle and prominence of the veins. (Gius, J. A.: *Fundamentals of General Surgery,* Chicago, Year Book Medical Pub. 1966)

shock; therefore, the treatment of the patient is in a general way almost identical to that described for shock, viz., (1) place patient in shock position (Fig. 9-20) and (2) administer morphine to keep the patient quiet. The wound always should be inspected to find out, if possible, the site of the bleeding. A sterile gauze pad and a snug bandage with elevation of the part, arm or leg, are indicated.

A transfusion of blood is the most logical therapeutic measure, and in the case of serious operation, the blood of the patient is typed and blood is secured beforehand. If blood is not available when needed, saline solution, plasma or a plasma volume expander (Dextran) may be given intravenously to tide the patient over temporarily until the blood can be secured (see pp. 85 to 98).

In giving fluids by vein in cases of hemorrhage, remember that too large a quantity or too rapid administration may raise the blood pressure enough to start the bleeding again, unless the hemorrhage has been well controlled.

Femoral Phlebitis or Thrombosis

This complication occurs most frequently after operations upon the lower abdomen or in the course of severe septic diseases, such as peritonitis and ruptured ulcer. An inflammation of the vein occurs associated with a clotting of blood; this may be mild or severe. The cause of the complication may be injury to the vein by tight straps or leg-holders at the time of operation, a blanket-roll under the knees, concentration of blood by loss of fluid or dehydration, or, more commonly, the slowing of the blood flow in the extremity due to a lowered metabolism and depression of the circulation after operation. It is probable that several of these factors may act together to produce the thrombosis commonly seen. The left leg is affected more

frequently. The first symptom may be a pain or a cramp in the calf (Fig. 9-21). Pressure here gives pain, and a day or so later a painful swelling of the entire leg occurs, often associated with a slight fever and sometimes with chills and sweats. The swelling is due to a soft edema that pits easily on pressure. There is marked tenderness over the anteromedial surface of the thigh, and frequently the vein itself may be palpated as a firm pencil-like mass that may be rolled under the fingers.

A milder form of the same disease is termed *phlebothrombosis,* to indicate intravascular clotting without marked inflammation of the vein. The clotting occurs usually in the veins of the calf, often with few symptoms except slight soreness of the calf. The danger from this type of thrombosis is that the clot may be dislodged and produce an embolus. It is believed that most pulmonary emboli arise from this source. (See also p. 153.)

Treatment

The treatment of thrombophlebitis or phlebothrombosis may be considered as (1) prophylactic and (2) active.

Prophylactic Treatment. Efforts are directed toward preventing the formation of a thrombus and include such measures as adequate administration of fluids after operation to prevent blood concentration, leg exercises, bandaging of the legs and getting the patient out of bed early to prevent stagnation of the blood in the veins of the lower extremity.

Leg exercises can be taught before surgery. If the patient recognizes their significance in preventing circulatory complications, he will often initiate his own exercises. Fastening leg straps in the recovery room should not be necessary, particularly with stretchers that are equipped with side rails. Not only does the patient dislike the restriction but straps can constrict and impair circulation.

Another important nursing measure is to avoid the use of blanket-rolls, pillow-rolls or the knee gatch, which can constrict vessels under the knees. Even the practice of "dangling" (having the patient sit on the edge of the bed with his legs hanging over the side) can be dangerous and is not recommended because pressure under the knees can cut off circulation.

Active Treatment. Some surgeons believe that ligation of the femoral veins is an important therapeutic method. The rationale behind this method of therapy is to prevent pulmonary embolism from the breaking off of thrombi.

Anticoagulant therapy has taken a prominent place in the prophylaxis and the treatment of phlebitis and phlebothrombosis. Heparin, given intravenously by the drip method or intramuscularly in an oily menstruum, reduces the coagulability of the blood rapidly and is used most often when an immediate effect is desired. Repeated checks of the coagulation time of the blood are necessary to control its administration. Dicumarol or similar acting drugs are used for the same purpose. It is given by mouth and does not become effective for about 24 hours. Its daily dosage is controlled by daily estimations of the prothrombin time of the blood (see also p. 334).

Both as a prophylactic and an active treatment of phlebitis and thrombosis, wrapping the legs from toes to groin with snug elastic adhesive bandages or wearing elastic stockings have much virtue. These bandages prevent swelling and stagnation of venous blood in the legs and do much to relieve pain in the phlebitic extremity.

Pulmonary Complications

Respiratory complications are among the most frequent and serious with which the surgical team has to deal. Experience has shown that they may be avoided in large measure by careful preoperative observation and teaching and by taking every precaution during and after the operation. It is well known that those patients who have some respiratory disease before operation are more prone to develop serious complications after operation. Therefore, only emergency operations are performed when acute disease of the respiratory tract exists. The nurse may aid by reporting any symptom, such as cough, sneezing, injected conjunctiva and nasal discharge, to the surgeon before the operation.

During and immediately after the operation, every effort should be made to prevent chilling. Aspiration of the nasopharynx in the recovery room removes secretions that would otherwise embarrass respirations in the postoperative period. Occasionally, when secre-

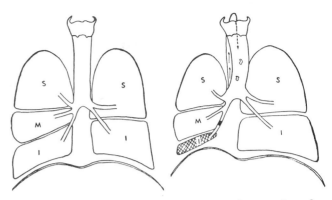

Fig. 9-22. Atelectasis. (*Left*) Normal expansion of all lobes of lungs. (*Right*) Plug of mucus or vomitus in bronchus leading to inferior lobe of right lung, with atelectasis of lobe. Arrows indicate the path followed by vomitus from the esophagus into the trachea before protective reflexes have returned following anesthesia. (Greisheimer, E. M.: The physiological effects of anesthesia, Am. J. Nursing 49:339)

tions form that cannot be coughed up by the patient, aspiration through the bronchoscope may be practiced, and, in very debilitated patients in whom retained secretions are a complicating factor, a tracheostomy may be performed that permits the nurse to aspirate the trachea directly through the tube as necessary.

The predisposing and exciting causes of pulmonary complications may be any of the following:

(1) Infections in the mouth, the nose and the throat

(2) The irritating effect of the anesthetic, especially ether, on the respiratory mucous membranes, with a resultant increase in mucous secretion

(3) The aspiration of vomitus

(4) Shallow respiration after operations, especially those on the upper abdomen, because of the pain in the wound that deep respiration causes

(5) A history of heavy smoking or chronic respiratory diseases

(6) Obesity, debilitation or being very old or very young.

Complications are described briefly here and in more detail in Unit 7, Chapter 14.

Atelectasis

When the mucous plug closes one of the bronchi entirely, there is a collapse of the pulmonary tissue beyond, and a massive *atelectasis* is said to result (Fig. 9-22). (See p. 238.)

Bronchitis

This pulmonary complication may appear at any time after operation, usually within the first 5 or 6 days. The symptoms vary according to the disease. A simple bronchitis is characterized by cough productive of considerable mucopus, but without marked temperature or pulse elevation.

Bronchopneumonia

Bronchopneumonia is perhaps the second most frequent pulmonary complication. Besides a productive cough, there may be considerable temperature elevation, with an increase in the pulse and the respiratory rates.

Lobar Pneumonia

Lobar pneumonia is a less frequent complication after operation. Usually it begins with a chill, followed by high temperature, pulse and respiration. There may be little or no cough, but the respiratory embarrassment, the flushed cheeks and the evident illness of the patient make a combination of clinical signs that are distinctive. The disease runs its usual course with the added complication of the operative wound.

Hypostatic Pulmonary Congestion

Hypostatic pulmonary congestion is a condition that develops too often in old or in very weak patients. Its cause is a weakened heart and vascular system that permit a stagnation of blood at the bases of both lungs. It occurs most frequently, perhaps, in elderly patients who have sustained a fractured femur and are not mobilized effectively. The symptoms frequently are not marked for a time—perhaps a slight elevation of temperature, pulse and respiratory rate, and also a slight cough. However, physical examination reveals dullness and rales at the bases of the lungs. If the condition goes untreated, the outcome may be fatal.

Pleurisy

Pleurisy is not an uncommon occurrence after operation. Its chief symptom is an acute, knifelike pain in the chest on the affected side that is particularly excruciating when the patient takes a deep breath. Also, there usually is some slight temperature and pulse rise, and respirations are rapid and more shallow than normal.

Medical and Nursing Management of Pulmonary Complications

Being aware of the many possible respiratory complications, the nurse is more likely to initiate the many preventive measures cited in the previous discussion (pp. 129-136). By recognizing the signs and symptoms, efforts can be directed to combating specific respiratory difficulties. Not only is the first postoperative day one of concern, but the first postoperative week of the patient's recovery requires close observation and careful management. The early signs of elevations in tempera-

ture, pulse, and respiration are significant. Chest pain, dyspnea, and cough may or may not accompany these elevations, however, the patient may seem to be restless and apprehensive. Such indications are important and should be reported to the surgeon.

Measures to Promote Full Aeration of the Lung

The prophylactic treatment of these conditions includes measures to promote full aeration of the lungs. The nurse should instruct her patient to take at least 10 deep inhalations every hour. Frequently, some surgeons recommend some apparatus (a spirometer, blow-bottle or Adler Rebreather) into which the patient blows in an effort to expand the lungs fully. Turning the patient from side to side results occasionally in coughing, with expulsion of the mucous plug, and recovery. At times the mucous plus may be removed by aspiration through a bronchoscope.

The increased metabolism, more complete pulmonary aeration and the general improvement of all body functions incidental to getting the patient up out of bed have led many surgeons to regard ambulation as one of the best prophylactic measures against pulmonary complications. When his wound or condition otherwise permits, it is not unusual to allow the patient to get up on the second or third day after operation, and even on the first day. This practice is especially valuable in preventing pulmonary complications in older patients.

Indications for Specific Measures

A most effective method of treatment of bronchitis is the inhalation of cool mist or steam, which may be administered by electric vaporizers. In using these the nurse must be careful to see that they are kept filled with water and are so placed that burning of the patient would be impossible. (See Chap. 15, p. 281.)

In lobar and bronchopneumonia, the patient is encouraged to take fluids, and expectorant and supportive drugs are given him. Distention should be watched for and prevented, if possible, so as to avoid added respiratory or cardiac embarrassment. Most of these patients are effectively treated by the use of antibiotics.

For pleurisy, a tight adhesive strapping, applied during full expiration, will relieve the pain almost at once. Aspirin, 0.6 gm. (gr. x), may be given if it is needed.

Pleurisy with effusion may result secondary to a primary pleurisy. In these patients aspiration of the chest frequently becomes necessary.

Many times the pulmonary complication of hypostatic pulmonary congestion becomes more serious than the original surgical condition, in which case the surgical condition may be disregarded in order to permit proper treatment of the hypostatic pneumonia.

Because of reduced aeration in many of the pulmonary complications, which means that less oxygen reaches the blood, many clinics employ an oxygen tent in treatment. This apparatus, which consists of a large hood that encloses the patient's face or head and shoulders, delivers oxygen in high concentration combined with a small amount of carbon dioxide. By this means the patient receives more oxygen with each respiration, cyanosis is lessened, and the general condition is improved. The nurse is required to see that the tent fits closely about the patient. (See p. 282.)

Pulmonary Embolism

An *embolus* is defined as a foreign body in the bloodstream. In most patients it is formed by a blood clot that becomes dislodged from its original site and is carried along in the blood. When the clot is carried to the heart, it is forced by the blood into the pulmonary artery, where it plugs the main artery or one of its branches. The symptoms produced are among the most sudden and startling in surgical practice. A patient passing an apparently normal convalescence suddenly cries out with sharp, stabbing pains in the chest and becomes breathless, cyanotic and anxious. The pupils dilate, cold sweat pours out, the pulse becomes rapid and irregular, then imperceptible, and death usually results. If death does not occur within 30 minutes, there is a chance of recovery.

This complication may arise at any time after operation. It is probable that movements of the patient dislodge the clot, because pulmonary embolism seems to occur most frequently immediately after the patient has been taken out of bed or put to bed again for the first time after operation. (See page 254.)

Treatment

If death does not occur at once, oxygen or fresh air should be given in abundance, with the patient in the sitting position to help respiration. Attempts should be made to quiet and reassure the patient, and drugs (morphine) should be given to prevent the panic that rapidly will wear out the overworked, dilating heart.

Urinary Problems

Urinary Retention

Urinary retention may follow any operation, but it occurs most frequently after operations on the rectum, the anus and the vagina, and after herniorrhaphies and operations on the lower abdomen. The cause is thought to be a spasm of the bladder sphincter.

Not infrequently patients are unable to void in bed but, when allowed to sit or stand up, do so without difficulty. When standing does not interfere with the operative result, male patients may be allowed to stand by the side of the bed or female patients to sit on the edge of the bed with their feet on a chair or a stool. However, many patients cannot be permitted this liberty and other means of encouraging urination must be tried. Some people cannot void with another person in the room. These patients should be left alone for a time after being provided with a warm bedpan or urinal.

Frequently the sound or the sight of running water may relax reflexly the spasm of the bladder sphincter. A bedpan containing warm water or an irrigation of the perineum with warm water frequently initiates urination for female patients. A small warm enema often is of value in such a situation. If the retention of urine continues for some hours, the patient complains of considerable pain in the lower abdomen, and the bladder frequently can be palpated and seen in outline distending the lower anterior abdominal wall.

When all conservative measures have failed, catheterization must be practiced. If the patient has voided just before operation, this procedure may be delayed in most cases for 12 to 18 hours. There are two reasons for wishing to avoid catheterization: (1) there is the possibility of infecting the bladder and producing a cystitis, and (2) experience has shown that once a patient has been catheterized, frequently he needs subsequent catheterizations.

Many patients may exhibit a palpable bladder, with lower abdominal discomfort, and still void small amounts of urine at frequent intervals. The keen nurse does not mistake this for normal functioning of the bladder. This voiding of 1 to 2 oz. of urine at intervals of 15 to 30 minutes is, rather, a sign of an overdistended bladder, the very distention being sufficient to allow the escape of small amounts of urine at intervals. The condition usually is spoken of as the "overflow of retention." A catheter usually relieves the patient by draining from 20 to 30 oz. of urine from the bladder. "Incontinence of retention" may be evidenced by a constant dribble of urine, yet the bladder remains overdistended. Overdistention injures the bladder; catheterization is indicated. There often is a definite psychic element in urinary retention.

At times, following extensive surgery, the surgeon may anticipate voiding difficulties and insert an indwelling catheter before the patient emerges from anesthesia. Usually the surgeon desires to be notified if less than 30 ml. of urine per hour are collected in the calibrated receptacle.

Urinary Incontinence

Incontinence of urine is a frequent complication in the aged, either after operation or after shocking injuries. It is due probably to weakness with loss of tone of the bladder sphincter. This symptom frequently disappears as the patient gains in strength and normal muscular tone is regained.

Treatment

Treatment of urinary incontinence is difficult. In many patients, an indwelling catheter may be inserted. In some individuals the giving of a bedpan hourly may be helpful (see p. 828 for management of neurogenic bladder). It is well to place a large pad under the patient to absorb the urine. Special pants for incontinent patients are available. The incontinent patient must be watched carefully to prevent the development of bedsores.

Gastrointestinal Problems

Intestinal Obstruction

Intestinal obstruction is a complication that may follow abdominal operations. It occurs most often after operations on the lower abdomen and the pelvis, and especially after those in which drainage has been necessary. The symptoms usually appear between the third and the fifth days. The cause is some obstruction of the intestinal current—frequently a loop of intestine that has become kinked from inflammatory adhesions or that has become involved in the drainage tract. A typical situation is that of a patient with a ruptured appendix, having pelvic drainage. He had his enema on the third day, and it was reported to be effective. He was fed a soft diet and, after a day or two, he complained of sharp, colicky, abdominal pains with a pain-free interval between. Usually there is no temperature or pulse elevation. At first the pains are localized, and this point should be noted by the nurse, because the localization of the early pains represents in a general way the loop of intestine that is just above the obstruction.

Usually, the patient continues to have abdominal pains, with shorter and shorter intervals between. If a stethoscope is placed on the abdomen, sounds may be heard that give evidence of extremely active intestinal movements, especially during an attack of pain. The intestinal contents, being unable to move forward, distend the intestinal coils, are carried backward to the stomach and are vomited. Thus, vomiting and increasing distention gradually become more prominent symptoms. Hiccup often precedes the vomiting in many patients. The bowels do not move, and enemas return nearly clear, showing that very little of the intestinal contents has reached the large bowel since the enema on the third day. Unless the obstruction is relieved the patient continues to vomit, distention becomes more pronounced, the pulse becomes rapid, and the end is a toxic death.

Treatment

Sometimes the distention of the intestine above the obstruction can be prevented by the use of the constant-suction drainage with the Miller-Abbott, Harris or Cantor tubes, in which case the inflammatory reaction of the bowel at the site of the obstruction may subside and the obstruction is relieved. However, at times it is necessary to relieve the obstructed intestine by operation. In addition, intravenous infusions of prescribed solutions usually are given. (See the section on intestinal obstruction for a more complete discussion of the treatment and the post-operative care, p. 493.)

Hiccup (Singultus)

Hiccup occurs not infrequently after abdominal operations. Often it occurs in mild transitory attacks that cease spontaneously or with very simple treatment. When hiccups persist they may produce considerable distress and serious effects such as vomiting, acid-base and fluid imbalance, malnutrition, exhaustion and possibly wound dehiscence.

Hiccup is produced by intermittent spasms of the diaphragm. It is associated with a coarse sound (an audible "hic"), a result of the vibration of the closed vocal cords as the air rushes suddenly into the lungs. The cause of the diaphragmatic spasm may be any irritation of the phrenic nerve from its center in the spinal cord to its terminal ramifications on the undersurface of the diaphragm. This irritation may be direct—such as a stimulation of the nerve itself by a distended stomach, peritonitis or subdiaphragmatic abscess, abdominal distention, pleurisy or tumors in the chest pressing on the nerves; or indirect—such as toxemia, uremia and so forth that stimulate the center; or reflex—such as irritations from a drainage tube, exposure to cold, drinking very hot or very cold fluids or obstruction of the intestines.

Treatment

The multitude of remedies suggested for the relief of this condition is proof that no one treatment is effective in every case. The best remedy, of course, is removal of the cause, which in some cases is simple, for example, gastric lavage for gastric distention, shortening or removal of drainage tubes causing irritation, or adhesive strapping in pleurisy. At other times the removal of the cause is almost impossible; then attention must be directed toward the treatment of the hiccup itself. Many simple remedies—such as drinking a half glass of water in which a teaspoonful of sodium bicarbonate has been dissolved, swallowing ice, stopping the patient from talking, sucking a lemon, taking a little vinegar, salt or sugar—have been used and often with success. Probably the most efficient of the older and simpler remedies is to hold the breath while taking large swallows of cold water.

After studying the problem recently, a group of anesthesiologists recommend treatment ranging from the simplest to the most drastic until relief is obtained. Their suggestions, in order, are:

(1) Finger pressure on the eyeballs through closed lids for several minutes

(2) Induced vomiting

(3) Gastric lavage

(4) Intravenous injection of atropine

(5) Inhalation of carbon dioxide (breathing in and out of a paper bag or more technical administration)

(6) Should these fail, a phrenic nerve block

(7) As a final resort, a phrenic nerve crush.

It has been suggested that an interruption of the reflex arc that results in the intermittent spasm of the diaphragm may be accomplished by the introduction of a rubber catheter 3 to 4½ inches into the pharynx. The catheter may be introduced either through the nose or through the mouth to tickle the pharynx. Dr. Salem of Chicago has reported cessation of hiccups in 99 of 100 patients in whom this procedure was used.

Wound Complications
Hematoma (Hemorrhage)

The nurse should know the location of the patient's incision so that she may inspect the dressings for hemorrhage at intervals during the first 24 hours after operation. Any undue amount of bleeding should be reported to the surgeon. At times concealed bleeding occurs in the wound but beneath the skin. This hemorrhage usually stops spontaneously but results in clot formation within the wound. If the clot is small, it will be absorbed and need not be treated. When the clot is large, the wound usually bulges somewhat, and healing will be delayed unless it is removed. After the removal of several stitches, the clot is evacuated, after which the wound is packed lightly with gauze. Healing occurs usually by granulation (see Fig. 9-14), or a secondary closure may be performed.

Infection

Staphylococcus aureus accounts for many postoperative wound infections. Other infections may result from *Escherichia coli, Proteus vulgaris, Aerobacter aerogenes,* and *Pseudomonas aeruginosa,* and, occasionally, other organisms. The most important area of prevention lies in meticulous wound management and surgical technique. In addition, housekeeping cleanliness and environmental disinfection are important. When the inflammatory process occurs, it usually begins to show symptoms in 36 to 48 hours. The patient's pulse rate and temperature increase, and the wound usually becomes somewhat tender, swollen and warm. At times, when the infection is deep, there may be no local signs. When the surgeon makes a diagnosis of wound infection, usually he removes one stitch or more and, under aseptic precautions, separates the wound edges with a pair of blunt scissors or a hemostat. The infection opened, he inserts a drain of rubber or gauze. In addition, many surgeons require some form of warm antiseptic solution with which to flush the wound. The surgeon may take a culture of the infected wound and prescribe specific antibiotics. It may be necessary to continue hot wet dressings if so ordered.

Rupture (Disruption, Evisceration or Dehiscence)

This complication is especially serious in the case of abdominal wounds. It results from the giving way of sutures and from infection; also, more frequently, after marked distention or cough. A 16-year study at the Mass. General Hospital[*] showed that the increase of incidence of wound dehiscence occurred because of increasing age and the presence of pulmonary or cardiovascular disease in abdominal surgical patients. The rupture of the wound may occur suddenly, with the escape of coils of intestine onto the abdominal wall. Such a catastrophe causes considerable pain and often is associated with vomiting. Frequently the patient says that something gave way. When the wound edges part slowly, the intestines may escape gradually or not at all, and the presenting symptom may be the sudden drainage of a large amount of peritoneal fluid into the dressings.

When rupture of a wound occurs, the attending surgeon should be notified at once. The protruding coils of intestine should be covered with sterile dressings.

A scultetus binder, properly applied, is an excellent prophylactic measure against an accident of this kind, and often it is used in the primary dressing, especially for operations on individuals with weak or pendulous abdominal walls. It is used often also as a firm binder when rupture of a wound has occurred. Vitamin deficiency or lowered serum protein or chloride may require correction.

Keloid

Not infrequently in an otherwise normal wound the scar develops a tendency to excessive growth. Sometimes the entire scar is affected; at other times the condition is segmented. This keloid tendency is unexplainable, unpredictable and unavoidable in some individuals. (See p. 645.)

Much investigation has been done along the lines of

[*] Guiney, E. J., *et al.*: Wound dehiscence. Arch. Surg., 92:47-51, Jan., 1966.

prevention and cure. Careful closure of the wound, complete hemostasis, pressure support without undue tension on the suture lines—all are reputed to combat this distressing wound complication.

Psychological Problems

Delirium

Postoperative delirium occurs occasionally in several groups of patients. The most common types are:

Toxic

Toxic delirium occurs in conjunction with the signs and the symptoms of a general toxemia. These patients are very ill, usually with a high temperature and pulse rate. The face is flushed, and the eyes are bright and roving. These patients move incessantly, often attempting to get out of bed and disarranging the bedclothes continually. They present a marked degree of mental confusion. These states are seen in surgical conditions, most often in patients with general peritonitis or other septic conditions.

In such patients elimination is promoted by encouraging the intake of fluids, and the causative condition is treated by antimicrobial therapy. At times, however, the outcome is fatal.

Traumatic

Traumatic delirium is a mental state resulting from sudden trauma of any sort, especially in highly nervous people. The malady may take the form of wild maniacal excitement, of simple confusion with hallucinations and delusions or of melancholic depression. Sedative drugs—chloral hydrate, paraldehyde and morphine—are used in treatment. Usually the state begins and ends suddenly.

Delirium Tremens

Individuals who have used alcohol habitually over a long period of time are very poor surgical risks. The alcohol has damaged practically every organ and in the event of accidents or serious surgical procedures their resistance is much below that of the average person. These patients always take anesthesia poorly.

After operation the patient may do well for a few days, but the prolonged abstinence from alcohol causes him to become restless, nervous and irritated easily by little things. His facial expression changes entirely. He sleeps poorly and often is disturbed by unreal dreams. When approached by the doctor or the nurse he appears to awake suddenly, asks "Who are you?" and, when he is told where he is, he will appear to be fairly normal for a short time. These symptoms should be watched for in patients who have been alcoholics, because active treatment at this stage may avoid the more violent delirium.

Active delirium tremens may come on suddenly or gradually. After a period of restless, nervous, semi-delirium, the patient finally loses entire control of his mental functions and "horrors reign supreme." His mind is a chaos of everchanging ideas. He talks incessantly, tries to get out of bed to get away from the hallucinations of fear and persecution that torment him continually. If attempts are made to restrain him, he may fight maniacally and often will injure himself and others. In this stage the patient is obviously sick. He is sleepless, he perspires freely and the limbs display a marked tremor. Finally, after many hours of torture, the patient becomes stuporous.

Treatment. When possible, the treatment of these patients should begin 2 or 3 days before operation by most thorough elimination from the kidneys, the bowels and the skin. These measures should be continued after operation, especially if any of the early signs of the condition develop. Sedative drugs and/or tranquilizers should be given in quantities to keep the patient quiet. Stimulation often is required, especially in the older alcoholics, in the form of whisky, strychnine and caffeine. The chief cause of the symptoms in chronic alcoholics has been shown to be a depletion of the carbohydrate stores of the body and an inadequate ingestion of vitamins. Therefore, glucose is given intravenously, and vitamins are administered in concentrated form by mouth and by injection.

RESTRAINT. In the postoperative care of patients, it is wise for the nurse to explain the necessity for the patient's remaining in bed until the surgeon permits him to get up. Often patients prefer to get out of bed to void or to get a drink of water rather than bother the nurse. This may lead to serious complications that a few words of explanation can prevent. However, in some patients it may be impossible for the patient to grasp this. This is true of patients who are disoriented, and especially of older individuals. In such patients, the simplest form of restraint is the use of a bed with siderails or side protection. This permits the patient to move about in bed but prevents him from getting out of bed easily and injuring himself.

To protect both patient and nurse, often it becomes necessary to apply some form of restraint in cases of delirium. In the milder forms, a restraining sheet may be used: an ordinary sheet folded lengthwise to be from about 12 to 15 inches wide, applied firmly over the thighs and held by wrapping each end round the bed frame.

Nursing Measures. The psychological effect of being restrained can be severe; therefore, any form of restraint should be applied *only as a last resort*. All other means of making the patient quiet should be tried first. If possible, he should be isolated from other patients. Any article in his vicinity that could be used harmfully should be removed.

When restraints are used, the patient should be in a comfortable and natural position and care should be taken that the part is not so constricted as to interfere with the circulation. Restraint to the chest should be avoided, if possible. The appearance of cyanosis in hand or foot indicates that the appliance is too tight. The appliances should be padded carefully and so used as to prevent chafing or pressure sores. The skin underneath them should be inspected frequently, bathed carefully and massaged at least every 2 or 3 hours. Even though restraints are applied, the patient never should be left unwatched. Any patient needing restraint should have constant and careful nursing attention.

BIBLIOGRAPHY

Balagot, R. C., and Bandelin, V. R.: Preoperative and postoperative inhalation therapy. Surg. Clin. N. Amer., 48:29-36, Feb., 1968.

Carnes, M. A.: Postanesthetic complications. Nurs. Forum, 4:46-55, No. 3, 1965.

Case, T. C., and Giery, R. A.: Surgery in patients between 80 and 100 years of age. J. Amer. Geriatrics Soc., 12:345-349, April, 1964.

Fenton, M.: What to do about thirst. Amer. J. Nurs., 69:1014-1017, May, 1969.

Knicely, K. H.: The world of distorted perception. Amer. J. Nurs., 67:998-1002, May, 1967.

Leithauser, D. J., Gregory, L., and Miller, S. M.: Immediate ambulation after extensive surgery. Amer. J. Nurs., 66:2207-2208, Oct., 1966.

Moore, S. W., et al.: Recurrent abdominal incisional hernia. Surg. Gynec. Obstet., 126:1015-1022, May, 1968.

Scully, H. F., and Martin, S. J.: Anesthetic management for geriatric patients. Amer. J. Nurs., 65:110-112, Feb., 1965.

Pain

Blaylock, J.: The psychological and cultural influences on the reaction to pain: A review of the literature. Nurs. Forum, 7:262-274, No. 3, 1968.

Chambers, W. G. and Price, G. G.: Influence of the nurse upon effects of analgesics administered. Nurs. Res., 16:228-233, Summer, 1967.

Gildea, J.: The relief of postoperative pain. Med. Clin. N. Amer., 52:81-89, Jan., 1968.

Halsell, M.: Moist heat for the relief of postoperative pain. Amer. J. Nurs., 67:767-770, April, 1967.

Jaffe, J. H.: Narcotics in the treatment of pain. Med. Clin. N. Amer., 52:33-46, Jan., 1968.

Jarratt, V.: The keeper of the keys. Amer. J. Nurs., 65:68-70, July, 1965.

Laver, J. W.: Hypnosis in the relief of pain. Med. Clin. N. Amer., 52:217-224, Jan., 1968.

McBride, M. A. B.: "Pain" and effective nursing practice. ANA Clinical Sessions. pp. 75-82. New York, Appleton-Century-Crofts, 1967.

————: The additive to the analgesic. Amer. J. Nurs., 69:974-976, May, 1969.

McCaffery, M., and Foss, M.: Nursing intervention for bodily pain. Amer. J. Nurs., 67:1224-1227, June, 1967.

Moss, F. T., and Meyer, B.: Effects of nursing interaction upon pain relief in patients. Nurs. Res., 15:303-306, Fall, 1966.

Pain, Part I—Basic concepts and assessment, Part II—Rationale for intervention (programmed instruction supplement. Amer. J. Nurs., 66:1085-1108, May, 1966; 66:1345-1368, June, 1966.

Quimby, C. W.: Preoperative prophylaxis of postoperative pain. Med. Clin. N. Amer., 52:73-80, Jan., 1968.

Sadove, M. S., and Albrecht, R. F.: Sedatives and tranquilizers in the treatment of pain. Med. Clin. N. Amer., 52:47-54, Jan., 1968.

Vomiting

Downs, H. S.: The control of vomiting. Amer. J. Nurs., 66:76-82, Jan., 1966.

Dumas, R. G., and Leonard, R. C.: The effect of nursing on the incidence of postoperative vomiting. Nurs. Res., 12:12-15, Winter, 1963.

McCarthy, R. T.: Vomiting. Nurs. Forum, 3:48-59, No. 1, 1964.

Shock

Ayres, S. M., and Giannelli, S.: Shock. In Care of the Critically Ill. New York, Appleton-Century-Crofts, 1967.

Bordicks, K. J.: Patterns of Shock. New York, Macmillan, 1965.

Connolly, J. E.: Practical approach to the diagnosis and treatment of shock. Hosp. Med., 4:4-13, April, 1968.

Eiseman, B., and Carnes, M.: Hemorrhagic and traumatic shock. In Randall, H. T.: Manual of Preoperative and Postoperative Care. Philadelphia, W. B. Saunders, 1968.

Maccannell, K. L., et al.: Dopamine in the treatment of hypotension and shock. New Eng. J. Med., 275:1389-1398, 1966.

Simeone, F. A.: The nature and treatment of shock. Amer. J. Nurs., 66:1287-1294, June, 1966.

Wound Care

Abramson, D. J.: A combined soft tissue and suction drain. Surg. Gynec. Obstet., 125:365-366, Aug., 1967.

Alexander, H. C., and Prudden, J. F.: The causes of abdominal wound disruption. Surg. Gynec. Obstet., 122:1223-1229, June, 1966.

Altemeier, W. A., Culbertson, W. R., and Hummel, R. P.: Surgical considerations of endogenous infections—sources, types, and method of control. Surg. Clin. N. Amer., 48:227-240, Feb., 1968.

Dorton, H. E.: Surgical tape trauma. Surg. Gynec. Obstet., 118:363, Feb., 1964.

Farnham, E. L.: et al.: The effect of early bathing on surgical incisions. J. Nat. Med. Ass., 59:15-16, Jan., 1967.

Foster, F. P.: Better management of severe postoperative infections. Hosp. Med., 1:12-15, June, 1965.

Ilfeld, F. W., and Field, S. M.: Silicone spray to waterproof adhesive taping. J.A.M.A., 201:208-209, 1967.

Pories, W. J., et al.: Acceleration of healing with zinc sulfate. Ann. Surg., 165:432-436, March, 1967.

Rockwood, C. A., Jr., and Chambers, G. H.: Use of portable wound suction units. So. Med. J., 60:498-501, May, 1967.

Pulmonary Problems

Adler, R. H., and Brodie, S. L.: Postoperative rebreathing aid. Amer. J. Nurs., 68:1287-1289, June, 1968.

CHAPTER **10**

Rehabilitation Nursing

- *Philosophy of Rehabilitation*
- *The Rehabilitation Team*
- *Psychological Implications of a Disability*
- *Principles and Practices of Rehabilitation Nursing*
- *Promoting Continuity of Patient Care*

PHILOSOPHY OF REHABILITATION

It is never how high one rises that determines one's merit, but rather how far one has come, considering his difficulties.

—ARCHIBALD RUTLEDGE

Rehabilitation is the process by which a disabled or ill patient is enabled to achieve his maximum possible physical, mental and social efficiency. How close he comes to achieving this goal determines the degree to which he becomes a socially and economically independent member of society. Rehabilitation has been called the third phase of medicine, the first being preventive, the second diagnosis and treatment, the third convalescence and rehabilitation. Morrissey defines modern rehabilitation as a process of wholesome adjustment to a handicap by educating the patient to integrate all of his resources and to concentrate more on existing abilities than on the permanent disabilities with which he must live.

In the interval between World Wars I and II, rehabilitation efforts developed significant meaning. The first comprehensive program in rehabilitation was started in 1947 at the Bellevue Hospital in New York City by Dr. Howard Rusk. Since then programs have been developed in most medical centers. Many hospitals have elaborate departments; however, a success-

ful program can be carried out even in a small hospital and with a minimum of personnel and equipment. A positive point of view plus dedication, patience and willingness to move through the many stages from inactivity to activity must be a part of the patient and of all those who work with him in achieving this goal.

Rehabilitation concerns not only the individual; it also concerns the nation. Early in 1962 the Department of Health, Education and Welfare launched a new approach in public welfare that stresses "services instead of support, rehabilitation instead of relief." The promotion of rehabilitation services and the family-centered approach is receiving particular emphasis.

The new Social and Rehabilitation Service (SRS) created in 1967 within the Department of Health, Education and Welfare combines the programs of Welfare Administration, the Vocational Rehabilitation Administration, the Administration on Aging, the Medicaid program and the Mental Retardation Division of the Public Health Service.

The federal funds to support state agency services have been increased to 80 per cent of the costs, thereby providing an incentive to the individual states to provide more rehabilitation services for the handicapped. The economic advantage of such an emphasis is readily apparent; instead of an individual receiving welfare aid, he will be rehabilitated into employment. Instead of being dependent on society, he will contribute to it. The effect on the individual is to change him from a hopeless dependent to an active self-sufficient citizen. But even more important, the person is helped to develop a satisfying way of life that preserves the uniqueness of his individuality. He gains inner strength from his own resources that makes it possible for him to partake of the joys and meet the problems of life in a meaningful way.

The trend in rehabilitation is to include not only the physically, mentally and emotionally handicapped, but to take in the aged and those who are disadvantaged from problems of poverty or social deprivation.

In the hospital setting, the patient and his problems are evaluated and a program is set up to enable him to achieve self-sufficiency within the level of his capabilities and desires. His abilities are stressed rather than his disabilities. Since each patient has a different level of capability, the program is individualized. Through such a program the patient is motivated and helped to attain social interdependence and greater economic security.

THE REHABILITATION TEAM

Rehabilitation requires a team of persons working together and contributing specialized services that may be required to assist the patient. The team members represent a variety of disciplines. They meet in group sessions at frequent intervals to evaluate the patient's progress and make the necessary program changes. His *physician* has the responsibility of making the diagnosis so that therapy can be directed toward realistic goals; he directs the patient's therapeutic program. The *physiatrist* is a physician who is a specialist in physical medicine and rehabilitation. He tests the patient's physical functioning and supervises his rehabilitation program. The *psychologist* assesses the patient's motivation, values and attitudes toward his disability. He also may talk with the family to help them to cope with the problems that have arisen as a result of the patient's disability.

Other counselors and therapists assist in this program. Vocational rehabilitation is the preparation of the disabled for useful employment. Through vocational rehabilitation the patient works toward economic independence. The *vocational counselor* tests him to determine his interests and aptitudes so that vocational training can be instituted. The *physical therapist* supports and supervises the patient during the prescribed exercise program. Using activities to develop skills that can be transferred to home and work situations, the *occupational therapist* devises practical projects for the patient to pursue that will develop his coordination and maintain his interest. The *social worker*, through contacts with the family, the

community and the employment situation, gives advice to facilitate the adjustment of the patient to his social environment.

The Nurse in Rehabilitation

The nurse has a unique function on the rehabilitation team, giving rise to the art of rehabilitation nursing.

The understanding nurse is a strong ally to the patient. She must support the therapy that is initiated by other members of the team. Her attitudes and understandings can either facilitate or hinder the rehabilitation program. Instead of doing things for the patient, the nurse's function is to *teach him to help himself.*

Rehabilitative nursing functions include:*

1. Developing a plan for nursing care services based upon nursing assessment of patient needs.

2. Providing direct nursing care services that will maintain optimum physical and mental health for the patient and will meet his medical treatment needs.

3. Applying nursing measures that prevent crippling and superimposed infections and insure the safety and comfort of the patient in his environment.

4. Establishing a sustained supporting relationship with the patient.

5. Participating in the retraining of the patient in self-care activities.

6. Providing health teaching and training that will meet the needs of the individual patient and his family.

7. Recording and reporting nursing observations of the patient's condition, progress and personal needs, and the action taken to meet the patient's nursing needs.

8. Assisting with patient discharge plans and providing for nursing referral of the patient for continued nursing services where needed.

9. Evaluating the nursing care in terms of the overall goals in patient care.

To overcome the patient's disability, the nurse helps him learn to care for his daily needs, to walk or employ some other method of transportation, to use ordinary toilet facilities, to communicate with others, and to apply and care for his own artificial prosthetic devices. These functions appear simple, but it may take many hours or many weeks of training to accomplish the patient's therapeutic goal.

Rehabilitation is an integral part of nursing and *should begin with the initial contact with the patient.* Every major illness carries with it the threat of disability. If the patient is hospitalized with a burn and develops a contracture deformity, his recovery time will be delayed greatly. Disabilities are not static but tend to become worse, and some complications of in-

* From Program Guide, G-8, of the Department of Medicine and Surgery, Veterans Administration.

activity can give the patient more pain and discomfort than the initial injury or disease.

The importance of rehabilitation often is underestimated. There are over 21.5 million disabled persons in the United States, and the aged population is steadily increasing. Every patient, regardless of his problem or diagnosis, has the right to rehabilitation services. Thus, rehabilitation is a large and increasing area of nursing responsibility. Though not all hospitals have departments of physical medicine and rehabilitation, *the principles of rehabilitation are basic to the care of all patients,* and the pages that follow point out how the nurse applies them.

PSYCHOLOGICAL IMPLICATIONS OF A DISABILITY

A physical disability often has a deep psychological significance to the patient. Physically a part of his body has deteriorated. He may have the shattering realization that he can do less than formerly. His shape and posture may have changed, as may have his state of mind. Even his position in society may be altered. He may classify himself as a member of a minority group. In short, he may feel that he is different.

Disability may spell hardship or even tragedy to the individual, depending on his occupation, cultural background and social status, and the support he receives from or provides for his family.

A person usually goes through a series of emotional reactions to a newly acquired disability. The first reaction may be that of denial. The patient may refuse to accept his new limitations and at times have an unjustified overconfidence in speedy recovery. His false hopes lead him to hear only what he wants to hear. He is likely to be self-centered and even childlike in his demands.

The patient may progress to a period of depression in which he appears to mourn for his lost function, or missing body part. This period of grief appears to be a necessary stage in making the required adaptations in living. He should not merely be encouraged blithefully to "cheer up." The nurse, simply with her attentive and ready-to-act presence, can transmit a feeling of caring to this patient.

In time the patient becomes more familiar with his condition and is able to tolerate it better. He revises his body image and modifies his former picture of himself. He is able to accept a degree of dependency and not resent being "waited upon." He begins to realize that hopelessness is futile and knows that he must adapt to the permanent aspects of the disability while relentlessly pursuing victory over temporary weaknesses.

The acceptance of the limitations imposed by the disability and the total investment of the patient in his rehabilitation program is basic to adjustment. It is from this point in rehabilitation that the patient begins to look ahead and develop realistic goals for his future.

Some patients do not accept their disability; they waste emotional energy in rebelling futilely against unalterable damage. Others ignore it and will not put forth any effort to adapt for everyday life the abilities that survive the disease or the treatment. Still others may over-react and build a false reputation for being "cheerful and courageous." Although "ignoring" may seem healthy, often it includes a total rejection of the disability, which keeps the patient from doing the small things that will be helpful to him. These patients may require assistance from either a psychologist or a psychiatrist. The nurse has the responsibility of watching patient reactions to disability and of reporting them to the physician. She has the privilege of listening to the patient, encouraging him and sharing in his satisfactions and triumphs as he progresses in his program. It is through the support and the inspiration of the members of the rehabilitation team that the patient becomes all that he is capable of being.

PRINCIPLES AND PRACTICES OF REHABILITATION NURSING

The most common complications that threaten a patient with a prolonged illness or disability are contractures, decubitus ulcers and bladder and bowel problems.

Lack of muscle use causes weakness. In addition, muscles that are not put through their full range of motion become shortened. Such a shortening (contracture) results in a deformity. These deformities may be prevented if the causal conditions are understood properly and preventive measures are instituted early.

When tissues do not receive adequate nourishment and exercise, they tend to deteriorate and to atrophy. By initiating deliberate and proper measures, tissue damage and decubitus ulcers can be combated and prevented.

Bladder and bowel difficulties may result from disease, injury or shock. In many patients, refunctioning can be accomplished through individualized teaching and persistent attention to the establishment of regular function.

The major responsibilities of the nurse in rehabilitation are: (1) to prevent deformities and complications, (2) to initiate, to teach and to support the patient (and his family when necessary) during the daily activities of living which include self-care, and (3) to refer the patient for proper follow-up care and supervision. Each of these categories will now be discussed in detail.

DEFINITIONS

Adduction—movement of a limb toward the body's center.

Abduction—movement away from midline of the body; turning outward.

Extension—when referring to an extremity means straightening out the joint.

Hyperextension—extension beyond the ordinary range.

Flexion—bending the various joints, such as the knee or the elbow, or the thigh on the trunk.

Dorsiflexion—bending backward.

Rotation—turning or movement of a part around its axis.

Internal: turning inward toward the center.

External: turning outward away from the center.

Pronation—turning downward.

Supination—turning upward.

Prevention of Deformities and Complications

Deformities and complications of illness or injury often can be prevented by proper body position in bed and by exercises.

Positioning

Unless contraindicated, the patient should be turned frequently. The reasons for changing body positions are these: (1)· to prevent contractures; (2) to stimulate circulation and to help to prevent thrombophlebitis, decubiti and edema of the extremities; (3) to promote lung expansion; (4) to promote drainage of respiratory secretions; (5) to relieve pressure on a body area.

The most common positions that the patient assumes in bed are the dorsal or supine, the side-lying or lateral, and the prone positions. The essential principles of body alignment necessary for maintaining these positions follow.

Dorsal or Supine Position

1. The head is in line with the spine, both laterally and anteroposteriorly.
2. The trunk is positioned so that flexion of the hips is minimized.
3. The arms are flexed at the elbow with the hands resting against the lateral abdomen.
4. The legs are extended with a small firm support under the popliteal area.
5. The heels are suspended in a space between the mattress and the footboard.
6. The toes are pointed straight up.
7. Small towel rolls are placed under the greater trochanters in the hip joint areas.

Side-lying or Lateral Position

1. The head is in line with the spine.
2. The body is in alignment and is not twisted.
3. The uppermost hip joint is slightly forward and supported in a position of slight abduction.

4. A pillow supports the arm, which is flexed at both the elbow and the shoulder joints.

Prone Position

1. The head is turned laterally and is in alignment with the rest of the body.
2. The arms are abducted and externally rotated at the shoulder joint; the elbows are flexed.
3. A small flat support is placed under the pelvis, extending from the level of the umbilicus to the upper third of the thigh.
4. The lower extremities remain in a neutral position.
5. The toes are suspended over the edge of the mattress.

Therapeutic Exercises

These exercises are prescribed by the physician and performed with the assistance and guidance of a physical therapist. If such a therapist is not available, the nurse may assist the patient. The objectives and goals of an exercise program are determined by the patient's condition. Exercise, when correctly done, assists in (1) maintaining and building muscle strength, (2) maintaining joint function, (3) preventing deformity, (4) stimulating circulation, and (5) building endurance. There are 5 types of exercise.

Passive. An exercise carried out by the therapist or the nurse without assistance from the patient.

PURPOSE. To retain as much joint range of motion as possible; to maintain circulation.

ACTION. Stabilize the proximal joint and support the distal part. Move the joint smoothly, slowly, and gently through its full range of motion. Avoid producing pain.

Active Assistive. An exercise carried out by the patient with the assistance of the therapist or the nurse.

PURPOSE. To encourage normal muscle function.

ACTION. Support the distal part and encourage the patient to take the joint actively through its range of motion. Give as little assistance as is necessary to ac-

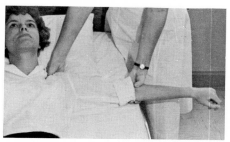

Abduction-adduction of the shoulder.

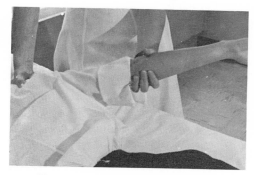

Hyperextension of the shoulder.

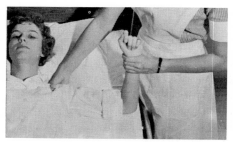

Internal-external rotation of the
shoulder (neutral position).

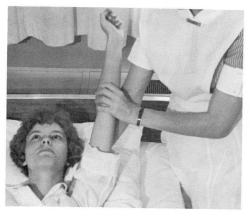

Flexion of the shoulder.

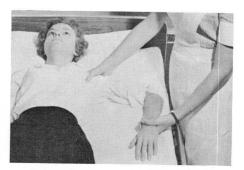

Internal rotation of the shoulder.

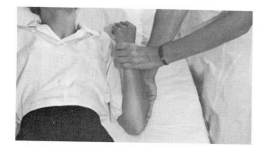

Flexion of the elbow.

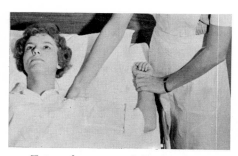

External rotation of the shoulder
(note: hand touches bed).

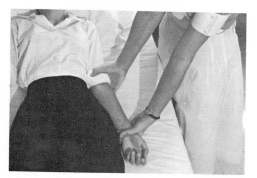

Extension of the elbow.

FIG. 10-1. Range of motion exercises.

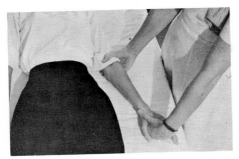

Pronation of the forearm.

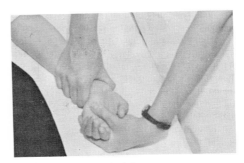

Ulnar-radial deviation.

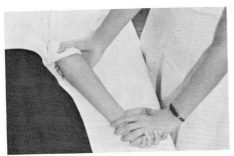

Supination of the forearm.

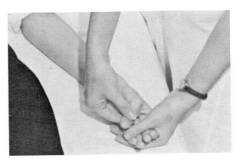

Thumb opposition.

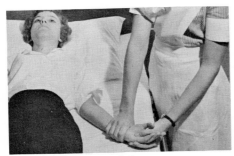

Extension of the wrist.

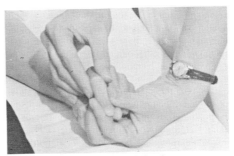

Flexion-extension of the fingers.

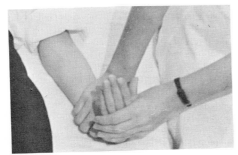

Flexion of the wrist.

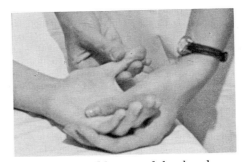

Abduction-adduction of the thumb.

FIGURE 10-1 (*Continued*)

complish the action. Short periods of activity should be followed by adequate rest periods.

Active. An exercise accomplished by the patient without assistance.

PURPOSE. To increase muscle strength.

ACTION. Active exercise when possible should be done against gravity. The joint is moved through full range of motion without assistance. (Make sure that the patient does not substitute another joint movement for the one intended.)

Resistive. An active exercise carried out by the patient working against resistance produced by either manual or mechanical means.

PURPOSE. To provide resistance in order to increase muscle power.

ACTION. The patient moves the joint through its

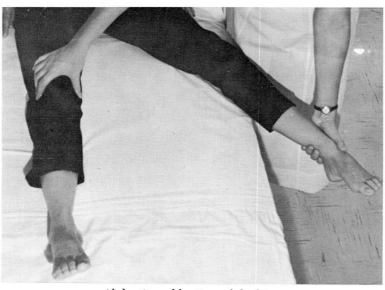

Abduction-adduction of the hip.

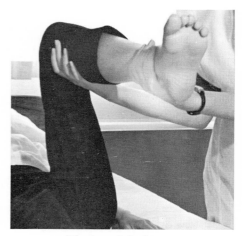

Flexion of the hip.

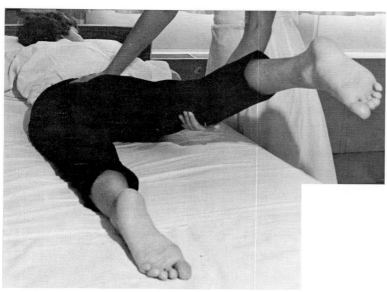

Hyperextension of the hip.

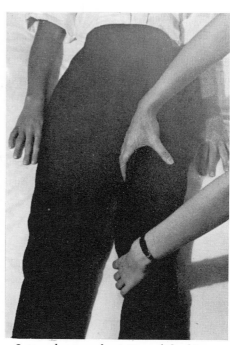

Internal-external rotation of the hip.

FIGURE 10-1 (*Continued*)

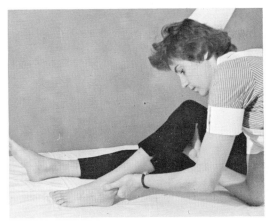

Flexion of the knee.

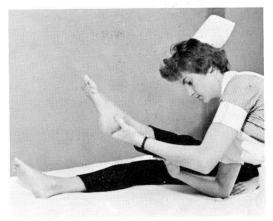

Extension of the knee.

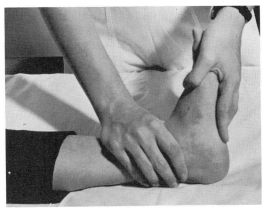

Dorsiflexion of the foot.

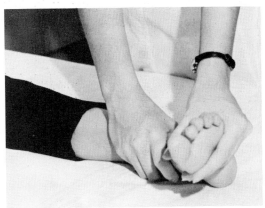

Inversion-eversion of the foot.

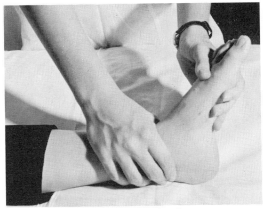

Plantar flexion of the foot.

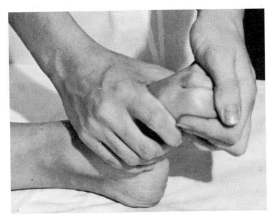

Flexion-extension of the toes.

FIGURE 10-1 (*Continued*)

TABLE 10-1. Passive range-of-motion exercises adapted for nursing

Joint	Normal Movement of Joint	Part to be Stabilized	Part to be Moved
Shoulder	Flexion Extension Abduction Adduction Internal rotation External rotation Hyperextension (done in prone position)	Shoulder girdle	Arm
Elbow	Flexion Extension Supination Pronation	Arm	Forearm
Wrist	Flexion Extension Ulnar deviation Radial deviation	Forearm	Hand
Thumb	Flexion Extension Abduction Adduction Opposition	Metacarpals and wrist	Metacarpophalangeal joint of thumb
Distal phalanx of thumb	Flexion Extension	Proximal phalanx of thumb	Distal phalanx of thumb
Joints of fingers Metacarpophalangeal joints	Flexion Extension Abduction Adduction	Metacarpals of hand	Fingers
Interphalangeal joints	Flexion Extension	Proximal or middle phalanx	Middle and distal phalanx
Toe Interphalangeal joints	Flexion Extension	Proximal or middle joint phalanx	Middle and distal phalanx
Metacarpophalangeal joints	Flexion Extension Abduction Adduction	Metatarsal	Proximal phalanx
Ankle	Dorsiflexion Plantar flexion Eversion Inversion	Leg	Foot
Knee	Flexion Extension	Thigh	Leg
Hip	Flexion Extension Abduction Adduction Internal rotation External rotation Hyperextension (done in prone position)	Pelvis	Thigh
Neck	Flexion Extension Rotation	Support head	Head

range of motion while the therapist resists slightly at first and then progressively with increasing resistance. Sandbags and weights can be used and are applied at the distal point of the involved joint. The movements should be done smoothly.

Isometric or Muscle Setting. An exercise performed by the patient.

PURPOSE. To maintain strength when a joint is immobilized.

ACTION. Contract or tighten the muscle as much as possible without moving the joint; hold for several seconds, then "let go" and relax. Breathe deeply.

Range-of-motion Exercises

Each joint of the body has a normal range of motion. In many musculoskeletal conditions the joints may lose their normal range, stiffen, and produce a permanent disability. If the range of motion is limited, the functions of the joint and the muscle that moves the joint are impaired. In order to prevent painful deformities, range-of-motion activities when permitted are carried out passively, with active assistance, or actively. Range-of-motion exercises are designed for either maintaining or increasing the maximal motion of a joint.

The patient must be in a comfortable position, lying supine with his arms to the side and his knees extended. Good body posture is to be maintained in each position assumed during the exercise. The bed should be high enough to permit the nurse to reach effectively the part to be exercised.

Unless otherwise ordered, a joint should be moved through its full range of motion about 3 times at least once every day. A joint should not be moved beyond its free range of motion. Therefore, the motion should be stopped at the point of pain. When muscle spasm is present, the joint should be moved slowly and to the point of resistance. Then a gentle steady pressure is exerted until the muscle relaxes.

In performing range-of-motion exercises, the bones above and below the joint to be moved are considered. For example, in taking the elbow through its range of motion, the humerus must be stabilized while the radius and the ulna are moved through their range of motion in the elbow joint.

Table 10-1 shows the normal movement of joints. To assist the nurse to learn logically the technique of range of motion, the name of the joint, the anatomic movements of the joint, the part to be stabilized, and the part to be moved are identified.

Fear and Pain. The ability of a patient to follow a pattern of exercises may be thwarted by *fear* and *pain*. These produce increased tensions and may result in muscle spasm and tightness of joint ligaments. If fear

FIG. 10-2. To make a trochanter roll: Take both ends of the towel (A) and bring them to the center. The towel is now folded in half with the edges at the center. Turn the towel over so that the ends (A) are facing downward. Turn the patient on his side with his upper leg flexed. Place one side (B) of the towel in the midline of the buttock. The towel should extend from the crest of the ilium to the midthigh. Then place the patient in a dorsal position with his leg extended. Grasp the remaining side (B) of the towel and roll it in an underneath fashion until the entire roll is well under the pateint's buttock. The roll should be taut and smooth. For the larger patient, a draw sheet or a bath blanket may be used.

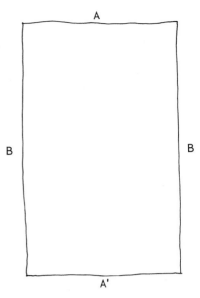

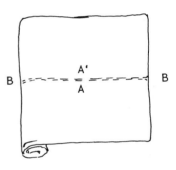

and pain are not relieved, they may lead to stiffness of joints, limitation in range of motion, muscle contractures and poorly coordinated muscle activity. For example: *pain* in the chest, as observed in chest and breast surgery, cardiac pain or burns of the thorax, frequently causes many patients to hold the arm close to the body, resting on the chest or abdominal wall with the elbow flexed. If permitted to continue for prolonged periods of time, this may result in tightness of the ligaments around the shoulder and elbow joints; and spasm of the large pectoral muscles and biceps may lead to adaptive shortening, tightening and contractures of these muscles. The weight of the arm on the chest and/or the abdomen restricts the expansive motion of the chest wall and muscles of respiration, which leads to inadequate ventilation.

Fear (as observed in patients who have had cardiac, chest or breast surgery, infections in the lungs and burns of the chest wall) often accounts for these individuals assuming protective positions that are restrictive in nature and prevent proper physiologic alignment.

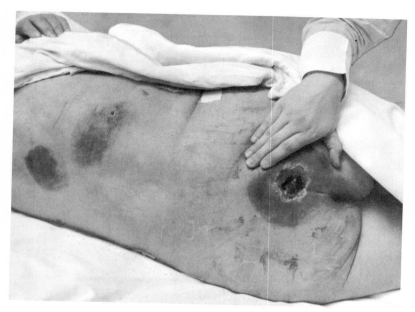

FIG. 10-3. Decubitus ulcer or bedsore over sacrum.

Preventing External Rotation of the Hip

Patients who are in bed for periods of time may develop external rotation deformity of the hip. The hip is a ball-and-socket joint and has a tendency to rotate outward when the patient lies on his back. A trochanter roll extending from the crest of the ilium to the midthigh will prevent this deformity. With correct placement, the trochanter roll serves as a mechanical wedge under the projection of the greater trochanter.

Preventing Foot Drop (Plantar Flexion)

This is a deformity in which the foot is plantar flexed (bending the ankle in the direction of the sole of the foot). If the condition continues without correction, the patient will walk on his toes without touching the ground with the heel of his foot. The deformity is caused by contracture of both the gastrocnemius and the soleus muscles. Prolonged bed rest, lack of exercise, incorrect positioning in bed, and the weight of the bedding forcing the toes into plantar flexion are factors that contribute to this crippling deformity. To prevent it, a footboard is used to keep the feet at right angles to the legs when the patient is in a supine position. The patient is encouraged to flex and then to extend (curl and stretch) his feet and toes frequently. The ankles should be moved clockwise and counterclockwise in a rotary motion several times each hour.

Preventing and Treating Decubiti

The prevention of decubitus ulcers (bedsores) is one of the most important considerations in the nursing care of patients. It is a complication that in most instances is due to poor nursing care. Such a sore is due to pressure that produces ischemia and consequently impaired nutrition to the tissues. This deprivation causes the cutaneous tissues to be broken or destroyed, and there is a progressive destruction of underlying soft tissue. The ulcer may be extremely painful and very slow to heal. Bacterial invasion and secondary infection are difficult to avoid. The lesion, if large enough, permits a continuous loss of serum, which may deplete the circulating blood and the entire body of essential protein constituents (Fig. 10-3).

Any patient who is stuporous, emaciated, incontinent, paralyzed, or whose treatment involves the immobilization of any portion of the body is in constant danger of developing a decubitus ulcer.

Essentials of Prevention

The best treatment of decubiti is prevention. The principles that underlie the nursing management are (1) *to relieve or to remove pressure,* (2) to stimulate the circulation, and (3) to keep the skin dry.

The patient needs frequent changes of position and the avoidance of positions that result in excessive local pressure. He should be turned every 2 hours. If possible, he should be taught and encouraged to turn himself. Turning helps the tissue to recover from pressure. Localized pressure, *for even a few hours,* may cause cessation of blood flow in the capillary bed. Redness and edema are seen. Then, within a few days ulceration and skin necrosis follow.

Bony prominences may be protected by inserting small pieces of sheepskin pads (preferably) or foam rubber beneath the sacrum, the trochanters, the heels, the elbows, the scapulae and the back of the head

ACTIVITIES OF DAILY LIVING (A.D.L.) SHEET

	EVALUATION OF THE PATIENT'S FUNCTIONING		
	Total Assistance	Partial Assistance	Independent

Prescribed Activities: *Functional Capabilities:*

Range of Motion

Positioning

Use of Tilt Table

  Degree

  How long

Exercises

  Breathing

  Balancing

  Crutch Training

  Parallel Bars

  Steps

Other Information:

Appliances or Prosthesis

Ambulation

Time Permitted Up

Bladder/Bowel Program

Bathing/Grooming Schedule

Speech Problems

Activities Being Learned

Name:

Diagnosis:

Doctor:

1. Flexes neck
2. Raises hand to head
3. Raises hand behind head
4. Reaches out at shoulder level to side (laterally)
5. Pronates/supinates forearm
6. Grasps objects
7. Begins grasp ability
8. Closes fist
9. Opens fist
10. Flexes and extends knee joint
11. Touches floor while seated
12. Crosses leg over opposite knee while sitting (with or without help of hands)
13. Transfers from sitting to standing (with or without holding to support)
14. Walks

FIG. 10-4. On the actual chart there is sufficient space left under each item for notes.

when there is pressure on these sites. The use of a footboard removes the pressure of the bedding from the feet and the extremities. The alternating pressure pad mattress covered with one-inch thick foam rubber is especially valuable in conditions in which the patient cannot turn. The alternating inflation and deflation of the pad produces a constriction followed by a dilatation of the superficial blood vessels of the skin. By such action, pressure on any one part is reduced and the blood supply is increased.

Since the stimulation of circulation relieves tissue ischemia, the forerunner of decubitus ulcers, the patient is encouraged to keep active. (Activity also stimulates the metabolic processes and helps to improve morale.) Frequent skin massage is useful as a means of stimulating the blood flow in the skin. A gentle circular motion is used around bony prominences and other vulnerable areas. If an abrasion is discovered, massage should be directed in ever-widening circles away from the lesion. Again, turning aids the circulation. The use of a rocking bed and a tilt table also aids in stimulating circulation.

Maceration of the skin by continuous moisture must be prevented by meticulous hygienic measures. The skin should be washed with a mild soap (or one containing hexachlorophene to reduce bacterial infection) and water and blotted dry with a soft towel. The skin then is lubricated with an emollient lotion to keep it soft and pliable. It is desirable that the patient assist in caring for his skin. He should be taught to inspect it at frequent intervals for evidence of pressure. Foreign bodies should be kept out of the bed because they serve to irritate the skin. Foundation sheets should be tightly stretched to prevent wrinkles.

Treatment

If a decubitus ulcer develops, the essentials of care are to remove the pressure and to keep the area clean and dry. The metabolic processes are stimulated by keeping the patient as active as possible. Blood flow may be improved by gentle massage to the adjacent area. The patient is placed on a high protein diet to promote healing.

Plasma, blood, sugar and other nutrients have been employed to encourage healing of the wound. Many clinicians and investigators feel that proteolytic enzymes have a significant place in the management of these wounds. However, 2 factors are always necessary for the successful healing of a decubitus ulcer: (1) avoidance of further pressure, and (2) keeping the wound well débrided and clean.

Flotation Therapy. A device recently developed to reduce pressure is the water bed. The patient is supported on a plastic tarpaulin. The tarpaulin rests on water and the patient floats freely in the water. The underlying principles are those of flotation and displacement: the body literally gives up its weight when it is partially submerged in water. Thus, the body weight is *lightened* and there is less pressure on body parts as the body floats in the water. Beds of varying designs are available; some permit the patient to assume a sitting position so he can carry out diversional and other activities. Flotation therapy has proved to be an effective and safe treatment for decubitus ulcers.

For deep decubiti that refuse to heal by conservative means, some advocate excision of the ulcer and often of the underlying bony prominence, with plastic closure by skin and fat flaps.

Supporting the Patient in Daily Self-Care

When a patient has a physical disability, the nurse helps him to make all types of adaptations in order to perform the self-care activities of daily living. This nursing practice requires common sense and a little ingenuity, for many patients do not perform these commonplace activities easily. Often a simple maneuver requires much concentration and the exertion of considerable effort.

Morrissey offers 3 *fundamental principles* which are relevant to all instruction *in self-care methods.** The first is that the nurse teaches and guides, but the patient is obliged to do the work. Secondly, motivation is an important factor; it is not possible to instruct and guide an unwilling patient. (However it behooves the nurse to use all her ingenuity to motivate the patient.) And third, there are individual differences in all people. Hence, self-care techniques should be flexible and easily adjusted to the patient's needs.

By using an "Activities of Daily Living (A.D.L.) Sheet" (Fig. 10-4) to evaluate the ability of a patient to perform certain activities, it is possible to determine his limitations. Another advantage of such a guide is to show the patient how he is progressing from one time to the next; this may be a valuable morale booster. When a patient's progress can be demonstrated, there is a tendency for such evidence to be a source of motivation.

Before initiating an A.D.L. program, the nurse must understand the patient's medical condition, his functional capacity and therapeutic goal. She also must be familiar with every detail of his care. It is wise to know the patient's family background in order to know how much support the family can give. An understanding of the educational background of the patient and the family members also will be helpful to the nurse.

* Morrissey, A. B.: Rehabilitation Nursing. p. 144. New York, G. P. Putnam's Sons, 1950.

The role of the nurse in A.D.L. is to teach, support and supervise the patient while he does these activities. An Activities of Daily Living program is started as soon as the rehabilitation process starts. The longer a muscle is in disuse, the weaker and more atrophied it becomes. The patient must learn that he will lose what he does not use.

Teaching the Activities of Daily Living

Since there are many ways to teach a task, the following is offered as a guide:

1. Ascertain what methods can be used to accomplish the task. (Example: There are several ways of putting on a given garment.)
2. Determine what the patient can do by watching him perform.
3. Ascertain the motions necessary for the accomplishment of the activity.
4. Encourage the patient to exercise the muscles necessary to perform the motions involved in the activity.
5. Select activities that encourage gross functional movements of the upper and lower extremities (e.g., bathing, holding larger objects).
6. Gradually include activities that use finer motions, e.g., buttoning clothes, eating with a spoon.
7. Increase the period of activity as rapidly as the patient can tolerate.
8. Perform and practice the activity in a real-life situation.
9. Encourage the patient to do every activity up to his maximal capabilities within the framework of his disability.
10. Support the patient by giving justifiable praise for effort put forth and for acts accomplished:

The A.D.L. Sheet is an information sheet for those who are taking care of the patient. The data on it serve to inform each member of the rehabilitation team what activities the patient can do. It also serves as an index of progress. For example, after it has been determined that the patient can bathe himself, this information is noted on the A.D.L. Sheet. The nurse who is responsible for the patient reviews this sheet at morning care time. She knows then what the patient is capable of doing and what activities he is learning. Thus the patient does not regress, because all members of the rehabilitation team are working toward the same goal.

The A.D.L. Sheet in Figure 10-4 is a guide to the assessment of the functions of the patient. These activities are key goals. If the patient can sit up and raise his hands to his head, he probably can begin to bathe himself. By asking the patient to do certain motions the nurse can determine what activities the patient will be able to do.

If the patient has difficulty in performing the activity, an adaptation will have to be made. Often a new method can be learned. If the patient cannot quite reach his head, perhaps he will be able to touch his head by leaning forward. Or, if the method cannot be changed, adaptive equipment (self-help devices) may be used—such as adding a long handle to a comb, "building up" the handle of a spoon, or a similar modification.

Assisting the Patient with Ambulation

Transfer Activities

As soon as the patient is permitted out of bed, transfer activities are started. While still confined to his bed, it is important that the patient practice "push-up" exercises to strengthen the arm and shoulder extensors. It is desirable that the patient be able to raise and move his body in different directions by means of these push-up exercises.

(1) Have the patient sit upright in bed.
(2) Place a book under each hand.
(3) Instruct the patient to push down on the book thus raising his body weight.

Since the nurse is so frequently concerned with getting weak and incapacitated patients out of bed, the following guidelines are offered for getting the patient out of bed into a chair.

Technique for moving the patient to the edge of the bed:

(1) Move head and shoulders of patient toward the edge of the bed.
(2) Move feet and legs to the edge of bed. (The patient is now in a crescent position that gives good range of motion to the lateral trunk muscles.)
(3) Nurse places both arms well under patient's hips. (Before the next maneuver the nurse should tighten [set] the muscles of her back.)
(4) Nurse straightens her back while moving the patient toward herself.

Technique for sitting patient on the edge of the bed:

(1) Place hand under shoulders of the patient.
(2) Nurse instructs the patient to push his elbow into the bed while she lifts his shoulders with one arm and swings his legs over the edge of the bed with the other. (Gravity pulls the legs downward, which aids in raising the patient's trunk.)

Technique for assisting patient to stand:

(1) Place patient's feet well under him.
(2) Face the patient with hands firmly grasping each side of his rib cage.
(3) Nurse pushes her knee against one knee of the patient.

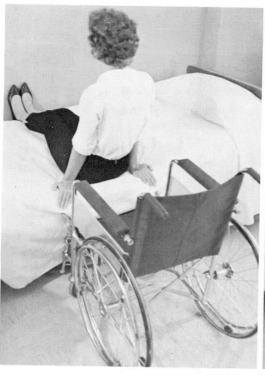 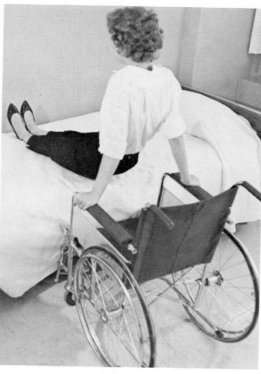

FIG. 10-5. Transfer technique for a paraplegic patient. The patient moves from her bed to a wheelchair. (*Left*) The wheelchair is placed facing the bed with the wheels locked and the pedals in the "down" position. (*Right*) The patient transfers her hands from the bed to the arms of the wheelchair, then lifts and pushes herself back into the chair.

(4) Rock the patient forward as he comes to a standing position. (The nurse's knee is pushed against the patient's knee as he comes to the standing position.)

(5) Ensure that the patient's knees are "locked" (full extension) while he is standing. (Locking the knees of the patient is a safety measure for those who are weak or have been in bed for a period of time.)

(6) Give the patient *enough time* to balance himself.

(7) Pivot the patient to position him to sit in the chair.

There are other methods of transferring from the bed to the wheelchair when the patient is unable to stand. Figure 10-5 shows the transfer for a paraplegic patient.

If the muscles that the patient uses to lift himself off the bed are not strong enough to overcome the resistance of body weight, a polished light-weight board may be used to bridge the gap between the bed and the chair, and the patient slides across on it. This board (or bench) also may be used to transfer the patient from the chair to the toilet or the bathtub.

Before the patient is taught to transfer, he is evaluated to determine his ability to transfer from one area to another. The nurse demonstrates the technique of transfer and the patient then is ready to practice and perform this activity (Fig. 10-5).

Preparation for Ambulation

Regaining the ability to walk is a prime morale builder. To be prepared for ambulation—whether with braces, cane or crutches—the patient must be strengthened and conditioned. *Exercise is the foundation of preparation.* By performing mat and parallel-bar exercises, the patient develops balance and coordination and strengthens his muscles. The following are preconditioning exercises that the nurse can teach and supervise.

To strengthen the muscles needed for ambulation, the *quadriceps setting* is used. The patient contracts the quadriceps muscle while attempting to push the popliteal area against the mattress and raising the heel. He maintains the muscle contracture until the count of five and relaxes for the count of five. He should repeat this exercise 10 to 15 times hourly. In the *gluteal setting*, he contracts or "pinches" the buttocks together until the count of five, relaxes for the count of five, and repeats.

To strengthen the muscles of the upper extremities, which are used for handling the cane, the crutches, and the walker employed in early ambulation, *sit-ups* are helpful. While in a sitting position, the patient raises his body from the chair by pushing his hands against the chair seat (or mattress). He also should be encouraged to do *push-ups* while in a prone position. Teach him to *raise arms* above his head and lower

FIG. 10-6. Crutch-walking. (*Left*) Note that the patient's weight is borne not in the axilla but on the palm of the hand, with the arm extended. The weight of the patient's body should be inclined forward to be supported by the crutches.

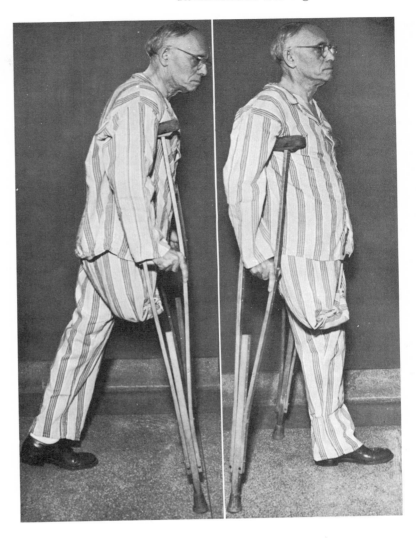

them in a slow, rhythmical manner while holding traction weights, gradually increasing the poundage of the weights. He can *strengthen his hands* by crumpling newspaper and squeezing a rubber ball. *Pull-ups* on a trapeze, lifting the body, is another effective conditioner.

Crutch-walking

In the treatment of most fractures of the lower extremity, of various forms of arthritis and after operations on the leg—especially after amputation—crutches provide a convenient method for getting from one place to another. Not an inherited skill, crutch-walking must be taught, and this learning process must begin early. It includes psychological preparation that can be developed long before the physical need is present. The individual needs of each patient must be considered and the methods of approach directed to them.

The patient's age, his interests and his future intentions, as well as his prognosis, are essential factors.

Adjustable crutches are practical because the disease may make changes in the muscles and the joints, or because the patient may improve and progress to a different crutch base and gait.

To measure a standing patient for crutches, measure 1½ to 2 inches from the axillary fold to a position on the floor 4 inches in front of the patient and 6 inches to the side of his toes. (This is merely an approximate measure. It is desirable to have a 2-finger width insertion between the axillary fold and the armpiece.)

If the patient has to be measured while lying down, measure from the anterior fold of the axilla to the sole of the foot, and then add 2 inches.

The handpiece should allow a 30° elbow flexion. The wrist should be extended, and the hand dorsiflexed. The patient should wear shoes that fit well and have firm soles. The crutches should be fitted with large rubber suction tips before measuring.

Good posture is essential to crutch walking. Before trying to use crutches, the patient should learn to stand by a chair on the unaffected leg in order to achieve balance. The nurse explains and demonstrates to the patient how he should manipulate his crutches before he attempts to do so.

The *tripod position* is the basic crutch stance. The crutches rest approximately 8 to 10 inches in front and to the side of the patient's toes. This gives the strongest and most balanced support. Since, to provide stability, a greater height requires a broader base, a taller patient needs a wider base and a shorter patient a narrower base.

The patient must be taught to support his weight on the handpiece. If the weight is borne on the axilla, the pressure of the crutch can damage the brachial plexus nerves and produce "crutch paralysis." A foam rubber pad on the underarm piece will relieve pressure on the upper arm and the thoracic cage.

Ability to shift body weight is the next step. The crutch gait selected depends on the nature of the patient's disability. The nurse must know how much (if any) weight can be placed on the affected side. She should know whether the crutches are being used for balance and support. The crutch gait should be prescribed by the physician.

All gaits begin in the tripod position. The more common gaits are:

The 4-point Gait. This gait can be used when supported weight-bearing is permitted for both legs. It is safe and gives maximal balance because there are always 3 points of contact with the floor; hence it is slow because it requires constant shifting of weight. The sequence is to advance (1) right crutch, (2) left foot, (3) left crutch, (4) right foot.

The 2-point Gait. This gait is faster, since there are only 2 points of contact with the floor at one time. Sequence: (1) right crutch and left foot, (2) left crutch and right foot.

The Swinging-to and Swinging-through Gaits. These gaits are more advanced. The patient bears weight on his good leg, places the crutches at an equal distance ahead of him and then swings to a position to or just ahead of the crutches. Weight is shifted to the palms of the hands and then back to the good leg. The elevation produced by a medium-heeled shoe on the good leg may permit the affected leg to swing through without touching the floor and without unnecessary flexion. It is desirable that the patient learn as many gaits as possible so that he may change his pattern when one gait tires him. The nurse should not permit patients to walk for too long, especially those who have been bedridden for a long time. Such signs as cyanosis, sweating or shortness of breath should be indications that

the lesson on crutches should be stopped and the patient permitted to rest or go back to bed.

Before a patient is sent home on crutches, it is important to ascertain whether or not he can dress himself, get in and out of chairs, on and off the toilet, in and out of doors, up and down stairs and ramps, and in and out of a car, a taxi or a public conveyance.

Some of the techniques of managing crutches have been standardized, as follows:

If the door is opened by pushing, the patient should get as close as possible to it, balance himself securely on crutches and feet so that the hand nearest the doorknob can be released, and turn the handle. The door is then pushed ajar and a crutch is quickly advanced to hold the gain. This operation is repeated until the patient, moving in progressive stages clears the door. Difficulties: getting close enough to the door; clearing the doorsill while advancing.

If the door must be opened by pulling, the above procedure is modified in that the patient stands to one side and pulls with the free hand.

Sitting down in and standing up from chair: These procedures are difficult. Soft, low chairs add to the difficulties. The technique should first be practiced with a fairly high chair equipped with arms and placed against the wall.

For sitting down, most techniques follow the practice of either falling or letting the body down into the chair, starting from a standing position with the patient's back to the chair. For the latter purpose, the crutches are grasped at the hand pieces for control; for the former method, the body is bent forward at the hips. Falling can be controlled to a certain extent, if muscular capacity allows, by gradually bending trunk forward, then knees, then placing hands on knees, and finally completing the forward bending of trunk until the body falls easily into the chair. Crutches may be previously placed against the chair, or be held passively during the change of position.

For standing up, one or both feet should be placed under the chair, not away from it. Grasping a hand piece of the crutch in each hand (or both hand pieces in one hand), the patient pushes down.*

The Use of the Tilt Table

Weight bearing on the long bones is essential to normal physiologic functioning. In order to prevent complications of inactivity, the upright position with weight bearing on the long bones is desirable at the earliest possible time. This position prevents decalcification of the bones, thus aiding in the maintenance of normal acid-base balance and the prevention of renal calculi; it also stimulates circulation to the lower extremities.

Some disabilities prevent patients from assuming an upright position by the usual methods. A tilt table or

* Gordon, E. E.: Multiple Sclerosis, Application of Rehabilitation Techniques (p. 29), National Multiple Sclerosis Society, New York, 1951.

bed is a device that permits this essential activity.

To assist the patient who has been in the recumbent position for a length of time, the nurse should consider the problems that may ensue when a standing position is assumed. The position should be assumed progressively and gradually. Evaluation of the patient's tolerance may be made by observation of blood pressure, pulse and general appearance. To prevent some of the more common complications, such as orthostatic hypotension and edema of the lower extremities, elastic compression bandages on the lower extremities may be indicated.

Assisting With Prosthetic and Orthotic Appliances

A *prosthesis* is an artificial replacement for a missing portion of the body. An *orthotic* device is an orthopedic appliance commonly termed a *brace*. A prosthetist or an orthotist fits these appliances only by prescription of the physician.†

Preprosthetic Care

The nurse performs a distinctive function in the preprosthetic phase of the patient's care. She sees the patient at the beginning of the disability and can help him to develop an attitude of realistic hopefulness. Her major function is prevent deformities so that the time between the healing of the tissues and the fitting of the prosthesis is kept to a minimum. In the amputation of an extremity, she is responsible for bandaging the stump correctly, so that proper shrinkage and shaping of the stump occurs and the patient can be fitted more effectively with a prosthesis (see pp. 865-868).

Braces

The patient should be fitted for a brace according to the prescription of the physician. A brace is a support that protects weakened muscles, prevents and corrects anatomic deformities and controls involuntary muscle movements. The essential parts of leg braces are frames, hinges, joints, straps, belts and lining. In the upright frames, the hinges and the joints usually are made of steel. Often a brace may appear to be heavy; yet its weight is necessary in order to be safe, durable and effective.

In caring for a patient wearing a brace, the major responsibility of the nurse is to make certain that the patient wears the brace and that it is not applied too

† Specific prostheses are described later in this book, when the clinical conditions calling for them are discussed, e.g., limb prostheses for the amputee and a breast prosthesis for the patient who has had a radical mastectomy. Information concerning prosthetic and orthopedic appliances may be obtained also from The American Orthotic and Prosthetic Association, 919 18th Street N.W., Suite 130, Washington, D.C. 20006.

tightly. The following are the main points in the care of braces:

(1) All locks should be opened once a week and cleaned with fine wire or a hairpin; place a drop of machine oil in each joint.

(2) Repair leather when necessary. Little can be done about perspiration stains; however, washing the leather in lukewarm water with saddle soap helps to preserve the leather.

(3) When not in use, it is well to lay the brace on a table or the floor in good alignment; hanging may cause it to distort its position.

(4) Twisting of the brace may occur with use; check alignment frequently. The joints should coincide with the body joints.

(5) Before putting a brace on, check carefully for worn areas, missing or loose screws and the condition of straps and buckles.

(6) Pressure areas may occur if metal rubs the skin. After removing a brace, check the skin immediately for reddened areas.

(7) Have the brace checked periodically.

Note: The patient himself should care for his brace when he is able.

Helping to Overcome Elimination Problems

Urinary and bowel incontinence in a patient is another problem that challenges the nurse's ingenuity. Bladder and bowel control are important functions of the body; social acceptance of the individual may be affected if he suffers from incontinence. Patients with various medical and surgical conditions have to be trained in regaining control of these functions.

Bladder Training

Tidal drainage, discussed on page 828, will condition or pretrain the bladder for activity that is not controlled by the central nervous system but is automatic. After tidal drainage is discontinued (or the indwelling catheter removed), the patient is ready for a bladder-training regimen. With the approval and the cooperation of the physician and with the willingness of the patient (who knows his habit patterns better than anyone else) a schedule is set up with definite times indicated for the patient to try to empty his bladder using either the bedpan or the toilet. The interval between voiding in the early phase of the training period is fairly short (1½ to 2 hours), but as the patient's bladder capacity increases, the interval is lengthened. A suggested procedure is to give a measured amount of fluid every 2 hours. After drinking, the patient waits for 30 minutes and then attempts to void. He gradually increases the period between voiding times. (It is best to give larger amounts of fluid at breakfast and to withhold fluids at bedtime.) The patient is encouraged

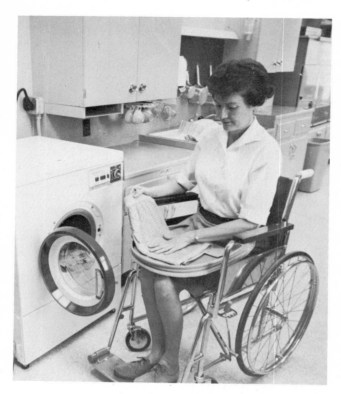

Fig. 10-7. Homemakers constitute the largest group among the disabled. Recognizing the economic and social values of homemakers, rehabilitation services have been expanded to include training women and men in homemaking. For the severely disabled person in a wheelchair, work surfaces should be low, continuous and open underneath with items within easy reach.

to hold his urine until the specified voiding time. Usually, there is a relationship between drinking, eating, exercising, and voiding, and the alert patient soon can determine his own intake schedule. Regularity is the key to success. Bladder training for the paraplegic or quadriplegic patient is discussed further in Chap. 34.

To assist in the act of voiding, the patient should either stand or sit with the thighs flexed and the feet and the back supported. Increasing intra-abdominal pressure by massage over the bladder or by leaning forward while sitting will help to initiate evacuation of the bladder. The patient must approve of the program and have a sincere desire to establish control. It may take weeks to accomplish; patience and persistence on the part of both nurse and patient plus expressions of approval for even slight gains are necessary. The use of a diaper at any time is discouraged, because its psychological effect is one of regression rather than progression.

Bowel Training

The first essential to bowel training that requires reflex assistance is the *establishment of regularity*. Any attempts at evacuation should be done within 15 minutes of the same time daily. An active aid toward bowel evacuation is the stimulation of peristalsis. Therefore, the patient should establish his bowel evacuation time after a regularly scheduled meal. One of the best times is after breakfast. However, if the patient has a previously-established habit pattern, it should be followed.

Physical activity is another helpful aid to peristaltic activity and bowel movement. Unless contraindicated by other existing conditions, the diet should include adequate roughage and a fluid intake between 2,000 to 4,000 ml. daily. Prune juice or fig juice taken at the same time daily may be beneficial when constipation is a problem.

The reflex habit should be established by regularity early in the course of the patient's illness. It may be aided by mechanical means. About 30 minutes before the scheduled bowel time, a glycerine suppository is inserted into the rectum. After the scheduled interval, the patient is encouraged to attempt to have a bowel movement. If at all possible he should assume the normal position for defecation. Instruct him to bear down and to contract his abdominal muscles. The patient may be taught to apply pressure to the abdominal wall to assist with his defecation.

After this routine is well established, mechanical stimulation with the suppository probably will not be necessary, and in a few weeks the patient will be having regular daily bowel movements.

PROMOTING CONTINUITY OF PATIENT CARE

The objective of a referral system is to maintain continuity of patient care as the patient is transferred from the hospital to his home or a convalescent home. Frequently the public health nurse is the case finder whose astute observations made the rehabilitation services possible to the patient. By visiting the patient in the hospital, the public health nurse is able to see what adjustments will have to be made in the home. She can help the family to select, to improvise, or to borrow the needed equipment from another agency. She determines what can be done to ease the family situation and can suggest ways in which adaptations in living arrangements can be made. After the patient returns to his home, the visiting or public health nurse makes sure that the patient does not "lose ground" and that he is able to maintain the independence that he gained in the hospital. The Activities of Daily Living Sheet is sent home with the patient so that the visiting nurse knows exactly what activities the patient can perform. The nurse continues to reinforce the teaching that has been done and helps the patient achieve attainable goals.

If the hospital has a home-care program, the home-care nurse acts as a liaison between the patient and the hospital to determine the need for continued nursing care.

The Rehabilitation Services Administration provides services whereby disabled persons or those disadvantaged by advanced age or other conditions obtain the help they need to engage in gainful employment. These services are provided by state agencies and include diagnostic, medical, surgical, psychiatric and hospital services, and assistance in securing prosthetic appliances. There is a counseling, training, placement and follow-up service available to help the patient to select and attain a vocational objective.

The following is a selected list of agencies and organizations, both governmental and private, that work with or for patients needing rehabilitation services.

AGENCIES

Federal:

The Rehabilitation Services Administration
    Dept. of Health, Education and Welfare
    Washington, D.C. 20201
President's Committee on Employment of the Physically
    Handicapped
    7131 Dept. of Labor Building
    Washington, D.C. 20210
V.A. Prosthetic Center
    Veterans Administration
    252 7th Avenue
    New York, New York 10001

Private:

American Federation of the Physically Handicapped, Inc.
    1376 National Press Building
    Washington, D.C. 20004
American Hearing Society
    817 Fourteenth Street, N.W.
    Washington, D.C. 20005
American Heart Association
    44 E. 23rd Street
    New York, New York 10010
American Legion, National Rehabilitation Committee
    1608 K Street, N.W.
    Washington, D.C. 20006
American Medical Association, Committee on Rehabilitation
    535 North Dearborn Street
    Chicago, Illinois 60610
American Occupational Therapy Association, Inc.
    250 West 57th Street
    New York, New York 10019
American Orthotic and Prosthetic Association
    919 Eighteenth Street
    Washington, D.C. 20006

American Physical Therapy Association
    1740 Broadway
    New York, New York 10019
American Psychiatric Association
    1700 Eighteenth Street, N.W.
    Washington, D.C. 20036
American Psychological Association
    1333 Sixteenth Street, N.W.
    Washington, D.C. 20036
American Rehabilitation Foundation, Inc.
    1800 Chicago Ave.
    Minneapolis, Minnesota 55404
Association of Rehabilitation Centers
    828 Davis Avenue
    Evanston, Illinois 60201
Comeback, Inc.
    16 West 46th Street
    New York, New York 10036
Goodwill Industries of America, Inc.
    744 N. Fourth Street
    Milwaukee, Wisconsin 53201
International Society for Rehabilitation of the Disabled
    219 East 44th Street
    New York, New York 10017
Institute for the Crippled and Disabled
    400 First Avenue
    New York, New York 10010
Institute of Rehabilitation Medicine
    400 East 34th Street
    New York, New York 10016
National Association for Mental Health
    10 Columbus Circle
    New York, New York 10019
National Association of Hearing and Speech Agencies
    919 Eighteenth Street, N.W.
    Washington, D.C. 20006
National Council on Rehabilitation
    1790 Broadway
    New York, New York 10019
National Foundation
    1790 Broadway
    New York, New York 10019
National Rehabilitation Association
    1522 K Street, N.W.
    Washington, D.C. 20005
National Research Council
    Committee on Prosthetics Education and Information
    210 Constitution Ave., N.W.
    Washington, D.C. 20418
National Society for Crippled Children and Adults, Inc.
    2023 West Ogden Avenue
    Chicago, Illinois 60612

BIBLIOGRAPHY

Books:

Colorado State Department of Health: Elementary Rehabilitation Nursing Care. Washington, D.C.: U.S. Dept. of H.E.W., P.H. Service Pub. #1436, 1966.
Covalt, N. K.: Bed Exercises for Convalescent Patients. Springfield, Charles C Thomas, 1968.

Fait, H. J.: Special Physical Education: Adaptive, Corrective, Developmental. Philadelphia, W. B. Saunders, 1966.

Garrett, J. F., and Levine, E. S.: Psychological Practices with the Physically Disabled. New York, Columbia University Press, 1962.

Hirschberg, G., et al.: Rehabilitation. Philadelphia, J. B. Lippincott, 1964.

Krusen, F. H. (ed.): Handbook of Physical Medicine and Rehabilitation. Philadelphia, W. B. Saunders, 1965.

Lawton, E.: Activities of Daily Living for Physical Rehabilitation. New York, McGraw-Hill, 1963.

National League for Nursing: Rehabilitative Aspects of Nursing; A Programmed Instruction Series. New York, 1966.

New York University-Bellevue Medical Center: Self-Help Devices for Rehabilitation. Dubuque, Iowa, William C. Brown, 1965.

Rusk, H. A.: Rehabilitation Medicine. St. Louis, C. V. Mosby, 1964.

Sorenson, L., et al.: Ambulation: A Manual for Nurses. Minneapolis, American Rehabilitation Foundation, Inc., 1966.

Viscardi, H.: A Letter to Jimmy. New York, Paul S. Erikssan, Inc., 1962.

Wright, B. A.: Physical Disability—A Psychological Approach. New York, Harper and Brothers, 1960.

Articles

Avedon, E. M.: The function of recreation service in the rehabilitation process. Rehab. Lit., 27:226-229, August, 1966.

Beavers, S. V.: Music therapy. Amer. J. Nurs., 69:88-92, Jan., 1969.

Burmeister, C. R.: Accent ability not disability. Amer. Assoc. Ind. Nurs. J., 15:16-20, Oct., 1967.

Christopherson, V. A.: Role modifications of the disabled male. Amer. J. Nurs., 68:290-293, Feb., 1968.

Dahlin, B.: Rehabilitation and the assessment of patient need. Nurs. Clin. N. Amer., 1:375-386, Sept., 1966.

Dasco, M. M.: Rehabilitation after major surgery and serious trauma. In Powers, J. H.: Surgery of the Aged and Debilitated Patient. pp. 552-579. Philadelphia, Saunders, 1968.

Elliott, J. E.: The nurse and rehabilitation. J. Rehab., 33:2, May-June, 1967.

Hallenbeck, P. N.: Special clothing for the handicapped. Rehab. Lit., 27:34-40, Feb., 1966.

Heinly, J. L.: The patient's need for recreation. In Bergersen: Current Concepts in Clinical Nursing. pp. 137-153. St. Louis, C. V. Mosby, 1967.

Hentgen, J. H.: Dressing activities for disabled persons. Nurs. Clin. N. Amer., 1:483-491, Sept., 1966.

Leavitt, L. A.: Decubitus ulcers. Hosp. Med., 2:76-85, Dec., 1966.

McDonald, G. B.: Surgery and rehabilitation in the management of decubitus ulcer. J. Rehab., 33:29-32, Sept.-Oct., 1967.

Meyer, G. G., et al.: Milieu therapy and the occupational therapist. Rehab. Lit., 27:106-109, April, 1966.

Neilson, N. J.: The clinical specialist in a rehabilitation center. Nurs. Clin. N. Amer., 1:365-373, Sept., 1966.

Olsen, E. V. (ed.): The hazards of immobility. Amer. J. Nurs., 67:779-797, April, 1967.

Park, W. E.: Patient transfer form. Amer. J. Nurs., 67:1665-1668, Aug., 1967.

Pfaudler, M.: Flotation, displacement, and decubitus ulcers. Amer. J. Nurs., 68:2351-2355, Nov., 1968.

Plaisted, L. M.: The clinical specialist in rehabilitation nursing, Amer. J. Nurs., 69:562-564, Mar., 1969.

Rodgiquez, A., and Wing, H.: Newer concepts of physical medicine and rehabilitation, Ind. Med. Surg., 36:802-805, Dec., 1967.

Rothberg, J. S. (ed.): Chronic disease and rehabilitation. Nurs. Clin. N. Amer., 1:355-519, Sept., 1966.

Sain, U.: The rehabilitation nurse. Rehab. Record, 8:39-40, May-June, 1967.

Saxon, J.: Techniques for bowel and bladder training. Amer. J. Nurs., 62:69-71, Sept., 1962.

Schwab, L. O.: The home economist in rehabilitation. Rehab. Lit., 29:130-135, May, 1968.

Spain, R. W.: Rehabilitation nursing for the long-term patient. Rehab. Lit., 25:130-138, May, 1964.

Spain, R. W.: Rehabilitative nursing. Nurs. Clin. N. Amer., 1:355-363, Sept., 1966.

Talbot, H. S.: A concept of rehabilitation. Rehab. Lit., 22:358-364, Dec., 1966.

Thornhill, H. L., and Williams, M.: Experience with the water mattress in a large city hospital. Amer. J. Hosp., 68:2356-2358, Nov., 1968.

Tiffney, H.: Guidelines for an inservice education program for general duty nurses in a rehabilitation unit. National League for Nursing, 1966.

Wahlstrom, E. D., and Weston, J. L.: Initiating referrals. Amer. J. Nurs., 67:332-335, Feb., 1967.

West, W. L.: Occupational therapy philosophy and perspective. Amer. J. Nurs., 68:1708-1711, Aug., 1968.

PATIENT EDUCATION

American Rehabilitation Foundation
1800 Chicago Avenue
Minneapolis, Minnesota 55404

Rehabilitative Nursing Techniques—1: Bed Positioning and Transfer Procedures for the Hemiplegic.

Rehabilitative Nursing Techniques—2: Selected Equipment Useful in the Hospital, Home, or Nursing Home.

Rehabilitative Nursing Techniques—4: Self-care and Homemaking for the Hemiplegic.

Toohey, P., and Larson, C. W.: Key to Joint Mobility. Booklet No. 703.

Sorenson, L., and Ulrich, P. G.: Ambulation: A Manual for Nurses. Booklet No. 707.

Nursing Education Department: Nursing Care of the Skin. Booklet No. 711.

Fahland, B.: More Than Choosing a Chair with Wheels. Booklet No. 713.

Bergstrom, D. A.: Care of Patients with Bowel and Bladder Problems: A Nursing Guide. Booklet No. 714.

Public Affairs Pamphlets
381 Park Avenue South
New York, New York 10016

Levitch, J. A.: Occupational Therapy—A New Life for the Disabled. Pamphlet No. 420.

CHAPTER **11**

The Patient with Cancer

- *The Nurse and the Cancer Patient*
- *Classification of Cysts and Tumors*
- *Incidence of Various Malignancies*
- *Treatment of Neoplasms*
- *Psychological Aspects of Nursing the Cancer Patient*
- *Terminal Nursing Care*
- *The Follow-Through*

THE NURSE AND THE CANCER PATIENT

The nurse is a very important member of any team fighting cancer. In the hospital her skill is a necessary adjunct to that of the surgeon, the radiologist and the internist. Within the community as a public health nurse, she regularly calls on the patient with cancer who is being treated at home. In industry, she not only must contend with illness of employees themselves but often worries about the health of their families as well. Directly or indirectly, her knowledge and influence supplement the doctor's plan of action for the diagnosis, the treatment, the rehabilitation or the terminal care of those who are cancer victims. (American Cancer Society, Inc.)

The hope of cure in malignant disease depends on treatment of the malignancy before it is spread beyond the possibility of removal. This means that treatment should be given as soon as possible after the malignancy is recognized, but it must also be understood that in some patients even by that time there may have been a spread of tumor, that would make it impossible to cure by our present methods of therapy. Rapid progress is being made in the education of the public as to the dangerous consequences of untreated tumors. The intelligent nurse is one of the most effective agents in the dissemination of such information. Not infrequently her patients or their friends will question her concerning "a lump that has formed" or a rapid loss of weight with increasing "indigestion."

In order to answer such questions she should remember that these symptoms and signs suggest malignant disease: *a swelling, usually painless, growing progressively larger; the abnormal appearance of blood from the stomach, the bowel or the pelvic organs; loss of weight; slowly increasing "indigestion"; or an ulcer that refuses to heal.* If these symptoms occur in a person past middle age, they are especially suggestive, because cancer occurs most frequently at that time of life.

Knowing that only early treatment can cure, the nurse should urge an immediate examination by a physician. The diagnosis is confirmed by the use of biopsy, cytologic test, endoscopy, roentgenogram, or blood tests.

The responsibility of the nurse begins in the early stages of cancer detection and progresses through the following roles: (1) supporting the patient undergoing diagnostic procedures; (2) recognizing the psychological and spiritual needs of the patient; (3) meeting the fluid and nutritional needs of the patient; (4) assisting in carrying out treatments of the malignancy itself; (5) assisting in the rehabilitation and convalescence of the patient; (6) assisting in the follow-up of all treated patients; (7) aiding in the collection of data

Benign	Malignant
Adult type of cell	Young type of cell
Closely resembles parent tissue	Tends to be anaplastic—less differentiated than the normal cells from which they are derived.
Slow growth	Rapid growth (usually)
Often encapsulated	Never encapsulated
Never grows into surrounding tissues	Invade surrounding tissues widely
Always remains localized at original site	Form secondary growths by metastasis through both the lymph and the blood stream
Does not tend to recur when removed	Tend to recur when removed
Harms the host only by pressure of growth on surrounding structures	Cause loss of weight and strength, anemia, cachexia and, eventually, death

for research; and (8) assisting in planning for the care of individuals whose disease has not been terminated.

In caring for patients with a malignant tumor, the nurse finds that the team of which she is a member never is limited to the surgeon, the patient and the nurse, but includes often the medical social worker, the nutritionist, the occupational and physical therapists, the psychiatrist and the clergyman. Over and above this, one cannot overlook the fact that the patient's family plays a significant role.

CLASSIFICATION OF CYSTS AND TUMORS

Cysts

A *cyst* is an abnormal collection of fluid within a definite sac or wall. Cysts may form in several different ways. When the outlet to a gland becomes blocked and the gland continues to secrete, a *retention cyst* is formed. The common sebaceous cyst or wen is an example. Remnants of fetal organs may secrete a fluid, often forming a cyst of considerable size especially when springing from the pelvic organs of the female. This is called an *epidermoid cyst*. An extravasation of blood in the tissues may become surrounded by a definite wall and form an *extravasation cyst*.

Cysts may be formed by parasites, especially the *Taenia echinococcus (Echinococcus granulosus)* or dog tapeworm. These cysts, spoken of as *hydatid cysts*, often are of considerable size and usually are found in the liver.

Treatment. Cysts of several types should be removed when possible because occasionally they change into malignant growths. They often may become infected; then incision and drainage are necessary.

Benign or Nonmalignant Tumors

Some tumors are surrounded by a definite capsule, remain localized in the tissue from which they spring, and disturb their host only by pressure on the surrounding structures and by robbing the normal tissues of their blood supply. These tumors usually grow rather slowly, and once removed they do not tend to recur. Such tumors are spoken of as *benign* or *non-malignant*.

Malignant Tumors

Other neoplasms are not surrounded by a capsule, but grow by invasion into the tissues surrounding them. They invade the blood vessels or the lymphatics and extend rapidly along these open channels. Often the tumor cells are broken off and carried by the blood and the lymph to other parts of the body, where they set up a secondary growth. Secondary growths are looked for at the nearest lymph filter, the lymph nodes. Here cells are caught and begin to form an independent tumor like the parent or primary growth. Thus, in every patient with cancer of the breast, the axilla is examined carefully for enlarged lymph nodes, because it is known that the lymph flow from the breast is through the axillary lymph nodes. Tumor cells invading the blood vessels are carried to organs where the venous blood passes through a capillary bed; thus we see secondary tumor appearing in the lung from a cancer of the breast or in the liver when the cells are carried by the portal venous system from a tumor in the abdomen. This property of these tumors is called *metastasis*, and the new or secondary growth is called a *metastatic growth*. The cells of these tumors grow rapidly and under the microscope resemble the rapidly growing cells found in the embryo. They invade the surrounding tissues in such a manner that it is nearly impossible to remove all the tumor cells and, therefore, they tend to recur after the main body of the tumor has been removed.

The rapid growth of the tumor and its secondary growths sap the vitality of its host, with the result that there is a rapid loss of weight and strength. These

Fig. 11-1. Forecast of cancer deaths. Note that the solid line through 1968 tells the actual number of deaths from cancer, while the dotted line is a statistician's prediction for the years to come—if present rates continue. It is hoped that some more effective means will be found to prevent deaths from cancer. (American Cancer Society)

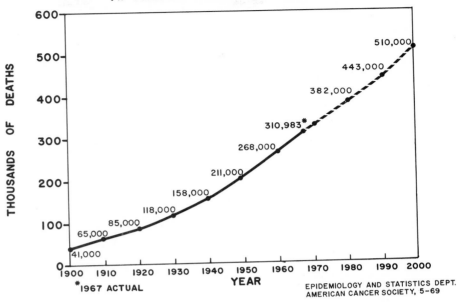

FORECAST OF CANCER DEATHS

(IF PRESENT TRENDS CONTINUE)

510,000
443,000
382,000
310,983*
268,000
211,000
158,000
118,000
85,000
65,000
41,000

THOUSANDS OF DEATHS

YEAR

*1967 ACTUAL

EPIDEMIOLOGY AND STATISTICS DEPT.
AMERICAN CANCER SOCIETY, 5-69

tumors bleed easily, producing a loss of the red cells in the blood—an anemia. The patient finally becomes thin, pale and weak, a shadow of his former self. This condition is spoken of as *cachexia*. The course of the disease frequently ends in death. These tumors are referred to as *malignant*.

At times a tumor that was at first benign may take on malignant characteristics. For this reason it is well to remove all tumors as soon as they are discovered in most instances.

Subdivisions on Basis of Tissue

Neoplasms are subdivided further according to the kind of tissue of which they are formed. In embryonic life there are 3 divisions of tissue from which all others are formed. These tissues are called (1) endoderm, (2) mesoderm and (3) ectoderm.

Endoderm is the tissue from which the lining membranes (mucosa) of the respiratory tract, the gastrointestinal tract and the genitourinary tract are formed.

Mesoderm is the tissue from which muscles, bones, fascia and connective tissue are formed.

Ectoderm is the tissue from which come the skin cells and the cells composing its hair follicles, sweat glands and the entire nervous system.

Complex Tissues. Some tumors, thought to arise from embryologic maldevelopment, contain more than one of the embryonal tissues. Those which contain two of the tissues, called *teratomas* or *dermoids,* are not infrequently seen in operations on the ovary or

Rank	Cause of Death	Number of Deaths	Death Rate Per 100,000 Population	Percent of Total Deaths
	ALL CAUSES	1,863,149	951.3	100.0
1.	Diseases of Heart	726,546	371.2	38.9
2.	Cancer	303,736	155.1	16.3
3.	Stroke (Vascular Lesions) . . .	204,841	104.6	11.0
4.	Accidents	113,563	58.0	6.1
	Motor-Vehicles Accidents .	53,041	27.1	2.8
	All Other Accidents	60,522	30.9	3.2
5.	Influenza and Pneumonia . . .	63,615	32.5	3.4
6.	Certain Diseases of Early Infancy	51,644	26.4	2.8
7.	Arteriosclerosis	38,907	19.9	2.1
8.	Diabetes Mellitus	34,597	17.7	1.9
9.	Cirrhosis of Liver	26,692	13.6	1.4
10.	Suicide	21,281	10.9	1.1
11.	Emphysema without mention of Bronchitis	20,252	10.5	1.1
12.	Congenital Malformations . . .	18,158	9.3	1.0
13.	Nephritis	11,540	5.9	0.6
14.	Homicide	11,606	5.9	0.6
15.	Hypertension without mention of Heart	11,380	5.8	0.6
	Other and Ill-Defined	204,791	104.6	11.0

Source: Vital Statistics of the United States, 1966

Fig. 11-2. Relation of cancer to leading causes of death (United States, 1966). (Courtesy of American Cancer Society)

TABLE 11-1. Classification of tumor cells

Type of Cell	Benign	Malignant
Epithelium:	Papilloma	Cancer—Carcinoma
Skin Epithelium	Wart (Verrucae)	
Gland Epithelium	Polyp	Basal Cell Carcinoma
	Adenoma	Adenocarcinoma
Endothelial Tissue:		Endothelioma
Blood Vessels		Hemangiosarcoma
Lymph Vessels	Hemangioma	Lymphangiosarcoma
Lymphoid Tissue	Lymphangioma	Lymphosarcoma
		Malignant
		Lymphosarcoma
Connective Tissue:	Fibroma	Fibrosarcoma
Fibrous Tissue	Fibroma	Fibrosarcoma
Adipose Tissue	Lipoma	Liposarcoma
Cartilage	Chondroma	Chondrosarcoma
Bone	Osteoma	Osteosarcoma
Muscle Tissue:	Myoma	Myosarcoma
Smooth Muscle	Leiomyoma	Leiomyosarcoma
Striated Muscle	Rhabdomyoma	Rhabdomyosarcoma
Nerve Tissue:		
Nerve Fibers	Neuroma	Neurogenic Sarcoma
Ganglion Cells	Ganglioneuroma	Neuroblastoma
Glial Cells	Glioma	Glioblastoma
Meninges	Meningioma	
Pigmented Neoplasms	Nevus-mole	Malignant Melanoma

the testicle. They may contain bone, teeth, muscle—all of which arise from the mesoderm—and hair, skin and subcutaneous glands, all of which develop from the ectoderm.

New growths often are composed of more than one tissue and are named accordingly—fibroadenoma, fibrolipoma, osteosarcoma and so forth.

INCIDENCE OF VARIOUS MALIGNANCIES

The importance of malignant growth to the nursing and the medical professions can be understood if some of the facts concerning its incidence are reviewed. It is estimated that in the United States malignancy annually exacts a toll of at least 325,000 lives, ranking second as the principal cause of death, being exceeded only by heart disease. More than 1 out of 6 deaths that occur in adults is caused by malignancy. It is estimated that more than 103,000 cancer patients might have been saved in 1969, for example, had they recognized early symptoms and sought prompt treatment. Cancer affects men and women of all ages and of all races. No organ of the body is exempt.

TREATMENT OF NEOPLASMS

It has been learned that malignant neoplasms usually lead to certain death if untreated, and that benign tumors may become malignant without warning. Therefore, it must be realized that the patient who is the host to tumors of any kind is the potential victim of a fatal disease. At present, 3 methods have proved their value in the treatment of cancer: surgery, radiation and chemotherapy.

Surgery of Cancer

Actually, surgery plays a part in the management of every growth that is suspected of being a cancer. When a piece of tissue is taken from a suspicious growth for examination under the microscope (*biopsy*), this procedure is a surgical one. Proof of malignancy can be definitely established by such a study. When the diagnosis is established, the surgeon removes the original growth, and in addition he removes the lymphatics that drain the area in which the growth is situated. Therefore, in operations for carcinoma of the breast, the overlying skin and the underlying muscles are removed with the breast, and the lymphatic chan-

Site	Estimated new cases 1969	Estimated deaths 1969	Warning signal. When lasting longer than two weeks, see your doctor	Safeguards	Comment
Breast	67,000	29,000	Lump or thickening in the breast.	Annual checkup. Monthly breast self-examination.	The leading cause of cancer death in women.
Colon and Rectum	73,000	46,000	Change in bowel habits; bleeding.	Annual checkup, including proctoscopy.	Considered a highly curable disease when digital and proctoscopic examinations are included in routine checkups.
Lung	65,000	59,000	Persistent cough, or lingering respiratory ailment.	Prevention: heed facts about smoking, annual checkup. Chest x-ray.	The leading cause of cancer death among men, this form of cancer is largely preventable.
Oral (including pharynx)	15,000	7,000	Sore that does not heal. Difficulty in swallowing.	Annual checkup.	Many more lives should be saved because the mouth is easily accessible to visual examination by physicians and dentists.
Skin	110,000	5,000	Sore that does not heal, or a change in wart or mole.	Annual checkup. Chest x-ray. exposure to sun.	Skin cancer is readily detected by observation, and diagnosed by simple biopsy.
Uterus	44,000	13,000	Unusual bleeding or discharge.	Annual checkup including pelvic examination and papanicolaou smear.	Uterine cancer mortality has declined 50% during the last 25 years. With wider application of the "Pap" smear, many thousand more lives can be saved.
Kidney and bladder	31,000	15,000	Urinary difficulty. Bleeding—in which case consult your doctor at once.	Annual checkup with urinalysis.	Protective measures for workers in high-risk industries are helping to eliminate one of the important causes of these cancers.
Larynx	6,000	3,000	Hoarseness—difficulty in swallowing.	Annual checkup, including mirror laryngoscopy.	Readily curable if caught early.
Prostate	35,000	17,000	Urinary difficulty.	Annual checkup, including palpation.	Occurs mainly in men over 60, the disease can be detected by palpation and urinalysis at annual checkup.
Stomach	18,000	16,000	Indigestion.	Annual checkup.	A 40% decline in mortality in 20 years, for reasons yet unknown.
Leukemia	19,000	15,000			Leukemia is a cancer of blood-forming tissues and is characterized by the abnormal production of immature white blood cells. Acute leukemia strikes mainly children and is treated by drugs which have extended life from a few months to as much as three years. Chronic leukemia strikes usually after age 25 and progresses less rapidly. Cancer experts believe that if drugs or vaccines are found which can cure or prevent any cancers they will be successful first for leukemia and the lymphomas.
Lymphomas	22,000	17,000			These diseases arise in the lymph system and include Hodgkin's and lymphosarcoma. Some patients with lymphatic cancers can lead normal lives for many years.

FIG. 11-3. Reference chart: leading cancer sites, 1969. (American Cancer Society)

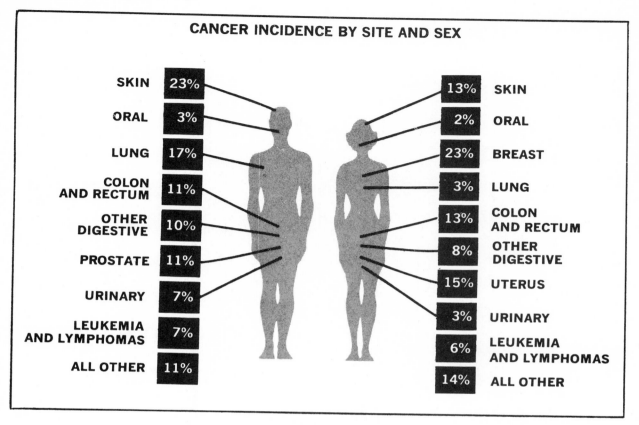

FIG. 11-4. (Courtesy of American Cancer Society)

nels of the axilla are dissected out carefully, along with any metastatic nodes that can be discovered.

Another type of cancer surgery may be called *preventive* or *prophylactic surgery,* which is of utmost importance in the control of cancer. This involves the removal of those lesions which, as known from past experience and study, are apt to develop into cancer if they are left in the body. An example would be the removal of small tumors (polyps) that often grow in the colon. These may be detected by roentgenograms or sigmoidoscopy.

Surgical removal of the entire cancer is regarded as the best method of cancer treatment. This often requires rather extensive operations and is only curative if the operation can be performed before the tumor has spread to areas that cannot be removed.

There is another field in which surgery aids in the control of cancer. This involves the removal of, or operations on, the different glands of the body which produce hormones that are known to affect the natural course of development of certain cancers. An example of this type of surgery is the removal of the ovaries in women who have had cancer of the breast and have not yet reached the menopause. The physician will do this if he thinks that by so doing he can increase his patient's chance of cure or reduce the rate of growth of the tumor.

Palliation of cancer is an attempt to relieve the complications of cancer; such complications may be ulcerations, obstruction of the gastrointestinal tract, pain produced by extension of the tumor to surrounding nerves, and bleeding and nutritional loss from the extensive tumor growth. Therefore, palliative surgery implies many sorts of operative procedures, depending on the complications present. Such operations are performed by the surgeon with the knowledge that he cannot produce a cure but with the hope that he can give the patient improved health and comfort for a longer period of time than would otherwise be the case. Thus, in bleeding or obstructing tumors of the stomach or the bowel, usually the tumor is resected in spite of the fact that the patient may have metastatic extension to the liver and with the knowledge that the operation is only a palliative rather than a curative one.

In addition to these attempts to remove the complications of tumors, sometimes other measures are employed, especially in an effort to relieve pain. These include radiation therapy with x-rays or radium and operations on nerves, the spinal cord or the brain to divide the pathways that carry pain sensation; the use of hormones in the case of tumors that are affected by hormone stimulation, such as those in the breast or the testes, and the removal of hormone-producing glands such as the pituitary, the adrenal, the ovary and the testis. None of these procedures can produce a cure for the cancer, but they may relieve pain and in some patients may produce a regression of the tumor for a time.

Chemotherapy of Cancer

The hope for a cancer cure by means of chemical agents (chemotherapy) depends on an understanding of the biochemical and metabolic differences between normal and neoplastic cells that enable tumor cells to be destroyed while healthy tissue remains intact. *In general it can be said that as yet no drugs have been discovered to cure malignant tumors;* however, cancer chemotherapy may (or may not) offer some help to patients for whom surgery and irradiation are no longer beneficial. Some of the drugs produce a regression of the tumor or its metastases, and the use of chemotherapeutic agents at the time of surgery may reduce or slow up the appearance of secondary growths. In some patients, pain and other symptoms are relieved for a time.

Chemotherapeutic agents are especially useful in the treatment of lymphomas and leukemias, diffuse tumors usually not amenable to surgical therapy. In such patients, the use of chemotherapeutic agents may prolong life for many years, with a remission but never a cure. In solid tumors the mass may become smaller, and surface ulcerations may heal for a time. Cure is not to be expected.

The rationale for administering these drugs is that they are capable of destroying young, rapidly multiplying cells; the cells comprising malignant tumors possess these characteristics. It is believed that these drugs interfere with the manufacturing of nucleic acids that are necessary for the building of genetic structures in cells. As a result, cellular growth and reproduction are inhibited.

There also are, however, normal cells in the body that have short life spans and compensate for this by rapid cell proliferation. The majority of these normal, rapidly reproducing cells are located in the bone marrow, the lining of the gastrointestinal tract, and the hair follicles.

Unfortunately, these drugs cannot differentiate between rapidly dividing cells that are normal and those that are abnormal. As a result of their effects on normal susceptible cells, toxic signs and symptoms may occur that constitute a major challenge to the nurse.

Specific Agents Used in Cancer Chemotherapy

1. **Polyfunctional alkylating agents** (cytotoxic or poisonous), of which the nitrogen mustards and the polysaccharides are examples. These poisons destroy both normal and tumor cells. It is believed that cells in mitosis (rapidly growing tumor cells) are more sensitive to toxicity than normal adult cells, and that tumors of well-differentiated cells are less sensitive to toxicity than those of less well-differentiated cells in some tumors. By acting with desoxyribonucleic acid in the nucleus, cell growth and division are hindered. The chief disadvantage of most of these drugs is their destructive effect on bone marrow, one of the body's chief sources of new blood cells. Other manifestations are nausea and vomiting, stomatitis and diarrhea.

2. **The antimetabolites,** folic acid and purine antagonists. These are synthetic substances similar to those that nourish the normal cell during its growth and development. However, they differ enough in their chemical composition so that, although the drugs are taken into the cell substance, they cannot be used by the cell. Thus, they deceive the cell, and act as a monkey wrench in the cellular machinery. The signs and symptoms indicating evidence of toxicity are similar to those of the alkylating agents.

3. **Steroid Compounds, ACTH, and Castration.** Alteration of the endocrine environment is a major approach in the chemotherapy of certain types of neoplastic disease: namely, tumors arising in organs usually under hormonal influence, such as the prostate (castration) and the breast (androgen and estrogen therapy). The patient receiving this form of therapy will need to be observed for toxicity signs such as fluid retention, increased libido and hirsutism, as well as nausea and vomiting. Oophorectomy, adrenalectomy and pituitarectomy represent similar forms of therapy.

4. **Miscellaneous Drugs.** Antibiotic drugs such as actinomycin D, mitomycin C and streptonigrin show therapeutic promise. Plant alkaloids, vinblastine (Velban) and vincristine (Oncovin) are derived from the flowering herb, periwinkle. Toxic manifestations of vinblastine (used in Hodgkin's disease) are nausea, vomiting, leukopenia and epilation. Vincristine given to children with acute leukemia may produce side effects of leukopenia and neuromuscular disturbances.

Note: None of these agents cures malignancy. They are efforts to make the physiology of the host less favorable for the growth of cancer.

Methods of Administration

The cancer chemotherapeutic drugs may be given orally, intravenously or intramuscularly into the systemic circulation or intra-arterially, depending on the drug and the carcinoma. In addition, efforts may be made to introduce the drug in high concentration into the tumor area by injection into its vascular supply. These efforts require complicated techniques that usually are carried out in specialized clinics.

Perfusion and Intra-arterial Infusion. Perfusion technique allows the administration of large doses of extremely toxic drugs to an isolated extremity, organ, or region of the body. Such a dose could not be tolerated by the entire body.

The usual vessels perfused for a lesion in the lower extremity are iliac, femoral and popliteal arteries and veins. The axillary artery and vein are injected in upper extremity perfusion. The abdominal aorta and the vena cava are used in pelvic perfusion.

On admission and preoperatively the patient is weighed, because the amounts of chemotherapeutic drug and heparin given are calculated on the basis of kilograms of body weight. Blood, urine, and x-ray studies also are done. Preparation of the patient for surgery includes the answering of his many questions, since perfusion is a relatively new procedure.

In the operating room by means of a pump-oxygenator, the patient's blood is circulated in a closed system for the involved part of the body. The chemotherapeutic drug is injected in concentrated doses. The duration of the perfusion depends on the drug, and the extent and the location of the growth. During the procedure, efforts are made by tourniquets and/or ligatures to prevent seepage of the drug into the systemic circulation. Obviously, it is easier to prevent leakage into the systemic circulation when an extremity is involved, but much more difficult when the torso is perfused.

With percutaneous introduction of the catheter into a major artery (intra-arterial infusion), it is necessary to use fluoroscopic guidance. This method has the chief advantage of not requiring major surgery and it can be repeated at intervals. The routes commonly used are brachial, axillary, carotid and femoral; this is determined by the location of the carcinoma.

Following the administration of the chemotherapeutic agent, blood tests are done frequently to check on bone marrow depression. Tissue in the local area is observed frequently for any reaction such as erythema, mild edema, blistering and petechiae. Any noticeable change is charted with full description. Pain usually is not a problem but if it is present, it may indicate severe injury to normal tissue.

The patient who has had an aortic perfusion should be observed for signs of malaise, nausea, vomiting, rising temperature, blood pressure and pulse (note signs indicative of a hypotensive reaction). Fluids are given intravenously for the first 48 hours; all the patient's total intake and output are recorded accurately. The patient is turned frequently, because pressure areas develop easily. These patients require emotional support; for those having surgery, the principles of effective postoperative care are followed.

Nursing Care of Patients Receiving Chemotherapeutic Agents for Neoplastic Disease*

The nurse should know the signs of toxicity from chemotherapeutic agents as well as the patient's reactions to them. She needs to understand that these signs may occur in different intensities in different patients and that they vary with different drugs. The multiplicity of toxic reactions that can occur can cause interference with the patient's basic needs for food, oxygen, fluid, and body protection as well as with his psychosocial needs, especially those relating to the acceptance of a change in self-image and body concept. The ingenuity of the nurse will sometimes be taxed in coping with the variety and complexity of the nursing problems that she encounters in striving to meet the needs of the patient.

Because certain cells are more vulnerable to chemotherapeutic agents than others, a common triad of symptoms related to the gastrointestinal tract occurs: stomatitis, nausea and vomiting, and diarrhea. As a result, the patient's nutritional status may be jeopardized, his fluid and electrolyte balance may be affected, and he may experience various feelings of discomfort.

The bone marrow depression caused by these drugs presents another triad of clinical manifestations. All cells produced by bone marrow, i.e., leukocytes, erythrocytes, and platelets, are affected, reducing the number available in the body to cope with metabolic and stress needs. The patient may develop anemia, bleeding tendencies, and decreased resistance to infection.

The patient receiving these drugs may experience signs and symptoms that are pronounced and enduring; common-place nursing care does not always suffice. The nurse often finds herself really challenged. For example, if the patient does develop inflammation of the oral mucosa, how does the nurse modify the manner in which oral hygiene is given so that the oral cavity does not become a breeding place for bacteria and so that the inflamed mucosa is not injured to a greater degree? What materials and agents does she use in giving mouth care? Frequent cleaning of the mouth with soft nonabrasive materials, followed by a soothing coating of the mucosa, would be pleasant to the patient and reduce the irritation.

The patient's nutritional state may be endangered because of nausea and vomiting so that the nurse must be instrumental in encouraging the patient to eat. However, in view of stomatitis, the nurse should regu-

* Joan A. Safko, R.N., M.S., Assistant Director, School of Nursing, Hospital of the University of Pennsylvania, Philadelphia.

Specific agents used in cancer chemotherapy

Agents	Principal route of administration	Usual dose	Acute toxic signs	Major toxic manifestations
Steroid Compounds				
Androgen				
Testosterone propionate	I.M.	50-100 mg. 3 x weekly	None	Fluid retention, masculinization.
Fluoxymesterone (Halotestin®)	Oral	10-20 mg./day		
Estrogen				
Diethylstilbestrol	Oral	1-5 mg. 3/day	Occasional N. & V.*	Fluid retention, feminization, uterine bleeding.
Ethinyl estradiol (Estinyl®)	Oral	0.1-1.0 mg. 3/day		
Progestin				
Hydroxyprogesterone caproate (Delalutin®)	I.M.	1 gm. 2 x weekly	None	
6-Methylhydroxyprogesterone (Provera®)	Oral I.M.	100-200 mg./day 200-600 mg. 2 x weekly		
Adrenal Cortical Compounds				
Hydrocortisone acetate Prednisone (Meticorten®)	Oral Oral	50-200 mg./day 20-100 mg./day	None	Fluid retention, hypertension, diabetes, increased susceptibility to infection.
Radioactive Isotopes				
Iodine (^{131}I)	Oral, I.V.	100-200 mc.	None	Myxedema, bone marrow depression, renal damage.
Phosphorus (^{32}P as sodium phosphate) (^{32}P as chromic phosphate)	Oral, I.V. Intracavitary	3-7 mc. 5-10 mc.	None None	Bone marrow depression.
Gold (^{198}Au)	Intracavitary	75-150 mc.	None	
Polyfunctional Alkylating Agents				
Methylbis (β-Chloroethyl) Amine HCl (HN2, Mustargen®)	I.V.	0.4 mg./kg. Single or Divided Doses	N. & V.	Therapeutic doses moderately depress peripheral blood cell count; excessive doses cause severe bone marrow depression with leukopenia, thrombocytopenia and bleeding. Maximum toxicity may occur two or three weeks after last dose. Dosage, therefore, must be carefully controlled. Alopecia and hemorrhagic cystitis occur occasionally with cyclophosphamide.
Chlorambucil (Leukeran®)	Oral	0.1-0.2 mg./kg./day 6-12 mg./day	None	
Melphalan (Alkeran®)	Oral	0.1 mg./kg./day x 7 2-4 mg./day maintenance	None	
Cyclophosphamide (Endoxan, Cytoxan®)	I.V. Oral	3.5-5.0 mg./kg./day x 10 (40-60 mg./kg. Single Dose) 50-300 mg./day	N. & V.	
Triethylenethiophosphoramide (TSPA, Thio-TEPA®)	I.V.	0.2 mg./kg. x 5 2-6 mg./day	None	
Busulfan (Myleran®)	Oral	2 mg./day maintenance	None	
Antimetabolites				
Methotrexate® (Methotrexate, Amethopterin)	Oral	2.5-5.0 mg./day	None	Oral and digestive tract ulcerations; bone marrow depression with leukopenia, thrombocytopenia, and bleeding.
6-Mercaptopurine (6-MP, Purinethol®)	Oral	2.5 mg./kg./day	None	Therapeutic doses usually well tolerated; excessive doses cause bone marrow depression.
6-Thioguanine (6-TG, Thioguanine®)	Oral	2.0 mg./kg./day		
5-Fluorouracil (5-FU, Fluorouracil®)	I.V.	15 mg./kg./day x 3 Smaller dose, 1-2 x weekly for maintenance	None	Stomatitis, nausea, GI injury, bone marrow depression.
Arabinosylcytosine (Ara-C, Cytarabine®)	I.V.	1.0-3.0 mg./kg./day x 10-20	N. & V.	Bone marrow depression, megaloblastosis, leukopenia, thrombocytopenia.
Miscellaneous Drugs				
Dactinomycin (Cosmegen®)	I.V.	0.01 mg./kg./day x 5 or 0.04 mg./kg. weekly	N. & V.	Stomatitis, GI disturbances, alopecia, bone marrow depression.
Vinblastine (Velban®)	I.V.	0.1-0.2 mg./kg. weekly	N. & V.	Alopecia, areflexia, bone marrow depression.
Vincristine (Oncovin®)	I.V.	0.015-0.05 mg./kg. weekly	None	Areflexia, muscular weakness, peripheral neuritis, paralytic ileus, mild bone marrow depression.
Procarbazine (Natulan,® N-Methylhydrazine)	Oral	50-300 mg./day	N. & V.	Bone marrow depression, leukopenia and thrombocytopenia, mental depression.
o,p'-DDD	Oral	2-10 gm./day	N. & V.	Skin eruption, diarrhea, mental depression, muscle tremors.
Quinacrine (Atabrine®)	Intrapleural	100-200 mg./day x 5	Local pain, fever	

* Nausea and Vomiting

Fig. 11-5. (From Karnofsky, D. A.: Cancer chemotherapeutic agents. CA—A Cancer Journal for Clinicians 18:72-79, 232-234, 1968)

Neoplastic diseases responding to chemotherapy

Diagnoses	Polyfunctional alkylating agents	Antimetabolites	Radioactive isotopes	Steroid hormones	Miscellaneous drugs	Results
Leukemia Acute, Children usually Lymphoblastic	Cyclophosphamide	6-MP, 6-TG Methotrexate Ara-C		Adrenal Cortical Hormones	Vincristine	80% bone marrow remissions; 60% live beyond one year.
Acute, Adults usually Myeloblastic		6-MP, 6-TG Methotrexate Ara-C		Adrenal Cortical Hormones	Vincristine	15-25% improved for several months or longer.
Chronic Myelocytic	Busulfan	6-MP, 6-TG	^{32}P			Patients maintained in good condition during major portion of disease; life occasionally prolonged.
Chronic Lymphocytic	Chlorambucil Thio-TEPA		^{32}P	Adrenal Cortical Hormones		Patients maintained in good condition during major portion of disease; life occasionally prolonged.
Hodgkin's Disease	Chlorambucil HN2 Thio-TEPA			Adrenal Cortical Hormones	Vinblastine Vincristine Procarbazine	Frequent favorable response, but no definite prolongation of life.
Lymphosarcoma	Chlorambucil Cyclophosphamide Thio-TEPA			Adrenal Cortical Hormones	Vincristine	Occasional favorable response; life occasionally prolonged.
Multiple Myeloma	Melphalan Cyclophosphamide		^{32}P	Adrenal Cortical Hormones		Symptomatic relief in about 50% of cases, and objective improvement in 35%.
Polycythemia Vera	Busulfan Chlorambucil		^{32}P			Prolonged clinical responses.
Carcinoma of Lung	HN2 Cyclophosphamide					Brief improvement in about 30% of cases.
Carcinoma of Ovary	Thio-TEPA Chlorambucil Cyclophosphamide	5-FU				30 to 50% of cases improved for one to three months, sometimes longer.
Carcinoma of Thyroid			^{131}I			Marked improvement in properly selected cases.
Carcinoma of Breast	Thio-TEPA Chlorambucil Cyclophosphamide	5-FU		Estrogens Androgens Adrenal Cortical Hormones		25 to 50% improved by hormonal therapy; life may be prolonged in some cases.
Carcinoma of Endometrium				Progestins		25% respond, chiefly pulmonary metastases.
Carcinoma of Prostate				Estrogens		80% of cases respond to hormonal therapy; definite prolongation of life.
Wilms' Tumor, Children	HN2 Cyclophosphamide				Actinomycin D Vincristine	Temporary regression; 50% pulmonary metastases respond with long survivors.
Neuroblastoma	Cyclophosphamide				Vincristine	About 50% temporary improvement with occasional prolongation of life.
Trophoblastic Tumors, Female		Methotrexate 6-MP			Actinomycin D Vinblastine	80% respond, of whom 70% show "permanent" regression.
Carcinoma of Colon		5-FU				15% respond for several months or longer.
Carcinoma of Adrenal					o,p'-DDD	Tumor regression and decrease in hyperadrenocorticism in selected cases.
Carcinoma of Testis	Chlorambucil*	Methotrexate*			Actinomycin D* Vincristine	35% of patients show a favorable and sometimes prolonged response.
Carcinoid	Cyclophosphamide				Actinomycin D	Symptomatic relief; occasional tumor regression.
Miscellaneous Carcinomas and Sarcomas	HN2 Thio-TEPA Chlorambucil* Cyclophosphamide	5-FU Methotrexate*		Adrenal Cortical Hormones	Actinomycin D*	In rare instances and in specific situations, favorable responses occur.

* Given in Combination

Fig. 11-6. (From Karnofsky, D. A.: Cancer chemotherapeutic agents. CA—A Cancer Journal for Clinicians 18:72-79, 232-234, 1968)

Neoplastic diseases responding to chemotherapy (*Continued*)

Diagnoses	Polyfunctional alkylating agents	Antimetabolites	Radioactive isotopes	Steroid hormones	Miscellaneous drugs	Results
		REGIONAL CANCER CHEMOTHERAPY				
Pleural, Pericardial and Abdominal Effusions (instillation into appropriate cavity)	HN2 Thio-TEPA		^{198}Au Cr^{32}PO$_4$		Quinacrine	About 50% of patients respond.
Carcinoma in Facial Areas (Intraarterial infusion)		Methotrexate 5-FU				Favorable response of tumors supplied by external carotid artery in selected cases.
Tumors of the Extremities (extracorporeal perfusion)	HN2					Response in selected cases.
Leukemic Involvement Central Nervous System (intrathecal injection)		Methotrexate				About 80% of children with CNS involvement respond temporarily.

FIGURE 11-6. (*Continued*)

late thermal, chemical, and mechanical factors to prevent further oral discomfort. She should convince the Italian patient that the spicy food that his family has prepared may cause his mouth to hurt more. For the patient with ill-fitting dentures, she should suggest that they be adjusted to prevent irritation. The patient who has had a ritual cocktail before dinner may have to give up the drink in order to decrease the severity of his oral symptoms. Smoking is discouraged. When a patient is discharged while he still has mouth problems, it is important that the nurse help him set up a pattern of care for good oral hygiene so that complications are minimized.

Perhaps the psychosocial need most affected by chemotherapeutic agents is the patient's need to have an acceptable self-concept and body image. As a result of the effect of these drugs on the hair follicles, the patient may develop alopecia. With the loss of hair, patients may become so depressed that they refuse to interact with others and may even have difficulty looking at themselves. The nurse can be very helpful with this by stressing the temporary aspect of the problem and the fact that there will be regrowth of hair. A wig may be the answer for the female patient if she can afford one. If the purchase of a wig is impossible, attractive scarves and roller caps can be used to deemphasize this problem. This is not purely a female problem, however, and the nurse must be ever cognizant of the impact that hair loss may have on the male patient.

Being well aware that these drugs are not curative and that they may make the patient more ill for a given period of time, it is imperative that the nurse contemplate, study, and explore her own feelings toward this mode of therapy. The personal attitude that she conveys to the patient and his family is of utmost importance and will affect the caliber of nursing care that she will be capable of giving to the patient.

In spite of the negative aspects of the therapy, the patient may experience a decrease in pain, an eventual increase in his feeling of well-being and develop a more hopeful attitude with ultimately a prolongation of life. The nurse should continually exert conscious efforts to broaden her perspective so that she is effective through attitude as well as through knowledge and skill to administer quality nursing care to patients receiving drugs for the treatment of cancer.

PSYCHOLOGICAL ASPECTS OF NURSING THE CANCER PATIENT

The Optimistic Approach

Because there are so many kinds of cancer (over 100), the diagnosis of cancer need not indicate a final outcome, and that, a hopeless one. Many forms of cancer are curable; many others achieve "cure" status if they are treated early.

Once the diagnosis of cancer has been established, a very effective and comfortable way to accept the illness is to live wholly for the present. To project thoughts to the future adds doubts and fears; to plan and live each day at it comes provides tangible means of achievement. The patient from this point of reference realizes he is still here; he acquires a feeling of extension of life. The opposite is true if his reference point is projected to a year from now; life from a more distant vantage point appears shortened and limited. Even dividing one's time into blocks of days walled in by visits to the doctor can be helpful. These units of time are quantities that can be appreciated and coped with by the patient.

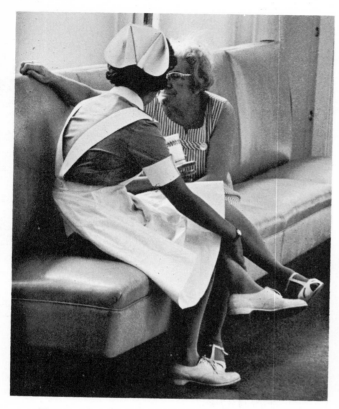

Fig. 11-7. The nurse by communicating with the patient helps her to verbalize and cope with her anxieties. (Courtesy of the Hospital of the University of Pennsylvania)

The physician responsible for the patient and the patient's family make the decision as to whether the patient should or should not be told that he has cancer. Any questions that may arise in this regard are to be directed to the physician. It is up to the nurse to find out from the physician what information he has given the patient and his family.

The manner in which a patient accepts the information that he has cancer often depends on his philosophy of life and his views of life and death. The greatest comfort may be spiritual consolation. The nurse should arrange to have those spiritual resources available that are most likely to meet his individual needs.

The prospect of a break-through in treatment is closer with each passing day. Hours of time, study and analysis are added daily to hundreds of thousands of dollars spent on research. Tomorrow could be the day that significant answers will come to the treatment of many kinds of cancer.

In modern cancer therapy it may happen frequently that extensive surgery and irradiation therapy may produce changes that are disfiguring or mutilating and not easily borne by the patient. The problems thus

created may be almost overwhelming. They begin before operation, when the question is raised as to how much the patient should be told about the details of his disease and his operation; they must be handled differently for each patient. It is probably best that the nurse should not be called on to divulge the details of diagnosis and treatment.

The adaption that has to be made to the therapeutic measures for the malignancy must begin in the preoperative period. The patients are particularly in need of support and reassurance in order to establish confidence in the skill of the surgeon and the hospital environment. When the patient approaches surgery with a sense of hopefulness and expectation, excellent results can be anticipated from a psychological point of view. If, however, he approaches surgery with the conviction that the operation is going to be painful, disfiguring and mutilating, it is almost to be expected that he should show depression and a marked sense of weakness postoperatively. The postoperative symptoms of depression may be sleep disturbance, loss of appetite, and other manifestations that may persist for an indefinite period. In their depression, patients may think there is hostility on the part of nurses, doctors and attendants.

Even when the physician is not blamed directly, often he is looked on unconsciously as the injuring party; hence, resentment may appear particularly toward nurses in the immediate environment, social workers, and even members of the family. The symptoms often take more demanding attention. The nurse must recognize this attitude as a part of the normal process of repair and should work through the anger and the resentment to win the patient over to a more normal attitude.

In other instances, patients may assume feelings of dejection accompanied by a sense of helplessness. Such anxiety often makes the patient turn to other people for help, advice, consolation and reassurance. This state is often only temporary, and the nurse, who is closest to him, can be of invaluable aid during this period of rehabilitation. Kindness and warmth give the patient the security he needs.

The nurse, of all medical personnel, has the most sustained and intimate contact with the patient during his hospitalization. Therefore, she is the person to whom the patient turns most often for kindness and support during the early postoperative period. If the nurse is able to meet these needs, not only will the pressure and the anxiety be alleviated, but also the patient's perception of his hospital experience will be modified.

In summary, the psychology of cancer patients is the psychology of a person who is facing a fundamental struggle with security and his self-value. Such problems can be met best by professional persons. The nurse is in a very advantageous position to aid the patient in his efforts to overcome depression and anxiety and to resume normal function after surgery.

Gravity of Prognosis

What is in the mind of a patient suffering from a fatal disease? What are his hopes and fears? How nearly does he suspect intuitively the truth of the situation, and, if he suspects the truth, by what psychological mechanisms is he saved from despair? How specifically and in what detail should he be informed regarding his illness and its probable outcome? If he demands an accurate appraisal of his status and a true estimate as to the prognosis, should this be supplied? What is his family to be told? What are the responsibilities of the nurse as regards the transmission of diagnostic and prognostic information to the patient's family?

These and similar questions regularly confront physicians and nurses responsible for the care of the seriously ill. Some of them may be answered without equivocation, with a reasonable degree of certainty and without important reservations, while others, depending on the personal philosophy of the physician, the family and the status of a particular patient, may be answered in generalizations which, although basically valid, are open to a variety of interpretations.

First, as regards the nurse-patient and the nurse-family relationship, it may be stated that whatever information is to be supplied concerning the diagnosis, whether or not it has been definitely established, never should be volunteered to the patient or his family by the nurse, except as planned as a result of mutual discussions with the responsible physician. By the same token, whatever prognostications are offered by the nurse should be precisely as specific as the physician's, and no more. Finally, any remarks of the nurse's that have a bearing on the possible implications of the diagnosis, prognosis or treatment should be made advisedly, in the light of the physician's known views and intentions. This admonition deserves considerable emphasis, for nothing is more destructive of confidence and morale than an impression of inconsistency, and nothing is more threatening to therapeutic success than confusion and distrust in the mind of the patient. Obviously, all of the statements and the actions of the nurse should be calculated to convey a sense of optimism; no matter how grave the situation or depressing the outlook, the nurse can lend a great deal of encouragement without exceeding either the bounds of reality or her professional responsibilities.

Normally, protective psychological mechanisms operate in patients with lethal disease, apparently to excellent effect, for very few such patients become acutely anxious or profoundly depressed, even when it is seemingly obvious that a fatal outcome is imminent.

The precise nature of these mechanisms presumably differs, depending on the individual and the situation. A conversion of the patient's will to live to a complete acceptance of the idea of death, even a desire for death, may be one aspect of this process of psychological adaptation in patients with prolonged and painful illnesses, although in most instances there is no sign of a death wish. On the contrary, the evidence would suggest that the desire to live persists with great tenacity, ideas of death apparently being altogether excluded from awareness.

The question regarding the degree to which the physician and the nurse are justified in supporting this false but benign optimism or, on the other hand, of clearing up the patient's misconceptions, in practice proves to be very much less difficult than one would anticipate. Patients become aware of an unfavorable prognosis far earlier than expected—in fact, almost as soon as its fatal character is established—probably because the reassurance received thereafter lacks its former conviction. However, provided that he is satisfied with the professional conduct of his case, as soon as he recognizes the truth of the situation, he promptly abandons his insistent questions regarding the precise prospects, and his anxieties become focused on problems that are completely irrelevant or only indirectly related to his personal affliction. Rarely does such an individual request a categorical answer concerning prognosis if he expects an unfavorable reply. Interest in the disease itself continues to be overt and lively, but its flavor is perhaps a little more academic in quality. The manifestations of the disease may be increasingly absorbing to the patient, but there is no apparent inclination on his part to discuss their real implications.

It is not often, therefore, that the physician or the nurse must decide how much of the tragic truth to tell; they seldom are asked. An occasional patient does persist in his direct questioning, apparently with logical reason, perhaps relating to his business plans or obligations to his family. Under these circumstances some physicians may feel justified in offering a complete evaluation of the case in detail and stating their conclusions in definite terms. The occasional result of this decision is a complete and unexpected shattering of the patient's morale.

Members of the patient's family and those of his associates who require explicit information, of course, must be made acquainted with the complete situation, and at least one member of the immediate family should be advised from the outset regarding all possible developments. If this is done, candid discussions concerning prognoses with the victims of hopeless disease are in no way justified. Optimism, valid or false, is to be strengthened, not destroyed, if the humane objective of patient care is to be served completely.

THE PATIENT WITH TERMINAL CARCINOMA—OBJECTIVES AND PRINCIPLES OF MEDICAL, SURGICAL, AND NURSING MANAGEMENT

I. To control the carcinogenic growth
   A. Prepare the patient for surgery, radiotherapy, and/or chemotherapy
      1. Assist with diagnostic tests to determine if metastasis has occurred
      2. Combat local and systemic infections
      3. Correct existing anemia and electrolyte imbalance
      4. Give the patient psychological support
         a. Explain the treatment
         b. Offer reassurance and support
         c. Listen to and observe the patient's anxieties
   B. Assist with the treatment as prescribed
      1. Surgical treatment
      2. Radiotherapy
      3. Chemotherapy
II. To treat auxiliary problems contributing to the patient's discomfort
   A. Radiation sickness
      1. Administer vitamin B as prescribed
      2. Give sedatives, antihistamines and antiemetic drugs as indicated
      3. Offer small, frequent feedings of high caloric, high protein foods
      4. Increase fluid intake
      5. Report patient's reactions
   B. Diarrhea
      1. Give low residue or bland diet
      2. Use anodyne suppositories
      3. Instill oil enemas to soothe rectal mucosa
      4. Give antidiarrhea medications as ordered
   C. Skin reaction
      1. Observe the skin for erythema
      2. Apply oil or bland cream to radiation site
      3. Protect skin from sunlight, heat, trauma, and tight clothing
      4. Avoid irritation with soap and water
      5. Observe for telangiectasis (a permanent, web-like dilatation of capillaries and small arteries)
   D. Blood cell depression
      1. Report results of laboratory evaluation
      2. Observe for evidences of bleeding
      3. Protect the patient from infection
III. To relieve the patient's pain
   A. Evaluate the quality, intensity and duration of pain as well as the patient's response to pain
   B. Promote the general comfort of the patient (i.e., turning, moving, ambulating)
   C. Administer agents to relieve pain when indicated
      1. Use specific drugs for the relief of nausea and vomiting
      2. Give ataractic agents to relieve fear and apprehension
      3. Utilize hot and cold compresses if indicated
      4. Give sedative and hypnotic drugs to induce sleep
      5. Apply local anesthetics
      6. Administer muscle relaxant drugs and antispasmodics; use non-narcotic drugs when possible; use the smallest amount of narcotic possible
      7. Give analgesic drugs for more intense pain
      8. Use tranquilizers to provide a sense of well-being
   D. Assist with surgical treatment for the relief of pain
      1. Prepare for alcohol injections to block nerve pathways
      2. Prepare for pre-sacral neurectomy when visceral pain is predominant
      3. Prepare for cordotomy when pain is intractable
   E. Assure patient that severe pain will be alleviated
IV. To control the odor
   A. Remove the odor at its source
   B. Encourage good personal hygiene
   C. Give normal saline irrigations (if indicated) to external lesions
   D. Administer prescribed vaginal irrigations when discharging vaginal lesions are present
   E. Keep perineal area shaved if malodorous discharge is present
V. To control the bleeding
   A. Observe for increasing pulse rate
   B. Observe for amount and color of blood
   C. Apply digital pressure if site is accessible
   D. Utilize vaginal or rectal packing as indicated
   E. Prepare patient for cauterization and ligation of exposed vessels if indicated
VI. To care for bladder frequency and incontinence
   A. Initiate a bladder control program
   B. Keep an accurate intake and output record
   C. Give meticulous skin care to perineal area
   D. Watch for formation of a vesicovaginal or rectovaginal fistula
   E. Insert an indwelling catheter if all other measures fail
VII. To prevent constipation
   A. Encourage fluids and regular meals
   B. Place patient on prune juice and glycerine suppository regimen
VIII. Reduce edema due to blocking of lymphatic vessels
   A. Encourage motion and exercise
   B. Elevate edematous extremity
   C. Utilize nursing measures to prevent decubiti
      1. Relieve the pressure
      2. Encourage circulation to the part
      3. Put extremities through range-of-motion exercises
IX. To assist the patient to cope with his situation
   A. Help patient to feel that he is understood
   B. Develop a supportive relationship with the patient
   C. Utilize all measures to keep the patient's ego intact
      1. Encourage him to make decisions and choices
      2. Answer his questions
      3. Listen to him

THE PATIENT WITH TERMINAL CARCINOMA—OBJECTIVES AND PRINCIPLES OF MEDICAL, SURGICAL, AND NURSING MANAGEMENT (*Continued*)

    4. Provide a daily schedule for the patient, including short daily rest periods
    5. Encourage the patient to keep active and to have interesting pursuits
X. To maintain the patient at optimal physical and emotional condition
    A. Give a high caloric, high protein diet (gavage feedings if indicated)
    B. Keep caloric intake up with between-meal feedings
    C. Give supplementary vitamins and hematemics

    D. Administer blood transfusions as ordered
    E. Encourage regular rest periods and periods in the outdoors
    F. Keep the patient as active as possible to build up endurance and avoid debilitation
    G. Alleviate the patient's anxiety and stress
    H. Maintain a cheerful and optimistic attitude
    I. Encourage verbalization
    J. Do little "extras" for the patient
    K. Include the family in the patient's care

TERMINAL NURSING CARE

Some authorities claim that the most important aspect in the care of the terminal patient is good nursing. Frequent changes of bed linen, cleanliness and keeping the patient warm are all comfort measures that can relieve a great deal of pain. During this care probably the most common emergency that the nurse should anticipate is hemorrhage, due to erosion of blood vessels by the malignancy itself, secondary necrosis or the sloughing of tissue following irradiation. In some instances, the nurse can control bleeding by digital pressure. In cases of hemorrhage that cannot be controlled by local measures, the patient should be kept quiet in the recumbent position, and the physician should be notified. The nurse should have the necessary equipment available for treating shock and hemorrhage (see pp. 146, 149).

Ambulation

The patient should be kept ambulatory as long as possible; however, the nurse must recognize when it is undesirable for him to get out of bed.

Nutrition and Hydration

The main limiting factor in attaining and maintaining a good nutritional level is anorexia. Specific food needs vary depending on the location of the tumor. For instance, the needs of a patient with cancer of the stomach may be quite different from those of a patient with cancer of the liver or the lungs. Small, frequent feedings are more likely to be accepted, together with protein supplementation and parenteral vitamin administration. Dehydration and electrolyte imbalance have to be prevented by correcting inadequate fluid intake and output.

Skin Care

Good skin care is imperative. Tissues do not repair so easily as in the normal individual; therefore, preventive measures may eliminate much discomfort. Back and body massages are helpful; in addition, they are conducive to relaxation and help to relieve pain.

Pain

The nurse must be able to judge whether her patient needs a soothing treatment, a sedative or a hypnotic. Usually, drugs can be given sparingly at first and then gradually increased in kind and amount. One must be cognizant of the effects of drugs on the debilitated and the older patient. These individuals have increased sensitivity and may have a chain-type reaction to narcotics. First, they are drowsy, take less food, become dehydrated, retain urine, and have gastrointestinal irritation, nausea and vomiting and ultimately develop a disturbed electrolyte and fluid balance. Of course, the treatment for such a condition would be to discontinue these medications or decrease their dosage.

Esthetic Factors

Facial tumors are often unsightly; the patient usually is very sensitive about his appearance. Such lesions should be covered if possible. Other features of the patient should be accented to detract attention from the tumor site. This can be done by careful grooming, attractive garments, etc. Bright lights in a room should be replaced by softer lights, inasmuch as shades of light and dark can tone down unsightly areas. The nurse can use her ingenuity in helping this individual to bear his burden more easily.

One of the most unpleasant features of cancer in exposed areas on the body is the foul odor that appears sooner or later. This is due to the sloughing of tissues. Every effort should be made to keep the patient and his room clean. Dressings should be changed frequently, removed quickly from the patient's room and deposited in a metal-covered container until they are sent to the incinerator. Bedclothes and the patient's clothing ought to be changed when soiled. The use of absorbent or oakum pads may help when drainage is present. The room should be ventilated properly. Deodorants may be necessary. Several of the essential oils, such as oil of geranium, oil of eucalyptus or oil of orange, will meet the situation. Neutroleum alpha is lasting and not unpleasant when 1 or 2 drops are applied to the dressing or to the bedclothing. Powdered charcoal in the dressing or potassium permanganate solution 1:2,000 as an irrigation often helps. Activated zinc peroxide is also effective in cleansing and deodorizing these wounds. Commercially prepared products can be disseminated from a bottle with a wick or by means of an electric deodorizer to absorb odors. These are quite successful.

The nurse should try to maintain a rational psychological approach toward death. She is often the person to whom the patient turns when he wants to talk about himself, his fears, his hopes, etc. To be able to listen and to offer encouragement are extremely important assets. Many times a patient demonstrates hostility and rebellion. In spite of this, the nurse, by remaining tolerant, shows her patient that she stands by him in spite of his unpleasant actions. In this manner, eventually she will be able to discover the reason for his outbursts and then help him to resolve them. (See "Psychological Aspects of Cancer Patient Care," above.)

Occupational and Recreational Therapy

Statistics reveal that the home is best suited for the care of this patient for several reasons. He is in a familiar environment and can see his friends and family. Many times, he can perform some household duties and thereby feel that he is helping. The financial burden on the family is reduced. The family knows what is happening to him, which often is not the case when he is in an institution. The home is more conducive for him to pursue his hobbies, such as caring for tropical fish, developing a miniature garden, etc. Much of the responsibility for his care rests with the family. The nurse and the physician can help them greatly in making the adjustment an easier one. For patients who do not have a home, the next best available environment should be sought. The nurse with sympathetic understanding can help her patient in making contact with the proper agencies for the adjustment of his social and economic problems. (See Objectives and Principles of Medical, Surgical and Nursing Management.)

Nursing in cancer of the various organs is discussed as each condition is studied in this text.

BIBLIOGRAPHY

Barckley, V.: The crisis in cancer. Amer. J. Nurs., 67:278-280, Feb., 1967.
————: Nursing the patient with cancer—an exercise in timing. CA 17:126-127, May-June, 1967.
Blakemore, W., and Ravdin, I. S.: Current perspectives in cancer therapy. New York, Harper and Row, 1966.
Bouchrad, R.: Nursing care of the cancer patient. St. Louis, C. V. Mosby, 1967.

Burt, A. L.: The role of the public health nurse in the care of the cancer patient. Nurs. Clin. N. Amer., 2:683-689, Dec., 1967.
Clark, R. L., et al.: Rehabilitation of the cancer patient. Cancer, 20:839-845, May, 1967.
Conference on Research Needs in the Rehabilitation of Persons with Disabilities Resulting from Cancer, U.S. H.E.W. Institute of Physiologic Medicine and Rehabilitation, New York U. Med. Center, 1965.
Craven, P. K.: A facade for fear. ANA Clinical Sessions, 28-33, 1966.
Fox, J. E.: Reflections on cancer nursing. Amer. J. Nurs., 66: 1317-1319, June, 1966.
Grant, R.: Nursing of the cancer patient. Nurs. Forum, 4:57-58, 1965. (No. 2)
Hammond, E.: Home care and improvisations. Nurs. Outlook, 12:49, April, 1964.
Leone, L. P.: The attack on heart disease, cancer and stroke. Is nursing ready? Amer. J. Nurs., 65:68-72, May, 1965.
Meinhart, N. T.: The cancer patient: Living in the here and now. Nurs. Outlook, 16:64-69, May, 1968.
Moore, G. E.: Cancer: 100 different diseases. Amer. J. Nurs., 66:749-756, April, 1966.
Nealon, T. F. (ed.): Management of the patient with cancer. Philadelphia, W. B. Saunders, 1966.
Ostendorf, M.: Emotional responses of patients to physical illness. ANA Clinical Sessions, 145-150, 1966.
Rogers, A.: Pain and the cancer patient. Nurs. Clin. N. Amer., 2:671-682, Dec., 1967.
Sr. F. X. Mangen, O. R.: Psychological aspects of nursing the advanced cancer patient. Nurs. Clin. N. Amer., 2:649-658, Dec., 1967.
Thornblad, I.: Hormonal ablative therapy for the premenopausal patient with advanced cancer. Nurs. Clin. N. Amer., 2:659-668, Dec., 1967.

Chemotherapeutic Agents

Donaldson, S. S. and Fletcher, W. S.: The treatment of cancer by isolation perfusion. Amer. J. Nurs., 64:81-88, Aug., 1964.
Ellison, R. R.: Treating cancer with antimetabolites. Amer. J. Nurs., 62:72-75, Nov., 1962.
Fox, S. A. and Bernhardt, L. C.: Chemotherapy via intra-arterial infusion. Amer. J. Nurs., 66:1966-1968, Sept., 1966.
Hilkemeyer, R.: Intra-Arterial Cancer Chemotherapy. Nurs. Clin. N. Amer., 66:295-308, June, 1966.
Karnofsky, D. A.: Cancer therapeutic agents. Cancer, 18:72-80, 1968.

PATIENT EDUCATION

American Cancer Society
    A wide variety of general and specific pamphlets, films and booklets are available. See your local American Cancer Society.
        The Hopeful Side of Cancer. Pamphlet.
        Cancer is a Lonely Business. Pamphlet.
Public Affairs Pamphlets
    381 Park Avenue South
    New York, New York 10016
        Ogg, E.: When a Family Faces Cancer. 1965.

CHAPTER 12

Radiation Nursing in Diagnosis and Therapy

- *Physical Aspects*
- *Biological Aspects and Clinical Application*
- *Radiation Detection, Control, and Precautions*
- *Roentgenologic Studies*
- *Radiation Therapy*

Generally, radiation is used in medicine in three ways—for diagnosis, therapy or research. For any of these, the available radiation sources can be listed simply as roentgenographic and fluoroscopic machines (x-rays), natural and artificial radioactive isotopes and the high energy particle machines.

Radiation is effective in destroying cancer cells and in preventing their spread. In the individual whose malignancy has spread to such an extent that other forms of treatment are ineffective, radiation may be used as a palliative measure in keeping the patient comfortable.

The nature of radiation needs to be understood in order to reduce the fears about it and to maintain the safety of all persons who come in contact with it.

PHYSICAL ASPECTS

Radioactivity

Everything in our universe, including man, has been subjected to radiation since the universe was formed. This ever-present radiation, called natural background, is a normal part of nature's balance and presents no hazard to ordinary living. However, about 1895, man discovered ways of creating artificially almost all of nature's natural forms of radiation and then went on to create new forms in infinite number, power and variety.

Upon examining the nucleus of an atom, the elements are considered stable because of the effect of neutrons on protons. In the heavier elements, this becomes increasingly difficult and such atoms are said to be unstable. In order to become more stable, nuclei give up energy in the form of rays or particles—alpha (α), beta (β), and gamma (γ). Such disintegration is referred to as *radioactivity*.

Radioisotopes

The atoms of each chemical element have the same number of protons, which means that ordinary physical and chemical properties of the element are similar in each of its atoms. However, a different form of the same chemical element may exist; this is called the isotope. An *isotope* is an element whose nucleus contains a constant number of protons but has a differing number of neutrons, thereby changing its weight. To indicate an isotope, the total number of neutrons and protons are appended, e.g., in cobalt-59 (^{59}Co), the isotope of cobalt has a total of 59 protons and neutrons. The optimal ratio between protons and neutrons in a chemical element is one that is stable—^{59}Co is an example. By using nuclear reactors and high speed particle accelerators, it is possible to bombard a stable isotope such as ^{59}Co with additional free neutrons. By absorbing an extra neutron, an unstable or radioactive isotope is formed, ^{60}Co. This isotope has valuable medical uses.

Most radioisotopes emit particulate radiation (small fragments of the nucleus having mass and size) and electromagnetic radiation ("rays" that have no mass). The basic radiation type is represented by *alpha* and *beta* particles, which are actual parts of radioactive atoms; these break away and travel at high speeds and with great energies.

X-ray is a good example of electromagnetic radiation, one of the basic types. It is made up of rays or waves of very high electric energy traveling at very high speeds. When electromagnetic radiation arises from natural or artificially created radioactive isotopes, instead of an x-ray machine, it is called *gamma radiation.*

All four of these types of radiation act on living tissue in the same way, by ionization or, in other words, alteration of atoms in the chemical systems of the cell. If the level of radiation and its resulting intracellular ionization is low enough, no irreversible damage is done to the cell or organism as a whole. However, if the level is high enough, the cell may be altered or even destroyed. When such ionization occurs in the cells of the gonads, genetic mutations may result. Radiation effect is cumulative; the ionization that occurs in cells is not reversible.

Alpha rays can be stopped by a sheet of paper, and most beta rays are hindered by a thin sheet of metal. In tissue, beta rays have a range up to 15 mm. Gamma rays are the most penetrating of the 3; they can penetrate the human body and can cause hazards to others near the patient. In summary, the amount of damage or destruction to tissue varies with dosage, intensity of radiation and the nature of the site to be irradiated.

Radioactive Decay or Disintegration

The rate at which atoms emit their radiation (disintegrate or decay) varies from isotope to isotope. The decay rate or *half-life* is the time (hours, days, months or years) required for one-half of the atoms of a particular radioactive material to decay or be reduced to half its initial activity. An example is iodine-131,

UNITS TO MEASURE AMOUNT OF ACTIVITY	
Curie (Ci)	the basic measure or unit to measure the amount of activity in a radioactive sample.
Millicurie (mCi)	one-thousandth of a curie
Microcurie (μCi)	one-millionth of a curie
Picocurie (pCi)	one-trillionth of a curie

UNITS TO MEASURE AMOUNT OF RADIATION TO WHICH A GIVEN SUBSTANCE IS EXPOSED OR ABSORBED	
Roentgen (R)	a standard unit of *exposure* (applicable to x-ray and gamma rays)
Milliroentgen (mR)	one thousandth of a roentgen
Rad	a unit to measure absorbed dose (1 rad—amount of radiation required to deposit 100 ergs of energy per gram of irradiated material)
Rem	a unit of measure of radiation dose equivalent which takes into account the relative biological effectiveness. ("roentgen equivalent man")

FIGURE 12-2

which has a half-life of slightly more than 8 days, where radium-226 has a half-life of over 1600 years. When a radioisotope is administered to a patient in open, unsealed form, it has a relatively short life and is essentially inactive after its therapeutic mission has been completed. Those isotopes of longer life are implanted in the patient in sealed containers and then removed for use at another time. An example of this is cobalt-60, which has a half-life of about 5 years.

BIOLOGICAL ASPECTS AND CLINICAL APPLICATION

Effect of Radiation on Tissue

Ionizing radiation is harmful to living tissue; therefore it requires good judgment in determining the benefit of radiation exposure versus risk of tissue damage. Factors that influence such risk are:

(1) The dose-rate—a prescribed dose causes less

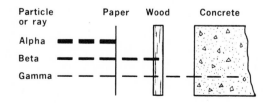

FIG. 12-1. Relative penetration of alpha, beta and gamma radiation. (U.S. Atomic Energy Commission)

TABLE 12-1. Summary of clinical effects of acute ionizing radiation doses*

Range	0 to 100 rems Subclinical range	100 to 1,000 rems Therapeutic range			Over 1,000 rems Lethal range	
		100 to 200 rems	200 to 600 rems	600 to 1,000 rems	1,000 to 5,000 rems	Over 5,000 rems
		Clinical surveillance	Therapy effective	Therapy promising	Therapy palliative	
Incidence of vomiting	None	100 rems: 5% 200 rems: 50%	300 rems: 100%	100%	100%	
Delay time	—	3 hours	2 hours	1 hour	30 minutes	
Leading organ	None	Hematopoietic tissue			Gastrointestinal tract	Central nervous system
Characteristic signs	None	Moderate leukopenia	Severe leukopenia, purpura, hemorrhage, infection, epilation above 300 rems		Diarrhea, fever, disturbance of electrolyte balance	Convulsions, tremor, ataxia, lethargy
Critical period post-exposure	—	—	4 to 6 weeks		5 to 14 days	1 to 48 hours
Therapy	Reassurance	Reassurance, hematologic surveillance	Blood transfusion, antibiotics	Consider bone marrow transplantation	Maintenance of electrolyte balance	Sedatives
Prognosis	Excellent	Excellent	Good	Guarded	Hopeless	
Convalescent period	None	Several weeks	1 to12 months	Long	—	
Incidence of death	None	None	0 to 80% (variable)	80 to 100% (variable)	90 to 100%	
Death occurs within	—	—	2 months		2 weeks	2 days
Causes of death	—	—	Hemorrhage, infection		Circulatory collapse	Respiratory failure, brain edema

* U.S. Dept. of Defense: The Effects of Nuclear Weapons. p. 591. Washington, D.C., Supt. of Documents, 1964.

tissue destruction if given in small amounts over a long period of time than when given all at once.

(2) Area of body exposure—the larger the area exposed, the greater the effect.

(3) Cell susceptibility—rapidly dividing cells with no specialized function are more sensitive than nondividing cells and highly differentiated cells (e.g., lymphocytes and germ cells are more sensitive than nerve or muscle cells).

(4) Biological variability—some individuals are more susceptible to radiation than others, e.g., the healthy person is more responsive than the malnourished. Although lymph cells are more radiosensitive, Hodgkin's disease continues to progress and is not cured by radiation. Noteworthy also is that the more radioresistant skin cells are cured of cancer when sufficient radiation is used.

The fact that the injury extends to all components of the exposed tissue and affects most severely the cells that are growing fastest, i.e., those engaged in tissue regeneration and repair, accounts for the slow healing and extensive scarring that are characteristic of radiation damage.

The skin is especially vulnerable to radiation injury by virtue of its exposed location. Healing is likely to be protracted and permanent changes are unusually extensive.

Bone marrow is one of the most radiosensitive of normal tissues, and damage to the marrow is potentially the most lethal of the complications of excessive irradiation. Interruption of marrow function results promptly in a fall in circulating platelets to thrombocytopenic levels, giving rise to a hemorrhagic diathesis for which there is, as yet, no adequate replacement therapy. Agranulocytosis develops concomitantly, causing a heightened susceptibility to bacterial infection that may prove to be as hazardous as thrombocytopenia. Fortunately, antibiotic therapy affords adequate protection against sepsis in the majority of patients. Radiation cataracts have been described from excessive exposure of the eyes to neutron or x-radiation, and diffuse, incapacitating fibrosis of the lungs may follow injudicious irradiation of the thorax. Damage to the fetus in utero, with production of congenital malformations, is apt to occur as a result of irradiation during the period from the second to the sixth week of gestation.

Short-term Effects. If a person has had a major portion of the body exposed to large doses of radiation (over 100 rems) in a short period of time, the symptoms of radiation syndrome will be apparent (see Table 12-1). This is manifested in 4 stages: (1) prodromal—nausea, vomiting, and malaise; (2) latent—symptoms subside; (3) illness—general malaise, epilation, hemorrhage (purpura, petechiae, nosebleeds, etc.), pallor, diarrhea, inflammation of mouth and throat; and (4) recovery or death.

Long-term Effects. This is an area of public health concern because it may involve large numbers of people who may be exposed to low levels of radiation over a long period of time. The classic example is of the women employed in the early 1920's to paint watch and clock dials with luminizing (radium-containing) paints. Years later, bone sarcomas resulted from the carcinogenic effect of the radium. Similarly, leukemia occurs more frequently in radiologists than other physicians. Another example is the Hiroshima survivors who have shown the effects of low levels of radiation.

When the gonads are exposed to radiation, the long-term effects may not be apparent in the individual but in his progeny. Genetic mutations can be transmitted to subsequent generations. Among the most serious of the late consequences of irradiation damage is the increased susceptibility to malignant metaplasia and the development of cancer at sites of earlier irradiation. Evidence cited in support of this relationship refers to the increased incidence of carcinoma of skin, bone and lung after latent periods of 20 years and longer following irradiation of those sites. Further support has been adduced from the relatively high incidence of carcinoma of the thyroid 7 years and longer following low-dosage irradiation of the thymus in childhood, and from the increased incidence of leukemia following total body irradiation at any age. Evidence for long-range damage from irradiation in the form of gene mutations in exposed germ plasm is derived almost entirely from observations on insects and small animals and is based on analogy. Statistical arguments and analogies aside, the potential capacity of radiation to produce gene mutations can scarcely be discounted; the existence of the threat cannot be denied. Accordingly, precautions against unnecessary or excessive exposure to radiation are appropriate, and every available safeguard against radiation damage is definitely indicated.

RADIATION DETECTION, CONTROL AND PRECAUTIONS

Radiation Detection and Control

While these radiations are very powerful, they cannot be directly seen, heard, smelled, tasted, felt or in any other way detected by ordinary human senses. So their characteristic ability to ionize matter through which they pass is utilized in designing instruments to detect and measure them. Simply, such instruments record the number of rays or particles of radiation that pass through the detecting unit in a given period of time. These instruments, such as Geiger counters, detect radioactivity and measure its general strength.

Radiation has an additional ability to affect the emulsion of photographic film as light does in a camera. Film badges can be worn while working with or near radiation. After development of the film from the badge, extent of exposure can be determined. This knowledge of total radiation exposure is very important. Within certain limits, cells live quite well while being constantly exposed—there is always a low continuous radiation background. At the other extreme, too much radiation exposure can cause physical damage and death.

In this country, and in much of the world, laws require that radiation sources and devices may be used only by persons trained in their theory and operation, who agree to abide by the specified standards and limits. Properly observed, they should enable anyone to work with or near radiation throughout his life without noticeable physical damage, shortening of life expectancy or genetic harm to future generations. Detailed specific dosage and exposure limits need not concern the average nurse, who is not working directly in a radiology department, so long as she does observe carefully the precautions outlined by the hospital radiologist for any particular case involving radiation. Her exposure ordinarily will be only occasional and, assuming proper precautions, very slight.

Prevention of Radiation Damage

Improvements in equipment for diagnostic radiology are clearly desirable and are constantly in progress. Policies have been recommended, more rigid than those of the past, regarding the extent to which diagnostic x-ray examinations should be carried out and the frequency with which they should be repeated. Prophylactic examinations for possible pregnancy or for purposes of pelvimetry, for example, are discouraged, as are all x-ray studies that are undertaken in the absence of disease. Perhaps the most important aspect of any program that might be designed for the prevention of radiation damage concerns the education of practitioners who are equipped with radiologic apparatus but are untrained in radiology.

Finally, it needs to be emphasized that the benefits of radiation therapy should never be denied to a patient with a radiosensitive neoplasm because of considerations regarding long-range radiologic safety. As a result of intensive publicity regarding the dangers of radioactive fallout and the complications of radiation damage in general, anxiety over the potential complications of radiotherapy, including x-ray irradiation and the use of radioisotopes, is prevalent among the laity. The nurse is very likely to be in a position to allay such fears in the minds of many patients for whom irradiation has been recommended but who are inclined to refuse it on the grounds of its inherent risks.

Roentgenologic Precautions

The safety of the patient, the therapist, the nurse, the x-ray technician and any other personnel who might be present during radiography, fluoroscopy or radiotherapy demands strict observance of certain precautions, including the following:

1. No one should be in the room with the patient who is undergoing x-ray therapy or roentgenography.

2. The fluoroscopic equipment and technique should be such as to prevent the leakage of radiation.

3. Each individual in the fluoroscopic room should protect himself from scattered radiation by wearing a lead apron and, if indicated, lead-impregnated gloves.

4. Complete protection of the patient's gonads during radiography and x-ray therapy should be assured by means of appropriate lead shielding.

The nurse should be familiar with these stipulations and their purpose so that she may explain them to the patient.

When a patient is receiving x-ray therapy, he ought to know why he seems to be left alone when receiving treatment and that a technician is always nearby, who can see him through a window. Also, the patient should know that there is an intercommunication system that allows him to talk to the technician. It is well to remember that external radiation will never cause any patient to become radioactive himself. He cannot possibly present any radiation hazard to himself, other patients or the nurse.

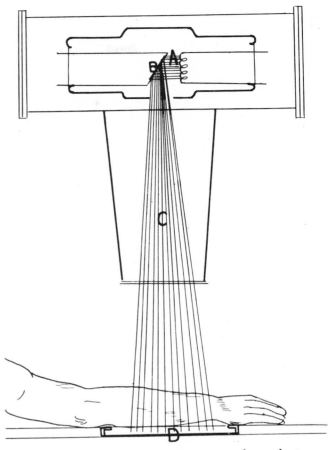

FIG. 12-3. Source of x-rays. X-ray tube at the top contains 2 electrodes in an air-evacuated glass tube. When the cathode is heated, electrons (A) are "boiled off" and hit the target (anode) at B; the electrons are absorbed and re-emitted as x-rays (C). These penetrate body tissues and register on film (D). (Flitter, H.: Physics for Nurses, St. Louis, Mosby)

ROENTGENOLOGIC STUDIES

Evaluation of the ill patient very often is aided by, or may require, a roentgenologic examination, for most systemic diseases produce structural or functional changes that are of diagnostic significance and are detectable by this means alone.

The American Public Health Service has shown concern not only about the numbers of diagnostic x-ray examinations made annually in this country (approximately 150 million) but whether proper safeguards are used and unnecessary exposure is eliminated. The reason for concern is that the genetically significant radiation dose received by the population in the U.S. is higher than in most other countries.

Basic procedures that are employed in various x-ray

studies are of immediate concern to the nurse (Fig. 12-3). In certain examinations she is a direct participant, their success or failure depending on the manner in which certain preliminary nursing measures have been carried out. Moreover, her familiarity with diagnostic roentgenology in general and her appreciation of the objectives of specific tests are essential to her understanding of her patients and their problems.

Any structure in the body can be visualized by roentgen rays if the molecular density of that structure differs sufficiently from that of the adjacent structures. Areas of lesser density, such as aerated lung tissue or gas-filled bowel, that transmit x-rays with less interferences appear relatively "radiolucent"; those of greater density, which absorb or refract the x-rays to a greater extent, are relatively "radiopaque." In order to achieve the necessary degree of inequality in density where no such inequality exists, it may be necessary to introduce either an artificial high-density "contrast medium," which will delineate the lumen of any tube or hollow viscus containing it, or injections of air in the vicinity of the structure to be examined, after which the latter can be delineated against a relatively translucent background. Roentgenologic study of the gastrointestinal tract, the gallbladder, the bronchi, the kidneys, the spinal canal, the genitourinary tract and the blood vessels depends in each case on the ingestion or the injection of an appropriate contrast medium.

Roentgenograms

The roentgenogram, or "x-ray plate," is analogous to the familiar photographic negative, consisting of a plastic sheet that has been coated with a light-sensitive emulsion. X-rays expelled from a cathode tube are directed through whatever anatomic structure or object may be under study, through a protective casing that encloses the film and protects it from exposure to light and, finally, through the film itself. Shortly thereafter, the film is developed and studied in the form of a negative print.

Fluoroscopy

This technique involves the continuous observation of an image reflected on a screen when exposed to x-radiation in the manner of a television screen that is activated by an electrode beam. Structures of differing densities that intercept the x-ray beams are visualized on the screen in silhouette. A permanent record of a fluoroscopic image may be secured by photography. Miniature photographs of this type, called "photofluorograms," are utilized by Public Health Chest Survey Units, hospitals and other organizations as a method of excluding lung disease rapidly and economically in large numbers of individuals. Fluoroscopic images, brightened and accentuated by electronic "image intensifiers," may be viewed either by the fluoroscopist through an optical system (intensifier fluoroscopy) or, preferably, by a television camera (video fluoroscopy) and relayed to a screen. Video fluoroscopy can be combined with motion picture filming of the output phosphor under the direct guidance and aim of the fluoroscopist at the monitor. A continuous video tape recording of the television signal can be made.

Angiography

See page 343.

Laminograms

The laminogram ("planogram" or "body section roentgenogram") furnishes sharply focused silhouettes of structures that lie within one plane only, other structures being obscured. This result is accomplished by means of a mechanical device that moves both the x-ray tube and the plate through a prescribed arc during exposure, the effect of which is to blur all outlines except those of structures that retain their original positions relative to both tube and plate. Multiple views of a body region, focused at successively deeper layers, visualize clearly some structures that would otherwise be obscured and localize accurately any lesions that might appear, as, for example, a tumor lying deep within the mediastinum, a lesion obstructing the bronchial lumen or a small area of bone destruction in a particular portion of the vertebrae.

Roentgenographic Examination of the Chest

The posterior-anterior (P.A.) view of the chest, commonest of all roentgenologic examinations, yields a wealth of information pertaining to the lungs and the pleura, locates the trachea and the bronchi, defines the position and the dimensions of the heart and the great vessels and determines the presence or the absence of abnormal mediastinal contents. Lateral and oblique views of the lungs are obtained for more precise localization of intrathoracic lesions. A posterior-anterior view of the chest taken with the tube at a standard distance (e.g., 6 or 7 feet) from the subject permits the quantitative measurement of certain cardiac dimensions that reflect the size of each individual atrium and ventricle. As indicated above, the cardiac examination may include, in addition, fluoroscopy for the detection and the measurement of abnormal movements in its pulsating walls or to differentiate a pulsatile mass, representing an aneurysm (p. 349), from one that does not pulsate, i.e., a solid tumor. Visualization of the small bronchi is accomplished with the aid of a contrast medium, Lipiodol, an iodized oil, which is instilled intratracheally an instant before the x-ray exposure is made. The resultant picture is called a "bronchogram." (See p. 231.)

Abdominal Roentgenograms

Anterior and posterior views of the abdomen, taken with the patient in horizontal position or sitting upright, are important in the diagnosis of intestinal obstruction. The presence, degree and location of gas and fluid levels within the intestinal lumen distinguish patients with obstruction from those with paralytic ileus. Stones (if radiopaque) in the gallbladder, the kidneys, the ureters or the bladder, as well as calcified blood vessels, lymph nodes, cysts and parasites, may be detected by this examination. Gastric or intestinal perforation may be discovered by the presence of free air under the diaphragm, observed in abdominal films. Depending on the amount of intestinal gas that is present, the spleen and one or both kidneys may be outlined in a flat abdominal film. The medial borders of the psoas muscles are usually apparent, their characteristics and location furnishing a clue as to the presence or the absence of tumors or other lesions in the retroperitoneal space.

Skeletal Roentgenograms

The roentgenographic appearance of the skeleton is of decisive importance in establishing and excluding the diagnosis of nutritional and endocrine disorders that are complicated by derangements of calcium and phosphorus metabolism. Abnormal radiolucency of the bones, indicating demineralization of the skeleton, is a characteristic of rickets, hyperparathyroidism and myelomatosis, for example. Specific changes are characteristic of rheumatoid hypertrophic arthritis, Paget's disease, osteosclerosis and other disorders of unknown etiology. The diagnosis of lead poisoning may be established by skeletal roentgenograms. Lymphomas and metastasizing carcinomas very often manifest themselves by localized osteolytic lesions in certain areas of the skeleton, the most common sites of involvement being the skull, the pelvis, the vertebrae and the ribs, i.e., where bone marrow is proliferating actively.

RADIATION THERAPY

Ionizing irradiation is the traditional alternative to surgery as a therapeutic approach to malignant diseases and remains the therapy of choice for most nonresectable tumors. Depending on the type of tumor to be treated, x-ray therapy may be preferred.

X-ray Therapy

X-rays and gamma rays are electromagnetic radiations. If the patient is to receive x-ray irradiation, the radiologist devises a program involving repeated exposures to fractional doses, directed in such a manner as to produce effective ionization within the tumor while avoiding unnecessary irradiation of normal structures. The course of therapy is individualized; the needs of the particular patient determine the rate at which radiation is given, the number of treatments and the frequency.

Low-voltage, high-voltage or supervoltage equipment is available for generating x-rays with energies that are appropriate for tumors of all sizes and in all locations. For low-voltage the unit of measure is KeV (thousand electron volts) and for super-voltage, MeV (million electron volts). The lesions most likely to respond to x-radiation are those originating from the reticuloendothelial tissues, i.e., leukemias and lymphomas, and from embryonal-type tissue, such as teratomas, for example. The least radiosensitive are tumors of nerve tissue, bone and muscle. X-ray therapy is notably successful in carcinoma of the larynx, the nasopharynx, the tongue, the lip, the skin, and in lymphomas, particularly Hodgkin's disease. Some regression is to be expected in most types of tumor so treated, especially if irradiated during phases of rapid growth. Postoperative irradiation of a tumor site is practiced commonly and is indicated, especially if the excised tumor is small and its histology is indicative of high-grade malignancy.

Nursing Support

Physical and Psychological Preparation. Having an x-ray for diagnostic purposes is so common that most patients have no questions about it. The person needs to know that he must be perfectly still and in proper position during the taking of the picture, or while receiving therapy. It may be necessary to use sandbags, pillows, or straps to maintain the correct position. Pins, buttons, pens or coins in the path of the x-ray will show up as opaque objects on the film, therefore one's clothing is usually replaced by a gown for body x-rays; hair pins and combs are removed from the hair for head x-rays. During the process of receiving x-ray therapy or pictures no sensation is experienced by the patient and it takes only a few minutes. The patient is in a separate room from the technician and all other individuals but is within hearing range; this precaution is taken to reduce the amount of exposure sustained by personnel.

The equipment used in x-ray therapy is often massive and may overwhelm the patient who is alone unless explanations have been given by the nurse. He ought to know that he will not feel the penetration of the rays. Following exposure, he is not considered radioactive and need not take special precautions in caring for his clothing or linens. It may be necessary for the radiologist to mark the exact area for radiation with indelible ink. This should not be washed off by

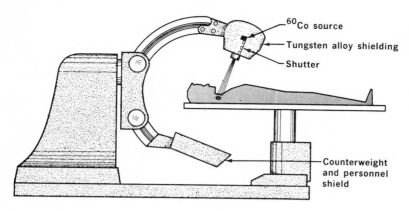

- ⁶⁰Co source
- Tungsten alloy shielding
- Shutter
- Counterweight and personnel shield

Fɪɢ. 12-4. Diagram showing position of patient receiving cobalt teletherapy. (U.S. Atomic Energy Commission)

the patient or nurse unless permission is given by the radiologist.

For the patient who has a malignancy, the thought of having x-ray therapy is often interpreted as terminal care and that all other forms of treatment are to no avail. The nurse should be aware of this possibility and direct her assessment and nursing plan accordingly. It may mean that the physician should be asked to clarify the purpose of the treatment to the patient.

The numbers of x-ray treatments vary with individuals, and so it is not usually possible to predict in advance how long or how many exposures will be necessary. This may prove discouraging to some patients and the nurse should be aware of it.

Skin Reactions. The patient undergoing radiation therapy may be told that he can expect some form of skin reaction; however, because it varies from person to person, the treatment of such a reaction must be individualized and is usually prescribed by the radiologist. No ointments, lotions, cosmetics or depilatories are applied to the site of radiation unless prescribed by the physician. Likewise, vigorous rubbing is discouraged because it can destroy skin cells. A bland ointment, such as one containing vitamins A and D, may be prescribed. Even long after a course of radiation therapy, the treated skin remains sensitive and the patient should be cautioned against irritation from friction, extremes in temperature and exposure to sunlight.

Systemic Reactions. Radiation may have a marked systemic effect upon the patient and lead to nausea, vomiting, fever, loss of appetite and a feeling of extreme malaise. Although this postirradiation upset may be only temporary, lasting from a few days to a week or more, it is during this period that good nursing care is most essential. The giving of sedatives, the careful selection of fluids and foods that will not induce or aggravate nausea and the constant reassuring attitude of the nurse are extremely helpful. Small frequent meals may be more acceptable than 3 larger

meals a day. Periods of normal activity should be interspersed with time for rest and relaxation. The nurse can often help the patient through these difficult days by showing him that she understands why he feels discouraged and experiences malaise.

Radioisotope Therapy

The use of radioactive isotopes affords a method of delivering ionizing radiation that is extraordinarily versatile, one that is applicable to most types of cases, is convenient to administer and is relatively inexpensive for the patient.

Teletherapy

Teletherapy (*tele* = distance) uses gamma rays emitted by a radioactive source that is kept in a shielded unit located at a distance from the patient. Radiation of a type similar to that delivered by a supervoltage x-ray apparatus is obtained from radioisotopes cobalt-60 (^{60}Co) and cesium-137 (^{137}Cs). A ^{60}Co teletherapy unit is roughly comparable, in beam energy and penetration, to a 2-million-volt (2 MeV) x-ray machine. A weak beta emission from this isotope is screened out by interposing a thin metal filter between the source and the target. Assuming that the quantity of ^{60}Co is adequate, it and its protective casing (i.e., the "cobalt bomb") can be located at a considerable distance from the patient. The machine resembles an x-ray machine; however, when the x-ray machine is turned off, rays are not emitted. With the ^{60}Co teletherapy unit, the radioactive source is continuously emitting radiation and must be shielded by heavy shutters or a retractable device. Even so, because gamma rays cannot be absorbed entirely, it is suggested that one spend as little time as possible in this room.

The advantages of a ^{60}Co unit over conventional x-ray equipment are: (1) undesirable skin effects are materially reduced; (2) there is little bone or cartilage involvement; and (3) the unit does not depend on

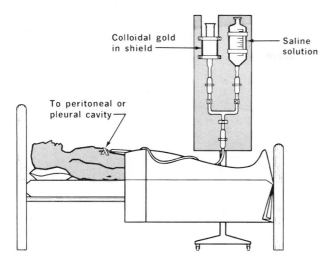

FIG. 12-5. Radioactive gold being injected into the peritoneal or pleural cavity. (U.S. Atomic Energy Commission)

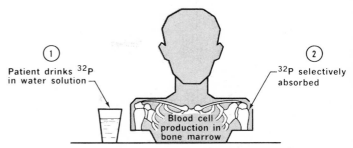

FIG. 12-6. Radioactive sodium phosphate has an affinity for thyroid tissue and bone marrow. (U.S. Atomic Energy Commission)

electronic circuits. The disadvantages are: (1) it is necessary to replace the ^{60}Co every 5 years (its half-life); (2) it is not possible to vary the radiation energy; and (3) the cost of room shielding is high.

External Molds

Cobalt-60 is employed also in external mold therapy, a method of irradiation in which the isotope, packaged and screened within an appropriate container, is applied directly to the skin surface. This method of application is of particular value in treating carcinomas of the lip, the ears, the scalp, the mouth, the larynx and the penis.

Another gamma emitter used in external molds is radioactive tantalum (^{182}Ta). Available in the form of flexible wire, this may be bent to conform to anatomic variations. For example, it may be applied in the form of a ring to the exterior surface of a retinoblastoma that involves the eyeball and the optic nerve. Radioactive strontium (^{90}Sr) and yttrium (^{90}Y), both pure beta emitters, are used in external molds for shallow irradiation of neoplasms in the eye. A most convenient method of applying beta radiation to superficial malignancies of the skin utilizes "plaques" consisting of bakelite, polyethylene plastic or blotting paper impregnated with radiophosphorus (^{32}P). These are cut and molded to size and shape, then taped in place over the lesion.

Intracavitary Isotope Therapy

Liquid radioisotopes—for example, solutions of radioactive colloidal gold (^{198}Au), radioactive sodium (^{24}Na) and bromine (^{82}Br)—have been placed in balloons within the bladder for beta irradiation of the

internal bladder wall to a depth of a few millimeters. Deeper penetration of the bladder is accomplished by gamma emission from a ^{60}Co source located in the center of a balloon that is distended within the center of the bladder. Capsules containing ^{182}Ta may be packed into the body of the uterus, the canal of the cervix or into a maxillary sinus.

Interstitial Isotope Therapy

Radioisotopes are available in the form of needles which can be implanted directly within the tumor tissue. These include cobalt-60, cesium-137, iridium-192, gold-198, radon-222, tantalum-182, and iodine-125. Such implants may be temporary or permanent and are frequently used as a supplement to surgery or to external beam irradiation. The implantation of radon seeds, needles, tubes or wires is done in the operating room under aseptic conditions. Interstitial irradiation also may be applied by injecting a radioisotope solution directly into the substance of the tumor and the surrounding tissue. Colloidal solutions of radioactive colloidal gold (^{198}Au) are especially suitable for this form of application. Radioactive colloidal gold also is injected into the pleural cavity, the colloid gradually precipitating onto the serosal surface, which is thereafter exposed to a pure beta emission (Fig. 12-5).

Internal Irradiation

Other clinical applications of radioisotopes include the treatment of myelogenous leukemia and polycythemia vera by intravenous injections of sodium phosphate (^{32}P). Solutions of radioiodine (^{131}I) are administered orally in patients with hyperthyroidism. The effectiveness of these measures is attributable to the fact that, in each instance, the target tissue has an affinity for, and concentrates within its substance, the therapeutic agent. Radioiodine becomes localized in the thyroid gland and metastatic thyroid tissue throughout the body, and radiophosphorus accumulates in the bones, where it is in close proximity to the proliferating marrow (Fig. 12-6).

Radioisotope Tests

Recent increases in the availability of isotope-tracer materials and improved methods of measuring radioactivity have opened entirely new approaches to the evaluation of the patient. Based on a variety of tracer techniques, several ingenious tests of organ function have been devised. The localization of certain malignant tumors has become possible, and, in some instances, methods are now available for observing and measuring biologic processes that hitherto have not been susceptible to direct demonstration. Representative tests, now in wide use and certain of general acceptance, are summarized below.

(See pp. 686 for Radioactive Iodine (^{131}I).

Radioactive Chromium (^{51}Cr) in Measurements of Blood Volume, Red Cell Longevity and Red Cell Sequestration in the Spleen

When sodium chromate-51 is added to samples of blood, the radioactive salt penetrates the red cell membranes, enters the erythrocytes and there becomes bound. These cells, for the remainder of their lifespan, are tagged with a radioactive label. Otherwise unaltered by the labeling process, the tagged cells can be used for a variety of in vivo tests, including measurements of the circulating red cell mass and red cell survival and for evaluating the role of the spleen in red cell destruction. The preliminary step in all of these tests is the collection of 10 to 50 ml. of venous blood into a sterile solution, to which is added sodium chromate-51. A red cell suspension is prepared and reinjected into the patient, an aliquot sample of the suspension being tested for "specific red cell activity," i.e., number of radioactive counts per ml. of red cells per minute. After a minimum of 1 hour following the injection of tagged red cells, a venous sample is obtained and likewise tested for specific red cell activity. The ratio of these values is inversely proportional to the volume of circulating red cells and the volume of red cells in the injected sample. The normal red cell volume ranges from 25 to 35 ml. per kilogram of body weight. The circulating plasma volume is calculated from the circulating red cell volume and the venous hematocrit, determined as described above. The plasma volume in normal individuals ranges from 40 to 50 ml. per kilogram of body weight.

The rate at which labeled red cells are eliminated from the circulation, based on successive changes in red cell radioactivity during the ensuing weeks, reflects the longevity of the mean red cell population. The normal lifespan may range from 110 to 130 days. In patients with hemolytic anemia, the lifespan of the red cells is relatively brief, e.g., 10 days or less, in the most severe cases. The degree to which the spleen is responsible for the destruction of red cells is often an important consideration in patients with hemolytic disease, for if there is evidence of excessive trapping of erythrocytes in that organ, its removal may be undertaken in the expectation of lessening hemolysis and correcting the anemia. Such evidence can be obtained by "external monitoring" over the splenic area and over a corresponding area on the opposite side (i.e., over the liver) after the patient has received an injection of ^{51}Cr-labeled red cells. The ratio of radioactive counts obtained simultaneously over these areas reflects the degree of red cell sequestration, hence, hemolysis in the spleen. If the splenic radioactivity exceeds liver radioactivity by a factor of more than two, splenectomy may be advised.

Radioactive [57]Co-Labeled Vitamin B₁₂, Absorption Test

Patients with pernicious anemia are constitutionally incapable of absorbing vitamin B_{12}, a characteristic that is unique. A radioactive tag ([57]Co) in the B_{12} molecule furnishes a simple means of detecting or excluding this absorption defect. The fasting patient receives a 1-microcurie oral dose of [57]Co-labeled B_{12} and the collection of urine is started. One to 3 hours later, a large quantity (1 mg., i.e., 1,000 micrograms) of nonradioactive B_{12} is injected intramuscularly for the purpose of saturating the tissues with B_{12}, thereby reducing the likelihood that any labeled B_{12} that may be absorbed from the intestine might be removed by the liver or stored elsewhere in the body. After this "loading dose" of unlabeled vitamin, whatever B_{12} may be contained in or enter the blood, including B_{12} absorbed from the intestine, is excreted in toto into the urine. Therefore, the proportion of the oral dose of [57]Co-labeled B_{12} that is absorbed in the blood of the patient can be calculated from the radioactivity of the urine that he excretes. This measurement is made 24 hours after the test dose.

As in the case of the ^{131}I excretion test of thyroid function (pp. 686) the measurement is valueless unless the 24-hour sample includes all the urine that has been voided during the test period. A second measurement may be made at the end of 48 hours, in which case a second loading dose of unlabeled B_{12} is injected intramuscularly at the beginning of the second day. Normal individuals excrete more than 10 to 20 per cent of the oral dose in 24 hours. The urinary excretion of less than 10 per cent is indicative of a malabsorption defect of some type, including pernicious anemia; the excretion of less than 3 per cent is presumptive evidence of pernicious anemia. Proof of this diagnosis may be secured by repeating the entire test, this time administering a preparation containing intrinsic factor along with the oral dose of [57]Co-labeled B_{12}. Under these conditions, the patient with pernicious anemia absorbs the labeled vitamin normally, and it will be detected in the urine in normal quantities. In patients with absorptive defects due to gastrointestinal disease, the absorption of B_{12}, hence its urinary excretion, is not increased by feeding intrinsic factor.

Radioisotopes: Nursing Precautions and Management

The receipt of a radioisotope in therapeutic dosage converts an individual temporarily into a radiation source, and the care of such an individual requires certain modifications if the nurse is to avoid the hazards of radiation exposure. The patient may wear a wristband with the radioactive symbol; his chart cover, doctor's and nurse's order sheets as well as special radiation instruction sheet should display the radioactive symbol in a prominent place. Such considerations do not apply, of course, in relation to patients undergoing radioisotope tracer tests, because of the relatively minute quantities of radiation that these involve.

The radiation instruction sheet includes the following information: type of radioactivity used, time of insertion, anticipated time of removal, precautions to be followed, and whom to notify when in doubt or in an emergency.

The location of the patient should be in an area that provides the greatest radiation safety to all personnel and other patients. By monitoring the area, the radiation safety officer is able to assure personnel that no undue radiation hazard exists. Psychologically, this has its advantages.

The amount of radioactivity that the nurse receives as she works near the patient depends on 3 factors: (1) her *distance* from the patient (doubling the distance from a radiation source cuts the intensity received to one fourth), (2) the amount of *time* spent in actual contact with him and (3) the degree of *shielding* provided. Such shielding usually is chosen according to the type of radiation in use, since alpha particles are absorbed by even a sheet of tissue paper, while gamma rays, on the other hand, may penetrate many inches of solid lead. During the first 24- to 72-hour period, which is the time of greatest radioactivity, actual nursing care must be limited to essential care. The patient should know why he must stay in bed or within his room during his course of treatment and why the nurse may not remain in his room longer than it takes to perform her nursing tasks.

Internal Use

The protective factors of time, distance and shielding help greatly with external radiation, but of these three, only time can be controlled when the radiation source has become internal through absorption, ingestion, injection, or other means.

All radioactive isotopes, by the very nature of their radioactivity, are destroying themselves at a rate that is constant but varies from one isotope to another. Each radiation particle or ray given off is the result of the destruction of one radioactive atom. So in time, all of the radiation disappears. Since this rate is constant, we can say that one half of the radioactivity is dissipated in a given time. For each isotope, we call this time the *physical half-life*.

In the body, any chemical substance is disposed of sooner or later by normal metabolic processes, so we can determine for any isotope how long it will take for one half to disappear from the body on a purely chemical and biologic basis. This we call the *biologic half-life*. Since both physical half-life and biologic half-life affect any internal isotope, the result is an *effective half-life* that is a combination of the other two.

In considering problems of internal radiation sources, it is extremely important to know the body's pattern of distribution, metabolism and excretion of each different isotope. An isotope that is completely dispersed throughout the body or a major portion of it is less hazardous to any one organ or tissue than another isotope concentrated by the body into a very localized organ or area. For instance, such concentration occurs with radioactive iodine in the thyroid gland, where most of the body's iodine is found. Naturally, an isotope that is excreted rapidly is less hazardous than one that is bound in the body for long periods of time.

It is easiest to consider the nursing problems of radiation sources in 2 major groups—those resulting from sealed sources, which are physically implanted in the patient, and those resulting from non-sealed sources that may be introduced into a patient.

Sealed internal radiation, such as radium, radon, iridium or gold seeds, is controlled from the moment of application in that the agent used is encased in a nonradioactive metallic covering so that it cannot directly contaminate any other object or tissue, even as it continues to radiate. The casing material absorbs all alpha radiation and most of the beta, so that the resulting hazard is one primarily of gamma radiation.

It is important that the nurse never fear such a patient. His internal radiation source cannot in any way be transferred to another person without actual contact. In addition, because the radiologist exercises safety controls, and as long as his orders and prescribed precautions are followed, the patient's internal radiation will not cause any other person to exceed normal exposure limits.

However, the radiation remains present, and, while

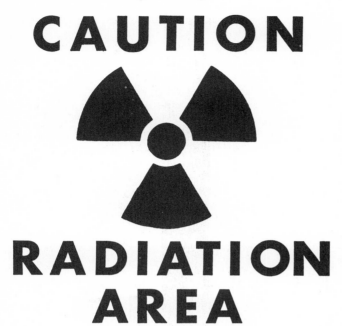

CAUTION

RADIATION AREA

Fig. 12-7. Radioactive symbol.[3]

giving the patient all the care that he needs and wants, the nurse should not linger with him unnecessarily.

If the implant is near the mouth, good oral hygiene is required. Before emptying the emesis basin, the nurse must check for dislodged implants.

In the unusual circumstance of a sealed source, such as a radium needle, becoming dislodged and perhaps falling on the bed or the floor, or being found in a dressing, it should be handled only with a long-handled forceps or tongs and reported immediately to the radiologist in charge.

The nurse should never discard a dressing or a bandage from such a patient until she is sure that it does not contain a radioactive source, which would not only become a hazard to others, but especially in the case of radium, also would be an expensive loss.

Although many patients are ambulatory, it is preferred that they remain within their own rooms. Usually, removal of implants is done in the radiology department. A check by radiograph or survey meter is made to be certain that all radioactive materials have been removed. Thereafter, radiation precautions are discontinued.

If the implant is permanent, such as is often the case in carcinoma of the bladder when radon seeds are used, the patient is on radiation precautions until the radiologist declares the hazard no longer existent. Meanwhile, all urine is collected and bed clothes are checked for possible lost seeds.

SUMMARY. (1) Follow directions on precaution sheet.

(2) Do not remain within 3 feet of the patient longer than is necessary to give required nursing care. Recognize the factors of time, shielding and distance.

(3) Never pick up dislodged radioactive sources with your hands. Use long-handled forceps. Notify the radiologist of such a dislodgement.

Unsealed Internal Radiation. The problems of *unsealed sources* are a bit more troublesome but when properly handled are no more dangerous. In these patients the radioactivity may be widely spread in the body, depending on a particular isotope's biologic distribution pattern. It may be localized or it may appear in any body tissue or fluid.

Probably the most widely used unsealed radioactive source is radioactive iodine, valuable in diagnosis and treatment of diseases of the thyroid gland. Of all the isotopes, it is the one most likely to be encountered by the nurse and is a good example for discussion of precautions to be followed with unsealed sources in general.

Except in unusual cases of large doses used for treatment, the radiation from a patient receiving iodine poses no important exposure hazard in ordinary nursing care; even with the largest dose, common sense observation of time and distance factors can control this problem.

However, since radioactive iodine, like most isotopes, circulates in the bloodstream and is excreted by the kidneys, both blood and urine of iodine patients contain radioactivity. In addition, it can be secreted by the sweat glands and is found in the vomitus of a patient who has recently taken an oral dose.

With iodine doses of the size used routinely for diagnostic purposes, the only major precaution is the careful handling and disposal of the patient's body fluids.

It is also wise to exercise extra care with bedpans as well as with any syringes and needles used, simply by seeing that all such contaminated objects are thoroughly washed before being returned to general use. The nurse's hands, especially, should be washed with extra care.

Wound dressings and bedclothes from patients who have received small tracer doses need only be wrapped well with paper or nonradioactive linens (so that no possible contamination is left exposed) and stored until safe for disposal.

In caring for patients who have received larger treatment doses, precautions must be somewhat more strict. With these individuals, items such as bedpans should be marked and used for that patient alone and never handled without rubber gloves. Dressings and bedclothes should also be handled with gloves during the first 2 or 3 days after administration of the dose, then treated as described above for tracer patients.

Because the radioactivity of iodine declines to one half in 8 days, and because the iodine is being removed constantly by the kidneys as well, all of these precautions become less important after the first 3 days and can usually be relaxed in 1 week.

Another radioactive isotope in general use is *radioactive phosphorus*. Essentially the same precautions apply here except that elimination is primarily in the feces instead of the urine. Since radioactive phosphorus emits no gamma radiation, as iodine does, phosphorus patients constitute no hazard as an external source.

Few nurses will encounter patients who have been treated with *radioactive colloidal gold*. In most instances, the gold is localized by injection into a single organ or body cavity. When gold is administered intravenously, the liver and the splenic tissue remove essentially all of the radioactive material from the blood within a very few hours. While direct contamination is less of a problem here, more attention must be given to the time spent with, and the distance from, the patient.

It is important to remember always that while the use of radiation may create new nursing problems, it is justified by its value to the patient. By understanding radiation and the problems of its use, regular nursing care can proceed safely, without worries of danger to the nurse and, most important, with no patient ever being neglected because of unreasonable fears or misunderstandings.

Radium. (See pp. 607 to 610)

BIBLIOGRAPHY

Augenstein, D.: Hyperbaric oxygen radiation therapy. Nurs. Forum, 7:324-335, No. 3, 1968.

Barnett, M.: The nature of radiation and its effect on man. Nurs. Clin. N. Amer., 2:11-22, March, 1966.

Bloedorn, F.: Principles—indication and prospects for preoperative irradiation. CA, 17:70-73, April, 1967.

Bouchard, R.: Nursing care of the cancer patient. pp. 42-49. St. Louis, C. V. Mosby, 1967.

Hilkemeyer, R.: Nursing care in radium therapy. Nurs. Clin. N. Amer., 2:83-95, March, 1967.

Hogerton, J. F.: Ionizing Radiation. New York, American Public Health Assoc., 1966.

Kautz, H. D., Storey, R. H., and Zimmermann, A. J.: Radioactive drugs. Amer. J. Nurs., 64:124-128, Jan., 1964.

Kendall, E. B.: Care of patients treated with sealed sources of radioisotopes. Nurs. Clin. N. Amer., 2:97-105, March, 1967.

King, Capt. E. R.: Survival in nuclear war. Clinical Symposia, Summit, N. J., Ciba Pharmaceutical, 14:3-33, Jan.-Feb.-Mar., 1962.

Schwartz, E. E. (ed.): The Biological Basis of Radiation Therapy. Philadelphia, J. B. Lippincott, 1966.

Wildermuth, O.: The care of hyperbaric oxygen radiotherapy. JAMA, 191:114-118, 1965.

U.S. Atomic Energy Commission, Division of Technical Information: Radioisotopes in Medicine. Oak Ridge, Tenn., 1966.

U.S. Dept. of Defense: The Effects of Nuclear Weapons. Washington, D.C., Supt. of Documents, 1964.

CHAPTER **13**

Nursing in Conditions of the Nose and the Throat

- *Anatomy of the Upper Respiratory Tract*
- *The Patient with Problems of the Nose*
- *Specific Infections of the Upper Respiratory Tract*
- *The Patient with Sinusitis*
- *The Patient with Problems of the Pharynx and Tonsils*
- *The Patient with Problems of the Larynx*
- *Aspirated Foreign Bodies*
- *Tracheotomy and Tracheostomy*

BASIC CONSIDERATIONS

The sole function of the respiratory system is to serve as a route of gaseous exchange between the atmosphere surrounding the body and the tissues within, so that the cells may have access to the oxygen that they require and a means of dissipating their waste carbon dioxide.

Any abnormality involving the respiratory system that interferes with its primary function is a potential threat to every organ, tissue and cell in the body, since it can easily result in a general state of oxygen deficiency complicated by carbon dioxide poisoning. A certain amount of interference of this sort, impairing aeration, is one of the most common and important complications of respiratory diseases.

Conditions that interfere with this mechanism result in an incomplete oxygenation of the blood, or *hypoxemia*. Arterial blood no longer has its bright red color; it is a dark purplish red. The patient's skin takes on a bluish pallor (cyanosis), which is best noted in the nail beds, the lips and the tongue.

Hypoxemia may occur from circulatory difficulties, such as cardiac failure, congenital cardiac or vascular defects, pulmonary embolism and so forth. Certain drugs interfere with the oxygenation of the blood (sulfanilamide, acetanilid) and produce cyanosis.

A very high proportion of respiratory diseases is infectious. In fact, infections of the upper respiratory tract, considered as a group, represent the most common of all illnesses. One reason may be that the external surface of the respiratory organs, including the alveolar walls, presents a very extensive area of exposure to the bacteria-laden atmosphere. Moreover, respiratory infections are spread far more readily than are other types of infections, owing to the rate at which virulent organisms are dispersed in the expired air of infected patients, with the obvious likelihood that these contaminants soon enter numerous other respiratory tracts in the vicinity.

Consideration is given in this chapter to both major and minor problems that cause interference with the normal function of the upper respiratory tract. In this unit, the major objectives of study are to understand the complications that may result from simple upper respiratory infections and to recognize the nurse's role in teaching individuals how to control the spread of upper respiratory infections. (See pp. 274 for physiology of respiration.)

ANATOMY OF THE UPPER RESPIRATORY TRACT

Nose

The nose has 2 passages, called *nares*, separated in the middle by the septum. These passages open ex-

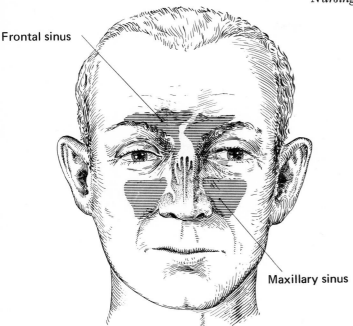

Frontal sinus

Maxillary sinus

Fig. 13-1. Position of nasal sinuses and their relation to facial structures.

ternally through the anterior nostrils and posteriorly into the nasopharynx. Between these 2 openings the air passages expand into broad chambers, on the lateral sides of which are 3 turbinate bones and into which open the paranasal sinuses, cavities within the hollow bones that surround the nasal passages.

Paranasal Sinuses

These include the frontal sinuses, located in the lower forehead between and above the eyes; the ethmoidal group of sinuses, both anterior and posterior, extending along the roof of the nostrils; the sphenoid sinuses, opening at the rear; and, located on either side of the nose, the maxillary sinuses, or antra. The same type of ciliated epithelium that lines the nasal passages also lines these paranasal sinuses.

A prominent function of the sinuses is to help give resonance and timber to speech. One notes how "nasal" the voice is when an individual has a head cold and sinusitis.

Turbinate Bones

The turbinate bones, the name of which was suggested by their shell-like appearance, are adapted by shape and position to increase the mucous membrane surface of the nasal passages and to obstruct slightly the current of air flowing through them. The sense organs of smell are located in the olfactory membrane, which covers the roof of the nose and the superior turbinate bones.

The current of air entering the anterior nostrils is deflected upward to the roof of the nose, describing a circuitous route before it reaches the nasopharynx. Therefore, it comes into contact with a large surface of moist, warm, mucous membrane that catches practically all dust and germs in the inhaled air. This air is moistened and warmed to body temperature and

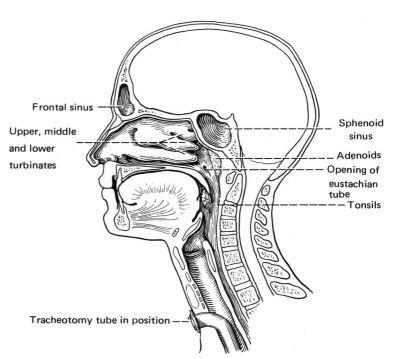

Frontal sinus

Upper, middle and lower turbinates

Sphenoid sinus

Adenoids

Opening of eustachian tube

Tonsils

Tracheotomy tube in position

Fig. 13-2. The parts of the upper respiratory tract and their relation to each other. In the lower part of the neck there is a tracheotomy tube in position.

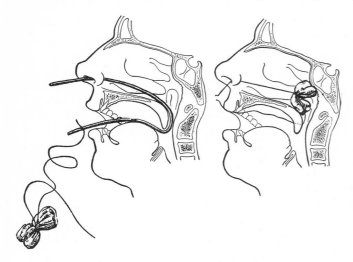

Fig. 13-3. Postnasal packing. (*Left*) The gauze pack is attached to a catheter with string. The catheter is then passed through the mouth and back out through the nose. (*Right*) After the pack is drawn into position, the ends of the string are taped to the cheek. (Pfizer Laboratories)

brought into contact with sensitive nerves, some of which detect odors and others of which provoke sneezing to expel irritating dust.

Pharynx

The pharynx is the throat. It is limited below by the larynx and the upper end of the esophagus. Its upper extension is the nasopharynx, into which open the posterior nostrils and the eustachian tubes from the middle ears. The nose and the nasopharynx are lined with the same type of ciliated epithelium as the trachea and the bronchial tree; but the pharynx, which serves as both a respiratory and an alimentary passage, is lined with squamous (flat-celled) epithelium.

Tonsils and Adenoids

The tonsils are 2 almond-shaped bodies, one on each side at the back of the throat. The adenoid, or pharyngeal tonsil, is located in the roof of the nasopharynx. The tonsils and the adenoids constitute only 2 of a ring of similar masses of lymphoid tissue that completely encircles the throat. These organs are important links in the chain of lymph nodes guarding the body from invasion by organisms entering the nose and the throat.

Larynx

The larynx is a cartilaginous epithelial-lined structure forming the upper extremity of the trachea. The vocal cords, controlled by muscular attachments, are mounted in its lumen. Over it, preventing the entry

of ingested food or liquid, is attached a valve flap called the *epiglottis*. The whole function of the larynx is to permit vocalization. It is the "voice box."

THE PATIENT WITH PROBLEMS OF THE NOSE

Epistaxis (Nosebleed)

Epistaxis may result from injury or disease. It is due to the rupture of tiny, distended vessels in the mucous membrane of the anterior septum and is not uncommon in normal young persons. The usual cause of small nosebleeds is "picking" of the nose. Other local causes are deviated septum, perforated septum, cancer and trauma. Epistaxis may also occur as a symptom of acute rheumatic fever, acute sinusitis, arterial hypertension and hemorrhagic diseases.

Treatment. In providing emergency care, remember that cessation of bleeding is aided by the maintenance of an elevated position of the trunk and by promoting vasoconstriction in the nasal mucous membrane. Instruct the patient to refrain from talking and to breathe through his mouth. The patient should compress the soft outer portion of the nose against the midline septum for 5 or 10 minutes continuously. The instillation of a local vasoconstricting drug, such as Neo-Synephrine, into the nostril may be helpful. Should these measures fail, the physician may find it necessary to apply Adrenalin or a cauterizing agent, such as silver nitrate solution or stick, to the bleeding point.

Often, however, the origin of the bleeding cannot be found. In these patients, after spraying the nose with cocaine and Adrenalin solutions, a rubber finger cot or the finger of a rubber glove may be inserted into the nostril, the open end being held with 3 or 4 hemostats while gauze packing is inserted (Fig. 13-3). This is postnasal packing. Pressure may be increased by moistening the gauze. The packing should be removed after 24 hours.

Rhinitis

Rhinitis is an inflammatory lesion involving the mucous membrane of the nose. It is sometimes a manifestation of allergy, in which instance it is referred to as "vasomotor rhinitis," but usually it is due to an infection. The most common variety of infection causing it is "coryza" (the common cold); it also is encountered with regularity in the early stages of measles and other specific viral infections.

In acute rhinitis, the nasal mucous membrane becomes congested, swollen and edematous. This quickly subsides, and the membrane returns to normal. After repeated attacks, however, particularly in cases which originate as a result of chronic sinusitis, this swelling

Fig. 13-4. Student securing bandage after submucous resection. (Loma Linda University)

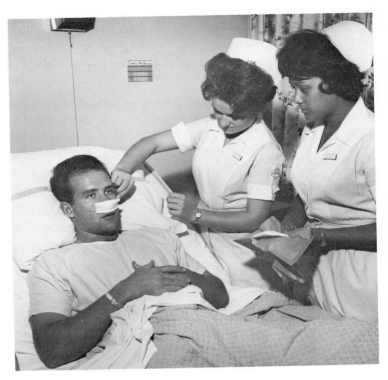

becomes obstinate, and the patient has a "chronic catarrh." These persons say that they are "subject to colds." The fact is that, excluding the recurring attacks of allergic vasomotor rhinitis, their attacks are acute exacerbations of the same "cold." If continued, chronic rhinitis leads to the deposition of abnormally large amounts of connective tissue in the nasal mucous membrane, which greatly thickens it, and causes the formation of spurs, polyps and hypertrophies on the nasal septum. Wasting or atrophy of the mucous membrane, the cartilage and the bones lining the nasal passages eventually may occur, with the result that these passages become large empty caverns, adhering to the walls of which is an abundant exudate emanating a disagreeable odor. This condition is called *ozena*.

The patient should be cautioned against blowing his nose too frequently or too hard. It should be done with the mouth open slightly while blowing through both nostrils to equalize the pressure.

Nasal Obstruction

Obstruction to the passage of air through the nostrils results frequently from a deflection of the nasal septum, hypertrophy of the turbinate bones or from the pressure of polyps—grapelike swellings that arise from the mucous membrane of the sinuses, especially the ethmoids. This obstruction also may lead to a condition of chronic infection of the nose and result in frequent attacks of nasopharyngitis. Very frequently the infection extends to the sinuses of the nose (mucous-lined cavities filled with air that drain normally into the nose). When sinusitis develops and the drainage from these cavities is obstructed by deformity or swelling within the nose, pain is experienced in the region of the affected sinus.

Treatment. The treatment of this condition requires the removal of the nasal obstruction, followed by measures to overcome whatever chronic infection exists. In many patients the underlying nasal allergy is the lesion requiring treatment. At times it is necessary to drain the nasal sinuses by radical operation. The operations performed depend on the type of nasal obstruction found. Usually they are performed with local anesthesia. This is obtained by introducing into the nostrils pledgets of cotton soaked in 10 per cent cocaine solution with Adrenalin. The nurse who assists the surgeon in operations on the nose and the throat must be extremely careful to identify the solutions of cocaine and procaine, for the toxic nature of cocaine when injected hypodermically would make the mistake a most serious one.

If a deflection of the septum is the cause of the obstruction, the surgeon makes an incision in the mucous membrane and, after raising it from the bone, removes the deflected bone and cartilage with bone forceps. The mucosa then is allowed to fall back in place and is held there by tight packing. Generally the packing used is soaked in liquid petrolatum to facilitate its removal in 24 to 36 hours. This operation is called commonly a *submucous resection* (Fig. 13-4).

Nasal polyps are removed by clipping them at their base with a wire snare. Hypertrophied turbinates may be treated by astringent applications to shrink them up close to the side of the nose.

After these procedures, the head of the bed is elevated to promote drainage and to help to alleviate the patient's discomfort due to edema. Frequent oral hygiene should be given because the patient breathes through his mouth.

Fractures of the Nose

Fractures of the nose usually result from direct violence. As a rule, they do not produce any serious consequences, but the deformity that may follow often gives rise to obstruction of the nasal air passages and to facial disfigurement.

Immediately after the injury there is usually considerable bleeding from the nose, both from the nostrils and into the pharynx. There is marked swelling of the soft tissues adjacent to the nose and, frequently, a definite deformity.

Treatment and Nursing Care. As a rule, the bleeding can be controlled by the application of cold compresses. A roentgenogram is helpful in determining the displacement of the fractured bones and in ruling out an extension of the fracture into the skull. With local cocainization of the nose or with intravenous anesthesia, it is possible usually to bring displaced fragments into alignment and then hold them by intranasal packing or external splints. The important points in the reduction of the fracture are to reform the nasal passages and to realign the bones so as to prevent disfiguring deformity. After reduction, the swelling that occurs may be decreased by the application of ice compresses with the patient in the sitting position.

Plastic Surgery of the Nose

The nose is such a prominent organ of the face that its deformity may cause the patient considerable embarrassment. The deformity may result from congenital causes, from disease or from injury.

Deformities resulting from congenital causes often may be corrected by simple operations in which the nose is straightened or lengthened by either removing offending bone or supplying new tissue (usually costal cartilage). The incisions are so placed as to be inconspicuous. In deformities resulting from injury or disease, various types of plastic surgery may be employed. Skin, tube or sliding grafts may be used to cover the defects left by scars, malignancy or injuries. In some instances, especially in older people with malignancy, artificial appliances may be modeled and held in place with the rims of glasses. (See Reconstructive Surgery, pp. 647-655.)

Nursing Care. After operation the patient usually is placed flat on his back with the head slightly elevated. Ice compresses are used frequently after operation to reduce bleeding, swelling and pain. Hemorrhage is the chief postoperative complication, and it must be remembered that the spitting up or the vomiting of blood that has run back into the pharynx is as much a symptom of nasal hemorrhage as is the flow at the nares. Frequent swallowing, followed by belching, often is indicative of bleeding that results in an accumulation of blood in the stomach.

In patients with whom local anesthesia has been used, the blood sometimes trickles down the throat, but the patient is not sufficiently aware of it to show a swallow reflex. If the bleeding is excessive or continuous, or if any of the constitutional signs of hemorrhage appear, the surgeon should be called, and the nurse should have ready for his use fresh packing, a light, a head mirror, a nasal speculum and packing forceps.

These patients may have a liquid diet on the day of operation and whatever they prefer after that. Sedatives often are necessary on the day and the night of operation, but after that there is little need of them. The patient is tempted often to blow his nose because of a full feeling, but if it is explained to him that this is because of the packing in his nose, he will be more patient. Packing is removed usually after 24 hours.

SPECIFIC INFECTIONS OF THE UPPER RESPIRATORY TRACT

Common Cold

The phrase "common cold" is a general term used by patients in different ways, usually referring to symptoms of upper respiratory infection. These symptoms are nasal discharge and obstruction, sore throat, sneezing, malaise, feverishness, chilliness and often headache and muscle aching. As the cold progresses, cough usually appears. Most specifically, the term means afebrile, infectious acute coryza. More broadly the term refers to acute upper respiratory infection and terms such as rhinitis, pharyngitis, laryngitis, chest cold and so on distinguish the sites of the major symptoms. The symptoms last 5 days to 2 weeks. If there is significant fever or more severe constitutional symptoms with the respiratory symptoms, we are no longer dealing with a common cold but with one of the other acute upper respiratory infections. Many different viruses (over 100) are known to produce the symptoms of the common cold and about 10 per cent of colds seem associated simultaneously with more than one virus. Also allergic conditions affecting the nose can mimic the symptoms of a cold. Colds are highly contagious and patients shed virus for about 2 days before the symptoms appear and during the first part of their symptomatic phase. Colds prevail among 15 per cent of the work population at any time during the winter and account for almost half of all work absences and one-quarter of the total time lost from work.

Three waves of colds appear yearly in the United States—in the fall just after the opening of school, in midwinter and in spring. Immunity after recovery is variable, depending on many factors including natural host resistance and which virus caused the cold in the first place. The major complication of a cold is the secondary bacterial infection in the ears, nose, sinuses, bronchi or lungs.

Treatment of the common cold consists of good fluid intake, rest, prevention of chilling, aqueous nasal decongestants, bronchodilators and expectorants as needed. Warm salt water gargles soothe the sore throat; aspirin relieves the general constitutional symptoms. Antibiotics are not indicated in the uncomplicated common cold. The use of disposable tissues and their hygienic disposal, covering of the mouth when coughing and avoidance of crowding are about all that can be offered in the way of prevention.

Streptococcal Sore Throat

Ranking high among the most uncomfortable, debilitating and dangerous of the upper respiratory tract infections are those produced by the Group A streptococcus. This type of infection is characterized by the abrupt onset of sore throat, chilly sensations or frank chills, temperature elevations above 38.3° C. (101° F.), headache and general malaise. Children may experience acute abdominal pain, nausea and repeated vomiting during the acute phase of this infection. The pharynx is diffusely reddened; the tonsils and the tonsillar nodes beneath the angles of the mandible enlarge; the uvula becomes edematous. A patchy or confluent exudate covers the tonsils and the pharynx. The face is flushed, and individuals who are not immune to the exotoxin of the Group A streptococcus (i.e., who are "Dick positive") are likely to develop the typical rash of scarlet fever. The blood leukocyte count generally exceeds 12,000.

Nursing Management and Chemotherapy. The nursing care of patients with acute pharyngitis, including the type due to the hemolytic streptococcus, is discussed in detail on pages 214 to 215. Early chemotherapy in patients with hemolytic streptococcal infection is of the utmost importance from the standpoint of preventing its most serious complications—acute rheumatic fever and acute glomerulonephritis. Penicillin is the drug of choice, given for 10 days, and the intramuscular route is the optimal method of administration. Antibiotics that may serve as adequate substitutes for penicillin in the event of sensitivity include erythromycin, tetracycline, chlortetracycline and oxytetracycline.

Adenovirus Infections

There are 31 human types in this group of viruses, of which 9 cause respiratory illnesses and another one keratoconjunctivitis. Acute respiratory disease (ARD), pharyngoconjunctival fever, febrile pharyngitis and some pneumonias in children are due to this group.

ARD shows the symptoms of a cold, sore throat, bronchitis, headache, malaise and high fever and, infrequently, pneumonia.

Pharyngoconjunctival fever shows the symptoms of a cold, exhibits a 1- to 10-day fever, sore throat and large tender cervical lymph nodes, hoarseness, headache, malaise and acute conjunctivitis. This infection is usually seen in the summer in children and is related to swimming pools.

Febrile pharyngitis exhibits the symptoms of a cold, pharyngitis, bronchitis, marked fever, prostration and occasionally pneumonia. Especially in young children, nausea and vomiting may also occur.

Rhinovirus infections, of which 53 types are known, are associated with the symptoms of the common cold and croup, bronchitis, bronchopneumonia and may cause as much as 40 per cent of acute respiratory illness in adults.

Respiratory syncytial virus infection can cause febrile upper respiratory infections and bronchopneumonia. There are no specific antibiotic therapies for any of the adenovirus groups.

Herpes Simplex Infection

The herpes simplex virus most commonly produces the familiar *herpes labialis* (cold sore, fever blister or canker), but in children who are reacting to this virus for the first time, the infection may take the form of an acute herpetic gingivostomatitis. Small vesicles, single or clustered, may erupt on the lips, the tongue, the cheeks and the pharynx. These soon rupture, forming sore, shallow ulcers that are covered with a gray membrane. Herpes infections appear often in association with other febrile infections, such as pneumococcus pneumonia, meningococcic meningitis and malaria. The virus remains latent in cells of lips or nose and is activated by febrile illnesses. The herpes virus does not yield in the slightest to any of the chemotherapeutic agents that have become available to date. Analgesics and codeine are helpful in relieving pain and discomfort. Applications of spirits of nitre may help dry the lesions.

Prevention of Upper Respiratory Infections

The prevention of most upper respiratory tract infections is difficult as their cause is legion. The responsible pathogen usually cannot be identified and vaccines are unavailable except in rare instances. Allergies, septum and turbinate pathology, emotional problems and various systemic illnesses may be predisposing factors in isolated cases. The following hygienic measures tend to support the body defenses and reduce susceptibility to respiratory infections:

(1) Practice good health measures to include a nutritious diet, appropriate exercise, adequate rest and sleep

(2) Avoid excesses in alcohol and smoking

(3) Correct air dryness by proper home humidification, especially during cold weather

(4) Avoid air contaminants (dust, chemicals) when possible

(5) Avoid unnecessary chilling of the skin especially the feet; chilling lowers resistance

(6) Obtain influenza vaccination if and when directed by the physician.

THE PATIENT WITH SINUSITIS

The sinuses are involved in a high proportion of upper respiratory tract infections. If their openings into the nasal passages are clear, the infections within them recover promptly; but if their drainage is obstructed by a deflected septum or by hypertrophied turbinates, spurs or polyps, the sinusitis may persist as a smoldering secondary infection or it may flare up into an acute suppurative process.

Acute Sinusitis

Acute sinusitis may be localized to one sinus or may involve several. If all are involved, the condition is called *pansinusitis.* The most prominent symptom of acute sinusitis is pain, the location of which is diagnostically important, and therefore should be noted by the nurse. In *frontal sinusitis,* the patient complains of frontal headache; in *ethmoidal sinusitis,* the pain is usually in or about the eyes; in *maxillary sinusitis,* pain is lateral to the nose and sometimes is accompanied by aching of the upper teeth of the corresponding side; in *sphenoidal sinusitis,* occipital headache may result. Nasal congestion and discharge are usually, but not necessarily, present. The patient feels generally miserable, quite apart from pain. Fever, however, if present at all, is usually mild. This may be the case even in the presence of an acute suppurative infection, or "empyema" of a sinus. The most dangerous variety of sinusitis is empyema of a frontal sinus, because it may rupture posteriorly, producing a brain abscess.

The treatment of acute sinusitis is bed rest and the establishment of free drainage of the sinuses involved.

This usually can be accomplished by nasal instillations or sprays of Neo-Synephrine (¼ per cent) or a similar vasoconstrictor drug. Depending on the type of infecting organism and the extent of the infection, the patient may be instructed to apply local therapy of this sort at intervals of 1 to 4 hours until drainage is established. The use of penicillin usually speeds recovery and definitely diminishes the chance of complications that follow the extension of a bacterial sinusitis. One of the antihistaminic agents (e.g., Pyribenzamine or thenylpyramine fumarate) in oral doses (25 to 50 mg.) may be beneficial, at least symptomatically, in very early cases.

Chronic Sinusitis

Chronic sinusitis usually manifests itself by persistent nasal obstruction, due to discharge and edema of the nasal mucous membrane. The patient experiences cough, due to the constant dripping of the discharge backward into the nasopharynx, and headaches, which are apt to be most pronounced on awakening in the morning.

The treatment of chronic sinusitis usually is the use of vasoconstricting drugs locally, in the form of sprays or nose drops, in an effort to establish proper drainage. The abuse of nasal decongestants by overuse or prolonged use may aggravate rhinitis and sinusitis by causing rebound congestion, thereby leading to further overuse. Oily nose drops are to be avoided. Sterile Ringer's solution used with a nasal douche can be obtained in any drugstore and is a soothing method of cleansing the nose. Structural deformities that obstruct the ostia of the sinus may require surgical attention: polyps may require excision or cauterization, a deflected septum may have to be removed or a narrowed ostium widened.

For drainage of the maxillary sinus, the incision is made along the upper gum line above the canine teeth (Caldwell-Luc operation). To drain the frontal sinus an incision is made through the inner third of the eyebrow.

Some victims of severe chronic sinusitis obtain relief only by moving to a dry climate.

THE PATIENT WITH PROBLEMS OF THE PHARYNX AND THE TONSILS

Pharyngitis

Acute Pharyngitis

Acute pharyngitis, caused by several viruses and bacteria, is a febrile inflammation of the throat. The pharyngeal membrane becomes fiery red; the lymphoid follicles of the throat and the tonsils become swollen and flecked with exudate, and there may be tender enlargement of the cervical lymph nodes. Uncomplicated virus infections usually recover promptly, within 3 to 10 days after the onset. But pharyngitis caused by certain of the more virulent bacteria, such as beta hemolytic streptococcus, hemolytic *Staphylococcus aureus*, influenza, or the diphtheria bacillus, is a more severe illness during the acute stage and far more important in the incidence of dangerous complications. These complications include sinusitis, otitis media, mastoiditis, cervical adenitis, rheumatic fever, nephritis and, in the case of infection by the diphtheria bacillus, paralysis. A throat culture is the chief means of determining the causative organism. When this is obtained, proper therapy can be prescribed.

Nursing Management. The patient should be kept in bed during the febrile stage of his illness. When he is ambulatory he needs periods of rest. Medical asepsis must be observed to prevent the spread of infection. Examine the skin once or twice daily for possible rash, because acute pharyngitis may precede some other communicable disease.

Aside from throat cultures, it may be necessary to secure nasal swabbings and blood cultures for further laboratory investigation to determine the nature of the causative organism.

Warm saline gargles or irrigations are employed, depending on the severity of the lesion and the degree of pain. Recognizing that the benefits of this treatment depend on the degree of heat that is applied, the nurse should ensure that the temperature of the solution is sufficiently high to be effective, i.e., approaching the limits of tolerance, which vary with each individual patient but never exceed 48.8° C. (120° F.). A throat irrigation, properly performed, is the most effective means available for reducing spasm in the pharyngeal muscles and relieving soreness of the throat. However, unless the principle of the procedure and its technique are understood clearly by the patient, the results may be less than completely satisfactory. Patients for whom the throat irrigation is a new experience should have it explained in advance by the nurse.

Symptomatic relief in patients with severe sore throat also may be afforded by the application of an ice collar and by means of analgesic drugs, e.g., aspirin or acetophenetidin in doses of 0.3 to 0.6 gm. given at 3 to 6-hour intervals and, if required, codeine sulfate, 15 to 30 mg. (0.25 to 0.5 gr.), 3 or 4 times daily. Antitussive medication, in the form of codeine, Hycodan or Toryn, may be required to control a persistent and painful cough that often accompanies acute pharyngitis. One of the barbiturates, e.g., Nembutal (0.1 to 0.2 gm.), may be prescribed for the patient as a soporific at bedtime.

If a bacterial etiology is suspected or demonstrated, treatment may include the administration of antimicrobial agents.

A liquid or soft solid diet is provided during the acute stage of the disease, depending on the patient's appetite and the degree of discomfort caused by swallowing.

The patient should be encouraged to drink to the limit of tolerance, the minimal intake during the febrile stage exceeding, if possible, 2,500 ml. each day. Success is often aided if the rationale of therapy is explained adequately to the patient. His personal tastes also need to be considered and indulged when possible.

Mouth care may add greatly to the patient's comfort and aid in preventing the development of fissures of the lips and pyoderma about the mouth in patients with bacterial infection.

Convalescent Care. Resumption of full activity should not be permitted until a period of time has elapsed that is at least equal to that of complete bed rest. Unusually conservative management is indicated in patients with hemolytic streptococcus infection in view of the possible development of complications such as nephritis and rheumatic fever, which may have their onset 2 or 3 weeks after the pharyngitis has subsided. Local extension of an apparently quiescent pharyngitis may develop in the form of sinusitis, otitis media, mastoiditis or cervical adenitis. Daily recording of morning and evening temperatures should be continued until convalescence is complete, and the patient or his family should be familiarized with symptoms that deserve investigation from the standpoint of a possible complication.

Chronic Pharyngitis

This disease is common in adults who work amid dusty surroundings, use the voice to excess and suffer from chronic cough. Its incidence also is high among habitual users of alcohol and tobacco.

Nasal congestion may be relieved by nasal instillations or sprays containing ephedrine sulfate, Neo-Synephrine or Tuamine sulfate in saline, and, in the early stages, one of the antihistaminic drugs such as Pyribenzamine, pyranisamine maleate or thenylpyramine fumarate in doses of 25 to 30 mg. every 4 to 6 hours by mouth. The attendant malaise is controlled effectively by aspirin or acetophenetidin. Contact with others should be avoided, at least until the fever has subsided completely, in order to prevent spreading the infection.

Three types of chronic pharyngitis are recognized: (1) hypertrophic, characterized by general thickening and congestion of the pharyngeal mucous membrane; (2) atrophic, probably a late stage of the above (this membrane is thin, whitish, glistening and, at times, wrinkled); and (3) chronic granular ("clergyman's sore throat"), with numerous swollen lymph follicles on the pharyngeal wall.

Patients with chronic pharyngitis complain of a

constant sense of irritation or fullness in the throat, of mucus collecting in the throat and expelled by coughing and of difficulty in swallowing. While chronic pharyngitis is annoying, it seldom disturbs the general health.

Treatment. The treatment of chronic pharyngitis consists of the avoidance of alcohol and tobacco, resting the voice and the correction of any upper respiratory, pulmonary or cardiac condition that might be responsible for a chronic cough.

Diseases of the Tonsils and the Adenoids

Tonsils

The tonsils are 2 groups of lymphatic tissue situated one on each side of the oropharynx. They are frequently the seat of acute infectious processes and of chronic infection, constantly giving off toxins in small amounts. Therefore, they are considered one of the most common sites of focal infection, producing chronic systemic diseases such as chronic arthritis, nephritis and so forth. Furthermore, they often grow to such a size as to interfere with normal respiration, a condition that is spoken of as hypertrophy of the tonsils.

Frequent acute infections, chronic infections, hypertrophy—all are regarded as indications for the removal of the tonsils.

Tonsillectomy may be performed under local anesthesia with the patient in a sitting position or under general anesthesia with the patient in the dorsal position. The tongue is depressed and the tonsil is grasped with tenaculum forceps. The tonsil is freed by blunt and sharp dissection sufficient to allow the snare to encircle the remaining attachment, which is crushed and the tonsil is removed. Hemorrhage usually is controlled by pressure with small gauze sponges. Occasionally it is necessary to clamp and ligate the bleeding vessel. Often the blood is swallowed, or, if the patient is unconscious, it will run down into the stomach and not be recognized until the patient vomits copiously.

Adenoids

Acute adenoiditis. A common accompaniment of acute tonsillitis, enlargement of the adenoid is responsible for the nasal obstruction and, to a certain extent, the vertical headache commonly experienced in this infection.

Chronic adenoiditis. This is of particular importance because the adenoid, when hypertrophied, is in a position to obstruct the posterior nares and the eustachian tubes (Fig. 13-2). Adenoid hypertrophy may cause (1) mouth breathing, tendency to facial deformities, and crooked teeth, (2) earaches, draining ears, and

mastoid infection, (3) frequent head colds, bronchitis, (4) fetid breath, voice impairment, snoring and noisy respiration.

Extension of the infection to the middle ears by way of the eustachian tubes may result in acute otitis media, the potential complications of which include spontaneous rupture of the ear drums and further extension into the mastoid cells, causing acute mastoiditis; or the infection may reside in the middle ear as a chronic, low-grade smoldering process that eventually may lead to permanent deafness.

Because enlarged adenoids are the cause of a long list of symptoms, adenoidectomy is recommended as soon as the condition is discovered, even if this is in infancy. The treatment, of course, is operative removal, which is done usually in conjunction with a tonsillectomy.

Nursing Care Following Tonsillectomy and Adenoidectomy

The chief danger after these operations is from hemorrhage; therefore, most surgeons require an evaluation of hemostasis before operation. Atropine always should be given before operation under general anesthesia to decrease the amount of mucous secretion. After operation, the patient should be placed in the dorsal or the sitting position, according to the postoperative orders. For patients who have had general anesthesia, the most comfortable position is prone, with the head turned to the side to allow for drainage from the throat. The airway should not be removed until the patient demonstrates that his swallowing reflex has returned.

An ice collar should be applied and a basin and gauze provided for the expectoration of blood and mucus. Children are treated best by placing them in the prone position with the head turned to the side, so that secretion may drain from the mouth and the pharynx.

Bleeding may be bright red if the patient spits it out at once. Often, however, it is swallowed and becomes brown in color immediately, due to the action of the acid gastric juice. If the patient vomits large amounts of altered blood or spits bright blood at frequent intervals, or if the pulse rate increases gradually, the attending surgeon should be notified. The nurse should have in readiness a light, a head mirror, gauze, curved hemostats and a waste basin. Occasionally it may be necessary to suture or ligate the bleeding vessel. In such cases the patient must be taken to the operating room and given anesthesia.

If there is no bleeding, water and cracked ice may be given the patient as soon as desired. Instruct the patient to refrain from too much talking and coughing, because this can produce throat pain. Alkaline mouth washes may be useful in coping with the thick mucus that may be present after a tonsillectomy.

The diet should be liquid or semiliquid for several days, excluding orange or lemon juice and other acids. Ice cream, ice sherbet, gelatin desserts, custards, and Junkets are very acceptable foods, especially for children.

Home Instruction. The patient may be discharged from the hospital the day after the operation, but he should convalesce at home for several days. This means getting plenty of rest and resuming activity gradually. Any bleeding should be reported to the physician; secondary hemorrhage may occur about a week after operation.

Sulfonamides and Antibiotics. In all of these acute infections of the pharynx, sulfonamides and antibiotics are used. They are given prophylactically, as well as therapeutically, before and after surgical procedures on the pharynx and the larynx.

Peritonsillar Abscess (Quinsy)

Peritonsillar abscess, or quinsy, is an abscess that develops above the tonsil in the tissues of the anterior pillar and soft palate (Fig. 13-5). As a rule, it is secondary to a tonsillar infection. The usual symptoms of an infection are present, together with such local symptoms as difficulty in swallowing (dysphagia), thickening of the voice, drooling and local pain. An examination shows marked swelling of the soft palate, often to the extent of half-occluding the orifice from the mouth into the pharynx.

Treatment. A considerable measure of relief may be obtained by throat irrigations or the frequent use of mouthwashes or gargles, using saline or alkaline solutions at a temperature of 40.6° to 43.3° C. (105° to 110° F.). This treatment hastens the pointing of the process.

The abscess should be evacuated as soon as possible. The mucous membrane over the swelling first is painted with 10 per cent cocaine solution; then, after a small incision has been made, the points of a blunt hemostat are forced into the abscess pocket and opened as they are withdrawn. This operation is performed best with the patient in the sitting position, as it is easier then for him to expectorate the pus and the blood that accumulate in the pharynx. Almost immediate relief is experienced. After-treatment is warm gargles at intervals of 1 or 2 hours for 24 to 36 hours.

Some laryngologists advocate bilateral tonsillectomy for acute peritonsillar abscess; they claim that this is necessary to prevent recurrences and eliminate unsuspected asymptomatic pockets of infection.

Antibiotics, usually penicillin, are extremely effective

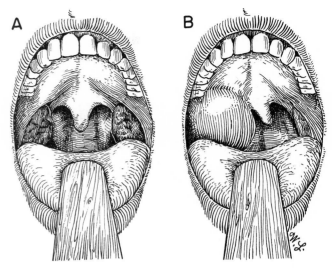

Fig. 13-5. Views of oral pharynx. (A) Showing enlargement of the tonsils. (B) Showing peritonsillar abscess on the right-hand side.

in the control of the infection in peritonsillar abscess. Given early in the course of the disease, the abscess may be aborted, and incision can be avoided. If antibiotics are not given until later, the abscess must be drained, but improvement in the inflammatory reaction is rapid.

THE PATIENT WITH PROBLEMS OF THE LARYNX

Laryngitis

Acute laryngitis is manifested by hoarseness or complete loss of the voice (aphonia) and by severe cough. The treatment is bed rest, steam inhalations and abstinence from talking and smoking. If the laryngitis is part of a more extensive respiratory infection due to a bacterial organism, or if it is severe, appropriate antibacterial chemotherapy should be instituted.

Chronic laryngitis, marked by persistent hoarseness, may follow repeated attacks of acute laryngitis. It is sometimes a complication of chronic sinusitis and chronic bronchitis. The condition also may be induced by the frequent inhalation of irritating gases, the excessive use of tobacco or alcohol or by the habitual overuse of the voice, as in the case of public speakers. Laryngoscopic examination is always indicated in a patient with chronic laryngitis in order to eliminate the possibility of tuberculosis or tumor of the larynx. The treatment of the condition is rest of the voice, elimination of any primary respiratory tract infection that may be present and restriction of smoking.

Laryngeal Obstruction

Edema of the Larynx

Edema of the larynx (or glottis) is a serious, often fatal, condition. The larynx is a stiff box that will not stretch, and the space within it between the vocal cords, through which the air must pass, is narrow. Swelling of the laryngeal mucous membrane, therefore, may close this orifice tightly, suffocating the patient. Edema of the glottis occurs rarely in patients with acute laryngitis, occasionally in cases of urticaria and more frequently in severe inflammations of the throat —for example, erysipelas and scarlet fever. It is an occasional cause of death in severe anaphylaxis (angioneurotic edema).

Laryngeal Tuberculosis

The larynx is not infrequently attacked by tuberculosis. Patients so affected become hoarse, have a most persistent cough and suffer acute pain when they attempt to swallow (dysphagia). Treatment entails complete rest of the vocal cords for a prolonged period of time and a course of antibiotic therapy with streptomycin, para-aminosalicylic acid or isoniazid. Direct destruction of the lesion by electrocautery may be undertaken if chemotherapy is unavailing.

Cancer of the Larynx

If detected early, cancer of the larynx is readily curable. It occurs about 10 times more frequently in males than females and most commonly in men from 50 to 65 years of age. It represents about 3 to 5 per cent of all cancers.

Early Symptoms

Dr. Jansen at first thought his voice became hoarse because he was giving more lectures. He noted some throat discomfort which was not relieved by lozenges, therefore he decided to reduce the number of cigarettes he smoked each day. When these symptoms persisted for 15 days, Dr. Jansen sought the advice of a laryngologist.

Dr. Jansen exhibited early symptoms that proved to be cancer. Later he might have had pain, obstructed respiration, difficulty in swallowing, bleeding or swelling of the neck from tumor growth. Certain factors seem to be related to the development of cancer of the larynx: heavy smoking, heavy drinking, vocal straining, chronic laryngitis, and family predisposition.

Medical Management

Precise determination of the exact location and involvement of the malignancy is done by indirect and direct laryngoscopy, biopsy, and x-ray before specific treatment by radiation or surgery is prescribed.

1. Radiation. When the lesion involves only one cord and it is normally mobile, that is, it moves with phonation, radiation therapy has produced good results. In addition, these patients retain a practically normal voice. A few may develop chondritis or stenosis; a small number may later require laryngectomy.

2. Laryngofissure (Thyrotomy). This is recommended in the early stages and has a cure rate of more than 80 per cent. It is recommended in intrinsic cancer of the larynx (limited to the vocal cords). In this operation, the thyroid cartilage of the larynx is split in the midline of the neck and the portion of the vocal cord that is involved with tumor growth is removed. Sometimes a tracheostomy tube (see p. 222) is left in the trachea when the wound is closed, in which event it is removed usually after a few days.

3. Laryngectomy. For extrinsic cancer of the larynx (extension beyond the vocal cords), the entire larynx is removed; this includes the thyroid cartilage, the vocal cords, and the epiglottis. Many surgeons recommend that a neck dissection be performed on the same side as the lesion even though no lymph nodes are palpable. The rationale for this position is that as many as 35 per cent of patients have had metastases to the cervical lymph nodes. Obviously there is an increased problem when a lesion involves midline structures or both cords. With or without neck dissection, a laryngectomy requires a permanent tracheal stoma (Fig. 13-7). The opening of the larynx is closed by sutures.

Nursing Assessment and Preparation for Surgery

Inasmuch as surgery of the larynx is done most commonly for a tumor that may be malignant, the nurse often has a patient who is worried for many reasons: Will the surgeon be able to remove all the tumor? Is it cancer? Will I die? Will I choke? Will I ever speak again? Therefore, the psychological preparation of the patient is as important as the physical. If he is going to have a complete laryngectomy, he should know that he will lose his natural voice completely but that, with training, there are ways in which he can carry on a fairly normal conversation. (He also will not be able to sing, laugh, or whistle.) Until he receives this training, the patient needs to know that the nurse can be reached by the call light and that he can communicate in the immediate postoperative phase by writing.

The physician describes the nature of the surgery and tells the patient that he will lose his ability to vocalize speech. He should be reassured that much can be done for him through a rehabilitation program, and he should be referred to a speech pathologist before surgery. The speech pathologist helps the patient to realize that with speech therapy his sound source can be replaced with either laryngeal or esophageal speech or one of the artificial larynx methods. It is ideal for the patient to begin to learn laryngeal or esophageal speech preoperatively if this is the method of choice. In this way the patient can hear his "new" voice and ask questions concerning speech training.

Mouth hygiene prior to surgery is imperative. Usually antibiotics are ordered to reduce further the possibility of infection. In men, preoperative shaving includes the beard and the hair on the neck and the chest down to the nipple line.

Nursing Management Postoperatively

Surgery can be done under local or general anesthesia. After operation the patient with a laryngofissure may have a tracheostomy tube which is later removed when the edema subsides. This may be in 2 or 3 days. (See p. 222.) The physician may insert a naso-esophageal catheter (No. 16 French urethral catheter), and feedings are given under the same precautions that prevail in gastrostomy feedings (see p. 469). Intravenous therapy may be given concurrently. Oral feedings often are started on the first day after operation if acceptable to the patient. Speaking is deferred until the physician permits whispering (2 to 3 days). This is followed by gradual resumption of the use of the voice.

In caring for a person with a total laryngectomy, it must be realized that the laryngectomy tube (which is shorter but has a larger diameter than the usual tracheotomy tube) is the only airway the patient has. The care of this tube is the same as for a tracheotomy tube (see p. 225). The patient should be observed for excessive coughing or hemoptysis. Communication can be done with a "magic slate." It is well to remember which hand the patient uses for writing; therefore the opposite arm is preferred for intravenous feedings.

A naso-esophageal catheter is passed by the physician after operation and liquid feedings are given. Thereafter the nurse is permitted to remove and pass this tube because there is no possibility of its getting into the trachea, the trachea now being sutured permanently to the skin as a tracheotomy. After a few days the patient can be taught to pass his own feeding tube. Good mouth hygiene must be followed rigidly. After about 7 days, when the incision has healed, the surgeon may allow the patient to begin oral feedings. Then he begins to develop his ability to belch. About an hour after he has eaten, the nurse can remind him to belch. Later this action, which at first is genuine, is transformed into simple explosions of air from the esophagus. At this point the speech pathologist progresses with him in an attempt to make his speech intelligible and as close to normal as is possible.

Antibiotics often are a part of treatment, as there is a possibility of incisional contamination. Vitamins may be given as supplemental feedings, and infusions often are necessary to keep up fluid, electrolyte and nutritional balance. The laryngectomy tube can be removed

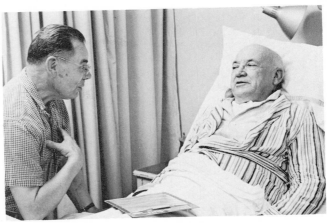

Fig. 13-6. A special kind of caller. During recovery, a former laryngectomee may visit the "new" laryngectomee. This caller will use esophageal speech and answer questions written by the patient. Such contact with a former patient has been very effective in encouraging the new patient when he needs it most. (Courtesy International Association of Laryngectomees)

when the stoma is well healed; usually this is from 3 to 6 weeks postoperatively.

Rehabilitation and Home Care of the Laryngectomized Patient

The patient should be reassured that much can be done for him through a rehabilitation program. Ideally, the speech pathologist sees the patient preoperatively for counseling and to augment what the doctor has told him. The speech pathologist reassures the patient that with speech therapy his sound source can be replaced with either alaryngeal or esophageal speech or by using one of the different types of artificial larynges.

The partially laryngectomized patient has little difficulty, because in a matter of a few days his voice will improve. However, the completely laryngectomized patient often is depressed and needs encouragement. The rehabilitative management of this patient requires a team that includes the surgeon, the nurse, the patient's family, persons who have had laryngectomies (Fig. 13-6), and the speech pathologist.

There are 2 methods of learning to speak after a laryngectomy. The first method is by the use of alaryngeal or esophageal speech. By this method the individual takes air into his mouth. By compression of the lips or by strong articulation of "plosive" speech sounds such as "p," "t," or "k," he can air charge or inflate his esophagus. By lip compression or the plosive sound method the air is sent posteriorly towards the esophagus. As air gets into the upper part of the esophagus, the increased pressure at that point will be released and will

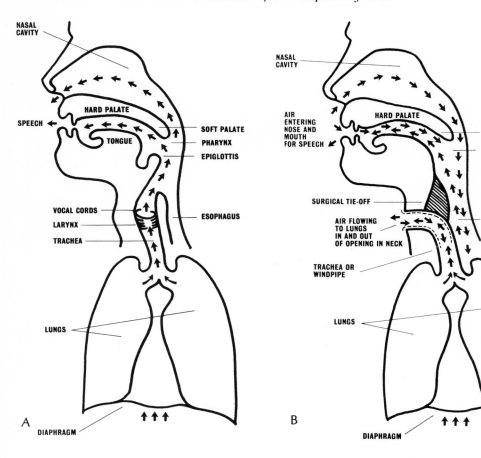

FIG. 13-7. Diagram showing direction of air flow before (A) and after (B) a total laryngectomy. (American Cancer Society)

produce a vibration or tone. This tone is made at the narrowing between the pharynx and esophagus. The resultant voice sounds low pitched because the neo-glottis from which the sounds are now emitted is indeed different from the normal vocal cords. In a few months time the new speech becomes automatic and the individual does not have to think about getting an adequate air charge before talking.

Another method of vocalization after a laryngectomy is by the use of an artificial larynx. Most laryngectomees are able to learn the esophageal method of voice production. However, if the patient is unable to attain esophageal speech due to various reasons (advanced emphysema, asthma, stenosis of esophagus, hearing loss, etc.) an artificial larynx can be used. A variety of artificial larynxes is available. One type is a vibrator powered by batteries, which is placed against the side of the neck. When it is turned on, the air inside the mouth is vibrated and the patient articulates in a somewhat normal fashion.

Another device, also battery-powered, utilizes a plastic tube that is inserted into the side and well to the back of the mouth. Similarly this device provides a continuous sound source in the mouth. The individual merely articulates this sound, shaping it in a normal

manner to form audible speech. The International Association of Laryngectomees is a voluntary organization that sponsors "Lost Chord" or "New Voice" clubs to encourage and give opportunities for laryngectomized persons to learn to speak again.

Patient Education. The nurse conveys optimism to the patient that he will be able to carry on most of the activities that he did before surgery. The patient needs specific information about his tracheostomy. He will frequently cough rather large amounts of mucus through this opening. Because the air passes directly into the trachea without being warmed and moistened by the respiratory mucosa, the tracheobronchial tree secretes excessive amounts of mucus to compensate. Therefore, the patient will have frequent coughing episodes. The brassy sounding, mucus-producing cough is troublesome to the patient, but these problems diminish in time as the tracheobronchial mucosa adapts to the patient's altered physiology. When he coughs, the orifice needs to be wiped and cleaned free of mucus. The skin around the stoma should be washed twice daily. If crusting occurs, the skin around the stoma can be lubricated with an ointment (prescribed by the physician) and the crusts removed with tweezers. It is necessary to wear a bib in front of the tracheostomy to keep the mucus from soiling the clothing. The bib may be a simple gauze flat taped over the neck or one made of other porous fabric.

One of the most important factors in decreasing cough and mucus production as well as crusting around the stoma is to have adequate humidification of the environment. Mechanical humidifiers, cool mist or steam vaporizers are excellent sources of humidification and are absolutely essential for the patient's comfort. Some system of humidification should be set up in the home *before the patient is discharged from the hospital.* An air conditioned atmosphere may be distressing to the newly laryngectomized patient, as the air may be too cool or too dry and thus too irritating.

The patient can expect to have a diminished sense of taste and smell for a period after the operation. Because he is breathing directly into the trachea, air is not passing through the nose to the olfactory end organs. Because taste and smell are so closely connected, his taste sensations are altered. However, in time the individual usually accommodates to this problem and his olfactory sensation adapts to meet his needs.

Special precautions need to be taken in a shower to prevent water from entering the stoma. A loose-fitting plastic bib or simply holding one's hand over the opening is effective. Swimming is not recommended, because this individual can drown without getting his face wet. Barbers and beauticians need to be cautioned so that hair sprays, loose hair and powder do not get near the stoma thereby causing blockage, irritation, and possibly infection.

Recreation and exercise are important. Golf, bowling, bridge, spectator activities and walking can be enjoyed safely. Moderation to prevent fatigue is important because, when tired, the laryngectomee has more difficulty speaking with his new voice. At such times, he can easily become discouraged and depressed.

It is important for the laryngectomee to visit his physician regularly for physical examinations and to obtain advice for any problems relating to his convalescent program.

Proper identification of a laryngectomee by means of a card carried on his person can alert a first-aider to the special requirements of resuscitation should this need arise (Fig. 13-8). On the back of the card can be included the name of a responsible person to notify in the event of emergency.

Problem Solving Activity. What can the nurse do to help the patient cope with the fears expressed in the following quotation?*

* Stoll, B.: Psychological factors determining the success or failure of the rehabilitation program of laryngectomized patients. Ann. Otol., 67:550-557, 1958.

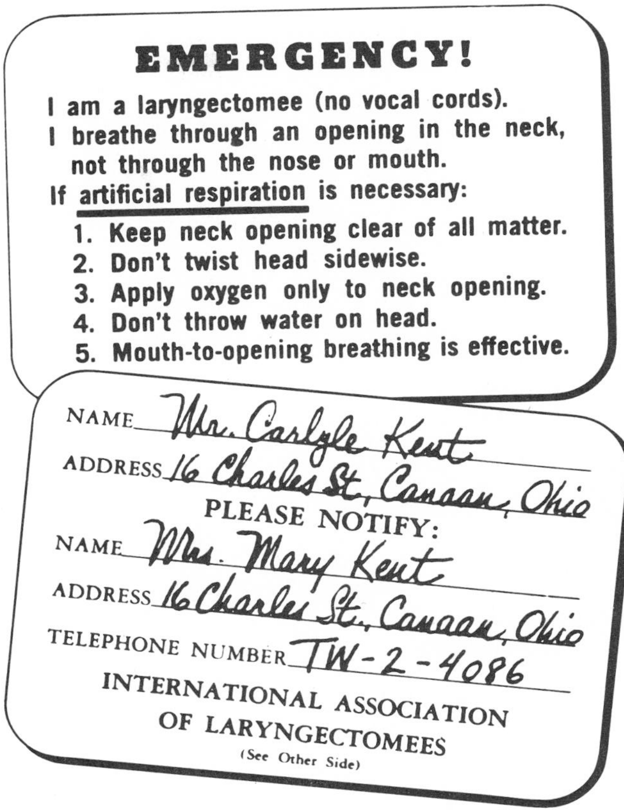
EMERGENCY!

I am a laryngectomee (no vocal cords).
I breathe through an opening in the neck, not through the nose or mouth.
If artificial respiration is necessary:
1. Keep neck opening clear of all matter.
2. Don't twist head sidewise.
3. Apply oxygen only to neck opening.
4. Don't throw water on head.
5. Mouth-to-opening breathing is effective.

NAME Mr. Carlyle Kent
ADDRESS 16 Charles St, Canaan, Ohio
PLEASE NOTIFY:
NAME Mrs. Mary Kent
ADDRESS 16 Charles St, Canaan, Ohio
TELEPHONE NUMBER TW-2-4086
INTERNATIONAL ASSOCIATION OF LARYNGECTOMEES
(See Other Side)

FIG. 13-8. Official identification cards may be obtained from the International Association of Laryngectomees, 219 E. 42nd St., N. Y. 10017.

The fears often experienced by patients postoperatively are as follows:

(1) The fear of the recurrence of the cancer, hence the continued fear of death.

(2) Fears due to the new physiological relationships resulting from the laryngectomy (the inability to lift heavy objects, the breathing and coughing from the tracheal stoma, the often impaired sense of smell and taste, the cosmetic liabilities of the tracheal stoma, etc.).

(3) The fear of old age which has been aggravated by the feeling of uselessness resulting from the loss of speech. The depression frequently observed often has its roots in this specific fear. The loss of earning power further contributes to this feeling of uselessness.

(4) Fear of being unable to re-establish old patterns of interpersonal relationships.

(5) The fears associated with the anticipation of failing to learn a new method of speaking.

ASPIRATED FOREIGN BODIES

Foreign bodies frequently are aspirated into the pharynx, the larynx or the trachea, especially by children. They cause symptoms in two ways: by obstructing the air passages they cause difficulty in breathing that may lead to asphyxia; later they may be drawn

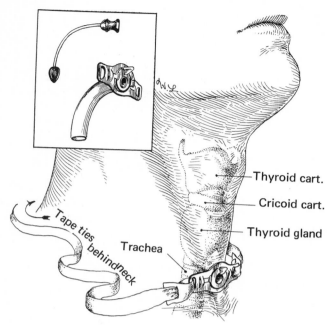

FIG. 13-9. Tracheostomy tubes in place. Note the method of holding the tube in place by tape ties, which are inserted through openings in the outer tube and passed through slits in the tape so as to make a flat connection. Tracheostomy tube and inner tube are shown in place. An obturator, which is introduced into the outer tube when the tracheostomy tube is inserted, completes the tracheostomy set.

farther down, entering the bronchi or one of their branches and causing symptoms of irritation, such as a croupy cough, bloody or mucous expectoration and paroxysms of dyspnea. The physical signs and roentgenograms confirm the diagnosis.

In emergencies, when the signs of asphyxia are evident, immediate treatment is necessary. Frequently, if the foreign body has lodged in the pharynx, it may be dislodged by the finger. If the obstruction is in the larynx or the trachea, an immediate tracheotomy is necessary.

TRACHEOTOMY AND TRACHEOSTOMY

A *tracheotomy* is an operation in which an opening is made into the trachea through which the patient may breathe (Fig. 13-9). It may be performed for any one of several reasons: (1) an inadequate upper airway, such as may be caused by tumors, foreign bodies, edema, nerve or vocal paralysis; (2) a need for effective removal of excessive tracheobronchial secretions; (3) shallow respirations resulting from unconsciousness or respiratory paresis; (4) problems resulting from poor gas transport across alveolar capillary membrane as may occur in severe pulmonary

edema or prolonged cardiac or lung surgery; and (5) the need to reduce dead space when tidal volume is impaired as in severe emphysema.

If the opening is a permanent one, the term *tracheostomy* is used.

Surgical Procedure

The patient is placed in supine position with the head in midline and the neck extended with chin pointing to the ceiling. Anesthesia may be local infiltration or general. A bronchoscope or endotracheal tube may be in place for oxygen and anesthesia. Depending on the surgeon's preference, a vertical or horizontal 3-cm. incision is made about 2 cm. above the suprasternal notch. The sternohyoid and sternothyroid muscles are separated in midline. Fascia along the trachea is dissected to allow insertion of small curved retractors that help in immobilizing the trachea. The trachea is incised with a vertical incision usually through tracheal cartilages 2 and 3. A tracheal dilator or forceps is used to spread the incision and the proper tube with obturator is slipped into the trachea. It is held in place by tapes fastened round the patient's neck (Fig. 13-9). Usually a square of sterile gauze is placed between the tube and the skin before the tape is tied.

Criteria for proper fitting of the tube: (1) the outer tube plate is flush with the skin of the neck (without pressure); (2) aspirating catheter can pass through the tube easily; and (3) the patient can breathe freely through the tube. Tubes are usually made of sterling silver (plastic is available). Each tube consists of 3 pieces: an outer cannula, to which the retaining tapes are fastened; an obturator, an olive-tipped, curved silver rod that is used to guide the cannula into the opening in the trachea; and an inner cannula that is inserted into the outer cannula after the withdrawal of the obturator (Fig. 13-9).

Therapeutic Regimen and Nursing Management

There is sufficient proof that both the incidence of complications and the death rate are increased many times by emergency tracheostomy. Therefore, the hope of the surgeon is that as indications for tracheostomy increase, the majority of operations can be done as elective procedures in the controlled environment of the operating room.

When emergencies arise in which a tracheotomy must be done, the life of the patient is at stake, and strict observance of aseptic technique and the psychological preparation of the patient are of secondary importance. However, there are instances in which there is time to explain the purpose of such surgery to the patient, with the result that he will adjust better to his situation after operation. He should realize that he will lose his voice temporarily, and that he will breathe by means of a tube in his trachea.

Immediate Postoperative Care. This patient requires nursing attention for at least the first 24 hours after operation. Surgery was done to relieve obstruction; *it is the responsibility of the nurse to keep the newly made opening patent.* Another objective in nursing care is *to alleviate the apprehension of the patient.* It is a new experience for him, and often he has a real fear of asphyxiation.

HUMIDIFICATION. Ordinarily the nose and pharynx moisten the inspired air and filter out the dust. This is not possible for the patient with a tracheotomy; therefore continuous moist air is necessary for at least the first 2 or 3 days. Heavily saturated mist can be provided in a tent, by ultrasonic fog, or by inhalation of nebulized water, saline or mucolytic agents. Adequate fluid intake also aids in humidification.

For a time after operation many surgeons cover the opening of the tube with a few layers of gauze moistened in warm saline solution. This tends to moisten the inspired air and to filter out dust, which function is performed in normal life by the nose and the phar-

ynx. However, it will be more to the patient's comfort if the air in the room is kept moistened with steam or cold vapor than if moist gauze is used as mentioned, as this tends to prevent the evacuation of secretions.

REMOVAL OF SECRETIONS. Slightly blood-tinged mucus usually is the first kind of secretion to come through the tracheotomy tube. As time passes, the amount of blood that comes through should diminish and disappear. If it does not, this may indicate hemorrhage, and it should be reported. All secretions should be wiped away carefully and quickly before they are aspirated by the patient.

Secretions are aspirated by a sterile rubber or polyethylene catheter (14 to 18 F.) connected to a suction machine. The catheter should be cut diagonally at the tip and have 2 or 3 holes along the side. To avoid irritation of the lining of the trachea, suction is turned off as the catheter is inserted. Suction (between 125 to 175 mm. Hg.) is adjusted to the type of secretion to be removed. A Y-connecting tube between the catheter and machine tubing provides a convenient means of regulating the suction by the nurse using her thumb on or off the Y-tube opening (Fig. 13-10). Apply

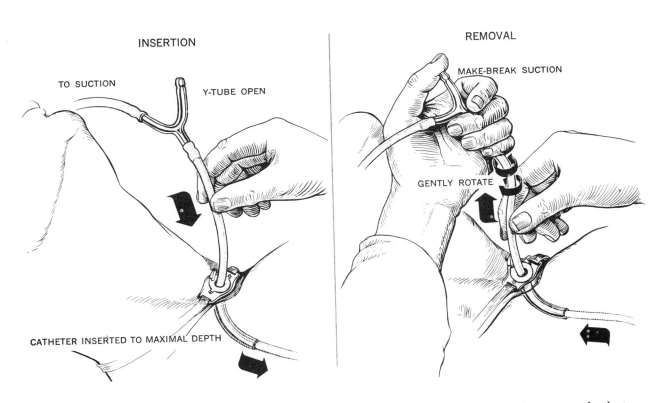

FIG. 13-10. Technique of catheter aspiration of tracheostomy. Slowly withdraw the catheter, completely turning it with a 360° rotating motion while suctioning the passageway. (Adapted from Samson, P. C.: Tracheostomy. Hospital Med. *1*:6, Dec. 1964)

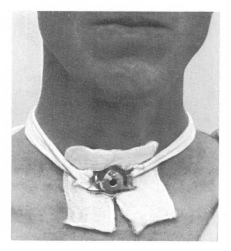

Fig. 13-11. Tracheotomy tube in use. After a few days the split dressing is changed to an unsplit one, and the tube is pushed through the dressing before it is inserted.

suction intermittently for periods of no longer than 5 seconds. Prolonged aspiration may produce a drop in the arterial oxygen concentration. Inefficient suctioning also irritates the mucosa of the trachea. The nurse usually is permitted to introduce the catheter up to 15 cm., but deeper aspiration may be done if she is properly instructed. If complete removal of mucus is not done at frequent intervals, the dried secretions may cause obstruction. A towel spread bib-fashion across the chest and below the tube may help to keep the patient neat when secretions are profuse.

It is recommended that sterile gloves be worn by the person doing the suctioning to prevent contamination of the suction tube. This tube can be exchanged for a sterile tube with each suctioning.

The inner cannula is removed gently by the nurse about every hour for the first day and less frequently after that. It is important to keep this tube clean to prevent encrustations and clogging. If the secretion is thick, instill about 5 drops of sterile water into the trachea through the tracheotomy tube before aspirating. (Care of the tube is explained later.) Before the inner cannula is replaced, the patient should be aspirated. *Generally, the outer cannula is not removed by the nurse.* However, if the patient has a tracheostomy, this may become her responsibility after about 10 days. Meanwhile, the surgeon changes the outer cannula as often as he feels that it is necessary.

A sterile dressing, 3 × 3 inches, is split to fit under the tapes and the shield of the tube so that the incision is covered (Fig. 13-11). This becomes soiled easily and should be replaced as often as is necessary. Care must be taken to prevent dislodging or moving the tube when this is done.

When a mechanical respirator is used, an adaptor of proper size can be fitted to the cannula. The adaptor varies with the equipment; it may be an integral part of the inner cannula or a separate unit with or without accordion tubing.

SUPPORTIVE AND PSYCHOLOGICAL CARE. The patient may have fluids during the day of operation and diet as tolerated after that if there are no other contraindications. Scrupulous mouth care is given before and after meals and whenever necessary. He may be placed in the semi-Fowler or sitting position. Morphine sulfate usually is not given as these patients are not in acute pain. Moreover, the drug is contraindicated because it depresses the cough reflex.

Paper and pencil or magic slate should be kept near the patient so that he has a means of communication. He needs reassurance, especially during the first night, for he may have a real fear that he will asphyxiate while he is asleep. A tap bell or electric cord signal should be within his reach.

Postoperative Complications. The nurse's responsibility to these patients lies not only in keeping a patent airway but also in recognizing untoward symptoms. Pulse and blood pressure should be checked at least every half hour during the first day to detect any signs of hemorrhage. This is not always evident by oozing from the tracheotomy tube; bleeding may occur inwardly.

Increasing apprehension and restlessness may indicate anoxemia. Perhaps the airway is becoming blocked and suctioning may relieve the symptoms. If not, call the physician. The character of respirations can be suggestive of difficulty. Any changes from the usual type of breathing may indicate a problem. If they are increasingly more rapid and seem to have concomitant wheezing or crowing, there may be an obstruction. *This also may be apparent if the patient has an indrawn appearance above the clavicles, in the suprasternal notch and in the epigastrium with each inspiration.* Color change from pallor to cyanosis is a symptom of respiratory embarrassment. If aspiration does not help, call the physician immediately.

Subcutaneous emphysema is a condition in which air escapes into the tissues. A puffiness is noted near the stoma as air escapes from the trachea. This may extend to the upper chest, the neck and the face. A crackling sensation may be detected on gentle pressure. With absorption of air by the tissues, this disappears in a few days. Wound infection can occur easily; therefore, good technique must be practiced in changing dressings and keeping the incision clean. If food or water leaks through the wound or the patient coughs or chokes immediately after eating or drinking, an esophageal fistula may have developed. This symptom should be reported to the surgeon at once. Occasionally, due to violent paroxysms of coughing or to poorly tied tapes, the tracheotomy tube may be expelled. The opening in the trachea will fall together

OUTLINE OF NURSING MANAGEMENT OF A PATIENT WITH AN UPPER RESPIRATORY OBSTRUCTION

Causes of obstruction:
Laryngeal foreign bodies
Injury or disease at or above the level of the glottis
Diseases of the pharynx, the mouth, the neck or the trachea
Inability of the patient to clear his air passages of secretions
Symptoms:
Hoarseness progressing to stridor
Inspiratory dyspnea with stridor

Suprasternal retraction
Indrawing of epigastrium, supraclavicular and intercostal spaces
Cough
Increasing pulse and respiratory rates
Restlessness, apprehension and struggling (late symptoms)
Hypotension
Progressive subcutaneous emphysema
Cyanosis (a late sign)

Nursing Objectives and Principles of Care

I. To open the airway until a permanent airway is established
  A. Assist with cricothyrotomy (incision through the cricoid and thyroid cartilages) if there is a complete airway obstruction
  B. Prepare for laryngoscopy to determine status of larynx
  C. Assist with bronchoscopy if larynx is clear
  D. Prepare patient for tracheostomy if indicated
II. To maintain a patent airway
  A. Keep the tube clear of secretions and crust formation by
    1. Suctioning efficiently to initiate vigorous coughing
    2. Suctioning less frequently as secretions diminish
    3. Cleaning the inner tube when indicated
    4. Humidification of the room with cold vapor, steam or a room humidifier
    5. Encouraging fluid intake to keep the patient well hydrated

    6. Keeping sedation at a minimum to avoid cough depression
  B. Observe constantly to ensure that the tube is in the trachea
III. To allay the apprehension of the patient and his family
  A. Explain the function of the tube
  B. Stay with the patient until he is able to communicate
  C. Teach the patient to suction his tube as soon as he is able to do so
IV. To prevent and treat complications such as
  A. Respiratory arrest and cardiovascular collapse
    1. Start artificial respiration
    2. Place patient in Trendelenburg position
    3. Administer vasopressor drugs as ordered
  B. Atelectasis
    1. Prepare the patient for roentgenogram
    2. Secure equipment for aspiration of pleural space

and, unless immediate treatment is given, the patient may die from asphyxia. The nurse must remember in such an emergency that the Trousseau dilator or a hemostat will spread the tracheal wound and allow the patient to breathe until the duplicate tube can be inserted by another person.

Care of Tubes. Cold running water removes much of the secretions from a tube. However, for more adherent mucus the following methods of cleaning are suggested:

Place the tube in a bowl with 2 per cent sterile soda bicarbonate solution. This will help to liquefy the secretions. Sterile saline also may be used. Pipe cleaners are effective; they are soft and will not injure the tube, yet the inner wire gives a degree of firmness. A 2-inch bandage on a piece of folded wire also can be used. Small test tube brushes are effective.

METAL TUBES. After a thorough cleaning, silver pol-

ish can be used to remove any tarnish. The cannula then is boiled or autoclaved and, finally, reinserted. Careful handling of tracheotomy tubes is important, because they are made of a soft metal and are damaged easily. A dented tube may fit poorly and cause trauma to the patient when an attempt is made to remove it. A part of one tube is not interchangeable with a similar part of another set of tubes. Therefore, each set of three parts must be kept intact.

PLASTIC NYLON TUBES. The care of these tubes is simplified, since they do not dent or tarnish. Furthermore, parts are interchangeable. Other decided advantages are that they are light in weight, do not frost in cold climates and can be boiled or autoclaved.

In preparing tapes for a tracheotomy tube, ¾-inch twill tape makes a strong set of ties. Each tie should be 16 inches long. About 1 inch from the end, a horizontal slit should be made. This end of the tie can be inserted through the side opening on the outer cannula, and the opposite end of the tie then can be threaded through the slit end and drawn tightly. This is more effective than to tie a knot to anchor the tape to the cannula, because a sizable knot can cause a pressure area on the neck of the patient (Fig. 13-9). Another method of securing a tape is to staple the short end to the long end.

Patient Education. The patient is taught to care for his own tracheotomy tube as soon as feasible. The nurse can instruct him concerning the parts of the instrument and how they function. With the use of a mirror, she can show him how to remove and how to insert the inner cannula. The care of this delicate instrument must be explained and demonstrated in detail, and the patient should repeat the demonstration to the nurse. If the patient is unable to care for himself, some member of the family will have to be taught before he is discharged.

Sometimes the insertion of a tracheotomy tube is a temporary procedure to tide the patient over an acute respiratory obstruction. In such cases the patient must return gradually to normal breathing. This is accomplished by producing a partial obstruction of the airway in the tracheotomy tube by the insertion of partial corks. When they are first inserted the patient must be watched constantly for signs of respiratory obstruction. If the patient tolerates a small cork, the opening may be decreased further by the use of larger ones until eventually the entire opening can be plugged. When the patient tolerates complete obstruction of the tracheotomy tube, it may be removed and the opening permitted to heal. This process is known as *decannulation*. During this process the nurse must inspect the corks carefully to see that they are not broken. As a rule, they are fixed to the tracheotomy tube with braided threads. The most suitable corks are those made of pure rubber ground down to fit the tube. In learning to talk, the patient may be permitted to use a cork to close the opening temporarily so that voice sounds will be produced more clearly. Often merely the placing of a finger over the tracheotomy opening will aid him when he talks. However, this must be cleared with the physician, for talking may be contraindicated if the larynx is to be at rest following disease or edema.

If the tracheotomy is permanent, the patient should be instructed regarding the danger of aspirating water. Therefore, he must not swim and he must exercise caution in taking a shower. So far as appearance is concerned, women can wear filigree made specially by a jeweler, or scarves, ties and so forth in such a way that the tracheotomy tube is not seen. Usually in a man the shirt will cover the tracheotomy opening.

BIBLIOGRAPHY

Upper Respiratory

Epistaxis. Canad. Nurse, *63*:37-39, Sept., 1967.

Guyton, A. C.: Textbook of Medical Physiology. ed. 3, pp. 765-768. Philadelphia, W. B. Saunders, 1966.

Lefkowitz, L. B.: The common cold syndrome. Amer. J. Nurs., *63*:70-74, Dec., 1963.

Tracheostomy

Betts, R. H.: Post-tracheostomy aspiration. New Eng. J. Med., *273*:155, 1965.

Dugan, D. J. and Samson, P. C.: Tracheostomy: present day indications and technics. Amer. J. Surg., *106*:290-306, 1963.

Jeffis, L., and Baker, C.: Nasopharyngeal and tracheal suctioning. Amer. J. Nurs., *67*:2361, Nov., 1967.

Lewis, B. J., and Gunn, I. P.: Tracheostomy, O_2 administration and expiratory air flow resistance. Nurs. Res., *13*:301-308, Fall, 1964.

Saunders, W. H., Havener, W. H., Fair, C. J., and Hickey, J. T.: Nursing Care in Eye, Ear, Nose, and Throat Disorders. ed. 2. Philadelphia, W. B. Saunders, 1968.

Totman, L. E., and Lehman, R. H.: Tracheostomy care. Amer. J. Nurs., *64*:96-98, March, 1964.

Work, W. P., and Smith, M. F. W.: Tracheotomy. Postgrad. Med., *34*:479-487, 1963.

Yanagisawa, E., and Kirchner, J. A.: The cuffed tracheotomy tube. Arch. Otolaryn., *79*:80-87, Jan., 1964.

Laryngectomy

Adler, S.: Speech after laryngectomy, Amer. J. Nurs., *69*:2138-2141, Oct., 1969.

Beattie, E. J., and Economou, S. G.: The current status of radical laryngectomy. Nurs. Clin. N. Amer., *3*:515-518, Sept., 1968.

Flowers, A. M.: Electronic mechanical aids for the laryngectomized patient. Nurs. Clin. N. Amer., *3*:529-532, Sept., 1968.

Gannon, R.: Recommendation: total laryngectomy. AORN J., *5*:39-43, Feb., 1967.

Hilkemeyer, R.: Meeting the nursing needs of the patient with total laryngectomy. ANA Technical Innovations in Health Care, *4*:5-16, 1962.

Holinger, P. H.: Laryngoscopy, bronchoscopy, and esophagoscopy. AORN J., *4*:61-67, May, June, 1966.

Levin, N. M.: Rehabilitation and speech therapy for laryngectomized patients. AORN J., *8*:55-62, Dec., 1968.

Locke, Cdr. B.: Psychology of the laryngectomy. Military Med., *2*:593-599, July, 1966.

Martin, H.: Rehabilitation of the laryngectomee. Cancer, *16*:823-841, July, 1963.

Murphy, G. E., and Ogura, J.: Rehabilitation following laryngectomy. Geriatrics, *22*:119-125, Dec., 1967.

Pitorak, E. F.: Laryngectomy. Amer. J. Nurs., *68*:780-786, April, 1968.

Rosenfeld, L.: Cancer of the larynx. Nurs. Forum, *4*:76-81, No. 3, 1965.

Stanley, L. M.: Meeting the psychologic needs of the laryngectomy patient. Nurs. Clin. N. Amer., *3*:519-527, Sept., 1968.

Sykes, E. M.: No time for silence. Amer. J. Nurs., *66*:1040-1041, May, 1966.

PATIENT EDUCATION

Superintendent of Documents
  U.S. Government Printing Office
  Washington, D.C. 20402
    The Common Cold. PHS Publication No. 106
    Sinus Infection (Sinusitis). PHS Publication No. 172
    Cancer of the Larynx. PHS Publication No. 1284
The DeVilbiss Company
  Somerset, Pennsylvania 15501
    Your Health—and Humidity.
International Association of Laryngectomees
  219 E. 42nd Street
  New York, New York 10017

Helping Words for the Laryngectomees. 1964.
The IAL News (a bi-monthly publication).
Laryngectomees at Work.
Rehabilitating Laryngectomees.
American Cancer Society
  (Contact your local chapter)
    First Aid for Laryngectomees. 1964.
    Waldrop, W. F., and Gould, M. A.: Your New Voice. (A
      32-page booklet containing 13 lessons on how to use your
      new voice.) rev. 1967.
    To Speak Again. (Film)
American Speech and Hearing Association
  9030 Old Georgetown Road
  Washington, D.C. 20014

CHAPTER **14**

Patients with Medical and Surgical Conditions of the Chest

- *Physiology of Respiration*
- *Pathophysiology of Respiration*
- *Diagnostic Studies in Thoracic Conditions*
- *Patients with Pulmonary Disorders*
- *Patients with Tumors of the Chest*
- *Tumors of the Mediastinum*
- *Patients with Aspirated Foreign Bodies in their Lungs*
- *Patients with Chest Injuries*

PHYSIOLOGY OF RESPIRATION

The cells of the body derive their necessary energy from the oxidation of food products transported by the bloodstream. For this process, as for any type of combustion, oxygen is required. As a result of oxidation in the body tissues, carbon dioxide is produced and must be removed from the cell as soon as formed. Deprived of oxygen and stifled by accumulated carbon dioxide, no body cell can survive.

Cells are supplied with oxygen and dispose of waste carbon dioxide through the medium of the circulating blood. No cell is far removed from a capillary, the thin walls of which present no barrier to the passage of water or dissolved gases. Interposed between the capillary and the cell membrane is a thin layer of tissue fluid, or lymph, from which the cells continuously extract oxygen. As a result, the oxygen tension outside the capillary is always lower than it is within, where it reflects the concentration of that gas passing inside the red blood cells. Thus, oxygen diffuses in solution from the capillary blood through the capillary wall, into the surrounding lymph, through the membrane of the tissue cell and into the contents of that cell. Diffusion of oxygen from blood to cells proceeds in this manner without interruption in all tissues of the body. The movement of carbon dioxide from cell to blood is accomplished by a similar process of diffusion, the dis-

solved gas moving continuously via the same route as the oxygen, but in the opposite direction. As a result of these exchanges the arterial blood loses approximately ⅓ of its oxygen, while its carbon dioxide content is increased by about ⅕. It has now become venous blood.

TABLE 14-1. Comparison of the gaseous content of both arterial and venous blood

	Arterial	Venous
Oxygen content, vols. per cent (ml. O_2/100 ml. blood)	18 to 21	12 to 14
Oxygen saturation, per cent (O_2 content/O_2 capacity X 100)	94 to 96	60 to 80
Carbon dioxide content, vols. per cent (ml. CO_2/100 ml. blood)	50 to 55	62 to 65

These relationships are demonstrated in Table 14-1, which shows the normal values for oxygen and carbon dioxide concentration in both arterial and venous blood.

The blood becomes oxygenated, i.e., its oxygen deficit is restored and its excess carbon dioxide is removed, in the capillaries of the lung. Here, following rapid diffusion of these gases through an extensive liquid-gas interphase, the blood approaches equilibrium with the air that we breathe.

The simplest type of lung is a narrow-mouthed sac lined with a thin membrane that contains an extensive network of capillaries. Gases diffuse easily and rapidly through this membrane. A simple structure of this type, although found in certain amphibians, is inadequate for man, who, because of his relatively large blood volume, requires a vast capillary system and a much more extensive respiratory surface.

The human lung is a composite organ, a collection of myriad tiny sacs, each of which is separate and complete in itself. Each has a tiny bronchus, called a *bronchiole* (a), opening into a group of air sacs or *alveoli* (b).

The alveoli furnish the respiratory surface. They are small air sacs scarcely visible to the eye. Their elastic walls are lined by thin alveolar epithelial membrane, a single layer of flat epithelial cells through which gases easily diffuse. Included within these walls is a network of pulmonary capillaries. So numerous are these alveoli that if their walls, the respiratory surface, were united to form one big sheet, it would cover an area of over 90 square yards.

The bronchioles through which air enters and leaves the alveoli are lined with an epithelial membrane composed of ciliated columnar cells, i.e., tall cells whose free ends are covered with short "hairs," called *cilia*. These cilia maintain a constant whipping motion, always in the same direction, sweeping out any foreign substance or excess of mucus. The bronchioles join to form larger and larger bronchi so that all the bronchi and bronchioles in one lung represent branches of one primary bronchus. The 2 primary bronchi then unite to form the trachea.

The lungs are elastic structures enclosed in an airtight chamber with distensible walls—the thorax. The movements of respiration involve the walls of the thorax and its floor, the diaphragm; their effect is alternately to increase and decrease the capacity of the chest. The lungs expand and contract passively, being so elastic that they can follow easily the changing volume of the thoracic cavity. The only open passage admitting air into the thorax is the trachea. When the capacity of the chest is increased, air must enter, due to the lowered pressure within. It passes through the trachea and the bronchi and inflates the lungs. When the chest collapses to its previous volume, the elastic lungs collapse with it, forcing the air out. In this fashion the entire lung is "ventilated," that is, each alveolus during inspiration receives a supply of fresh air that is expelled during the next expiration.

The outer surfaces of the lung are enclosed by a smooth, slippery membrane called the *pleura*—which also extends to cover the interior wall of the thorax and the superior surface of the diaphragm. The pleura is always moistened by lymph, which allows the opposing pleural surfaces, i.e., the "parietal pleura" lining the thorax and the "visceral pleura" covering the lungs, to rub together freely and painlessly during respiration.

The mediastinum is the wall that divides the thoracic cavity into 2 halves. It is composed of 2 layers of pleura between which lie all of the thoracic structures except the lungs.

PATHOPHYSIOLOGY OF RESPIRATION

Deficient Aeration

Interference with aeration, resulting in a reduction in blood oxygen and an abnormal increase in its carbon dioxide content, can be caused by abnormal respiratory movement, obstruction of the respiratory tract or a reduction in the area of "respiratory surface," the area of alveolar epithelium where the blood-gas exchange occurs. Laboratory studies in such cases would reveal an abnormally low oxygen content of both arterial and venous blood in proportion to its oxygen capacity, whereas its carbon dioxide content would be elevated abnormally.

Symptoms and signs that immediately strike the nurse's attention and represent to her the picture of oxygen lack include, an increasing pulse rate, drowsiness or restlessness and, often, confusion as well as the appearance of cyanosis. Carbon dioxide retention, if only moderate in degree, may or may not be accompanied by clinical manifestations, depending on the length of time this situation has existed and on the degree to which base (e.g., sodium) is available to neutralize the excess carbonic acid. If sufficient sodium has been retained to keep the blood acidity within the physiologic range, i.e., at a pH level between 7.35 and 7.40, no symptoms referable to the excess carbon dioxide are to be expected. Such a patient is said to have "compensated acidosis."

In uncompensated respiratory acidosis the blood acidity is increased, i.e., the pH falls below 7.35. The most prominent sign associated with this metabolic disturbance in its early phases is hyperpnea, characterized by rapid, deep breathing. Long-standing carbon dioxide retention eventually reduces or eliminates altogether the sensitivity of the respiratory center to an elevation of carbon dioxide concentration in the blood, or to a lowering of the blood pH. Under these circumstances, oxygen deficiency becomes the principal respiratory stimulus. Such patients may display no hyperpnea; on the contrary, if their hypoxia is relieved by oxygen inhalation therapy their respiratory rate may decline to dangerously low levels. An excess of carbon dioxide in the blood of any patient, regardless of his earlier status, is capable of producing coma and death.

TABLE 14-2. Ventilatory function tests*

Term Used	Symbol	Description	Remarks and Clinical Application
Vital capacity	VC	The largest volume measured on complete expiration after the deepest inspiration without forced or rapid effort.	This may be normal or even high in chronic obstructive pulmonary disease and is of little value by itself.
Forced vital capacity	FVC	The vital capacity performed with expiration as forceful and rapid as possible.	This volume is often significantly reduced in chronic lung disease due to air trapping, and is an important standard of measurement.
Forced expiratory volume (qualified by subscript indicating time interval in seconds)	FEV_T ($FEV_{1.0}$)	Volume of gas exhaled over a given time interval during the performance of a forced vital capacity.	If below predicted normal values, this is a valuable clue to the severity of the expiratory airway obstruction.
Percentage expired (in T seconds)	$FEV_T\%$	FEV_T expressed as a percentage of the forced vital capacity: $$\frac{FEV_T}{FVC} \times 100$$	This time-volume relationship is another way of expressing the presence or absence of airway obstruction.
Forced expiratory flow	$FEF_{200-1200}$	The average rate of flow for a specified portion of the forced expiratory volume, usually between 200 and 1200 ml.	Formerly called maximum expiratory flow rate (MEFR). A slowed rate is an early manifestation of chronic obstructive pulmonary diseases.
Forced mid-expiratory flow	$FEF_{25-75}\%$	Average rate of flow during the middle half of the forced expiratory volume.	Formerly called mid-expiratory flow rate. This is slowed early in the course of ventilatory impairment.
Maximal voluntary ventilation	MVV	Volume of air which a subject can breathe with voluntary maximal effort for a given time.	Formerly called maximum breathing capacity. Another valuable test, usually correlating well with the patient's complaint of dyspnea.

* National Tuberculosis Association: Chronic Obstructive Pulmonary Disease. p. 24. 1966.

Hyperventilation

An increase in the respiratory rate is a common finding in patients suffering from a wide variety of disorders, in most of which the respiratory center is hyperstimulated as a result of acidosis, hypoxia or by nervous reflexes from the lungs or elsewhere. In the vast majority of patients, an increased respiration serves a definite physiologic need by restoring an oxygen deficit or reducing an excess acidity by increasing carbon dioxide excretion; in such instances the term "hyperventilation," which suggests excessive respiration, is hardly applicable. True hyperventilation is encountered in patients with hysteria. Whatever its psychiatric implications in these individuals, it is certainly without physiologic benefit to the patient, its principal effect being to "wash out" carbon dioxide, with the result that the blood becomes too alkaline. This immediately induces a train of symptoms, including sensations of numbness, tingling of the arms and the legs, dizziness, faintness and abnormal contractility of the muscles, evidenced by spasmodic twitchings of the facial muscles and the extremities. These effects are entirely reversible, lasting only for the duration of the alkalosis, namely, until the hyperventilation has ceased.

Therapeutic measures that effectively restore the normal blood acidity, despite continuance of overbreathing, are inhalations of carbon dioxide-oxygen mixtures containing 10 per cent carbon dioxide, or having the patient inhale and exhale in a paper bag, causing him to rebreathe some of the carbon dioxide in his own expired air. If possible, the patient should be helped to understand how anxiety can produce the hyperventilation syndrome.

DIAGNOSTIC STUDIES IN THORACIC CONDITIONS

Ventilatory Function Tests

These tests are done with a spirometer and are designed to determine how well the lung "ventilates," that is, its ability to take in oxygen and release carbon dioxide. The various categories described in Table 14-2 measure lung volumes and time-volume relationships. (See also Table 15-2, p. 278.)

These tests usually are done only on chest patients having borderline respiratory reserve. As a rule, no special preparation is required for these tests; the nurse can tell her patient that he is to have a breathing test. He follows the instructions of the physician as to whether to breathe normally, inhale deeply, etc.

Blood Gas Analysis

A very important determination in patients with chronic lung disease or those being ventilated by mechanical means is the partial pressure of oxygen and carbon dioxide in the arterial blood, along with the pH of the same sample.

The blood may be obtained by direct puncture of the femoral, brachial, or radial artery with a small gauge needle or drawn from a catheter previously placed in one of these arteries. The sample must be heparinized, drawn without contamination by air bubbles, and immediately placed in a container of ice. Machines are available to perform these determinations on small samples of blood (less than 5 ml.).

Obviously, the partial pressure of oxygen (pO_2) shows how efficient the lung is in transmitting inspired oxygen to the blood. The partial pressure of carbon dioxide (pCO_2) is a good index of the degree of ventilation. If a patient is overventilated, or if alveolar walls are thickened so gas exchange cannot occur properly, CO_2 is blown off and the pCO_2 decreases. If underventilation is taking place, CO_2 accumulates in the blood and the pCO_2 rises. The pH is responsive both to the metabolic state of the patient and to the influence of respiration (particularly to the carbon dioxide content of the blood). (See Table 15-2, p. 278.)

Roentgenograms

Roentgenograms and sectional roentgenograms (laminogram, planogram or strategram) are a real aid to the physician and the surgeon in recognizing lung function, the relationship of the vital structures and suggestions of pathology (see page 200). Patience and cooperation on the part of the patient are desirable, and the nurse should endeavor to obtain them.

Bronchogram. A bronchogram is an x-ray examination of the bronchial tree after a radiopaque dye is instilled. Before the procedure, a sedative and atropine are given, and usually a meal is withheld to prevent aspiration from regurgitation. Cocaine or pontocaine in the form of a spray through the nose and the mouth help to prevent gagging and coughing when the tube is passed nasally. After such a roentgenogram, food and fluids are withheld until the effects of the local anesthetic have worn off. The patient is placed on a regimen of postural drainage to allow the oily dye to be removed. Often because of the hazards of oil in the respiratory passages, he is sent home for 2 months before surgery is done.

Bronchoscopy and Esophagoscopy

When a foreign body enters the smaller air passages in the lungs, it may obstruct the bronchi with a resulting obstruction of air in the portion of the lung supplied by them. This produces a partial collapse of the lung with pulmonary symptoms of cough, expectoration and so forth. Secondary infection often occurs with resultant formation of chronic pulmonary suppuration or abscess.

In many cases it is possible to remove the foreign body and to relieve the patient's symptoms by means of *bronchoscopy*. By this method of treatment, a lighted rigid tube is inserted through the pharynx and the trachea into the bronchus containing the foreign body. After aspiration of the secretions, the foreign body may be removed with forceps. Many brilliant cures have been effected by this method of therapy, which demands the highest degree of skill and adequate equipment (Fig. 14-1).

Bronchoscopy also is used in the diagnosis and the treatment of many intrathoracic diseases. By means of this lighted tube, tumors of the air passages can be viewed and biopsied, secretions can be aspirated for cytologic and bacteriologic study and medication is applied at times. In the study of some diseases of the lungs, such as bronchiectasis, radiopaque liquids are injected to outline the air passages on the x-ray film (*bronchogram*).

Esophagoscopy is the viewing of the interior of the esophagus through a lighted tube. It is used to remove foreign bodies, to inspect lesions of the esophagus,

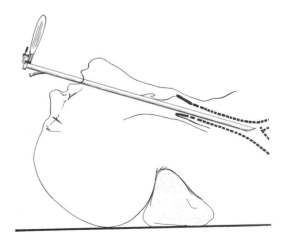

Fig. 14-1. Introduction of the bronchoscope.

THE ROLE OF THE NURSE IN ASSISTING THE PATIENT HAVING A THORACENTESIS

Guidelines for Nursing Action

A thoracentesis (aspiration of fluid or air from the pleural space) is done on patients with various clinical problems. It may be a diagnostic or therapeutic procedure for:
  (1) removal of fluid and air from the pleural cavity
  (2) diagnostic aspiration of pleural fluid.

The responsibilities of the nurse in relation to the patient having a thoracentesis and the rationale of her participation are summarized below.

Nursing Activities	Rationale
Ascertain in advance if chest roentgenograms have been ordered and completed.	Posteroanterior and lateral chest x-rays are used to localize fluid and air in the pleural cavity and facilitate in determining the puncture site.
Determine if the patient is allergic to the local anesthetic agent to be used. Give sedation if ordered.	

Inform the patient about the procedure and indicate how he can be helpful. Explain
  (1) The nature of the procedure
  (2) The importance of remaining immobile
  (3) Pressure sensations to be experienced
  (4) That no discomfort is anticipated after the procedure
	An explanation helps orient the patient to the procedure, assists him to mobilize his resources and gives him an opportunity to ask questions and verbalize anxiety.

Make the patient comfortable with adequate supports. If possible, place him upright and
  (1) Sitting on the edge of the bed with the feet supported and his arms and head on a padded over-the-bed table, or
  (2) Straddling a chair with his arms and head resting on the back of the chair, or
  (3) Lying on his unaffected side if he is unable to assume a sitting position.
	The upright position facilitates the removal of fluid that usually localizes at the base of the chest. A position of comfort assists the patient to relax.

Support and reassure the patient during the procedure.
  (1) Prepare the patient for cold sensation of antiseptic solution and of pressure sensation from infiltration of local anesthetic agent.
  (2) Encourage the patient to refrain from coughing.
	Sudden and unexpected movement by the patient can cause trauma to the visceral pleura with resultant trauma to the lung.

Expose the entire chest.	If fluid is in the pleural cavity, the thoracentesis site is usually in the 7th or 8th intercostal space in the posterior axillary line.
	If air is in the pleural cavity, the thoracentesis site is usually in the 2nd or 3rd intercostal space in the midclavicular line.
	(The density of the air is much less than the density of liquid.)
The procedure is done under aseptic conditions. After the skin is disinfected, a local anesthetic is injected slowly with a small caliber needle into the intercostal space by the physician.	An interdermal wheal is raised slowly; rapid interdermal injection causes pain. The parietal pleura is very sensitive and should be well-infiltrated with anesthetic before the thoracentesis needle is passed through it.
The physician advances the thoracentesis needle slowly and maintains constant suction on the syringe so it will be immediately apparent when the fluid pocket is reached. (1) A 50-ml. syringe with a 3-way adapter (stop cock) is attached to the needle (one end of the adapter is attached to the needle and the other to the tubing leading to a receptacle receiving the fluid being aspirated).	When a large quantity of fluid is withdrawn, a 3-way adapter serves to keep air from entering the pleural cavity.

THE ROLE OF THE NURSE IN ASSISTING THE PATIENT HAVING A THORACENTESIS (*Continued*)

Nursing Activities (*Continued*)	Rationale (*Continued*)
(2) If a considerable quantity of fluid may be removed, the needle is held in place on the chest wall with a small hemostat.	The hemostat steadies the needle on the chest wall. Sudden pleuritic chest pain or shoulder pain may indicate that the visceral or diaphragmatic pleura are being irritated by the needle point.
After the needle is withdrawn, pressure is applied over the puncture site and a small sterile dressing is fixed in place.	
Place the patient on his unaffected side for approximately 1 hour.	This permits the pleural puncture site to seal itself and thus prevents fluid seepage from cough or from gravitational forces.
Record the total amount of fluid withdrawn and the nature of the fluid, its color and viscosity. If ordered, prepare samples of fluid for laboratory evaluation.	The fluid may be clear, serous, bloody, purulent, etc.
Evaluate the patient at intervals for faintness, vertigo, tightness in chest, uncontrollable cough, blood tinged frothy mucus and a rapid pulse.	Pneumothorax, tension pneumothorax, subcutaneous emphysema or pyogenic infection may result from a thoracentesis. Pulmonary edema or cardiac distress can be produced by a sudden shift in mediastinal contents when large amounts of fluid are aspirated.

such as ulcers, diverticuli and tumors, and often to make a positive diagnosis by removing small bits of tissue for microscopic examination (biopsy).

Nursing Management. Before bronchoscopy or esophagoscopy the patient must take nothing by mouth for at least 6 hours. Morphine sulfate or a similar drug usually is given adults. All removable dentures must be removed. The patient should be told what to expect so as to gain his cooperation. Many times, such a patient fears that he is to undergo real surgery. When he sees physicians and nurses garbed in operating masks and gowns, he may reasonably be upset.*

When the patient returns from the operating room the local anesthetic used in the throat may interfere with swallowing and cause him to choke. After the return of the cough or gag reflex, cracked ice and later liquids may be given and, if the hypodermic does not cause nausea, the patient is permitted to return to the preoperative diet in about 6 hours. Difficulty in breathing, particularly in children, is looked for and reported promptly.

Until the local anesthesia has disappeared after esophagoscopy, care should be exercised in giving liquids. Determine whether the patient can cough before offering any fluids. Then, they may be given, if they are tolerated, and the patient is permitted to return to the preoperative diet in about 6 hours. Some discomfort on swallowing may occur, but marked discomfort should be reported promptly.

---

* The procedure may be done under local anesthesia using cocaine, Butyn Sulfate or Xylocaine or under a general anesthetic. During a bronchoscopic examination the nurse may assist the patient by "vocal anesthesia," informing him of the progress of the procedure and praising him for his helpful participation.

Sputum Studies

Sputum may be obtained to determine the organisms present or to see if malignant cells can be discovered; the patient should be instructed to cough deeply so that a true specimen may be obtained for the sterile Petri dish. Often a qualitative study is done to determine whether the secretions are saliva, mucus or pus. Usually they separate into layers that are seen readily when a conical glass container is used. For quantitative studies, the patient is given a special container in which to expectorate. This is weighed at the end of 24 hours, and the amount and the character is described and charted. In disposing of such a specimen, it is well wrapped in paper and taken to the incinerator. To prevent odors, all sputum containers should be covered and concealed. Malodorous discarded mouth wipes should be removed, and there must be good ventilation in the room.

Thoracentesis

The aspiration of chest fluid may be a therapeutic or a diagnostic procedure. Frequently a needle biopsy of the pleura is taken at the same time. The preceding chart concerns the nurse's responsibilities in assisting the patient who is having a thoracentesis.

PROBLEMS OF PATIENTS WITH PULMONARY DISORDERS

Certain problems are encountered frequently in the care of patients with chest conditions. These relate to the occurrence of cough and expectoration, the necessity for mouth care, symptoms of dyspnea, chest pain and hemoptysis, and the presence of air or fluid in the pleural cavity.

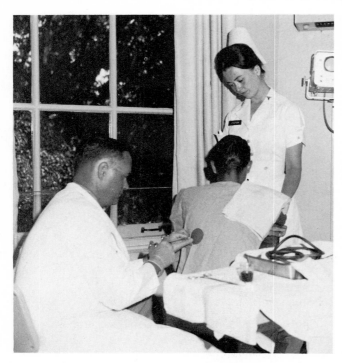

Fig. 14-2. The patient is having a diagnostic thoracentesis performed. The nurse is in a position to evaluate his response to the procedure and afford him support. (Armed Forces Inst. of Pathology Photograph)

Cough, Expectoration and Mouth Care

The stimulus producing a cough may arise from an infectious process or from an air irritant, such as smoke, smog, dust or a gas. "The cough is the watchdog of the lungs" and is the patient's chief protection against the accumulation of secretions in the bronchi and bronchioles. On the other hand, the presence of cough may indicate serious pulmonary disease. For example, it is one of the prominent symptoms of bronchogenic carcinoma. If the cough is harsh and loud, the patient probably has a disease of the trachea or large bronchi, while the presence of a painful, short, dry cough may indicate a lesion of the parenchyma or pleura.

A patient who coughs long enough will almost invariably expectorate. The production of sputum is the reaction of the lung to any constantly recurring irritant. The nurse should determine whether the sputum is associated with a nasal discharge. If there is a profuse amount of purulent sputum, the patient may have an infectious process; whereas a gradual increase of sputum over a period of time may reveal the presence of chronic bronchitis or bronchiectasis. Pink-tinged mucoid sputum is suggestive of a lung tumor, and profuse frothy pink material may indicate pulmonary edema.

The nurse's charting should be specific with respect to the amount, the odor, the character, and, if known, the source of the sputum.

The patient's appetite may be lessened because of the odor and the taste in his mouth that result from the frequent raising of sputum. Adequate mouth hygiene, proper environment and wise selections of food will stimulate his appetite. After careful cleansing and rinsing of the mouth, sputum cups and emesis basins should be removed before his meal arrives. Some foods, such as citrus juices, make the mouth feel fresher and the patient is then more receptive to the rest of the meal.

Promotion of an Effective Cough Routine. Effective coughing is necessary for the mobilization and the removal of bronchial secretions and exudates. The promotion of vigorous coughing is essential for the patient undergoing thoracic surgery. Preoperatively he should be assured that coughing postoperatively will not "break his incision open" and informed that he will be assisted to cough every hour.

If possible, the patient should be in a sitting position while coughing, and the nurse should stand behind him. The patient should be taught to cough into 2 tissues. Either of the following techniques may be used:

1. The nurse's hands should support the chest incision anteriorly and posteriorly. The patient is instructed to take several deep breaths, inhale, and then to cough forcibly.

2. With one hand, exert downward pressure on the shoulder of the affected side while firmly supporting beneath the wound with the other hand. The patient is instructed to take several deep breaths, inhale, and then cough forcibly.

Dyspnea

Dyspnea, as discussed on page 22, is a symptom common to many pulmonary conditions, including tracheal or bronchial obstruction by inflammatory processes, pleurisy, tumors of the mediastinum or aspirated foreign bodies. Dyspnea can also be observed in cardiac conditions, anemia, and even psychiatric disorders, such as anxiety. Parenchymal lesions of the lung, as well as pulmonary atelectasis, reduce the vital capacity and therefore predispose to dyspnea. Respiration becomes shallower and more rapid if the lungs become congested or inflamed. In general, the acute diseases of the lungs produce a more severe grade of dyspnea than do the chronic diseases.

Therapeutic control of dyspnea depends on the success with which its cause can be eliminated. Alleviation of the symptom is achieved by placing the patient at rest and, in severe cases, by the administration of oxygen inhalation therapy.

Chest Pain

Chest pain associated with pulmonary conditions may be sharp, stabbing and intermittent, or dull, aching and persistent. It usually is felt on the side where the pathology is located, but it may be referred elsewhere, for example, to the neck, the back or the abdomen. Chest pain is experienced by most patients with pneumonia and pleurisy, and it is a common symptom of bronchogenic carcinoma.

Pleuritic pain is sharp and catching on inspiration; patients describe it "like a knife stabbing." They are more comfortable when they can be persuaded to lie on the affected side, a posture that tends to "splint" the chest wall, restrict the expansions and the contractions of the lung and reduce the friction between the injured or diseased pleurae on that side. Pain associated with cough may be lessened by manual splinting of the rib cage, as illustrated in Figure 14-3.

Analgesic and antitussive medication in the form of codeine sulfate and Hycodan alleviate the harrassing cough and reduce the pain of pleurisy. If the pain is severe, meperidine hydrochloride may be given intramuscularly in doses of 50 to 100 mg. at intervals of 4 to 6 hours. On the other hand, because of its suppressive action on the respiratory center, morphine is used rarely or only with extreme caution in patients with chest disorders. For relief of extreme pain the physician may resort to regional anesthetic block, which is achieved by injecting procaine along the intercostal nerves supplying the painful area.

Hemoptysis

When a patient expectorates blood, the question at once arises as to its source. Has it come from the gums, the nasopharynx, the lungs, or the stomach? Careful observation by the nurse, who may be the only witness to the episode, may be of great value in determining this point. The following points should be borne in mind as she makes and records her observations.

In patients whose bloody sputum originates from the nose or the nasopharynx expectoration is usually preceded by considerable sniffing and blood may appear in the nares. Blood from the lung is usually bright red, frothy and mixed with sputum. Initial symptoms include a tickling sensation in the throat, salty taste, burning or bubbling sensation in the chest and perhaps chest pain with a tendency for the patient to splint the bleeding side. The term *hemoptysis* is reserved for the coughing of blood arising from a pulmonary hemorrhage. This blood has an alkaline pH.

In contrast, if the hemorrhage is in the stomach, the blood is vomited rather than coughed up (*hematemesis*). Blood that has been in contact with gastric juice is sometimes so dark that it is referred to as "coffee-ground" material. This blood has an acid pH. (See p. 461.)

Hemoptysis occurs in many lung diseases, notably bronchogenic carcinoma, lung abscess, pulmonary infarcts, bronchiectasis, tuberculosis and pneumonia. It is also a symptom of mitral stenosis due to rupture of a blood vessel somewhere in the congested pulmonary

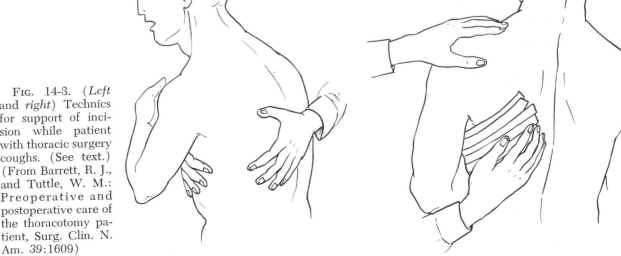

FIG. 14-3. (*Left* and *right*) Technics for support of incision while patient with thoracic surgery coughs. (See text.) (From Barrett, R. J., and Tuttle, W. M.: Preoperative and postoperative care of the thoracotomy patient, Surg. Clin. N. Am. *39*:1609)

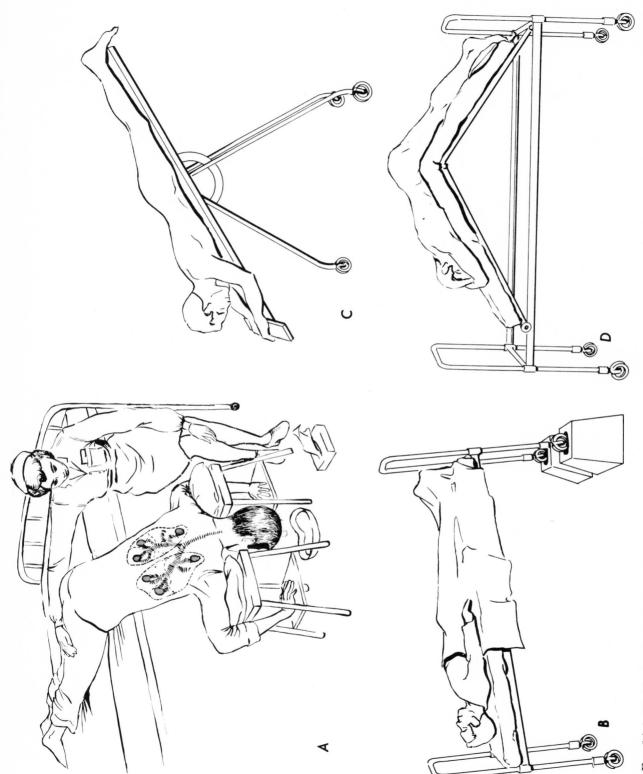

Fig. 14-4. Positioning for postural drainage. (A) This position for postural drainage is good for the lowest lobes, fairly good for the middle lobe but inadequate for the upper lobes. (B) This head-low position is good for drainage from the lower halves of each lung. (C) A tilt table can be used for draining the lower halves of each lung and is particularly useful in draining posterior lesions. (D) When the patient's bed can be adjusted to provide this position, it is a comfortable one; however, it is effective in draining the lower lung only and inadequate for the upper lobes.

circuit. A careful history and physical examination are necessary to establish a diagnosis of the underlying disease, whether the bleeding produced a fleck of blood in the sputum or a massive hemorrhage. The seriousness of cause is not necessarily in positive correlation with the amount of blood produced. Roentgenologic examinations are indicated, which may include fluoroscopy, planograms and bronchograms. If the nature of the process is not evident, bronchoscopy should be performed without delay in order to rule out an early tumor growth, bronchiectasis, an abscess or a foreign body.

Medical and Nursing Management. A patient who has experienced a hemoptysis, whatever its cause, should be placed immediately at complete bed rest and his respiratory movements reduced to a minimum by every available means, including oxygen inhalation therapy and morphine sedation. Sandbags may be applied to the anterior chest to restrain its motion.

Transfusion may be required if peripheral vascular collapse ensues or if shock results from the loss of blood. Equipment for performing an emergency laryngoscopy and bronchoscopy should be in readiness for the removal of blood clots from the respiratory passages if the patient shows the initial signs of asphyxia. If the hemorrhage is not controlled by these measures, an artificial pneumothorax may be induced in an effort to prevent as much mechanical expansion and contraction of bleeding lung tissue as possible.

The nurse must realize that hemoptysis is one of the most frightening of all the symptoms that patients experience. Fright promotes hyperventilation, which is the opposite desired, namely, a minimum of thoracic movement. Therefore, it is of the utmost importance that she avert panic and maintain emotional equilibrium in her patient by presenting the appearance of untroubled calm herself, functioning swiftly, efficiently and with utmost assurance, betraying no hint of alarm, but expressing confidence and optimism. Sedation, either barbiturates or tranquilizers, may be ordered to quiet the patient without unduly suppressing his ability to cough. When intractable cough threatens to perpetuate bleeding, codeine or other narcotic cough inhibitors may be given as a temporary measure.

Collections of Fluid in the Lungs

Postural drainage is the attempt to drain collections of fluid in the lung by gravity. These collections, which usually occur in pockets in the lung tissue, such as those seen in pulmonary abscess or in bronchiectasis, are drained by positioning the patient so that the collection is higher than the trachea and mouth. The expectation is that if the collections are sufficiently fluid, they drain by gravity through the bronchi, trachea to the pharynx so that they can be coughed up.

Postural drainage is most effective for collections that appear in the lower lobes of the lung. For those that occur in the upper lobes, postural drainage is less effective.

The Promotion of Postural Drainage. This is accomplished by placing the patient in a position so that the head and the thorax are dependent in relation to the rest of the trunk. The patient may simply flex his body over the side of the bed, head and shoulders hanging as close to the floor as possible, while his legs, held by the nurse, remain supported on the bed. A chair or a foot-stool of the proper height beside the bed provides a stable support. Resting his weight on his hands or elbows, the patient can maneuver himself into an optimal position, namely, the position that has been found by the patient to yield a most prompt and copious expectoration. Evacuation of the abscess is aided by coughing, which, therefore, should be encouraged. The frequency and the duration of postural drainage are decided on the basis of the volume of sputum ejected on each occasion, averaging from 5 to 10 minutes every 2 to 4 hours, and taking into account the patient's need for rest and his resistance to fatigue. Because of the exhausting character of the procedure, no period of drainage should exceed 10 minutes. During each performance the patient's color and pulse should be examined repeatedly by the nurse for signs of suffocation or peripheral circulatory collapse requiring immediate resumption of the horizontal position.

Satisfactory drainage can be accomplished in some patients with less arduous effort. For example, the patient may lie prone, with head and shoulders dependent, on a bed that has been elevated at one end to an angle of 20° from the horizontal. Or, the patient may lie prone, with head at the foot of a bed angulated to the maximum knee-rest position (Fig. 14-4).

If the sputum is foul-smelling, this procedure may well be carried out in a room away from other patients. Deodorizers should be used. Paper wipes and a bag for their disposition must be available. After postural drainage, it is refreshing for the patient to brush his teeth and use a mouthwash; he then should rest in bed for a half hour.

The effectiveness of postural drainage is estimated on the basis of the clinical signs: the course of the fever, pulse and respiration; the changes in appetite; the alterations in the body weight and the patient's sense of well-being. Its efficiency is best determined by estimating the proportion of exudate remaining in the abscess cavity at the conclusion of the drainage, as seen by roentgenograms, or as actually obtained by direct suction through a bronchoscope. If suction through a bronchoscope proves to be a rewarding procedure, it too should be scheduled routinely at intervals of from 1 to 3 days.

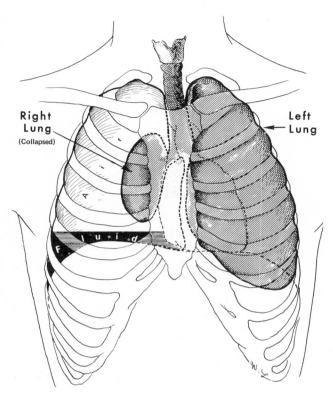

Right Lung (Collapsed)

Left Lung

Fig. 14-5. Chest cavity showing hydropneumothorax on the right side with atelectasis (collapse) of the right lung.

Atelectasis

Pulmonary atelectasis, or collapse, may result from pressure on the lung tissue, confining its normal expansion on inspiration. Such pressure may be caused by fluid accumulation within the thorax (pleural effusion), by air in the pleural space (pneumothorax), by an extremely large heart or a pericardium distended with fluid (pericardial effusion). It may be due to a tumor growth within the thorax or to an elevated diaphragm displaced upward as the result of abdominal pressure. In such circumstances there is a crowding of the intrathoracic contents, and, since the spongy lung tissue is most compressible, it collapses without resistance. Where it is compressed it becomes airless, or atelectatic, and the efficiency of pulmonary function is reduced accordingly. Atelectasis of this type is encountered most often in patients with pleural effusion due to cardiac failure, or in pleural infection.

Another form of atelectasis is caused, not by external pressure, but by obstruction of a bronchus, the effect of which is to impede the passage of air to and from the alveoli communicating with it. The alveolar air thus trapped soon becomes absorbed into the blood-

stream, and, all external communication having been blocked, its replacement from the outside air is impossible. The net result is that the portion of lung so isolated becomes airless: it shrinks in size causing the remainder of the lung to overexpand (compensatory emphysema). Bronchial obstruction, in this way causing atelectasis, may follow inhalation of a foreign body. It may be due to a plug of thick exudate that is not, or cannot be, expelled by coughing. Thus, it occurs in severe bronchial asthma, due both to bronchiolar spasm and to plugging of the bronchi by a thick tenacious secretion. This is the usual mechanism producing the "massive collapse" occasionally observed postoperatively and in debilitated bedridden individuals. In these people there is likely to be long-continued respiratory depression, together with inadequate depth of respiratory excursion, and perhaps unusually profuse or poorly expectorated bronchial secretions. Tumors of the bronchi often make their presence known first by an atelectasis resulting from their obstructive growth.

Symptoms. If collapse occurs suddenly, and if sufficient lung tissue is involved, the following may be anticipated: marked dyspnea, cyanosis, prostration and pleural pain which usually is referred to the lower chest. Fever commonly occurs. Tachycardia and dyspnea are unusually prominent. The patient characteristically sits bolt upright in bed, his expression anxious, his color cyanotic and his respirations labored. The chest wall on the affected side moves little, if at all, whereas on the opposite side the excursion appears excessive. Examination reveals signs of displacement of all intrathoracic organs toward the side of the collapsed lung, which lacks resonance on percussion and radiance by roentgenograms. Lungs that have collapsed due to the obstruction of a bronchus should be re-expanded as rapidly as possible to avoid the common complications of pneumonia or lung abscess.

Therapeutic Regimen and Nursing Management. If atelectasis has resulted from a pleural effusion or pressure pnemothorax, the fluid or air may be removed by needle aspiration. If bronchial obstruction is the cause, the nature of the obstruction must be ascertained and it should be relieved, if at all possible. To accomplish this, the respiratory center is stimulated to the maximum by means of carbon dioxide inhalations that may be administered at the bedside by the nurse, and also caffeine—particularly if morphine, a respiratory depressant, is to be used for the control of the pleural pain. The patient should be turned frequently in an effort to stimulate coughing. If these measures do not relieve the obstruction, prompt recourse should be had to bronchoscopy, which affords a most effective means of bronchial drainage and also of accurate diagnosis, both as regards location and nature of the obstructive lesion—exceedingly important in view of the possible presence of an aspirated foreign body. Antibiotic therapy should be given prophylactically in all cases of atelectasis, the objective being to forestall the development of a bacterial infection in the collapsed portion of the lung.

The incidence of postoperative pulmonary atelectasis has been reduced significantly as a result of the more conservative and judicious use of preoperative and postoperative sedation and by early ambulation of postoperative patients. Another important factor in its prevention is the stimulation of ventilation during and following operation by means of carbon dioxide inhalations, the purpose of which is to cause hyperventilation and, therefore, more adequate drainage of bronchial secretions. All stuporous, debilitated and heavily sedated patients should be turned frequently in bed, a procedure that affords increased respiratory excursion on the uppermost side. Judicious use of nasopharyngeal and nasotracheal suction is also of great help in stimulating patients to cough and to assist in removing tenacious secretions (see p. 263).

Collections of Air and Fluid in the Pleural Cavity

Hydrothorax. Serous (nonpurulent) effusions may occur in such medical conditions as cardiac or renal failure, lung and pleural tumors and so forth. The presence of the fluid may so embarrass respiration as to require aspiration (thoracentesis).

Pneumothorax and Hemothorax. Air in the pleural cavity may occur spontaneously from rupture of a lung alveolus; it may be induced deliberately to collapse cavities and set the lung at rest, as in the treatment of tuberculosis; or it may arise from trauma, the air entering the pleural cavity through the resulting wound or from the injured lung. Bleeding usually accompanies such trauma, so that a hemopneumothorax results. Aspiration of the blood and air permits re-expansion of the lung and a return to a more physiologic state. These patients usually respond to bed rest. If the pneumothorax is sudden and massive, the trachea and mediastinum shift to the opposite side due to air pressure causing respiratory embarrassment. This situation requires intubation of the hemothorax attached to a water seal to let the air out.

Chylothorax. Injury to the thoracic duct or to other lymphatic radicals in the chest may permit the escape of lymph into the pleural cavity. The lymph from the thoracic duct, rich in fat absorbed from the intestines, is called *chyle*, and the condition is called *chylothorax*. Injuries to the lymphatic radicals may arise from trauma or from operations in the posterior thorax, such as esophagectomies or sympathectomies. Small leaks may heal spontaneously, but thoracentesis may be required to relieve respiratory embarrassment. If the leak continues, operative intervention is required to suture or ligate the injured vessel. Continued loss of chylous fluid ends fatally.

THE PATIENT WITH A PULMONARY INFECTION

Acute Tracheobronchitis

An acute inflammation of the mucous membranes of the trachea and the bronchial tree, acute tracheobronchitis often follows infections of the upper respiratory tract. A patient with a viral infection has a lessened resistance and can readily develop a secondary bacterial infection. The adequate treatment of upper respiratory infections is one of the major factors in the prevention of acute bronchitis. Inhalation of physical and chemical irritants, gases, or other air contaminants is also an important cause of acute bronchial irritations.

The patient's symptoms result from the mucopurulent sputum that is secreted by the hyperemic edematous mucosa of the bronchi. The patient has a dry, irritating cough and expectorates a scanty amount of mucoid sputum at first. He complains of sternal soreness from coughing, has fever, headache and general malaise. As the infection progresses, the sputum is more profuse and purulent, and the cough becomes looser. Acute tracheobronchitis can be a serious disease in very young children. The child is acutely ill and may have noisy strident respirations with intercostal retraction. Strict nursing vigilance and prompt action are required if these symptoms of respiratory obstruction appear.

Medical and Nursing Management

The treatment is largely symptomatic. Therefore, the nurse's observations are important in determining the therapeutic plan. The patient is placed on bed rest. Moist heat to the chest will relieve the soreness and pain, and hot drinks may prove soothing. Cool vapor therapy or steam inhalations are beneficial in relieving the laryngeal and tracheal irritation. Increasing the vapor pressure (moisture content) in the air will reduce irritation.

Cough depressants should not be given, or given only with caution, when the cough becomes productive. An expectorant, such as potassium iodide, may be given and the fluid intake increased to "thin" the viscous and tenacious secretions. Usually recovery ensues within 7 to 10 days. Antibacterial chemotherapy may be ordered if the patient does not improve promptly.

A primary nursing function is to caution the patient against overexertion and chilling, which can induce a relapse or extension of the infection. Aged individuals are prone to develop bronchopneumonia as a complication. They are not always able to cough effectively and therefore tend to retain the mucopurulent exudate. These patients should be turned and should assume the sitting position at frequent intervals. Adequate opportunity for convalescence should be provided after the acute infection subsides, in order to avoid its recurrence.

Chronic Bronchitis

Chronic bronchitis is a progressive and potentially serious disease. The patient's major problem is the protracted and abundant production of inflammatory exudate that fills and obstructs his bronchioles and is responsible for his persistent, productive cough and shortness of breath. Alveoli adjacent to the affected bronchioles may become damaged and fibrosed. In time, irreversible lung changes may occur, with resultant emphysema or bronchiectasis.

This disorder may follow an acute respiratory infection, such as pneumonia or influenza. It is encountered in individuals whose occupation exposes them to irritating gases and smoke. Heavy tobacco smokers exhibit a high incidence of chronic bronchitis. The disease is most prevalent among middle-aged and elderly men—individuals who are especially vulnerable to recurrent attacks of acute bronchitis.

Because of the disabling nature of chronic bronchitis, the nurse should direct every effort toward its prevention. All patients with acute upper respiratory infections should receive proper treatment and adequate convalescence. Symptomatic individuals should stop smoking; air irritants of other types should be avoided whenever possible.

The main objective in the treatment of chronic bronchitis is the control of acute infections that threaten the lungs. Patients who are especially vulnerable should receive appropriate antimicrobial chemotherapy in the early stage of every febrile respiratory infection. To facilitate the removal of bronchial exudates, and to supply aerosolized medication most effectively, intermittent positive pressure breathing (page 252) may be instituted. In some cases that are complicated by an underlying bronchiectasis, postural drainage is beneficial. Basically, the medical treatment and the nursing management of patients who have chronic bronchitis or pulmonary emphysema (page 249) are very similar.

Pneumonia

The term *pneumonia* refers to a partial solidification of the lung, due to the filling of the alveoli with an inflammatory exudate in response to an infection or, less commonly, to a chemical irritant. Pneumonia is classified according to its causative agent, if known: for example, as a *bacterial, viral,* or *lipid pneumonia;* also, there is a *chemical* pneumonia, such as that seen after ingestion of kerosene or inhalation of irritating gases. If a substantial portion of one or more lobes is involved, the disease is referred to as *lobar pneumonia. Bronchopneumonia* implies that the pneumonic process is distributed in patchy fashion, having originated in one or more localized areas within the bronchi and extended to the adjacent lung parenchyma.

Prevention

The nurse should be acquainted with various factors and circumstances that commonly predispose to the development of pneumonia, so that she may be alert to the possibility of its occurrence and assist most effectively in its prevention. Aged individuals, patients with chronic bronchitis or emphysema, patients with cardiac failure and pulmonary congestion, and patients who are debilitated are prime candidates for pneumonia. Individuals who are intoxicated chronically are peculiarly susceptible to this infection and, if acquired, the course of pneumonia in the alcoholic patient is likely to be unusually severe.

Any patient who is permitted to lie passively for prolonged periods in bed, relatively immobile and breathing shallowly, is highly vulnerable to the risk of bronchopneumonia. The likelihood of its development is increased markedly if the patient is unable to cough effectively because of debility, prostration or shock, or as a result of sedation with a cough-suppressing drug. Any condition that promotes the retention of secretions in the bronchi predisposes to pneumonia. Aspiration of foreign material into the lungs during a period of unconsciousness, e.g., during anesthesia, is very likely to be followed by bronchopneumonia.

Bronchopneumonia, as a postoperative complication, is a potential threat in every case. There is a danger that the patient's cough reflex may be overly suppressed by drug sedation, or that coughing may be inhibited by the production of pain at the operative site. In the latter instance, the patient should be encouraged to cough as vigorously as possible while the nurse "splints" his incision in the manner illustrated in Figure 14-3. Any patient scheduled to receive a sedative drug, particularly one of the opium alkaloids, should be observed closely from the standpoint of respiratory rate and depth before the drug is given; and its administration should be withheld if respiratory depression is apparent, because respiratory depression predisposes to the pooling of bronchial secretions and, therefore, to the development of pneumonia. Postoperative pneumonia should be anticipated in the elderly patient and its development forestalled by frequent changes of his position. The observation of slow and shallow breathing may warrant the repeated administration, to such a patient, of carbon dioxide at hourly intervals or oftener. An important prophylactic measure, which is widely applicable, is the frequent suctioning of secretions from the mouths of patients who are unconscious or otherwise helpless, thereby reducing the likelihood that this material may be aspirated, accumulate in the lungs and induce bronchopneumonia.

Bacterial Pneumonia

Etiology. Bacterial pneumonia is most prevalent during the winter and spring months, when upper respiratory infections are most common.

The infecting agents most often responsible for this disease are the *pneumococci*, capsulated diplococci, of which there are at least 35 distinct immunologic types. Some of these predominate in certain localities at certain seasons, some are almost certain constant inhabitants of the normal upper respiratory tract. Organisms much less frequently involved include *Staphylococcus aureus, Klebsiella pneumoniae (Bacillus mucosuscapsulatus,* Friedländer's bacillus), *Streptococcus hemolyticus,* and *Hemophilus influenzae.* In recent years with the use of immunosuppressive drugs, antileukemic drugs or corticosteroids over long periods of time, an increase in the incidence of pneumonia due to more unusual organisms such as fungi has occurred.

Symptoms and Signs. The onset of acute pneumococcal pneumonia is precipitous. Previously well, the patient is suddenly prostrated by a sharp pain in the chest that prevents him from taking a deep breath. He is seized with a severe chill. The temperature rises rapidly and within a few hours reaches a level of 40.0° to 41.1° C. (104° to 106° F.). The pulse is rapid and bounding. The cheeks are flushed, the eyes bright and the lips cyanotic. The respiration is rapid; the nostrils dilate with each inspiration, and each expiration is punctuated with a grunt. The dyspnea may become extreme, and, although not truly orthopneic, the patient prefers to be propped up in bed because of his cough, which is short, painful and incessant.

The mental symptoms may be so pronounced as to overshadow all others, dominating the clinical picture completely. The patient may exhibit a restless, excited delirium. In such patients, who can least afford a delay in treatment, the diagnosis of pneumonia may be overlooked for a time, unless the nurse is unusually observant and alert to spot whatever clue might be at hand, such as a fleck of bloody sputum on the bedclothes or a transient chill.

Initially, the sputum may be clear; occasionally it is frankly bloody. But eventually, in most patients, it becomes rusty in color and so tenacious that it can be expectorated only with such difficulty that the nurse may be obliged to wipe it from the mouth. (The nurse is reminded to adhere to the principles of medical asepsis in caring for these patients.) Bacteriologic examination of this material reveals the infective agent.

The blood leukocyte count usually becomes elevated during the first or second day, ranging during the acute stages from 20,000 to 30,000 per cubic millimeter, a finding which is a great help in diagnosis. In very severe infections the white blood count may be depressed—a serious sign. The blood culture frequently is positive in the early stages before therapy is begun.

Treatment and Nursing Management. If the patient with bacterial pneumonia is treated promptly and appropriately, the infection, in most cases, is controlled quickly. Antimicrobial chemotherapy is instituted without delay, usually in the form of penicillin administered by intramuscular injection. Depending on the identity of the infecting organism isolated from the sputum, throat or blood cultures, and its drug sensitivity, as determined in vitro in the microbiology laboratory, another antibiotic or a sulfonamide drug may be substituted for penicillin.

The patient is placed on bed rest until the infection shows signs of clearing. Although specific isolation precautions generally are unnecessary, visitors should be restricted to members of the immediate family. The arrangement of the bed should provide maximum comfort and optimal respiratory efficiency, the orthopneic or semi-orthopneic position being preferred if dyspnea is severe. The least possible disturbance should attend the treatments and examinations that are carried out during the early, acute stage of the illness. The patient must be protected from drafts and, as a further precaution against chilling, dry linen should be substituted at once for garments or bedding dampened by perspiration.

OXYGEN. Oxygen inhalation therapy is indicated if the patient is cyanotic, dyspneic, or complains of pain on breathing, or if breathing appears to require undue effort. Under these conditions an oxygen tent or mask offers more than physiologic support: It brings both relief from pain and rest.

ANALGESIC AND ANTITUSSIVE MEDICATION. Codeine sulfate or Hycodan will alleviate the harrassing cough and reduce the pain of pleurisy. If pain is severe, Demerol may be given subcutaneously in 50- to 100-mg. doses at intervals of 4 to 6 hours; morphine, on the other hand, because of its suppressive action on the respiratory center, generally is considered as being contraindicated in patients with acute pneumonia.

The antipyretic drugs are useful in controlling general malaise and muscular pains; on the other hand, if the temperature is markedly elevated, the diaphoretic (sweat stimulating) action of these agents may only add to his discomfort. It must not be forgotten that numerous physical devices are available that may be as efficacious as the analgesic drugs and at the same

THE PATIENT WITH BACTERIAL PNEUMONIA
Objectives, Principles and Rationale of Care

I. To assist with collection of laboratory data for the identification of the causative bacteria:

A. Bacteriological study of sputum
1. Instruct patient to cough productively so that specimens will be of bronchial secretions.

Specific antimicrobial therapy depends upon the nature and sensitivity of organisms isolated from the culture and sensitivity tests of the sputum specimen.

2. If patient is too ill to raise sputum, aspirate trachea with catheter.

Tracheal apiration can produce a paroxysm of coughing productive of sputum.

3. Collect sputum in sterile containers.
B. Hemogram and urinalysis
C. Bacteriological study of blood
D. Posteroanterior and lateral chest x-rays

II. To provide specific therapy to eradicate the organism:

A. Give prescribed antibiotic at correct time intervals
1. Penicillin 600,000 to 1,200,000 units daily I.M.
   (a) Subsequent dosages may be ordered orally.
   (b) Penicillin treatment usually continued 3 to 4 days after clinical symptoms have improved.

Pneumococci are highly susceptible to the action of penicillin.

2. Tetracycline, cephlothin, or erythromycin can be given if patient is allergic to penicillin.

These antimicrobials are effective against pneumococcal infections in penicillin-sensitive patients.

B. Observe patient for nausea, vomiting, diarrhea, anal pruritis, skin rash and soft tissue reactions

III. To evaluate the patient's response to therapy:

A. Take T.P.R. and B.P. at regular 4 hour intervals and more frequently if indicated

The temperature curve provides an index of the patient's response to therapy and of his progress.

Hypotension occurring early in the course of the illness may indicate hypoxia or bacteremia.

Salicylates should be given with caution as they produce a drop in temperature and thus interfere with evaluating the temperature curve.

B. Evaluate for evidences of peripheral vascular collapse
1. Combat shock immediately and vigorously with pressor amines, I.V. fluids and blood.
2. Give penicillin I.M. if shock is present.

If hypotension is present, there is a decrease in coronary and brain oxygenation, which may produce serious effects.

C. Assess patient for evidences of delirium

Delirium is considered a grave prognostic sign.

IV. To provide supportive care and relieve the patient's discomfort:

A. Assist the patient to cough productively
1. Splint the patient's chest while coughing.

Depression of the cough reflex may produce retention of pulmonary secretions and lead to atelectasis.

2. Give codeine (64 mg. every 4 to 6 hours) as ordered.

Elderly patients have a diminished cough reflex and may require vigorous measures (suctioning, bronchoscopy) for removal of secretions.

B. Use measures to reduce pleuritic pain
1. Use hot and cold applications as ordered.
2. Spray ethyl chloride to site of pain as ordered.
3. Assist with intercostal nerve block with procaine.
4. Use analgesics with caution to prevent depression of cough reflex.

Pain and cough result from pleuritic invasion by pneumococci. The discomfort of pleuritic pain can interfere with the mechanics of ventilation. Pleuritic pain causes shallow breathing; the aeration of the pulmonary alveoli is diminished and this contributes to the development of cyanosis and serious respiratory problems.

THE PATIENT WITH BACTERIAL PNEUMONIA (Continued)

IV. To provide supportive care and relieve the patient's discomfort (*continued*)

    C. Maintain fluid and electrolyte balance
        1. Offer 2,000-3,000 ml. of fluids daily.
        2. Administer I.V. fluids and electrolytes if patient is seriously ill or vomiting.
    D. Give oxygen as indicated for dyspnea, circulatory disturbance or delirium

With lobar pneumonia there is arterial desaturation and the CO_2 content of the blood is increased.

A patient suffering from pneumonia who has pre-existing chronic obstructive pulmonary disease (bronchitis, emphysema) is apt to develop CO_2 narcosis when receiving oxygen (see pp. 229-231). A mechanical respirator may be required.

V. To be alert for complications:

    A. Pleural effusion
    B. Delayed resolution
    C. Superinfection
        1. Pericarditis
        2. Bacteremia
    D. Delirium

Approximately 15 to 20 per cent of patients with pneumonia develop complications.

VI. To educate the patient concerning prevention of pulmonary disease:

One episode of pneumonia appears to make the individual susceptible to recurring respiratory infections.

    A. Obtain influenza vaccine at prescribed times
    B. Avoid overfatigue, chilling and overindulgences, which lower resistance to pneumonia

Influenza increases susceptibility to secondary bacterial pneumonia.

    C. Report any signs and symptoms of a respiratory infection to the physician
    D. Urge patients to have follow-up examinations after recovery and dismissal from the hospital

Pneumonia frequently coexists with other pulmonary pathology, namely, cancer of the lung.

---

time lack their undesirable side-effects; for example, the febrile patient with pneumonia may obtain quite as effective relief from tepid sponges as with any of the drugs previously enumerated.

The combination of oxygen deficiency, high fever and toxicity associated with pneumonia may precipitate an acute anxiety state, delirium or disorientation. Should the patient develop these symptoms, sedation, possibly in the form of intramuscular paraldehyde (6 to 10 ml.) may be ordered. Tepid sponges exert a quieting effect and tend to reduce the fever. Restraints should be avoided; an excited patient will resist these vigorously, with the result that he may become thoroughly exhausted and severely febrile. Quiet conversation with the patient, arranging for a member of his family to stay with him or allowing him to sit in a chair often will help him through this phase.

ANTIDISTENTION THERAPY. Abdominal distention is a frequent complication of pneumonia in severely toxic patients. It is not merely a source of great discomfort,

but it impairs the efficiency of respiration by elevating the diaphragm and limiting its excursion. Measures indicated for its relief include the repeated administration of small saline enemas (1000 ml.), the insertion of a rectal tube, the application of moist heat to the abdominal wall and the subcutaneous injection of Prostigmin methylsulfate or Prostigmin bromide (0.5 to 1.0 mg. given at 4-hour intervals).

SOPORIFICS. Chloral hydrate is perhaps the least objectionable of all hypnotic agents in treating patients with acute pneumonia; mental aberrations due to cerebral hypoxia are less apt to occur in patients treated with this soporific than with other drugs in common use. The barbiturates are efficacious and likewise without ill effect in the majority of patients.

NUTRITION. The food selection for patients with pneumonia is limited to liquids and soft solid foods of high caloric value until the appetite is restored and a more liberal regimen is possible.

HYDRATION. Adequate hydration is important during the febrile period, when evaporation of moisture from the skin is increased. Adequate hydration is also of value in the stimulation of respiratory tract secretion. Milk, because of its nutritious qualities, is especially recommended; its caloric value may be increased by the addition of lactose, which cannot ferment in the gastrointestinal tract and, therefore, does not contribute to abdominal distention.

Patients with pneumonia complicated by congestive heart failure must not receive an unlimited quantity of fluids, and the sodium intake must be curtailed. Hydration of these patients demands the most careful supervision, for there is grave danger that fluid will accumulate to dangerous excess in the tissues, particularly in the lungs, producing pulmonary edema and, quite possibly, death.

ELIMINATION. The use of cathartics is rarely warranted in pneumonia, fecal retention being avoided quite readily in most patients by means of low saline enemas.

MOUTH CARE. Cleansing of the mouth, with particular attention to the tongue and the lips, should be performed conscientiously as long as the patient is febrile and dehydrated and the sputum is purulent. The importance of oral hygiene is even greater if there are herpetic sores about the mouth, which cause a great deal of discomfort in a high proportion of pneumonia patients.

COMMUNICABLE DISEASE PRECAUTIONS. Measures to prevent the spread of the patient's infection should be carried out by the nurse with all due sense of responsibility. The infective organisms can become disseminated by means of air-borne droplets or through contact with articles contaminated by the patient's respiratory secretions. The hands should be washed thoroughly after each manual contact with the patient or his immediate environs. Mouth wipes, paper bags and disposable sputum cups should be used exclusively and should be wrapped securely and burned without delay. The patient should be instructed to turn away from those at his bedside while coughing. The risk of contagion, regardless of the type of pneumonia or the stage of treatment, cannot be neglected as long as fever persists.

In so far as it is possible, visitors should be excluded during this phase, and any who are admitted should receive instructions regarding protective measures to be adopted.

Clinical Evaluation and Records. The temperature, the pulse and the respiration should be examined at 4-hour intervals, and the blood pressure should be measured at least once daily during the acute stage; these data should be charted promptly. Included on the chart should be data relative to the daily fluid intake and the number of stools each day.

Diagnostic Tests. In addition to routine blood, urine and stool examinations, blood cultures are taken and sputum specimens collected for bacteriologic study. It is essential that the sputum obtained for laboratory examination consist of material that is coughed from the depth of the bronchial tree and diluted as little as possible by saliva. If coughing is inhibited by pleural pain, the maneuver may be assisted by turning the patient on the affected side. An x-ray examination of the chest is indicated in every patient as soon as it can be performed. Personnel assigned to take portable bedside roentgenograms should be acquainted with the risk of infection and properly versed in the protective methods to be followed. An electrocardiogram also may be requested if the character or the rate of the pulse is abnormal or if there is any evidence of heart disease from the past history or the physical examination.

Complications. A spread of the pneumonic process or its failure to resolve may occur if the lungs are invaded by a species of bacteria against which the patient has not acquired an adequate immunity. Another explanation for these complications is the development, by the bacteria, of an acquired resistance to the particular agent that is employed in therapy, the effectiveness of which for that organism is, therefore, lost. Fortunately, however, bacterial resistance does not extend to all drugs and antibiotics that are available, and cure usually can be obtained by means of a suitable substitution of another agent.

Empyema, an accumulation of infected fluid in the pleural space, is now a relatively uncommon development with the advent of modern therapy. Its treatment and prevention are accomplished by chemotherapy alone, unless the empyema fluid is unusually viscid, in which case thoracotomy and mechanical drainage may also be required. Sterile pleural effusion may develop instead of a purulent empyema. Staphylococcal or Klebsiella infections are prone to destroy lung tissue, form lung abscesses and are very slow to resolve. They leave a good deal of scarring of the lung.

Septicemia following invasion of the bloodstream may result in meningitis, endocarditis, purulent arthritis or other localized infections. A pneumococcal infection may invade one of the paranasal sinuses, causing acute sinusitis, or it may enter the middle ear, resulting in acute otitis media. All infectious complications of pneumonia, as mentioned above, are entirely preventable and responsive to treatment with the same type of specific therapy that is effective in clearing the antecedent pneumonic process.

Atelectasis, "collapse" of the lung, is perhaps the most important of the noninfectious complications of pneumonia. It is caused by the obstruction of a bronchus with accumulated secretions that fail to be expelled before all of the alveolar air in the distal portion of the lung has been absorbed completely by the bloodstream. This complication is prevented by avoiding unnecessary sedation of the patient, so that the cough reflex never is greatly impaired, and by wisdom in the restriction of his activity so that he is never too immobile or immobilized for too long a period while acutely ill.

The appearance of *shock* in a patient with pneumonia is an ominous development. This complication is encountered chiefly in patients who have received no specific treatment, have been treated too little or too late, have received chemotherapy to which the infecting organism is resistant, or whose pneumonia is complicated by another debilitating illness. To combat peripheral collapse and maintain the arterial blood pressure, a vasoconstrictor agent such as Metaraminol bitartrate is given intravenously in the form of a constant infusion, and at a rate that is readjusted constantly in accordance with the pressure response. Corticosteroid drugs, such as hydrocortisone or dexamethasone, may be administered parenterally to combat shock and toxicity in patients with pneumonia who are extremely ill and in apparent danger of succumbing to the infection.

Primary Atypical Pneumonia (Viral pneumonia; acute interstitial pneumonitis)

Primary atypical pneumonia is now known to be caused by the Eaton agent (mycoplasma pneumonia organism). This agent is responsible for over 25 per cent of atypical pneumonias in adolescents and young adults. It is probably spread by infected respiratory droplets, that is, person-to-person contact. Often these patients develop positive cold agglutinin titers in their serum.

The inflammatory process spreads throughout the entire respiratory tract, including the bronchioles. Generally it has the characteristics of a bronchopneumonia.

Usually the patient has had an upper respiratory infection, and the onset of his pneumonic symptoms is gradual. The predominant symptom is a harassing and nonproductive cough. After a few days, mucoid or mucopurulent sputum is expectorated. The patient complains of headache that is aggravated by the cough. Malaise, chilliness, and fatigue are present.

The objective of nursing care is to promote the patient's rest and comfort. He should be placed in a single room and protected from activities that produce fatigue. Eaton agent pneumonia responds to the tetracycline drugs. Other "atypical" pneumonias are viral in origin and do not respond to antibiotics. The nursing care and treatment (with the exception of antibacterial therapy) is the same as that given to the patient who has a bacterial pneumonia.

Pleurisy

Pleurisy, or pleuritis, is the inflammation of the pleura, visceral and parietal, and the rubbing together of these inflamed membranes with respiration causes severe, sharp, "knife-like" pain. Later, as pleural fluid develops, the pain lessens. In the early dry period, the pleural friction rub can be heard with the stethoscope, only to disappear later as fluid appears to separate the roughened pleural surfaces. Pleurisy may develop at the onset or during the course of pneumonia or tuberculosis, after trauma to the chest or pulmonary infarction, in the viral disease known as epidemic pleurodynia and after thoracotomy. Careful x-ray and sputum examinations are indicated in order to discover the underlying condition.

Treatment and Nursing Approach

The patient should be kept at bed rest until the fever subsides and is made as comfortable as possible with such agents and devices as those discussed in relation to the bacterial pneumonias, depending on the specific indications in each particular case. Inasmuch as this patient has real pain on inspiration, the nurse can offer suggestions to make him more comfortable. Instruct him to lie on the affected side in order to splint the chest wall; this will lessen the stretch of the pleura. The nurse or the patient can use the hand to splint the rib cage when the patient must cough. Often he is apprehensive and needs empathy and the comfort measures that the nurse can provide. Patients with an apparently spontaneous fibrinous pleurisy should be treated with a view to preventing the further development of any tuberculosis present.

Pleural Effusion

Pleurisy with effusion sometimes begins as a fibrinous pleurisy, but in the majority of patients the onset is so insidious that the patient scarcely realizes its presence. Gradually he becomes pale, short of breath, easily fatigued, loses weight and strength and, sometimes, but not always, has a slight dry cough. Many a person with such symptoms continues at work until he is so tired that he must stop, whereupon the doctor often finds one of the pleural cavities almost full of fluid.

This type of pleurisy is usually tuberculous, but a few cases are due to infections by other organisms that cause empyema.

Symptoms

On inspection, the affected side looks distended, does not move on respiration and is flat on percussion. The heart is visibly moved to the more normal side, which is seen to make unusually wide respiratory excursions, since one lung must do the work of both. The presence of the fluid is demonstrated clearly on roentgenograms. Some of it should be removed at once by thoracentesis (p. 233) for examination. Of the fluid that is aspirated, some should be cultured on the usual bacteriologic media, some injected into a guinea pig to demonstrate the presence or absence of tubercle bacilli and some studied (cytologically) in a search for possible tumor cells indicating carcinoma of the pleura. The fluid may be clear, straw-colored and sterile on culture. Such findings suggest tuberculosis as the cause of the pleurisy. Fluid containing blood may be found in patients with tuberculous pleurisy, patients with malignant tumors involving the pleura and patients who have a pulmonary infarction. Sufficient fluid should be removed often enough through a large needle to keep the patient comfortable. The patient should be guarded against further progress of any tuberculous lesion present.

Nursing Care

Care of patients with pleural effusion entails the encouragement of bed rest with restriction of physical activity as long as fever persists and the provision of a nutritious diet reinforced with dietary supplements, as indicated. It is the nurse's responsibility to prepare the patient, mentally and physically, for thoracentesis (p. 232) and to assist the physician in its performance.

Empyema Thoracis (Pyothorax)

Acute empyema thoracis is a collection of pus in the pleural cavity. It occurs as a result of pneumonia or injury to the chest wall, and is most frequent in children. The usual history is of an acute pneumonia, in which a septic temperature persists or develops after the crisis has occurred. The patient is extremely ill, often with sufficient dyspnea to require a sitting posture (orthopnea) in order to obtain relief. Roentgenograms, which are of considerable aid to the surgeon, must be taken in the upright position.

Treatment

The causative organisms are identified, and the appropriate antibiotic is administered. A regimen of intermittent aspiration and instillation of antibiotics is tried. The use of fibrinolytic enzymes such as trypsin, streptokinase and streptodornase seems to be effective in dissolving fibrin clots and decreasing the viscosity of pus. However, if the patient still has a temperature elevation after a week or 10 days, and the cavity is not well on the way to obliteration, surgical drainage is done.

Operations. The operations are of 2 types. In the first type, an effort is made to drain the pleural cavity without permitting the entrance of air into it. This is spoken of often as *closed drainage*. In the second type,

drainage of the empyema cavity is accomplished by the removal of a section of rib, which permits an opening into the pleural collection. This is spoken of as *open drainage* or *thoracotomy*, and is used in cases with thick pus.*

When the pus is thick, indicating an empyema of long duration, the pus cavity usually is fairly well walled off, and the danger of collapse of the lung is not so great.

After an operation for empyema, the chief consideration in the recovery of the patient is the collapse of the empyema cavity by expansion of the lung. To this end the patients are instructed to breathe deeply every hour; they are urged to blow into a spirometer or a blow bottle, using the increased intrapulmonary pressure thus developed to expand the lung.

These patients should be allowed out of bed as soon as possible, usually after 7 to 10 days. They may sit in a wheelchair and outdoors in the sun if this is possible. A high caloric diet is given, especially high in carbohydrates, protein and vitamins. The chief nursing challenge is to encourage this patient to meet his nutritional needs. Attractive trays with small servings offered frequently and any other ways of tempting him to eat should be employed.

As soon as the drainage has decreased sufficiently, the tube may be removed from the chest and the wound is covered by simple gauze dressings. The convalescence should be passed as much as possible in the open air and sunlight.

Lung Abscess

This term refers to a localized necrotic lesion characterized by cavity formation. In the initial stages this cavity in the lung may or may not communicate with a bronchus; eventually, however, it becomes surrounded or "encapsulated" by a wall of fibrous tissue, except at 1 or 2 points where the necrotic process extends until it reaches the lumen of some bronchus or the pleural space and establishes, thereby, a communication with the respiratory tract, the pleural cavity or both. In the first instance, its purulent contents are evacuated continuously in the form of sputum, whereas if a pleural exit is accessible, empyema results; if both types of communication are furnished, the case becomes one of "bronchopleural fistula."

Etiology

A lung abscess may occur as the sequela of an infected pulmonary infarct, of bacterial pneumonia and in tuberculosis. There are many situations, however,

---

* If the inflammation has been long-standing, an exudate can form over the lung and interfere with its normal expansion. This will have to be removed surgically (decortication).

FIG. 14-6. Lungs affected by bronchiectasis.

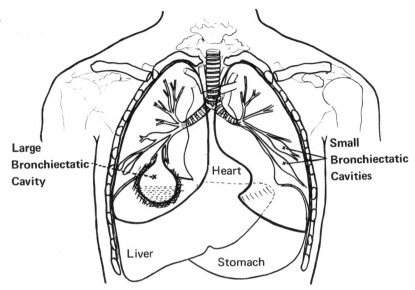

Large Bronchiectatic Cavity

Heart

Small Bronchiectatic Cavities

Liver

Stomach

in which bacterial infection plays no etiologic role, the origin instead being a lung tumor or an aspirated foreign body impacted in a bronchus.

Prevention

All individuals who are responsible for the care and training of children should be taught to recognize the importance of lung abscess as a dangerous disease, but one that is preventable inasmuch as its most important cause in childhood is the careless handling of small objects, such as coins, whistles, thimbles, buttons, etc., which should be kept out of the mouths of children as much as possible. If aspiration of a foreign body occurs, it is imperative that medical advice be sought at once so that bronchoscopic examinations may be conducted at the earliest possible moment.

Course

Many patients experience fever at first, and, for a time, this is their only symptom, but as soon as a bronchial communication is established, allowing the abscess to drain, the symptoms are progressively more severe and the infection is increasingly productive of sputum that is both purulent and foul. Fever mounts, emaciation becomes pronounced, and, unless therapy is effective, death soon may intervene.

Symptoms

After the early, relatively asymptomatic stages have passed, the diagnosis of lung abscess is fairly self-evident from the course it runs. In addition to the physical findings in the chest, clubbing of the fingers (hypertrophic pulmonary osteoarthropathy) may supply a helpful clue. Confirmation may be obtained from

the x-ray examination or by direct bronchoscopic visualization, a procedure that is almost always indicated because the possibility of a foreign body in the lung cannot be excluded otherwise.

Drug Therapy

A combination of drugs usually is employed in the treatment of lung abscess in recognition of the fact that a variety of organisms may be involved, some of which may be relatively unresponsive to any single agent. Drug selection depends on cultures and sensitivity studies, and use may be prolonged. An acceptable combination, for example, is sulfadiazine by mouth and penicillin by parenteral injection or in combination with streptomycin. A more important consideration, however, is the adequacy with which drainage is accomplished, whatever the means employed. Bronchoscopy and bronchial aspiration may have to be done repeatedly. Terpin hydrate or hydriodic acid syrup (only if tuberculosis has been excluded) may be used. Codeine should be given only if definitely indicated, and only on a temporary basis to relieve an exhausting cough.

Surgical Intervention

Surgery is indicated only when medical therapy has been proved inadequate by repeated failures to empty the cavity completely.

Preoperative Treatment and Nursing Care. A lung abscess will heal if the cavity can be emptied of its contents completely and at frequent intervals. This objective may be accomplished by means of postural drainage (p. 237), by aspiration through a bronchoscope or by open drainage through a chest wall incision, i.e., thoracotomy. The first method suffices in the majority of patients.

Patients with chronic lung abscesses whose lungs have become honeycombed with multiple fibrotic hard-walled cavities after a prolonged putrid infection can be restored to health only by the complete removal of the process by lobectomy or pneumonectomy. Before the operation the patient must be prepared adequately with antibacterial chemotherapy, blood transfusions and dietary measures in order to reduce the operative risk to a minimum.

Postoperative Nursing Care. After surgery there is usually a somewhat prolonged period of drainage before the wound closes entirely. In many cases, it may be necessary for some person in the family to change the simple dressings frequently enough to prevent excoriation of the skin and an offensive odor. Therefore, it is advisable frequently to give instructions in the method of dressing the wound and to demonstrate it. If possible, these patients are placed under the supervision of a public health nurse or some community agency that will help the family to meet any problems that may arise as a result of the care and the needs of these patients.

Bronchiectasis

Bronchiectasis is the permanent dilatation of one or several bronchi (Fig. 14-6). Some cases are congenital, more result from chronic bronchitis, and many cases originate in attacks of severe influenza or whooping cough, especially if the attacks occur in adult life. In the majority of patients several bronchi, usually of the lower lobes, are affected. The dilatation may be cylindrical—that is, tubular—or there may develop one or more saclike cavities containing several ounces of pus.

The condition results from weakening of the bronchial walls by chronic infection. The walls become permanently distended by severe coughing. The infection extends to the peribronchial tissues, so that in the case of saccular bronchiectasis each dilated tube virtually amounts to a lung abscess, the exudate of which drains freely through the bronchus.

Symptoms

Characteristic symptoms of bronchiectasis include chronic cough and the production of foul sputum in copious amounts. A high percentage of patients with this disease experience hemoptysis. Clubbing of the fingers is very common. The patient is likely to be subject to repeated episodes of pulmonary infection.

Most cases of bronchiectasis pass unrecognized, being mistaken for simple chronic bronchitis. A definite clue is offered by the prolonged history of productive cough, with a sputum consistently negative for tubercle bacilli. The diagnosis is established on the basis of the roentgenogram of the chest taken after the instillation of Lipiodol (a radiopaque iodide in an oil base) through the trachea into the bronchi. Direct bronchoscopy occasionally is valuable in determining the location and the extent of the disease.

Medical and Surgical Management

Patients may be put on a year-round regimen of antibiotics, alternating the type at intervals of several months. Some physicians use antibiotics throughout the winter or if acute upper respiratory infections occur.

Postural drainage is helpful, as are expectorants and bronchodilators. Good nutrition is a must because these patients tend to lose weight. Correction of chronic sinus infections should be undertaken. Of course, smoking is contraindicated.

There is really no satisfactory method available for collapsing a bronchiectatic cavity; therefore, the cavity often fails to heal on conservative therapy. The only definitive therapy is surgical removal; it may be necessary to remove a segment of a lobe (segmental resection), a lobe (lobectomy) or an entire lung (pneumonectomy).

Segmental resection is the removal of an anatomic subdivision of a pulmonary lobe. The chief advantage is that only diseased tissue is removed, with greater conservation of healthy lung tissue. Bronchography aids in the delineation of the segment.

Postoperatively, 2 tubes from the chest of the patient are connected to water-seal controlled suction. Air from air leaks following segmental resection is removed by this method, and the remaining lung is maintained in a more expanded state. Suction is discontinued in 2 or 3 days. (Preoperative and postoperative nursing care for segmental resection is the same as for any chest surgical patient, as discussed on p. 258.)

The immediate prognosis with surgical treatment is good, even in the case of bilateral operations, and with recovery the patient is cured completely of a most disagreeable and often incapacitating chronic disease. The operation is preceded by a period of preparation, which is exceedingly important. The object of this is to eradicate as far as possible the pulmonary infection and to improve the general condition of the patient, who may be extremely debilitated as a result of the disease. The infection is treated by frequent drainage of the cavity. This is accomplished by means of postural therapy or, if the abscess is suitably situated, by direct suction through a bronchoscope. A course of anti-bacterial chemotherapy should be started before the operation and continued in the postoperative period. The patient's general condition is improved by a liberal nutritious diet. If anemia is present, transfusions of whole blood are indicated.

Prevention of bronchiectasis depends on the avoidance of pertussis, accomplished by prophylactic immunization in childhood, on adequate management of chronic bronchitis, and on the successful treatment of pneumonia.

THE PATIENT WITH PULMONARY EMPHYSEMA

Now ranking second only to heart disease in causing disability, emphysema has also been listed among those diseases showing the greatest rise in the rate of fatalities. The large majority of patients are men; it is estimated that as many as one man in 10 over the age of 45 may have some degree of the disease. The incidence in women is also increasing each year. This increase is noticed particularly among urban dwellers who smoke cigarettes and have frequent respiratory infections.

Pathophysiology

In emphysema there is dilatation of all of the finer air passages and dilatation and coalescence (fusing together) of the alveoli with loss of inherent elasticity. The alveolus is the site in the lung where venous blood and environmental air complete the process of gas exchange. In order for gas exchange to be effective, the alveoli must be adequately ventilated with air. Interference with alveolar ventilation may occur if there is bronchial obstruction or in conditions in which there is uneven expansion of the lungs with poor air distribution.

The person with emphysema has a chronic obstruction (marked increase in airway resistance) to the inflow and to the outflow of air from the lungs. The lungs are in a state of chronic hyperexpansion. In order to get air into and out of the lungs, negative pressure is required during inspiration and an adequate level of positive pressure must be attained and maintained during expiration. The rest position is one of inflation. Instead of being an involuntary act, expiration becomes a muscular act. The patient becomes increasingly short of breath, the chest becomes rigid, and the ribs are fixed at their joints. This accounts for the "barrel chest" of many of these patients (Fig. 14-7). There is a continuous reduction of the vital capacity. Full deflation becomes increasingly difficult, and finally impossible. The total vital capacity may be normal, but the 1-second vital capacity is low (FEV_1). The patient moves air more slowly and inefficiently and has to work hard to do it.

The alveoli, long distended, begin to break down, a process accelerated by recurrent infections. As the walls of the alveoli are destroyed, the internal surface of the lungs, i.e., the area available for the exchange of oxygen and carbon dioxide between the atmosphere and the blood, continually decreases. There is interference with carbon-dioxide diffusion and the increased carbon-dioxide concentration stimulates respiratory activity in lungs that are already overworked and handicapped. This causes a mild to severe *pulmonary acidosis*. There is also impairment of oxygen diffusion with inadequate oxygen saturation of the venous blood. The increased CO_2 level within the affected alveoli is so increased that the partial pressure of O_2 and CO_2 in the alveoli is the opposite of normal; hence, little if any diffusion takes place in the affected areas of the lung (i.e., O_2 does not enter the blood and CO_2 does not leave it).

As the alveolar walls continue to rupture, the pulmonary capillary bed is reduced. The pulmonary blood flow is speeded and the right ventricle is forced to maintain a higher blood pressure in the pulmonary artery. Right-sided heart failure is one of the complications of emphysema. The presence of leg edema (dependent edema) or pain in the region of the liver suggests the development of cardiac failure.

Secretions are increased and retained because of inability to make a forceful enough cough to expel

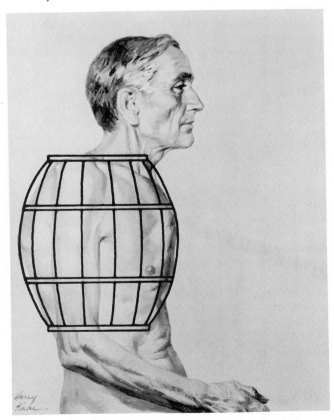

Fig. 14-7. The common "barrel chest" condition of the patient with emphysema. (Knoll Pharmaceutical Company)

them. Chronic and acute infections thus take hold in the emphysematous lungs, adding to the air transfer problem.

Patient Symptoms

A common pattern of symptoms is presented in the following case history of Mr. James, who had emphysema with respiratory acidosis.

> For 38 years, Mr. James, 62, smoked 2 packs of cigarettes a day. Only during the past 12 years had he noticed the "usual smoker's cough." On occasion he noticed shortness of breath, especially in association with respiratory infections. Now even the slightest exertion, such as bending over to tie his shoelaces, produces dyspnea and fatigue.

The emphysematous lung is not contracted on expiration, and the bronchioles are not effectively emptied of their secretions. The patient readily develops inflammatory reactions and infections due to the pooling of these secretions.

> After each heavy cold, Mr. James has been aware of prolonged wheezing expiration. He appears to hold his chest in a permanent inspiration position with shoulders elevated. He does not seem to be able to get rid of a productive cough. Many times he complains of a dull headache. He breathes more and more through his mouth. He looks anxious and speaks in jerky phrases.

Diagnostic Evaluation and Nursing Assessment

The patient's symptoms and the findings of the physician on physical examination provide the initial clues to the individual's problem. Other aids in helping the physician to arrive at a diagnosis include roentgenography, ventilatory tests and blood studies, as well as the electrocardiogram.

The nurse's observations and charting should reveal an understanding of the patient and his disease. How long has he had respiratory difficulty? What are the pulse and the respiratory rates? Are the respirations even? Does the patient contract his abdominal muscles during inspiration? Are the accessory muscles of respiration used? Does exertion increase the dyspnea? What are limits to his exercise tolerance? Is cyanosis evident? Are the patient's neck veins engorged? Is he coughing? What is the color and consistency of the sputum? What is the status of the patient's sensorium? Is there increasing stupor and apprehension? At what times during the day does he complain most of fatigue and shortness of breath? Have his habits of eating or sleeping been affected? What does he know about the disease and his condition?

Medical and Nursing Management

There is a multidisciplinary approach to the treatment and rehabilitation of the patient with emphysema. A desirable program for the care of individuals with emphysema is one that begins with an accurate diagnosis. This is followed by (1) prevention and prompt treatment of infection, (2) maintenance of proper environmental conditions to facilitate breathing, (3) use of pharmacological and physical aids to conserve and increase pulmonary ventilation, (4) prescribed activity and exercises, (5) supportive and psychological care, and (6) teaching and home care.

Prevention and Prompt Treatment of Infection. Preventive measures designed to forestall the development and progression of this disease must be recognized by the nurse. Obstructive adenoids and chronically infected tonsils should be removed in early youth, and all attacks of bronchitis and bronchial asthma should be treated adequately. Effective mouth hygiene is an essential part of preventive care.

For the emphysematous patient, infections are a constant threat. Some physicians keep their patients on prophylactic antimicrobial therapy, whereas others administer antibiotics only when the individual has been exposed to upper respiratory infections. Reverse isolation may be modified as a means of protecting this patient from infection. The cough associated with acute bronchitis introduces a vicious cycle, with further trauma and damage to the lungs, further progression of symptoms and further increase in susceptibility to bronchial infection. The patient should be instructed to report to the physician immediately if his sputum becomes discolored, because purulent expectoration is evidence of infection. He should be taught that any worsening of his symptoms—for example, increased tightness of the chest or increase in dyspnea—also is suggestive of infection and should be reported.

Maintenance of Proper Environmental Conditions to Facilitate Breathing. The patient should be instructed to avoid excessive heat and cold. Heat increases the body temperature, hence raises the oxygen requirements of the body; cold tends to promote bronchospasm. High altitudes aggravate the hypoxia. Bronchospasm may be initiated by such air pollutants as fumes, smoke, dust and even talcum and lint.

Patients with emphysema should be informed unequivocally that, for them, smoking is contraindicated. Cigarette smoking profoundly affects the ciliary cleansing mechanism of the respiratory tract, the function of which is to keep the breathing passages free of inhaled irritants, bacteria and other foreign matter. This is one of the major defense mechanisms of the body. When this cleansing mechanism is damaged by smoking there results obstruction to airflow and air becomes trapped behind the obstructed airway. The air sacs greatly distend and the individual's lung capacity is diminished. Cigarette smoking also irritates the goblet cells and mucous glands, causing an increased accumulation of mucus. The mucous accumulation produces more irritation, infection and damage to the lung capacity. Frequently the patient is unaware of what is happening until he notices that extra physical effort produces respiratory distress. At this point the damage may be irreversible. Therefore, patients with emphysema should definitely refrain from smoking.

Patients with emphysema should restrict themselves to a life of moderate activity, ideally in a climate with minimal shifts in temperature and humidity. Stress situations that might trigger a coughing episode or emotional disturbance need to be avoided. In her contacts with the family, the nurse can emphasize the importance of this.

Pharmacologic and Physical Aids to Conserve and Increase Pulmonary Ventilation. *Bronchodilating Drugs.* Oral preparations containing ephedrine or similar bronchodilating drugs are beneficial to certain patients. Epinephrine 1:1000 (0.5 to 1 ml.) subcutaneously may afford relief. Other adrenergic dilators that may be used are isoproterenol hydrochloride and methoxyphenamine (Orthoxine). Aminophylline (500 mg.) is effective orally or in rectal suppositories. If the patient is too dyspneic and ill to tolerate oral medication, aminophylline (250 to 500 mg.) is given slowly intravenously. The nurse must be aware of the fact that when this drug is given too slowly, it may fail to produce bronchodilatation, whereas too rapid administration may cause cardiovascular or central nervous system toxicity.

Aerosol solutions of bronchodilator drugs given by intermittent positive pressure on inspiration produce maximal bronchodilatation in many patients. Intermittent positive pressure breathing (p. 252) assists in reducing airway resistance, relieving bronchospasm, mobilizing bronchial secretions, and increasing alveolar ventilation with little effort by the patient. Oxygen is forced into the lungs and accumulated carbon dioxide is flushed out of the residual air spaces. The improvement of the oxygen saturation of the arterial blood and a reduction of its carbon dioxide content assists in relieving the patient's hypoxia and gives considerable relief from constant respiratory fatigue.

Humidification and Mucolytic (Mucus-Dissolving) Agents. Water is regarded by many as the best liquefying agent. It may be given by mouth, steam inhalation or nebulizer. Wetting agents or detergents such as acetylcysteine and propylene glycol aid in decreasing the surface tension of the water. A more recent humidifier is fog created by the ultrasonic nebulizer; a cup of water is bombarded with high-frequency sound waves that produce pure droplets far smaller (millionths of an inch in diameter) than ordinary nebulizers.

If the sputum is thick and purulent, *enzymes* such

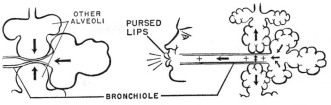

FIG. 14-8. Effect of positive pressure breathing. (National Tuberculosis and Respiratory Disease Association)

as trypsin, streptokinase or chymotrypsin liquefy the secretion by digestion. Careful observation by the nurse and prompt removal of liquefied secretions is necessary to prevent the patient from "drowning" in his own fluids.

Expectorants. The iodides aid in lessening the viscosity of sputum. Other medications are glyceryl guaiacolate and ipecac syrup.

Postural Drainage. This is prescribed to induce gravitational flow of sputum (see p. 237).

Because the patient is usually in an upright position, his secretions are likely to accumulate in the lower part of the lung. By using postural drainage exercises, the patient assumes various positions that help the force of gravity to drain the secretions from the smaller bronchial airways to the main bronchi and trachea. The secretions are then removed by coughing. Inhalation of the prescribed bronchodilators before postural drainage assists in draining the bronchial tree. To aid in the removal of thicker secretions, the chest may be tapped with cupped hands. A therapist (or nurse) gently taps in front and back of the chest simultaneously from the lower ribs upward. The vibration produced by the tapping helps loosen bronchial secretions and mucous plugs (see p. 279). The best time for performing postural drainage exercises is early in the morning, before meals, and at bed time.

Prescribed Activity and Exercises. In many instances, breathing exercises succeed in improving pulmonary ventilation. These are designed to alter the patient's breathing pattern from the thoracic type, characteristic of emphysema, to the lower costal and diaphragmatic type, favoring efficiency and conserving effort (see pp. 265-269).

Pursed-lip breathing exercises after a full deep breath allow slow exhalation with the lips partly closed. This encourages increased effort of the muscles between the lower ribs and upper abdomen. One method is blowing against a flame of a candle causing the flame to bend but not extinguish. The candle is

GUIDELINES IN ASSISTING THE PATIENT TO USE INTERMITTENT POSITIVE PRESSURE BREATHING (IPPB)

The intermittent positive pressure breathing (inspiration) unit is a piece of equipment that supplies air or oxygen under increased pressure during inspiration.

Nursing Activities	Rationale Underlying the Nursing Management and Treatment
Explain the procedure to the patient.	Proper explanation of the procedure helps to ensure the patient's cooperation.
For patients using bronchodilator drugs for the first time, take the blood pressure and pulse before and after inhalation.	Bronchodilators accelerate cardiac action. They may produce precordial distress, palpitation, dizziness, and nausea.
Instruct the patient to sit or be in a semi-Fowler's position.	The diaphragmatic excursion is greater in this position.
Turn on the oxygen cylinder.	This is a pressure-operated machine whose source of pressure may be supplied from a cylinder of oxygen, a cylinder of compressed air, a pipe line, or a motor-driven air compressor.
Place the prescribed medicine in the nebulizer.	The volume of medication is gauged to give a treatment lasting 15 to 20 minutes. Notify the doctor if the medication is nebulized too quickly.
Select the pressure prescribed (usually 15 to 20 cm. H_2O). Cover the mouthpiece with a paper towel to ascertain when the predetermined pressure is reached.	Each unit should be tested to see whether the predetermined setting is accomplished before treating the patient.
Turn on the nebulizer control to produce a fine spray.	Adequate fog and particle size is essential to sufficient medication distribution.
Adjust the mask or the mouthpiece on the patient. If the patient objects to the nose clip, instruct him to hold his nose. After several treatments, the patient can train himself to do without the nose clip.	The mask or mouthpiece must constitute a closed circuit, if the unit is to cycle. (If the patient exhales through the nose while using the mouthpiece, the unit will not reach the desired pressure.)
Have the patient place his hands on his diaphragm while breathing, concentrating on causing motion with the diaphragm rather than with the chest muscles.	This type of breathing encourages good diaphragmatic motion and reduces residual air volume.
Instruct the patient to make only a slight inspiratory effort, i.e., breathe as passively as possible.	A slight inspiratory effort will activate the positive pressure phase, and the lungs will be inflated with a rapid rate of flow until the predetermined pressure is reached.
Remind the patient to exhale using a gently forced expiration.	After the lungs are inflated, the flow of gas ceases and allows the patient to exhale without any assistance from the machine.
Encourage the patient to continue this type of breathing until all the medication is given.	The medication should be completely nebulized to ensure treatment effectiveness.

placed 6 inches from the person and each day the distance is increased 2 to 4 inches until a distance of 36 inches is reached. The exercise is done for 5 minutes once or twice daily. Other exercises of this nature include blowing ping-pong balls, and bubble-blowing using a straw in ½ glass of water.

The patient may be ambulant and active within the limits of his ability, unless otherwise ordered. Ambu-

lation prevents weakness and loss of muscle tone and aids morale.

A patient with emphysema has definite periods of the day when his exercise tolerance is decreased. This is especially true on arising in the morning, because bronchial secretions and edema collect in the lungs during the night while he is lying supine. He often will be unable to shave or to wash. Activities requir-

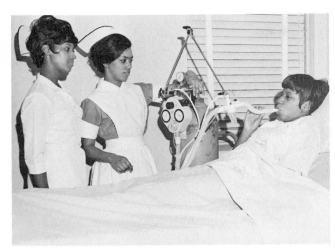

FIG. 14-9. The instructor and student are assisting the patient, who has chronic obstructive lung disease, with an IPPB treatment. During the treatment the nurse encourages the patient to breathe slowly and evenly to facilitate maximum ventilation of the lungs. (Freedmen's Hospital School of Nursing)

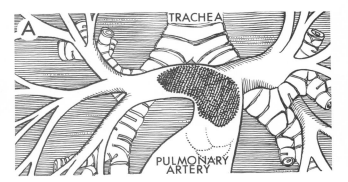

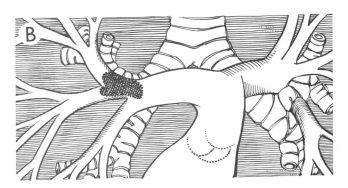

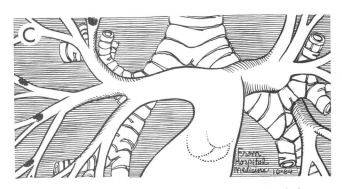

FIG. 14-10. (A) A massive thrombus at the bifurcation of the pulmonary artery may prove to be fatal. (B) Pulmonary artery branch thrombus. (C) Thrombi in terminal branches. (Adapted from Hospital Medicine, October, 1964)

ing the arms to be supported above the level of the thorax may produce distress. These activities may be tolerated better after he has been up and moving around for an hour or more. Therefore, he has the right to participate in planning his nursing care with the nurse and determining the best time for bathing and shaving. A hot beverage on arising will assist him to expectorate and will shorten the period of disability noted on arising.

Another period of increased disability occurs immediately after meals, particularly the evening meal. Fatigue from the day's activities coupled with abdominal distention combine to limit his exercise tolerance. The patient's chief complaint at this time is fatigue. This is another way of saying, "I am dyspneic": dyspnea is the underlying cause of his fatigue.

Supportive and Psychological Care. Any factor that interferes with normal breathing quite naturally induces anxiety and apprehension. By demonstrating nursing competence and concern as well as including him in the planning and execution of his care, this patient is more likely to develop a positive and optimistic outlook.

Give the IPPB treatment before meals to improve lung ventilation and thus reduce the fatigue that accompanies eating. Gas-producing foods are to be avoided because they hamper abdominal breathing. Fluids taken frequently prevent dehydration. Small frequent feedings also help to lessen pulmonary fatigue and serve to maintain adequate caloric intake. Activi-

ties and exercises (p. 251) tend to promote a general feeling of well-being.

Teaching and Home Care. One of the major teaching factors is to help the patient to accept realistic long-range goals. If he is severely disabled, the objective of treatment is to preserve his present pulmonary function and relieve his symptoms as much as possible. If his disease is mild, the objective is to increase his exercise tolerance and prevent further loss of pulmonary function. The patient has to be told what to expect. He and those caring for him need patience to achieve these goals.

THE PATIENT WITH PULMONARY EMBOLISM

Pulmonary embolism refers to the lodgement in one or more pulmonary arteries of a thrombus (or thrombi) originating somewhere in the venous system or in the heart. This commonly produces an infarction of lung tissue due to interruption of its blood supply. This problem is seen with increasing frequency and is often associated with advanced age.

The majority of thrombi originate in the deep veins of the legs. Other sources include the pelvic veins and the right atrium of the heart. Sometimes irritating solutions given intravenously in the veins of the arms produce thrombosis and embolism. Although blood clots usually compose the thrombus, air, fat, bone marrow, and septic material may occasionally be involved in embolization. Fat emboli may follow fractures of large bones.

The *symptoms* of pulmonary emboli depend upon the size of the thrombus and the area of the pulmonary artery occluded. A large embolus occluding the bifurcation of the pulmonary artery (Fig. 14-10A) can produce sudden substernal pain, pronounced dyspnea, rapid and weak pulse, shock, syncope and sudden death. If one or more branches of the right or left pulmonary arteries are obstructed (Fig. 14-10B) the patient experiences dyspnea, mild substernal pain, weakness and tachycardia. Usually these symptoms are the result of pulmonary infarction. There may also be fever, cough and hemoptysis. The patient's respiratory rate is accelerated out of proportion to the degree of fever and tachycardia. If the terminal pulmonary arteries are occluded (Fig. 14-10C), a pleuritic type of pain develops together with cough and hemoptysis. Multiple small emboli can lodge in the terminal pulmonary arterioles producing multiple small infarctions. The clinical picture may simulate that of bronchopneumonia.

Any condition that produces slowing of blood flow can produce a thrombus and resultant embolization. Immobilization per se is a predisposing factor. Thus pulmonary embolism is an ever present danger in patients after surgery, obstetrical delivery or prolonged bed rest. Many so-called postoperative pneumonias are now known to be due to pulmonary emboli. This is especially true in the aged individual who may be inactive and have diminished muscle tone. A pulmonary embolism is likely to occur in patients with congestive heart failure or with atrial fibrillation. The nurse should be on guard for occurrence of sudden pleuritic pain, increasing dyspnea or hemoptysis in any patient for whom she is caring.

In *diagnosis,* patients with pleurisy, cough, hemoptysis, tachycardia, pallor, perhaps signs of shock are suspect especially if phlebitis is present in the legs or if the patient is postoperative. Certain electrocardiogram changes (i.e., of right heart strain) and discrete shadows or patches of "pneumonia" on the chest x-ray are helpful diagnostically. Often treatment must be made on presumption rather than proof in order to prevent further large and fatal emboli.

Management

The ideal method of treatment is prevention. Effort is directed towards preventing venous stagnation in patients on bed rest by ambulation or by active and passive leg exercises. By moving the legs in a "pumping" exercise, the leg muscles assist in increasing venous flow. Patients with conditions predisposing to slowing of venous return (varicosities, polycythemia, fractures, congestive heart failure) should wear elastic stockings or bandages.

If the patient has a large obstructing pulmonary embolus, the objective of therapy is to combat shock, hypoxia and ensuing heart failure. This is a true medical emergency. The blood pressure is maintained with transfusions and intravenous administration of vasopressor solutions. Oxygen is given as a supportive measure. Digitalization is begun if the patient is in right ventricular failure. The patient is observed for symptoms of cardiac arrhythmia and cardiac arrest. An important aspect of treatment is the prevention of further immediate embolization. The patient is usually given anticoagulants initially with heparin and then given coumadin derivatives for several weeks following the embolic episode.

Surgical Treatment. The surgical treatment of pulmonary embolism may be divided into 2 kinds. Because of the not infrequent complication of phlebitis after surgical procedures, much attention is given to prophylactic treatment. This involves measures to prevent emboli from reaching the right heart once phlebitis has developed. Experience has shown that emboli that causes serious and often fatal pulmonary embolism arise most often from clots that form in phlebitis in the leg, and less often in the pelvis. Hence, to prevent pulmonary emboli in patients with phlebitis of the legs, the veins are ligated high in the thigh, sometimes only on the side with phlebitis or often on both sides. In those patients who have already had pulmonary embolism, the vena cava itself may be ligated to prevent the passage of a massive embolus to the heart. This is discussed more fully in Chapter 18, page 352.

The second type of surgical treatment for pulmonary embolism is a direct attempt to remove the embolus

THE PATIENT WITH EMPHYSEMA; PATIENT EDUCATION EMPHASIS

Teaching the emphysematous patient is one of the most important aspects of his care. The patient becomes an active participant in planning his care when he understands the objectives of his therapy and has guidelines set forth to achieve them.

I. To delay the progression of the disease process:

A. Understand the importance of preserving existing lung function.
 1. Become familiar with the nature of the disease and the reasons for the therapeutic regimen.
 2. Accept the fact that therapy and medical supervision must be continued for a lifetime.
 3. Secure vocational rehabilitation services if a job change is indicated.

B. Avoid activities that produce excessive dyspnea.
 1. Live within the limitations that emphysema imposes.
 2. Learn to relax and work at a slower pace.
 3. Adjust activities according to individual fatigue patterns.
 4. Breath in a slow and relaxed manner during periods of physical activity.
 5. Avoid emotional stresses or cope as positively as possible with those that trigger attacks of dyspnea.

C. Avoid exposure to respiratory irritants (fumes, dust, smoke, cold, etc.).
 1. Stop smoking (see p. 249).
 2. Stay out of extremely cold weather or keep a scarf over nose and mouth to warm inspired air.
 3. Avoid sudden changes in environmental temperatures.

II. To prevent and eliminate bronchial infections:

A. Report any evidence of respiratory infection to the physician promptly.
 1. Observe sputum and notify physician if there is any change in amount, character or color.
 2. Take prescribed antibiotic as directed.

B. Maintain general health in as optimal a condition as possible.
 1. Follow good habits of nutrition.
  (a) Have rest periods before and after meals if eating produces dyspnea.
  (b) Avoid excessively hot or cold fluids and foods that may provoke irritating cough.
 2. Avoid overfatigue, which is a factor in producing respiratory distress.
 3. Use good oral hygiene frequently to prevent respiratory infections.
 4. Avoid contact with persons having respiratory infections.
 5. Obtain immunization with Asian flu vaccine at prescribed times, if advised by physician.

III. To reduce bronchial secretions:

A. Prevent and control respiratory infections.
B. Maintain an adequate fluid intake (12-15 glasses daily).
C. Use home humidifier (especially if home has hot air heat).
D. Follow postural drainage procedures as directed.
E. Take medications prescribed for cough and expectoration.
F. Take bronchodilators as ordered.

IV. To increase pulmonary ventilation:

A. Use nebulization treatment consistently and faithfully.
 1. Do the procedure immediately upon arising in the morning and before meals when indicated.
 2. Learn how to assemble and disassemble equipment.
 3. Use the proper amount of medication ordered by the doctor.
 4. Inhale and exhale as evenly as possible during the treatment.
 5. Try to cough *productively* after the treatment.
 6. Observe oral hygiene after each treatment.
 7. Wash the mouthpiece and nebulizer after each use.

B. Do breathing exercises to strengthen muscles of expiration.
 1. Learn the importance of slow and relaxed breathing.
 2. Practice diaphragmatic breathing (see p. 251).
 3. Practice pursed-lip breathing.
 4. Do resistive exercises (candle- and bottle-blowing).
 5. Consciously use pursed-lip breathing during episodes of dyspnea.
 6. Maintain muscle tone of the body by regular exercise.

from the pulmonary artery. Obviously, when a large clot is pushed into the pulmonary artery from the right side of the heart, large enough to block the main pulmonary artery or the main branches of that artery, the sudden blockage would produce an increasing dilatation of the right heart that would lead to death, often in a matter of minutes or hours. The ideal surgical treatment is to operate and remove the embolus from the pulmonary artery. This requires the facilities of an operating room prepared for cardiac surgery, including facilities for open heart surgery (see p. 394), and a skilled cardiac surgeon. The operation cannot be delayed long if it is to be successful. These ideal circumstances cannot always be found in large hospitals and

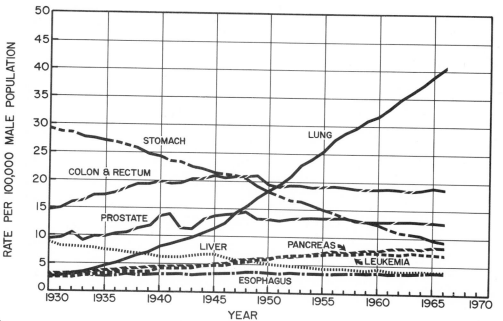

FIG. 14-11. Cancer death rates by site. The lung cancer death rate for males rose from 3.6 per 100,000 population in 1930 to approximately 37.6 in 1965, while death rates for other sites remained fairly level or actually decreased. It is estimated that about 55,000 Americans, 46,000 men and 9,000 women, will die of lung cancer in 1968. (Adapted from: 1968 Cancer Facts and Figures, p. 10, New York, American Cancer Society)

*Rate for the male population standardized for age on the 1940 U.S. population.
Sources of Data: National Vital Statistics Division and Bureau of the Census, United States.

EPIDEMIOLOGY AND STATISTICS DEPT. AMERICAN CANCER SOCIETY, 7 – 68

even more rarely in smaller hospitals. In some larger hospitals pulmonary emboli teams are organized. These teams attempt to reduce time lost before the patient can be operated upon. Most successful results have occurred with those patients in whom the clot did not completely block the pulmonary arteries or its larger branches, and who live long enough to permit operation. The successful cases are usually younger patients, who do not have complicating cardiorenal disease.

In addition to these surgical measures, attempts are being made to treat pulmonary embolism by trying to "dissolve" the clot in the pulmonary vessels. This is done by injecting fibrinolysin into the pulmonary artery through a vascular catheter introduced into the right heart through a vein at the elbow or neck. In other patients, the solution may be injected intravenously. Other drugs such as urokinase have been used, but these are not yet available for general use.

The clots of pulmonary emboli spontaneously disappear in about 50 per cent of the patients who live long enough (a period of 2 to 3 weeks).

PATIENTS WITH TUMORS OF THE CHEST

A chest tumor may be *primary*, that is, it may arise within the lung or the mediastinum; or it may represent a metastasis from a primary tumor site elsewhere. Metastatic tumors of the lungs are not rare, because

the bloodstream brings to them free cancer cells from primary cancers elsewhere in the body. Such tumors grow in and between the alveoli and the bronchi, which they push apart in their growth, often for a long time causing few or no symptoms. If, however, a nodule grows just beneath the pleura, the affected pleural cavity fills with fluid (often bloody), which, if removed, quickly collects again.

Primary tumors of the lung may be benign or malignant. In the majority of patients, at least, they arise from the bronchial epithelium. If they are benign they are known as *bronchial adenomas;* if malignant, *bronchiogenic carcinomas.* The effects they produce on the patient are exceedingly variable, depending entirely on their location and the nature of their growth. Benign adenomas are apt to bleed, giving rise to repeated hemoptyses. Also, by obstructing a bronchus, they may cause emphysema or atelectasis of the lobe with which the bronchus communicates. Tumor growth in the bronchus causes coughing. Pain is determined by the structures the tumor involves. The malignant carcinoma, in addition to causing bleeding and bronchial obstruction, spreads to involve other portions of the lung tissue, and frequently other organs as well, notably the lymph nodes of the mediastinum and the neck, the liver, the adrenal glands and the bones. By direct extension it may invade a pulmonary vein, a portion of the vena cava or the heart itself, giving rise to symptoms attributable to the resultant circulatory disturbance.

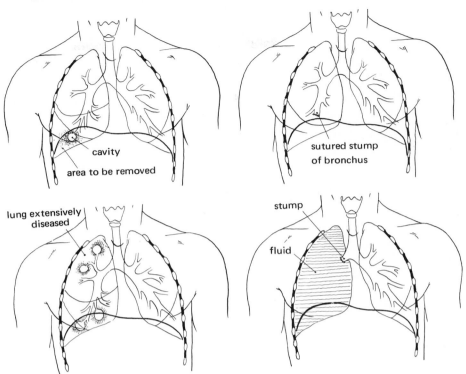

FIG. 14-12. Lobectomy and pneumonectomy for lesions of the lung. The lesions shown are abscesses or tuberculous cavities, but the same operations may be done for bronchiectatic cavities or for lung tumors. (*Top, left*) Lesion in the lower lobe of the right lung and (*top, right*) appearance after lobectomy. (*Bottom, left*) Multiple areas of disease in the right lung. These may be tuberculous cavities, an abscess cavity, a bronchiectatic cavity, or a lung tumor. (*Bottom, right*) Appearance after removal of the entire lung—pneumonectomy.

Cancer of the Lung

Cancer of the lung is an increasingly common tumor in the male population, and statistically it now is a leading cause of death in white males (Fig. 14-11).

All studies agree that the lung cancer death rate among men with a history of regular smoking for at least 20 years is approximately 10 times greater than that of men who never smoked. The lower incidence of lung cancer in women is explained by the fact that the proportion of regular smokers is less in women than in men, the female smoker starts later in life and smokes for fewer years, and female smokers inhale much less than men. Actually, as smoking has increased in women, so has their incidence of cancer of the lung increased.

There is obviously an asymptomatic period in the development of cancer of the lung, when, like the proverbial submerged iceberg, it cannot be recognized by presently available diagnostic methods. Every person who has smoked cigarettes for 15 or 20 years should be suspected of harboring such a cancer and deserves to have periodic roentgenography of the chest every 3 or 4 months, and a yearly physical examination, even though he is asymptomatic. Although it is not always practical to do so, such a patient would probably also benefit from periodic examination of the sputum and bronchoscopy.*

* Ochsner and Ochsner: Cancer of the lung. Surg. Clin. N. Amer., *46*:1411, Dec., 1966.

Lung tumors appear to arise from the lining membrane of the large air passages in men of 40 years and beyond. The earliest symptom of lung cancer is cough, which is present in about 80 per cent of patients. It begins as a hacking nonproductive cough, and later progresses to produce a thick purulent sputum as secondary infection occurs. A wheeze in the chest is noted in about 20 per cent of cases, and spitting of blood or blood streaks in the sputum is common. In a few patients, recurrent fever due to a persisting infection in an area of pneumonitis distal from the tumor is the early symptom. Pain is usually a late manifestation of lung cancer. The diagnosis is made by a combination of diagnostic studies. Usually the roentgenogram shows a definite tumor mass, and by bronchoscopy one may remove sections of the tumor or examine the secretions for tumor cells. Such cells may also be found in fresh sputum.

Medical Management. Surgical removal of the lung tumor, and of areas of spread to the mediastinum is looked upon as the best hope for cure. The best results seem to occur when preoperative irradiation is given before surgery. The surgery performed varies with the finding at operation. In early cases, only one lobe may have to be removed (lobectomy); in patients with more extensive tumors, the entire lung may have to be removed (pneumonectomy). (See Fig. 14-12.) Such operations are performed under endotracheal anesthesia; as a rule, a wide incision is made between the ribs to expose the pedicle of the lung. After the diseased tissue is removed, the chest wall is closed tightly and often a drainage tube is inserted into the pleural cavity. This tube may or may not be used for airtight suction or water-seal drainage but, in any event, it must be kept airtight unless otherwise ordered. The surgeon may make an intrathoracic injection of penicillin and/or streptomycin in the post-pneumonectomy patient for a few days.

The outlook for patients operated upon for lung cancer is poor. The overall 5-year survival rate is about 5 per cent. However, if the operation is performed while the tumor is localized, the 5-year survival rate is 40 to 50 per cent. When the tumor has spread to the regional lymphatics, it drops to 15 to 20 per cent. The operative risk is 25 per cent for localized tumors.

Irradiation has a very definite place in the treatment of inoperable lung cancer. It often relieves pain and makes life more tolerable for a time for these unfortunate patients.

NURSING MANAGEMENT OF THE PATIENT HAVING CHEST SURGERY

In addition to a skillful operation, the success of chest surgery depends on good preparation before operation and intelligent observation and nursing care after operation.

Preoperatively, the emphasis is on (1) assisting the patient who is undergoing diagnostic studies, (2) reducing the number of organisms in the upper respiratory tract, (3) preparing the patient mentally and physically for the surgical program ahead and (4) acquainting the patient with some of the postoperative problems, such as coughing.

Postoperatively, the major objectives are (1) maintaining a patent airway, (2) providing for maximum expansion of the remaining lung tissue, (3) recognizing early symptoms of untoward complications and (4) providing supportive and rehabilitative measures.

Preoperative Management

Psychological Aspects

Usually, several days are allotted to the preoperative phase, which provides time for the nurse to talk with her patient. By listening to him, she may be able to discover how he really feels about his illness and the proposed treatment. He may reveal significant reactions: the fear of hemorrhage because of bloody sputum, the discomfort of a chronic cough and chest pain, the social stigma attached to a foul-smelling sputum, the fear of death because of dyspnea—all contribute to his psychological status. The nurse can help him to overcome many of his fears by correcting any false impressions, by offering reassurance in the capability of the surgical team and by reporting special problems to the appropriate services available.

General Preparation

This is a general evaluation of the patient to determine and to correct any associated problems, such as metabolic disturbances, dehydration, cardiac impairments, etc. If he is malnourished and has a history of weight loss, naturally he will be placed on a high-caloric, high-protein diet reinforced with vitamins. He is encouraged to be up and about to maintain good muscle tone. Blood tests, including sedimentation rate, are done. The patient is told that he will be required to cough postoperatively and that it may hurt to do so. He is also taught how to cough; the nurse emphasizes the importance of bringing up secretions. She also can tell him that he may be receiving oxygen therapy, and that this is routine to facilitate breathing. Also, blood transfusions may be given. He should know that such treatment does not necessarily mean that his condition is precarious.

Reduction of Organisms in Upper Respiratory Tract

Mouth Hygiene. Inasmuch as the mouth is a portal of entry for organisms into the respiratory tract, good oral care is a necessity. If the patient needs dental care, this should be reported to the physician. Brushing of the teeth must be done on rising in the morning, after each meal and before retiring.

Postural drainage may be indicated in bronchiectasis and other chest conditions to bring up excess secretions (see pp. 236-237).

Antibiotics and Chemotherapy. In addition to the above methods for reducing the number of organisms present, systemic antibiotic therapy and chemotherapy are used.

Immediate Preoperative Preparation

The night before surgery, the patient is given a mild sedative, after he has had the operative area shaved (see Fig. 9-6), and an enema, if ordered. The usual preparation immediately before surgery is done. In patients with suppurative diseases, atropine is withheld until postural drainage is done. Usually, chest surgical patients receive a larger amount of atropine than do abdominal surgical patients, so that secretions are minimized.

The anesthetic is administered by the endotracheal technique, and one anesthetic or a combination of anesthetic agents is used.

Operative Procedures

Pneumonectomy

The removal of an entire lung is done chiefly for cancer, but may be performed for extensive unilateral tuberculosis, multiple lung abscesses or bronchiectasis. A posterolateral or anterolateral thoracotomy incision is made with resection of 1 or 2 ribs. The pulmonary artery and the pulmonary vein are ligated and severed.

The main bronchus is divided and the lung removed. The bronchial stump is sutured and no drains are used because the accumulation of fluid in the empty hemithorax is the desired end result. The phrenic nerve on the involved side is crushed to allow the diaphragm to rise on the affected side so that the cavity that is left may be reduced.

Lobectomy

A lobe of lung is removed when the pathology is limited to this one area. This operation may be done for cysts, abscesses, benign tumors, tuberculosis or bronchiectasis and local carcinomas. A thoracotomy incision is used, its exact location depending on the lobe to be resected. When the pleura is entered, the involved lung collapses and the main vessels and the bronchus are ligated and divided. After the lobe is removed, the remaining lobes of the lung are re-expanded. This patient usually has 2 chest catheters for drainage. The upper tube is for the removal of air; the lower one is for drainage of fluid.

Segmental Resection

Some lesions are confined to a segment of lung. Bronchopulmonary segments are subdivisions of the lung that function as individual units. They are held together by delicate connective tissue; disease processes may be limited to a single segment. Such an area can be removed, thereby allowing healthy functioning pulmonary tissue to remain. This is especially important in patients who have limited cardiorespiratory reserve; they need their undiseased segments.

A lingular segment of the upper lobe of left lung may have to be removed, in which case the operation is called a *lingulectomy.*

Wedge Resection

This resection of a small, well-circumscribed lesion may be done without regard for the location of the intersegmental planes. The pleural cavity usually is drained because of the possibility of an air leak.

Postoperative Management

Reception of the Patient

During transfer of the patient to the recovery room or the intensive care unit, it is extremely important to note that a patent airway is maintained. The patient usually is supine with his head turned to the side to allow for secretions to drain. Blood pressure, pulse and respirations are taken every 15 minutes for 2 or 3 hours, then at 30-minute intervals for the next several hours. Usually, these vital signs are taken hourly during the first night. Oxygen therapy is administered by tent or oropharyngeal catheter. It is used only as long as necessary. Beyond this time, it retards early ambulation and discourages coughing.

Position of the Patient

After the stabilization of the vital signs and the patient's return to consciousness, the head of his bed is elevated 30° to 45°. It is preferable not to use the Trendelenburg position, because the elevation of the diaphragm may interfere with ventilation. Adequate blood replacement usually takes care of shock. However, some surgeons feel that the Trendelenburg position should be used but to facilitate postural drainage; therefore, the best advice is to check with the surgeon responsible for the particular patient.

The patient with a pneumonectomy should be turned hourly from the back to the operated side and not turned directly onto his unoperated side. Turning to the unoperated side is contraindicated primarily because of the possibility that the bronchial stump might open and allow the accumulated fluid to "drown" the remaining lung. The patient should be advised to wait at least 6 months after operation before attempting to sleep with the remaining lung in a dependent position.

The patient with a lobectomy usually can be turned from the back to either side; however, some surgeons prefer that the patient not lie on the operated side so that optimal lung expansion can take place on that side.

For individuals who have had a segmental or a wedge resection, lying on the operated side is contraindicated, since it is desirable to have the remaining lung tissue on this side expand as much as possible.

Pain and the Use of Narcotics

Narcotics are used judiciously for these patients. Certainly their use must be individualized, for the threshold of pain varies from person to person. Some clinicians prefer not to give morphine to postoperative thoracic patients. On occasion, some of the intercostal nerves are injected or cut during the operation, thus reducing the problem of pain. The important point for the nurse to remember is that she wants her patient to be as comfortable as possible but does not want his cough reflex to be dulled.

Fluids and Nutrition

The patient usually receives a blood transfusion during the operation or immediately after it, and this is followed by infusion. The rate of flow should not be greater than 50 to 60 gtt./min. (unless otherwise ordered by the physician) because of the danger of pulmonary edema. The early symptoms of such a complication are cyanosis, dyspnea, rales and bubbling sounds in the chest, as well as frothy sputum. Such a condition must be reported to the physician immediately. Clear fluids may be given when the patient has responded to treatment and when no nausea is present. The next day and thereafter he may have solid foods as desired.

THE NURSE'S ROLE IN THE MANAGEMENT OF THE PATIENT WITH WATER-SEALED CHEST DRAINAGE

Guidelines for the Use of Water-Sealed Chest Drainage (Figs. 14-13 and 14-14)

PURPOSE: An intrapleural drainage tube is used after some intrathoracic operative procedures. One or more chest catheters (usually No. 28 Fr. rubber tubes) are held in the pleural space in the posterior axillary line by suture to the chest wall. The purpose is:

(1) to remove air and fluid from the thoracic cavity; and,

(2) to facilitate re-expansion of the lung after surgery or trauma.

Nursing Activities

Attach the drainage tube from the pleural cavity to tubing that leads to a long glass tube that ends under sterile water.

The glass tube should be approximately one inch below the water line. Mark the original fluid level on the bottle.

Fasten the tubing to the draw sheet so flow by gravity will occur. The tubing should not loop or interfere with movements of the patient.

Encourage good body alignment. When the patient is in the lateral position, place a sandbag on each side of the tubing to protect it from the weight of the patient's body.

Put the arm and the shoulder on the affected side through range-of-motion exercises several times daily.

"Milk" the tube at prescribed intervals.

Make sure that there is oscillation of fluid level in the tube:

(1) The oscillation of fluid level in the tube will stop when the lung has re-expanded.

(2) There may be cessation of oscillation before re-expansion due to blood clots and fibrin sealing off the tube.

Tape the part of the tube entering the drainage bottle to a tongue blade.

Encourage the patient to cough and breathe deeply.

Observe and report symptoms of respiratory embarrassment, pressure in the chest and symptoms of hemorrhage immediately.

Stabilize the drainage bottle within wooden blocks on the floor or in a special holder.

Caution visitors and personnel against handling equipment and/or displacing the bottle.

Clamp the patient's chest tube (close to the chest) immediately if the apparatus is damaged. Have this clamp available at the bedside at all times.

Rationale Underlying Nursing and Treatment Measures

Water-sealed drainage provides for the escape of air and fluid into a drainage bottle. The water acts as a seal and keeps air from being drawn back into the chest.

If the tube is submerged too deeply below the water level, a higher intrapleural pressure is required to expel air.

Kinking or looping or pressure on the drainage tubing can produce retrograde pressure, thus forcing drainage back into pleural cavity.

The patient's position should be changed frequently and the body kept in good alignment to prevent postural deformities and contractures.

Exercise helps to avoid ankylosis of the shoulder and assists in minimizing postoperative pain and discomfort.

"Milking" the tubes prevents them from becoming plugged with clots and fibrin.

Oscillation of the water level in the glass tube shows that there is effective communication between the pleural cavity and the drainage bottle.

Constant attention to maintain the patency of the tube will facilitate prompt expansion of the lung and minimize later complications.

This prevents kinking of the tube and resultant obstruction of drainage.

Coughing and deep breathing assist in raising the intrapleural pressure and in clearing the bronchi, expanding the lung and preventing atelectasis.

If any part of the apparatus is damaged, the closed system of drainage will be destroyed and the patient will be endangered by the attainment of atmospheric pressure in the pleural space and the resultant collapse of the lung.

THE NURSE'S ROLE IN THE MANAGEMENT OF THE PATIENT WITH
WATER-SEALED CHEST DRAINAGE (*Continued*)

Nursing Activities (*Continued*)	Rational Underlying Nursing and Treatment Measures (*Continued*)
If the patient has to be transported to another area, place the drainage bottle below the chest level if he is lying on a stretcher and in his lap if he is in a wheelchair.	The negative intrapleural pressure is not great enough to pull the fluid into the pleural cavity if the bottle is kept below the chest level.
When assisting in removal of the tube: (1) Give the analgesic as ordered as this is a moderately painful procedure. (2) Ask the patient to exhale. The tube is withdrawn and a 2 × 2 gauze sponge is applied quickly and made air tight with snug-fitting adhesive.	During removal of the tube, the chief precaution is to avoid the entrance of air into the pleural cavity.
Wash hands thoroughly before and after handling the equipment.	Introduction of organisms during treatments can produce contamination of the pleural cavity.

Adequate Air Exchange

Immediately after operation, many of these patients receive oxygen as a supportive measure. This is essential because of the diminished respiratory reserve due to decreased lung volume, blood loss and reduced blood pressure. The quality of respirations must be noted by the nurse. Dyspnea, cyanosis and acute chest pain suggest a tension pneumothorax and they should be reported immediately. The treatment would be an aspiration of the chest or thoracentesis, for which the nurse should be prepared.

The use of the blow bottle can be dangerous to a patient who has had extensive surgery because of the possibility of blowing out a ligated section of the bronchial tree. Therefore, a blow bottle should be used only when it has been ordered specifically by the physician.

Suction and Drainage

Catheters are positioned strategically in the chest for postoperative connection to drainage bottles for 2 chief reasons: (1) to allow for the escape of air that otherwise might produce a pneumothorax, a shift of the mediastinum to the unoperated side or an emphysema and (2) to allow for the withdrawal of serosanguineous fluid.

The important aspect of nursing attention is this: Be certain that the system is airtight and the tubes open. "Milking" the tubes will prevent plugging with clots or fibrin. Only enough suction tubing should be used to bridge the bottles and to extend to the wall and the patient, allowing leeway for the patient to turn. Excess tubing can be tripped over and often is caught behind the bed. A safety pin or a clip is effective in securing drainage tubing to the draw sheet; make sure that there are no kinks in the tubing. A

trough can be made with the draw sheet so that the tubing is nestled and the safety pin does not constrict the tubing. Abdominal pads or small pillows around the tube to make a trough also help.

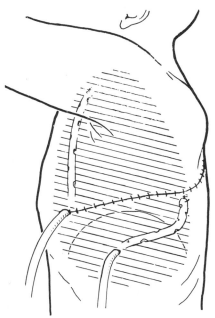

FIG. 14-13. Postoperative drainage of the chest. The upper drainage tube is used for the escape of air from leaks in the resected lung. The tip is anchored in the parietal pleura near the apex and brought out through the anterior end of the incision. The lower tube is usually for serosanguineous drainage. (Johnson, Julian, and Kirby, C. K.: Surgery of the Chest, p. 99, Chicago, Yr. Bk. Pub.)

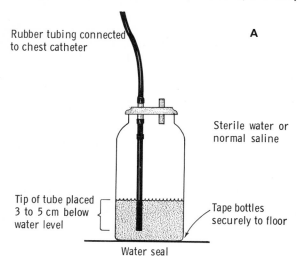

A

Rubber tubing connected to chest catheter

Sterile water or normal saline

Tip of tube placed 3 to 5 cm below water level

Tape bottles securely to floor

Water seal

FIG. 14-14. Methods of water seal chest suction. (A) Water seal drainage alone has been found to be adequate in most patients. (B) Two-bottle water seal suction may be used when a persistent air leak is present and cannot be controlled by drainage alone. (C) Three-bottle suction. This demonstrates a useful arrangement for chest suction. The first trap bottle permits visualization of the fluid drainage. The second, in combination with the first bottle, can operate as a simple water seal. When the third bottle is added, the amount of suction can be measured by the depth of the tube under water. (Parts A & B are from: Blades, B.: Surgical Diseases of the Chest, p. 63, St. Louis, Mosby, 1961; (C) is from Roe, B. B.: The use and abuse of chest drainage, West. J. Surg., *61*:708, December, 1953)

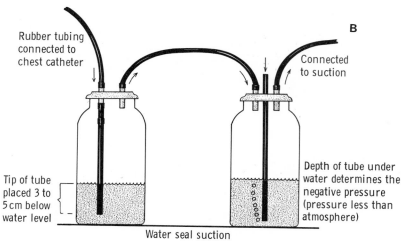

B

Rubber tubing connected to chest catheter

Connected to suction

Tip of tube placed 3 to 5 cm below water level

Depth of tube under water determines the negative pressure (pressure less than atmosphere)

Water seal suction

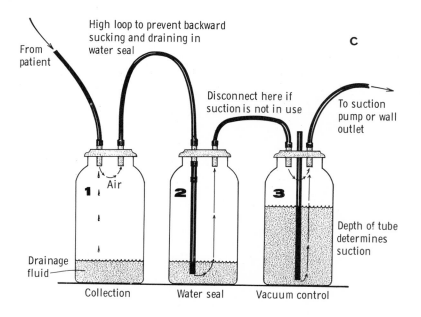

C

From patient

High loop to prevent backward sucking and draining in water seal

Disconnect here if suction is not in use

To suction pump or wall outlet

1 Air

2

3

Depth of tube determines suction

Drainage fluid

Collection   Water seal   Vacuum control

The color, the consistency and the amount of drainage should be charted at least every 8 hours. In patients with large losses, especially after heart surgery, hourly volume determinations should be performed.

In closed suction it is important to clamp the suction tubing before removing the drainage bottle to measure the contents.

Usually the catheters are removed in 2 or 3 days, providing that the remaining lung tissue is well expanded, that air leaks are eliminated and that the total fluid drainage is less than 75 ml. daily. Pneumonectomy patients usually do not have chest suction and drainage; however, if used, it is similar to that described above.

Another method of chest drainage is that of using a *flutter valve* to replace the underwater drainage bottle apparatus.

A flutter valve consists essentially of a single piece of rubber tubing, one end of which is compressed and retains a flattened shape. The 2 flat sides of the tubing remain in contact with each other. The length of contact of the 2 sides permits the valve to be functionally closed to reflux even while fluid, air, or clots are traversing it (peristaltic-like motion). This security against reflux, plus the minimal resistance it offers to the passage of drainage, makes the flutter valve most suitable for draining the chest.*

The disposable valve is attached to the chest catheter and the drainage flows into a plastic container (Fig. 14-15). By this method, the patient may be ambulatory because the valve prevents reflux of air and fluid into the chest and functions with the patient assuming any position. Although this method is relatively simple, the patient requires the same meticulous care and observation that he would receive if he were having the conventional type of chest drainage.

The Removal of Retained Secretions

This is undoubtedly the most important aspect of postoperative nursing care in the chest patient. It is imperative that he cough strongly enough to bring up secretions. He usually is taught to do this preoperatively and knows that he will have discomfort. The danger in retaining secretions is that of atelectasis and pneumonia. When mucus is thick and tenacious, inhalations of steam or bronchodilator aerosols may help. If the nurse is unsuccessful in getting her patient to bring up secretions or if he refuses to cough, an endotracheal aspiration must be done. Usually the surgeon does this; however, in many hospitals, this is becoming a nurse's responsibility.

Endotracheal Aspiration. A No. 16 rubber catheter,

*Heimlich, H. J.: A flutter valve to replace underwater drainage bottles. JAMA, 192:262, 1965.

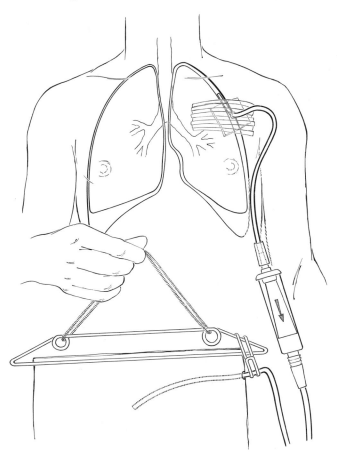

FIG. 14-15. Ambulatory patient with a flutter-valve in place. Note that the valve prevents reflux of air and fluid into the chest.

wall or electric suction, a square of gauze, tissue wipes and an emesis basin are all that is required for this procedure. The patient is instructed to sit upright. When he protrudes his tongue, it is grasped with a dry piece of gauze and pulled forward gently. Next, the tube is advanced through the nose until it reaches the glottis. Then the patient is instructed to inhale or cough, and the catheter is passed quickly into the trachea. Inability of the patient to produce vocal sounds distinctly is the best evidence that the catheter is in the trachea. Then the catheter is connected to gentle suction. The catheter should be moved slowly up and down the trachea. The chief value of endotracheal aspiration is that it stimulates the cough reflex and produces violent coughing.

Complications

The nurse should be alert for atelectasis, emphysema, and tension pneumothorax. In patients from

NORMAL RESPIRATION

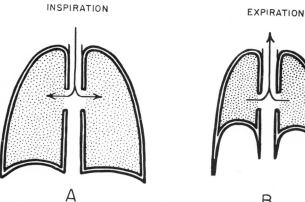

INSPIRATION   EXPIRATION

A   B

PARADOXICAL MOTION

INSPIRATION   EXPIRATION

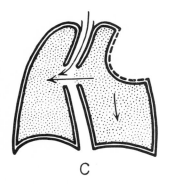

C   D

FIG. 14-16. Comparison between normal respiration and paradoxical motion. (A and B) Normally, on inspiration all portions of the thoracic cage move outward, and the diaphragms move downward. Motion is in the opposite direction on expiration. (C and D) When a portion of the chest wall becomes flexible as a result of losing its bony support, motion of the flexible area is controlled by the changing intrapleural pressures and is in a direction opposite to that of the normal positions of the chest wall. (Johnson, Julian, and Kirby, C. K.: Surgery of the Chest, p. 21, Chicago, Yr. Bk. Pub.)

whom 3 or more ribs have been removed, there is a possibility of paradoxical chest motion.

Paradoxical chest motion (Fig. 14-16) can occur when the integrity of any portion of the thoracic bellows is lost, such as multiple rib fractures or removal of several ribs as in a thoracoplasty. The nurse should observe chest movements of her thoracic surgical patients. When she detects paradoxical motion, she should report it immediately, for if uncorrected, it

may result in serious respiratory and circulatory impairment. Treatment usually consists of firm adhesive strapping of the chest with the application of pads or a sandbag for further support. In some instances a type of skeletal traction may be employed to keep the chest wall from collapsing.

In general, the signs and the symptoms that should be reported to the surgeon immediately are cyanosis, dyspnea, pallor, acute chest pain, increase in pulse and respiratory rates, temperature elevation over 37.2° C. (99° F.), systolic blood pressure reading below 90 mm. and evidence of hemorrhage on the dressings.

Ambulation and Convalescence

If shock has been prevented adequately and the patient does not have heart disease or a limited cardiovascular reserve, he may get out of bed the evening of or the day after surgery. Drainage tubes and bottles may hinder this somewhat.

Breathing and postural exercises recommended by the surgeon and the physical therapist are begun a day or 2 after surgery to produce better lung ventilation, to restore motion and muscle tonus in the shoulder girdle and trunk and to maintain normal posture.

Roentgenograms are taken frequently to determine the patient's progress. If air or fluid accumulates in the chest, it will be necessary to aspirate by means of a thoracentesis.

For patients who have had surgery for lung cancer, refer to the chapter on cancer nursing, p. 179.

Rehabilitative plans are made by the surgeon, the nurse, the patient, his family, the physical therapist and the medical social worker. The nurse will find the following points helpful in her suggestions to the patient:

(1) Practice deep breathing exercises for the first few weeks at home.

(2) Practice good body alignment by standing up straight with shoulders held back (preferably in front of a full-length mirror).

(3) Practice exercises that were done while in the hospital.

(4) Practice good oral hygiene by brushing teeth well and visiting the dentist frequently.

(5) Remain away from crowds during upper respiratory epidemics.

(6) Seek medical attention at the onset of an upper respiratory infection.

(7) Avoid areas where the air is filled with dust, smoke, and irritating chemicals.

(8) Avoid anything that may cause spasms of coughing.

(9) Maintain good nutrition.

(10) Obtain adequate rest. A good plan should

TABLE 14-3. Exercises designed to restore function following thoracic surgery

Muscle Affected by Thoracotomy	Function	Activities to Restore Function
Trapezius	Promotes arm extension, abduction and reach extension.	Extend the arm up and back, out to the side and back, down at the side and back.
Rhomboideus major	Adducts and slightly elevates scapula.	Place hands in small of back. Push elbows as far back as possible.
Latissimus dorsi	Depresses the shoulder.	Sit erect in an armchair; place the hands on the arms of the chair directly opposite either side of the body. Press down on hands, consciously pulling the abdomen in and stretching up from the waist. Inhale while raising the body until the elbows are extended completely. Hold this position a moment, and begin exhaling while lowering the body slowly to the original position.
Serratus anterior	Rotates scapula and fixes it against the rib cage.	Reach over head and "push" in an upward and outward motion.

include an early afternoon nap for the first few post-hospital weeks.

Usually, patients having had pulmonary resections are able to return to sedentary occupations about 2 to 3 weeks after discharge and to heavy labor in about 6 to 8 weeks after discharge. Some individuals, usually with pre-existing lung disease and after extensive resection, may experience a significant reduction in their exercise capacity. This is usually permanent, and their tolerance at 8 to 12 weeks post-hospitalization is about the level at which it will remain. Social and occupational counseling may be necessary.

Rehabilitation of the Chest Patient

Rehabilitation should begin when the patient seeks help; consequently, rehabilitation measures are an integral part of his therapeutic program. Basic rehabilitation measures that are applicable to most patients with pulmonary conditions include (1) the promotion of an effective cough routine (see p. 234); (2) activities to improve the efficiency of pulmonary function; and (3) skeletal exercises for the retraining of injured muscles and the prevention of deformities. The rehabilitation program is designed and adjusted to meet the needs of each individual patient. The nurse or the therapist observes the patient closely during his exercise program in order to evaluate his ability to tolerate the prescribed activity and evaluate his progress.

Promotion of Respiratory Efficiency. Patients with pulmonary problems should be maintained in correct recumbent, sitting and standing postures. Only one pillow should be permitted. The shoulders should be level, the hips and the shoulders aligned to prevent scoliosis.

Breathing Exercises. The rate, the depth and the rhythm of respirations are affected by the patient's emotional state. Many of these patients are anxious and apprehensive. Their tension causes further respiratory impairment because tension and muscular stress increase metabolic demand. Assisting the patient to relax is part of the therapeutic program. Instruct him to contract and relax his muscles consciously without moving the part. (This is a form of isometric exercise: muscle relaxation and contraction affected without joint movement.) For example: "Contract the muscle of your left hand, let go, relax."

The purpose of breathing exercises is to obtain full movement of the diaphragm and to assist in lung re-expansion.

EXAMPLE: Place the patient in a recumbent position. Place one of his hands on his abdomen and the other on his upper chest. Instruct him to inhale through his nose, raising his abdomen against his hand. Exhale while pursing the lips and contracting the abdominal muscles, moving the abdomen inward. The chest should not move.

The contraction of the abdomen and the expiratory muscles against increased pressure obtained from pursed-mouth breathing assists in emptying the lungs and in the elevation of the diaphragm. As the patient is increasingly able to tolerate this exercise, 8 to 10 pounds of sandbags can be placed on his abdomen to increase the intra-abdominal pressure. This aids exhalation. The exercise is repeated 10 to 15 times and is performed at least 3 times daily.

Patients with emphysema have air trapped in the alveoli. Therefore they are encouraged to inhale quickly and exhale slowly. Raising the arms during

FIG. 14-17. Muscles affected by thoracotomy. Rehabilitation should be planned in relation to the action of the muscle involved.

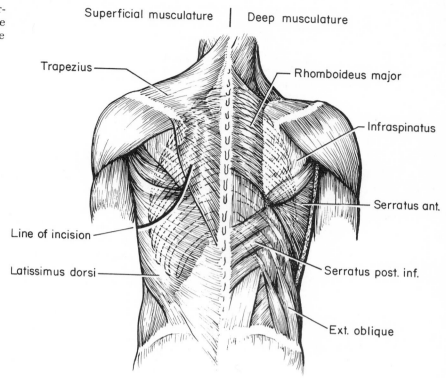

Superficial musculature | Deep musculature

Trapezius

Rhomboideus major

Infraspinatus

Serratus ant.

Line of incision

Serratus post. inf.

Latissimus dorsi

Ext. oblique

inspiration and returning them to the sides while tightening the abdominal muscles during exhalation will also improve expiration.

The patient's shoulder should be taken through a full range of motion on the operative side in order to pre-

vent frozen shoulder. The nurse should do this several times daily. It is desirable for the patient to participate in this activity at least 6 times daily as soon as his condition permits.

The exercises may be done by the patient as soon as

FIG. 14-18. At Valley Forge General Hospital, four exercises are taught for initial use after thoracic surgery. Others are added as a patient can tolerate and remember them. The initial exercises are as follows:

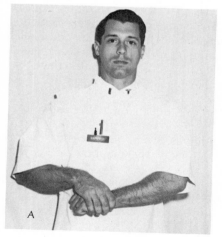
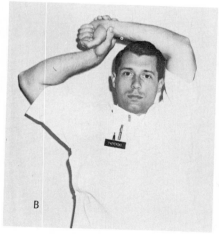
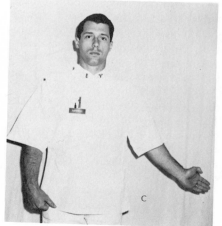

(A, B, C) Arms at side, palm in, raise arm straight forward upward overhead deep breathing simultaneously, 5 times. This exercise requires flexion of the operative arm. The patient is instructed to take a deep breath while raising the arm, therefore fulfilling two goals of treatment.

the surgeon permits. They should be stopped as soon as pain and fatigue begin. Other activities may be added as the patient's condition improves and he is ready for them. (Example of exercises are shown in Fig. 14-18.)

When the patient is able to perform these exercises without shortness of breath, he can progress from lying to sitting, then to standing and walking posture. Bending forward while walking helps forced expirations. Each procedure is introduced in sequence. The patient

Fɪɢ. 14-18. (*Continued*)

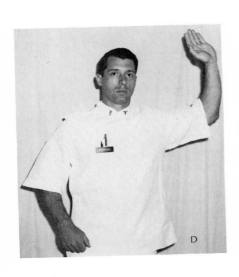
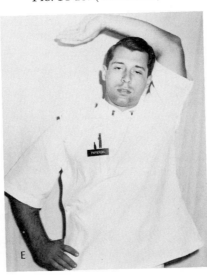
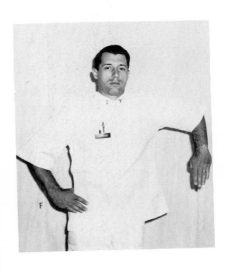

(D, E, F) Arm at side, palm up, raise arm sideward upward overhead, 5 times. Performance of this exercise necessitates abduction of the operative arm. Assistance is not usually needed here, for the patient can slide the arm along the bed while supine.

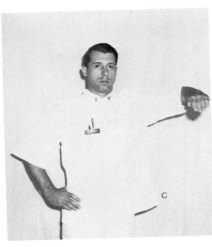
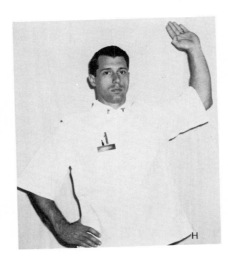
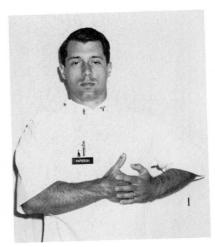

(G, H, I) Arm to side, shoulder level and elbow bent; rotate shoulder by moving forearm back to touch bed, then forward to touch bed, 5 times. This provides for rotation of the shoulder on the operative side.

Segmental breathing is accomplished by using hand for educational counter pressure on inhaling; abdominal breathing, both inhaling and exhaling, 10 times. This increases the depth of respiration and enables the patient to feel this depth. (U.S. Army photograph. From Baskfield, M. M.: Preoperative and Postoperative care of the patient with cancer of the lung. Nurs. Clin. N. Amer., 2:609-622, 1967) should be shown the exercise, encouraged to practice it with supervision, and then instructed to rest. A patient with a productive cough should evacuate his sputum before beginning the exercises. Breathing exercises not only strengthen the diaphragm, the lower rib cage and the abdominal muscles, but also help the patient to increase his activities gradually without shortness of breath. The emphasis on any breathing exercises should be placed on improving expiration.

Skeletal Exercises. Figure 14-17 shows the muscles that are affected by the most common thoracic surgical procedures. In order to perform chest surgery, the

---

SUMMARY OF THE MEDICAL AND NURSING MANAGEMENT OF THE THORACIC-SURGERY PATIENT

PREOPERATIVE OBJECTIVES: To ensure optimal patient condition for surgery.

I. *To improve ventilatory function*

   A. Institute breathing exercises to improve respiratory efficiency.

   B. Improve condition of patients who have impaired pulmonary function.
     1. Administer intermittent positive pressure breathing treatment (p. 252) and bronchodilating drugs.
     2. Control infections with antibiotics.

II. *To minimize pulmonary secretions*

   A. Eliminate smoking to reduce pulmonary irritation.

   B. Maintain schedule of oral hygiene to reduce bacterial flora in mouth.

   C. Treat existing infections if present.
     1. Antibiotic therapy.

     2. Postural drainage to facilitate removal of secretions.

   D. Provide adequate hydration to reduce viscosity of secretions.

III. *To prepare the patient for the surgical experience by reassurance and explanation*

   A. Orient the patient to the postoperative period.
     1. Function of the chest tube.
     2. Cough routine.
     3. Type of incision.
     4. Breathing and exercise program.
     5. Control of pain.
     6. Oxygen tent.
     7. Blood transfusion.

   B. Encourage expression of psychological and safety needs.

POSTOPERATIVE OBJECTIVES: To restore normal function as early as possible.

I. *To ensure proper expansion of the lung*

   A. Promote coughing to clear airway.

   B. Water-sealed chest drainage to remove air and fluid from chest.

   C. Frequent changing of position to mobilize secretions.

   D. Breathing exercises to aid lung re-expansion.

   E. Careful pain control to facilitate coughing and deep breathing.

   F. Removal of tracheobronchial secretions if patient is unable to clear airway
     1. Nasotracheal suction (mechanical stimulation of cough).
     2. Bronchoscopy.
     3. Tracheostomy.

II. *To restore normal range of motion and function of shoulder and trunk*

   A. Skeletal exercises to promote abduction and mobilization of shoulder.

   B. Breathing exercises to mobilize the thorax.

   C. Ambulate as soon as pulmonary and circulatory systems are compensated.

   D. Encourage progressive activities according to development of fatigue.

III. *To anticipate and forestall possible complications*

   A. Hypotension (during immediate postoperative period).
     1. Evaluate blood pressure and pulse carefully.
     2. Measure urinary volume.
     3. Have blood replacement available.

   B. Cardiac arrhythmias.
     1. Apical and radial pulse measurements.
     2. Have digitalis or quinidine available.

   C. Hemorrhage.
     1. Evaluate vital signs.
     2. Evaluate chest drainage.
     3. Have blood replacement available.

   D. Atelectasis.
     1. Prepare for bronchoscopic aspiration.
     2. Have oxygen available.

   E. Acute pulmonary edema.
     1. Careful regulation of intravenous fluids.
     2. Have parenteral digitalis, diuretics, and rotating tourniquet setup available.

   F. Respiratory insufficiency.
     1. Place patient in respirator for assisted ventilation.
     2. Prepare for tracheostomy.

muscle groups that make up the shoulder girdle and maintain trunk posture are transected. If the muscles on one side of the body are affected, the contralateral muscles (those on the other side) become stronger and can produce deformity.

The patient's joint range should be measured pre-operatively to help to determine the postoperative goal. The patient needs to be reassured that the exercises will help to prevent deformity of the trunk and the upper extremities. Other objectives of skeletal exercises before and after thoracic surgical procedures are to assist in maintaining a normal range of motion of the involved joints, to gain maximal pulmonary function and to improve the patient's posture.

TUMORS OF THE MEDIASTINUM

Benign mediastinal tumors, comparatively rare, include the following types: adenoma of the thyroid, fibroma, lipoma, chondroma, myoma and cysts. The majority of *primary mediastinal malignant tumors* are sarcomas which arise in the thymus or mediastinal lymph nodes. The carcinomas found in this region usually are secondary to those of the breast or the gastrointestinal tract, but rare primary ones arise in the esophagus, the trachea, a bronchus, the thymus or an accessory thyroid gland.

Cysts of the mediastinum usually are small when benign. Dermoid cysts occasionally develop, and these may ulcerate into the air passages.

Symptoms

Nearly all the symptoms of mediastinal tumors are due to the pressure of the mass against important intra-thoracic organs. Among these pressure symptoms are bulging of the chest wall; orthopnea, an early sign due to pressure against the trachea, a main bronchus, the recurrent laryngeal nerve or the lung; cardiac palpitation, anginal attacks and various other circulatory disturbances; cyanosis; swelling of the face, the neck and the upper extremities, and the marked distention of the veins of the neck and the chest wall, evidence of the closure of large veins of the mediastinum by thrombi; and dysphagia, due to pressure against the esophagus. The fingers may become clubbed.

Diagnostic Studies

Roentgenograms are of great value in the diagnosis of mediastinal tumors and cysts, yet even with the aid of the fluoroscope and roentgenokymogram it may be difficult to distinguish between a mediastinal abscess, tumor and aortic aneurysm. The biopsy of an enlarged lymph node removed from above the clavicle or in the axilla may reveal the diagnosis. Blood studies are of value in excluding leukemia, and sputum examinations aid in ruling out tuberculosis, while the presence of teeth and hair in the sputum indicates that the tumor is a dermoid cyst.

Treatment

With the exception of intrathoracic goiters and cysts, few mediastinal tumors can be removed by operation. Fibroid tumors occasionally are removed by x-ray irradiation. This irradiation also often retards the growth of carcinomas, yields quite favorable results in cases of lymphosarcoma and usually gives prompt but temporary relief in cases of Hodgkin's disease, Hodgkin's sarcoma or lymphatic leukemia.

THE PATIENT WITH AN ASPIRATED FOREIGN BODY IN THE LUNG

Foreign bodies not infrequently are aspirated into the lung, especially by children. The object lodges more commonly in the right main bronchus, as it is more vertical than the left. The complete closure of a bronchus by a foreign body may result in sudden death. However, the usual result is that the lobes communicating with the occluded bronchus collapse as the air contained in them becomes absorbed in the bloodstream.

A small solid object such as a pin, a tack or a tooth in a bronchus causes trouble, not from the obstruction of a bronchus, but from infection. For a short time following the aspiration there may be symptoms of choking, gagging and coughing. But these symptoms, often mild, abate and for a time become forgotten. For weeks the only suggestion of trouble may be a persistent cough. Such substances as peanuts, grains of corn, etc., on the other hand, produce a severe bronchitis with high irregular fever and all the symptoms and signs of a severe pneumonitis. Whether the foreign body is composed of organic or inorganic material, signs of obstructive emphysema, atelectasis or lung abscess eventually appear.

Treatment

The prognosis is serious unless the foreign body is removed early, for rarely is it coughed up spontaneously. Therefore, bronchoscopy is indicated when this diagnosis is suspected. When removed early, aspirated foreign bodies rarely give rise to complications.

Prevention

This is of the utmost importance and consists in teaching children not to put small toys, coins, buttons, pencil caps and such articles in their mouths. Open safety pins should never be put on a pillow near a baby, nor should a child be permitted to play with a button box. Parents require considerable education in such details of child training, and no small part of their responsibility in this regard is the example that they set for their offspring.

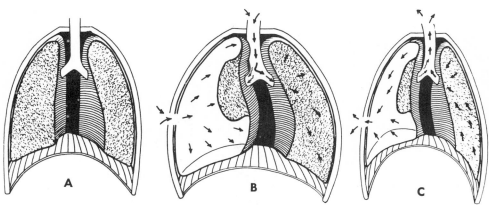

FIG. 14-19. Open pneumothorax and mediastinal flutter. (A) Normal lung. (B) The mediastinum shifts toward the unaffected side on inspiration and, as noted by arrows, air rushes into pleural cavity. Air may enter the unaffected lung through the trachea, but the collapsed lung can take little or no air. (C) On expiration, the reverse is true. The mediastinum swings back toward midline and air escapes through the thoracic wound. Air also can leave the normal lung on expiration, but the collapsed lung contributes very little to either phase of respiration. (Streider, J. W.: GP *13*:75-85)

THE PATIENT WITH CHEST INJURIES

Injuries to the chest may cause minor or serious disturbance of cardiorespiratory function, depending on which part of the complex mechanism is involved. Thus, a fall against the side of a bathtub may fracture 1 or 2 ribs with painful but rather slight disturbance of respiratory function, whereas an automobile accident in which the driver of the car is thrown against the steering wheel may cause a crush of the chest with cardiac and lung injuries that may be rapidly fatal. In the treatment of injuries to the chest, efforts are made to correct the disturbances of cardiorespiratory function caused by the trauma.

Closed or Crush Injuries

Simple fracture of 1 or 2 ribs is a painful injury, and because of pain with respiration, there is some degree of limitation of respiratory excursion. Pain can be relieved occasionally by chest strapping, but more commonly a local anesthetic is injected at the fracture site, or is used to block the intercostal nerves that transmit painful sensations from that area. Tracheostomy and/or assisted ventilation are used in the management of the very severe crush injuries with flail chest.

When the chest is crushed between 2 objects, multiple fractures of each of several ribs may occur, so that one portion of the chest wall no longer has a bony connection with the rest of the rib cage. This is called "stove-in" or "flail" chest. During attempted respiration, the detached part of the chest wall shows a paradoxical movement, being pulled in on inspiration and blown out on expiration (Fig. 14-16). This impairs the normal mechanics of respiration enough to jeopardize ventilation seriously. Various methods of stabilizing the chest wall may be used to overcome the paradoxical movement of the injured area during respiration. These may include traction with weights and pulleys applied

through wires, or towel clips applied to the broken portions of the ribs.

In addition, these more severe injuries usually are accompanied by the collection of blood in the chest cavity (hemothorax) from torn intercostal vessels or from lacerations of the lungs, or the escape of air from the injured lung into the pleural cavity (pneumothorax). Often, both blood and air are found in the chest cavity (hemopneumothorax). The lung on that side of the chest is compressed, thus interfering with its normal function. Needle aspirations or chest tube drainage of the blood and/or air allows the lung to re-expand and again perform its function in respiration.

Tension Pneumothorax

In some patients, air may be drawn into the pleural space from the injured lung, or through a small hole in the chest wall. In either case, the air that enters the chest cavity with each inspiration is trapped there: it cannot be expelled through the air passage or small hole in the chest wall. A tension thus is built up in the chest, which produces a collapse of the lung and even may push the heart and the great vessels toward the normal side of the chest, thus not only interfering with respiration but also with the circulatory function. Relief of this "tension pneumothorax" must be looked on as an emergency measure. A tube must be inserted into the chest to which suction is applied, to withdraw the air in the pleural space and thus relieve the tension.

Sucking Wounds

Open pneumothorax implies an opening in the chest wall large enough for air to pass freely in and out of the thoracic cavity with each attempted respiration. The rush of air through the hole in the chest wall produces a sucking sound, and such injuries are termed "sucking wounds" of the chest. In such patients not only is the lung collapsed, but the structures of the mediastinum (heart and great vessels) are pushed toward the uninjured side with each inspiration and in the opposite direction with expiration (Fig. 14-19). This is termed "mediastinal flutter," and it produces serious embarrassment of circulatory function. *To stop the flow of air through the opening in the chest wall is lifesaving.* In such an emergency, anything may be used that is large enough to fill the hole—a towel, handkerchief, or the heel of the hand may be used. If the patient is conscious, tell him to inhale as deeply as possible and strain against a closed glottis. This action assists in the re-expansion of the lung and pushing out the air in the thorax. In the hospital, the opening is plugged by sealing it with gauze impregnated with petroleum jelly.

Wet-Lung Syndrome

Almost every major injury to the thorax is associated with the "wet-lung" syndrome. This syndrome is due to several factors, all of which interfere with the normal passage of air into the lung. They include an increase in tracheobronchial secretions, blood in the tracheobronchial tree, an inability to cough up these secretions because of pain, and ineffectual cough due to the mechanical effects of the injury. In addition, atelectasis of a lung or part of a lung often occurs as a result of the obstructed airway, all of which adds to the difficulty of blood oxygenation. Cyanosis and dyspnea with rattling, labored respiration are associated symptoms. If the airway cannot be cleared by catheter suction or bronchoscopy, a tracheostomy often is performed. This permits the frequent aspiration of retained secretion that is a most important part of the nursing care of these patients (see p. 222).

Cardiac Tamponade

Blows on the anterior chest, stab wounds and crush injuries may cause bleeding into the pericardial sac, with resultant compression of the heart. When the heart is unable to function normally, the patient exhibits cyanosis and dyspnea, the pulse becomes weak, the blood pressure falls, and there may be loss of consciousness from lack of cerebral circulation. Decompression of the pericardium by needle aspiration or by operation permits heart action to be resumed. If the bleeding is due to a wound of the heart, the wound must be closed by suture.

Subcutaneous Emphysema

When the lung or the air passages are injured, air may enter the tissue planes and pass for some distance under the skin. The tissues give a crackling sensation when palpated, and the subcutaneous air produces an alarming appearance with face, neck, body, and scrotum misshapen by subcutaneous air. Fortunately, subcutaneous emphysema is of itself not a serious complication. The subcutaneous air is spontaneously absorbed, if the underlying air leak is treated or stops spontaneously.

General Principles of Care

Most patients with severe chest injuries are in a state of shock for a time. This is treated by intravenous fluids, blood, etc. (see p. 146).

Pain must be treated cautiously to avoid a depression of the cough reflex. Perhaps meperidine hydrochloride (Demerol) rather than morphine is better in this regard. Older people are especially prone to respiratory depression from morphine or other depressants. Nerve block may be used effectively.

Many injuries involving the chest may have associated abdominal and other injuries that require treatment and close observation by both the doctor and the nurse.

Principles of nursing care are essentially those discussed on pages 258 to 269.

BIBLIOGRAPHY

Books

Baum, G. (ed.): Textbook of Pulmonary Disease. Boston, Little and Brown, 1965.

Bendixen, H. H., *et al.*: Respiratory Care. St. Louis, C. V. Mosby, 1965.

Blades, B. (ed.): Surgical Diseases of the Chest. St. Louis, C. V. Mosby, 1966.

Blum, H. L., and Keranen, G. M.: Control of Chronic Diseases in Man. U. S. Public Health Service, 1966.

Bunn, P. A.: Treatment of bronchopulmonary infections. *In* Advances in Cardiopulmonary Diseases. Vol. II. Chicago, Year Book Publishers, 1964.

Diedrich, W. M., and Youngstrom, K. A.: Alaryngeal Speech. Springfield, Ill., Charles C Thomas, 1966.

Gibbon, J. H.: Surgery of the Chest. Philadelphia, W. B. Saunders, 1962.

Gius, J. A.: Fundamentals of General Surgery. Chicago, Year Book Publishers, 1966.

Guyton, A. C.: Textbook of Medical Physiology. ed. 3, pp. 545-620. Philadelphia, W. B. Saunders, 1966.

Hinshaw, H. C., and Garland, L. H.: Diseases of the Chest. Philadelphia, W. B. Saunders, 1963.

Johnson, J., and Kirby, C. K.: Surgery of the Chest. ed. 2. Chicago, Year Book Publishers, 1958.

Pulaski, E. J.: Common Bacterial Infections. Philadelphia, W. B. Saunders, 1964.

Pullen, R. L.: Pulmonary Diseases. Philadelphia, Lea & Febiger, 1965.

Reid, L.: The Pathology of Emphysema. Chicago, Year Book Publishers, 1967.

Rubin, E., and Rubin, M.: Thoracic Diseases. Philadelphia, W. B. Saunders, 1961.

Smoking and Health. Report of the Advisory Committee to the Surgeon General of the P.H.S., P.H.S. 1103, 1964.

Snidecor, J. C.: Speech Rehabilitation of the Laryngectomized. Springfield, Ill., Charles C Thomas, 1962.

Medical Clinics of North America: Modern Management of Respiratory Diseases. Vol. 51, No. 2, March, 1967. (entire volume)

Articles

Cooley, D. A., and Beall, A. C., Jr.: Embolectomy for acute massive pulmonary embolism. Surg. Gynec. & Obstet., *126*:805-810, April, 1968.

Crocco, J. A., *et al.*: Massive hemoptysis. Arch. Int. Med., *121*:495-498, June, 1968.

Dittbrenner, Sr. M., and Hebert, W. M.: Regimen for a thoracotomy patient, Amer. J. Nurs., *67*:2072-2075, Oct., 1967.

Douglas, R. G., Lindgren, K. M., and Couch, R. B.: Exposure to cold environment and rhinovirus common cold: No effect. New Eng. J. Med., *279*:742-747, 1968.

Haas, A., and Rusk, H. A.: Rehabilitation of patients with obstructive pulmonary diseases. Postgrad. Med., *39*:612-620, June, 1966.

Hanamey, R.: Teaching patients breathing and coughing techniques. Nurs. Outlook, *13*:58-59, Aug., 1965.

Hedges, J. E., and Bridges, C. J.: Stimulation of the cough reflex. Amer. J. Nurs., *68*:347-348, Feb., 1968.

Horowicz, C.: Bronchoscopy as an outpatient procedure. Amer. J. Nurs., *63*:106-107, May, 1963.

Kurihara, M.: Postural drainage, clapping and vibrating. Amer. J. Nurs., *65*:76-79, Nov., 1965.

——: Assessment and maintenance of adequate respiration. Nurs. Clin. of N. Amer., *3*:65-76, March, 1968.

Larson, E. L.: The patient with acute pulmonary edema. Amer. J. Nurs., *68*:1019-1021, May, 1968.

Levine, E. R.: Inhalation therapy—aerosols and intermittent positive pressure breathing. Med. Clin. N. Amer., *51*:307-321, Mar., 1967.

——: Mechanisms of improvement in bronchopulmonary disease. Dis. Chest, *49*:610-624, June, 1966.

Massuml, R. A.: Pulmonary thromboembolism. Postgrad. Med., *41*:315-326, March, 1967.

McArdle, K. H.: The patient and the Bennett. Nurs. Clin. N. Amer., *1*:143-152, March, 1966.

McCallum, H. P.: The nurse and the respirator. Nurs. Clin. N. Amer., *1*:597-610, Dec., 1966.

Nett, L. M., and Petty, T. L.: A new IPPB device for bronchial hygiene. Amer. J. Nurs., *68*:2570-2571, Dec., 1968.

Pruitt, C. V., Westbury, E. L., and Hairston, P.: Nursing care of patients with surgery of the chest. Nurs. Clin. N. Amer., *2*:513-520, Sept., 1967.

Rodman, T.: Management of tracheobronchial secretions. Amer. J. Nurs., *66*:2474-2477, Nov., 1966.

Turner, H. G.: The anatomy and physiology of normal respiration. Nurs. Clin. N. Amer., *3*:383-401, Sept., 1968.

PULMONARY INFECTIONS

Bradford, J. K., and DeCamp, P. T.: Bronchiectasis. Surg. Clin. N. Amer., *46*:1485-1492, Dec., 1966.

Chapman, J. S.: The atypical mycobacteria. Amer. J. Nurs., *67*: 1031-1037, May, 1967.

Donovan, C.: Making theory work in patient care (pneumonia). Amer. J. Nurs., *66*:2204, Oct., 1966.

Harkins, H. P.: Aspiration pneumonia. Hosp. Med., *4*:52-60, Nov., 1968.

Petty, T. L., and Mitchell, R. S.: Suppurative lung diseases. Med. Clin. N. Amer., *51*:529-540, Mar., 1967.

Pickar, D. N.: Pulmonary abscess: a medicosurgical problem. Hosp. Med., *2*:7-15, Oct., 1966.

Reiman, H. A.: Acute nonbacterial pneumonias. Hosp. Med., *3*:104, Mar., 1967.

——: Viral versus bacterial and other pneumonias. Hosp. Med., *4*:36-54, Sept., 1968.

Schepers, G. W. H.: Pneumoconiosis. Amer. J. Nurs., *64*:109-114, Feb., 1964.

Sykes, E. M.: No time for silence. Amer. J. Nurs., *66*:1040-1041, May, 1966.

Turch, M.: Current therapy of bacterial pneumonias. Med. Clin. N. Amer., *51*:541-548, March, 1967.

EMPHYSEMA

Bates, D. V.: Chronic bronchitis and emphysema. New Eng. J. Med., *278*:546, 1968.

Chronic Bronchitis and Pulmonary Emphysema—Rehabilitation Manual, PHS, Bureau of Disease Prevention and Environmental Control, National Center for Chronic Disease Control, Arlington, Va., 1968.

Chuan, H.: Impaired pulmonary circulation due to pulmonary emphysema. Nurs. Clin. N. Amer., *1*:39-45, March, 1966.

Friedman, A. H.: The patient with chronic obstructive lung disease and his care at home. Nurs. Clin. N. Amer., *3*:437-451, Sept., 1968.

Hargreaves, A. G.: Emotional problems of patients with respiratory disease. Nurs. Clin. N. Amer., *3*:479-487, Sept., 1968.

Helming, M. G.: Nursing care of patients with chronic obstructive lung disease. Nurs. Clin. N. Amer., *3*:413-422, Sept., 1968.

Hoffman, F. P.: Rehabilitation of chronic obstructive lung diseases. Rehab. Lit., *29*:34-39, Feb., 1968.

Lyons, H. A.: Treatment of emphysema. JAMA, *194*:1234-1236, 1965.

Management of Chronic Obstructive Lung Diseases, Conclusions of the Eighth Aspen Emphysema Conference, U. S. Dept. of Health, Education, and Welfare, P.H.S. Washington, D. C. 20201, May, 1966.

Miller, W. F.: Treatment of chronic pulmonary emphysema. Postgrad. Med., *39*:230-239, March, 1966.

National Tuberculosis Association: Chronic Obstructive Pulmonary Diseases. New York, 1966.

Nett, L. M., and Petty, T. L.: Effective treatment for emphysema and chronic bronchitis. J. Rehab., *33*:10-11, 53-56, Sept.-Oct., 1967.

Rie, M. W.: Physical therapy in the nursing care of respiratory disease patients. Nurs. Clin. N. Amer., *3*:463-478, Sept., 1968.

Robinson, F. N.: Nursing care of the patient with pulmonary emphysema. Amer. J. Nurs., *63*:92-96, Sept., 1963.

Scott, B. H.: Tensions linked with emphysema, Amer. J. Nurs., *69*:538-540, Mar., 1969.

Secor, J.: The patient with emphysema. Amer. J. Nurs., *65*:75-81, July, 1965.

CANCER OF THE LUNG

Bailey, A. J.: Lung cancer and smoking. Canad. Nurse., *61*:285-286, April, 1965.

Baskfield, M. M.: Preoperative and postoperative care of the patient with cancer of the lung. Nurs. Clin. N. Amer., *2*:609-622, Dec., 1967.

Boucot, K. R., Cooper, D. A., and Weiss, W.: Detection of lung cancer. Hosp. Med., *1*:28-32, Sept., 1965.

Ochsner, A., Jr., and Ochsner, A.: Cancer of the lung: recognition and management. Surg. Clin. N. Amer., *46*:1411-1425, Dec., 1966.

Parnell, J. L., Anderson, D. C., and Kinnis, C.: Cigarette smoking and respiratory infections in a class of student nurses. New Eng. J. Med., *274*:979-984, 1966.

Shaw, R. L.: The surgical management of bronchogenic carcinoma. AORN J., *2*:55-65, Nov-Dec., 1964.

Watson, W. L., and Loucks, E.: Oat-cell lung cancer. Amer. J. Nurs., *65*:113-115, Feb., 1965.

Wolf, J.: Management of the patient with inoperable bronchogenic carcinoma. Med. Clin. N. Amer., *51*:563-572, Mar., 1967.

PERIODICALS

The American Review of Respiratory Diseases. Official Journal of the American Thoracic Society, published by the National Tuberculosis and Respiratory Disease Association, New York, New York.

Diseases of the Chest. The official periodical of the American College of Chest Surgeons.

Journal of Thoracic and Cardiovascular Surgery. C. V. Mosby Co., St. Louis, Missouri.

Medical Bulletin on Tobacco. Published quarterly by the American Public Health Association, American Heart Association, American Cancer Society and the National Tuberculosis and Respiratory Disease Association, Room 1410, 1740 Broadway. New York, New York 10019.

PATIENT EDUCATION

Institute of Physical Medicine and Rehabilitation
New York University Medical Center
400 East 34th Street
New York, New York 10016

  Haas, A.: Essentials of Living with Pulmonary Emphysema. A Guide for Patients and Their Families.

National Tuberculosis and Respiratory Disease Association
1740 Broadway
New York, New York 10019

  The FACTS: Air Pollution
              Bronchiectasis
  (series)   Chronic Bronchitis
              Chronic Cough
              Cigarette Smoking
              Dust Diseases
              Pleurisy
              Pneumonia
              Shortness of Breath
              Emphysema
  Introduction to Respiratory Diseases
  What Can You Do About Your Breathing?

Public Affairs Pamphlets
381 Park Ave. South
New York, New York 10016
  Saltman, J.: Emphysema, When the Breath of Life Falters. Pamphlet No. 326. $.25.

Riker Laboratories
19901 Nordhoff Street
Northridge, California 91324
  Living with Asthma, Chronic Bronchitis and Emphysema. A Guide to Self Care.

Superintendent of Documents
U.S. Government Printing Office
Washington, D.C. 20402
  Common Cold. PHS Publication No. 106
  Emphysema. PHS Publication No. 1414 ($.05)

Also:
  Murray, D.: Our fastest-growing health menace. Reader's Digest, *90*:111-114, Jan., 1967. Pleasantville, New York. reprint.

  Petty, T. L., and Nett, L. M.: For Those Who Live and Breathe With Emphysema and Chronic Bronchitis. Springfield, Ill., Charles C Thomas, 1967.

Information also available from:
Chronic Respiratory Diseases Branch
  Division of Chronic Diseases
  Public Health Service
  Washington, D.C. 20201

CHAPTER **15**

Respiratory Intensive Care Nursing

- *Physiology*
- *Respiratory Failure*
- *Recognition of Respiratory Failure*
- *Chest Physical Therapy*
- *Respiratory Therapy*
- *Artificial Ventilation*
- *Cardiopulmonary Resuscitation*

Excellent nursing care is the absolute prerequisite for successful management of a patient with acute respiratory failure. The nursing care program must include prevention, recognition and treatment of the problem. To care adequately for a patient in respiratory failure a nurse must know something of disease processes that result in respiratory failure. She must know and recognize the signs and symptoms of respiratory failure and understand their limited reliability. She must have a working knowledge of pulmonary physiology and the interpretation of blood gas measurements. Finally, she must be highly skilled in the measures to treat and, more importantly, to prevent respiratory failure.

PHYSIOLOGY

The function of the lung is to supply body tissue cells with oxygen and to remove carbon dioxide formed by cell metabolism. Inspiration brings fresh air to the alveoli of the lung, thereby increasing the partial pressure of oxygen above that in venous blood entering pulmonary capillaries. The pressure difference between alveoli and pulmonary capillaries transfers oxygen by diffusion to red cell hemoglobin, loading the blood with oxygen. This oxygenated blood is then distributed by the left ventricle of the heart to the body tissues. Ventilation of alveoli with fresh air also causes elimination of carbon dioxide from venous blood by lowering the pressure of carbon dioxide in the alveoli below that in venous blood.

pO$_2$ and pCO$_2$

A "p" indicates pressure; pO$_2$, the pressure of oxygen, and pCO$_2$, the pressure of carbon dioxide. More correctly, these are referred to as partial pressures, since the pressure these gases exert is a part of total atmospheric pressure. The total atmospheric pressure is 760 mm. Hg. Partial pressures in alveolar gas are approximately as follows:

Partial pressure of nitrogen	= 573 mm. Hg
Partial pressure of H$_2$O vapor	= 47 mm. Hg
Partial pressure of O$_2$	= 100 mm. Hg
Partial pressure of CO$_2$	= 40 mm. Hg
Total of partial pressures	= 760 mm. Hg

The terms "partial pressure" and "tension" are often used interchangeably. Thus, paO$_2$, the partial pressure of oxygen in arterial blood and "arterial oxygen tension" mean the same thing; similarly paCO$_2$, the partial pressure of carbon dioxide in arterial blood and "arterial carbon dioxide tension" mean the same thing.

To obtain a specimen, blood is drawn into a heparinized syringe, bubbles expelled, and the syringe capped tightly to prevent exposure to air. The sample

Total ventilation = Dead space + Alveolar
ventilation ventilation

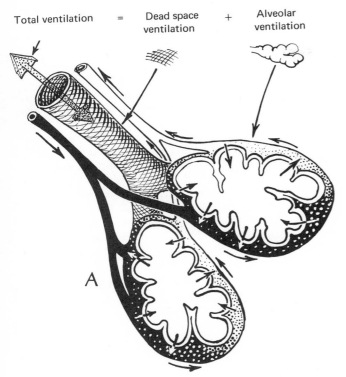

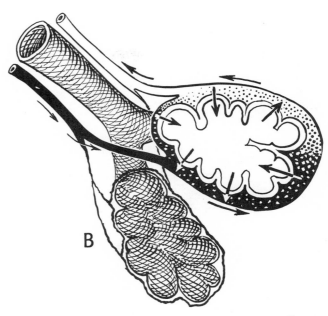

FIG. 15-1. (A) Normal relation of ventilation to blood flow. Venous blood is pumped to the lung (pulmonary capillaries) by the right ventricle. Oxygen diffuses from alveoli in the lung to capillary blood; carbon dioxide diffuses from capillary blood to alveoli. Oxygenated arterial blood returns through the pulmonary veins to the left atrium and is pumped by the left ventricle to supply oxygen needed for body tissue metabolism. Ventilation of alveoli with fresh air (alveolar ventilation) removes carbon dioxide and maintains alveolar oxygen tension; that fraction of ventilation which fills the tracheobronchial tree (dead space ventilation) does not participate in gas exchange.

(B) Increased dead space. Cessation of capillary blood flow to an alveolus which remains ventilated increases the proportion of total ventilation which does not participate in gas exchange. This increase in dead space requires that the patient breathe at a larger total ventilation to maintain the same amount of alveolar ventilation; if he is unable to do so (and alveolar ventilation falls) arterial carbon dioxide tension will also rise.

should be iced unless the measurements will be done in minutes. Simultaneous with blood sampling, the patient's tidal volume, respiratory rate, body temperature and inspired oxygen concentration must be measured to allow adequate evaluation of the laboratory results. An intra-arterial cannula and 3-way stopcock may be used in patients who require frequent blood-gas determinations.

Ventilation

Tidal volume is the total volume of each breath, i.e., the depth of breathing: it moves in and out like the tides. Not all of each tidal volume reaches the alveoli to participate in the exchange of oxygen and carbon dioxide. The portion that remains in the conducting airways from the nose and mouth to bronchioles, and which does not participate in gas exchange, is known as "dead space." Dead space is approximately 150 ml. in the normal adult.

The total volume of air entering the nose and mouth each minute is referred to as "minute ventilation." Minute ventilation is subdivided into alveolar ventilation and dead space ventilation, the normal distribution being ⅔ to alveoli and ⅓ to dead space (Fig. 15-1A).

Increased Dead Space

In some patients the flow of venous blood through the capillaries to some alveoli may have ceased. Alveoli that have lost their blood flow do not participate in blood-gas exchange; functionally, therefore, they act as increased dead space. Clinical conditions that lead to increased dead space are pulmonary embolism, hemorrhage, hypotension and emphysema.

The presence of increased dead space requires a patient to breathe at greater than normal minute ventilation to achieve normal alveolar ventilation. If he is unable to do this the rate of carbon dioxide elimination decreases and arterial carbon dioxide tension (Pa_{CO_2}) rises (hypercarbia) (Fig. 15-1B).

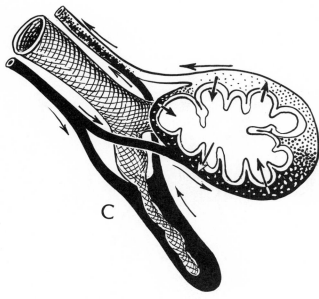

C

(C) Increased shunting. Cessation of ventilation to a pulmonary capillary (due to atelectasis, pneumonia, pulmonary edema) in which blood flow continues results in the bypassing or "shunting" of venous blood through the lung to mix with oxygenated blood from ventilated alveoli. The resulting arterial blood contains less oxygen per unit volume of blood (decreased oxygen content); arterial oxygen tension is also decreased. In order to maintain the same rate of transport of oxygen to body tissues the patient must increase cardiac output (the volume of blood pumped by the heart each minute). If circulatory compensation is not possible (i.e. due to heart disease) hypoxia may cause tissue damage or death. Oxygen administration will increase alveolar oxygen tension and therefore increase arterial oxygen tension and content; this is the primary reason for oxygen therapy.

Increased Shunting

Normally, about 2 per cent of the blood pumped to the lung by the right ventricle bypasses alveoli and does not participate in blood-gas exchange. This blood is returned unoxygenated to the left heart as venous blood and mixes with arterial blood. That fraction of pulmonary blood flow that bypasses ventilated alveoli is called the "shunt."

Atelectasis, pneumonia, and pulmonary edema all produce nonventilation of some alveoli. When blood flow to these alveoli continues, an increase in shunting occurs, more venous blood returns to the right heart and arterial oxygen tension (Pa_{O_2}) falls (hypoxemia) (Fig. 15-1C). Thus, areas of the lung where blood flow stops (e.g., pulmonary emboli) but ventilation continues function as increased dead space; the reverse

circumstance, cessation of ventilation to areas where blood flow continues, causes an increase in shunt.

Ventilation Pattern

The normal pattern of ventilation includes about 6 to 10 deep breaths or sighs, considerably larger than tidal volume, per hour. If no breaths are larger than tidal volume, alveolar collapse occurs, because not all alveoli are opened with each breath. Alveolar collapse (atelectasis) produces unventilated areas with continued blood flow and this increase in shunt causes arterial oxygen tension to fall. Periodic deep breaths serve to keep all alveoli open. This is the reason for encouraging postoperative patients to take deep breaths, and also is the rationale for using intermittent positive pressure breathing to increase tidal volume.

Vital Capacity

Vital capacity is a measure of the patient's ability to take a deep breath. It is defined as the maximal volume of gas that can be expelled from the lungs by forceful effort following a maximal inspiration. Vital capacity is measured by asking the patient to take the deepest possible breath and exhale it fully through a gas meter (respirometer). The normal vital capacity is about 70 ml./Kg. body weight; the normal tidal volume is about 5 ml./Kg. body weight. Reduction in vital capacity is an important index of respiratory failure. Indeed, patients with vital capacity of 10 ml./Kg. body weight or lower develop progressive alveolar collapse and shunting.

Vital capacity may be decreased by postoperative pain following abdominal or thoracic surgery, pulmonary disease, obesity, abdominal distension, and muscular weakness.

Inspiratory Force

Deep breaths may be decreased or eliminated by central nervous system depression, disease, or drugs; in this group of patients vital capacity is not a useful measurement because a conscious cooperative effort is required for the test. In the unconscious or uncooperative patient the measurement of inspiratory force is substituted for vital capacity. Inspiratory force is the maximal negative pressure that the patient can exert against an occluded airway. The minimal safe value is 25 cm. H_2O. Lower values indicate insufficient muscle strength for deep breaths or effective coughing.

Effect of Pain-Relieving Drugs

Drugs that relieve pain depress ventilation and coughing. Morphine changes the ventilation pattern in postoperative patients by eliminating spontaneous deep breathing. However, morphine may increase the

TABLE 15-1. Causes of respiratory failure*

Physiologic Abnormalities	Causes
A. Central nervous system depression	Drugs (opiates, barbiturates, anesthetics) Intracranial disease or trauma
B. Weakness	General debility Neuromuscular disease (myasthenia gravis, infectious poly- neuritis, poliomyelitis, tetanus) Neuromuscular block (curare, succinylcholine, neomycin)
C. Increased work of breathing 1. Increased airway resistance	Asthma, bronchitis, emphysema Airway tumor, stenosis, foreign body Retained secretions
2. Increased tissue resistance (lungs and chest wall)	Atelectasis, pneumonia, pulmonary edema Pulmonary fibrosis Obesity, kyphoscoliosis Pneumothorax, hemothorax Abdominal distension

D. Increased respiration requirement
    1. Increased dead space
      (causing increased ventilation requirement)
	Hemorrhage, hypotension
	Pulmonary emboli
	Emphysema, atelectasis

2. Increased shunt (increasing inspired oxygen requirement)	Atelectasis, pneumonia Pulmonary edema, pneumothorax Obesity
E. Increased metabolic rate (causing increased oxygen con- sumption and increased carbon dioxide production)	Fever Restlessness, shivering, seizures Thyrotoxicosis

* Modified from H. H. Bendixen: Prevention and management of postoperative respiratory problems. American Society of Anesthesiologists 18th Annual Refresher Course Lectures, New York, American Heart Association, 1967.

patient's ability to take a deep breath when he is requested to do so, by relieving pain that previously limited his vital capacity.

RESPIRATORY FAILURE

Definition

Respiratory failure exists whenever the exchange of oxygen for carbon dioxide in the lungs cannot keep up with the body tissue metabolic rate of oxygen consumption and carbon dioxide production. This results in a fall in arterial oxygen tension (hypoxemia) and a rise in arterial carbon dioxide tension (hypercapnia). To return arterial gases to normal, the inspired oxygen concentration and the total ventilation must be increased.

Causes of Respiratory Failure

Disease and other factors that cause respiratory failure act by producing neurologic depression or muscle weakness, by increasing the work of breathing, by increasing the ventilation or inspired oxygen requirement, or by increasing metabolic rate (see Table 15-1).

RECOGNITION OF RESPIRATORY FAILURE

Clinical Signs

Hypoxia and hypercarbia may produce changes in central nervous system and circulatory functions with consequent clinical signs. Cyanosis may result from decreased arterial oxygen tension or decreased cardiac output; however, some patients may die from hypoxia without ever showing cyanosis. Absence of cyanosis does *not* indicate adequate oxygenation.

Both hypoxia and hypercarbia increase sympathetic nervous system activity in healthy persons and as a result produce tachycardia and hypertension, signs of increased cardiac output. However, many patients are incapable of increasing cardiac output in response to hypoxemia; they will respond with bradycardia and hypotension.

Dyspnea, restlessness, irritability and coma may result from hypoxia or hypercarbia. These signs when present are important, but again, their absence does not exclude respiratory failure; consequently, objective measurements plus close observation are necessary.

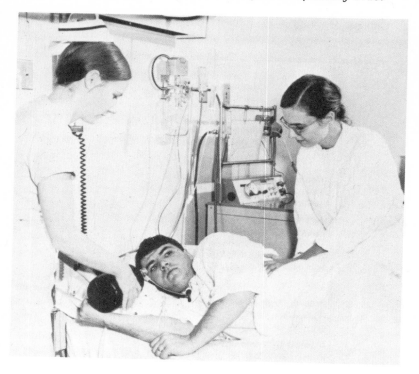

FIG. 15-2. Chest physical therapy. Vibration of the chest wall mobilizes secretions from the periphery of the lung to the large bronchi from where they drain by gravity to to the trachea and are removed by coughing or sterile catheter aspiration. Deep inflations may be provided manually for patient with decreased vital capacity by means of a self-inflating bag.

TABLE 15-2. Measurements of respiratory function

Vital capacity	normally 3500-5500 ml.	
	1000 ml.	needed for effective deep breathing, coughing
	below 700 ml. :	usually leads to respiratory failure and requirement for artificial ventilation (low values indicate decreased muscle strength *or* increased tissue resistance)
Tidal volume	normally 300-400 ml.	
Inspiratory force	25 cm. H_2O	minimal safe level
	below 25 cm. H_2O	indicates inadequate muscle strength
Timed vital capacity (or forced expiratory volume in one second)	normally 75% of measured vital capacity	
	below 75%	indicates increased airway resistance
Arterial Gases		
Arterial oxygen tension (Pa_{O_2})	normally above 600 mm. Hg. . .	breathing 100% oxygen
	normally 90-100 mm. Hg. . .	breathing room air
	below 70 mm. Hg. . .	requires increase in cardiac output to maintain oxygen transport to tissues
Arterial carbon dioxide tension (Pa_{CO_2})	normally 40 mm. Hg.	
	above 40 mm. Hg.	alveolar hypoventilation
	below 40 mm. Hg.	alveolar hyperventilation
Ventilation/Blood Flow Relationships		
Dead space	normally ⅓ of tidal volume	
	above ⅓ of tidal volume . . .	requires increase in total ventilation to avoid hypercarbia (alveolar hypoventilation)
Shunt	normally 2% of cardiac output	
	above 2% of cardiac output	requires increase in inspired oxygen concentration to avoid hypoxemia

FIG. 15-3. Positioning a patient to maintain an open upper airway. The patient is positioned semi-prone; the head is tilted backward. Oxygen is administered by mask. Immediately at hand are suction, an oral airway, and a bag and mask for positive pressure ventilation.

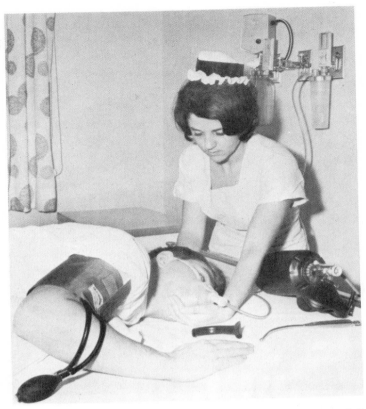

Measurements

Objective determinations of respiratory function are listed in Table 15-2. (See Table 14-2, p. 230.)

Prevention of Respiratory Failure in Surgical Patients

Two-thirds of patients with acute, and therefore reversible, respiratory failure are postoperative surgical patients. The commonest cause is abdominal, not thoracic, surgery. Preoperative preventive measures include chest physical therapy, the administration of aerosols, intermittent positive pressure breathing, cessation of smoking, and the obtaining of sputum for bacteriologic examination. Additional preventive measures employed in the postoperative period include frequent position change, assistance with intermittent deep breaths and coughing, knowledgeable administration of narcotics, accurate fluid balance and daily weighing, and monitoring of circulatory and respiratory function. These nursing care measures are discussed in the following sections.

CHEST PHYSICAL THERAPY

Frequent repositioning of patients is essential for the prevention of respiratory failure. The patient who spends long hours on his back tends to develop atelectasis of the lower lobes, pulmonary infection and respiratory failure. Perhaps the most frequent cause of preventable death in hospitalized patients is immobilization in the supine position. Sick patients must be repositioned from side to side (or better, semiprone to semiprone) to prevent this chain of complications.

In addition to frequent repositioning, a program of *segmental postural drainage* is used to promote gravity drainage of the secretions in the tracheobronchial tree. The nurse or chest physical therapist places the patient in a sequence of specific positions that promote gravity drainage of each bronchial segment. In each position the chest wall overlying the involved bronchial segment is percussed with cupped hands to loosen secretions. It is more comfortable for the patient if a terry cloth towel is placed over the chest wall. This technique is contraindicated if an acute inflammatory process, pain, or cardiac disease is present. *Vibration* of the chest wall during expiration will then mobilize secretions from the periphery of the lung toward the larger bronchi, from which they are expelled by coughing or sterile aspiration. Vibrations are produced by placement of the hands on the chest wall and tensing of the arm and shoulder muscles (see Fig. 15-2).

RESPIRATORY THERAPY

The equipment and methods used in respiratory therapy (inhalation therapy) perform 4 functions: maintenance of an *open airway* from nose and mouth

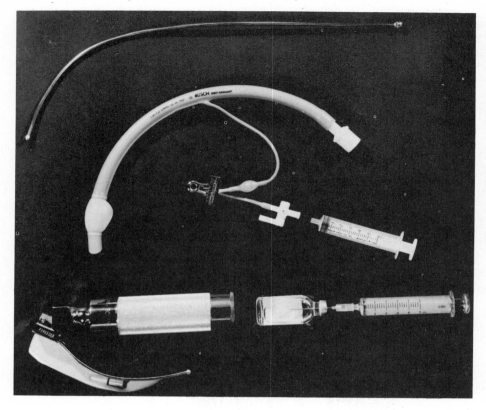

FIG. 15-4. Equipment for intubation of the trachea. An oral-endotracheal tube (*Center*) is shown with the cuff inflated. The larynx is visualized with a laryngoscope (*Bottom left*), which lifts the tongue and jaw and provides light. The tip of the endotracheal tube is passed through the vocal cords of the larynx and the cuff inflated by syringe to make a seal between tube and tracheal wall. A bendable copper stylette (*Top*) may be necessary to provide rigidity to the tube during intubation. Intravenous use of a muscle relaxant drug (*Bottom right*) may facilitate intubation.

to alveoli, and provision of *oxygen, humidity,* and *controlled ventilation* to meet the patient's requirements.

Maintaining a Clear Airway

The most frequent cause of *upper airway obstruction* is the posterior surface of the tongue resting on the back wall of the pharynx. Two factors promote obstruction from this cause: decrease in consciousness and the force of gravity. Consequently, an obtunded patient should never be left supine unless control of the airway has previously been secured by endotracheal intubation or tracheotomy. Drowsy patients should be nursed in the semiprone position with the neck flexed forward and the head tilted backward to help maintain an open upper airway (Fig. 15-3). Occasionally an oral airway is necessary to further aid in lifting the posterior tongue off the wall of the pharynx.

Use of a *cuffed endotracheal tube* (Fig. 15-4) inserted through the mouth or nose provides several advantages: the upper airway is maintained with greater certainty, the tube provides an easy avenue for aspiration of secretions by a sterile catheter, and the cuff provides a seal between the tube and tracheal wall and helps to prevent aspiration of pharyngeal and regurgitated gastric contents. The cuff also furnishes

a leakproof means of administering controlled positive pressure ventilation. Disadvantages of prolonged endotracheal intubation are several: (1) effective coughing is eliminated because the tube keeps the vocal cords open; (2) a break in sterile technique may introduce bacteria into the lower respiratory tract; (3) pressure from the tube or cuff may cause erosion and subsequent stricture of the larynx or trachea; (4) not all conscious patients will tolerate an endotracheal tube without sedation; and (5) good mouth care must be given and the tube repositioned frequently to prevent pressure ulceration of the lip.

When endotracheal intubation is required for more than about 2 days, tracheotomy is usually performed. *Tracheotomy* offers several advantages. The hazard of laryngeal damage is eliminated, and the shorter tube length makes the removal of retained secretions by the use of a sterile suction catheter easier. Patients tolerate tracheostomy tubes better than endotracheal tubes. More importantly, turning the patient to the semiprone position is facilitated, provided that the tube is fitted with appropriate connections (see Fig. 15-5).

The primary cause of *lower airway obstruction* is retained secretions (bronchospasm and bronchiolar collapse are also important causes in patients with chronic pulmonary disease). Mucous secretion from

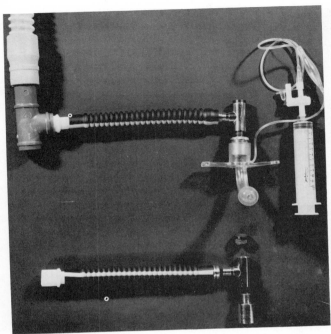

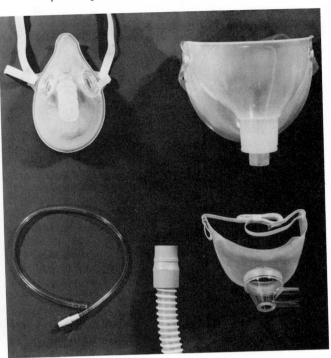

Fig. 15-5. The swivel connector. Use of a threaded swivel connector which turns freely in both the horizontal and the vertical planes allows the turning of patients into the semiprone position without dislodging the tracheostomy tube (or endotracheal tube). Removal of the threaded swivel cap permits aspiration of the trachea with a sterile catheter without disconnecting the patient from his oxygen supply. Humidified oxygen should be delivered to patients during weaning from the ventilator. A plastic T-piece provides easy connection of the oxygen supply to the swivel connector. A plastic cuffed tracheostomy tube is shown.

Fig. 15-6. Equipment for administration of oxygen and mist. A face mask (*Upper left*), face tent (*Upper right*), nasal catheter and tracheostomy mask are shown. Wide-bore tubing is necessary for delivery of water aerosols by face mask, face tent, or tracheostomy mask.

the tracheobronchial tree is normally transported up to and out of the larynx by ciliary activity. When cilia are damaged or are overloaded by copious or thick mucus, the primary means of clearing the tracheobronchial tree is by coughing. Effective coughing requires adequate inspiratory volumes and sufficient expiratory force to produce the high air flow rate required to propel mucus up the tracheobronchial tree. More force is required to dislodge thick mucus that is low in water content and high in viscosity. Methods are available to deal with each of these problems. Administration of water mist to the tracheobronchial tree increases the water content of secretions; intermittent positive pressure breathing increases the inspired volume, and percussion and vibration of the chest wall increases the forcefulness of expiration. Intermittent positive pressure breathing with a pressure-limited ventilator, particularly in patients with decreased vital capacity, is useful to increase tidal volumes for more effective coughing. The diameter of small bronchioles

is increased during peak inspiration and this further promotes effective coughing by lowering resistance to air flow. If additional bronchodilator effect is needed, drug aerosols (isoproterenol, phenylephrine) may be administered with the same apparatus.

Humidity and Nebulization Therapy

Water may be added to the tracheobronchial tree in 2 forms, as a gas (water vapor, humidity) or as a liquid (aerosols, mist). The most efficient *humidifiers* provide inspired gas fully saturated at body temperature. That is, the water content of the gas delivered to the tracheobronchial tree is precisely the same as that delivered by the nose under normal circumstances. This is usually sufficient to maintain secretions at normal viscosity. However, patients with thickened secretions (decreased water content) require a higher water content in the inspired gas to return sputum viscosity to normal. To increase water content above full saturation, water must be added in the liquid phase as a mist or aerosol.

Devices designed to generate aerosol mists are *nebulizers*. Jet-type nebulizers produce relatively large water particles that are deposited primarily in the tra-

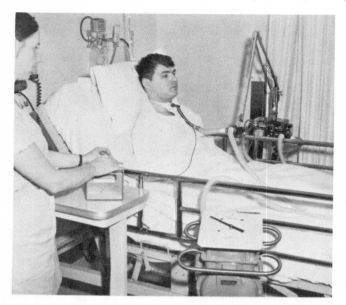

FIG. 15-7. Measurements to control artificial ventilation. Regardless of the type of ventilator used, several variables must be known and frequently measured: tidal volume, ventilator rate, and inspired oxygen concentration. To measure tidal volume a gas meter is connected to the expiratory valve of the ventilator and the expired volume from the patient noted. Ventilator rate is counted with the aid of a watch. The nurse is measuring the inspired oxygen concentration by means of an oxygen analyzer.

chea and the large bronchi. Use of a heated water reservoir with these nebulizers provides a much higher water content. Ultrasonic aerosol generators yield mists of the highest water content and of a particle size small enough to reach the smallest bronchioles.

Nebulizers have 2 potential disadvantages: (1) bacteria contaminating the water reservoir are efficiently transmitted in water droplets to the patient's airway, and (2) some of the excess water added to the tracheobronchial tree is absorbed, a hazard to patients with alveolar or interstitial pulmonary edema.

Oxygen Therapy

Arterial hypertension, arterial hypotension and increase in respiratory rate are all indications for measurement of arterial oxygen tension and, usually, the administration of oxygen.

Commonly used devices for the administration of oxygen include the nasal catheter, the face mask, and the face tent (Fig. 15-6). The *nasal catheter* should be inserted to the nasopharynx. At an oxygen flow of 6 to 8 L./minute, an inspired oxygen concentration of 30 to 50 per cent is provided. If the catheter is inserted too far, it enters the esophagus and gastric distension occurs. If the patient breathes predominantly through

his mouth, the inspired oxygen concentration will fall.

A higher oxygen concentration (35 to 70 per cent) is provided by the *face mask* at an oxygen flow of 6 to 12 L./minute. Inspired oxygen concentration varies with oxygen flow rate and mask fit. With high flow rates and a reasonable fit, an inspired oxygen concentration of about 60 per cent can be reliably maintained.

The *face tent*, a device that cradles the chin and directs oxygen flow upward across the face, is the most comfortable alternative for most patients. It is ideal for providing extra humidification or aerosols, but is less reliable than the face mask for maintaining high inspired oxygen concentration. Oxygen flow of 4 to 10 L./minute by way of the face tent provides approximately 30 to 50 per cent oxygen.

The adult oxygen tent is primarily of historical interest; it is costly to operate and considerable effort is necessary to maintain significant elevation in the inspired oxygen concentration.

Intermittent Positive Pressure Breathing

Intermittent positive pressure breathing therapy (IPPB) has several applications in patients who may develop or who are recovering from respiratory failure. Patients demonstrating marked reduction in vital capacity (less than 1,200 ml.) may require periodic deep breaths to prevent atelectasis. To ensure that the tidal volume introduced by the IPPB apparatus is greater than the patient's vital capacity, tidal volume must be measured. This is done by connecting a *gas meter* (respirometer) to the *expiratory valve*. This method of measuring expired tidal volume is identical to that used during artificial ventilation (Fig. 15-7).

Providing increased tidal volume for the patient with decreased vital capacity may also promote more efficient coughing, which assists in the removal of secretions. In addition, IPPB may act as a mechanical bronchodilator, since the bronchioles are more widely open with deeper inspirations. Dilated bronchioles allow higher air flow rates and permit more efficient coughing.

Water aerosols decrease the viscosity of thickened secretions; bronchodilators such as isoproterenol and phenylephrine relax bronchial smooth muscle and thereby decrease the resistance to air flow. Both may be administered by IPPB. (See also pp. 251-254.)

ARTIFICIAL VENTILATION

Indications

Artificial ventilation is indicated when the patient is unable to maintain safe levels of arterial carbon dioxide or oxygen by spontaneous breathing. Respiratory failure with progressive arterial hypercarbia and hypoxia, if uninterrupted, produces circulatory failure and cardiac arrest. Thus, the treatment of respiratory failure by artificial ventilation may be begun as part of an attempt at resuscitation. Patient survival is far higher when the course of developing respiratory failure is documented by serial measurement of vital capacity and arterial blood gases, and when artificial ventilation is instituted earlier. Most patients with a vital capacity less than 10 ml./Kg. of body weight develop progressive atelectasis and respiratory failure.

Alveolar hypoventilation results in carbon dioxide accumulation and causes respiratory acidosis. An elevation of carbon dioxide tension that yields an arterial pH below 7.25 is an indication to begin artificial ventilation.

Hypoxia, despite the efficient administration of oxygen, is another reason for instituting controlled ventilation. In practical terms, this corresponds to an arterial oxygen tension of 80 mm. Hg or less while the patient is breathing oxygen at high flow rates through a face mask—about 60 per cent oxygen is then being inspired.

Ventilators

Ventilators may be grouped into 2 types: those that inflate to a preset pressure and those that inflate to a preset volume. Whether a pressure-limited or volume-limited ventilator is in use, the nurse must be aware of the 3 variables that control ventilation and oxygenation (Fig. 15-7):

(1) The ventilator rate, measured with a watch;

(2) The tidal volume, measured as expired volume with a gas meter;

(3) The inspired oxygen concentration, measured with an oxygen analyzer.

Tidal volume and rate together control the elimination of carbon dioxide. The inspired oxygen concentration is controlled to produce normal arterial oxygen tensions.

The duration of inspiration should not exceed expiration. The elevation of intrathoracic pressure during prolonged inspiration may decrease the return of venous blood to the heart. The heart can only pump out that blood that returns in the veins. Hence obstruction of venous return by prolonged inspiration lowers cardiac output and decreases the rate of oxygen transport to body tissues.

The inspired gas delivered to the patient must be fully saturated with water to prevent thickening of tracheobronchial secretions. Water is added by either a humidifier or a nebulizer.

Preventive Therapy

To prevent and treat atelectasis and pneumonia, chest physical therapy must be continued during artificial ventilation. Of primary importance is frequent repositioning of the patient. Connections between the ventilator and the patient must be so designed to permit full turns to the semiprone position (Fig. 15-5).

Complications

The complications of artificial ventilation include: airway obstruction, endobronchial intubation, damage to the trachea, infection, pulmonary edema, gastrointestinal bleeding, tension pneumothorax, inability to wean and pulmonary oxygen toxicity.

In a patient undergoing artificial ventilation, *total airway obstruction* may occur from a plug of thickened secretions, from overinflation or displacement of the cuff, or from partial dislodgement of the tube. An extra sterile tube should be kept at the patient's bedside at all times. The patient will die unless the airway is promptly opened. Passage of a suction catheter should be attempted. The cuff should be deflated to rule out obstruction by the cuff. If this does not open the airway, the tracheostomy tube is removed and replaced with a fresh one. If the tube cannot be readily replaced, the tracheostomy stoma is covered by hand and the patient must be ventilated by bag and mask with oxygen or mouth-to-mouth.

The nurse should listen frequently to both sides of the chest with a stethoscope, not only to note secretions but to ensure air entry. Absence of air entry to one hemithorax usually means that the tip of the endotracheal or tracheostomy tube has descended into one main stem bronchus, usually the right. Atelectasis of the unventilated lung occurs rapidly.

Excellence in nursing care minimizes the incidence of most complications.

Nursing Care of the Patient in Respiratory Failure

Successful management of the patient in respiratory failure is only possible if a well-defined program is established that continues 24 hours each day. The patient should never be left unattended or unobserved.

The first 8 of the following measures should be carried out at approximately hourly intervals:

1. Position Change. The patient's position is alternated from side to side. Lateral turns of 120° are desirable, from right semiprone to left semiprone. At regular intervals the patient should be placed sitting upright for better ventilation of the lower lobes. Postural drainage is substituted several times daily for segmental bronchial drainage. Adequate postural drainage decreases the need for deep tracheobronchial catheter aspiration by preventing retention of secretions in the periphery of the lungs.

2. Deep Breaths. The patient's spontaneous tidal volume or tidal volume on the ventilator is periodically augmented by giving at least 6 to 8 deep breaths with a self-inflating bag and valve. Periodic sighing with greater than normal tidal volumes helps to prevent alveolar collapse. The inspired oxygen concentration

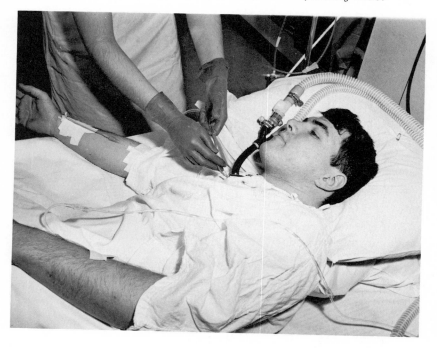

FIG. 15-8. Sterile aspiration of tracheal secretions. The sterile suction catheter is passed through the tracheostomy tube into the trachea until resistance is met. Then intermittent suction is applied and the catheter rotated as it is withdrawn. The patient should be ventilated with oxygen before a second passage of the catheter is attempted. Sterile gloves and a different sterile catheter are used for each suctioning episode. The nurse should examine the amount, color and consistency of the secretions obtained and inform the physician of any change.

should not be decreased during this maneuver. An oxygen flow rate of 10 L./minute to the self-inflating bag usually is adequate; however, patients requiring continuous ventilation with 100 per cent oxygen must be provided with a system that delivers that concentration.

Provision of deep breaths by hand also helps to promote coughing and reveals the presence of retained secretions (Fig. 15-2).

3. Aspiration of Secretions. If secretions are present, they are aspirated from the trachea using sterile technique. Sterile gloves and catheters are used for every tracheal aspiration (Fig. 15-8). The patient should be preoxygenated for 1 to 2 minutes prior to each suctioning episode. The suction catheter is inserted gently, as far as possible, withdrawn 1 to 2 cm., and intermittent suction is applied while slowly rotating the catheter. Aspiration must never be prolonged for more than 15 seconds, because cardiac arrest may ensue in patients with borderline oxygenation. Prior to a second passage of the catheter the patient should again be ventilated with oxygen for about 10 breaths. The nurse should note the amount, color and consistency of tracheal secretions obtained and inform the physician if there is appreciable change.

4. Breath Sounds. The nurse should listen to the chest from bottom to top on both sides with a stethoscope. Since the nurse is the patient's primary observer, she is responsible for noticing changes in breath sounds that may indicate increased secretions, pulmonary edema, atelectasis or other pulmonary pathology.

Sophistication is hardly necessary; it is sufficient to note whether breath sounds are present or absent, normal or abnormal, and whether a change has occurred.

5. Humidification. For the patient receiving humidified gas from a ventilator or wall humidifier, certain precautions are necessary. Water condensing in the delivery tubing must be periodically emptied, to prevent obstruction of gas flow and sudden flooding of the trachea. The level of water in the reservoir must be frequently checked to ensure that the patient is never ventilated with dry gas.

6. Airway Pressure. For patients on volume-limited ventilators the airway pressure gauge should be checked at frequent intervals. Since these ventilators deliver a fixed volume, a sudden drop in pressure indicates a leak in the system, and a sudden rise in pressure indicates obstruction of the delivery of gas to the patient.

7. Tidal Volume. For patients on pressure-limited ventilators, tidal volume should be frequently measured with a respirometer. An abrupt fall in tidal volume should be reported to the physician, because this indicates either increase in airway resistance (e.g., bronchospasm or other obstruction), or increase in tissue resistance (e.g., pulmonary edema).

8. Cuff Inflation. The cuff of an endotracheal tube or tracheostomy tube should be periodically deflated. It is important that the cuff not be deflated until the pharynx and larynx have been cleared of accumulated secretions by either suction or postural drainage. Air is released from the cuff slowly using a syringe while

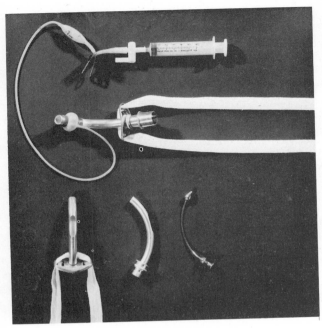

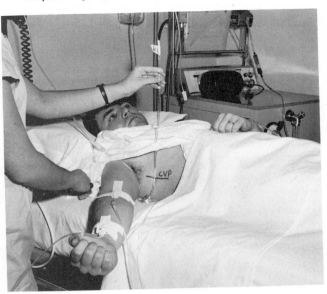

Fig. 15-10. Central venous pressure measurement. The water manometer is connected to a plastic intravenous catheter which has been threaded through an arm vein until the tip lies in the superior vena cava. The zero point of the manometer is held at the mid-axillary line (marked to insure a constant base line). The manometer is filled with fluid from the intravenous bottle. When the stopcock is switched to connect the manometer to the intravenous catheter, fluid in the column falls until it balances the central venous pressure in the superior vena cava. The fluid level indicates the central venous pressure in cm H_2O. (See text for interpretation.)

Fig. 15-9. Tracheostomy tubes. (*Center*) an assembled cuffed silver tracheostomy tube. Note the rubber cuff which, when inflated, provides an airtight seal between the tube and tracheal wall to allow positive pressure ventilation. The cuff is inflated with a syringe and sealed by a stopcock or clip. The fixed metal flange (through which the cloth tape passes) prevents descent of the tube into a main-stem bronchus. The tape, which is tied around the neck, prevents dislodgement of the tube. (*Bottom*) a disassembled uncuffed fenestrated tracheostomy tube with inner cannula and stylette which facilitates insertion. The neck orifice of this tube may be plugged to evaluate the patient's ability to raise his secretions by coughing.

positive pressure is maintained from the ventilator or a self-inflating bag. This maneuver blows accumulated secretions in the upper trachea and larynx into the mouth and prevents their aspiration into the lungs. The cuff should be reinflated with *just enough air to prevent gross leak* when positive pressure is again applied to the airway. Under no circumstances should the cuff be overinflated. The nurse should record the volume of air required in the cuff to achieve an airtight seal. If increasing amounts of air are required, the patient's physician should be informed. Overdistension of the trachea is probably the primary cause of erosion of tracheal mucosa and cartilage and of subsequent tracheal stenosis.

9. Tracheostomy Care. Tracheostomy care should be done every 4 hours and more frequently if needed. Some patients with a tracheostomy are managed with a double-wall tracheostomy tube (Fig. 15-9). Double-wall tubes are so designed that the nurse may remove and clean the inner cannula. At this time the soiled tracheostomy tape and dressing are changed and replaced with sterile ones. To continue ventilation while the inner cannula is removed, a sterile substitute inner cannula or adaptor should be inserted into the outer cannula and connected to the ventilator. The tracheostomy stoma and surrounding skin should be washed with hydrogen peroxide or suitable soap solution and dried at this time. Redness or inflammation around the tracheostomy stoma should be brought to the physician's attention. (Also see pp. 222–226.)

10. Swivel Connector. The flexible connection from tracheostomy tube to ventilator lines (e.g., Mörch swivel) is cleaned or replaced by a sterile one at the same time tracheostomy care is given.

11. Bacteriologic Specimens. Shortly after endotracheal intubation or tracheotomy, and twice a week thereafter, tracheal secretions should be aspirated into a sterile container and sent to the lab for culture and sensitivity tests. Each day tracheal secretions should be obtained and smeared on a glass slide for staining by the gram method. This technique allows the earliest detection of infection or change in infecting organisms in the tracheobronchial tree.

12. Circulatory Measurements. Pulse rate and arterial blood pressure are checked and recorded frequently. Arterial pressure may be measured by the usual method using a blood pressure cuff and stethoscope or by *intra-arterial pressure monitoring*. In the latter method a catheter is introduced into an artery, usually the radial or femoral, and the pressure at the catheter tip is transmitted to a *pressure transducer* that converts the pressure wave into an electrical signal that is displayed for continuous visual observation on an oscilloscope.

The measurement of *central venous pressure* is frequently indicated. A plastic catheter is threaded, usually through an arm or neck vein, into the superior vena cava just before it enters the right atrium of the heart. Measurement of the pressure at the tip of this catheter provides an index of right atrial filling pressure. This measurement may provide a guide to the administration of blood and other intravenous fluids, and also is a criterion to determine the presence of right ventricular failure. Central venous pressure may be monitored by a transducer and oscilloscope. More often it is measured intermittently by balancing a water column (manometer) against the pressure in the catheter. To do this, the zero point of the manometer is levelled with the right atrium by placing the patient supine and flat and holding the zero point of the manometer at the midaxillary line. The height of the water column above this point equals the central venous pressure, usually measured in centimeters of water (Fig. 15-10).

To ensure that the measurement obtained is in fact central venous pressure, several observations are helpful:

(1) The length of catheter threaded intravenously should be sufficient to reach the superior vena cava.

(2) When the manometer is filled and then connected to the catheter, the fluid level falls rapidly to the balance point.

(3) Fluid level fluctuates with respiration and rises sharply with coughing.

(4) Blood can be aspirated from the catheter.

(5) The catheter tip is visualized in the superior vena cava upon chest x-ray.

Abrupt rise in the central venous pressure may indicate the onset of a cardiac arrhythmia or passage of the catheter tip into the right ventricle. Both intra-arterial catheters and central venous catheters require frequent flushing with dilute solutions of heparin to prevent obstruction by blood clotting.

13. Sedation and Muscle Relaxants. Patients undergoing controlled ventilation may require sedation or muscle relaxation with such drugs as morphine or curare to eliminate spontaneous breathing efforts between ventilator cycles, or to reduce oxygen consumption. Both morphine and curare, and some similar drugs, produce vasodilation. Arterial pressure should be measured frequently after their administration, since hypotension may ensue. The nurse caring for a patient who is paralyzed by muscle relaxants must constantly remember that the patient may be fully awake although not capable of any motor response. All procedures must be explained to the patient before their initiation, and an extra measure of reassurance provided. The nurse must also remind others of this necessity.

14. Fluid Balance. Positive fluid balance resulting in increase in body weight and interstitial pulmonary edema is a frequent problem in patients requiring artificial ventilation. This is better prevented than treated. Prevention requires early recognition of fluid accumulation, which can only be achieved with *precise recording of fluid intake and output* and the obtaining of *accurate daily body weights*. It is most important that no patient be considered too sick or too encumbered with tubes and other apparatus to be weighed. Failure to weigh patients because it is inconvenient results in errors in fluid management and, in some patients, death from interstitial pulmonary edema and resulting hypoxia. The average adult who is wholly dependent on parenteral nutrition can be expected to lose about ½ pound each day, since maintenance nutritional requirements cannot be completely supplied by the intravenous route. Thus, under these circumstances, *constant body weight* indicates *positive fluid balance*.

15. Nutrition. Starvation is a frequent and serious complicating disease in patients with respiratory failure. Many patients with a tracheostomy tube in place and some patients with endotracheal tubes can swallow sufficiently well to maintain an adequate oral intake. Aspiration of food is a significant hazard, however, and should this occur feeding should be stopped, the patient placed in the semiprone position with head-down tilt and chest physical therapy instituted to remove aspirated material.

If oral intake is not adequate, nasogastric feedings should be promptly substituted. Patients wholly dependent on parenteral nutrition may be benefited by the use of high caloric intravenous solutions.

16. Abdominal Complications. About ¼ of patients requiring artificial ventilation develop gastrointestinal bleeding, and of those about half require transfusion. To detect this problem when it first occurs, all stools and gastric drainage should be tested for the presence of occult blood.

Abdominal distension occurs frequently with respiratory failure, and further hinders respiration by elevation of the diaphragm. Daily measurement of abdominal girth provides objective assessment of the degree of distension.

17. Weaning. Artificial ventilation is discontinued by permitting the patient to breathe on his own for gradually-increasing periods of time, a process referred to as "weaning." During this period, which may initially be only a few minutes, the patient must be provided with high inspired oxygen concentrations and must never be left alone. Weaning should be discontinued by the nurse if there is marked change in vital signs or if the patient becomes restless. It is usually wiser to provide artificial ventilation each night until the patient can safely maintain spontaneous breathing throughout the day.

Weaning usually progresses through 4 stages: from artificial ventilation, from the tracheostomy tube cuff, from the tracheostomy stoma and finally from supplementary inspired oxygen. The patient should be seated upright and the tracheostomy tube cuff should usually be deflated during periods of spontaneous breathing. Before oral feedings are given with the cuff deflated, the patient's ability to swallow without aspiration should be tested: The patient is seated upright and the trachea, nasopharynx, and oropharynx are cleared by sterile aspiration before the cuff is deflated. While the cuff is deflated, the patient drinks a glassful of dilute methylene blue solution (0.5 ml in 60 ml water). The trachea is aspirated immediately. Absence of blue dye in the tracheal aspirate indicates the ability to swallow without aspiration.

After artificial ventilation has been discontinued, a fenestrated tracheostomy tube may be used (Fig. 15-9). These are uncuffed tubes with a fenestration, or window, cut in the greater curvature to decrease resistance to air flow. When the external orifice of the fenestrated tracheostomy tube is plugged, one can evaluate the patient's ability to breathe spontaneously for long periods, and his ability to cough and mobilize secretions without the aid of tracheal aspiration. In addition, he can now talk easily because all expired air passes through the larynx. This is no small boost to morale. If secretions cannot be coughed up, the plug is removed and secretions aspirated by sterile catheter as before. When tracheal aspiration has been unnecessary for 24 hours, the tube is usually removed and the stoma is covered with a sterile dressing and allowed to close. Supplementary inspired oxygen by face mask may be required for an additional period until arterial oxygen tension during breathing of room air reaches safe levels.

18. Communication. The patient in respiratory failure requiring artificial ventilation has many anxieties that are common to other sick patients. In addition, he has one unique source of frustration—the inability to talk. The simple provision of a writing pad and pencil may help solve the problem for some. For others, too

sick to write, some form of nonverbal communication can usually be established if the nurse is sufficiently kind and patient. Both the patient and his family must be reassured each day; it is particularly important that the reason for the tracheostomy tube and the inability to speak be explained frequently to both patient and family along with reassurance that normal speech will return when the tube can be removed.

Even though the nurse is always in close proximity, the patient should be given the call light cord and instructed in its use.

CARDIOPULMONARY RESUSCITATION

Cardiac arrest is the sudden and unexpected cessation of respiration and effective circulation. It is particularly important that the nurse be skilled in the techniques of resuscitation from cardiopulmonary arrest, because she frequently is the only person attending the patient at the time this emergency occurs. Useful brain function is preserved only if ventilation and circulation are re-established within 2 to 3 minutes. Within seconds the nurse must make the diagnosis, call for help, and provide initial effective ventilation and circulation (see p. 418).

Make the Diagnosis

The patient who sustains cardiopulmonary arrest loses consciousness and stops breathing, often with gasping respiration that proceeds to apnea. The nurse should immediately check the neck (carotid) or groin (femoral) pulses. If these are not palpable, cardiac output is inadequate for effective circulation of blood. Next, the pupils of the eye are quickly checked. Dilation of the pupils begins in about 45 seconds and is complete within another minute. Sudden absence of pulses and dilation of pupils requires immediate institution of artificial ventilation and external cardiac compression. The nurse should call for help, both to aid her in initiating resuscitation and to summon a physician or the hospital emergency team. She should note the time of arrest (writing this on the bed sheet is useful) and begin resuscitation.

Artificial Ventilation

The most reliable means of emergency artificial ventilation is mouth-to-mouth ventilation with expired air. The first step is to open the airway. The mouth is rapidly cleaned of any foreign material. The head is then tilted backward as far as possible by lifting the neck with one hand and pushing back on the forehead with the other. (This tends to lift the tongue off the back wall of the pharynx and open the airway.) The patient's lungs are inflated by forceful expiration of a full breath through a mouth-to-mouth airtight seal. The nose is pinched shut to prevent a leak. About 12 breaths per minute are provided. The patient's chest must visibly expand with attempted inflation. Absence of chest expansion indicates airway obstruction, which may be relieved by placement of the resuscitator's thumb in the patient's mouth and pulling the lower jaw forward during ventilation. Alternative methods of emergency artificial ventilation include the use of an S-tube (which is a more difficult technique but may be more aesthetic to some), and the use of a bag and mask (which requires additional equipment and skills).

Artificial Circulation

External cardiac compression is necessary to circulate blood that has been oxygenated by artificial ventilation. To accomplish this the patient must be placed supine on a hard surface. Manual pressure is applied to the sternum, which squeezes the heart between the sternum and the spine, forcing out blood with each compression. The heel of one hand is placed on the lower half of the sternum and the opposite hand placed on top of the first hand. Firm heavy pressure is applied with each compression. For adequate circulation the sternum must be depressed 1.5 to 2.0 inches, which in the average adult requires 80-100 pounds pressure. This requires considerable effort and can best be done by positioning oneself with knees on the bed beside the patient, keeping the elbows straight and letting the back and body weight do the work. Sixty to 80 compressions per minute are necessary. Constriction of the pupils and the presence of a palpable carotid pulse are evidence of effective circulation of oxygenated blood. One deep breath should be delivered for each 5 cardiac compressions, without interruption of compression rhythm.

Drugs Administered

Cardiotonic and peripheral vasoconstrictor drugs are used, both to stimulate myocardial activity and to elevate the perfusion pressure that results from cardiac compression. Epinephrine, which has both cardiotonic and vasoconstrictor action, is the preferred drug. It is administered either directly into the heart by way of a long needle or, preferably, intravenously if an intravenous route is already available.

Marked metabolic acidosis occurs at the time of cardiac arrest and persists during cardiopulmonary resuscitation, since perfusion of body tissues is far below normal. Acidosis both depresses the myocardium and renders it less responsive to the cardiotonic effects of epinephrine. Sodium bicarbonate is administered to correct metabolic acidosis and restore pH to normal. The nurse should prepare and label the following drug solutions:

(1) One ml. epinephrine (1:1000) diluted with 9 ml. isotonic saline in a 10-ml. syringe with a 3.5 inch, 22 gauge needle;

(2) Sodium bicarbonate 44.6 mEq. (3.75 gm.) in a 50-ml. syringe.

She should always have these drugs ready in separate syringes, because the usual timing of drug administration is epinephrine every 5 minutes and sodium bicarbonate every 10 minutes.

Equipment

An electrocardiographic monitor and defibrillator are next obtained. If the electrocardiogram demonstrates the presence of ventricular fibrillation, electrical countershock must be applied by the defibrillator.

Following restoration of heart function, artificial ventilation should be continued until measurement of vital capacity and arterial blood gases indicates that spontaneous breathing will result in safe oxygenation and ventilation. Intra-arterial and central venous pressure monitoring are usually indicated. Monitoring of the electrocardiogram should be continued for 72 hours. Hypothermia and intravenous urea may be employed to treat cerebral edema.

BIBLIOGRAPHY

Books

American Heart Association: Cardiopulmonary Resuscitation: A Manual for Instructors, New York, 1967.

Bendixen, H. H., *et al.*: Respiratory Care. St. Louis, C. V. Mosby, 1965.

Comroe, J. H.: Physiology of Respiration. Chicago Year Book Publishers, 1965.

Safar, P.: Respiratory Therapy. Philadelphia, F. A. Davis, 1965.

Articles

Abram, H. S.: Psychological aspects of the intensive care unit, Hosp. Med., 5:94-95, Dec., 1969.

Betson, C.: Blood gases, Amer. J. Nurs., 68:1010-1012, May, 1968.

Didier, E. P., and Helmholz, H. F.: Principles in the selection and use of mechanical ventilators and assistors. Med. Clin. N. Amer., 48:867-876, July, 1964.

Eckenhoff, J. E.: Care of the unconscious patient. JAMA, 186: 541-543, 1963.

Egan, D. F.: Inhalation therapy in the general hospital. G.P., 33: 99-104, March, 1966.

Fitzwater, J.: Planning an intensive care unit. Amer. J. Nurs., 67: 310-314, Feb., 1967.

Hammes, H. J.: Reflections on "intensive care." Amer. J. Nurs., 68:339-340, Feb., 1968.

Hedley-Whyte, J., and Winter, P. M.: Oxygen therapy. Clin. Pharmacol. Ther., 8:696-737, 1967.

Kornfeld, D. S., Maxwell, T., and Momrow, D.: Psychological hazards of the intensive care unit. Nurs. Clin. N. Amer., 3: 41-51, March, 1968.

Minckley, B. B.: The multiphasic human-to-human monitor (ICU model). Nurs. Clin. N. Amer., 3:29-39, March, 1968.

Murphy, E. R.: Intensive nursing care in a respiratory unit. Nurs. Clin. N. Amer., 3:423-436, Sept., 1968.

CHAPTER **16**

Patients with Pulmonary Tuberculosis

- *Clinical Manifestations*
- *Miliary Tuberculosis*
- *Pathophysiology of Chronic Pulmonary Tuberculosis*
- *Management of Pulmonary Tuberculosis*
- *Public Health and Prevention*
- *Atypical Mycobacteria*

Tuberculosis is defined as "that infectious disease caused by one of several closely related mycobacteria, including *M. tuberculosis, M. bovis,* and *M. avium.* It usually involves the lungs, but it also involves and sometimes produces gross lesions in other organs and tissues."*

CLINICAL MANIFESTATIONS

Since tubercle bacilli can establish themselves in almost every type of human tissue, and since there is no organ system that they cannot colonize, the clinical manifestations of tuberculosis are extremely numerous and varied. Commonest, by far, of all variants of this infection is pulmonary tuberculosis, in which there is involvement of some portion of the lung parenchyma, together with the bronchi and the bronchioles within it, the mediastinal nodes that drain it and the pleura that covers it. In other patients the principal site of involvement is in the upper respiratory tract, as in cases of tuberculous tonsillitis and laryngitis. The most prominent lesion may be a tuberculous laryngitis. Lymph nodes that guard the lymphatic drainage may become infected, producing the picture of tuberculous adenitis. Organisms that are swallowed and later ab-

sorbed from the small bowel may localize in the mesenteric or retroperitoneal lymphatic system, giving rise to tuberculous mesenteric adenitis or peritonitis and later tuberculous ileitis or splenitis or renal tuberculosis. The infection may spread from retroperitoneal to mediastinal nodes, producing tuberculous mediastinitis, pleuritis or pericarditis. From lymph nodes in the neck, the mediastinum or the retroperitoneum the infection may extend to the spine, causing tuberculous osteomyelitis with resultant vertebral collapse and deforming kyphosis, or it may enter the spinal canal and infect the meninges, producing tuberculous meningitis. Transported by way of the blood stream, which it has many opportunities to enter, the tubercle bacillus finds access to and may localize within the brain, forming a "tuberculoma"; cause tuberculous uveitis; or when in a joint, produce tuberculous arthritis. Or it may implant and grow simultaneously in hundreds of sites throughout the body, which is the situation in "miliary tuberculosis."

Mycobacterium tuberculosis, the tubercle bacillus, can be recognized partly from its size and shape, but particularly from the color-fast quality that it exhibits when stained by a certain method, i.e., its "acid-fast" quality.

The strain, *M. tuberculosis* var. *hominis,* is responsible for almost all tuberculous infections in humans in

---

* National Tuberculosis Association: The Diagnostic Standards and Classification of Tuberculosis. 1961.

Fig. 16-1. Diagrammatic representation of tuberculosis pathology. (National Tuberculosis and Respiratory Disease Association)

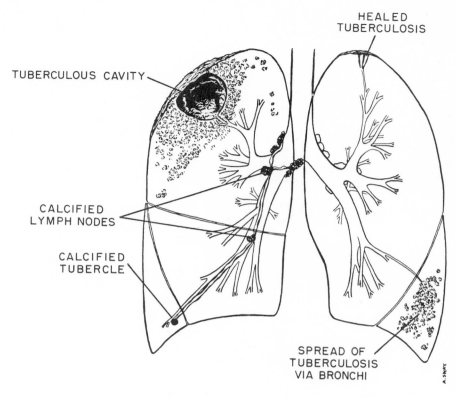

HEALED TUBERCULOSIS

TUBERCULOUS CAVITY

CALCIFIED LYMPH NODES

CALCIFIED TUBERCLE

SPREAD OF TUBERCULOSIS VIA BRONCHI

the United States. Another strain, *M. tuberculosis* var. *bovis,* exhibits similar morphologic criteria and is responsible for producing tuberculous infections in cattle. The latter strains may produce human infections, especially of the tonsils, cervical lymph nodes, and gastrointestinal tract, after ingestion of infected milk. Infections with the bovine strain of tubercle bacillus still remain a significant problem in underdeveloped countries. Public health control measures have almost completely eradicated bovine tuberculosis in cattle and dairy herds in the United States.

In contrast with the majority of infectious diseases, the germ of tuberculosis, once it has gained a foothold in the body, is likely to remain there quiescent for years after the forces of immunity have controlled the original infection. If, during this quiescent period, the resistance of the host is weakened, the germ at once begins to multiply, causing any one of many tuberculous diseases. If the patient's body proves able to recover from this illness, then the tubercle bacilli again become dormant.

Pathology

Tuberculosis is one of the so-called *granulomatous* diseases; that is, when the organism invades normal tissues, these form in response to it a new tissue, masses of which are called *infectious granulomas*. The tubercle (little tumor), the characteristic lesion of tuberculosis,

is a tiny spherical infectious granuloma just large enough to be seen with the naked eye. Another more diffuse and equally characteristic tissue reaction also occurs in response to the tubercle bacillus.

Tubercle bacilli, swept along by the lymph and bloodstream, lodge in susceptible tissues in small clumps. The neighboring tissue cells quickly accumulate around each of these, forming a protective wall that checks their further spread and may kill them. If immunity is successful, after a long time the germs die, and the tubercle becomes transformed into a tiny mass of fibrous tissue. At the same time, the tissue of the tubercle may become necrotic and transformed into a cheesy mass, a process known as *caseation.* If this occurs, the germs are liberated from the imprisonment and lymph sweeps them into the surrounding tissues, which respond by enclosing these freed germs in new tubercles. In this way, the original miliary (like millet seeds) tubercle grows into larger and larger irregular masses, some as large as a fist.

The fate of the patient depends on which of these two processes prevails. If the tissue barriers survive, then the imprisoned tubercle bacilli cease to multiply and may die. Lime salts from the blood are deposited in the dead caseous material, and scar tissue forms around the infected area, which remains throughout life as a healed calcified mass. However, if the germs survive and are freed from the tubercle, they multiply and are swept along by the lymph stream into the neighboring tissues and by the bloodstream into other organs, where they lodge and repeat the same process.

MILIARY TUBERCULOSIS

Miliary tuberculosis is the result of bloodstream invasion by the tubercle bacillus. It is the most serious form of tuberculosis. The origin of the bacilli that flood the bloodstream is either some chronic focus that has ulcerated into a blood vessel or multitudes of miliary tubercles lining the inner surface of the thoracic duct. The germs, poured from these foci into the bloodstream, are carried throughout the body and locate throughout all tissues, everywhere inducing tubercle formation. Definite evidence of this tubercle formation almost always is found on x-ray examination of the lungs. Another location of diagnostic importance is the choroid of the eye, where these tubercles become visible on ophthalmic inspection.

The clinical course of miliary tuberculosis is varied, depending on which organs are involved earliest and most severely. The usual picture is one of prolonged high, irregular fever without chills and gradually progressive inanition, weight loss and prostration. At first there may be no localizing signs except for splenomegaly, anemia and leukopenia, or at least the absence of leukocytosis, which distinguishes it from most other bacteremias. Within a few weeks, however, a roentgenogram of the chest reveals small densities scattered diffusely throughout both lung fields; these are the miliary tubercles, which gradually increase in size. Very few physical signs may be elicited on physical examination of the chest, but at this stage the patient suffers from a severe harassing cough, dyspnea and cyanosis. Treatment is precisely as described for pulmonary tuberculosis.

PATHOPHYSIOLOGY OF CHRONIC PULMONARY TUBERCULOSIS

Tissues respond to the invading tubercle bacillus in different ways, depending on the degree of immunity possessed by the patient and the degree of inflammatory reaction provoked by the organism and its products. Let us assume that a few tubercle bacilli, recently inhaled, have lodged and gained a foothold in the wall of one of the bronchi. It is usually one of the smaller bronchi near the periphery of the lung that is infected. The usual reaction is the prompt formation of clusters of tubercles around these bacterial clumps. Some of the organisms escape into the lymph ducts that drain this area of lung and are trapped in the hilar lymph node with which the duct communicates. The imprisoned bacteria gradually die, the tubercles in the lung tissue and in the infected lymph node become necrotic, and calcium becomes deposited in the caseous tissue.

The end-result is a healed primary tuberculosis, manifested by a calcified nodule (the Ghon tubercle) at the site of the original infection and a calcified node at the corresponding hilus, a combination known as the *Ghon complex.* Subsequent invasions by the tubercle bacillus will be met more promptly, and, in most cases, unless the infecting dose is large, the organisms will never have a chance to multiply or spread. In America, a large, although decreasing, percentage (less than 20 per cent) of all persons contract such a lesion. The infection rarely gives rise to a single symptom or sign other than x-ray evidence of the Ghon complex.

Individuals who have experienced a primary tuberculous infection are sensitized or allergic to the chemical constituents of the organism. Henceforth, contact with the bacillus, whether it is alive or killed, produces an acute local tissue inflammation. This is the basis of the tuberculin test, in which a suspension of ground-up killed tubercle bacilli obtained from a culture is injected into the skin. If the patient is allergic—that is, has at one time had a tuberculous infection—a local skin inflammation results (p. 292); whereas if there is no allergy, no reaction whatever is obtained.

A similar inflammatory reaction develops in the lung of a person who has been sensitized previously to the tubercle bacillus, if this lung is invaded later by more organisms than his immune processes can handle at the time. In contrast with the relatively bland, silent, primary type of pulmonary tuberculosis, the course of the reinfection type is complicated by necrosis with resulting ulceration of the infected lung tissue. Clusters of tubercles, as in the primary type of tuberculosis, form at once around the nests of organisms, but now, due to the tissue sensitivity, these become surrounded by zones of inflammatory reaction. The alveoli in the area become filled with exudate; in other words, a tuberculous bronchopneumonia develops. The tuberculous tissue in this area gradually becomes caseous and ulcerates into a bronchus, causing a cavity. At the same time, as the ulcerations heal, considerable scar tissue forms locally, especially around the cavities. The pleura over the infected lobe, more often an upper lobe, becomes inflamed, then thickened and retracted by scar tissue.

This cycle of inflammatory bronchopneumonia proceeds to ulceration with cavitation, followed by scarring. Unless the process can be arrested, it spreads slowly downward toward the hilum and later extends into adjacent lobes. The activity of the process may be very prolonged and characterized by long remissions, when the case may appear to be arrested, only to be followed by periods of renewed activity.

Depending on whether the predominant pathologic feature of the infection is ulceration or fibrosis, a case is designated as *chronic ulcerative pulmonary tubercu-*

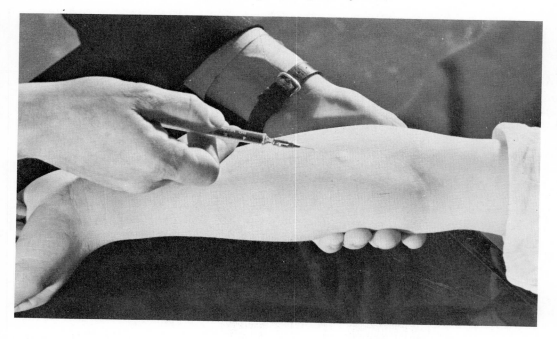

FIG. 16-2. The Mantoux Test. Using a tuberculin syringe and a subcutaneous needle with the bevel up tubercle bacillus extract has been injected into the skin of the forearm. (National Tuberculosis Association, New York, N.Y.)

losis or *chronic fibroid tuberculosis*. Fibroid tuberculosis is that form of the infection in which the healing process is sufficient to prevent gross caseation of the tuberculous areas yet cannot halt the infection. The result is a gradual transformation of a lobe, or of the entire lung, into a mass of fibrous tissue. The pleurae become thick and adherent, and the bronchi dilated, their walls pulled apart by the contracting scar tissue in the lung, while the chest on the affected side becomes shrunken, the spine curved laterally.

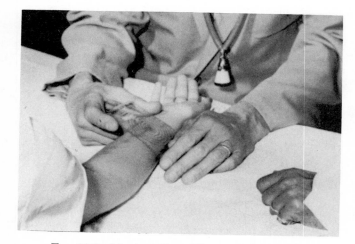

FIG. 16-3. Mantoux Test. The area of induration is measured more accurately with the aid of a plastic ruler containing concentric circles of specific diameters. (National Tuberculosis Association)

Symptoms and Course

Chronic pulmonary tuberculosis is insidious in its onset and course—so insidious that its diagnosis may be missed for a long time. The early symptoms seldom suggest the lungs as the seat of the disease. Often the patient notices first that he is losing weight; that, although he feels very well on rising in the morning, he fatigues a little more easily than previously, especially in the afternoon. He becomes a trifle pale, his appetite gradually fails, and he may suffer from "indigestion." He gradually acquires a cough, or at any rate he "clears his throat" every morning. His temperature, although normal in the morning, is definitely elevated each afternoon. He may think he has a cold that is just "hanging on."

With the progress of the disease, the anorexia and the "indigestion," may be marked. Abdominal pain or even vomiting may occur after meals. The cough, for weeks passed off as bronchitis or a cigarette cough, gradually becomes more troublesome, and the sputum increases. There is no longer doubt as to the afternoon fever; the patient has night sweats. Loss of weight and strength is rapid.

Hemoptysis (hemorrhage from the lungs) is frequent in pulmonary tuberculosis. It may be the first symptom noticed by the patient. These hemorrhages are usually only slight in quantity but when due to ulceration of an artery rarely may be profuse or even fatal. They occur unexpectedly and quite independent of exertion or activity. In fact, they may occur during sleep. On the other hand, there may just be slightly blood-streaked sputum.

Since the advent of specific tuberculosis chemotherapy, the prognosis for the patient has greatly improved. Over 90 per cent of patients with early tuberculosis can be cured with current available treatment, and those with far advanced tuberculosis have a better prognosis than heretofore. However, the course of the patient with chronic untreated pulmonary tuberculosis is marked by ups and downs. Now the healing process gains the ascendancy and the patient feels better; now the ulcerative process progresses and he feels worse. So it goes for months and years, until either the disease stops or an acute exacerbation of the trouble, such as tuberculous bronchopneumonia, enters the scene. Many are the cases of chronic tuberculosis in which the cavity formation is arrested and the patient is able to continue at his occupation for many years. In the past such patients were largely responsible for the spread of this disease.

DIAGNOSTIC EVALUATION OF THE PATIENT

All patients with a history of unexplained weight loss, fatigability, fever, chronic cough or chest pain deserve careful study to rule out pulmonary tuberculosis. The added history of contact with tuberculous individuals, previous pleurisy or hemoptysis is extremely suggestive. The physical signs, if present at all, may be those of pneumonitis, perhaps with contraction, of one or both upper lobes.

The most important single examination is roentgenography of the chest, by which means even minimal tuberculous lesions can be identified and their activity gauged to a certain extent. The sputum, especially the morning sputum, and the fasting gastric contents should be examined repeatedly, both microscopically, after concentrating them and applying the acidfast stain to the concentrate, and by special methods of culture that favor the growth of the tubercle bacillus in an artificial medium. The intraperitoneal inoculation of guinea pigs with concentrated sputum and gastric washings also is recommended as an additional check in the bacteriologic "screening" investigation.

Tuberculin Testing

The *Mantoux test* involves the inoculation of tubercle bacillus extract ("tuberculin") into the skin of the forearm on its inner aspect. The material is injected as superficially as possible beneath the skin surface, with needle bevel up (Fig. 16-2). Either of 2 substances may be used: "Purified Protein Derivative" (PPD) or "Old Tuberculin" (OT). After a lapse of 48 to 72 hours the site of injection is examined for the presence or absence of an inflammatory response, which is evaluated on the basis of the extent of induration (see Figs. 16-3, 16-4). An area of induration mea-

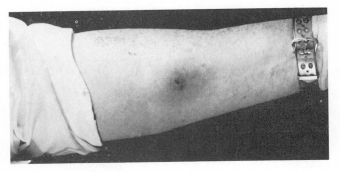

FIG. 16-4. Mantoux Test. The site of injection is obviously indurated to 10 mm. or more. Note also the surrounding area of erythema. (National Tuberculosis Association)

suring 5 mm. or more in diameter is interpreted as a positive reaction. This reaction in a patient with active tuberculosis may be very intense; therefore, if a patient is suspected of having an active infection it is customary to initiate the test with an injection of very dilute ("first strength") PPD, repeating the procedure with successively higher doses of the material if negative reactions are obtained. The Mantoux test is the preferred tuberculin test because it is precisely measured and accurate.

For testing large groups, a multiple puncture skin test (Tine or Heath test) is utilized. *The Tuberculin Tine test* (Fig. 16-5) is a multiple puncture test that consists of a disc attached to a plastic handle. The disc has 4 tines projecting from it that have been dipped in concentrated Old Tuberculin, dried and redipped and dried again. One of the drawbacks of this test is the lack of accurate dosage control. However, the Tuberculin Tine test is valuable for clinical screening on a large scale. It is convenient and easy to administer. The tines are pressed into the prepared and stretched skin of the patient's forearm for a full second. The unit is then withdrawn and discarded. The test is read on the third day after administration. A negative reaction is an area of induration less than 2 mm. in diameter, whereas a positive reaction is recorded when there is confluence (meeting) of 2 or more puncture sites. If the patient has a "doubtful positive" or positive reaction, he should be immediately tested with the Mantoux test and have a chest X-ray.

A positive tuberculin test indicates that a patient has had contact with the tubercle bacillus, but yields little information regarding the activity of the infection. In general, the more intense the reaction, the greater the likelihood of an active infection. A negative test is even more valuable diagnostically, for it practically rules out the presence of active tuberculosis except in patients with miliary tuberculosis, who may lose their

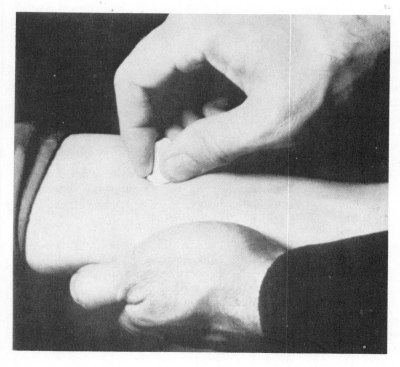

Fig. 16-5. The tine test is simple to apply, is accurate and economical, and compares favorably with other forms of tuberculin testing. (Lederle Laboratories Division, American Cyanimid Company)

capacity to react to tuberculin, and in patients who are receiving one of the corticosteroid drugs, whose tests may become negative in the face of an active infection.

The value of tuberculin skin testing for the finding of cases of tuberculosis has increased considerably in the past 20 years. Whereas, previously, the majority of adult patients gave positive tuberculin reactions, only 20 per cent or less of adults now have positive tuberculin reactions. Since the majority of new cases of active tuberculosis arise from previously quiescent lesions that have become reactivated, this test serves to identify the group at greatest risk of developing active disease. In addition annual tuberculin tests are of value for identifying the time of initial tuberculous infections in children. Treatment of such primary infections in children has been shown to decrease the risk of progressive pulmonary tuberculosis and more severe disease such as miliary and meningeal tuberculosis.

MANAGEMENT OF PULMONARY TUBERCULOSIS

Basic Concepts and Objectives

The recent advent of effective chemotherapy has resulted in a complete reversal of earlier concepts regarding the treatment, the nursing care and the rehabilitation of patients with tuberculosis. Before drugs became available, the therapeutic keynote was rest—physical, mental and emotional rest for the patient, and immobility for his diseased lung. The average hospital stay was well over 400 days. Now it is approximately 180 to 200 days, and many patients have little (2 to 3 months) or no hospitalization. The psychological complications that are inherent in "rest," not to mention the physical deterioration that it induces, created a tremendous problem of rehabilitation, which was complicated further by the economic and vocational problems that were the inevitable product of very prolonged hospitalization.

The situation now is very different. Hospitalization of patients with active pulmonary tuberculosis still is highly desirable, although no longer an absolute prerequisite of adequate care. However, complete bed rest has been eliminated as an essential part of the program. Similarly, surgical procedures and other maneuvers designed to immobilize and collapse the tuberculous lung have largely been abandoned, including artificial pneumothorax, phrenicotomy and phrenic nerve crush operations. Tuberculosis surgery now is more important than before, but it is of a different design and done with different intent: to remove cavities and lesions that have succeeded in harboring viable tubercle bacilli in the face of vigorous chemotherapy and to re-expand lungs that are compressed and collapsed by contracted pleura.

The rationale of the new surgical approach and the changed concepts regarding rest in tuberculous patients are primarily the result of the tremendous effectiveness of antituberculous chemotherapy. There are factors that modify the effectiveness of chemotherapy, which must be understood for its proper utilization. (1) Whereas the tubercle bacillus is susceptible to several drugs, there are no drugs to which it cannot develop resistance. Such resistance results from genetic mutations of the organism. This is the reason for using 2 drugs in treatment, because the second agent destroys those mutants resistant to the other drug. (2) There is a tendency for blood vessels in tuberculous tissue to become thrombosed and obliterated, with the result that the involved tissue becomes ischemic and necrotic—an excellent nutrient medium for the tubercle bacillus and, moreover, one that isolates it from the bloodstream and all of the antituberculous drugs except INH. (3) Although the organisms are ingested by tissue macrophages, they are not digested and destroyed; on the contrary, the tubercle bacilli find themselves in the safest possible place, i.e., enclosed within a membrane that is impenetrable to streptomycin. (4) The pathologic changes associated with tuberculosis are such as to cause stricture and finally complete stenosis of the smaller bronchi and the bronchioles; as a result, the necrotic lung tissue cannot evacuate itself, i.e., spontaneous drainage of these lesions becomes impossible.

The virtue of limited activity, as opposed to complete bed rest, then, is to promote drainage of the necrotic lesion, to mobilize the infective organisms, to flush them from their shelters into the open, so to speak, where the drug concentration is high—not allow them to remain sequestered in areas of low drug concentration, where they may survive long enough to acquire drug resistance. The justification for radical resection of a lesion that fails to heal promptly in response to chemotherapy is clear; namely, failure to heal, under these circumstances, may be construed as evidence that the organisms contained in it have succeeded in becoming resistant, thus implying that the tissue that sheltered the organisms when they were more vulnerable would afford no less protection in the future, should a different drug be tried, and that intensification of chemotherapy would have no effect other than to improve bacterial resistance.

Hospitalization and Communicable Disease Precautions

Tuberculosis patients should be hospitalized for proof of diagnosis, evaluation of the extent of pathology and determination of the responsiveness of the tubercle bacillus to chemotherapy. Further objectives of hospitalization are to protect the patient from serious drug toxicity or allergy, to isolate him while he is contagious and to perform surgery as soon as the indications are clear.

If patients are physically able, they should have bathroom privileges and walk to meals, assuming that there are dining-room facilities for ambulant patients. At other times their activities should be reduced to a minimum as long as tuberculous activity is manifest.

Patients with "open" tuberculosis, i.e., active and communicable because of the production of infective sputum, must be segregated, preferably in a sanatorium, and cared for by individuals trained in the practice of isolation techniques. Instructions must be provided regarding the precautions that are necessary for the protection of others, including the necessity for covering the mouth and the nose while coughing or sneezing, for disposing carefully and quickly of tissues contaminated by sputum or other secretions, for making use of a paper bag pinned to the bed and for depositing the sputum in a closed sputum cup. One of the most important considerations in preventing the spread of tuberculosis is *adequate ventilation to reduce the number of droplet nuclei in the air.* Salivary secretion should not be spread over pens, pencils, bobby-pins or stamps. Those individuals who are obliged to expose themselves to the risk of infection through contact with actively infected patients or materials that are contaminated by infective secretions never should relax their precautions for their own protection. They should use well-designed masks worn properly when in the vicinity of these patients and take pains to avoid unnecessary contact with the patient or objects in their immediate vicinity; when such contact is necessary, they should use a protective gown during the period of contact, and carefully wash their hands after the removal of the gown and the conclusion of the contact.

Visitors must be educated thoroughly in the practice of these precautions.

Nursing Management of Patients With Pulmonary Tuberculosis

The activity of a tuberculous infection is gauged by changes in the body temperature, the pulse rate, the body weight and changes in x-ray findings. Therefore, all of these must be measured at appropriate intervals and charted.

The malaise attending high fever may be relieved effectively by the application of cool sponge baths. The discomfort of night sweats is reduced by the wearing of flannel night clothes, which should be replaced at once when damp.

Cough may be alleviated by steam inhalations. Sedation should not be employed with the view of abolishing cough altogether, for a certain amount of coughing is necessary for the removal of exudate from the infected lung. Moreover, the use of narcotic agents, even codeine, in chronic tuberculosis as in any chronic disease, is hazardous because of the danger of addiction.

TABLE 16-1. Chemotherapeutic agents used in the treatment of tuberculosis

Drug	Customary Dosage	Therapeutic Considerations	Nursing Implications
Isoniazid (INH)	300 mg., or 4 to 5 mg./Kg. of body weight—daily by mouth	INH may be used alone in treatment of mild infections, e.g., asymptomatic primary tuberculosis when cultures are negative and there is no clinical evidence of activity. When INH is prescribed in high dosage, pyridoxine usually is given as an adjunct to prevent peripheral neuritis.	Observe patient for symptoms of numbness, tingling and weakness in the extremities, which are indicative of a complicating polyneuritis.
Para-aminosalicylic acid (PAS)	12 gm. daily in divided doses—by mouth	Enhances effectiveness of INH and streptomycin.	Drug should be given with meals. Epigastric distress and diarrhea are common. Fever and skin rash may develop. For dyspepsia, offer milk (not antacids, which inactivate PAS). Stress importance of continuing PAS in face of minor complications.
Streptomycin	1 gm. 2 or 3 times weekly—intramuscularly	Highly effective during febrile, exudative stage of pulmonary tuberculosis, but effective for only limited period of time.	Be alert for, and report promptly, symptoms indicating ototoxicity: i.e., tinnitus, deafness, vertigo, or an unsteady gait. Watch for allergic skin reaction.
Viomycin Pyrazinamide Cycloserine Ethionamide Ethambutol Capreomycin		Used in different combinations when the patient does not respond to standard chemotherapy. These are secondary drugs used in case of resistance.	These drugs are all toxic and the patient should be observed for varying manifestations of toxicity.

Management of Hemoptysis. If hemorrhage occurs, the patient, if up and about, should be put to bed at once and immobilized as completely as possible. He should lie on the infected side, and the thoracic movement should be confined with sandbags or whatever device is immediately available. Morphine sulfate, 12 to 16 mg. (⅙ to ¼ gr.), may be given at 4-hour intervals if necessary to control pain, dyspnea and anxiety, and oxygen inhalations should be started on the appearance of cyanosis or dyspnea of increasing severity. If hypotension or "shock" appears, blood transfusions should be administered.

The color of the blood produced during the hemorrhage should be noted by the nurse and described carefully to the physician in the event that she is reporting the occurrence by telephone. If it is bright red, the bleeding is probably venous in origin and very likely will cease spontaneously. Under these conditions, sedation is not only unnecessary but also undesirable, for it impairs the evacuation of the blood from the bronchi. Blockage of the bronchi leads to the development of atelectasis, with the danger of fatal pneumonia in the collapsed lung.

Antituberculosis Chemotherapy

Isoniazid (INH), para-aminosalicylic acid (PAS) and streptomycin are the antimicrobials used most often in the treatment of tuberculosis at the present time. The following principles govern their use:

1. Two of these agents, or all 3, usually are given in combination in an effort to prevent the development of drug resistance.

2. Whatever drug combination is selected, Isoniazid usually is included because it is by far the most effective agent. (INH and PAS are generally considered to represent the combination of choice.)

3. Antituberculous chemotherapy, barring complications, is administered without interruption for a

minimum of at least 12 months, or even for 24 months, in order to prevent relapse.

Table 16-1 gives the details concerning the administration of the antituberculous drugs as well as the nursing implications associated with each of these agents.

Other agents (cycloserine, viomycin, pyrazinamide, ethionamide, ethambultol, and kanamycin) also are sometimes used in the treatment of tuberculosis. These are often termed "second line," because their lesser effectiveness and greater toxicity have usually limited the use to the treatment of patients with infections resistant to INH, streptomycin and PAS.

Surgery in Pulmonary Tuberculosis

Segmental resection (removal of a portion of a lobe), lobectomy (removal of a complete lobe) and rarely pneumonectomy (removal of an entire lung) are carried out for the purpose of eliminating solid or cavitary lesions that have ceased to decrease in size after several months of therapy. Such lesions are particularly apt to contain resistant bacilli or to reactivate at a future date. Other indications for surgery would be irreversible structural changes such as bronchiectasis or bronchial stenosis (see p. 248), or the necessity of removing a pleura that had become contracted following pleural effusions, or an earlier pneumothorax by a procedure known as "decortication" (described later), in order to permit the lung to re-expand and resume normal function.

Operative Procedures. *Thoracoplasty with Pulmonary Resection.* When lobectomy or pneumonectomy is performed for tuberculosis, some surgeons prefer to do a thoracoplasty in 3 to 6 weeks. In unusually good operative risks, these procedures can be done at the same time. The purpose of doing a rib resection is to prevent overdistention of the remaining lung tissue. The possibility of bronchopleural fistula and tuberculous empyema is lessened. Usually 4 ribs are removed following lobectomy and 6 or 7 following pneumonectomy.

Drainage Operations. Drainage procedures are used for palliation in patients who are quite ill. The *Monaldi* method is performed by inserting a catheter into the abscess or cavity through a cannula. After insertion, the catheter is attached to water-seal drainage. A *cavernostomy* is done by resecting a rib and incising the chest wall into the lung. Open wound drainage means that the dressings must be changed at least daily. *Empyema drainage* also can be done. This is described on page 246.

Decortication of the Lung. Decortication is the surgical removal of fibrinous deposit on the pleura that prevents re-expansion of the lung and has resulted from prolonged pneumothorax and tuberculous empy-

ema. It is done in selected cases when there is little likelihood of reactivation of the disease and where healthy lung tissue can be re-expanded. The care preoperatively and postoperatively is the same as that described on pages 258-269.

Preoperative Nursing Emphasis. An understanding of the mental problems of this patient is essential. When one realizes that he usually has a history of illness of a year or more, that he may have been in a sanatorium for a long while, and that he probably has had his hopes raised innumerable times only to be blasted when therapy failed, one is more tolerant of his reactions. He must be made to realize that a thoracoplasty is not an immediate cure, and that convalescence is slow. The socioeconomic factors cannot be neglected. In addition, the patient usually is on isolation precautions. Some physicians prefer to have their patients raise as much sputum as possible about 30 minutes before operation. This may be done by postural drainage or by coughing voluntarily. The shaving of the chest and the remaining preparation is the same as that for other chest surgical patients.

Postoperative Nursing Care. Postoperative care is directed toward preventing many possible complications—for example, shock, hemorrhage, respiratory and circulatory collapse, paradoxical motion, the spread of infection, wound infection and deformity. The patient is kept in the Trendelenburg position until he is conscious and his vital signs are satisfactory. He should be turned from his back to the operated side every second hour and encouraged to cough in an effort to bring up secretions. Often the tight adhesive strapping is not sufficient to allay the patient's fears when he coughs, and it is necessary for the nurse to splint the wound with the palm of her hand or her forearm. During this postoperative period, the nurse must be on the alert for signs that suggest a retention of secretions such as "wet" inspirations and expirations after coughing, increasing dyspnea and a temperature elevation. If this occurs, the physician should be notified and an endotracheal aspiration tray made available. Every effort must be exerted to prevent atelectasis, not only because of the resultant obstruction of a portion of the lung but also because of the likelihood of spread of infection.

Paradoxical motion is one of the complications that can occur in the postoperative thoracoplasty patient (see Fig. 14-16). By applying external pressure, this phenomenon can be controlled. Sandbags that weigh about 5 lb. can be applied beneath the clavicle. Unfortunately, they are cumbersome and difficult to keep in place. Some surgeons prefer to apply thick gauze pads beneath the clavicle and in the axilla. They are held in place by 2-inch adhesive strips applied over the back and the shoulders so that skin tension is distributed widely. Blistering from adhesive must be guarded against.

Physical Therapy. Passive and then active movements of the arm on the affected side should be started on the day of operation and continued after that on instructions from the physician and the physical therapist. Proper body posture with adequate support of the back, the shoulders and the arm must be maintained. A Balkan frame with a trapezelike bar provides an excellent means for the patient to move in bed with a desirable amount of exercise. Often the patient favors the operated side by lifting the arm with the opposite hand, by rotating the trunk instead of the head and by drooping his shoulder protectively. Without a doubt this leads to scoliosis and a crippling posture, and it must be prevented. In all efforts at rehabilitation, the patient must express a desire and a willingness to help himself. After the second or the third stage of thoracoplasty, a small, firm pillow may be placed in the axilla on the operated side. This will increase collapse of the thoracic wall and prevent scoliosis. Some physicians prefer to have the patient use a chest sling, which is a piece of canvas about 12 to 15 inches wide and 3 feet long. A hammock is formed to encase the patient as he lies on his operated side. By counteracting weights (pulley system) he is lifted from the bed, thus utilizing body weight to produce further collapse. He remains in this position for only a few minutes at first, after which the time gradually is increased to 30 minutes 3 times a day.

The successful care of this patient includes special emphasis on good mouth hygiene, plenty of fresh air, adequate nutrition, proper exercise and an optimistic frame of mind. Diversional occupational therapy that is prescribed carefully is essential because of the long period of essentially inactive convalescence. Frequently, this rehabilitative and "resting" stage can be spent at home.

Convalescent Management of the Patient With Tuberculosis

One of the most important aspects of nursing care in pulmonary tuberculosis is guiding the patient through his convalescence. A program of convalescence and rehabilitation is designed for each individual patient, tailored to meet his specific and unique requirements, and subject to constant readjustment as progress permits or circumstances require. Among the many controlling factors in this program are the course of his body temperature, pulse rate and respiratory rate, the amount and character of his sputum, his appetite and weight, his general health, and his sense of well-being.

One of the most important, and perhaps most difficult, of the nurse's responsibilities in relation to the convalescent care of the patient with pulmonary tuberculosis is to assist in combating the psychological invalidism that is so apt to result from any prolonged illness. The patient's interest in outside pursuits and activities should be stimulated and his self-reliance encouraged.

Education of the Patient. The patient should be instructed in reading a thermometer and in the correct method of measuring body weight. He must understand the importance of a complete physical examination, including roentgenograms of the chest, every 6 months for a minimum of 2 years after his discharge. *He must have medical supervision for his lifetime.* Literature concerning tuberculosis should be made available to the patient in order to improve his insight and knowledge of the disease. A major reason for treatment failure is that patients do not take their medications regularly and for the long period of time prescribed. One of the teaching functions of the public health nurse is to stress the importance of uninterrupted and long-term chemotherapy.

The patient and his family should be instructed carefully in regard to possible complications, including hemorrhage, pleurisy and other untoward symptoms that are indicative of a possible recurrence of tuberculous activity.

PUBLIC HEALTH AND PREVENTION

The emphasis in tuberculosis eradication is on prevention, case detection, sanitation and public education. *Chemoprophylaxis* holds tremendous potential for the prevention of tuberculosis. Persons who have close contact with patients suffering from active tuberculosis and persons who become positive reactors to tuberculin tests (with a familial history of tuberculosis) are considered special risks. The administration of Isoniazid daily for at least a year is advocated to prevent many of these individuals from developing tuberculosis.

Children exposed to individuals with active tuberculosis should be examined annually. Positive reactors should have annual tuberculin tests and roentgenograms of the chest. Vigilance must be doubled during adolescence when they are most vulnerable—when old infections are particularly apt to become reactivated and new ones acquired. Examinations should be arranged on the development of any suggestive symptom, such as unexplained weight loss, anorexia, pain in the chest or cough.

Due to the tuberculin testing of cattle and the pasteurization of milk, infection by drinking contaminated milk has been almost completely eliminated.

Whereas the death rate from tuberculosis has declined at a gratifying rate, the number of new cases developing per annum has not changed very much in recent years. There are an estimated 250,000 known as well as unknown active cases of tuberculosis in the United States today. Moreover, the new cases are just as far advanced as they were before the advent of chemotherapy. Although children, particularly in adolescence, are susceptible to the disease, age is no barrier to its development; frequently, tuberculosis of the lungs and other organs is acquired in later life. Therefore, the necessity for careful examination, preferably on a routine basis, is obvious.

Important advances in tuberculosis prophylaxis are the increasing value of tuberculin skin testing and the increasing availability of roentgenographic examinations of the chest without cost; this is accomplished on a mass scale by means of photofluorograms, entailing the photographing of the fluoroscopic image while the chest is irradiated. X-ray surveys are especially valuable in communities known to have a high tuberculosis rate. With facilities of this type available, failure to be examined cannot be excused on the grounds of economy, or, in fact, on any other basis.

Tuberculosis associations and health departments are working diligently to eradicate tuberculosis. It has been their experience that certain groups should receive top priority in case detection programs, among them persons with positive tuberculin skin tests and those who are or have been closely associated with patients with tuberculosis. A recent public health study revealed the incidence of tuberculosis in this group to be almost 40 times greater than that observed among the general population.

Another susceptible group is comprised of known suspects who have symptoms suggesting tuberculous activity. Inactive cases should be followed for a lifetime, because they may become active again. Patients newly admitted to hospitals should be screened routinely for tuberculosis. Foodhandlers, a notoriously transient group, show a high tuberculosis rate. Tuberculosis testing in schools and child health clinics and community surveys for tuberculosis also are valuable in case finding. The vaccine BCG (bacille Calmette-Guerin) is given sometimes to nonreactors to tuberculin. Its use is restricted to persons who are tuberculin negative, because it does not benefit persons who have already been infected and thus are positive tuberculin reactors. It is infrequently used in the United States, because the medical and socioeconomic conditions are more favorable here and there are better methods of control and prevention. However, on a world-wide basis there are between 15 and 20 million infectious cases of tuberculosis. Eighty per cent of these sufferers are in the developing countries. It has been found that BCG gives substantial protection against tuberculosis in these countries (Fig. 16-8).

The National Tuberculosis Association is a voluntary

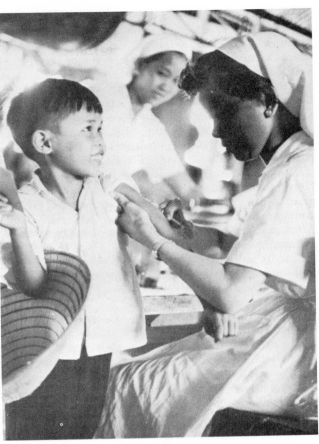

Fig. 16-6. At the end of the war a campaign was started to give BCG vaccination to people threatened by tuberculosis. This work is still going on in many countries with assistance from WHO and UNICEF. Ninety million have been vaccinated. BCG vacine is available in the freeze-dried state from WHO. (World Health Organization Photo)

nonprofit public health agency dedicated to the eradication of tuberculosis and control of other respiratory diseases. The Association's official publications are the *Bulletin*, which disseminates information about tuberculosis and respiratory diseases to lay and professional groups, and *The American Review of Respiratory Diseases*, a journal for professional readers.

ATYPICAL MYCOBACTERIA

In recent years, it has been recognized that some bacteria, which give a staining reaction similar to that of *Mycobacterium tuberculosis*, but which have distinctly different growth and cultural characteristics, may produce an infection that is clinically indistinguishable from tuberculosis. When tuberculosis was a much more common disease than at present, and when more sophisticated bacteriologic techniques were not used, these infections were overlooked or the organisms discarded as contaminants. Today, these strains of mycobacteria, termed anonymous or atypical mycobacteria, are classified more precisely. In some localities, infections with these atypical mycobacteria comprise 10 per cent of cases of suspected tuberculosis. These organisms not only produce infections indistinguishable from tuberculosis, but because of their chemical similarity to the tubercle bacillus, infected patients often have a positive tuberculin skin test.

These organisms have been divided into 4 groups. Group one organisms are often termed "photochromogens." When grown in the dark, these bacteria produce nonpigmented colonies resembling tubercle bacilli. After exposure to light, the colonies develop a bright yellow pigmentation. Group 2 organisms show bright yellow to orange pigmentation when grown in the dark and are termed "scotochromogens" (from skotos, the Greek word for darkness). Group 3 organisms are referred to as "nonchromogens" or "Battey bacilli" (after Battey State Hospital in Georgia where they were first identified). Group 4 bacilli are termed "rapid growers," because they produce visible colonies within a few days of culture, whereas 3 to 4 weeks are usually required for cultivation of *M. tuberculosis*. None of these bacilli are pathogenic for guinea pigs and this characteristic is used to distinguish them from *M. tuberculosis*. In addition, other laboratory procedures are used to distinguish these strains from *M. tuberculosis* and from one another.

Of these atypical mycobacteria, Group 1 and 3 bacilli are pathogenic for man and often produce pulmonary infections indistinguishable from pulmonary and less often, other forms of tuberculosis. Organisms belonging to Group 2 "scotochromogens" rarely cause pulmonary disease but often produce suppurative infections in the lymph nodes of the neck. The Group 4 "rapid growers" rarely produce human infection. In addition, organisms of all 4 groups may be isolated from healthy people with no evidence of disease, and their isolation alone is not always indicative of disease.

Little is known about the epidemiology of infections with "atypical mycobacteria." Available evidence suggests that there is little hazard of person-to-person transmission. Treatment of infections with these "atypical mycobacteria" is often quite difficult, since they are usually resistant to INH, streptomycin and para-amino-salicylic acid.

BIBLIOGRAPHY

Books

Allen, J. C. A psychodynamic approach of the nurse in combating denial of the disease—tuberculosis. Nursing Approaches to Denial of Illness, No. 12, American Nurses Assoc., 1962.

Future of Tuberculosis Control—A Report to the Surgeon General of the Public Health Service. PHS Publication No. 1119, 1965.

Harrison, T. R. (ed.): Principles of Internal Medicine. pp. 1604-1621. New York, McGraw-Hill, 1966.

Moyer, C. A., *et al.*: Surgery. Principles and Practice. pp. 1339-1360. Philadelphia, J. B. Lippincott, 1965.

National Tuberculosis Association: Chronic Obstructive Pulmonary Disease (A Manual for Physicians). 1966.

——: Safer Ways in Nursing: To Protect Against Airborne Infections. 1962.

——: Tuberculosis Handbook for Public Health Nurses. ed. 4. 1965.

NLN and National Tuberculosis Association: The Circle Back. League Publication No. 45, 1967.

Articles

A new NTA-ATS statement: Infectiousness of tuberculosis. Bull. Nat. Tuberculosis Assoc., 53:6-8, Nov., 1967.

B.C.G. Bull. Nat. Tuberculosis Assoc., 53:8-9, Jan., 1967.

Curry, F. J.: A new approach for improving attendance at tuberculosis clinics. Amer. J. Pub. H., 58:877-881, May, 1968.

Darrah, W.: Tine testing in the home. Nurs. Outlook, 13:38-41, Dec., 1965.

Ferebee, S. H.: An epidemiological model of tuberculosis in the United States. Bull. Nat. Tuberculosis Assoc., 53:4-7, Jan., 1967.

Holgwin, A. H.: The vast potential for prevention of tuberculosis. Bull. Nat. Tuberculosis Assoc., 52:4-6, May, 1966.

Hopewell, P. C.: Chemoprophylaxis for the prevention of tuberculosis. Amer. Rev. Resp. Dis., 97:721-722, April, 1968.

Jones, J. M.: Tuberculosis: present day concepts of management. Hosp. Med., 3:76-93, June, 1967.

Koonz, F. P.: Nursing in tuberculosis. Nurs. Clin. N. Amer., 3:403-412, Sept., 1968.

Lego, S.: A consideration of conflict in the psychological approach to tuberculosis nursing. ANA Regional Clinical Conferences, 4:47-52, 1966.

Martin, C. J., *et al.*: Tuberculosis, emphysema and bronchitis. Amer. Rev. Resp. Dis., 97:1089-1094, June, 1968.

Meyers, J. A.: The changing face of tuberculosis—a lifetime study. Postgrad. Med., 44:166-171, Oct., 1968.

——: Tuberculosis in the aged. Postgrad. Med., 41:214-222, Feb., 1967.

Moulding, T.: Newer responsibilities for health departments and public health nurses in tuberculosis—Keeping the patient on therapy. Amer. J. Pub. Health, 56:416-427, March, 1966.

Mushlin, I., and Amberson, J.: Tracking down tuberculosis. Amer. J. Nurs., 65:91-94, Dec., 1965.

Report on the thousands who took part in the U.S. chemoprophylaxis trials. Bull. Nat. Tuberculosis Assoc., 54:6, Feb., 1968.

Rosenthal, S. R.: The tuberculin tine test. GP, 34:116-121, Nov., 1966.

Shaw, R. F., *et al.*: An assessment of the tuberculin tine test. Dis. Chest, 51:162-165, Feb., 1967.

Stead, W. W.: Pathogenesis of the sporadic case of tuberculosis. New Eng. J. Med., 277:1008-1012, 1967.

Stead, W. W., *et al.*: The clinical spectrum of primary tuberculosis in adults. Ann. Int. Med., 68:731-745, April, 1968.

Film

The Special Universe of Walter Krolik. Nursing education film co-sponsored by the National Tuberculosis Association, ANA and NLN, 1966.

AGENCIES

National Tuberculosis and Respiratory Disease Association
    1740 Broadway
    New York, New York 10019
Tuberculosis Nursing Advisory Service
National League for Nursing
    1740 Broadway
    New York, New York 10019
U. S. Department of Health, Education and Welfare
    Public Health Service
    Washington, D. C. 20201
World Health Organization
    Avenue Appia
    Geneva, Switzerland

N.B. Tuberculosis nursing materials are available from the National Advisory Services of the National Tuberculosis and Respiratory Disease Association and the National League for Nursing, 10 Columbus Circle, New York, New York 10014.

PATIENT EDUCATION

National Tuberculosis and Respiratory Disease Association
    1740 Broadway
    New York, New York 10019
        Be Safe, Be Sure.
        Climate and TB.
        Gambling with TB.
        How to Guard Against Hidden TB.
        How to Kill TB Germs.
        How Your Body Fights TB.
        Introduction to Respiratory Diseases.
        The Tuberculin Test.
        TB Facts in Picture Language.
        TB from 18 to 80.
        TB Respects No Age.
        The You in TB.
Superintendent of Documents
    U. S. Government Printing Office
    Washington, D. C. 20402
        The Future of Tuberculosis Control. PHS Publication No. 1119.
        The Development of Present Knowledge About Tuberculosis. PHS Publication No. 33A.
        Tuberculosis Today. PHS Publication No. 30.

CHAPTER **17**

Patients with Hematologic Disorders

- *The Cellular Components of Normal Blood*
- *The Anemic Patient*
- *Patients with Hereditary Hemolytic Disorders*
- *Patients with Acquired Hemolytic Disorders*
- *Patients with Polycythemia*
- *Patients with Leukopenia and Agranulocytosis*
- *Patients with Leukemia*
- *Patients with Malignant Lymphoma*
- *The Patient with a Bleeding Disorder*
- *Splenectomy*

THE CELLULAR COMPONENTS OF NORMAL BLOOD

Erythrocytes

The red cells, or *erythrocytes,* comprise the vast majority of all blood cells and are chiefly responsible for the color of this liquid tissue. Approximately 5 million erythrocytes are contained in one cu. mm. of blood, i.e., a drop about the size of the head of a very small pin. The normal red cell is a biconcave disk, its configuration resembling that of a soft ball compressed firmly between two fingers. The principal function of this cell is to transport oxygen. This is accomplished through the agency of an iron-containing pigment, *hemoglobin,* which accounts for 95 per cent of the mass of the cells, and the total concentration of which is normally about 15 gm. per 100 ml. of whole blood. Hemoglobin has a great tendency to combine with oxygen, this affinity being such that when the two are in brief contact they unite to form *oxyhemoglobin,* the pigment accounting for the bright red color of arterial blood. However, this combination is a weak one, for oxyhemoglobin readily releases its oxygen when exposed to concentrations of oxygen lower than its own. The affinity of hemoglobin for oxygen, and the reversible nature of their combination, together explain the

mechanism of oxygen transport in the body and the role of the red cell in this mechanism.

The red blood corpuscles are produced in red bone marrow, the tissue that also provides the blood with most of its leukocytes and all of its platelets. In infants the marrow of all the bones is red, but as the child grows older, about the time of puberty, fatty tissue (fat marrow) replaces the red marrow of the long bones. Hence, the red corpuscles of normal adults are formed only in the short and flat bones, such as the ribs, the sternum, the skull, the vertebrae and the bones of the hands and the feet. In certain types of anemia accompanied by an increased rate of blood production, great increases occur in the amount and the activity of the red bone marrow, which may replace, temporarily or permanently, the fatty marrow.

Red blood corpuscles in normal blood have no nuclei. From the primitive stem cells in red bone marrow arise *erythroblasts,* nucleated cells that in the process of maturing accumulate hemoglobin. The nucleus becomes small and dark (*normoblast*), then disappears, and the cell is known as a *reticulocyte.* The final step in maturation consists in the loss of all darkly staining substances and shrinkage to normal size.

Differentiation of the primitive multipotential stem cells of the marrow into erythroblasts is stimulated by a humoral substance in the blood known as *erythropoietin.* Under conditions of prolonged hypoxia, as in the case of individuals dwelling at high altitudes and patients with chronic heart or lung disease and impaired pulmonary ventilation, erythropoietin is increased, more red blood cells are produced, the red cell mass expands and erythremia results (see p. 315).

For normal erythropoiesis the bone marrow requires a number of nutrients, including iron, vitamin B_{12}, folic acid and pyridoxine. Iron is needed for hemoglobin formation. If the amount of iron absorbed from the gastrointestinal tract is insufficient to meet the increased requirements imposed by growth, or to compensate for the loss as incurred as a result of bleeding, red cell maturation becomes faulty at the normoblast stage. Many of these cells, unable to incorporate hemoglobin in their cytoplasm, fail to develop further and never leave the marrow but disintegrate in situ; those that do mature fully and succeed in entering the circulating blood are abnormally small and contain less than the normal complement of hemoglobin. Vitamin B_{12} is absorbed from the gastrointestinal tract following the ingestion of certain foods, especially skeletal muscle, milk and eggs, by individuals possessing normal gastric juice. This vitamin is necessary for the evolution of red cells, granulocytes and platelets from their precursor cells in the marrow. B_{12} deficiency is responsible for a disease called "pernicious anemia," characterized by abnormally large and misshapen red cells in reduced number, granulopenia and thrombocytopenia (see p. 307). Provided that the genetic constitution of the red cell precursors is normal and that all requisite marrow nutrients are in adequate supply, a healthy, nonanemic human adult produces between 16 and 20 cc., or about 200 billions of new red cells each day. Moreover, his marrow is capable of increasing this rate of production at least six- to eightfold on demand, for example, following an episode of bleeding or hyperhemolysis.

The normal life expectancy of a red cell is between 115 and 130 days, at which time it is eliminated by phagocytosis somewhere in the reticuloendothelial system, most probably in the spleen or liver.

Normal Values. The concentration of circulating red cells, or red cell count, varies in normal adult males from approximately 4.5 to 5.4 million and, in normal females, from 4.0 to 4.8 million per cu. mm. of blood. The space occupied by these cells, represented by the packed red cell volume (measured in a tube after fast centrifugation and expressed as the "hematocrit reading") in males is between 42 and 52 and, in females, between 38 and 48 per cent of the whole blood volume. The blood hemoglobin concentration establishes the presence or absence of anemia, on the one hand, or of polycythemia on the other. Values less than 14.0 gm.

per 100 ml. in an adult male, or less than 12.0 gm. per 100 ml. in an adult female, represent anemia; one above 17.0 gm. in either sex represents polycythemia.

Leukocytes

The leukocytes, or white blood cells, normally are present in a concentration of between 5,000 and 10,000 cells in each cu. mm. of whole blood; in other words, there is one white cell for every 500 to 1,000 red cells. The leukocytes, unlike adult erythrocytes, contain no hemoglobin, but they do possess a nucleus; moreover, they are capable of active movement. Major categories of leukocytes include the granulocytic series, lymphocytes, monocytes and plasma cells.

When the white cell count is over 10,000, the condition is called a *leukocytosis;* when it is below 5,000, a *leukopenia.* Inflammations anywhere in the body and diseases with abscess formation often cause a rise in the count, due to an increase in the polymorphonuclear leukocytes. In pneumonia, for example, the leukocyte count may be as high as 10,000 or more per cu. mm. In certain infections the white cells may fail to increase, and actually may become reduced in number. Not only the total count but also the relative count of these diverse varieties of leukocytes is an important aid in diagnosis.

Granulocytes. Leukocytes produced in the marrow, i.e., the "myeloid series," comprise about 70 per cent of all the white cells and are termed *granulocytes,* because of the abundant granules contained in their cytoplasm, or *polymorphonuclear leukocytes,* since their nuclei, when mature, are of a highly irregular configuration.

Lymphocytes, most numerous of the "mononuclear" cells, comprise about 25 per cent of the circulating white cells. They are produced in lymph nodes throughout the body and to a lesser extent in the bone marrow. This cell is responsible for the immunologic competence of an individual. It is involved in the rejection of foreign tissue transplants and in sensitivity reactions of the tuberculin (delayed) type. *Monocytes* account for about 5 per cent of the white cell count. They are derived from components of the reticuloendothelial system, i.e., the total aggregate of tissue histiocytes to be found in various locations, particularly spleen, liver and lymph nodes. Monocytes constitute a ready source of mobile phagocytes, congregating and performing their scavenging function at sites of inflammation and tissue necrosis, wherever these may develop. *Plasmacytes,* representing approximately one per cent of the blood leukocytes, are formed both in lymph nodes and bone marrow, principally the latter. They are the main and probably sole source of the circulating immune globulins.

Platelets

Blood platelets, or *thrombocytes*, the smallest and most fragile of the formed blood elements, are small particles devoid of nuclei that arise as a result of a fragmentation process, or "budding," from giant cells in the bone marrow called *megakaryocytes*. There are approximately 250,000 to 500,000 platelets per one cu. mm. of blood.

The prime function of platelets is to halt bleeding. This they accomplish by congregating and clumping at all sites of vascular injury and by plugging with their own substance the lumens of the bleeding vessels. As they disintegrate they release a constituent (platelet Factor 3), which initiates clot formation in their immediate vicinity, thereby checking the flow of blood through and the leakage of blood from the lacerated vessel. Platelets cause blood clots to shrink (retract), the effect of which is to draw together the margins of vascular defects, reduce their size and further stem the leakage. Platelet deficiency (thrombocytopenia), if profound, leads to multiple spontaneous small vessel hemorrhages in the skin, mucous membranes and internally throughout the body; it is the basic defect in an important hemorrhagic disorder called "idiopathic thrombocytopenic purpura" (see p. 323). Increased platelets (thrombocytosis) is a characteristic feature of the so-called myeloproliferative disorders, including granulocytic leukemia and polycythemia vera (pages 315 and 316).

THE ANEMIC PATIENT

The term *anemia* implies an abnormally low number of circulating red cells or a decreased concentration of hemoglobin in the blood. The appearance of anemia reflects either marrow failure or excessive red cell loss, or both. Marrow failure, i.e., reduced erythropoiesis, may occur as a result of a nutritional deficiency, toxic exposure, tumor invasion or, as in many instances, from causes unknown. Red cells may be lost through hemorrhage or hyperhemolysis (increased destruction). In the latter case the problem may be rooted in some red cell defect that is incompatible with normal red cell survival, or is explainable on the basis of some factor extrinsic to the red cell that promotes red cell destruction.

Red cell lysis occurs mainly within the phagocytic cells of the reticuloendothelial system, notably in the liver and spleen. As a by-product of this process, bilirubin, formed within the phagocyte, enters the bloodstream, and any increase in hemolysis is promptly reflected by an increase in plasma bilirubin. (This concentration normally is 1.0 mg. per cent or less; levels above 1.5 mg. per cent produce visible jaundice of the sclerae.) If, as happens in certain specific hemolytic disorders, red cells are destroyed within the circulating bloodstream, hemoglobin itself appears in the plasma (hemoglobinemia) and, if its concentration there exceeds the capacity of the plasma haptoglobin to bind it all, i.e., if the amount is more than about 100 mg. per cent, then this pigment is free to diffuse through the renal glomeruli and into the urine (hemoglobinuria). Thus, the presence or absence of hemoglobinemia and hemoglobinuria is most informative with respect to the location of abnormal blood destruction in a patient with hyperhemolysis, and a possible clue to the nature of the hemolytic process.

A conclusion as to whether the anemia in a particular patient is caused by hyperhemolysis or by inadequate erythropoiesis usually can be reached on the basis of the reticulocyte count in the circulating blood, from the degree to which young red cells are proliferating in the bone marrow and the manner in which they are maturing as observed on biopsy, and on the presence or absence of hyperbilirubinemia and hemoglobinemia. Moreover, one can actually quantitate erythropoiesis by measuring the rate at which injected radioactive iron is incorporated into circulating erythrocytes, and one can measure the lifespan of the patient's red cells (ergo, the hemolytic rate) by tagging a portion of these with radioactive chromium, reinjecting them and following their disappearance from the circulating blood over the course of the ensuing days or weeks. Methods by which one particular type of marrow failure may be distinguished from another type of marrow failure, and one hemolytic disease from another, are specified in relation to each of the conditions discussed.

The effect on the patient of severe anemia *per se*, irrespective of its cause, is to render him pallid, accelerate his heart and respiratory rates, increase his cardiac output, limit his capacity for physical exertion, reduce his muscular efficiency, predispose him to attacks of angina pectoris, congestive heart failure, or both, and disturb his cerebration. All of these symptoms and signs are reversible; with correction of the anemia, they may be expected to disappear altogether.

Several factors affect the anemic patient, aside from the severity of his anemia, which tend to influence the severity of his symptoms and on which depends their existence in the first place: (1) the speed with which the anemia has developed, (2) its prior duration, i.e., its chronicity, (3) the metabolic requirements of this particular patient, (4) any other disorders or disabilities with which the patient is currently afflicted, and (5) special complications or concomitant features of the condition that has produced this anemia.

The more rapidly an anemia develops, the more severe its symptoms. An otherwise normal individual can tolerate as much as a 50 per cent gradual reduction in hemoglobin, red count or hematocrit without pronounced symptomatology or significant incapacity, whereas the rapid loss of as little as 30 per cent may precipitate profound vascular collapse in the same individual. A person who has been anemic for a very long period of time, having hemoglobin levels between 9 and 11 gm. per cent, experiences few or no symptoms other than slight tachycardia on exertion; exertional dyspnea is likely to occur below, but not above, 7.5 gm. per cent; weakness, only below 6.0 gm. per cent; dyspnea at rest, below 3.0 gm. per cent; and cardiac failure, only at the profoundly low level of 2.0 to 2.5 gm. per cent! Patients who customarily are very active are more likely to experience symptoms, and symptoms that are more pronounced, than a more sedentary individual. A hypothyroid patient, requiring, as he does, less than the usual amount of oxygen, may be perfectly asymptomatic without tachycardia or increased cardiac output, at a hemoglobin level of 10 gm. per cent. Contrariwise, at any given level of anemia, patients with underlying heart disease are far more apt to experience angina or symptoms of congestive failure than someone without heart disease. Finally, as will emerge in the discussions that follow, many anemic disorders are complicated by various other abnormalities—abnormalities that do not depend on the anemia but that are inherently associated with these particular diseases. These abnormalities may give rise to symptoms that completely overshadow those of the anemia, as exemplified by the painful crises of sickle cell anemia. See page 311.

Clearly, then, to discuss anemia as an isolated therapeutic problem would be inappropriate and unprofitable. Rather, we will consider a number of hematologic disorders in which anemia is the presenting problem, or the problem of paramount concern and which, as a group, exemplify all of the etiologic factors that have been discussed and pathogenic mechanisms that have been formulated to date in relation to anemia.

Patients With Deficiency Anemia

Iron Deficiency

In individuals who are iron deficient, the blood hemoglobin and the red blood cell count are reduced. The hemoglobin is reduced more than is the number of red cells, and for this reason the latter tend to be small and relatively devoid of pigment, i.e., "hypochromic." Hypochromia is the hallmark of iron deficiency. The cause of this deficiency is failure of the patient to ingest, or absorb, sufficient dietary iron to compensate for the iron requirements associated with body growth or for the loss of iron that attends bleeding, whether the bleeding is physiologic (e.g., menstrual) or pathologic.

Of all the deficiency states to which human beings are subject, iron deficiency is by far the commonest, and the hypochromic anemia of iron deficiency is more than twice as prevalent as all other types of anemia combined. This is true despite the fact that the total loss of iron from all sources (in the sweat and the bile, and in cells desquamated from the lining of the gastrointestinal tract) in the normal individual who is not bleeding is exceedingly small in amount: between 0.5 and 1.5 mg. per day; and it is true even though the average diet furnishes from 10 to 15 mg. of iron each day. The reason becomes clear in the light of the following facts.

Less than 10 per cent of all iron that is ingested, including food iron plus any iron supplements that might be taken, is absorbed. This means that the diet alone, however well-rounded and ample, is unlikely to supply the body with more than 1.0 to 1.5 mg. of the mineral each day, which is little more than enough to satisfy the requirements of a normal male who is experiencing no blood loss (and is not subject to menstrual bleeding), has incurred no iron deficit from hemorrhages in the past and who is not in a period of rapid growth. Iron loss due to bleeding is calculated on the basis of one mg. iron per ml. of red cells, or one ml. per approximately 2.5 ml. of whole blood. Thus, the menstrual bleeding of a normal woman, which averages between 35 and 70 ml. every 28 days, adds 0.5 to 1.0 mg. to her average daily iron loss, and the total amount lost equals or exceeds the amount she is absorbing from her diet. Small wonder that the majority of growing adolescent girls are iron deficient! During childbearing the mother contributes approximately 400 mg. of iron to the fetus and 150 mg. to the placenta, and loses an additional 175 mg. through postpartum hemorrhage; in other words, she loses an average of about 2.7 mg. of iron per day throughout pregnancy. The additional iron requirement imposed by growth averages about 0.5 mg. per day from infancy to age 20.

It follows from these data that the normal male should subsist satisfactorily, from the standpoint of his iron needs, on a normal diet alone, without benefit of iron supplements. The development of iron-deficiency anemia in a male is prima-facie evidence of either (1) faulty diet during childhood or adolescence, (2) a gastrointestinal disorder leading to malabsorption, or (3) most likely of all, recent or past blood loss. As for the female, the development of iron-deficiency anemia during adolescence is almost inevitable and, as a result of pregnancy, entirely inevitable in the absence of iron therapy.

Symptoms of iron-deficiency anemia, if mild, may be limited to pallor, fatigue and dyspnea on exertion. If severe, e.g., with hemoglobin values of less than 8 gm. per 100 ml. of blood, the patient may complain of

COMMON PROBLEMS OF PATIENTS WITH BLOOD DISORDERS

The Problem	Nursing Management
Fatigue and weakness	Plan nursing care to conserve the patient's strength. Give frequent rest periods. Encourage ambulation activities as tolerated. Avoid disturbing activities and noise. Encourage optimal nutrition.
Hemorrhagic tendencies	Keep the patient at rest during the bleeding episodes. Apply gentle pressure to the bleeding sites. Apply cold compresses to the bleeding sites when indicated. Do not disturb clots. Use small gauge needles when administering medications by injection. Support the patient during transfusion therapy. Observe for symptoms of internal bleeding. Have a tracheostomy set available for the patient who is bleeding from the mouth or the throat.
Ulcerative lesions of the tongue, the gums, and/or the mucous membranes	Avoid irritating foods and beverages. Give frequent oral hygiene with mild, cool mouthwash solutions. Use applicators or soft-bristled toothbrush. Keep the lips lubricated. Give mouth care both before and after meals.
Dyspnea	Elevate the head of the bed. Use pillows to support the patient in the orthopneic position. Administer oxygen when indicated. Prevent unnecessary exertion. Avoid gas-forming foods.
Bone and joint pains	Relieve pressure of bedding by using a cradle. Administer either hot or cold compresses as ordered. Provide for joint immobilization when ordered.
Fever	Administer cool sponges. Give antipyretic drugs as ordered. Encourage fluid intake unless contraindicated. Maintain a cool environmental temperature.
Pruritus and/or skin eruptions	Keep the patient's fingernails short. Use soap sparingly. Apply emollient lotions in skin care.
Anxiety of the patient and his family	Explain the nature, the discomforts and the limitations of activity associated with the diagnostic procedures and treatments. Offer the patient the service of listening. Have an empathetic attitude. Promote the patient's relaxation and comfort. Remember the patient's individual preferences. Encourage the family to participate in the patient's care (as desired). Create a comfortable atmosphere for the family to visit with the patient.

marked weakness and fatigability, breathlessness and cardiac palpitation. The tongue may become sore, and the nails brittle and spoon-shaped. Sometimes extreme difficulty in swallowing (Plummer-Vinson syndrome) is experienced, due to pharyngeal edema and ulceration. The diagnosis is based on the morphology of the red cells, which are hypochromic, microcytic and reduced in number; and on the finding of a low serum iron (hypoferremia), which may be as little as 10 micrograms per 100 ml. of blood or less, as compared with a normal value of between 50 and 150 micrograms. Just as important as confirming the diagnosis of iron deficiency is establishing its cause, which means, unless the cause is self-evident, a search for a source of blood loss, especially gastrointestinal bleeding.

Treatment. In the absence of active bleeding, infection, some inflammatory process or uremia, iron deficiency can be corrected and the blood picture restored to normal by the administration of an iron salt in adequate amount. Among the preparations used most commonly are ferrous sulfate, given in a daily dose of 0.9 to 1.2 gm. (15 to 20 gr.); ferrous gluconate, 1.5 to 2.0 gm. (24 to 30 gr.) daily; and ferric ammonium citrate, 6 gm. (90 gr.) each day. Iron preparations suitable for parenteral injection include a dextran complex (Imferon) and a polysaccharide of iron (Feojectin).

Nursing Responsibilities in Iron Therapy. With respect to the oral feeding of iron salts, it is important to recognize that all of these, without exception, are gastric irritants. Therefore, they should be given in divided doses with, or shortly after, meals rather than on an empty stomach. The nurse should educate the patient who is receiving large doses of iron to anticipate a certain amount of dyspepsia from time to time and impress him with the fact that such symptoms carry no serious implications, but rather serve as a guide in the regulation of dosage and schedule of treatment.

Since ferrous sulfate (which is extremely black) is formed in the intestines, iron salts alter the color of the stools, contributing a tarry color that suggests the presence of digested blood. The patient should be informed with regard to the color changes to be expected and reassured as to their benign character.

Ferrous sulfate is apt to deposit on the teeth and the gums. Hence, the nurse should urge the patient to cleanse the teeth frequently and with regularity, and those receiving liquid preparations of iron should be advised to use a straw for that purpose.

Pernicious Anemia (Vitamin B_{12} Deficiency)

Pernicious anemia is a disease of adults that has a definite familial incidence and is characterized by macrocytic anemia, gastrointestinal disturbances, neurologic abnormalities typical of combined system disease, gastric achylia, a course marked by progressively severe relapses and ultimate death, without specific therapy, and the capacity to respond to the parenteral administration of vitamin B_{12}. The basic cause of this deficiency state is a defect in the gastric secretory function, the gastric juice being devoid of a material (intrinsic factor) that is necessary for the absorption of B_{12} (extrinsic factor) from the lower portion of the ileum, the only site where B_{12} can be absorbed. The basic defect in pernicious anemia appears to involve the synthesis of nucleoprotein (DNA) required for nuclear division.

Symptoms. Physical weakness during its entire course is one of the most conspicuous features of this disease. Usually it is the first symptom and finally it dominates the picture. This weakness is due to the anemia, which also causes the pallor, dyspnea, orthopnea, palpitation, angina pectoris and edema of the legs that are usually present. Gastrointestinal symptoms (sore mouth with smooth red "beefy" tongue, loss of appetite, indigestion, abdominal pain and recurring diarrhea or constipation) are conspicuous. Neurologic symptoms develop in a high proportion of untreated patients. These include tingling, numbness or burning pain involving the hands and feet (paresthesias), loss of position sense leading to disturbances in gait, disturbances of bladder and bowel function, irritability, amnesia, depression, paranoia and delirium, anorexia and weight loss.

Laboratory Findings. The bone marrow exhibits very active, but qualitatively defective, erythropoiesis and granulopoiesis.

Gastric analysis demonstrates a low volume of gastric contents with a high pH (neutral or alkaline, rather than normally acidic, i.e., 7.0 units or more). The volume, moreover, is increased little, if at all, and the pH lowered not at all by histamine stimulation, a lack of response that is virtually unique. Bioassay of the serum B_{12} concentration demonstrates a level well below the normal range (200 to 800 picograms* per ml.), while the serum folate level is normal (8 to 15 nanograms** per ml.) or above normal. The most definitive single test, however, is a test of B_{12} absorption conducted first without, then with, supplemental intrinsic factor. One of the most widely used of these tests is the "Schilling test," which is carried out as follows:

The fasting patient receives a 0.5 to 2.0 microcurie oral dose of ^{57}Co-labeled B_{12} and the collection of urine is started. About an hour later a large dose (i.e., 1 mg., or 1,000 micrograms) of nonradioactive B_{12} is injected intramuscularly for the purpose of saturating the tissues with B_{12}, thereby reducing the likelihood that any labeled B_{12} that may be absorbed from the intestine might be removed by the liver or stored elsewhere in the body. After this "loading dose" of unlabeled vitamin, whatever B_{12} may be contained in or enter the blood, including B_{12} absorbed from the intestine, is excreted in toto into the urine. Therefore, the proportion of the oral dose of ^{57}Co-labeled B_{12} that is absorbed in the blood of the patient can be calculated from the radioactivity of the urine that he excretes. This measurement is made 24 hours after the test dose.

As in the case of the ^{131}I excretion test of thyroid function, the measurement is valueless unless the 24-hour sample includes all the urine that has been voided during the test period. A second measurement may be made at the end of 48 hours, in which case a

---

* A picogram is one trillionth of a gram, i.e., 0.000000000001 or 1×10^{-12} gm.

** A nanogram is one billionth of a gram, i.e., 0.000000001 or 1×10^{-9} gm.

second loading dose of unlabeled B_{12} is injected intramuscularly at the beginning of the second day. Normal individuals excrete more than 10 to 20 per cent of the oral dose in 24 hours. The urinary excretion of less than 10 per cent is indicative of a malabsorption defect of some type, including pernicious anemia; the excretion of less than 3 per cent is presumptive evidence of pernicious anemia. Proof of this diagnosis may be secured by repeating the entire test, this time administering a preparation containing intrinsic factor along with the oral dose of ^{57}Co-labeled B_{12}. Under these conditions, the patient with pernicious anemia absorbs the labeled vitamin normally, and it is detected in the urine in normal quantities. In patients with absorptive defects due to gastrointestinal disease, the absorption of B_{12}, hence its urinary excretion, is not increased by feeding intrinsic factor.

A therapeutic trial of parenteral B_{12} remains a valid, reliable and definitive diagnostic test for pernicious anemia, and frequently is very useful. The procedure is to administer 1 to 5 micrograms of B_{12} intramuscularly daily for ten days. By this time, if the patient does indeed have pernicious anemia, the reticulocyte count will have peaked to an appropriate level, depending on the original hemoglobin level, and the latter will have started to rise.

Therapeutic and Nursing Management. Pernicious anemia, untreated, is inevitably fatal. Contrariwise, adequate treatment corrects the anemia completely and ensures a normal life expectancy. Treatment consists in the administration, by parenteral injection, of vitamin B_{12} (cyanocobalamine).

Patients in full relapse customarily receive B_{12} in doses totaling between 100 and 1,000 micrograms each week during the first month, the vitamin being injected into the deltoid at daily (or weekly) intervals in the form of a solution containing 100 or 1,000 micrograms per ml.

Maintenance therapy, in the form of regular injections of vitamin B_{12}, must be continued throughout the remainder of the patient's life. One hundred micrograms, supplied at monthly intervals, satisfies completely the requirements of most patients for this vitamin, full hematologic remission being maintained and neurologic complications failing to appear, or existing lesions to progress, on this regimen. A small proportion of patients require more frequent injections in order to remain in optimal status; for such patients, from 100 to 200 micrograms may be injected at 2-week intervals.

Special Nursing Emphasis. A patient with pernicious anemia who is sufficiently ill to require hospitalization, whose red count, for example, is less than 1.5 million, should be placed at bed rest until a satisfactory response to therapy has begun. A certain amount of activity outside the bed, including bathroom privileges and brief periods of sitting in a chair each day, usually is permissible and is to be recommended unless there is severe neurologic involvement of an incapacitating sort. Patients with this disease are unusually sensitive to cold, requiring extra blankets and obtaining comfort from flannel bedclothes. Footboards or cradles likewise may be an aid to comfort by protecting the extremities from the pressure of weighty linen.

The use of mechanical devices to prevent the patient from falling out of bed are to be recommended if there is evidence of mental deterioration due to combined system disease. Sensory disturbances, such as numbness of the hands and the feet, necessitate caution in applying hot-water bottles. Close observation of such patients by the nurse, as in any case of advanced cerebral disease, is an obvious necessity.

The mouth, especially the teeth and the gums, requires careful attention in elderly patients and those with severe glossitis. Special mouth care is supplied at regular intervals to maintain cleanliness of the oral cavity.

Involvement of the bladder and the rectal sphincters may complicate the problems of nursing care in cases of advanced combined system disease. If there is neurogenic paralysis of the bladder, tidal drainage may be instituted in an effort to stimulate spontaneous evacuation of that organ.

The temperature, the pulse and the respirations are taken and charted at least twice each day, and, until the red count decidedly improves or exceeds 2.0 million per cu. mm., a blood pressure examination is indicated each day.

A well-balanced diet is offered in which muscle meat, fish, milk and eggs are provided amply.

Transfusions of whole blood or red cells may be required in order to increase the red cell count to safe levels during the interval between the start of the treatment and the onset of remission. The patient should be observed continuously during transfusion, since pyrogenic reactions may be extraordinarily violent and have proved to be fatal in severely anemic individuals. The nurse should report immediately any change in pulse rate or arterial pressure, as well as any evidence of chilling, fever or unusual symptoms of any type during or following transfusion. If a reaction occurs during the procedure, the infusion should be halted immediately by the nurse without waiting for instructions. She should then report the event to the physician and proceed to assemble equipment for whatever specimens he might desire to obtain.

A patient having a chill should be made as comfortable as possible with extra blankets, warm fluids and whatever analgesic drugs may be prescribed.

Dyspepsia, if present, may be treated by means of hydrochloric acid given after meals, well diluted in a glass of water and sipped through a drinking tube, a treatment to be omitted as soon as a therapeutic response has been obtained, when this symptom can be expected to disappear spontaneously.

Convalescent Care. As soon as a therapeutic remission is well under way, i.e., approximately 3 weeks after treatment is started, and the red cell count is well over 2 million, an increasing amount of activity is permitted, its limits depending chiefly on the patient's cardiovascular status and the degree of neurologic disability. Various degrees of flaccid and spastic paralysis may be present, for which appropriate physiotherapy is indicated, including massage, passive exercises and a complete program of progressive muscle re-education.

Patient Education. The one educational problem of prime importance in connection with this disease is that of teaching patients the need for continued medical observation and treatment, apparent cure notwithstanding. The risks of therapeutic neglect should be stressed with conviction but without occasioning unnecessary alarm. Assurance can be offered that the prognosis is excellent when therapy is adequate, although the complete reversal of severe neurologic disabilities already present cannot be guaranteed. The patient treated early and without interruption should not only live out his normal life expectancy but also should enjoy as good health as he might have in the complete absence of pernicious anemia.

Other Megaloblastic Anemias

B$_{12}$ Deficiency from Causes Other than Pernicious Anemia. B$_{12}$ deficiency, together with the complete P.A. syndrome, has been observed following surgical removal of most or all of the stomach, following extensive ileal resections and surgically created blind intestinal loops, and in patients with diverticula of the small bowel. All of the above situations favor the luxuriant growth of intestinal bacteria to such an extent that the bacteria compete successfully with their host for all ingested B$_{12}$. Fish tapeworms likewise compete avidly for this vitamin, as illustrated by many patients with *Diphyllobothrium latum* infestation and megaloblastic anemia. B$_{12}$ deficiency on a purely dietary basis is rare in the U.S., but has been described in India and elsewhere. Such a dietary deficiency should respond to 25 micrograms by mouth daily. B$_{12}$ deficiency due to defective gastrointestinal absorption should be treated with 100 micrograms of B$_{12}$ daily by intramuscular injection for 10 days, followed thereafter by 100 micrograms monthly intramuscularly. Patients with infected, infested and otherwise diseased bowels as the basis for their B$_{12}$ deficiency clearly require correction of those abnormalities, plus parenteral B$_{12}$ therapy.

Folate Deficiency. Nutritional macrocytic anemia based on folate deficiency usually is associated with inadequate food intake, food faddism or poverty. Other factors, operative in some cases, include pregnancy, lactation, chronic liver disease, and the long-term use of certain anticonvulsant drugs (phenylhydantoin, phenobarbital and primidone), which may interfere with folate absorption. A serum folate level of 7 nanograms per ml. or less is highly suggestive of folate deficiency. Diagnostic confirmation is obtained by means of a therapeutic trial with 50 to 100 micrograms of folic acid injected intramuscularly each day for 10 days. Adequate therapy in most cases of folate deficiency can be accomplished with as little as one mg. of the vitamin daily by mouth.

Patients With Marrow Failure (Aregenerative Anemia)

An aregenerative anemia, as the designation implies, is one that is attributable basically to failure by the bone marrow to release new red cells at a rate sufficient to maintain the red cell count and hemoglobin concentration at normal levels, assuming red cell loss to be within normal limits (i.e., approximately one per cent per day through senescence) or only moderately increased (as a result of hemorrhage or hemolysis).

Anemia of this type may result from physical injury to the bone marrow, such as occasionally occurs in chronic exposure to x-ray or radioactive materials. Sometimes it is caused by mechanical interference with blood formation (myelophthisic anemia), for example, by leukocyte-forming bone marrow tissue such as is encountered in the leukemias, plasmoma and myeloma; by bone marrow invasion by metastatic carcinoma; by Hodgkin's disease of the bone marrow; or by infiltration with abnormal lipoid accumulations with cells containing abnormal lipoid accumulations (xanthomatoses). Bone marrow function may be disturbed or destroyed by overgrowth of the surrounding bone cortex (osteosclerotic anemia), which results in fibrosis of the blood-forming organs. Bone marrow fibrosis is the end stage of many bone marrow disturbances, and occasionally it occurs without known cause.

Anemia of Chronic Disease (Relative Marrow Failure)

An aregenerative anemia of intrinsic origin occurs in patients with chronic infection. It is regularly associated with inflammatory states, such as active rheumatoid arthritis, and with neoplastic disease of all types, even in its early stages.

Red cell production, while normal for a nonanemic individual or even a little faster, is still far below the potential maximum, hence the term "relative marrow failure." Medications of all types are ineffective in correcting this anemia until the infectious or inflammatory process has been controlled or the tumor eradicated. Nor, conversely, will a deficiency anemia due primarily to lack of iron or some other specific nutrient respond adequately to this material as long as infection, inflammation or neoplasia persists.

The anemia of uremia represents another common example of aregenerative anemia. Again, no response to hemopoietic stimulants can be expected until renal function has improved.

Aplastic Anemia

Aplastic anemia of the type encountered in adults usually proves to be the expression of a toxic myelopathy, that is, bone marrow depression or destruction by a drug or chemical, or the result of radiation damage. Agents that regularly produce marrow aplasia in sufficient dosage include benzene and benzene derivatives, antitumor agents, such as nitrogen mustard and its congeners, the periwinkle alkaloids, etc., the antimetabolites, including methotrexate and 6-mercaptopurine, and certain toxic materials, such as inorganic arsenic. Other agents occasionally responsible for aplasia or hypoplasia include certain antimicrobials, anticonvulsants, antithyroid drugs, antidiabetic agents, antihistamines, analgesics, sedatives, phenothiazines, insecticides and heavy metals. The most common offenders in this respect are the antimicrobials chloramphenicol and the organic arsenicals, the anticonvulsants Mesantoin and Tridione, the anti-inflammatory analgesic drug phenylbutazone, and gold compounds. Only a relatively small minority of persons who have received these drugs in their recommended dosage have developed a blood dyscrasia. The cases we are describing, therefore, may be considered a type of idiosyncratic drug reaction in persons who are hypersusceptible for reasons as yet unknown. Provided that their exposure is terminated early (i.e., on the first appearance of reticulocytopenia, anemia, granulopenia or thrombopenia), a prompt and complete recovery may be anticipated. (Unfortunately, one cannot be so optimistic in the case of chloramphenicol recipients. Reactions in individuals hypersusceptible to this drug may be completely unrelated to dosage, may develop without premonitory changes in the hemogram long after the drug has been discontinued, and progress to a complete and fatal aplasia despite all available therapy.) Whatever the offending drug, if exposure is allowed to continue after signs of hypoplasia have appeared, bone marrow depression almost certainly progresses to the point of complete and irreversible failure —hence the importance of frequent hemograms on every patient receiving a drug or exposed regularly to any chemical that has been implicated in the production of aplastic anemia.

The onset of aplastic anemia characteristically is a gradual one, marked by weakness, pallor, breathlessness on exertion and other manifestations of anemia. A presenting symptom in about a third of the patients is abnormal bleeding due to thrombocytopenia. When the granulocytic series is involved as well, the patient is likely to present with fever, acute pharyngitis or some other form of sepsis, in addition to bleeding. Physical signs, save for pallor and skin hemorrhages, are unremarkable. The hemogram is marked by variable degrees of pancytopenia.

Management and Prognosis. The most important aspect of treatment is, of course, prevention. As indicated above, this is accomplished through frequent laboratory observations on every individual exposed to a potentially dangerous drug and prompt withdrawal of such a drug, upon the discovery of a drop in the granulocyte, platelet or reticulocyte count. In an effort to hasten the recovery of a depressed marrow, the corticosteroids are generally prescribed and a course of androgens may be recommended. Antibiotics should be reserved for patients with demonstrable infections and their selection based on bacteriologic criteria.

The chances for recovery from aplastic anemia are most favorable if the toxic agent has been identified with certainty and the patient's exposure terminated promptly, completely and permanently. If marrow damage at the time of termination has been limited to erythroid hypoplasia alone, the chances of complete recovery are 20 per cent or better. In cases with pancytopenia, i.e., combined anemia, granulopenia and thrombocytopenia, the mortality rate by the end of one year is over 20 per cent and by the end of 5 years, 80 per cent. Death, when it occurs, is usually the result of systemic infection or of diffuse, uncontrollable bleeding due to thrombocytopenia.

Patients With Hemorrhagic Anemia

Chronic Blood Loss

The most important complication of chronic bleeding is depletion of the body iron stores leading to all of the complications, specified earlier, of iron deficiency. Principal among these is a microcytic, hypochromic anemia. The serum iron level is low (usually less than 10 to 15 mcg. per cent) and the total iron binding capacity, high. There is normoblastic proliferation in the marrow but the normoblasts are abnormally basophilic, reflecting their defective hemoglobinization, and there is no stainable iron to be seen.

The main concern in this case is the source of bleeding and the prime goal is to find it. If the patient has been unaware of any hemorrhage, its probable location has been somewhere in the gastrointestinal tract. With this consideration in mind, a complete radiologic study of that tract plus a series of stool tests for melena should be undertaken without delay.

PATIENTS WITH HEREDITARY HEMOLYTIC DISORDERS

Sickle Cell Disease

The term "hemoglobinopathy" refers to a condition in which normal, adult hemoglobin ("A"), owing to a genetic defect, has been supplanted by another molecular species of hemoglobin, with results that are detrimental to health. The hemoglobin molecule is comprised of two fractions or "moieties": (1) the "heme" portion, an iron-porphyrin complex, which accounts for hemoglobin's color and its ability to enter into reversible combinations with oxygen; and (2) the "globin" moiety, which provides a framework or stabilizer for the heme. Globin is a small protein, consisting merely of 2 pairs of identical polypeptide chains (in hemoglobin A, 2 "alpha" and 2 "beta" chains made up of 141 and 146 amino acids, respectively). These amino acids are arranged quite precisely as to type and sequence; the patterns are standard, not varying from one normal individual to another. Apparently these patterns are ideal for hemoglobin, from the standpoint of optimal physical properties and optimal behavior as a respiratory pigment. Hemoglobin S differs structurally from hemoglobin A only to the extent that one single amino acid out of 146 amino acids in the beta chain of A has been replaced by another, but this single substitution—this miniscule chemical difference—proves to be extremely important. Because of it, the hemoglobin polymerizes, becomes insoluble and virtually crystallizes at low oxygen tensions, the consequences of which, so far as those who possess hemoglobin S in lieu of A are concerned, are truly staggering. Several dozen types of abnormal hemoglobin have been identified, the vast majority of which likewise are marked by a single amino acid substitution in the alpha or beta chains of hemoglobin A. The functional efficiency and physical properties of these deviants for the most part are quite unimpaired and, but for a few exceptions—most notably, hemoglobin S —these alterations are of little or no consequence clinically. We will now consider the exceptions.

Hemoglobin S disease, or "sickle cell disease," is a condition confined almost exclusively to Negroes. Its name derives from the fact that red cells containing this variant of hemoglobin acquire a rigid, crescentic or boat-shaped form when exposed to low oxygen tensions. Sickle cell disease most often occurs in the heterozygous state, that is, based on a single defective gene inherited from one parent only. If the corresponding gene from the other parent is for hemoglobin A, the individual produces both varieties of hemoglobin, S and A, in approximately equal amounts, and is said to have the *sickle cell trait*. Each of his red cells contains both, and because the S is diluted with normal A hemoglobin, these red cells have considerably less tendency to sickle than cells containing S exclusively (i.e., the cells of patients with the homozygous defect—SS hemoglobin and *sickle cell anemia*). Sickle cell trait, affecting between 8 and 11 per cent of American Negroes, is completely devoid of symptoms and causes no ill-health or disability throughout life except under conditions of extraordinarily severe hypoxia, such as might develop in the course of a severe pneumonia, or might occur in a high-flying aircraft without pressurized cabin or supplemental oxygen.

Sickle cell anemia, based on a pair of defective S genes (one from each parent), is a familiar disease entity and one of major importance. This disease, which affects about 1 in 500 American Negroes, is featured by chronic, severe anemia, unremitting jaundice and so-called crises: recurring attacks of abdominal, muscular and joint pains that presumably result from obstruction of the microcirculation with rigid, sickled red cells. Among the many complications of sickle cell anemia are: cholelithiasis, i.e., the formation of bilirubin gallstones, which is almost inevitable in these cases and is apt to occur at an early age; ulcerations of the skin, especially of the lower extremities, which often are deep, extensive and slow to heal; bony resorptions, which may occur at various sites; and multiple, recurrent infarctions of any or all organs, especially the spleen, kidneys, lungs, and bowel, occasionally the myocardium and less often, the brain. All of this patient's tissues and all of his organs are constantly vulnerable to microcirculatory interruptions by the sickling process and therefore are susceptible to hypoxic damage or true ischemic necrosis at any time.

Treatment

Treatment of sickle cell crises is purely palliative. These episodes generally last 2 to 4 days and may require liberal doses of analgesic medication. If a hyperbaric oxygen chamber were available, its use would be a logical means of reversing the sickling process and re-establishing free blood flow throughout the body, thereby terminating the crisis.

Blood transfusion is indicated only rarely in sickle cell anemia, and in any event it should be used most sparingly, in view of the extra iron load that it contributes. Certain circumstances, to be sure, do compel the transfusion of packed red cells, e.g., the need—sometimes vital—to compensate for temporary marrow failure caused by an acute infection. Renal infarction and hemorrhage may respond to alkalinization with intravenous sodium bicarbonate, the effect of which is to elevate the pH in the renal medulla and therefore inhibit sickling in that location. Splenectomy sometimes is undertaken for the purpose of reducing the hemolytic rate in children with sickle cell anemia, splenomegaly and manifestations of hypersplenism (see p. 325).

Other Hemoglobinopathies

Approximately 100 variants of hemoglobin A have been discovered and characterized to date, but in most instances, as pointed out previously, the alteration has not proven detrimental to health. Certain variants, however, including those designated C, D and E, although far less injurious than S, are not altogether benign, especially when they occur in combination with hemoglobin S. Most common of the variants in the U.S. is hemoglobin C, which, in the heterozygous form, affects 2 to 3 per cent of American Negroes. Double heterozygotes involving S and one of these other defective hemoglobins (e.g., patients with SC and SD disease), although less handicapped by hematologic and vascular complications than patients with SS disease, are considerably more handicapped than individuals with sickle cell trait, i.e., AS hemoglobin. Homozygous C disease, present in about 1 in 6,000 Negroes, is comparable in severity and similar in its manifestations to moderately severe sickle cell disease.

Thalassemia

Thalassemia also stems from a biochemical abnormality affecting the formation of either the alpha or the beta polypeptide chains of globin. In this instance, the chain in question simply is not produced in adequate quantities and the production of hemoglobin is correspondingly inadequate. In patients with so-called *beta-thalassemia,* whose beta (not alpha) chains are in short supply, the bone marrow attempts to compensate for the shortage by reverting to or increasing the production of two other chains to take its place. One of these, the so-called "gamma" chain, normally is made during fetal life but not to any significant extent thereafter, being discontinued and replaced at birth about 99.8 per cent by beta chains. The combination of alpha and gamma chains represents "fetal hemoglobin," or "hemoglobin F." "Hemoglobin A_2," composed of alpha and "delta" chains and normally comprising only 1.5 to 3.0 per cent of the total adult hemoglobin, likewise shows a compensatory increase, e.g., to 6 per cent or more, in beta-thalassemia.

Thalassemia major. The clinical and hematologic features of homozygous thalassemia (thalassemia major, or Cooley's anemia) include a severe chronic hemolytic anemia, marked enlargement of the liver and the spleen, and jaundice. The red cells are small and hypochromic, as in severe iron deficiency; however, in contrast with the latter, serum iron values are normal or high in thalassemia. Diagnostic signs in this disease include the finding of an increased concentration of fetal hemoglobin and hemoglobin A_2 on electrophoretic analysis. No treatment is available, other than symptomatic replacement of red cells by transfusion.

Thalassemia minor, or "Cooley's trait," is devoid of symptoms or signs except for the laboratory findings of defective red cells, the latter being abnormally small and the concentration of intracellular hemoglobin markedly reduced. This deficiency of hemoglobin sometimes is compensated for by a proportionate increase in the red cell count, the level of which may constantly exceed 6 or 7 million per cu. mm. When the condition exists merely as a trait, it is presumed to have been transmitted from one parent only, whereas Cooley's anemia presumably reflects the inheritance of this defect from both parents.

Hereditary Spherocytosis

Included among the more common varieties of chronic hemolytic anemia is a type known as hereditary spherocytosis, or congenital hemolytic jaundice. This condition is caused by an inherent defect in the red cell membrane, which is reduced in area relative to the volume of cell contents and is equipped with a relatively inefficient "sodium pump," i.e., the membrane is less able to exclude sodium (hence water) from the exterior, especially under conditions of stasis. As a result, these cells become increasingly spheroidal in shape as they age, and these abnormally thick and relatively inflexible "spherocytes" tend to become trapped in the splenic sinusoids where they are destroyed by phagocytes.

The condition is characterized clinically by anemia, reticulocytosis, jaundice, splenic enlargement and a family history of a hemolytic anemia. The diagnosis of hereditary spherocytosis depends on the detection of spherocytes in the blood smear and on the demonstration of an abnormal fragility test (see p. 970), which reflects their spheroidicity. Blood destruction is reduced to normal and the patient cured symptomatically by removal of the spleen.

Red Cell Enzymopathies

The absence, partial or complete, of one or another red cell enzyme, due to a genetic defect, accounts for the premature destruction of red cells in the so-called red cell "enzymopathies." Two examples of enzymopathy are described: a rare hemolytic disorder attributable to the absence, genetically determined, of any one of several glycolytic enzymes of the red cell, and a relatively common disorder, based on a deficiency involving a key enzyme, glucose-6-phosphate dehydrogenase (G-6-PD), which is manifested by hemolytic reactions to drugs of a certain type. These reactions, although drug-induced, occur exclusively in persons who are vulnerable to that particular class of drugs because of a specific genetic defect in their red cells. Such persons may be said to have an idiosyncrasy toward those drugs, and reactions of this type are designated *idiosyncratic.*

G-6-PD Deficiency and Idiosyncratic Drug Hemolysis

G-6-PD deficiency, inherited as a sex-linked characteristic, is found in 13 per cent of Negro males and 3 per cent of Negro females. About 1.5 per cent of American Caucasians are similarly affected. The effect of this enzymopathy is to render the red cell unduly susceptible to hemolysis by a number of chemical oxidants, including many drugs that are completely devoid of any such effect for other individuals. With glucose metabolism interrupted or curtailed, no chemical defense can be marshalled by the cell to absorb the oxidative effects of these drugs. Among those drugs that are hemolytic for G-6-PD deficient individuals are antimalarial drugs, sulfonamides, nitrofuran, the common coal tar analgesics (including aspirin and acetophenetidin), the thiazide diuretics, the oral hypoglycemic agents, chloramphenicol, para-aminosalicylic acid (PAS), vitamin K and, for certain individuals subject to "favism," the fava bean.

Exposure to one of these drugs on the part of a susceptible individual is followed by a 7- to 12-day period of acute intravascular hemolysis, marked by hemoglobinemia and hemoglobinuria. The serum bilirubin rises and Heinz bodies appear (representing granules of oxidized, degraded hemoglobin within the cell). Thereafter the hemogram proceeds to improve, reticulocytes appear in increasing numbers and the hemoglobin rises as new cells emerge from the marrow. These new cells, relatively well-supplied with G-6-PD and hence relatively unsusceptible to the oxidant drug, survive for a time even if drug exposure continues. Thereafter, unless the contact is broken, follows a prolonged period of chronic hyperhemolysis that lasts until the drug is discontinued.

The essence of treatment, of course, is the identification and removal of the offending drug, and the prevention of future exposure to the same or a comparable agent. It is important to realize that abnormal vulnerability to oxidants poses a threat to a great many individuals and will continue to do so for the foreseeable future. Screening tests are available for the detection of this enzymopathy. These should be employed widely, possibly on a mass scale, so that those who are affected will be aware of their vulnerability and therefore in a position to protect themselves from noxious exposures.

Congenital Nonspherocytic Hemolytic Anemia

This disorder represents another manifestation of a red cell enzymopathy, involving in many instances the same enzyme we have been discussing, namely G-6-PD. In these cases, however, the deficiency is not partial but complete. Enzymes other than G-6-PD that have been implicated in this disorder include pyruvate kinase, glutathione reductase and others. Thus far the condition has been reported exclusively in Caucasian males. Most patients with congenital nonspherocytic hemolytic anemia have been jaundiced since birth, and most give a history of anemia and jaundice following infections as well as after drug ingestion. More often than not their anemia is relatively mild, in fact, the hyperhemolysis may be compensated completely, manifested solely by persistent hyperbilirubinemia and reticulocytosis. The spleen may be enlarged. Splenectomy, however, is not helpful in these patients and should not be undertaken.

PATIENTS WITH ACQUIRED HEMOLYTIC DISORDERS

Traumatic and Toxic Hemolysis

Intravascular hemolysis induced by physical injury to the erythrocyte is exemplified most dramatically by the hemoglobinemia, hemoglobinuria and anemia that promptly follow extensive thermal burns. Physical trauma doubtless is responsible for the hyperhemolysis that frequently follows the introduction of prostheses into the vascular system for the repair of cardiac septal defects or the replacement of heart valves with ball valves or plastic cups. At any rate, the blood of such patients is likely to contain a large and varied assortment of red cell fragments, or "schizocytes," whose survival in the circulation is brief.

Microangiopathic Hemolytic Anemia

This term has been applied to a condition featured by anemia, signs of hyperhemolysis and the presence of fragmented red cells in the blood of patients with serious systemic disease, such as widespread bacterial sepsis, malignant hypertension, widespread cancer, or following massive injuries. It is speculated that red cells intimately exposed to the products of tissue necrosis or inflammation may incur membrane damage of a type that is incompatible with normal survival.

Toxic Hemolysis

As noted previously, many drugs possessing mild oxidant properties, while harmless for the majority of people, regularly produce hemolysis in those whose red cells are G-6-PD deficient. Certain other chemicals and drugs are capable of producing a similar hemolytic reaction in anyone, including individuals whose red cells are perfectly normal. Such compounds include phenylhydrazine, hydroquinone, phenol and arsine. Their potency, as oxidants is such that normal red cells, despite a full complement of protective GSH, are irreversibly damaged in their presence. After brief exposure to these compounds the membrane ceases to function properly as a selective barrier, the hemoglobin is degraded to methemoglobin and sulfhemoglobin, and the cells soon hemolyze.

Immunohemolytic Disorders

The term "immunohemolytic" implies a process of red cell destruction involving an immune reaction in which the red cell is the target of an antibody. Two clinical disorders based on this mechanism have already been described: namely, the hemolytic transfusion reaction (p. 95) and hemolytic disease of the newborn (erythroblastosis fetalis). In both of these instances, red blood cells are destroyed by antibodies from another individual, i.e., the antibodies of the transfusion recipient reacting with the donor red cells, or maternal antibodies destroying fetal red cells. Such reactions between antigens and antibodies from different sources within the same (human) species are called "isoimmune reactions." Other immunohemolytic disorders, now to be described, appear to represent disorders of "autoimmunity," the hemolytic agent in each case being a serum protein of the immune globulin type, like an antibody, and producing the same destructive effect on red cells as a blood group-specific isoantibody, but these hemolytic agents have their origins in the patient himself.

Autoimmune Hemolytic Anemia (Acquired Hemolytic Jaundice). This disease is generally regarded as the product of an abnormal and a damaging immune reaction in which the patient's reticuloendothelial system is stimulated to produce antibodies that react with his own erythrocytes. The latter become coated with globulins and as a result clump together. Aggregate masses of these cells become trapped in the sinusoids of the spleen, where they are easy prey for the phagocytic cells that are so abundant in that organ and are cannibalized en masse.

Clinically, acquired hemolytic jaundice is characterized by periods of exacerbations and remissions occurring over months or years. Its course often is marked by "crises" when massive blood destruction occurs, with death sometimes resulting from a precipitous and profound anemia.

The diagnosis of autoimmune hemolytic anemia is based on a positive Coombs' test (see Appendix), i.e., by the demonstration that the patient's red cells, after multiple washings with saline, are agglutinable with antiglobulin serum, implying that these cells are coated with a firmly attached globulin—presumably antibody globulin.

Treatment. Splenectomy is indicated as soon as the hemolytic rate has been reduced to normal by steroids. In the absence of the spleen, the site at which a large proportion of the destructive antibody is produced and hemolysis takes place, a prolonged remission is likely. Subsequent recurrences are not uncommon, but the severity of these attacks is relatively mild and their control, by steroids, relatively easy.

Paroxysmal Nocturnal Hemoglobinuria (PNH)

This disease, one of the most incapacitating of the acquired hemolytic disorders, is encountered in both sexes and may start at any age. Its onset may be abrupt, with chills, fever, rapidly progressive anemia and striking hemoglobinuria, or it may start insidiously with manifestations that are more characteristic of an aplastic than a hemolytic anemia. The disease, when fully developed, is featured by chronic fatigue, scleral icterus, splenomegaly, complaints of episodic pains in the back, abdomen and chest, and the passage, consistently for days or weeks on end, of brown- or port-wine-colored urine.

The diagnosis of PNH is established on the basis of the "acid-hemolysis" (Ham) test, which demonstrates partial lysis of the patient's red cells after their acidification and incubation at 37° C. in the presence of complement. Those cells that are susceptible to hemolysis, under these conditions and in vivo, appear to possess defective membranes, although the precise nature of the membrane lesion is as yet unknown.

In the majority of patients PNH proves to be a lifelong, debilitating illness, but one with a reasonable life expectancy. In addition to hemolytic anemia these patients are subject to thromboembolic disease, the commonest causes of death in this group being cerebral, portal, mesenteric, renal and femoral thrombosis, and the complications thereof.

Treatment. The only useful and effective therapy in PNH is blood transfusion, preferably given in the form of washed red cells. In view of the magnitude of iron loss by way of the urine in PNH, an occasional course of iron salts may be prescribed.

Hypersplenism

A spleen that is grossly enlarged from any cause, be it lymphoma, sarcoid, portal hypertension, tuberculosis, or whatever, may function as a filter for the formed blood elements, constantly trapping and destroying red cells, platelets and granulocytes in substantial numbers. The resultant panhematopenia is the hallmark of the condition designated *hypersplenism*. The destructive role of the spleen in a patient who presents such a picture may be suspected on the basis of a marrow biopsy that displays erythroid, granulocytic and megakaryocytic hyperplasia (i.e., panhyperplasia) and that excludes the possibility of leukemia, another important cause of pancytopenia. The obvious treatment for hypersplenism, circumstances permitting, is splenectomy.

PATIENTS WITH POLYCYTHEMIA

Polycythemia Vera

This disorder is characterized by a persistent and marked erythremia, with elevation of the red cell count to between 7 and 10 million, an equally marked expansion of the circulating red cell mass, leukocytosis, thrombocytosis, and splenomegaly. In a typical patient its course is marked by gouty arthritis secondary to chronic hyperuricemia, recurrent peptic ulcer, and thromboembolic complications that are favored by the high blood viscosity and reduced blood flow. The cause of polycythemia vera is unknown; it is generally classified as a myeloproliferative disease, i.e., malignant overgrowth of the bone marrow, especially, in this instance, its erythroid elements. Males middle-aged and older are predominantly affected. Their complaints include headaches, indigestion, leg pains and periodic mental confusion. They are prone to have peptic ulcers that bleed, as well as multiple intravascular thromboses in various locations. Splenic infarcts are common and myocardial infarction is the commonest cause of death in these patients. A substantial proportion of those who survive 10 years or longer develop hematologic changes typical of acute granulocytic leukemia and succumb shortly thereafter.

Treatment. The basic objective of therapy is reduction of the high blood viscosity, the most hazardous feature of polycythemia vera and the source of most of its complications. This may be achieved by repeated phlebotomies supplemented, in many instances, by the administration of a myelosuppressant agent, such as radioactive phosphorus (^{32}P) or busulfan (Myleran). For those patients who regularly exhibit a high blood uric acid and are therefore susceptible to gout (p. 713) and the development of renal calculi (p. 566), allopurinol may be prescribed on a chronic prophylactic basis.

Secondary Polycythemia

This condition, likewise characterized by erythremia and hypervolemia, occurs as a complication of chronic hypoxia, the effect of which is to stimulate the production of erythropoietin and increase erythropoiesis. Thus, it is seen characteristically in association with congenital heart disease of the cyanotic type, and in patients with severe pulmonary emphysema. It is also encountered occasionally in patients with certain malignant tumors, notably renal carcinoma, presumably due to the overproduction or excessive activation of erythropoietin by the tumor tissue. Red cell counts and blood volumes in secondary polycythemia are comparable to those found in polycythemia vera but, in contrast to the latter, the leukocyte and platelet counts are normal and the spleen is not enlarged. All of the other symptoms, signs and complications of polycythemia vera, including thromboembolism, are associated with secondary polycythemia as well, and the prime objective of therapy in both conditions—namely, normalization of the hematocrit—is the same.

PATIENTS WITH LEUKOPENIA AND AGRANULOCYTOSIS

The term "leukopenia" is applicable when the white cell count is less than 5,000. This can occur from many causes, including viral infections, overwhelming bacterial sepsis and neoplastic diseases of the bone marrow, particularly leukopenic or "aleukemic" leukemia. However, the most common etiology is drug toxicity, because numerous chemical agents, including some used in medical treatment, are capable of suppressing bone marrow activity and decreasing the production of white cells. Among these are included benzene, amidopyrine, sulfapyridine, Mesantoin, gold (given by injection), nitrogen mustard, urethane, radioactive phosphorus (^{32}P) and many others. No clinical manifestations are to be expected as a result of leukopenia per se unless the reduction in the granulocytes is extremely marked; in this event the patient becomes susceptible to bacterial infections. Infection of the throat, or "agranulocytic angina," is the most dangerous of these complications; the throat becomes increasingly sore and eventually gangrenous, accompanying which are all of the manifestations of a systemic infection. Without treatment, death may be anticipated within 1 to 3 days, but with appropriate antibacterial chemotherapy the process usually can be controlled. The nature and gravity of the threat may be ascertained from a bone marrow examination, which might demonstrate total aplasia or merely a maturation arrest in the granulocytic series. In the latter event, the outlook for recovery is reasonably good, assuming complete withdrawal of the offending drug and effective application of the measures specified below.

Treatment and Nursing Care

Patients with profound leukopenia, e.g., with granulocytes numbering less than 500 per cu. mm. or approaching that figure, should be placed on reverse precautions, their hemograms should be checked and their throats cultured at frequent intervals. Upon the advent of fever, vigorous antibacterial chemotherapy should be applied, utilizing whatever agent or combination of agents are appropriate in the light of the bacteriologic findings then available or, in the absence of such data, some combination of agents with a broad spectrum of antibacterial activity.

Hot saline irrigations of the throat are employed to

keep it clear of necrotic detritus and exudate. Comfort is provided by supplying an ice collar and whatever analgesic, antipyretic and sedative drugs may be indicated. The essence of treatment, apart from eradicating the infection, is to eliminate, if possible, the factor responsible for the bone marrow depression. Spontaneous restoration of marrow function, except in the case of neoplastic diseases, often occurs in time, i.e., within 2 or 3 weeks, if death from infection can be averted.

PATIENTS WITH LEUKEMIA

Leukemia (white blood) is a term that originally was applied to a few cases in which the blood appeared milky at necropsy. Since such a condition can arise only when the leukocyte count almost equals that of the red cells, it means that the leukocyte count must be about 1,000,000 per cu. mm. and the anemia profound. Only one disease can produce it, the one we still call *leukemia*. (However, in the great majority of cases of this disease the blood is red, since the leukocyte count seldom rises above 500,000 per cu. mm.)

Several varieties of leukemia are recognized; they all are characterized by the presence of immature leukocytes of one type or another in the peripheral blood and by extensive hyperplasia (overgrowth) of the tissue producing that particular cell. The most common are granulocytic, lymphocytic and monocytic leukemia, these terms referring in each case to the cell type that is involved.

The clinical course of leukemia may be fulminating, progressing to a fatal termination usually within a period of a few weeks or months.

Whether acute or chronic, every leukemic process is a manifestation of malignant neoplasia—the uncontrolled, destructive proliferation of a blood cell that has acquired through some genetic alteration a biologic advantage over other cells, enabling it to outgrow them, even in their native tissues, their optimal environments, and freeing it from the physiologic restraints that usually prevent overgrowth.

Acute Leukemia

Acute leukemia may occur at any age, but is encountered most frequently in children and young adults. Regardless of the cell type, i.e., whether one is dealing with an acute lymphoblastic, myeloblastic, monoblastic or stem cell leukemia, these patients exhibit many characteristics in common. The onset is typically very sudden, manifested by an acute tonsillitis, furunculosis or the appearance of an abscess in the mouth or the skin. The total course may be limited to a few days or weeks and is marked by a high fever. Hemorrhagic features appear early and may include bleeding from the gums, the nose, the stomach and the rectum, as well as hemorrhages into the skin and into the fundus of the eyes. Swelling and gangrenous ulceration of the gums, the cheeks, the jaw and the tonsils likewise are common. Bone pain may become a prominent symptom and neurologic manifestations may appear. Enlargement of lymph nodes, liver and spleen may occur, but these findings are less common and less prominent than in chronic leukemia.

Acute leukemia is an important disease to keep in mind, since it may be mistaken for an acute infection, acute rheumatic fever, idiopathic thrombocytopenic purpura or some specific type of anemia. The diagnosis usually, but not invariably, can be made from an examination of the peripheral blood, with findings of primitive leukocytes in the smear, anemia and thrombocytopenia. The most important diagnostic criterion, however, is the presence of numerous blast cells in the patient's bone marrow. The prognosis in all cases is poor. Without treatment the illness lasts an average of 3 or 4 months; with treatment, adults with acute leukemia survive about a year, on the average, and children, somewhat longer.

Treatment. Of prime importance in the treatment of acute leukemia is chemotherapy, for which several effective agents are available for use alone, sequentially or in combination. These include the purine antimetabolite 6-mercaptopurine (6-MP, Purinethol), 2.5 mg./Kg./day orally; a folic acid antimetabolite, amethopterin (Methotrexate), 2.5 to 5.0 mg./day orally; a periwinkle plant derivative with growth inhibiting properties, vincristine (Oncovin), 0.015 to 0.05 mg./Kg./week I.V.; and an adrenal cortical hormone, prednisone, 20 to 100 mg./day orally. Platelet transfusions may be required to control bleeding due to thrombocytopenia, and transfusions of packed red cells to maintain an adequate hemoglobin level. Antibacterial chemotherapy, selected on the basis of bacterial cultures and sensitivity tests, is required by many patients with acute leukemia who, because of their white cell defects, are exceedingly susceptible to infections of all types.

Chronic Leukemias

Chronic Granulocytic (Myelogenous) Leukemia. This is a condition characterized by white cell counts ranging from 100,000 to 1,000,000 per cu. mm.; a high percentage of these leukocytes are immature cells. The condition is associated with a great enlargement of the spleen and the liver but little swelling of the lymph nodes. Chronic myelogenous leukemia may appear at any period of life, most often between the ages of 25 and 40. The onset of this disease is usually gradual and insidious. Many patients accidentally discover a tumor (the spleen) in the abdomen, or complain of dragging sensations due to the weight of this organ. The long bones (the tibias, the ribs and the sternum, in particular), due to their invasion by the abnormal marrow, often become spontaneously painful and tender on pressure.

Treatment usually includes the administration of an alkylating agent, busulfan (Myleran), either intermittently in doses of 2 to 6 mg./day or on a chronic maintenance schedule of 2 mg./day. The patient may receive in addition radioactive phosphorus (^{32}P) intravenously or by mouth in doses of 3 to 7 millicuries, or splenic irradiation from an external, preferably supravoltage (e.g., ^{60}Co), source. The antimetabolites 6-mercaptopurine (6-MP) and 6-thioguanine (6-TG) have been prescribed with benefit in doses of 2.5 mg./Kg./day and 2.0 mg./Kg./day, respectively. With or without treatment death usually ensues within a period of 3 to 5 years following the onset of symptoms, caused in most cases by thromboembolism, thrombocytopenic purpura or infection.

Chronic Lymphatic Leukemia. Occurring most frequently between the ages of 45 and 60, this leukemia is characterized by a greatly increased leukocyte count, over 90 per cent of the cells being mature lymphocytes. The onset is typically insidious, with symptoms that closely resemble those of the myelogenous type. For months the only significant physical sign may be the gradual appearance of a generalized lymph node enlargement. Subsequent developments include the appearance of anemia, fever, cachexia and hemorrhagic features, all of which are apt to be more pronounced than in myelogenous type leukemia.

Leukemic infiltrations appear in the retinae of the eyes and in the skin, which may become pruritic and bronzed. Ascitic and pleural effusions are not uncommon, the latter occasionally chylous because of the pressure of enlarged nodes on the thoracic duct.

With judicious chemotherapy and appropriate supportive treatment, patients with chronic lymphatic leukemia can be maintained in good physical condition throughout most of the duration of their disease, and their lives, moreover, may be prolonged significantly. The chemotherapeutic agents most often selected in these cases include the alkylating agents chlorambucil (Leukeran), 6 to 12 mg./day by mouth, and Thio-TEPA, given in five intravenous doses, 0.2 mg./Kg. body weight each, plus an adrenal cortical hormone equivalent to 20 to 60 mg. of prednisone daily or every other day by mouth.

Survey of the Patient's Problems. From the above discussion one sees that the patient with leukemia has complex problems due to pathologic disturbances in major organ systems. His fatigue, anorexia, bleeding tendencies, neurologic involvement, dyspnea and fever all require specific therapy and nursing support. The major goal of therapy and nursing management is to help that patient live as normal a life as possible by maintaining him in a state of remission for as long as possible. (A remission is a temporary arrest of a disease.) Various chemotherapeutic agents are used to obtain a remission. These all produce rather severe toxic effects which cause considerable discomfort. They include ulceration of the mouth, depression of bone marrow resulting in leukopenia, thrombocytopenia and anemia. Adrenal steroids used in the treatment of leukemia may cause rapid and dramatic improvement but these drugs have toxic effects including sodium and fluid retention, decreased resistance to infection, hypertension, cerebral edema and hyperglycemia. The alkylating agents can produce partial or complete loss of hair (alopecia). It is ironical that the drugs used against leukemia can produce so many complications. In caring for each patient the nurse should seek to know: *What is the toxicity of the drug(s) being used?*

Supportive Nursing Therapy

Although there are several varieties of leukemia the principles of care are similar. Patients who are battling against fatal illnesses often exhibit admirable resources of courage and fortitude. When adequate medical and nursing support are given they will endure much discomfort associated with their treatment. Each patient is a unique individual with his own specific needs and possesses his own way of coping with his physiologic and emotional stresses. The understanding nurse is sensitive to these needs and endeavors to assist the patient to accept and participate in his therapeutic regimen as effectively as possible.

As with every other patient, the individual with leukemia seeks relief of his pain and discomfort. There are many nursing measures that can be used to make his life more endurable. In controlling pain, it is wise to begin with aspirin and a sedative (if needed) and then change to a milder then stronger narcotic as the patient's condition requires. Phenergan or Thorazine enhance the effect of narcotics. Appropriate antiemetic drugs given one-half hour before meals may help assuage the patient's nausea. Small bland feedings may be a partial answer to his aversion to food. If vomiting and diarrhea are present, intravenous fluids are given. The oral fluid intake must be maintained between 3 and 4 liters daily to prevent precipitation of uric acid crystals in the kidneys. Overproduction of uric acid (causing uric acid stones, obstruction, pain and infection) is due to the tremendous proliferation of blood cells and the destruction of these cells by antileukemic agents. Alkalinization of urine may be achieved with sodium bicarbonate given every 4 to 6 hours during the day.

General measures to combat fever include increasing the fluid intake, fever sponges and administration of antipyretic drugs. Ulcerations in the mouth are very painful and contribute to the patient's disinterest in food. Frequent mouth care will remove old dried blood and combat mouth odors. Alternate solutions of mouth wash, dilute hydrogen peroxide solution and glycerine may be used for cleaning and lubricating the mouth. Cotton applicators, used instead of a toothbrush, can prevent further irritation. The nostrils also require gentle cleansing. Applications of petroleum jelly on the lips will prevent drying and cracking. The diet should be soft to reduce mechanical irritations to the gums.

Due to the disease process itself and to bone marrow depression by chemotherapy, infection is an ever present threat. Reverse isolation procedures may be carried out during periods of hemopoietic depression to protect the patient. Hexachlorophene soap is used on the skin to reduce bacterial flora. Any evidences of infection (chills, fever, skin lesions) should be promptly reported. Appropriate antibiotics are usually given.

These patients have marked bleeding tendencies manifested by petechiae, areas of ecchymosis and more grossly by hematuria, melena, etc. Transfusions of fresh whole blood are given to maintain the hemoglobin over 8 grams per 100 ml. of blood. Transfusions of platelet concentrations have also proved useful. There are hazards attending every transfusion. (See p. 94 for the nursing management of patients having transfusions.) The nurse should handle the patient gently to prevent further trauma. Observe the body orifices and skin for signs of bleeding. Hemorrhage, a major complication and cause of death, is treated by placing the patient on bed rest, and administering transfusions and steroids.

When the patient no longer responds to his therapeutic regimen his course may be a rapid downhill one. He is hospitalized for supportive care. He has "lived with his disease,", its remissions and exacerbations and with hope and despair. He is very tired and very ill. He requires knowledgeable nursing assessment and support and expert physical care. The reader is referred to "The Patient with Terminal Carcinoma" in chapter 11 for a review of the salient principles of nursing care. The demonstration of the nurse's concern for his welfare does much to comfort this patient. Other aspects of supporting the dying patient are discussed in Chapter 3.

PATIENTS WITH MALIGNANT LYMPHOMA

The term *lymphoma* refers to a primary tumor of lymphatic tissue caused by the neoplastic overgrowth of one of its cellular components. Lymphomas generally originate in lymph nodes where most lymphatic tissue is located and, as they grow and spread, they show a definite predilection for other lymph nodes. Thus, the most characteristic clinical feature of lymphoma is lymph node enlargement. But lymphatic tissue is not confined exclusively to lymph nodes: numerous lymph follicles are present in the walls of the respiratory and gastrointestinal tracts, and their cellular ingredients, comprising the "lymphoreticular system," are to be found in many locations elsewhere, including the spleen, liver, bone marrow, lungs and skin. These organs and tissues, as well as lymph nodes, occasionally become primary sites of malignant lymphomas and can be expected ultimately to participate in most lymphomatous processes, including those of lymph node origin.

Three principal cell types are represented in lymphatic tissue: lymphocytes, reticulum cells and histiocytes. Each of these may undergo neoplastic transformation leading to the cell production of a malignant lymphoma, the variety of lymphoma produced being determined by the particular cell type that is involved. Lymphocyte neoplasia, for example, gives rise either to lymphosarcoma, lymphatic leukemia or both, depending on the relative extent to which the neoplastic lymphocytes aggregate to form solid tumor masses, or become dispersed throughout the body as discrete elements. Reticulum cell neoplasia causes reticulum cell sarcoma, and neoplastic proliferation of the histiocytic series presumably is the basis of Hodgkin's disease. Summarized below are the outstanding features of various lymphomas and some of the more important details regarding their therapeutic management.

Hodgkin's Disease

Hodgkin's disease, like other lymphomas, is a malignant disease of unknown etiology that originates in the lymphatic system and involves predominantly the lymph nodes. It occurs at all ages and in both sexes equally.

The malignant cell of Hodgkin's disease, its pathologic hallmark and its essential diagnostic criterion is the "Reed-Sternberg cell," a gigantic, atypical tumor cell, morphologically unique and of uncertain lineage, which many regard as an aberrant histiocyte. Patients with Hodgkin's disease are customarily classified into subgroups based on pathologic criteria that reflect the grade of malignancy and suggest the prognosis.

Hodgkin's paragranuloma, for example, with fewest Reed-Sternberg cells and least disturbance of nodal architecture, carries a much more favorable prognosis than *Hodgkin's sarcoma,* in which the lymph nodes are virtually replaced by tumor cells of the most primitive type. The majority of patients, with so-called *Hodgkin's granuloma* (which includes 2 conditions currently designated "nodular sclerosis" and "mixed cellularity") are in an intermediate position as regards the density and destructiveness of tumor cells, therapeutic responsiveness and overall outlook.

Hodgkin's disease usually begins as a painless enlargement of the lymph nodes on one side of the neck, which becomes increasingly conspicuous. However, for months generalized pruritus may be the first and only symptom and later is often a most distressing one. The individual nodes remain firm and discrete (that is, they do not soften and do not fuse) and they are seldom tender and painful. Soon the lymph nodes of other regions, usually the other side of the neck, also enlarge in the same manner. The mediastinal and retroperitoneal lymph nodes may also enlarge, causing severe pressure symptoms: pressure against the trachea causing dyspnea; the esophagus, dysphagia; the nerves, laryngeal paralysis, and brachial, lumbar or sacral neuralgias; the veins, edema of one or both extremities and effusions into the pleura or peritoneum; and the bile duct, obstructive jaundice. Later the spleen may become palpable, and the liver may enlarge. In some patients the first nodes to enlarge are those of one axilla or of one groin. Occasionally, the disease starts in mediastinal or peritoneal nodes and may remain limited to them. In still other cases the enlargement of the spleen is the only conspicuous lesion.

Sooner or later a progressive anemia develops. A leukocytosis often is observed with an abnormally high polymorphonuclear and an elevated eosinophil count. About half the patients have a slight fever, but with a temperature seldom above 38.3° C. (101° F.). However, the patients with mediastinal and abdominal involvement present a remarkable intermittent fever. The temperature goes as high as 40.0° C. (104° F.) for periods of 3 to 14 days, returning to normal within a few weeks. Untreated, this disease is progressive in its course; the patient loses weight, becomes cachectic, the anemia becomes marked, anasarca appears, the blood pressure falls, and in 1 to 3 years death is likely to ensue.

The diagnosis of Hodgkin's disease hinges on the identification of its characteristic histologic features in an excised lymph node. A diagnosis having been firmly established on the basis of the requisite criteria, it becomes necessary to assess as accurately as possible the total extent of tumor involvement and to define the manner in which it is distributed. In other words, one attempts to pinpoint the location of every tumor lesion inside and outside the lymphatic system and to exclude the presence of a tumor in organs and tissues that are not yet involved. This is a difficult, expensive and uncertain undertaking but an extremely important one, since these are the very considerations on which treatment is to be based.

Current concepts of treatment stem from the following observations and premises:

(1) Hodgkin's disease spreads from its original location (usually a single node) by way of the lymphatic channels to contiguous lymph nodes, which in turn become the site of tumor growth; it rarely skips lymph nodes en route to more distant sites of metastasis.

(2) Rarely does Hodgkin's disease spread beyond the lymphatic system to involve other organs and tissues until late in the disease.

(3) Hodgkin's disease is completely and permanently eradicated from any site that has received 4,000 to 4,500 rads within the space of about 4 weeks. Megavoltage radiation techniques permit the delivery of such a dose to one or more entire lymph node chains.

(4) Areas of the body in which the lymph node chains are located can tolerate doses of this magnitude without serious damage (as can the area of the spleen and the oronasopharynx, both of which may become involved in Hodgkin's disease), so far as vital structures such as the lungs, liver, gastrointestinal tract, kidneys and bone marrow are protected by carefully shaped lead shields.

From the foregoing it is postulated that Hodgkin's disease is potentially curable by radiotherapy, provided it has not extended beyond the lymph node chains, spleen and oronasopharynx. Failing signs of such extension, patients with this disease should have the benefit of "curative" radiotherapy in which tumoricidal doses are delivered not only to obvious tumor nodes but to all adjacent nodes and lymph node chains as well. Conversely, any signs of spread beyond the treatable areas automatically disqualifies the Hodgkin's patient from such a program, in which case a combination of chemotherapy and palliative radiotherapy would be indicated.

Staging of Hodgkin's Disease. For the sake of simplicity, uniformity and convenience in categorizing Hodgkin's patients with respect to the extent and activity of their disease, hence their eligibility for curative radiotherapy, the disease generally is classified or "staged" as follows:

Stage I: disease limited to a single node and contiguous structures;

Stage II: disease involves more than a single node

or group of contiguous nodes, but is confined to one side of the diaphragm only;

Stage III: disease is present both above and below the diaphragm, but does not extend beyond lymph node chains, spleen or the oronasopharynx;

Stage IV: disease has extended to the bone marrow, lung parenchyma, pleura, skin, gastrointestinal tract or liver.

Stage II and stage III patients are further subdivided on the basis of the presence or absence of constitutional symptoms: those without, being designated IIA or IIIA; those with, IIB or IIIB. Therapeutic programs vary in different institutions, but most would agree that all stage I and stage II patients should receive "curative" radiotherapy. Some would also include stage IIIA patients in this program, whereas others would be inclined to substitute a combination of chemotherapy and palliative radiation. For stages IIIB and IV the use of cytostatic and antimetabolite drugs generally is regarded as the therapeutic mainstay, radiation being reserved for the palliative treatment of local lesions that are especially damaging or painful.

Among the chemotherapeutic agents useful in Hodgkin's disease, nitrogen mustard (Mustargen; HN_2) has been employed most extensively. This drug is administered in a single intravenous dose of 0.4 mg./Kg. of body weight, or in 2 to 4 divided doses totalling this amount. Each such course is followed by a 3- to 4-week period of bone marrow depression, which limits the frequency with which this treatment may safely be repeated. Other agents commonly used include chlorambucil (Leukeran), 4 to 10 mg./day by mouth; vinblastine (Velban), 0.1 to 1.2 mg./Kg./week I.V.; procarbazine (Natulan), 50 to 300 mg./day by mouth; and adrenal cortical hormones. Should one drug prove ineffective initially, or when it loses its original effectiveness, another is substituted.

The mean survival in Hodgkin's disease, adequately treated, tends to be somewhat longer than in other lymphomas; the 5-year rate is in the range of 20 to 25 per cent, and the 10-year rate, about 10 per cent. Some patients have survived with their disease for as long as 20 to 30 years and a few have ostensibly been cured. To what extent radical radiotherapy of the type outlined above may modify the outlook in this disease remains to be seen.

Lymphosarcoma and Reticulum Cell Sarcoma

These closely related lymphomas, together with Hodgkin's disease, account for most of the solid tumors of the blood-forming organs. Lymph node tumor is their most outstanding and usually their presenting feature but ultimately, or even originally, as in Hodgkin's disease, any lymphoid tissue may become in-

volved. With respect to grade of malignancy, the "giant follicle lymphoma," or "follicular lymphoma," is one of the least aggressive and most responsive to treatment of all lymphomas, whereas reticulum cell sarcoma, like Hodgkin's sarcoma, is one of the most destructive and carries the least favorable prognosis. Lymphosarcoma, like chronic lymphatic leukemia, is commonly featured by such immunohemolytic complications as autoimmune hemolytic anemia. Marrow damage, manifested by anemia and thrombocytopenia, and immune dysfunction, with heightenend susceptibility to bacterial and mycotic infections, are also especially pronounced in patients with lymphosarcoma.

Treatment. The practice of staging patients with lymphosarcoma and reticulum cell sarcoma in the manner described for patients with Hodgkin's disease is becoming increasingly widespread, and therapy for these patients is often planned on a similar basis. Radiotherapy is generally selected as the treatment of choice, except for patients with widely disseminated disease who, as in the case of Hodgkin's patients, are candidates for chemotherapy. Moreover, allowing for relatively minor differences in drug preference or in sequence of drug use in different clinical centers, the same agents tend to be applied in all of these lymphomas. Nitrogen mustard and vinblastine, to be sure, are used relatively little and chlorambucil, cyclophosphamide and vincristine (0.015 to 0.05 mg./Kg./week intravenously) are used much more frequently in lymphosarcoma and reticulum cell sarcoma than in Hodgkin's disease. Moreover, corticosteroids are likely to prove more effective, at least for a time, in these patients and are very specifically indicated, of course, in those patients with immunohemolytic complications.

Myeloma (Myelomatosis; Multiple Myeloma)

This disease, like the lymphomas described above, is a solid tumor arising in blood-forming tissue, the malignant proliferating cell being a plasmacyte or a precursor thereof. Unlike the other lymphomas, however, this tumor, like chronic granulocytic leukemia or like any of the acute leukemias, has its origin and principal location in the bone marrow, with involvement of lymph nodes, liver, spleen, kidneys, etc., occurring as a later development and less prominent feature. There may be only one solitary tumor or very few discrete tumors comprised of these cells, in which case the lesions are designated "plasmacytomas." By far the most common form of the disease, however, is one in which there is widespread proliferation of immature plasma cells in the cancellous bone within the marrow cavity throughout the skeleton. Numerous areas of localized bone destruction may be visible on skeletal x-ray examination. About one-quarter of the patients show evidence of diffuse demineralization of the skeleton. Spontaneous fractures of long bones and compression fractures of vertebrae are common in this disease. Back pain is one of the most characteristic symptoms of myeloma. Anemia is almost universally present, due to replacement of the marrow with neoplastic plasma cells. Associated with this anemia may be a marked thrombocytopenia and granulopenia, the basis of 2 common complications of myeloma: abnormal bleeding and susceptibility to bacterial infections.

Bone marrow aspiration biopsy is diagnostic for this condition, the neoplastic cell comprising 30 per cent to 95 per cent of the entire marrow population (in contrast to a normal representation of 5 per cent plasmacytes or less). These cells are directly responsible for other diagnostic features of myeloma and for a very potent source of its complications: an abnormally high concentration of one or another immune serum globulin and the presence in the urine of a polypeptide fragment of this globulin (Bence-Jones proteinuria).

In advanced, symptomatic and untreated myeloma, life expectancy does not exceed a year or two, but the duration of the disease in its preliminary asymptomatic stages may extend for as long as 5 or 10 years. Treatment includes specific measures directed to the tumor itself and a number of supportive treatments. The only useful chemotherapy presently available for the control of myeloma is the administration of phenylalanine mustard (Alkeran; Melphalan), which is given in 2 to 8 mg.-doses daily by mouth. This drug exerts a depressive effect on all marrow elements; its dosage, therefore, must be controlled closely on the basis of frequent hemograms. Localized bony involvement often responds to radiotherapy with symptomatic improvement. Other measures frequently indicated in myeloma include the application of orthopedic supports to stabilize a damaged spine; alkalinization of the urine to prevent precipitation of Bence-Jones protein in the urine, with consequent uremia; the administration of sodium phosphate, sodium fluoride or both to favor remineralization of the bones; and, in an occasional case, plasmapheresis to reduce extremely high levels of serum globulin.

Mycosis Fungoides

Mycosis fungoides is regarded as a variant of the lymphoma group of diseases, most closely allied with Hodgkin's granuloma. Although the lymph nodes, the liver and the spleen are involved as well, the skin is the site of its most prominent manifestation throughout the entire illness.

The course of this disease, like that of the other lymphomas, is characterized by remissions and exacerbations. It begins as a generalized severe itching that may last for years; this is followed by a stage of eruptions of erythematous, urticarial, eczematous or psoriasislike lesions. These eruptions come and go, possibly for years, before any of the typical tumors appear, and they also continue to some degree throughout the entire course of the disease. The swellings characteristic of this disease arise from some of the above-mentioned lesions, which become indurated and more and more fungoidal until they are mushroom-like growths, vivid scarlet or purplish in color, varying in size from that of a cherry to that of an egg, or even an orange. The body may be covered with such lesions. At first these appear and disappear alternately, but later they become more permanent, more or less confluent. Some of them break down, forming crateriform ulcers. For years the patient's general health seems unaffected, although the skin manifestations appear tempestuous; later the patient becomes weaker, cachectic and dies, usually with overt manifestations of a systemic lymphoma.

Treatment. X-ray irradiation, electron beam therapy and nitrogen mustard chemotherapy generally succeed in inducing remissions that last for several months.

Nursing Management of Patients with Hematologic Neoplasms

Supportive and protective measures are very important in the treatment of patients with the lymphomas including the correction of anemia and the control of infection, to which these patients are peculiarly subject. The instructions issued to the patient by the nurse regarding the prevention of infection can be extremely helpful in accomplishing this objective. The only effective antianemic therapy in these patients is the transfusion of whole blood or red cell concentrates. Infections are treated by chemotherapy and other auxiliary measures according to their type and location. The hemorrhagic complications of bone marrow disease, mainly due to platelet deficiency, are responsive, temporarily at least, to transfusions of fresh blood or platelet concentrates.

Relief of Symptoms. The malignant disorders under discussion are capable of producing any and all types of symptoms demanding therapeutic measures for their relief. Pain may originate in soft tissues anywhere in the body, due to the encroachment of glandular swellings that are associated with most lymphomas. If superficial and well localized, these pains may respond to simple measures, such as the application of cold compresses, but chief reliance usually must be placed on the analgesic drugs, such as codeine sulfate or phosphate in doses of 15 to 60 mg. (0.25 to 0.5 gr.); morphine sulphate, 10 to 30 mg. (0.17 to 0.5 gr.); or one of the more effective morphine substitutes, such as meperidine hydrochloride (50 to 200 mg.) or methadon hydrochloride (amidone hydrochloride), the latter being given orally in doses ranging from 2 to 10 mg. at 3- to 4-hour intervals, as required.

Respiratory difficulties that are caused by tumors in the neck and the mediastinum may be ameliorated by placing the patient in a semi-orthopneic position, oxygen inhalations being required in patients with marked obstruction of the trachea or the bronchi. Control of a distressing or intractable cough may necessitate the use of sedatives, such as codeine, Hycodan or other opiates, depending on the indications. Areas of the skin that have been exposed to x-ray irradiation may be sensitive and should be protected from unnecessary pressure or friction. If a patient complains of pruritus or exhibits excoriations, his nails should be trimmed and an antipruritic lotion, e.g., Quotane Hydrochloride, applied.

Hydration and nutrition must be furnished by parenteral routes to a considerable proportion of patients, and the value of these measures as symptomatic therapy is incalculable, especially in patients who are extremely ill. Patients suffering from abdominal lymph node enlargement are especially prone to lose their appetites completely, posing an almost insurmountable problem from the standpoint of oral feeding. Hygienic measures are mandatory in the care of these, as in all, sick patients; the details of these measures depend on the nature of the patient's problems and on the ingenuity of the nurse.

THE PATIENT WITH A BLEEDING DISORDER

Protection of the body against excessive and lethal blood loss is afforded by several mechanisms. Thus, hemorrhage from a large lacerated vessel is retarded as a result of an abrupt lowering of the arterial blood pressure, i.e., "shock," which reduces the rate of blood flow throughout the body and, therefore, reduces the rate of its escape. Further protection also may be furnished by compression of the leaking vessel by the swelling mass of blood (hematoma) surrounding the vessel. Complete and permanent sealing of the latter, however, is accomplished through the clotting of the blood which results in the production of an adherent gel-like mass, that effectively controls most types of hemorrhage. Another phenomenon of protective value, occurring before clotting, is the aggregation of platelets at the point of vascular rupture. Masses of these tiny, sticky blood elements apparently form a temporary plug at this site, mechanically impeding the escape of blood while liberating the material responsible for starting the formation of a clot precisely where a clot is needed most urgently. Finally, a factor of great importance in the prevention of bleeding is the normal resistance of blood vessels to mechanical rupture, i.e., by the pressure of blood exerted from within the vessel or traumatic pressures exerted from the outside.

Based on a disturbance of one or another of these factors—the clotting properties of the blood, the availability of platelets and the stamina of the blood vessels—a variety of disorders are encountered that are characterized by an abnormal tendency to bleed. These will be discussed in three major categories: those classed as vascular purpura, marked by the spontaneous rupture of small vessels that presumably are defective or injured; those attributable to a deficiency of platelets; and those that are related to the existence of a clotting defect.

Vascular Purpuras

Purpura is the term applied to small hemorrhages in the skin and the mucous membranes; they occur spontaneously as an isolated phenomenon or as an accompaniment of obvious disease. The smallest hemorrhages, pinhead in size, are called "petechiae," whereas larger hemorrhagic lesions are described as "ecchymoses." Both types occur as the result of vascular rupture, permitting the leakage of blood into the subcutaneous tissue of the mucous membranes. In one type, called "symptomatic" or "secondary" purpura, this bleeding is quite unrelated to any intrinsic defect of the blood vessels; certain types of bloodstream infections (e.g., meningococcemia and subacute bacterial endocarditis) exhibit this phenomenon due to direct damage to the vascular walls by the infectious agent. Another group of patients exhibiting this type of purpura are those with severe arterial hypertension and "easy bruisings," perhaps due to an abnormal degree of pressure in the fragile capillary circuits when the blood flow within these vessels is increased, as may occur as a result of a blow, exposure to heat or following the release of a tourniquet on an extremity. Other examples of vascular purpura, the mechanism of which is even more obscure, are found in cachectic individuals and in patients with uremia.

Anaphylactoid Purpura

This represents yet another type of vascular purpura, the clinical features of which are somewhat more complex and comprise a distinct entity. Among its numerous manifestations are various skin lesions, purpuric and otherwise, and episodes of arthritis, abdominal pain, hematuria, gastrointestinal hemorrhages and fever. These attacks recur for years, and each attack lasts for several weeks. The leakage of blood vessels at localized points throughout the system apparently is responsible for the principal complications of anaphylactoid purpura, the basic cause of which, however, is obscure. Generally it has been regarded as an allergic disorder. Steroid therapy often is effective.

Familial Hemorrhagic Telangiectasia

This is a hereditary disorder manifested by an abnormal tendency to bleed and become bruised. Localized aggregations of dilated capillaries may be observed in the skin and in the mucous membranes of the nose or the mouth. They also may be present in the gastric mucosa, explaining certain cases of gastrointestinal bleeding. Whether the characteristic lesions are present or absent, there may be a generalized decrease in capillary "resistance," as evidenced by the abnormal ease with which the vessels are ruptured by minor traumas. However, the precise nature of the defect is obscure, and the condition does not respond to any proved method of treatment.

Toxic Purpura

This condition has been observed after exposure to certain drugs and poisons, including aniline, certain arsenicals, Sedormid (a soporific) and snake venom. Some of these toxic cases present the features of thrombocytopenic purpura, but others are explained more readily on the basis of blood vessel damage.

Platelet-Deficiency Disorders

Thrombocytopenic Purpura

A reduction in the number of circulating platelets (thrombopenia) below a critical level (approximately 20,000 per mm.) inevitably is followed by the appearance of spontaneous hemorrhages in the skin, the mucous membranes and the internal organs and is responsible for prolonged bleeding from small lacerations on the body surface. Death may occur as a result of hemorrhage in the brain. Thrombopenia, as a complication of certain diseases, already has been discussed, e.g., in relation to toxic depression and neoplastic invasion of the bone marrow. Cases of this type are labeled "secondary thrombocytopenia."

Treatment of secondary thrombocytopenia often is not rewarded by improvement unless the basic defect can be corrected. A transient increase in circulating platelets may follow transfusions of fresh blood or platelet concentrates. Donor platelets may survive for 5 or 6 days at first, but their life expectancy is shorter after each succeeding transfusion, so that replacement therapy becomes ineffective and must be abandoned. Splenectomy is similarly without benefit in the majority of these patients, whose fundamental problem is failure of the marrow to produce platelets whether the spleen is present or absent.

Idiopathic Thrombocytopenic Purpura

This disease, like acquired hemolytic jaundice, represents a disorder of immunity. Present evidence indicates that the mechanism responsible for the platelet deficiency in these patients is based on the presence of a platelet antibody. The condition is characterized clinically by its early onset, which usually precedes puberty; its sex distribution, occurring most commonly in females; and the manner in which it progresses, its course being marked by remissions and exacerbations over periods of many years. It responds to steroid therapy and to splenectomy precisely as does acquired hemolytic jaundice. Steroids enable a patient with either disease to be subjected to splenectomy with equal impunity and equally favorable prognosis.

The role of these formed elements in the mechanism of clot formation has been well established, but whether or not the clotting defect associated with thrombocytopenia can explain all of its hemorrhagic manifestations is debatable. Most of these suggest that some abnormality of the blood vessels themselves causes a structural weakness of their walls. This "weakness" is presumed to reflect not a structural defect in the vessels themselves, but the absence of a mobile defense barrier that the platelets provide. The barrier consists of plugs and films that normally are constructed with great rapidity by platelets and form by a process of agglutination at sites where the vessel wall is lacerated or damaged by distention.

Clotting Defects

Hemophilia and Hemophilic States

The hemorrhagic disorders now to be discussed are attributable solely to defective clotting, the basis of which, in each instance, is the lack of some blood constituent that is involved specifically in the process of coagulation.

Hemophilia is a rare disorder, limited almost exclusively to males. Whenever and wherever these individuals are struck, a large bruise is apt to appear, and any small cut or scratch of the skin may result in a hemorrhage that may last for several hours or days. They may bleed to death as a result of epistaxis following a blow on the nose, or from hemorrhage of the gums following a tooth extraction. Purpuric hemorrhages of the type observed in thrombocytopenic purpura are unusual, but internal hemorrhages are common, one of the characteristic bleeding sites, for example, being the weight-bearing joints, the result of which is an ankylosing type of arthritis, one of the most constant features of this disease. Hematuria, gastrointestinal bleeding and hematoma formation between muscle groups likewise are characteristic of hemophilia. The abnormality usually manifests itself in early childhood and lasts throughout life.

Blood clotting is retarded greatly in this disease, the coagulation time being prolonged far beyond the maximal limits of normal (10 to 12 minutes), often to as long as an hour or longer. The bleeding time, measured by the duration of blood oozing from a small prick in the skin, however, is within the normal range (3 to 6 minutes), and the number of circulating platelets is likewise normal. The clotting defect is attributable to the absence of one of the plasma proteins required for normal clotting, namely one of the thromboplastin precursors, AHG (antihemophilic globulin) or PTC (plasma thromboplastin component). Its absence is an inherited abnormality that invariably is transmitted from mother to son: the inherited trait, in other words, is sex-linked. For example, if Mr. A. is a bleeder, none of his children, either his sons or daughters, will be bleeders; his sister's sons, on the other hand, may be affected. The disease is transmitted only through the women of the family.

Treatment. Definitive treatment consists of replacing the missing factor by transfusions of fresh whole blood or plasma or of intravenous injections of purified "antihemophilic globulin" extracted from normal human plasma. As a result of these procedures, the clotting time is reduced to near normal for several hours, and the hemorrhagic tendency consequently is abolished for a time. The same treatment is indicated as a prophylactic measure in these patients preparatory to any operative procedure that may be contemplated, including dental extractions. This form of replacement almost always is effective; however, hemophiliacs have been encountered who are apparently "sensitized" (i.e., produce antibodies) against the clotting factor that they lack and, therefore, are completely unresponsive to treatment, just as Rh-negative individuals, lacking the Rh factor themselves, can be sensitized by repeated transfusions of Rh-positive blood and, as a result, eliminate Rh-positive donor cells almost as rapidly as they are injected.

It rarely happens that an individual, usually an adult female, develops a condition that is precisely similar to hemophilia in all respects except for its etiology and pathogenesis. The cause of this hemophilia-like disorder is related to the production of an autoimmune antibody that has a specific neutralizing effect on thromboplastin. This development occurs spontaneously, for reasons unknown, sometimes in close relation to parturition during the postpartum period. Treatment is highly inefficient because of the destructive effect of the antibody on therapeutic agents containing antihemophilic globulin, and the prognosis is quite unpredictable. Deaths have occurred in these patients, despite massive doses of this substance and vigorous treatment with steroids.

Hypoprothrombinemia

Prothrombin, as previously discussed, likewise is essential for the clotting process. This substance is produced in the liver from one of the fat-soluble vitamins, vitamin K. Our main supply of K is synthesized by the bacteria that reside in the intestine. Normal prothrombin activity in the blood depends on adequate absorption of this vitamin from the gastrointestinal tract and on adequate liver function for its conversion. Therefore, prothrombin deficiency may arise as a result of diarrhea, from a lack of bile in the gastrointestinal tract (necessary for normal fat absorption) due to biliary tract obstruction, from a gastrointestinal disorder of any other type that interferes with the digestion or absorption of food products or as a result of liver disease. The principal manifestation of prothrombin deficiency, as observed in patients with hemophilia, is prolonged hemorrhage from blood vessels that are damaged by trauma or disease, which explains the characteristic occurrence of ecchymoses, hematuria, gastrointestinal bleeding and postoperative hemorrhages.

Dicumarol Toxicity. Dicumarol is a drug that is often employed medicinally for the express purpose of inducing a partial depression of prothrombin activity, its action blocking the conversion of vitamin K to prothrombin by the liver. Properly applied, Dicumarol therapy need never give rise to a hemorrhagic disorder but should merely inhibit, as intended, the formation of clots within blood vessels. In excessive dosage, however, it produces the complete picture of prothrombin deficiency, with consequences that often prove to be extremely dangerous.

Treatment. Hypoprothrombinemia, if due to vitamin K deficiency, responds to treatment with any of several preparations that are available for oral or parenteral administration. However, when corrective measures are urgently required, particularly in patients with liver disease or Dicumarol toxicity, the effective treatment requires the direct replacement of prothrombin by means of transfusion, purified preparations of prothrombin being unavailable as yet.

Deficiency of Prothrombin Conversion Accelerators

Hemorrhagic disorders have occurred as a result of deficiency states involving both factors responsible for accelerating the conversion of prothrombin to thrombin, i.e., the stable factor, or "serum prothrombin conversion accelerator" (SPCA) and the labile factor. The net result of such a deficiency is precisely equivalent to that caused by a lack of prothrombin itself. Treatment consists in the injection of plasma (or whole blood). Unless it can be established that the stable, rather than the labile, factor is involved, it is wise to employ fresh blood in these transfusions, since the labile compound rapidly becomes inert during storage.

Hypofibrinogenemia

Fibrinogen, the precursor of fibrin (the substance of the clot), may be deficient due to an inherited trait (congenital fibrinopenia), eclampsia or prolonged surgical procedures attended by massive hemorrhages that deplete the available supply of this factor in the circulating blood. The result, as in other clotting defects, is a hemorrhagic diathesis with uncontrollable bleeding from all sites where there is blood vessel damage, traumatic or otherwise. Effective treatment is possible by means of whole blood or plasma transfusions, or, preferably, by injections of purified fibrinogen fractionated from human plasma.

Fibrinolysis. A phenomenon in which clots form and then spontaneously dissolve, fibrinolysis is responsible for a serious hemorrhagic disorder, one clinically identical with that of fibrinogen deficiency, which, in effect, this is. Its occurrence, fortunately rare, is observed in the course of prolonged surgical operations in patients who have severe blood loss and have experienced oligemic shock or following trauma. Solution of the clot is due to the action of a proteolytic enzyme, "plasmin," a normal blood constituent, the enzymatic properties of which normally are held in check and never released except under certain circumstances, when efficient removal of thrombi or hematoma obviously requires the liquidation of fibrin. However, in this hemorrhagic disorder plasmin activity, instead of being confined to a restricted area, extends throughout the body. The only treatment of possible avail is the intravenous injection of large quantities of concentrated fibrinogen, since whole blood or plasma cannot possibly be administered in sufficient quantities or with sufficient speed to compensate for its rapid destruction by the abnormal enzymatic activity.

SPLENECTOMY

The spleen, the largest lymphoid organ in the body, is situated in the upper left portion of the abdomen under the diaphragm. It becomes of interest surgically when it is injured or diseased. Not infrequently splenic rupture is produced with severe injury to the left loin and the upper left abdomen. In such patients, rapid hemorrhage from the highly vascular organ makes splenectomy necessary. In hemolytic jaundice and in some other diseases of the blood (purpura, splenic anemia, leukemia and so forth, removal of the spleen often is of value as a therapeutic measure.

Splenectomy is not a difficult operation when the spleen is small but, when the organ is hypertrophied and surrounded by many adhesions, its removal is more difficult. Hemorrhage and abdominal distention are the most frequent postoperative complications. The nursing care of such patients is the same as for those who have undergone laparotomy. It should be remembered that surgery for disease of the spleen is fraught with much danger because of the serious associated diseases of the liver and the blood. Rupture of the spleen is associated frequently with other severe injuries that increase the gravity of the case. After splenectomy, the majority of patients have a constant temperature that at times is as high as 38.3° C. (101° F.) for ten days or so. Occasionally deficient wound healing and dehiscence of the wound follow the operation.

Enlarged spleen (splenomegaly) often causes such discomfort or disability as to justify its removal. In these patients a snugly fitted abdominal binder helps to prevent postoperative overdistention of the stomach and the intestines. Prostigmine or Pitressin administered hypodermically is of value in this connection.

BIBLIOGRAPHY

Crosby, W. H. (ed.): Hematologic disorders. Med. Clin. N. Amer., 50: Nov., 1966.
Crosby, W. H.: Iron and Anemia, Disease-A-Month (January, 1966). Chicago, Yearbook Medical Publishers, 1966.
Dacie, J. V., et al.: Haemolytic Anemias. Seminars in Hematology. Vol. VI, No. 2, 1969.
Gardiner, F. H., et al.: Polycythemia. Seminars in Hematology. Vol. III, No. 3, 1966.
Geller, W.: Hodgkin's disease. Med. Clin. N. Amer., 50:819-832, May, 1966.
Gurski, B. M.: Rationale of nursing care for patients with blood dyscrasias. Nurs. Clin. N. Amer., 1:23-30, March, 1966.
Hall, C. A.: The Blood in Disease. Philadelphia, Lippincott, 1968.
Herbert, V.: The Megaloblastic Anemias, Disease-A-Month (August, 1965). Chicago, Yearbook Medical Publishers, 1965.
Jacobs, M.: Malignant Lymphomas and their Management. New York, Springer, 1968.
Krakoff, I. H.: The management of myeloproliferative disorders. Med. Clin. N. Amer., 50:803-817, May, 1966.
Leavell, B. S. and Thorup, O. A.: Fundamentals of Clinical Hematology. Philadelphia, Saunders, 1966.
Lunceford, J. L.: Leukemia. Nurs. Clin. N. Amer., 2:635-647, Dec., 1967.
Mollison, P. L.: Blood Transfusion in Clinical Practice. 4th ed. Philadelphia, Davis, 1967.
Platt, W. R.: Color Atlas and Textbook of Hematology. Philadelphia, J. B. Lippincott, 1969.
Ratnoff, O. D.: Treatment of Hemorrhagic Disorders. New York, Hoeber, 1968.
Zarafonetis, C. J. D.: Proceedings of the International Conference on Leukemia and Lymphoma. Philadelphia, Lea and Febiger, 1968.

CHAPTER **18**

Patients with Vascular Disorders

- *Introduction to Peripheral Vascular Disease*
- *Vascular Anatomy, Physiology and Pathophysiology*
- *Assessment of Effects of Deficient Blood Supply to Tissues*
- *Therapeutic Measures to Increase Blood Supply to Tissues*
- *Management of the Patient with a Peripheral Vascular Problem*
- *Patients with Disorders of the Veins*
- *Patients with Diseases of the Arteries*
- *Patients with Lymphatic Conditions*

INTRODUCTION TO PERIPHERAL VASCULAR DISEASE

Peripheral vascular diseases include all conditions that affect the circulatory system excluding the heart. In particular, these include problems of the arteries, veins, lymphatic system and tissues directly affected. (Conditions of the great or major vessels are discussed in Chap. 19.) Anatomically it is fairly easy to identify the circulatory system and consider it separately; however, physiologically this major network of vessels cannot be considered alone because it operates interdependently with the rest of the body. Likewise, any peripheral vascular problem that an individual may have cannot be considered by itself but must be treated and understood in its complex association with the whole person.

Prevention of vascular problems must be considered when caring for all persons, whether they are sedentary office workers, young mothers, diabetics, postoperative patients, or the "average" individual. The teaching that the nurse is obligated to do may help to prevent much suffering from chronic peripheral vascular disorders. Although there is no specific way to prevent these difficulties, much can be done to promote rather than hinder circulation.

VASCULAR ANATOMY, PHYSIOLOGY AND PATHOPHYSIOLOGY

Blood Vessels

Blood vessels are of 3 types: arteries, capillaries and veins.

Arteries. The arteries carry the blood from the left heart to all parts of the body. Their walls, necessarily thick and strong since the blood within them is under high pressure, are made up of three layers. The inner layer, the intima, is a thin membrane covered by a single layer of flat endothelial cells and provides a surface suitable for contact with the flowing blood. The middle layer, the media, on which the strength and caliber of the vessel depend, is a thick strong coat made up of muscle fibers mingled with strands and sheets of strong elastic tissue. The outside coat, the adventitia, is a thick layer of connective tissue that binds the artery to the structures through which it courses.

Capillaries. As the artery, by dividing, becomes smaller and smaller, first the adventitia disappears, and the media becomes progressively thinner. Finally, after repeated divisions, the tiny artery, called an *arteriole*, breaks up into a group of tiny tubes with walls composed of a single layer of cells. Such a vessel

Fig. 18-1. Schematic drawing of systemic circulation. (Start at bottom of diagram.) Loaded with carbon dioxide, blood from the body capillaries goes through venules and veins into the right chamber of the heart (dark blue arrows). It is pumped into the two lungs. Having dropped carbon dioxide and picked up oxygen, it goes back to the left chamber of the heart (light blue arrows). From there it is pumped through the aorta into the body circulation (arteries and arterioles) until it reaches the body capillaries, where it gives up oxygen and picks up carbon dioxide. (National Tuberculosis and Respiratory Disease Association)

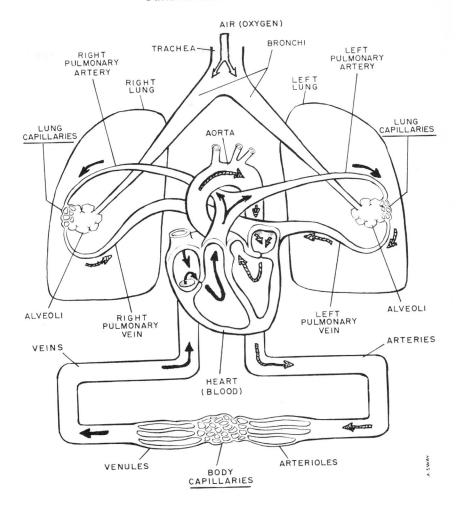

is a capillary, a tube about 1/32 inch long and just wide enough for red corpuscles to pass through in single or double file.

The nourishment and oxygen carried by the blood cannot pass through the walls of the arteries and the veins, but it can pass through those of capillaries, which consist of one layer of intimal cells. During the brief second that the blood slowly traverses the capillary, there is a quick exchange of gases and dissolved substances between the blood in this vessel and tissue lymph. In this way the tissue cells receive a fresh supply of food and oxygen and rid themselves of their special products, as well as all waste matter resulting from their cellular metabolism.

There are myriad capillaries in the tissues. Could all the capillaries in the body be joined end to end to form one single tube, it would stretch for thousands of miles. Several are in the near vicinity of each tissue cell; in fact, each actively functioning cell is literally surrounded by capillaries. Not all of the same group are open at the same time; the number of such vessels open and functioning in a given area is closely related to the needs of that area. The functioning of capillaries appears to depend on the concentration of certain cellular products in the vicinity and also on the activity of the autonomic nerve fibers, which have an important influence on their caliber.

Veins. At the distal ends of the capillaries begin the smallest veins (*venules*). These, by uniting, become larger and larger and their walls thicker although even the largest veins are relatively thin. The 3 layers are present, but the smooth muscle layer is inconspicuous compared with that in the walls of arteries of the same size; there is no need for such a heavy muscle layer because the blood within the veins is under much lower pressure. The larger veins are equipped with valves to prevent pooling and backflow of blood into areas that they drain.

The Systemic Circulation

If we trace a blood cell in its journey starting at the aortic valve, we find that when it leaves the heart it enters the aorta, passes into one of the many branches of this, thence through smaller and smaller arteries until it enters a capillary—in a muscle, for example. After passing through this capillary, it enters a small vein, whence it moves on through larger and larger veins until finally it enters the vena cava, which carries it to the right atrium of the heart, and thence into the right ventricle.

Pulmonary Circulation. From the right ventricle, the red cell then enters the pulmonary circulation. The right ventricle pumps it through the pulmonary artery into the lungs, where it passes through one of the capillaries in the wall of an alveolus and then enters a pulmonary vein, thence into the left atrium, and from this into the left ventricle, where is located the aortic valve whence it started.

Portal Circulation. Other corpuscles take a somewhat more complex route. From the aorta they enter the mesenteric arteries, and through their branches finally reach the capillaries of the intestinal wall. Passing through them they enter mesenteric veins, and then on into the portal vein, which carries them to the liver. Here they must pass through a second capillary, and then on into the hepatic vein, to the vena cava and to the right side of the heart. The journey of this second corpuscle has included a trip through the portal system.

Pathophysiology

Metabolic activity of a part of the body is accelerated (1) when that part is physically active, as occurs in exercise, (2) when heat is applied, or (3) when an infection is present. Each of these factors causes dilatation of arterioles and an increase in the blood velocity in the veins. The metabolic rate is decelerated (1) when significant cold or chilling occurs, and (2) during rest, when less demands for blood are made by tissues. With these conditions, arterioles constrict and blood flow is reduced somewhat. The usual cause of arterial insufficiency is atherosclerotic narrowing of the artery. Less often, acute thrombosis or an embolus blocks the vessel.

ASSESSMENT OF EFFECTS OF DEFICIENT BLOOD SUPPLY TO TISSUES

Local and temporary deficiency of blood to the tissues due to constriction of vessels is called *ischemia*. Each of us has experienced the effects of a constricting blood pressure cuff. In the instance of arterial blood flow ceasing with an inflated pressure cuff, pain does not occur for 3 or 4 minutes; however, if the forearm is exercised, severe muscle spasm occurs in a matter of seconds. This spasm is fairly common in impaired circulation of the legs, such as in Buerger's disease (p. 347). The man so afflicted may walk a few hundred feet and be forced to stop because of severe aching calf muscles. Rest relieves the problem, but it occurs when similar conditions are present (intermittent claudication). The degree of such claudication is measured by the distance a patient can walk before pain forces him to stop and rest. The cause of ischemic pain is unknown; however, it is relieved by supplying oxygenated blood. Some suggest that pain is caused by the accumulation of large amounts of lactic acid in the tissues; others believe that histamine or other chemicals stimulate pain nerve endings.

In addition to the pain of intermittent claudication is rest pain. This may occur as a result of thrombus or embolism causing arterial occlusion or because of severe arterial insufficiency. Metabolic or ulcerative changes and stasis may be responsible; some relief may be obtained by massage, warm compresses or placing the extremity in a dependent position. Nocturnal leg cramps is a common form of rest pain and may be relieved by taking Benadryl or quinine before retiring.

Coldness, numbness, pallor, loss of hair and trophic skin changes are also observed as a result of a deficient blood supply. Even in a warm environment, the extremity affected may feel cool to the patient and to the nurse's touch. Healthy flesh color is blanched in appearance as superficial vessels are constricted.

With a prolongation of blood impairment, skin tissue can reflect a darker reddish color suggesting damaged, dilated vessels. .This may result from injury due to cold or anoxia; it suggests impaired rather than improved circulation. Cyanosis occurs when there is a concentration of deoxygenated hemoglobin. Of course, skin pigment and skin thickness affect the degree of apparent discoloration.

Elevation of the extremity with impaired arterial circulation produces cadaveric pallor and lowering it to a dependent position thereafter is accompanied by delayed return of normal color and finally dependent rubor. The pulsations in the affected area are weak or absent and application of the oscillometer shows impaired arterial oscillations (pulsations).

Arterial insufficiency may affect any area of the body, but the most common areas are the lower extremities. Mesenteric arterial insufficiency leads to abdominal pain, especially after meals and may result in mesenteric thrombosis. Carotid artery, basilar or vertebral or cerebral artery narrowings lead to cerebral symptoms such as dizziness, blurred vision, blackouts (transient ischemic attacks) and finally to strokes (see Chap. 19).

THERAPEUTIC MEASURES TO INCREASE BLOOD SUPPLY TO TISSUES

Arterial blood supply to a part can be enhanced when that part is lower than the level of the heart. For the lower extremities, this can be accomplished by elevating the head of the bed or allowing the patient to be in a sitting position with his feet resting on the floor. To promote circulation, particular exercises including walking may be recommended.

Postural Exercises

If postural exercises are prescribed, the patient should elevate the extremities for a minute and then place them in a dependent position until the rubor or cyanosis becomes maximal, then lie with the extremities in the horizontal position for a minute. These time intervals may be changed according to the disease, the condition of the patient and his ability to continue them. Again, it is important to emphasize that if the leg is to be elevated, the object (such as a bed cradle or an inverted chair) on which the part is resting must be padded to prevent injury to the limb.

The Oscillating Bed. A method of administering passive postural exercises to allow for the intermittent filling and emptying of capillaries, venules and arterioles is the use of the oscillating bed. The bed is set on a rocker operated by a motor so that it tilts on its long axis at regular intervals. The intervals may be adjusted according to the needs of the patient and the wishes of the physician. Proper orientation regarding the function and purpose of such a bed will assist the patient in adapting to it. The patient can be taught to operate the switch; he may stop the bed for his meals or treatments. Gradual introduction will help eliminate the discomfort of dizziness, headache or nausea. Should these occur, the motion can be stopped. This method of administering passive postural exercises may be carried out day and night. Should the patient slip downward, the feet can be protected and supported by means of a padded footboard. This device is claimed by some to have produced relief of the pain resulting from being in one position too long and of the pain associated with ulcers and gangrene. It may be used in the treatment of arteriosclerosis, thromboangiitis obliterans and, in minor degree, of arterial embolism.

Buerger-Allen Exercises. With the patient lying flat in bed, the legs are elevated above the level of the heart for 2 minutes. Then sitting on the edge of the bed with the legs dependent, he exercises the feet for 3 minutes. He then lies flat for 5 minutes. This exercise may be repeated about 5 times and performed 3 times a day. Some physicians prefer not to time the exercises, but to have the patient or nurse observe the extremity for blanching when it is elevated, then shift to the dependent position until redness appears and lastly, rest in the supine position.

Temperature Changes

Warmth. Although the application of external heat to an extremity possessing normal tissue will increase circulation, such a measure is used very cautiously with diseased tissue. By increasing tissue metabolism where the vessels are unable to function properly, further tissue destruction results. Impaired function may block sensations; this could result in a damaging burn or tissue necrosis.

Warm baths and light-weight warm clothing are effective measures to maintain a good body temperature. Heat to the abdomen of the patient lying in bed will assist in promoting warmth to the extremities.

Contrast Baths. In some instances, circulation is stimulated by the use of contrast baths. Cold water is placed in one tub and warm water in another. The temperature of the water in each tub should be prescribed by the doctor, and the tubs should be large enough to immerse both extremities at once to the middle of the leg. The feet and the legs are immersed in the water in each container alternately for one minute during a period of about 15 minutes. This procedure may be repeated 2 or 3 times a day. After the prescribed time of treatment, the feet are dried carefully and lubricated with a bland cream, such as lanolin.

Pharmacotherapy

Drug therapy consists mainly of vasodilators to dilate blood vessels and anticoagulants to lessen the tendency of the blood to coagulate. Vasodilators are given to combat vasospasm, relieve obstruction in an artery due to a thrombus, or to aid circulation when vessels are narrowed by disease, e.g., by arteriosclerosis. Anticoagulants are used in the treatment of thrombosis and prophylactically in patients who are suspected of developing thrombosis or thrombophlebitis. Antibiotics would be prescribed to combat infection.

Prevention of Vasoconstriction

Measures to prevent vasoconstriction include restricting the use of tobacco, avoiding exposure to cold, and eliminating practices such as crossing the legs, or the wearing of tight garters or clothing.

Vasodilatation may be accomplished by interrupting sympathetic impulses. The use of alcohol injections or even cutting of the nerves (sympathectomy) has been used to improve circulation in superficial vessels. Surgical measures include lumbar sympathectomy to relieve vasoconstriction to lower extremities and replacement of occluded arteries by grafts of plastic material or autogenous veins. If an arterial occlusion can be operated upon quickly, the clot may be removed surgically and the artery preserved. The technique consists of surgical "reaming out" of the narrowed vessel lumen to enhance blood flow.

NURSING INSTRUCTION AND MANAGEMENT OF THE PATIENT WITH A PERIPHERAL VASCULAR PROBLEM

Psychosocial Problems

Much of the progress made by patients with peripheral vascular conditions depends on nursing care. The problems of these individuals may appear minor compared with those of other patients, and, as a result, often they are neglected; yet they may have long histories of circulatory difficulties and are depressed and greatly in need of help.

Treatment may be a long slow process; there are frequent setbacks and this in itself can become discouraging. Usually this patient is past 50 and perhaps has other physical problems. Peripheral vascular diseases are chronic or soon become chronic. The patient may have concerns about his employment, financial insecurity, or the risk of being a burden to his family. All avenues that may be sources of worry to this person should be explored and relieved inasmuch as emotional disturbances aggravate vascular disturbances.

The patient's stay in the hospital may be reduced if the physician is convinced that someone is able to take care of him at home. Many restrictions must be observed and precautions taken as described in the following paragraphs. To be cared for adequately at home requires the nurse to teach the patient and the person responsible for his care. His special problems and needs may be relayed to the visiting nurse.

Physical Problems

Effect of Temperature. Changes in atmospheric temperature have greater effect on a patient with a vascular disease than on the healthy person. Warmth is desirable in order to provide or maintain optimal circulation to the extremities and to promote comfort. This should be achieved by warm clothing or a warm bath rather than by the use of hot water bottles, electric pads or hot baths. The effect of these physical measures may be damaging before the individual is aware of it, because of impaired nerve function. This is why it is desirable to check the temperature of the bath with the elbow before stepping into the tub. Excessive heat increases metabolism, which in turn requires oxygenated blood; perhaps this cannot be supplied because of an occlusion. Too much heat injures the poorly oxygenated tissues, and even slight physical trauma may set the stage for the development of gangrene.

Exposure to chilling must be avoided, because this can cause vasoconstriction and result in further restriction of the circulation to a diseased extremity. Therefore, in cold weather adequate clothing should be worn.

Cleanliness and Prevention of Infection. By practicing sound hygienic habits and keeping the body clean, many problems can be avoided. However, as one ages, skin and vascular changes indicate that changes in care are needed. Vigorous rubbing of the skin after a bath must be replaced by gentle rubbing or patting. Since dryness occurs more frequently, superfatted soaps with a mild detergent action are preferred over harsh soaps (see p. 631). After a warm bath, softening lotions or creams are effective when applied gently to the skin. The patient is discouraged from scratching itching areas; calamine lotion may be effective in relieving pruritis.

Care of the Feet. The nurse and the physician are responsible for instructing the patient in foot care. It must be realized that the chief objective is to protect him from foot trauma. The feet should be washed daily with neutral soap and warm water. They must be dried thoroughly, but not roughly. Lanolin or petrolatum can be used to prevent drying and cracking of the skin. Lamb's wool placed between the toes helps to prevent irritation. Woolen socks can be worn in winter and white cotton socks in warm weather. A clean pair should be available every day. Bed socks may be worn, but hot-water bottles or electric heating pads should not be used. The patient must be instructed not to use strong antiseptics, such as tincture of iodine, Lysol and so forth. Corns and calluses require expert care. The trimming of toenails is done best after a footbath; they should be trimmed straight across. The patient also should be instructed not to cross his knees when sitting. Circular garters, constricting girdles or belts are to be avoided. Any signs of blister, ingrowing toenail, infection and so forth must be reported to the physician. The older person with impaired vision may need to have someone examine his feet periodically for signs of trauma or circulatory impairment.

Walking in bare feet or stocking feet is discouraged because of the possibility of injury from a bump or splinter. Shoes should provide support, be comfortable and nonconstricting; new shoes should be broken in gradually and alternated with another pair. Leather soles are preferred to rubber soles because the latter interferes with proper ventilation. Wet or damp shoes are allowed to dry slowly on shoe trees to help retain their shape.

Prolonged standing is to be avoided. Frequent changes of position and alternating between walking and sitting will prevent stasis. Moderate exercise is desirable. Good posture is recommended for sitting, standing or lying. When sitting, the body should be upright with proper support to the back and thigh. Compression at the popliteal space constricts posterior vessels supplying the lower leg and causes stasis.

Because of the individual nature of vascular problems, it is necessary for the nurse and patient to obtain specific instruction regarding elevation of the legs. A general rule cannot be followed, but instructions need to be individualized to meet each patient's requirements.

At night, bed clothing can be loosened at the foot-end to prevent constricting the feet. A foot board will assist in maintaining proper position of the feet. A firm mattress ensures even distribution of body weight.

Maintaining Proper Nutrition. A diet high in protein is desirable to prevent tissue breakdown. Vitamins, particularly B and C, also are needed. Obesity should be avoided, inasmuch as excess weight increases congestion and affects proper functioning of the heart, which, in turn, affects circulation. Elevated blood lipids indicate that the diet should be low in saturated fat. A balanced and varied diet that maintains a desirable weight for the patient, provides less fat, more protein and a good selection of fruits and vegetables is recommended. The patient with diabetes mellitus requires special dietary care.

Dressings and Wound Care. If it is desirable to treat an extremity with moist dressings and there are no open wounds, this can be done with surgically clean gauze and solution. However, if there is an ulcer or an open infection, strict asepsis must be followed. In this case, use sterile gloves rather than attempt to change or apply dressings with forceps. The extremity must be supported adequately when bandage dressings are removed or applied. Often the surgeon débrides necrotic tissue and irrigates the wound. Petrolatum gauze or plain dressings moistened with saline at room temperature may be applied. If only some parts of an extremity are to receive moistened dressings, the best way to prevent areas from becoming wet is to apply petrolatum. A plastic wrapping can secure the dressings in place, but it should not be held in place with a constricting bandage.

Smoking. As a rule, tobacco in any form is denied these patients. Vessel spasm definitely is related to smoking. A major nursing problem is to help the physician to convince many avid smokers of the need to stop this habit. Otherwise, there is little hope for improvement of the vascular condition.

THE PATIENT WITH PERIPHERAL VASCULAR PROBLEMS

Objectives and Principles of Medical and Nursing Management

SYMPTOMS

Intermittent claudication
Differences in skin temperature, size and color of the extremity
Tingling and numbness of toes
Trophic changes

THE PROBLEM

1. Peripheral arterial insufficiency of the extremities represents only one part of the disease that affects other parts of the body.
2. A patient's arteriosclerosis is usually advanced before his symptoms become apparent.
3. The end-result of uncontrolled circulatory impairment is gangrene.

MANAGEMENT AND THERAPEUTIC GOALS

I. To remove all vasoconstricting factors:
  A. Encourage the patient to abstain completely from tobacco.
  B. Instruct the patient to avoid wearing circular garters and constricting girdles or belts.
  C. Avoid experiences that are emotionally upsetting to the patient.
  D. Keep the patient as comfortable as possible with the prescribed analgesic drugs.

II. To increase peripheral blood flow to the extremities:
  A. The patient should sleep with the head of the bed elevated.
  B. Encourage the patient to take warm baths.
  C. Teach the patient that heat to the feet by means other than warm clothing is contraindicated.
  D. Give vasodilating drugs as ordered.
  E. Increase collateral circulation:
    1. Engage in passive and active exercises as indicated.
    2. Progressively increase walking time.

III. To decrease the metabolic demands of the body; it is necessary for the patient to:
  A. Prevent injury and infection.
  B. Learn hygienic care of his feet.
  C. Remain on bed rest if ulceration or gangrene is present.
  D. Avoid exposure to cold.
  E. Reduce physical activity to allowed limits.

IV. To prepare for surgical procedures that will increase circulation (when indicated):
  A. Sympathectomy.
  B. Bypass graft procedures.
  C. Thrombo-endarterectomy.

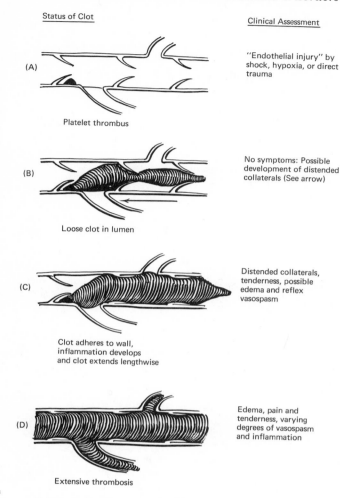

Status of Clot

(A)

Platelet thrombus

(B)

Loose clot in lumen

(C)

Clot adheres to wall,
inflammation develops
and clot extends lengthwise

(D)

Extensive thrombosis

Clinical Assessment

"Endothelial injury" by
shock, hypoxia, or direct
trauma

No symptoms: Possible
development of distended
collaterals (See arrow)

Distended collaterals,
tenderness, possible
edema and reflex
vasospasm

Edema, pain and
tenderness, varying
degrees of vasospasm
and inflammation

Fig. 18-2. Deep venous thrombosis showing parallel development of pathologic conditions and clinical symptoms. (Adapted from Barker, W. F.: Surgical treatment of Peripheral Vascular Disease. New York, McGraw-Hill, 1962)

PATIENTS WITH DISORDERS OF THE VEINS

Pathophysiology: Thrombus, Thrombosis, Embolism

A *thrombus* is a blood clot formed within the lumen of a blood vessel, which it partly or completely closes (Fig. 18-2). If it occurs on the wall of one of the cavities of the heart it is called a mural thrombus. The vessel thus occluded is said to be thrombosed, and the condition is called *thrombosis*. It is believed that the blood will not clot spontaneously within a vessel unless the intimal surface has sustained some damage. The intima may be injured by trauma, degenerated by arteriosclerotic changes or inflamed. Inflammation may result from direct infection. On the spot of injured intima, platelets first collect (Fig. 18-2). These disintegrate and liberate substances that cause fibrin formation, which entangles the blood cells and causes a thrombus. A thrombus is likely to form at the infected point; also, thrombosis not due to infection often is the reason for the development of secondary phlebitis where previously there had been none.

An *embolus* is usually a thrombus or a fragment of a thrombus that breaks away from the point where it formed, is swept on in the bloodstream through the arteries, comes to one too small for it to pass through and plugs it tightly. This process is called *embolism*. The majority of emboli are fragments of thrombi formed on the walls of the cavities of the heart and on the edges of the heart valve. Others are fragments of thrombi in veins, especially from thrombi laden with germs, as in cases of infectious phlebitis. An embolus from a vein or from the right heart may travel to the lungs and occlude a branch of the pulmonary artery; an embolus from a pulmonary vein may occlude the left heart; and an embolus from a large artery will plug a small systemic artery. Where the embolus stops, it again becomes a thrombus. Apart from thrombi, emboli may consist of bubbles of air (air embolism), plugs of fat (fat embolism) or, in short, any foreign body in the bloodstream.

The effects of embolism depend on what vessel is closed and on what tissues become deprived of their blood supply.

There are two types of arteries: those that communicate (anastomose) with some of the finer branches of nearby arteries, and those that do not, the latter termed end-arteries. If an end-artery becomes plugged, all circulation along that channel stops, and the tissue that that artery feeds becomes necrotic. But if the vessel closed is not an end-artery, then when it is closed, the arteries that anastomose with it will send blood through the communicating branches into the artery beyond the obstruction, and so keep alive the tissues that the closed artery formerly fed. The small anastomosing arteries at once begin to grow larger and larger until they are able to carry all the blood necessary. Then we say a sufficient collateral arterial circulation has been established.

Phlebothrombosis (Postoperative)

It is not unusual for a nurse to have a patient who during his convalescence complains of pain in the calf of the leg that is aggravated when the foot is dorsiflexed (Homan's sign). She must be aware of the fact that this may be a symptom of *phlebothrombosis*, and that, to avoid dislodging a thrombus, she should not massage the part. She should keep the patient in bed and notify the physician.

When a ligation is to be done or a clot is to be removed, the nurse must know what area or areas are to be prepared. A common method employed by some surgeons to indicate the site is to make an X on the skin with an applicator stick dipped in methylene blue. For a femoral ligation, the inguinal and, possibly, the pubic areas should be shaved on the side that is affected.

Prevention

The use of anticoagulant drugs for the prevention of thromboembolic diseases or to limit their extension if already present, has been discussed. The importance of early ambulation and systematic exercises for the patient at bed rest, as a means of avoiding venous stasis in the lower extremities, has been emphasized.

Deep-breathing exercises are beneficial, as they produce in the thorax increased negative pressure, which assists in emptying the large veins.

One further approach to prophylaxis is the use of elastic stockings, which are prescribed for patients on a regimen of restricted activity, particularly those who are confined to bed. These stockings, by exerting a sustained, evenly distributed pressure over the entire surface of the calves, reduce the caliber of the superficial veins of the lower extremities, with the results that deeper venous blood flow is speeded and any tendency toward stagnation or pooling of blood in that area is reduced or abolished. It is important for the nurse to note that any type of stocking, including the elastic type, can be converted into a tourniquet if applied incorrectly, i.e., rolled tightly at the top, and consequently produce stasis instead of reducing it. Obviously, this must be avoided, and the nurse must satisfy herself that her patients so understand.

These stockings should be removed for a brief interval at least twice daily. While they are off, the nurse should inspect the skin for signs of irritation and examine the calves for possible tenderness. If any skin changes or signs of tenderness are observed, these should be reported at once.

Phlebitis and Thrombophlebitis

Inflammation of the walls of veins (*phlebitis*) occurs following direct injuries (such as a perforating wound or a bruise) to a vein, as an extension of an infection of the tissues surrounding the vessel, as a result of continuous pressure against the vein by a tumor or aneurysm, and as a common complication of varicose veins. The condition is apt to arise in circumstances that promote stasis in the leg veins. Thus, it is not an uncommon complication of late pregnancy and should be anticipated in all patients who must be in bed for a prolonged period. For each bedfast patient, whether postoperative, postpartum or ill with any condition that significantly reduces muscular movement, provision must be made for adequate venous drainage from the lower extremities, whether by active or passive leg exercises or by postural changes.

Phlebitis may occur after unusual activity in a person used to a sedentary life, or even without apparent cause. It is probable that stagnation of venous blood resulting from infrequent movement of the muscles may be a causal factor. It is for this reason that people are urged to move about intermittently when sitting for long periods of time, as when riding in a car or plane or when watching television. The simple act of walking contracts muscles that press upon veins to empty them, and so start up venous circulation and prevent venous stasis.

Thrombophlebitis is the term applied to the condition in which a clot forms in a vein, either secondary to phlebitis or due to partial obstruction of the vein. The danger in this situation is that the clot, or a portion of it, may become detached and be swept into the pulmonary circulation, producing embolism.

Phlebitis and thrombosis occur most often in the veins of the leg, but also occur in veins of the femoral pelvis, and less often in other areas of the body. The symptoms may be minimal, consisting of stiffness and soreness in the calf, progressing to swelling (edema), which may become quite marked in some cases. Pain in the upper posterior calf on dorsiflexion of the foot with the knee extended or slightly flexed is referred to as *Homan's sign*. At times, it is confused with sore musculature that results from wearing flat-heeled slippers postoperatively.

When the veins under the skin are involved, the area is red, hot and tender. There is usually a slight elevation of temperature and pulse rate; in fact, this finding may be the first to draw attention to the possibility of a phlebitis in a postoperative patient.

Medical and Nursing Management

In spite of the complaint of aching or stiffness in the calf, the nurse must avoid rubbing or massage of the part, because of the danger of breaking off a piece of clot to form an embolus. In most instances, the patient is put to bed with the leg elevated. Since there are differences of medical opinion regarding elevation of the extremity and the extent of activity allowed, it is necessary for the nurse to clarify these matters with the patient's physician. Arguments in favor of elevation point to the reduction of venous congestion and edema, whereas others are fearful that the greatest risk when a leg is elevated is the possible release of emboli.

Often heat is applied to the affected area in the form of hot wet dressings or a heat cradle. Antibiotics are not usually given, because there is little evidence that phlebitis is due to an infection. On the other hand, anticoagulants such as heparin are given to prevent further growth of the clot in the vein. Since growth of the clot often produces a thrombus that floats free in the lumen of the vein and that can be easily broken off, depression of the blood's tendency to clot is a method of decreasing the probability of embolism. As a rule, bed rest is enforced until the swelling, pain and soreness are gone for several days.

Anticoagulant Therapy. Anticoagulant therapy is used almost routinely in these patients, the administration of both heparin and Dicumarol being started at the earliest possible moment after the thrombotic process is discovered. Heparin or Dicumarol may be given with the object of delaying clotting of the blood, both as a preventive measure in postoperative patients and to forestall the extension of a thrombus once it has formed.

Measures for the prevention or reduction of blood clotting within the vascular system are indicated in patients with thrombophlebitis, pulmonary embolism, coronary thrombosis and, in fact, for any active thrombotic or embolic process. The usual treatment consists of the administration, singly or in combination, of heparin or Dicumarol, which reduces the normal activity of the clotting mechanism. Heparin interferes with the clotting reaction at many points, but primarily it acts as an antagonist to thrombin; Dicumarol blocks the formation of prothrombin from vitamin K, a conversion normally taking place in the liver.

As a therapeutic agent, each of these drugs has its advantages and disadvantages. Heparin is prompt and predictable in its effects but requires an injection technique for its administration. Dicumarol, on the other hand, although far more economical in expense and effort and suitable for oral administration, frequently is disadvantageous because of the prolonged lag period (2 to 3 days) between its ingestion and the appearance of its effect and because of the unpredictable duration of its anticoagulant action, the latter sometimes persisting for as long as 3 weeks. An alternative agent that resembles Dicumarol in its effect on prothrombin formation but achieves this effect more rapidly and is more amenable to close regulation is phenindione or Hedulin.

Patients to be "heparinized" first are tested for clotting efficiency by a determination of the clotting time. Heparin then is injected, preferably by the intramuscular route, in a dosage of 50 to 100 mg. Four hours later the clotting time is determined again; if it is prolonged, the test is repeated after 2 hours. If no residual heparin effect is demonstrable at that time, the

initial dose is considered suitable for continued repetition at intervals of 6 hours thereafter. If, on the other hand, no clotting delay is discovered 4 hours after the initial injection, a larger quantity of the drug is given promptly; the effectiveness of this, from the standpoint of duration, again is tested as described above. This measure of "heparin tolerance" is repeated until the proper dosage is established, e.g., one that maintains a prolonged clotting time for a 5- to 6-hour period and permits, therefore, a convenient scheduling of injections.

Dicumarol is given orally in an initial dose of 200 to 300 mg., the patient previously having been tested for prothrombin activity by a measurement of the prothrombin clotting time. A second dose, somewhat smaller, is given on the following day. Subsequent doses are adjusted on the basis of daily prothrombin determinations, the average dosage requirement being from 50 to 100 mg. per day.

The principal complication of anticoagulant therapy with either drug is the occurrence of spontaneous bleeding anywhere in the body. The earliest evidence of such a predisposition is obtained on routine examination of the urine, evidence of bleeding from the kidneys (microscopic hematuria) being one of the first signs of danger. The effects of heparin can be abolished very promptly by the intravenous injection of protamine sulfate, the dosage of which should be approximately double that of the heparin given on the previous dose. The elimination of Dicumarol or Hedulin activity is relatively more difficult and will continue to be so until purified injectable human prothrombin is available generally. The most effective measure is the transfusion of fresh whole blood or plasma. Vitamin K_1 (Mephyton) is also capable of restoring the prothrombin activity to normal.

Surgical Management. Although anticoagulants and prophylaxis (ambulation and elastic stockings) are the first line of defense against phlebitis and venous embolism, there are times when surgery is required in the management of these patients.

The surgical approach is necessary when (1) the patient cannot be given anticoagulants; (2) the danger of pulmonary embolism is extreme; (3) the venous drainage is so severely compromised that permanent limb damage will probably result; and (4) rarely, to remove life-threatening pulmonary emboli already present.

In those patients (groups 1 and 2 above) in whom pulmonary emboli are to be prevented, venous interruption is performed. Most commonly, the inferior vena cava is ligated or plicated (narrowed from one large channel to 3 or 4 small channels—usually by a Teflon clip) but, in some cases, the femoral veins may be ligated. These procedures prevent large clots from traveling to the lung and causing blockade of the pulmonary artery.

In those patients with severely compromised venous drainage (group 3), venous thrombectomy is performed. This can be accomplished by incising the vein (usually the femoral) and passing specially designed balloon catheters (Fogarty thrombectomy catheters) in both directions. The catheter is initially passed with the balloon deflated; when it is properly situated, the balloon is inflated and the catheter withdrawn. This pulls the clot in the vessel to the place where the vein has been incised and it can easily be removed. The vein is then closed by suture. This procedure can be done under local anesthesia.

Following a thrombectomy, the patient's limb is bandaged with a 4-inch elastic bandage extending from the metatarsal heads to below the knee, and then a 6-inch bandage continues to midthigh. In order to maintain a plane elevation above-the-heart for the legs between the knee and toes, the foot of the bed is elevated 6 inches. Ambulation begins the first or second postoperative day as determined by the comfort of the patient. Heparin therapy is initiated on the day of surgery and later followed by warfarin sodium. The continuation of the latter depends upon the patient's needs. He may require it for 3 months or be on the medication indefinitely. The elastic support may be discarded while the patient is still in the hospital if the thrombectomy has been complete; otherwise, if there is residual swelling, a heavy-weight elastic stocking is fitted. The first pair may be thigh-length and later a below-the-knee stocking may be sufficient.

Finally, those patients who already have *life-threatening* pulmonary emboli (group 4) may have a pulmonary embolectomy performed. Cardiopulmonary bypass is necessary since the main pulmonary artery must be opened to remove emboli from both the right and left pulmonary arteries.

Postphlebitic Syndrome

Recovery from an attack of phlebitis is not always a complete cure. Because the main channel for the return of blood from the leg to the heart has been blocked by the thrombus, smaller vessels dilate, especially the long superficial saphenous vein, to take up the burden of the increased venous flow in them. The clot in the vein that was the original site of the phlebitis gradually reduces in size, so that blood can flow around the clot (channelization of the clot). However, as a result of the phlebitis, the valves of the veins become diseased and no longer can prevent back-flow in them. This results in chronic venous stasis, with swelling and edema, and a further difficulty, viz., varicose superficial veins. The lower leg becomes discolored due to venous stasis and pigmentation, and

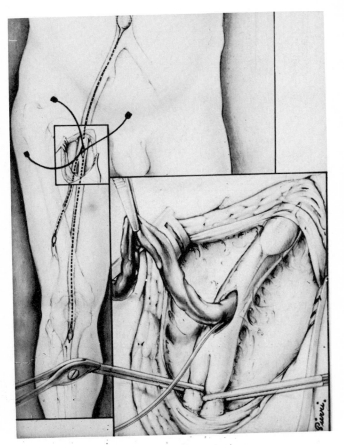

FIG. 18-3. The larger diagram shows the positioning of 3 Fogarty catheters in the femoral artery. (A Fogarty catheter is especially designed with an inflatable balloon at its tip.) Following positioning, the catheter is carefully inflated and gradually withdrawn as it pushes the clot toward the incisional opening. In the enlarged diagram at the left, the surgeon has grasped the clot with an instrument and the inflated balloon is approaching the incisional exit. (Edwards Laboratories, Inc.)

there frequently develops an ulceration on the inner side of the leg, just above the ankle. This type of ulcer is really a stasis ulcer, but a large part of the stasis is due to the phlebitis, and such ulcers are called *postphlebitic ulcers*. They differ from the common "varicose ulcer" only in the fact that the venous stasis results from disease of the deep veins, and not wholly from the dilated varicose superficial veins (see p. 341).

Postphlebitic syndrome results in a chronic venous stasis with associated changes: discoloration, swelling, ulceration, pain, venous congestion and recurrent thromboses. The treatment of this type of venous stasis is much more difficult than that resulting from vari-

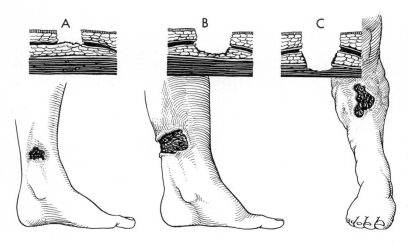

Fig. 18-4. Common types of leg ulcers and their relative depth of penetration. (A) Varicose ulcer. Ulcers are usually shallow; regional changes may not be marked. Varicosities are prominent. (B) Postphlebitic ulcer. Ulcers may be deep, irregular and extensive. Local skin changes consist of edema, induration and pigmentation. Varicosities may or may not be present. (C) Arteriosclerotic ulcer. Ulcers are deep, irregular and usually located over the tibial area. Associated changes are due to arterial insufficiency rather than to venous stagnation. (Gius, J. A.: Fundamentals of General Surgery. ed. 3. Chicago, Yearbook Medical Publishers, 1966)

cosities of only the superficial veins. In some patients there may be no superficial venous enlargement visible or palpable.

Much depends on which veins are affected and the extent of the problem. Gravity imposes overwhelming stress on the postphlebitic system. With increased pressure and stagnant blood in the dependent channels, edema results. Fibrosis follows each bout of edema. In addition, cutaneous reaction to chronic venous hypertension becomes critical. Itching, skin cracking, microscopic superficial infections, and reactions to medicaments used in treating the skin problem result. There is increasing pigmentation and the skin begins to atrophy and becomes susceptible to injury.

Various measures have been suggested in the attempt to remove the venous stasis. These include ligation of the superficial femoral veins and ligation of the saphenous (long and short), if these are varicosed. Most often a more conservative method of therapy is applied, consisting largely of methods to prevent venous stasis by providing external pressure and gravity drainage of venous blood. In order to impress the patient with the necessity for thwarting venous stasis and swelling of the legs, certain rules have been suggested for the patient with phlebitis. These are:

(1) Prevent edema by wearing elastic stockings. Details of care have been described on p. 333.

(2) Mere standing or sitting produces increased venous stasis; therefore, some slight exercise should be attempted, such as walking, moving the toes in the shoes, etc. During the year following the attack of phlebitis, the legs should be elevated to a horizontal position on a chair at least 5 minutes out of every 2 hours.

(3) At least 2 or 3 times a day the legs should be elevated above the head by lying down. With the leg elevated on the back of a sofa or even against the wall while the patient is lying on his back, the venous blood is drained by gravity from the part. Whenever possible, the leg should be elevated on another chair when sitting down.

(4) At night, the foot of the bed should be elevated 6 or 8 inches to permit venous drainage by gravity to take place.

(5) Patients with irritation of the skin of the leg should apply bland, oily lotions to prevent scaling and dryness.

(6) Constricting bandages and indiscriminate use of tourniquets must be avoided.

(7) Finally, the patient should be careful to avoid all trauma, bruising, scratching or other forms of injury to the skin of the leg and the foot.

If these suggestions are carried out repeatedly, it is possible to avoid many of the complications that otherwise appear in the postphlebitic leg.

Leg Ulcer

The evidence of chronic leg ulcers continues to increase simply because the age group in which they are found is increasing. It is estimated that of all leg ulcers, postphlebitic and varicose ulcers (see Fig. 18-4) account for about 70 per cent; the remaining 30 per cent are of nonvenous origin such as those caused by burns, sickle-cell anemia and neurogenic disorders. Of the 70 per cent, about three-quarters are postphlebitic. Diabetic patients are prone to develop arterial vascular insufficiency and leg ulcers.

The nursing challenge in caring for these persons is great whether the older person is in the hospital or at home. The physical problem is often long-term and causes substantial drain on the patient's physical, emotional and economic resources.

Because there are many causes of ulcers, it is important that a proper causative diagnosis be made so that the proper therapy can be prescribed. A diagnostic aid used by some physicians is *phlebography*. A radi-

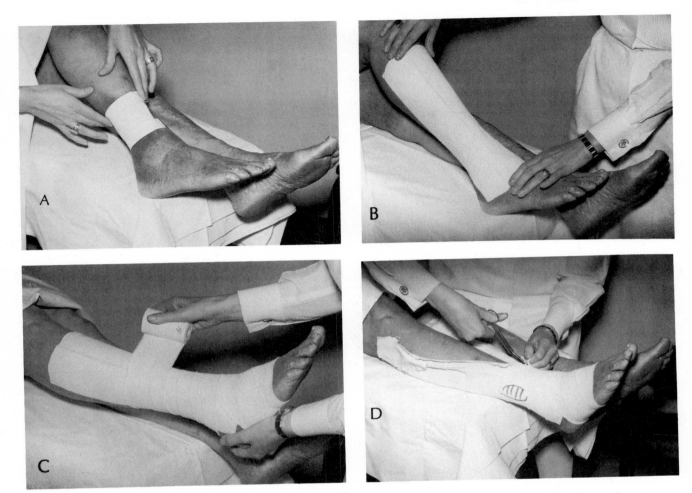

FIG. 18-5. Elastoplast bandage: (A) After ointment has been applied, ulcer is covered with a Telfa or other non-adherent bandage, secured with non-allergic tape if plain adhesive irritates the patient's skin. (B) Strips of Elastoplast gives support and protection. (C) Starting with a turn around foot, bandage is spiraled upward with firm, even pressure and fastened securely below knee. (D) Removing bandage after several days, nurse uses special care; even slight trauma could cause injury. (Wilson, S.: Chronic leg ulcers, Amer. J. Nurs., 67:98, Jan., 1967)

opaque substance (50 per cent Hypaque) is injected into a foot or ankle vein and forced into the deep system by a proximal tourniquet; films are taken before and after exercises. A normal phlebogram reveals an intact deep venous circulation and the presence of good valves. After exercise, the dye is cleared from the deep veins.

Therapeutic Management

Immediate objectives of therapy include (1) reduction of inflammation by proper cleansing and removal of devitalized tissue, and (2) stimulation of healing by reducing infection and providing physiological and nutritional support.

Cleansing requires very gentle handling; a mild soap, lukewarm water and cotton balls are used.

Flushing out of necrotic material can be done with hydrogen peroxide. Enzymatic débridement is helpful in reducing the amount of necrotic accumulation. Effective ointments are fibrinolysin and desoxyribonuclease, combined-Bovine (Elase) and proteolytic enzymes with neomycin (Biozyme). An ointment with neomycin and hydrocortisone (Chymar) acts as an enzyme and treats secondary infection. Other hypoallergic agents for treating infections are bacitracin ointment and tetracycline powder (Achromycin).

The surrounding skin is as important to treat as is the ulcer. If the area is inflamed and oozing, sterile saline compresses are effective. One clinic recommends compresses of cool normal saline for an hour twice daily. At other times, a dry gauze pad is used, on top of which sponge-rubber is placed and held with an

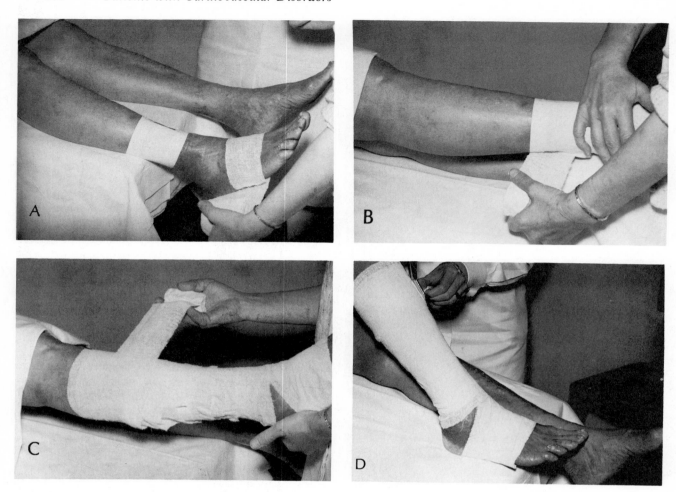

FIG. 18-6. Unna's boot: (A) Application of wet bandage (Gelocast or Dome-Paste) is begun with a circular turn around the foot. (B) Bandage goes over the protective dressing, on up to just below knee. Boot may remain in place as long as two weeks. (C) Ruffles are pressed flat with gentle downward motions. Boot is allowed to dry at room temperature. (D) Boot is removed just as any dry gauze bandage would be. It is removed at once if patient has discomfort. (Wilson, S.: Chronic leg ulcers, Amer. J. Nurs., 67:99, Jan., 1967)

elastic bandage (Fig. 18-5). For the home patient unable to do this, a Gelocast boot (Unna paste) may be applied and changed in the physician's office twice weekly (Fig. 18-6). (Also see p. 341.)

Gold leaf may be used directly over the ulcer site because it appears to stimulate the formation of granulation tissue. The very thin gold leaf is packaged in a small booklet and is of the type used for application on glass. It adheres by electrostatic attraction. Every 2 to 4 days, it is replaced after the area has been thoroughly cleansed.

If a relatively small venous ulcer does not heal during ambulatory conservative treatment in a reasonable period of time, radical excision with skin grafting may be considered.

The value of nursing care is not to be underestimated with these patients. There is a strong tendency for the patient at home to try different medications in his attempt to treat the "sore." Teaching and proper guidance are necessary to point out the pitfalls of such practice and to urge the patients to follow the instructions of a physician. Patience and conscientious care may be required over a long period of time. Then when the ulcer finally heals, the problem of maintaining healthy tissue is another real challenge.

Varicose Veins

The Problem, Its Incidence and Symptoms

Varicose veins (varicosities) are abnormally dilated veins. Most commonly this condition occurs in the lower extremities or the lower trunk; however, it can occur elsewhere in the body, e.g., esophageal varices (p. 523). The blood flow in the veins is directed

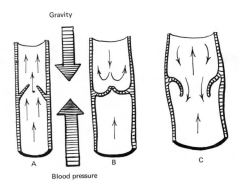

FIG. 18-7. (A, B) *Competent* valves allow blood to flow against gravity. (C) With faulty or *incompetent* valves, the blood is unable to move toward the heart.

toward the heart and its flow in the reverse direction is prevented by a series of cup-shaped valves (Fig. 18-7). A deficiency of these valves may be produced by disease, as in phlebitis, or by long-standing distension due to back pressure on the veins, as in pregnancy, obesity, or prolonged standing. A hereditary weakness of the vein wall may also contribute to the difficulty.

It is estimated that of persons over the age of 40, one-half of all women and one-fourth of all men have varicose veins. Occupation may be a factor in that the incidence of this problem is higher in sales people, barbers, beauticians, elevator operators, nurses, and dentists than in individuals who sit most of the day. However, sit-down workers need to walk at periodic intervals to prevent stasis in the lower leg.

The veins most commonly affected in the lower extremities lie in the subcutaneous fatty tissues, especially the long saphenous vein. The dilatation of this vein produces a venous stasis with secondary edema, replacement fibrosis in the subcutaneous fatty tissue, pigmentation of the skin and, because of these changes, a lowered resistance to infection and to trauma. The symptoms produced most often are disfigurement due to the large size of the vein, easy fatigue of the part, a heavy feeling, cramps in the legs at night and, often, pain during the menstrual period. The darkened, tortuous, swollen veins are more prominent when the patient stands, and a common reason for their treatment in women is that of disfigurement which they cause. If varicose veins are untreated, the changes in the lower leg mentioned above may appear. Repeated attacks of inflammation are not uncommon and ulceration may develop.

FIG. 18-8. Trendelenburg test. (A) With the patient supine, the extremity is elevated to 65°. The veins empty by gravity. A tourniquet is applied to the thigh tight enough to constrict the superficial vein but not the deep veins. (B) With tourniquet in place, veins fill slowly from below in 20 to 30 seconds. The rate of filling is not accelerated by removal of tourniquet. This indicates that although there is some vein dilatation, the valves are competent. (C) With tourniquet in place, veins fill rapidly from below. In lower legs, "blowouts" may be evident. The rate of filling is not accelerated by tourniquet removal. This indicates that communicating veins of the lower leg are incompetent but those above are functioning normally. (D) Upon tourniquet removal, there is a rapid flow of blood down the saphenous vein. Since the veins fill rapidly from above, this indicates that the saphenofemoral valve and the valves of the superficial veins are incompetent. (Blood flow in superficial veins is completely reversed.) (E) Before tourniquet removal, the veins fill rapidly from below as in (C). After tourniquet removal, filling is accelerated from above. This indicates incompetency of saphenofemoral veins, valves, superficial veins, and valves of the communicating veins.

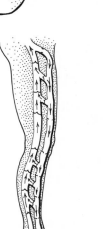
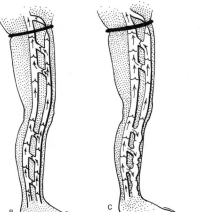
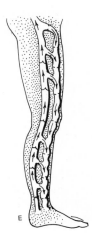

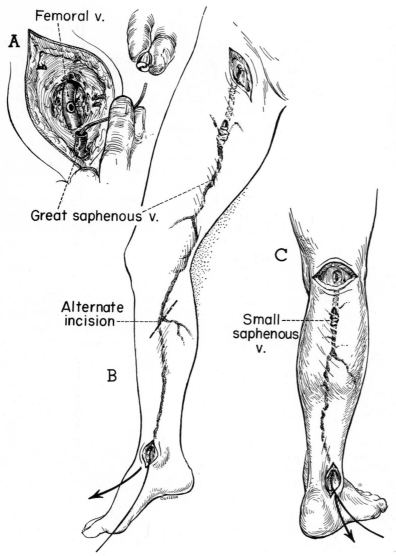

Fig. 18-9. Ligation and stripping of the great and the small saphenous veins. (A) The tributaries of the saphenous vein have been ligated, and the saphenous vein has been ligated at the saphenofemoral junction. Vein stripper has been inserted from the ankle superiorly to the groin. (B) The vein is stripped from above downward. A number of alternate incisions may be needed to remove separate varicose masses. (C) The small saphenous vein is stripped from its junction with the popliteal vein to a point posterior to the lateral malleolus. (Rhoads, *et al.*: Surgery, Principles and Practice, Ed. 4, Philadelphia, J. B. Lippincott, 1970)

Patient Assessment.

A common diagnostic test for varicose veins is the *Trendelenburg test* (Fig. 18-8). This is a test to demonstrate competence of the valves of the superficial veins and of their branches that communicate with the deep veins of the leg. With the patient lying down, the leg is elevated to empty the veins. A tourniquet is then applied about the upper thigh and the patient is asked to stand. If the valves of the communicating veins are incompetent, blood flows into the superficial vein from the deep veins; if then the tourniquet is released and blood flows rapidly from above into the superficial vein, the inference is that the valves of the superficial vein are also incompetent. This test is used to deter-

mine the type of treatment to be recommended for the varicose veins.

A test done less commonly is the *venography;* the veins are injected with a radiopaque substance and blood flow and valve action are observed by x-ray.

Prevention, Treatment and Nursing Implications

Those activities that cause venous stasis should be avoided, e.g., wearing tight garters, or a constricting girdle that obstruct venous flow, particularly when the wearer is sitting, crossing the legs at the thighs, and sitting or standing for long periods of time. Frequent changes of position, elevating the legs when they are tired, and getting up to walk several minutes of every hour promote circulation. For primary varicose veins, it may be necessary to wear support hose or elastic stockings that are specifically prescribed by the physician. The overweight patient needs to be guided in a weight-reduction plan.

In the treatment of secondary varicose veins, it is essential to remove the hydrostatic pressure of the column of blood in the veins. This can be done by a ligation of the saphenous vein in the upper part of the thigh. The procedure is considered a minor surgical one, however, the patient receives a general anesthetic.

The dilated saphenous vein with its incompetent valves is removed by a procedure called "stripping" (Fig. 18-9). A metal or plastic stripper is inserted into the lower end of the vein in the groin and is threaded down the leg toward the knee and the ankle. If the vein is not too tortuous (twisted) it may be possible to thread the stripper through the entire vein down to the ankle. In other patients the stripper may be caught in vein pockets in the thigh or the leg. An incision is made at the lowermost point of the stripper, and the end of the stripper is pulled out of the vein. By tying the vein to the stripper and pulling downward, the vein is pulled out of its location in the subcutaneous tissues. Pressure along the course of the vein is all that is necessary to control bleeding. After several incisions are made, excision of tortuous veins may be necessary in addition. The legs are dressed with gauze and elastic adhesive bandages.

Postanesthetically, the patient is encouraged to walk. He is permitted analgesics and needs the support and encouragement of the nurse. Circulation is observed to detect the possibility of hemorrhage or a dressing that may be too constricting. Posthospital instruction is given to have the patient realize that varicosities may recur and that conservative measures practiced preoperatively must be continued.

By injecting into the vein a chemical that is an irritant and that produces thrombosis, the vein lumen is obliterated. This treatment may be carried out alone for small veins or in combination with ligation or stripping. When done alone, it is usually done in the clinic or the physician's office. The patient may require support as he stands for the treatment; small dressings are applied and he is instructed not to scratch or injure the site. Sclerosing drugs are sodium tetradecyl sulfate (Sotradecol sodium), and 50 per cent glucose, 30 per cent sodium chloride and many others. Because some of these solutions may cause allergic reactions in some individuals, an antihistaminic should be available.

Varicose Ulcers

The prolonged venous stasis and edema seen in patients with varicose veins result in a gradual replacement of subcutaneous fatty tissue by fibrous tissue.

The skin becomes discolored and, on pressure, is firm and brawny. These tissues have a poor resistance to infection, so that minor trauma and abrasions result in ulcerations that tend not only to remain but to enlarge and progress. The ulcers are surrounded by an area of hard edema and frequently are characterized by a burning pain. In advanced cases, the ulcers may progress to involve the entire circumference of the leg. They are seen most often in patients who have had a previous phlebitis.

When varicose veins have progressed to ulceration, supportive therapy of some type is of value, in addition to the treatment of the veins themselves. This support may be given by elastic bandages or stockings, but can probably be accomplished best by the use of a gelatin impregnated roller bandage (Fig. 18-6, Unna's boot). A sterile dressing is laid over the ulcer. The skin from the metatarsals to the knee is painted with the paste, using a 3-inch brush; a layer of 2- or 3-inch bandage is applied, followed by more paste and more bandage until the desired thickness is obtained, usually 2 or 3 layers. After application, the patient should remain for a half hour to permit drying and to have the circulation checked. If the toes are warm, normal in color and show no signs of edema, he may be discharged. The boot is changed every 14 to 21 days. With this treatment most ulcers will heal.

The thin epithelium that eventually heals the ulcer is traumatized easily, and recurrence of ulceration is not infrequent. In many patients, a better and more permanent healing may be obtained by excision of the fibrous subcutaneous tissue and the application of skin grafts.

It is recognized that the underlying cause for the ulcer is venous stasis due to varicose veins. Therefore, after the ulcer has been "cleaned up" by appropriate treatment, a definite attack usually is made on the varicose veins, and by ligation and/or stripping, they are removed. Rapid healing of the ulcer usually takes place as soon as the venous stasis is removed.

PATIENTS WITH DISEASES OF THE ARTERIES
Arteriosclerosis and Atherosclerosis

Arteriosclerosis is a disease of the arteries producing a loss of elasticity and a hardening of the vessel wall, primarily the middle (media) layer. *Atherosclerosis* is a type of arteriosclerosis and is characterized by the formation of deposits containing cholesterol, fatty acids and other substances along the inner wall (intima) of the artery.

Arteriosclerosis is the disease that indirectly kills the majority of all men beyond middle life. Its symptoms do not arise from the diseased arteries themselves, but

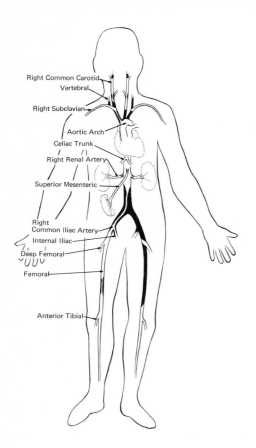

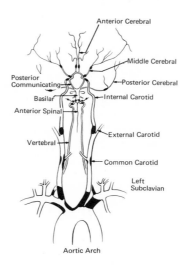

Fig. 18-10. Common sites of atherosclerotic obstruction in major arterial systems of the body. (Left, Redrawn from Crawford, E. S., and DeBakey, M. E.: Surgical treatment of occlusive cerebrovascular disease. Mod. Treat., 2:36, 1965. *Right,* Beeson, P. B., and McDermott, W.: Textbook of Medicine. Philadelphia, W. B. Saunders, 1971)

from the heart, the kidneys, the brain, etc., whose functions are disturbed because of circulatory impairment.

Pathophysiology and Etiology

The most common direct results of arteriosclerosis are the narrowing, the closure by thrombosis and the rupture of the smaller arteries. Its indirect results are malnutrition, with subsequent fibrosis of the organs that the sclerotic arteries supply with blood. All actively functioning tissue cells require an abundant supply of food and oxygen and are sensitive to any reduction in the supply of these. If such reductions are severe and permanent, these cells undergo ischemic necrosis and are replaced by fibrous tissue, which requires much less food. Hence, malnourished organs become sclerotic and, in time, since scar tissue contracts, more or less contracted. Thus arise the degenerative areas in the brain, in the heart's weak myocardium and in the small contracted kidneys.

Arteriosclerosis affects the entire arterial tree in varying degrees, with some organs developing more fibrosis than others. Since the myocardium and the kidneys furnish the most significant symptoms of this malady, the majority of patients are grouped under the term cardiovascular-renal diseases.

When the long arteries of the extremities are affected by arteriosclerosis, the blood supply may be insufficient to maintain the tissues in a viable state, and gangrene (complete death of the tissue) occurs. This change usually affects the toes and the feet. Usually gangrene is of the dry type, a mummification. Frequently, however, the gangrenous area becomes infected secondarily and produces marked systemic, as well as local, symptoms.

A moderate degree of arteriosclerosis is considered by some authorities as an inevitable consequence of the aging of the vessels, almost as normal for elderly persons as is white hair. However, this is not a fair statement of the case. Many an elderly person has soft vessels, and a few young men have marked arteriosclerosis. It commonly is associated with diabetes mellitus, chronic nephritis and arterial hypertension.

The tendency to arteriosclerosis is a definitely inheritable condition. The statement has been made that almost 70 per cent of all patients who develop this condition early in life give a history of the disease among several generations of their family. At present the factors most stressed are a hereditary tendency, metabolic disturbances and factors related to arterial hypertension.

The arteriosclerotic vessel is often characterized by the deposition of calcium in the media of the vessel wall, and therefore causes a loss of elasticity (pipe-stem vessels); but this does not necessarily produce symptoms due to an impairment of circulation because other vessels (collaterals) may provide an effective circulation. Arteriosclerosis most often affects the peripheral arteries.

Atherosclerosis on the other hand affects the large vessels of the trunk and the larger vessels of the extremities. It consists of plaque-like deposits containing fatty substances, mostly cholesterol, fatty acids, and often calcium which form in the intima or inner wall of an artery. There may be hemorrhage underneath the plaques from small vessels in the arterial wall, which pushes the deposit into the lumen of the vessel, or the rough edge of the plaque may produce a clot (thrombus) as the blood passes over it. Any one or combination of these complications may produce a gradual or sudden block in the vessel.

Research being carried out to prevent or treat atherosclerosis has been largely directed toward the diet. A diet high in fats is often associated with a high level of cholesterol in the bloodstream, and for this reason fats are restricted in the diet. The type of fat in the diet may influence the amount of cholesterol in the body. Fats are classified according to their chemical structure as *saturated* or *unsaturated*. The saturated fats are those of animal origin, such as in meat, milk, butter and eggs, as well as the solid vegetable oils. Unsaturated fats, such as corn oil, cottonseed oil, safflower oil, and the fats in fish, may be capable of reducing the blood cholesterol level. Therefore, many physicians may prescribe a diet in which unsaturated fats are substituted for saturated fats in the treatment of patients with atherosclerosis. All fats in the diet are reduced in such cases. However, these measures do not solve the problem, since it is known that cholesterol is manufactured in the body, even in the walls of the blood vessels themselves.

Certain drugs are being used to reduce the blood level of cholesterol. Among these are clofibrate, cholesytramine, dextrothyroxine and large doses of nicotinic acid. It is still too early to evaluate the long-term efficacy of these agents.

Tests Used Primarily to Determine Arterial Insufficiency

In order to assess the degree of vascular impairment produced by the arteriosclerosis, various tests are employed, depending upon the vessel under investigation.

Oscillometry. The level of arterial occlusion may be determined by the use of an oscillometer, which measures pulse volume. An inflatable cuff is wrapped about the extremity; a sensitive diaphragm transmits arterial pressure to an indicator on a dial. The units of measurement are recorded as the *oscillometric index.* Normals for these are:

Lower Extremity:	Midthigh	4-16 mm./Hg.
	Upper third of leg	3-12 mm./Hg.
	Above ankle	1-18 mm./Hg.
	Foot	0.2- 1 mm./Hg.
Upper Extremity:	Upper arm	4-16 mm./Hg.
	Elbow	3-12 mm./Hg.
	Wrist	1-10 mm./Hg.
	Hand	0.2- 2 mm./Hg.

Skin Temperature Studies. The objective skin temperature is a valuable index of circulatory function that can however, be affected by vasomotor control. For example, by placing an individual in a new environment, his hands and feet may become cold not because of arterial insufficiency, but because of vasomotor response. Significance is attached to differences noted between two extremities whether they are temperature or color variations.

Another way of measuring the amount of arterial impairment of the legs is by measuring the skin temperature. For accurate measurements the patient must be tested in a special room maintained at a constant temperature and humidity. By immersing one leg in a bath of water heated to 42° to 44° C. (107° to 112° F.), the skin temperature of the opposite leg should increase perceptibly within one half hour. If there is little temperature rise, it must be concluded that the leg vessels cannot dilate, and that vascular impairment is marked.

A simple clinical test that gives almost the same information is carried out by placing an electric heating pad on the abdomen. After a period of about 30 minutes, a skilled physician can tell by feeling the lower leg whether there has been enough vasodilation to increase the temperature of the legs; i.e., whether there is little or much vascular disease.

Angiography. Angiography is a test that gives the most definite information about the state of the vessels. This is an x-ray visualization of the vascular tree performed in the x-ray department. Renografin or Hypaque solutions are injected into the artery to be studied, and during the last few seconds of the injection, serial x-rays are taken. The test demonstrates the site of vascular blocks and the information is of great value in deciding upon the type of surgical treatment that may be attempted, e.g., if the block is short and in one vessel, a vascular shunt around the block may be worthwhile.

Angiography is not done without discomfort. At the time of injection, an intense burning sensation can be noted in the area where the injected solution extends. This lasts for only a few seconds, as the solution runs into the vessel. A second type of reaction for which the nurse must be alert is a reaction to the injected solution. Those solutions containing iodine may cause a severe allergic reaction in some patients, causing dyspnea, nausea and vomiting, sweating, rapid heart rate, and numbness of the extremities. The reaction may appear at the time of the injection, or it may be delayed for a time and appear after the patient has left the x-ray department and has returned to his room. Any such reaction should be reported at once. Usually these reactions are treated by epinephrine (Adrenalin, by injection), antihistaminic drugs, and occasionally by oxygen inhalations.

The nurse should observe the site of the dye injection for signs of local irritation (redness or swelling), which may occur if some of the dye has escaped into the surrounding tissues; or there may be a local thrombosis at the site of the arterial injection, which produces similar findings. These complications are usually treated by the application of warm moist packs.

Test to Determine Intermittent Claudication. Chronic occlusion of the arteries, particularly the lower extremities, is often determined by a test for intermittent claudication (see p. 347). At rest, the blood supply is adequate to meet tissue needs; however, after activity such as walking, running or climbing stairs, a severe cramping pain develops in the muscle groups that are not adequately supplied with blood. Upon resting, pain is relieved as soon as the metabolites are removed from the tissues and a balanced ratio of work to blood supply is restored. This is difficult to measure; some physicians ask the patient to count the number of steps he walks and record the time it takes before pain occurs. Another method is a foot-pedal device that the patient presses down, which in turn lifts a weight. Normally, this activity can be done 120 times a minute for 5 to 10 minutes before fatigue occurs. The person with chronic arterial occlusion develops pain in less than a minute.

Lumbar Sympathetic Block. A final test used to evaluate the peripheral circulation of the legs is the *lumbar sympathetic block.* In this test, a local anesthetic is injected into the retroperitoneal space, so that the sympathetic ganglionic cord that sends fibers to the leg is blocked by the anesthetic, or the solution may be injected as a spinal anesthetic, to block the sympathetic nerves that go to the legs. Since the sympathetic nerves control the tension in the muscles of the blood vessels, block of these nerves should produce vasodilation and increased temperature in the legs if the vessels are normal. Arteriosclerotic vessels are incapable of vasodilation; hence there is no, or only slight, increase in temperature in the legs. This test is often used to determine whether or not sympathectomy would be of benefit to the patient with impaired circulation of the legs.

Patient Assessment and Prognosis

Arteriosclerotic patients, as a rule, have a variety of symptoms attributable to several organ systems, as one might expect in the case of a generalized vascular disease. Of the organ systems that suffer most as a result of generalized arteriosclerosis and whose dysfunction gives rise to the most disagreeable and dangerous symptoms, five feature most prominently: the brain, the heart, the gastrointestinal tract, the kidneys and the muscles of the extremities. The proportionate involvement of each organ system varies widely from patient to patient, and the therapeutic problems to which each gives rise are discussed in detail in the sections of the book devoted to the patient with diseases of that particular system. The prognosis for the patient depends on the location of the weakest spot in his arterial tree.

Arteriosclerosis Obliterans

Arteriosclerosis obliterans is the name given to that condition in which the arteries of the leg become so blocked that they are unable to transport enough blood to the leg and foot to nourish these tissues and supply them with oxygen. As a result, symptoms appear which may be gradual in onset, consisting of skin temperature changes (coldness), decrease in size of the legs, and a change in color of the leg. Men are more frequently affected than women. A characteristic symptom is intermittent claudication (see above). Later, the patient may experience pain even at rest ("rest pain"). This usually appears at night, and the patient usually knows that getting out of bed and walking will relieve it. Excruciating cramps in the muscles of the calf and thigh are common, probably due to tissue ischemia. These are often relieved by Benadryl, 50 mg. before going to bed. Tingling and numbness of the feet and toes are common complaints. Since the blood supply is barely able to keep the tissues alive, it is not surprising that ulcers of the feet and toes develop, especially after slight trauma, even after such minor injuries as might be obtained from cutting the toenails. The nurse must be careful to avoid burns that may occur when hot water baths are used to treat the coldness of the feet.

Medical and Nursing Management

The management of the patient with arteriosclerosis must be individualized since no 2 patients are affected alike. Because this is a chronic progressive disease, medical and nursing measures are directed toward "caring" for the patient, since "curing" is not likely. Adequate nutrition is emphasized, exercise to stimulate collateral circulation is recommended and diversional activities are suggested. All along the way, encouragement and understanding must be given. Although a damaged artery cannot be repaired, nevertheless, by early treatment, the destructive processes often can be reduced, and the organ dysfunctions already created may be relieved in part. The patient should avoid strenuous or fatiguing efforts, should rest each day at noon, should retire early, take long vacations and treat all minor illnesses as serious.

When the toes and the feet are involved, preventive measures, such as practicing good foot hygiene and wearing proper shoes, should be taken. There is rarely any treatment of any value for the arteriosclerotic patient with gangrene, except removal of the gangrenous parts. In these patients it may be necessary to perform a high amputation, usually through the thigh, in order to obtain a wound that will heal (see p. 864).

Surgical Intervention

Because the ischemia produced by the arteriosclerosis of the larger vessels is associated often with a spasm of the smaller, less-involved peripheral vessels, attempts have been made to increase the peripheral circulation by dividing the sympathetic nerve supply to these vessels. This procedure, *sympathectomy*, releases the contraction of the arterioles and permits an increased peripheral blood supply.

Other types of surgery helpful to many patients with arteriosclerosis (or thromboembolism) are discussed on page 334.

The Patient Having a Sympathectomy. Sympathectomy (a severing of ganglionic nerve fibers) has been performed for several decades, but there still exists little unanimous agreement regarding indications for its use and its specific mode of action. Lumbar sympathectomy increases blood flow to the lower extremities as a result of decreased peripheral resistance from dilatation of the vascular tree distal to the popliteal artery. It is a useful adjunct in increasing blood supply to reconstructed segments after grafting or endarterectomy. Sympathectomy is also performed as an emergency treatment following severe vasospasm due to arterial embolism in a major vessel supplying an extremity, or due to freezing of an extremity.

When it is possible or desirable, procaine is injected into the ganglia to determine whether the benefits of a sympathectomy are possible.

Upper Cervical Sympathectomy. This is performed to remove the superior cervical ganglion, which then increases the blood in internal carotid thrombosis. Since a ptosis of the eye occurs as a result of the facial paralysis, this operation enhances the blood supply by way of the ophthalmic artery.

Thoracic and Cervicothoracic Sympathectomy. This is less frequently performed than lumbar sympathectomy probably because lasting improvement is not often accomplished. Primarily, it is done for vascular insufficiency in the arm. The approach may be anterior or posterior. Depending upon the individual problems, ribs may or may not be removed. The type of incision and nature of the operation determines the postoperative nursing measures to be initiated. The principles of chest surgical care are followed in the posterior approach, in which case ribs are usually removed. In the anterior cervical approach, local anesthesia may be used. Postoperative position changes from lying to sitting must be done gradually to allow for circulatory adjustment. Failure to do this may cause the patient undue dizziness.

Sympathetic denervation of the upper extremity and heart is accomplished in this procedure. Intractable angina pectoris is benefitted with this operation and the vasospasm of Raynaud's disease may be relieved.

Lumbar Sympathectomy. The incision is an oblique one, similar to an extended McBurney incision (done for appendicitis) on either or both sides of the lower abdomen. Usually the peritoneum is not entered, but a retroperitoneal muscle-splitting approach provides adequate exposure under spinal anesthesia. The desired segments of ganglia are excised. Postoperatively, the nurse observes for the appearance of neuritis, which may result from manipulation during surgery. It may occur during hospitalization, or it may be a delayed type, occurring about the tenth postoperative day. The signs of such a complication are pain in the hip, anterior thigh and medial leg area. The patient needs reassurance that the condition will remit spontaneously. He should be told to refrain from tiring activities, to develop hobby interests, and to avoid daytime naps in order to ensure night sleeping.

The patient may note a slight temperature increase in his feet and legs and perhaps a feeling of fullness. An elastic stocking offers relief. Abdominal distention due to lessened peristalsis can be relieved in the initial postoperative period with neostigmine and a flatus rectal tube. On the affected extremity, the patient will notice that his foot does not perspire.

Operations for Arteriosclerosis Obliterans. Modern methods of diagnosis (aortogram, arteriogram) have demonstrated that the disease of arteriosclerosis obliterans shows a definite tendency to involve only a segment of the arterial tree. The commonest areas that are involved are the aorta at its bifurcation, the iliac arteries, and the superficial femoral arteries. Other sites commonly involved are the popliteal artery, the coronary artery, and the cerebral vessels. The segment showing severe degeneration of the artery is often found adjacent to other segments showing only minor pathology. These facts have made it possible to treat arteriosclerosis surgically by one of several ways.

(1) The obstruction in the vessel may be removed by making an incision into the artery after clamping

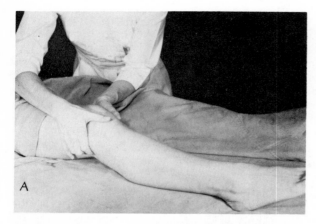

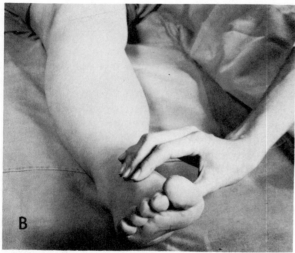

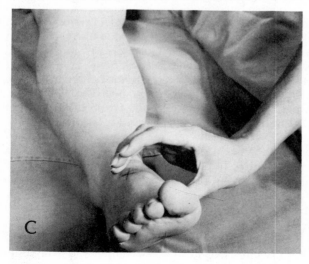

FIG. 18-11. (A) Popliteal pulse. (B, C) Pedal pulse. (From Ajemian, S.: Bypass grafting for femoral artery occlusion. Amer. J. Nurs., 67:565, March, 1967)

above and below the plug in the vessel. By the use of special instruments, it is possible to shell out the atheromatous plug, which involves the intima and part of the media. The opening in the vessel is closed with fine silk sutures. The roughened lining of the reformed vessel becomes smooth after a very short time, and circulation is restored through the previously obstructed vessel.

(2) The circulation may be restored by the use of vascular grafts. In some cases of segmental occlusion, it may be possible to cut out the degenerated segment of artery, and to suture a graft in place end-to-end to replace the excised diseased segment. More often, grafts are implanted to "bypass" the obstructed diseased segment of vessel. The bypass graft has the advantage of reducing the amount of surgical trauma because it is not necessary to remove the obstructed segment of artery. The grafts commonly employed are autogenous vein grafts, usually the saphenous vein, or prosthetic vessels of woven Dacron or Teflon yarns. The artificial vessels are becoming the preferred graft material because they serve well as substitute vessels and are easily available.

(3) Patch grafts are used to increase the lumen of small areas of narrowing in arteries. The artery is clamped above and below the short narrowed area, and is then incised in the long axis of the vessel. A patch of woven Teflon material is sewed to the edges of the incision, thus increasing the diameter of the artery with a minimum of trauma. At times a piece of vein may be used for the patch graft instead of the Teflon material. Sympathectomy is often performed in addition to the arterial surgery.

At the time of surgery, heparin solution is sometimes used to prevent clotting locally after endarterectomy, but the nurse should be alert to watch for color and temperature changes in the legs after aortic surgery, and should be taught to look for and record pulses in the feet and legs (Fig. 18-11). The disappearance of a pulse may indicate a thrombosis or obstruction of the artery by a clot, and the surgeon should be notified at once. Another complication for which the nurse should watch is paralysis of the lower extremities after operations upon the aorta. Prolonged occlusion of this vessel may produce ischemia of the spinal cord. This complication should be reported to the surgeon at once.

A further complication seen after operations on the lower aorta is the intense muscle spasm in the region of the abdominal incision. These spasms usually appear a day or two after operation and seem to be brought on by movement of the patient. The spasms usually subside in a short time if the patient lies quietly in bed. He should not be turned. Blood pressure readings should be made, but they rarely show a fall in pressure during these painful spasms, thus ruling out more serious complications at the operative site. The spasms should also be called to the attention of the surgeon.

Thromboangiitis Obliterans (Buerger's Disease)

Buerger's disease is a recurring inflammation in the arteries, veins, and adjacent nerves of the extremities, usually of the lower extremities, and results in thrombus formation and occlusion of the vessels. The cause of the condition is not known, but it is believed by many to be of bacterial origin because of the acute stages of the disease.

It occurs primarily in Jewish men between the ages of 20 and 45, and there is considerable evidence that smoking is a factor, if not in the etiology at least in the progress of the disease. As a rule, the patient appears for treatment when the disease has affected so many of the vessels of the extremity as to reduce the peripheral arterial circulation. At this point, the collateral circulation, which has been called upon more and more to take over the work of the damaged vessels, is being overtaxed. The patient complains of cramps in the legs after exercise, which are relieved by inactivity (intermittent claudication); often there is considerable burning pain that is aggravated by emotional disturbances, smoking or chilling. Frequently, the patient notices painful red lumps under the skin; these heal and move to nearby areas in a migrating fashion as the phlebitis shifts.

As the disease progresses, definite cyanosis of the part appears when it is dependent, and ulceration with gangrene occurs, especially about the nails and the toes.

Medical and Nursing Management

The main objectives of patient care are to improve circulation to the extremities, prevent the spread of the disease and protect the extremities from trauma and infection, to which they are dangerously susceptible. All attempts to help this patient end in failure if he continues to smoke; hence it is necessary to convince him of this most important facet of treatment. In addition, he should have sufficient rest and maintain adequate hydration.

Scrupulous attention to cleanliness is essential; daily washing of the feet with bland soap and warm water is desirable. After washing, the feet are dried, patted with a soft nontraumatizing towel and powdered. Clean socks or stockings should be worn each day or changed as often as necessary. The patient should massage the extremities with a bland lubricating oil each day. Circumstances predisposing to trauma and infection must be strictly avoided. Shoes and stockings should be fitted accurately, and the feet protected adequately from cold and, similarly, from the incautious exposure to heat provided by mechanical warming devices or hot water.

Caustic antiseptics, such as iodine or phenol and its derivatives, never should be applied to the feet if the peripheral circulation is inadequate, for tissue necrosis develops easily under these conditions. The patient must refrain from performing feats of minor surgery on corns and calluses. Caution must be exercised in the cutting of the toenails, which should be trimmed squarely. Circular garters and rolled stockings are to be avoided. Medical attention is indicated on the initial appearance of color changes in the feet, the development of a blister, an abrasion or infection, or changes in sensation, such as tingling, burning, numbness or pain. Vasodilators are usually prescribed.

For patients with peripheral vascular disease with intermittent claudication, exercises are prescribed that are designed to promote the development of collateral circulation in the affected limbs. These exercises involve alternate raising and lowering of the legs in timed cycles, the rate and the duration of the exercises being regulated specifically for each individual patient on the basis of changes in skin color and subjective sensations of discomfort.

It is important to remember that in no case of acute local circulatory insufficiency, whether due to an embolus or to intrinsic arterial disease, should heat be applied to the affected extremity. Heat merely increases tissue metabolism and raises the requirement for oxygenated blood, which demand cannot be fulfilled. Some clinics even pack the extremity in ice, reporting resultant relief of pain and occasional halting of a gangrenous process.

It has been found worthwhile, in many types of peripheral obliterative arterial disease involving the legs, to perform a temporary sympathetic block by injecting the lumbar sympathetic ganglia and cord with procaine (see also p. 345). The proportion of patients who respond to this abolishment of the vasoconstricting influence of the sympathetic nervous system has been striking. Cold, cyanotic, painful legs with circulation impaired as a result of arteriosclerosis, as well as by inflammatory arterial disease, occasionally have returned to a much more normal state immediately after this test procedure. If definitely favorable, a lumbar sympathectomy may be performed for a more permanent effect. In the late stages of the disease, after gangrene has appeared because of deficient circulation, amputation may be necessary. Occasionally, conservative measures may be practiced after desensitization of the part involved by injecting alcohol into the sensory nerves. However, the disease is a progressive one, and often the amputation of a single toe must be followed by amputation of another, until eventually it is necessary to amputate a foot or a leg (p. 616).

Aortic Diseases

Aortitis

Aortitis is arteritis of the aorta, its arch being particularly affected. There are two types of this disease —the arteriosclerotic and the luetic. Both cause pain, dilatation or aneurysm of this vessel and aortic-valve insufficiency.

Arteriosclerotic Aortitis

Aortitis of the arteriosclerotic type, which is only a part of general arteriosclerosis, usually appears after the age of 60. In this, the entire surface of the intima degenerates and becomes sclerosed.

Luetic Aortitis

Luetic aortitis, unlike the arteriosclerotic type, usually begins before the age of 50. It starts at the root

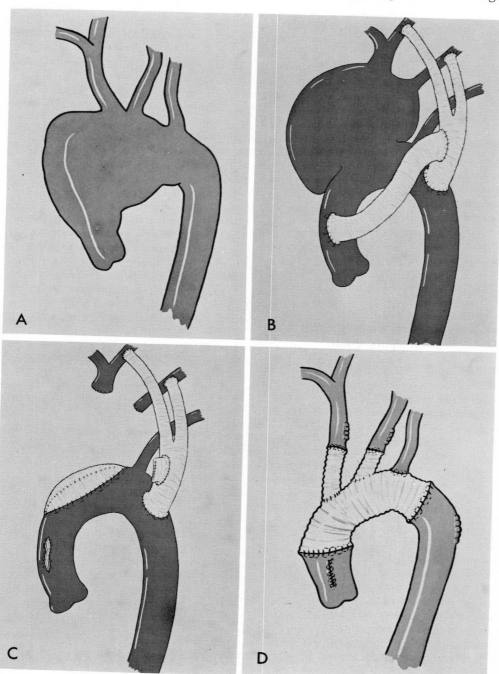

Fig. 18-12. (A) Location and extent of aortic aneurysm. (B) Method of treatment utilizing temporary bypass graft to maintain normal aortic circulation during excision of aneurysm. (C) Completed procedure with patch graft angioplasty to repair excised segment of aortic arch and conversion of temporary bypass graft to innominate and left common carotid arteries into the permanent graft. (D) Temporary bypass grafts used to maintain normal aortic circulation during excision and graft replacement of aneurysm has been completely removed and aortic graft inserted. (De-Bakey, M. E.: Changing concepts in vascular surgery, Figs. 12B, 12E, 13C and 13D, J. Cardiov. Surg., *1*:3-44)

of the aorta and spreads in the form of a few discrete patches scattered over an otherwise normal intima. Its symptoms often are unusually severe, yet in some patients they are entirely absent.

Symptoms. The most common symptoms of luetic aortitis are sensations of substernal oppression or weight, or viselike feelings of constriction of the chest, or attacks of pain, often agonizing. There are characteristic sudden attacks of dyspnea (often called *asthma*), which start abruptly, are agonizing, last from 5 to 15 minutes and are accompanied by rapid pulse rate, high blood pressure, deep cyanosis and profuse sweating.

Luetic aortitis leads to aortic insufficiency with the same symptoms and findings as described under rheumatic aortic insufficiency.

Diagnosis. Luetic aortitis should be thought of in all cases of lues, even though no symptoms suggest its presence, and especially if vigorous antiluetic treatment has failed to reverse a positive serologic reaction. The condition often is discovered unexpectedly on roentgenograms. The presence of aortic insufficiency without an associated mitral lesion, paroxysmal dyspnea, anginal attacks and the development of an aortic aneurysm all suggest this diagnosis.

Prognosis. Of untreated patients, over two thirds die within 1 year after the characteristic symptoms appear. While luetic aortitis in large measure can be prevented by early and adequate antiluetic therapy, and can be arrested by specific treatment, the damage never can be repaired entirely.

Aortic Aneurysms

Nature and Classification of Aneurysms

Since arteries are elastic tubes filled with blood flowing under high pressure, should the wall of a vessel gradually become weak and yet not burst, it becomes distended at the weakened point. Such local distention is described as an *aneurysm*. Very small aneurysms due to local infection are designated as *mycotic aneurysms*. An aneurysm which is somewhat larger, but still limited in extent, projecting from one side of the vessel only is called a *saccular aneurysm*. If the whole artery becomes dilated, a *fusiform aneurysm* develops (Fig. 18-12). A wall of scar tissue at once begins to form around the developing aneurysmal sac, but never quite rapidly enough, hence there arises a slowly growing, pulsating tumor filled with blood communicating with the lumen of the vessel.

Possible causes for local weakness of the arterial wall that may result in aneurysm include local trauma by knife or missile, a local infection either pyogenic or luetic, and arteriosclerosis. Some spots may have been congenitally weak. This is true in the case of most cerebral aneurysms.

About 90 per cent of aortic aneurysms are located within the thorax, and the majority of these are on the aortic arch. The cause in most patients is syphilis, though a certain percentage of aneurysms of the fusiform type are due to arteriosclerosis.

Subjective Symptoms. Some aortic aneurysms give symptoms so slight that for a time the condition is not suspected, but all eventually make their presence known by symptoms of congestive heart failure or the pressure that the pulsating tumor exerts against other intrathoracic organs. Pain is the most prominent pressure symptom. This may be constant and boring in character, due to the erosion of a vertebra or rib by the pressure of the pulsating sac, or intermittent and neuralgic, due to pressure against nerves. Other conspicuous symptoms are dyspnea, the result of the pressure of the sac against the trachea, a main bronchus or the lung itself; cough, frequently paroxysmal and with brassy quality ("goose cough"); hoarseness, weakness of the voice or complete aphonia (evidences of pressure against the left recurrent laryngeal nerve); and dysphagia, due to impingement against the esophagus. In cases of luetic aneurysm, the patient is also likely to suffer from angina and paroxysmal dyspnea, a consequence of the luetic aortitis that caused the aneurysm.

Objective Symptoms. Dilated superficial veins on the chest, the neck or the arms, edematous areas on the chest wall and often cyanosis are evidence that large veins in the chest are being compressed. The pupils of the eyes may be unequal because of pressure against the cervical sympathetic chain.

Tracheal tug is due to adhesions between the sac and the trachea. The pulses at the 2 wrists differ markedly if the aneurysm impedes the blood flow into the left subclavian artery. An abnormal pulsation usually can be seen on the chest wall over the aneurysm, and occasionally the sac itself protrudes as a tumor under the skin, which means that it has eroded through the ribs.

Diagnosis. The diagnosis of most aneurysms is made readily on fluoroscopic examination, which reveals a pulsating tumor. Nevertheless, mediastinal tumor, lung tumor and enlarged mediastinal lymph nodes occasionally are difficult to exclude. In such cases a positive serologic reaction is a great help.*

Treatment. The prognosis for the patient with an advanced aneurysm is poor, and death from the serious effects of compression or from rupture is inevitable without treatment. However, with modern surgery it is now possible to remove the aneurysm and restore vascular continuity. Aneurysms of the aortic arch are the most complicated and difficult to treat.

---

* A more accurate diagnosis is made by injecting radiopaque solution into the heart or the aorta. This angioaortogram permits a visualization of the vessels and of the aneurysm.

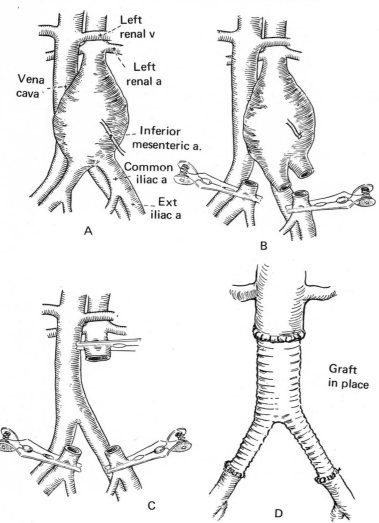

Left
renal v

Left
renal a

Vena
cava

Inferior
mesenteric a.

Common
iliac a

Ext
iliac a

A

B

C

D

Graft
in place

Fig. 18-13. Resection and homologous artery graft replacement of aneurysm of abdominal aorta. (A) Usual location of aneurysm below renal arteries and involving bifurcation to a varying degree. (B) Proximal and distal control with clamps is followed by removal of the aneurysm. The defect left in (C) is restored by the implantation of the graft (D). (Rhoads, *et al.*: Surgery, Principles and Practice, Philadelphia, J. B. Lippincott, 1970)

Aneurysm of the Abdominal Aorta

This aneurysm presents a palpable mass with a definitely expansile pulsation, produces a constant, severe, boring pain and causes a number of other pressure symptoms as well. The pressure of the pulsatile mass may erode the vertebral bodies. Untreated, the eventual outcome is rupture and sudden death. Medical treatment has nothing to offer these patients.

Surgery for aneurysm of the abdominal aorta is rapidly becoming the accepted method of treatment. When time permits, the aneurysm is outlined by injecting into the aorta a radiopaque dye (aortogram). The roentgenogram taken after the injection shows the size and the extent of the aneurysm. Surgical excision of the section of the aorta involved in the aneurysmal disease is carried out with replacement of the excised segment by a homograph or an artificial Teflon vessel.

This type of surgery is not always successful because most of the patients are in the older age group and the vascular tract is widely diseased in addition to the area of aneurysm. However, since no other treatment offers any benefit, the patient is compelled to take the risk. Surgeons even are attempting to remove recently ruptured aneurysms. It is understandable that the risk is much greater in such patients and the prognosis less favorable.

Dissecting Aneurysm of the Aorta

On rare occasions an aorta diseased by arteriosclerosis develops a tear in its intima. This permits blood to dissect its way into the substance of the aortic wall. This wall then may be split apart by the blood, which of course is under pressure, with the resultant formation of a large hematoma in the wall, the layers of which may be ripped apart for a considerable dis-

Fig. 18-14. Common sources of peripheral arterial emboli. (A) Composite showing sources of emboli within the heart. (B) Aneurysm with mural thrombus as source of emboli. (C) Arteriosclerotic plaques with thrombus formation. (Rhoads, *et al.*: Surgery, Principles and Practice, 4th ed., J. B. Lippincott, 1970)

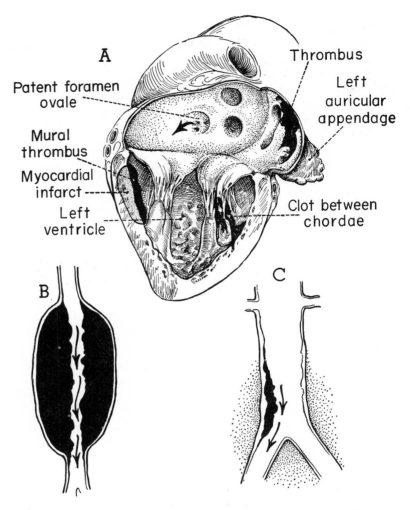

tance. Such dissection leads to compression and occlusion of the arteries branching from the aorta in the area involved by the process. The rip occurs most commonly in the region of the arch. The dissection of the aorta may progress backward in the direction of the heart, closing off the mouths of the coronary arteries and leading to hemopericardium. Or, it may extend in the opposite direction, causing occlusion of the arteries supplying the gastrointestinal tract, the kidneys, the spinal cord and even the legs. This is one of the most catastrophic accidents that can involve the cardiovascular system, and recovery from it is rare. It is diagnosed on the basis of signs and symptoms closely resembling those of coronary occlusion (p. 373), but with signs in addition due to multiple occlusions of the aortic branches. In this type of aneurysm, as well as in cases of the syphilitic variety, a definitive diagnosis is made by aortography.

Surgical Therapy. Although the prognosis is not good, the lives of many patients with dissecting aneurysms of the aorta may be saved by excising the aorta involved in the aneurysm and replacing the segment of vessel with the Teflon graft.

Aneurysms may also arise in peripheral vessels, most often due to arteriosclerosis. These may be found involving such vessels as the renal artery, the subclavian artery, but most frequently the popliteal artery in the area of the knee. The aneurysm produces a pulsating mass and a disturbance of peripheral circulation distal to it. Pain and swelling develop due to pressure upon adjacent nerves and veins. Surgical repair of such aneurysms is now carried out with replacement grafts.

Aortic Thrombosis (Leriche's Syndrome)

Gradual occlusion of the abdominal aorta and the iliac arteries was first described by Leriche and has been recognized in recent years by the injection of radiopaque dye into the aorta (aortography). This occlusion of the distal aorta is more common in men and results occasionally from an embolus but more often from gradually increasing arteriosclerotic changes in the lower portion of the aorta. The symptoms occur characteristically in early middle age; because of the poor circulation in the extremities, there is extreme fatiguability in the lower extremities and loss of sexual function. Atrophy of the lower extremities is a late symptom.

Treatment consists of excision of the diseased portion of the aorta, with replacement of this area by a graft.

Arterial Embolism

Most arterial emboli arise from thrombi that develop in the chambers of the heart due to atrial fibrillation or to myocardial infarction secondary to occlusion of the coronary artery. These thrombi may become detached and carried from the left side of the heart by way of the aorta to plug an artery that is too small to pass it. Emboli may also develop in advanced arteriosclerosis of the aorta due to roughening and even ulceration of the atheromatous plaques that form. Thrombi may form in such cases and break off to form emboli that lodge in the arterial system, most often where vessels divide (Fig. 18-14).

The symptoms of acute arterial embolism are acute pain and loss of function. The pain is severe and the loss of function is both motor and sensory. The patient shows a sudden paralysis and anesthesia of the part; the part shows pallor and is cold. These symptoms are due not only to the block of the artery by the embolus, but also to an associated vasomotor reflex that affects the arterial tree distal to the embolus. To relieve the vasoconstriction, the sympathetic ganglia may be blocked with procaine, and heparin is often given intravenously to reduce the tendency for a clot in the ves-

sel to form and extend. These measures may be sufficient to prevent death of tissue in embolism of small arteries, but in embolism of larger arteries, such as the aorta or the iliac arteries, surgery is usually undertaken as an emergency procedure. The artery is exposed, and after controlling the vessel above and below the site of the clot lodgement with clamps or tapes, an incision is made into the vessel and the clot removed. The opening in the vessel is closed with a fine silk suture, and as closure is made, a small amount of heparin solution is injected into the lumen of the vessel to minimize the tendency to thrombosis as the vessel is being closed. In some cases, it may be necessary to flush out clots that have migrated below the primary embolus into the distal arteries of the leg (Fig. 18-15).

Postoperatively, every effort is made to encourage motion in the leg to prevent stasis, and the nurse should get specific instructions regarding this. Anticoagulants (heparin) are given carefully, not only to prevent thrombosis of the operated artery, but also to diminish the development of thrombi at the original source of the embolus. The nurse must be constantly on guard to note bleeding from the surgical wounds, which might occur from an overdose of heparin. She should also remember that the primary difficulty in these patients is cardiac—atrial fibrillation or coronary thrombosis—either of which of itself demands careful nursing attention.

Arterial Thrombosis is another type of acute arterial occlusion that may develop in association with coronary occlusion. In the phase of depressed blood pressure, there is a reduced peripheral circulation, especially showing itself by arterial thrombosis in the degenerated vessels of the legs. The symptoms of arterial thrombosis are somewhat similar to those of acute arterial occlusion due to embolus, but the treatment is made more difficult by the fact that the arterial occlusion has occurred in a degenerated vessel, requiring more extensive surgery (endarterectomy or graft), which can only be performed if the patient's arterial blood pressure can be restored.

Vasospastic Disease

Raynaud's Disease

Raynaud's disease is found most often in young women between the ages of 18 and 30; it is characterized by a blanched, dead white appearance of symmetrical parts of the extremities—that is, fingers on both hands, then both hands. This may be followed by local asphyxia, which produces a marked purplish color in the extremities involved. These phenomena are brought about by an abnormal sensitivity of the vasoconstrictor influence to cold and emotional disturbances. When such spasms occur frequently, they

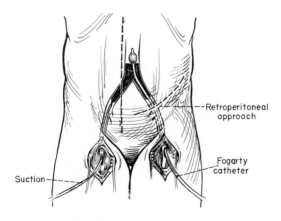

Fig. 18-15. Aortic bifurcation embolectomy may be approached directly through the abdomen or in a retrograde fashion via the femoral arteries by suction or Fogarty catheter. (From Rhoads, *et al.*: Surgery, 4th ed., J. B. Lippincott)

cause nutritional changes in the part and gangrene appears in areas, most often the fingertips, and sometimes large parts of the member are involved. Some patients with Raynaud's disease eventually develop scleroderma or other collagen disease.

Medical Treatment and Nursing Management. Avoidance of the particular stimuli that provoke vasoconstriction is the prime objective in controlling Raynaud's disease. First, an effort is made to avoid situations that may upset the patient. The need for a therapeutic environment is as important to this individual as insulin may be to the person who has diabetes. Secondly, exposure to cold must be minimized. In areas where the fall and winter months are cold, the patient should remain indoors, which means no hiking or participation in winter sports. For those occasions when it is necessary to go outdoors, warm clothing must be worn. Attractive fleece-lined boots, gloves, and hooded jackets are effective as well as fashionable. Leotards and slacks can keep the legs warm. Heated automobiles and heated shopping centers also help in reducing exposure to cold. The homemaker can avoid placing her hands in cold water by always using tepid or warm water. Oven mittens may be worn to remove frozen packages and articles from the refrigerator. Cold beverages can be handled in insulated glasses or tumblers partially covered with knitted "pants."

A third aid in controlling this disease is the systemic administration of peripheral vasodilators. Fourthly, since ulceration can easily develop following trauma to the digits, it is necessary for the patient to handle knives, needles, and other sharp objects carefully.

In severe cases, however, an interruption of the sympathetic nerves by removal of the sympathetic ganglia or division of their branches is the only method of affording much improvement. These ganglia are located either in the upper part of the thorax and lower neck for the upper extremity or along the vertebral column behind the peritoneum for the lower extremity. The operation for removal of these ganglia is spoken of as a *sympathetic ganglionectomy.* This operation produces only comparative relief by reducing the frequency of the attacks and increasing the stimulus required for their production.

Hypertensive Vascular Disease (The Patient with Hypertension)

Incidence and Etiology

About 20 per cent of the population develop hypertension (defined as persistent levels of blood pressure above 150 systolic and 90 diastolic)—95 per cent of these have essential hypertension (i.e., of no known cause), and the remainder develop blood pressure elevation from some specific etiology such as renovascular narrowing, aldosterone-producing adrenal tumor, pheochromocytoma or other rare conditions.

Elevated blood pressure is associated as a part of many disease states, such as thyrotoxicosis or preeclampsia, and it is corrected when the basic disease is corrected.

Essential hypertension usually begins as a labile intermittent process in the late thirties to early fifties and gradually becomes "fixed." Occasionally it may appear abruptly and severely and take an accelerated or "malignant" course with rapid deterioration of the patient. Overstimulation with coffee, tobacco, and stimulatory drugs, as well as emotional disturbances and obesity play a role, but the disease is strongly familial. It affects more women than men, but men, especially Negroes, tolerate the disease more poorly. Prolonged elevation of blood pressure eventually damages blood vessels throughout the body, and this is most notable in the eyes, heart, kidneys and brain, so that failing vision, coronary occlusion and congestive heart failure, renal failure and strokes are the usual consequences of prolonged, uncontrolled hypertension.

Increased peripheral resistance controlled at the arteriolar level is the basic cause for the elevated blood pressure, but the causes of increased resistance are poorly understood. Drug therapy is aimed at reducing peripheral resistance, thus lowering the blood pressure and thereby lessening the stresses on the vascular system.

Signs and Symptoms

The symptoms may be none or severe with morning headaches, easy fatigue, a sense of nervousness, irritability; if the heart is involved, dyspnea, edema or the anginal syndrome and palpitations may appear. Nocturia and other signs of renal damage occur as the kidney becomes involved. There may be transient ischemic attacks such as giddiness and blackouts, indicating central nervous system involvement. On physical examination no abnormalities may be found other than high blood pressure, but there may be eye changes in the retinae with hemorrhages, exudates, narrowed arterioles and in severe cases, papilladema. Cardiac enlargement and arrhythmias may be found, along with signs of congestive heart failure. In the older patient, evidences of arteriosclerosis may be manifest, because prolonged hypertension seems to increase the rate of development of the arteriosclerotic processes.

Diagnosis

Laboratory findings depend on the target organ damage. Electrocardiographic abnormalities, enlarged heart by x-ray, proteinuria, inability to concentrate the urine and increase in the blood urea nitrogen may all be present. Special studies such as renogram, intravenous pyelogram, renal arteriograms and split renal function studies and the determination of renin levels are made to distinguish those patients with renovascular occlusion. VMA (vanilmandelic acid) and catecholamine determination and the Regitine test detect the rare pheochromocytoma (see p. 976). Elevated aldosterone levels and decreased renin levels are highly suggestive of primary aldosteronism.

Treatment including Pharmacotherapy

Treatment is aimed at lowering the blood pressure to normal levels with the hope of alleviating symptoms and preventing the development or arresting the progress of vascular damage. In accelerated or malignant hypertension, where the natural history of the disease is relatively short and the life-span limited, drug therapy has produced a greatly improved outlook, especially if kidney damage is not severe when treatment gets underway. Most physicians today believe that even milder instances of hypertension should be treated.

In all instances there are general measures to be followed. Overweight is corrected. Overuse of stimulants and tobacco is curbed. Patients are urged and educated to promote a more tranquil outlook upon life and its problems and to alter their habits so as to lead a well-balanced life with proper proportions of work, play and rest. This is not easy, because many of these patients are tense, hard-driving individuals for whom relaxation is difficult. Dietary salt intake should be reduced. Other disease states such as anemia, thyrotoxicosis and renal infection should be corrected.

In mild cases, the foregoing general measures plus mild sedation with barbiturates, perhaps in the form of phenobarbital, 15 mg. (¼ gr.) 3 times a day or reserpine, 0.25 mg. daily, is all that is needed. Other patients require the addition of a thiazide diuretic, such as Diuril, 500 mg., or Hydrodiuril, 50 mg. daily or every other day.

If the foregoing combinations of drugs do not control the blood pressure, another drug is added, such as hydralazine (Apresoline), and this triple combination is given conveniently as Ser-Ap-Es (Serpasil, Apresoline and Esadrix containing reserpine, hydralazine and hydrochlorothiazide), one tablet 2 to 4 times daily. For still more severe hypertension, one may use reserpine, thiazide and guanethidine. Guanethidine is an adrenergic blocking agent and produces a postural drop as well as a supine lowering of the blood pressure. The intensity of the postural drop is the limiting factor in dosage level. Too much guanethidine leads to giddiness or blackout. Guanethidine has largely replaced the old ganglionic blocking agents such as hexamethonium, Inversine, and Ansolysen, which caused rather marked effects on bowel and bladder.

Methyldopa (Aldomet) is another useful hypoten-

sive agent in doses of 500 mg. to 2 gm. per day, and is usually combined with a thiazide diuretic. The thiazides cause salt and water excretion and have allowed patients to have somewhat less severely salt-restricted diets.

The acute crises of hypertension, such as encephalopathy, eclampsia and malignant phase of the disease, require parenteral therapy at the outset. Intramuscular reserpine 2 mg., repeated in 3 to 6 hours as needed, provides a satisfactory fall in blood pressure in about 85 per cent of the patients. Others may need quicker results, for which Arfonad, 150 mg., may be given intravenously, but its effect is rather short-lived and repeated doses are needed. Occasionally *Veratrum viride* preparations such as Veriloid are used parenterally, but the therapeutic-toxic range for veratrum products is very narrow, making their satisfactory use difficult and therefore not very frequent. A newer agent, Hyperstat (diazoxide 300 mg.) seems promising for intravenous use for emergency lowering of the blood pressure without severe side-effects. This drug, given orally, is not very useful because it tends to raise the blood sugar.

Side-effects of hypotensive agents must be kept in mind because of their frequent and sometimes severe occurrence. Rauwolfia preparations may cause recurrence of peptic ulcer in the susceptible patient, often increases the appetite with consequent weight gain and may cause severe mental depression. It has a pulse-slowing effect that is not a side-reaction but a pharmacologic action of the drug. It also causes nasal stuffiness. Thiazide diuretics may deplete the body of potassium, with development of muscle weakness, for which potassium supplements may be needed. If sodium is lost quickly or excessively through thiazide diuresis and saluresis, muscle cramping and weakness may occur, especially in hot weather. Hydralazine given by itself may cause headaches, tachycardia and increased cardiac output; these latter 2 events are not desired in patients with coronary disease. In combination with rauwolfia, the side-effects of hydralazine are lessened and small dosages may be used. In daily doses over 200 mg. for prolonged periods, hydralazine may provoke the lupus erythematosus syndrome and symptoms of rheumatoid arthritis. Guanethidine may cause diarrhea in many patients, and if the postural drop is too great, central nervous symptoms (as mentioned previously) occur. The ganglionic blocking drugs, now little used, may cause severe constipation, bloating, ileus and urinary retention and visual blurring. Methyldopa occasionally causes a drop in hemoglobin, bizarre feelings of being unwell, dizziness, nasal stuffiness, dry mouth and rarely jaundice.

Patient Education. Generally patients on an anti-hypertensive program have some sense of sedation, and this may be too great for comfort. Many of these symptoms pass away as the patient becomes adjusted to the medications or if adjustments are made in dosage levels. At times, but not often, patients are taught to measure blood pressure at home. The disadvantage of this is the development of a neurotic focus and preoccupation with the blood pressure levels. It is difficult to convince many patients that the blood pressure is a normally variable thing and does not stay fixed at one number. Patients must be encouraged to stick to their treatment program. The disease is controllable but not curable and treatment at the present time must continue indefinitely. About 20 to 25 per cent of patients who stay faithfully on treatment and have good control for a period of 2 or 3 years may find that they are able to go without medication thereafter for a period of time. However, no one can predict in advance which patients will have this happy outcome.

Surgery. Thoracolumbar sympathectomy was formerly a commonly performed procedure for the hypertensive individual, but with the advent of potent drugs, it is now rarely done. Also, the subtotal adrenalectomy has become a thing of the past. Surgery at present is focused on the correction of renovascular occlusion by either correcting them with a graft or by removing the involved kidney if a revascularization procedure cannot be done. With the injection of a radiopaque dye into the aorta (aortography), it is possible to demonstrate a narrowing of the renal artery and reduction of renal blood flow in about 20 per cent of the patients with severe hypertension. Revascularization of the kidney by means of synthetic grafts from the aorta to the renal artery beyond the obstruction has restored the blood pressure to normal in about half the patients who were operated on by Dr. DeBakey and his group at Baylor College of Medicine. In another 8 to 10 per cent the hypertension was reduced. As noted earlier, this group makes up a small percentage of all cases of hypertension. Furthermore, many of the patients with unilateral renovascular occlusion may have evidence of vascular disease elsewhere or other diseases that make them poor candidates for surgery. In such instances it has been found that medical therapy with antihypertensive drugs has given acceptable results. On the other hand, if the previously described tests show a unilateral renovascular lesion that is functional (i.e., causing the high blood pressure) and the patient is in otherwise good condition, surgery may give excellent results. Surgery is also the treatment for the hypertension of pheochromocytoma and aldosteronoma and consists of the removal of the tumor. In reference to the pheochromocytoma, the nurse must be highly attentive to the patient once the tumor is removed, because frequently the patient goes into a hypotensive state and may actually require a pressor agent in the form of Levophed for a period of time postoperatively.

Nursing care relating to hypertensive vascular disease is discussed in detail in those sections devoted to the treatment of coronary heart disease and congestive heart failure.

PATIENTS WITH LYMPHATIC CONDITIONS

The Lymphatic System

The lymphatic system is a set of tubes that spread throughout most of the body. The vessels of this system start as lymph capillaries draining tissue spaces. These unite to form the lymph vessels, which in turn pass through the lymph nodes and finally empty into the large thoracic duct which joins the jugular vein on the left side of the neck. The lymphatic system of the abdominal cavity maintains a steady flow of digested fatty food (chyle) from the intestinal mucosa to the thoracic duct. In other parts of the body its function is more regional; the lymphatic vessels of the head, for example, empty into clusters of lymph nodes located in the neck, and those of the extremities, into nodes in the axillae and the groin.

Assessment by means of Lymphangiography

Radiologic visualization of the lymphatic system is possible after the injection of contrast medium directly into lymphatic vessels in the hands and the feet. This technique affords a means of detecting lymph-node involvement by metastatic carcinoma, lymphoma or infection in sites that are otherwise inaccessible to the examiner except by the direct surgical approach—for example, in the pelvis, the retroperitoneum and deep in the axillae.

The first step in this procedure is the location of a lymphatic vessel in each foot (or hand) by injecting Evans blue dye intradermally between the first and the second digits and then, 15 to 20 minutes later, incising the skin proximal to the injection site. A blue lymphatic is identified, isolated, cannulated with a 25- to 30-gauge needle and infused very slowly with a contrast medium containing iodine and oil (Ethiodol). Approximately 10 ml. of this material is injected into the foot (or 5 ml. into the hand) at a rate not exceeding 7 ml. per hour. Appropriate x-ray pictures are taken at the conclusion of the injection, 24 hours later and periodically thereafter, as indicated. Injection of the feet delineates, for about an hour, the lymphatic channels in the legs and the thoracic duct and, for many weeks, the inguinal, abdominal and supraclavicular lymph nodes. Similar delineation of lymphatic vessels in the upper extremity, and of the axillary and the supraclavicular nodes, follows injection of the hand.

Apart from its diagnostic value in cases of unsuspected lymph-node disease, lymphangiography offers a means of evaluating the presence and the extent of metastases in patients who are known to have cancer. Moreover, since lymphomatous lymph nodes retain the contrast medium for 4 to 6 weeks after the injection, any change in their size that may occur in response to irradiation or chemotherapy can be measured and used as a criterion of therapeutic effect.

Tuberculosis of Lymph Nodes

The local spread of tuberculosis almost entirely is through the lymph channels. Hence the nodes that filter the lymph flowing from the portals of entry for tubercle bacilli are the first tissues actually to become infected, and the condition that arises in them is called *tuberculous adenitis.* Lymph nodes thus diseased often swell to the size of Lima beans or larger, and, since these nodes nearly always are arranged in groups, large swellings may develop. These nodes may heal and return to their normal size, but always with a caseated area at their center which eventually becomes impregnated with lime salts. (Such calcified nodes bear witness throughout life that once they were tuberculous.) Occasionally, this tuberculous inflammation extends to tissues surrounding the infected nodes, matting them together into one caseous necrotic mass—a tuberculous abscess.

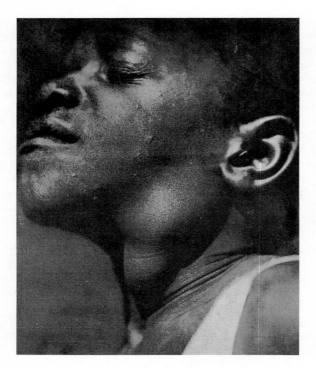

Fig. 18-16. Tuberculous cervical adenitis.

Tuberculosis can involve simultaneously practically all the lymph nodes of the body, but this condition is rare. Usually it is a regional condition, only those nodes that receive the germs through some portal of entry or that drain some tuberculous focus being infected. The groups of nodes most frequently involved in primary infections are the cervical, the mediastinal and the mesenteric glands.

Tuberculous Cervical Lymphadenitis. This is the most common form of tuberculosis of children between the ages of 3 and 7. The portal of entry of the germs usually is the tonsils. Early in the disease the individual nodes in the group may be distinguishable by palpation, but later they become matted together and often become necrotic. Such abscesses, breaking through the skin, explain the running sores in the neck that remain open for months and leave, as they heal, the ugly scars so conspicuous throughout life.

Tuberculous Mediastinal Lymphadenitis. The tracheobronchial (mediastinal) lymph nodes, draining the tracheal and bronchial mucous membranes, when tuberculous cause few or no local symptoms unless an abscess forms or unless they become sufficiently large to exert pressure. When they exert pressure on the trachea, they cause paroxysms of coughing; when on the blood vessels or nerves in the mediastinum, they cause distention of the veins of the chest wall and other symptoms.

Tuberculous Mesenteric Lymphadenitis. Tuberculosis of the lymph nodes of the mesentery and of those behind the peritoneal cavity draining the intestines is a common disease of young children infected by milk from tuberculous cows. In some patients these nodes suppurate; in others, they form large masses in the abdomen (mesenteric tabes). In all, if extensive, they produce a gradual loss of weight and strength, a distention of the abdomen and diarrhea, with passage of thin, offensive, fatty stools.

Necrosis of tuberculous mesenteric lymph nodes produces tuberculous peritonitis.

Treatment and Nursing Care. The treatment of tuberculous lymphadenitis, in whatever region it develops, employs the same general measures and embodies precisely the same principles as those prescribed in connection with pulmonary tuberculosis. Tuberculous abscesses involving the cervical nodes are incised or aspirated. Chemotherapy employing streptomycin with para-aminosalicylic acid as an adjunct has proved to be effective in many types of lymph node tuberculosis.

Lymphangitis and Lymphadenitis

Lymphangitis is an acute inflammation of the lymphatic channels. It arises most commonly from a focus of infection in an extremity. Usually it is caused by the streptococcus. The characteristic red streaks that extend up the arm or the leg from an infected wound outline the course of the lymphatics as they drain toward nodes in the elbow or the axilla in the arm or the knee or the groin in the leg. The presence of a lymphangitis indicates that the infection has not become localized, but is extending at least to the lymph nodes, and, in some patients, it may progress and involve the bloodstream (septicemia). The absorption of toxins produces high fever, often chills, in addition to the local symptoms of pain, tenderness and swelling along the lymphatics involved. The lymph nodes in the course of the lymphatic channels also become enlarged, red and tender (acute lymphadenitis), and often become necrotic and form an abscess (suppurative lymphadenitis). The nodes involved most often are those in the groin, the axilla or the cervical region. Also lymphadenitis occurs frequently without any signs of a preceding lymphangitis, due to bacteria that have lodged in the lymph nodes from lymph drained from a focus of infection. The same signs (redness and swelling) and symptoms (pain, tenderness and fever) as already mentioned for acute lymphadenitis are present. Here, again, abscess formation may take place.

Lymphangitis and acute lymphadenitis now are not of serious import, because these infections are caused nearly always by organisms (streptococcus and staphylococcus) that are brought under control rapidly by the sulfa drugs and the antibiotics. The part affected is treated usually by rest, elevation and the application of hot moist dressings, but the rapid response to penicillin and/or sulfadiazine usually make this treatment unnecessary after a very short time. If necrosis has resulted in abscess formation, incision and drainage become necessary.

Acute Cervical Adenitis. This acute infection of the lymphatic glands of the neck is usually secondary to an infection in the mouth, the pharynx or the scalp.

This condition occurs very frequently in children, and the prophylactic treatment should be directed toward preventing infection in these areas or removing it should it occur. School nurses and public health nurses especially should inspect the teeth and the tonsils of children under their care and should recommend appropriate prophylactic treatment. Pediculosis of the scalp (lice) is a very common cause of infection of the posterior group of glands. These parasites should be looked for in every patient with "glands of the neck," and parasiticides should be applied in all positive or suspicious cases.

The patients develop a swelling of one side of the neck that is markedly tender and edematous. The systemic signs, which in the case of children usually are marked, are those of an acute infection. The process often goes on to abscess formation and spontaneous rupture if the swelling is not incised.

Treatment. The treatment in the early stages comprises attention to the focus of infection, the use of penicillin intramuscularly and the application of warm moist dressings or poultices. If an abscess forms, incision and drainage are required. Frequently the hot moist applications are continued for several days after operation.

Lymphedema—Elephantiasis

An obstruction to the lymph flow in the extremities produces a chronic swelling of the part, especially if it is in a dependent position. The obstruction may be in both the lymph nodes and the lymphatic vessels, and at times it is seen in the arm after a radical mastectomy for carcinoma, and in the leg in association with varicose veins or a chronic phlebitis. In the latter case the lymph block usually is due to a chronic lymphangitis. Lymph block due to a parasite (filaria) is seen frequently in the tropics. When chronic swelling is present, there are frequent bouts of acute infection characterized by high fever and chills. These lead to a chronic fibrosis and a thickening of the subcutaneous tissues and hypertrophy of the skin. To this condition of chronic swelling of the extremity, which recedes only slightly with elevation, is given the name *elephantiasis*.

The swelling of lymphedema may be prevented by the application of elastic bandages or stockings. Often elephantiasis produces such marked disability that surgical relief is sought. The thickened fibrosed subcutaneous fat and much of the excess skin are cut away, along with the fascia overlying the muscles. Skin grafts are cut from the tissue removed and applied to the exposed muscles. By removing the subcutaneous tissue in which the fluid collects, the part is brought back to normal size and to normal function.

In the postoperative care of these patients, pressure dressings are applied to hold the skin grafts in place until they attach themselves to the underlying muscles.

Nursing Care. A block to the lymphatic flow in an extremity means that the part involved may be traumatized easily. Before operation, the arm or the leg is supported on a pillow and bandaged. Some surgeons order diuretics to help in reducing edema. Sulfa drugs and penicillin may be given prophylactically. The part is washed carefully with soap and water before surgery. In the postoperative care of these patients, transfusions usually are necessary to prevent the shock that may arise from the long operative procedure and rather profuse blood loss. The extremity is elevated for at least 2 weeks and then is lowered gradually. If it is a leg, weight is borne only with support. Precautions to avoid injury must be observed carefully.

BIBLIOGRAPHY

General

Barker, W. F.: Treatment of Peripheral Vascular Disease. New York, McGraw-Hill, 1962.

Breslau, R. C.: Intensive care following vascular surgery. Amer. J. Nurs., 68:1670-1676, Aug., 1968.

DeBakey, M. E. (ed.): Symposium on vascular surgery. Surg. Clin. N. Amer., 46:825-1071, Aug., 1966.

DeBakey, M. E., *et al.*: Basic biologic reactions to vascular grafts and prostheses. Surg. Clin. N. Amer., 45:477-497, April, 1965.

Fulcher, A. J.: The nurse and the patient with peripheral vascular disease. Nurs. Clin. N. Amer., 1:47-55, March, 1966.

James, G.: A stop smoking program. Amer. J. Nurs., 64:122-125, June, 1964.

Julian, O. C., and Dye, W. S.: Peripheral vascular surgery. *In* Moyer *et al.*: Surgery. pp. 1246-1316. Philadelphia, J. B. Lippincott, 1965.

Olwin, J. H., and Koppel, J. L.: Anticoagulant therapy. Amer. J. Nurs., 64:107-110, May, 1964.

Sr. Mary Elizabeth: Occlusion of the peripheral arteries. Amer. J. Nurs., 67:562-564, March, 1967.

Embolism and Thrombosis

Chassin, J. L.: Improved management of acute embolism and thrombosis with an embolectomy catheter. JAMA, 194:845-850, 1965.

Conn, J., Jr., and Bergan, J. J.: Treatment of arterial embolism: The conservative approach. Surg. Clin. N. Amer., 48:163-176, Feb., 1968.

Israel, H. L., *et al.*: Fibrinolysin treatment of thromboembolism. JAMA, 188:628, 1964.

Arterial Problems

Ajemian, S.: Bypass grafting for femoral artery occlusion. Amer. J. Nurs., 67:565-568, March, 1967.

Bergersen, B. S.: Detection of peripheral arterial disease and instruction of patients. *In* Bergersen: Current Concepts in Clinical Nursing. pp. 43-56. St. Louis, C. V. Mosby, 1967.

Davis, R. W.: Carotid endarterectomy with regional hypothermia. AORN J., 6:50-53, Dec., 1967.

Eastcott, H. H. G.: Arterial Surgery, Phila., Lippincott, 1969.

Fogarty, T. J., and Cranley, J. J.: Catheter technique for arterial embolectomy. Ann. Surg., 161:3:325, 1965.

Lord, J. W., Jr.: Cigarette smoking and peripheral atherosclerotic occlusive disease. JAMA, 191:249-251, 1965.

Venous Problems

Dionne, P.: Varicose veins of the lower limbs. Canad. Nurs., 63:39-42, Jan., 1967.

Hafner, C. D., *et al.*: Venous thrombectomy: current status. Ann. Surg., 161:411-417, 1965.

Latham, H. C.: Thrombophlebitis. Amer. J. Nurs., 63:122-126, Sept., 1963.

Schairer, A. E., and Pesek, I. G.: Aids in the treatment of varicose veins. Surg. Clin. N. Amer., 48:111-120, 1968.

Leg Ulcers

Dale, W. A.: Management of chronic leg ulcers. Hosp. Med., 2:26-30, Jan., 1966.

Dubuque, T. J., Jr.: Stasis ulcer of the lower extremity. Arch. Surg., 96:508-511, 1968.

Horvath, P. N.: Chronic leg ulcers, medical management. Amer. J. Nurs., 67:94-97, Jan., 1967.

Kanof, N. M.: Gold leaf and the treatment of cutaneous ulcers. J. Invest. Derm., 43:441-442, Nov., 1964.

Wilson, S.: Chronic leg ulcers, nursing management. Amer. J. Nurs., 67:96-99, Jan., 1967.

PATIENT EDUCATION

American Heart Association
(Local chapter) or
44 East 23rd St.
New York, New York 10010

> High Blood Pressure. (pamphlet)
> Varicose Veins. (pamphlet)

U.S. Dept. Health, Education & Welfare:
Supt. of Documents
Washington, D.C. 20402

> Varicose Veins—What can be done about them. PHS Publication No. 154.

Patients with Conditions of the Heart

THE NURSE AND THE CARDIAC PATIENT

Cardiovascular disease, heart disease in particular, is the number one health problem of our society, ranking first as a cause of death in the United States. The public is both aware and naturally deeply concerned about the implicatons of a personal diagnosis of heart disease. Indeed, there is even an exaggerated fear in many people, much of which can be alleviated by well-informed nurses.

Safe and effective nursing care in cardiac conditions requires a thorough appreciation of the pathologic and physiologic processes that are involved. And, if the nurse is to contribute materially toward the recovery of her cardiac patients, she must understand clearly the rationale of the treatment that is prescribed for them.

The symptoms of heart disease vary from patient to patient. However, most cardiovascular symptoms are likely to be included in this brief list: fatigue, chest pain, dyspnea, orthopnea, cough, palpitation, edema and cyanosis. Symptomatic relief is a major objective of nursing, but objectives change as the patient's problems and needs change. With the passage of time therapeutic priorities must be revised in accordance with these needs. Facets of nursing care to be considered, apart from observation, identification, inter-

pretation and relief of symptoms, include the teaching of methods for the prevention of symptomatic recurrences, and the instruction of patients regarding health measures that are designed to retard the progression of heart disease. One important nursing goal is to equip the patient with knowledge and inspiration to participate effectively in his own plan of care.

The nursing care of the patient with heart disease is never routine because there are too many variables in heart disease. In making modifications in the nursing management of these patients, the nurse must ask herself, "Which is easier for *this* patient?" Will it be less stressful for the patient to feed himself or to be fed? Will the patient become more upset by being shaved, not being shaved or by receiving help? In giving the cardiac patient the nursing support he requires, the nurse demonstrates to him that she is interested in him as a person and gives him the feeling of being understood. This is so important in helping the patient to cope with his anxiety. The relief of anxiety is a major factor in caring for any patient with a cardiac condition.

To provide the nurse with a sound factual basis for her concepts regarding various cardiac conditions she is likely to encounter, and to acquaint her with some of the many specific nursing problems that will confront her in connection with patients with heart disease, this chapter has been designed.

359

ROLE OF THE NURSE
IN PREVENTING HEART DISEASE

In the course of her contacts with patients and their families, the nurse is likely to encounter many individuals with cardiovascular symptoms who have not sought, but obviously need, diagnostic, therapeutic or preventive services. As an informed case-finder she should be particularly alert for symptoms of edema and shortness of breath. Whenever she hears an individual blame his exertional dyspnea on a "cold," "too many cigarettes" or "old age," the nurse, who realizes that dyspnea never is normal, should attempt to convince him of the importance of securing immediate medical attention.

The nurse should instruct parents regarding the potential dangers that are associated with tonsillitis and pharyngitis. Were every patient with streptococcal pharyngitis to receive prompt and adequate treatment with penicillin, rheumatic fever would virtually cease to exist. The nurse has an important role in the instruction of patients who have had rheumatic fever, which should stress the purpose and the importance of continuing antibiotic prophylaxis for an indefinite period of time.

How may the nurse be a case-finder of persons with congenital heart disease? It is important that she serve in this role, for by so doing she can make a major contribution to its early diagnosis. Early diagnosis is the key to the successful treatment of congenital heart disease, which is most likely to be accomplished by early surgery: i.e., surgery carried out before the patient develops pulmonary hypertension. With the school nurse and the public health nurse continually on the lookout for children who become cyanotic or unduly breathless on exertion, this diagnostic possibility is not likely to be overlooked. Moreover, familiar as she is with the normal patterns of body growth and development, the nurse should be quick to perceive the possibility of congenital heart disease in a child who appears not to be developing normally. Should she encounter an individual who is in the first trimester of pregnancy and has just been exposed to German measles (Rubella), she should advise an immediate visit to the doctor for prophylactic injections of gamma globulin, for the evidence indicates that if this particular infection is contracted at this stage of pregnancy the offspring is more likely to be afflicted with congenital defects than otherwise would be the case. There are active vaccines now available for both rubella (German measles) and Rubeola (measles). With the widespread use of these vaccines the prevention of measles should be possible in the future.

Syphilitic aortitis and aortic aneurysm are prevent-able. The nurse who participates in the treatment of patients with early syphilis must educate these individuals concerning the potential long-range effects of this infection that are avoidable if the disease is eradicated completely by adequate therapy. She should stress to the patient the desirability of complete cooperation with his physician, throughout the follow-up period, and until such time as he may receive his final discharge from the clinic.

Even with improvement in therapy there is a high mortality rate for patients with coronary heart disease. Risk factors to identify individuals who are coronary-prone have now been formulated. These include an elevated serum cholesterol, increasing levels of blood pressure, cigarette smoking, electrocardiogram abnormalities, obesity and a low vital capacity. The nurse can help identify these susceptible individuals and encourage them to seek medical assistance for appropriate prophylactic measures and a program for prevention.

There is also a definite relationship between habitual lack of exercise and cardiac morbidity and mortality. Sedentary work and living habits are common in this country and may well be a serious challenge to preventive medicine in the future. Physical exercise is beneficial because it increases cardiac output and coronary blood flow. It behooves the nurse to participate in a daily program of exercise and to encourage this activity in others.

Study has shown that the serum cholesterol level is the best predictor of the development of coronary heart disease. Serum cholesterol concentrations can decline when the diet is modified in total calories and total fats and low in fatty acids and cholesterol.

Of course, obese individuals should be encouraged to correct their nutritional status. Weight reduction assumes an over-riding importance for the individual who is overweight if, in addition, he has arterial hypertension or coronary artery disease—and he should be instructed accordingly. Convincing evidence has accumulated that points to an association between cigarette smoking and deaths from the complications of coronary heart disease. Any cigarette smoker with symptoms of angina pectoris or with a history of myocardial infarction should be informed of this relationship in no uncertain terms, and strongly urged to discontinue the use of tobacco. It has been demonstrated that men who quit smoking before the development of overt coronary disease will have a lower rate of disease incidence than do the men who continue to smoke. Whatever success the nurse may have in assisting the patient toward this objective represents an exceedingly important contribution to the prevention of heart disease.

Patients who repeatedly return to their physician or hospital in a recurrent state of cardiac decompensation need continuing reevaluation and repeated preventive teaching. A detailed description of the previous day's meals should be requested on the occasion of each visit, in order to determine to what extent the patient has been adhering to his low-sodium diet. Although meticulous about his diet, does he relieve his dyspepsia with antacid powders that contain sodium? Is he keeping track of his weight to detect water retention and to control edema? These and many other considerations bear repeated discussion. Repetition is essential to the process of learning; it likewise is an important principle in preventive teaching.

NORMAL CARDIAC FUNCTION

The heart is a hollow muscular pump that forces the blood on by contractions, called *beats* or, better, *systoles*. The only visible evidence of these is a slight outward thrust of the apex of the left ventricle, called the *apex beat*, usually seen at a point just below the medial to the left nipple in the fourth or fifth costal interspace. Each systole is followed by a period of rest, called its *diastole*, during which the heart wall is relaxed. So that the blood may always be pumped in the right direction, the heart is provided with valves. Thus, when the right ventricle contracts, it forces the blood through the pulmonic orifice into the pulmonary artery, since the tricuspid valve prevents its regurgitation into the right atrium, whence it came. The heart contraction over, the blood in the pulmonary artery cannot flow back into the right ventricle, now in diastole, since the pulmonic valve closes to prevent this. In a similar manner, on the left side of the heart, the mitral valve prevents any backflow from the left ventricle into the atrium, and the aortic valve, its return into the left ventricle. These valves are membranes of wonderful strength, yet almost as thin as heavy paper. The edges of the mitral and tricuspid valves are anchored by fine but very strong threads called *chordae tendineae*.

The ability to contract is inherent in all parts of the heart wall (myocardium). If the ventricles were cut entirely free from the rest of the heart, under proper conditions they would contract regularly, about 28 times per minute. The walls of the atria also can beat independently and do so at a faster or occasionally slower rate than the walls of the ventricles.

The Conduction System of the Heart

The heart has a pacemaker, the sino-atrial node, located in the right atrial wall near the opening of the superior vena cava, where, normally, all its beats start. It is through this node that certain nervous centers in

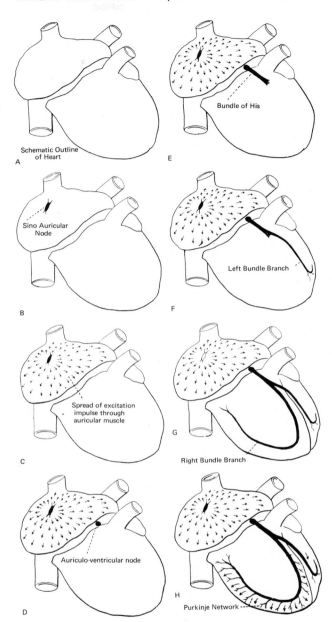

Schematic Outline
of Heart
A

Sino Auricular
Node
B

Spread of excitation
impulse through
auricular muscle
C

Auriculo-ventricular node
D

Bundle of His
E

Left Bundle Branch
F

Right Bundle Branch
G

Purkinje Network
H

Fig. 19-1. Component parts of the conduction system of the heart in sequence A to H. (Leaman: *Management of the Cardiac Patient*, J. B. Lippincott Co.)

the brain control the rate of the heartbeat. Through sympathetic nerve fibers they hasten it, and through fibers in the vagus nerve they slow it. It is the balance of these two nerve systems controlling the sino-atrial node that determines the rate of the heartbeat.

Normally every muscular contraction of the heart, therefore every heartbeat and pulse wave, occurs specifically in response to a single electrical impulse that has been generated by, and originated in, this node, serving as the *pacemaker*. Each of these impulses travels simultaneously through the atrial walls, exciting their immediate contraction, to the atrioventricular (AV) node, and then through a special bundle of nerve fibers ("bundle of His"). Here transmission is delayed for about fifteen-hundredths of a second. The pathway divides shortly beyond the AV node, two separate nerve-like bundles (the right and left bundle branches) and their communicating fibers conducting the impulse from the node to the right and the left ventricles, respectively, distributing it throughout their walls and stimulating them to contract (Fig. 19-1).

Thus, entailed in each heartbeat is an orderly, precisely timed sequence of events, as follows: an electrical discharge emanates from the sino-atrial (SA) node, in immediate response to which the 2 atria contract and empty their contents into the corresponding ventricles, which at that instant are in a state of relaxation. After an interval of 0.10 to 0.15 seconds, the 2 ventricles contract simultaneously: the right ejects its contents (systemic venous blood from the superior and inferior vena cavae, via the right atrium) into the pulmonary arterial circuit; and the left ejects oxygenated blood from the pulmonary circuit (delivered from the pulmonary veins by the left atrium) into the aorta and the systemic circulation.

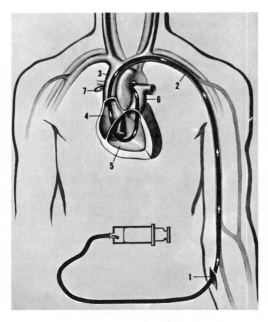

FIG. 19-2. Route of cardiac catheter.

NURSING ASSESSMENT OF THE CARDIAC PATIENT

When a patient is hospitalized for a cardiac condition, it often indeed is a life-threatening situation. The nurse's observations are important for the patient's diagnostic and therapeutic regimen. No symptom is unimportant. Although there are some exceptions (angina pectoris and certain arrhythmias), the symptoms of heart disease usually correlate with the degree of heart disease present. The following is an outline of salient observations that have first priority in patient evaluation. This knowledge helps the nurse to determine the patient's primary problems and gives direction in establishing objectives and planning nursing care.

1. Skin color and temperature.
   Pallor, flushing, cyanosis, petechiae.
   Sweating, cold, clammy, warm and dry.
2. Heart Rate
   Apical and radial rates
   Description of rate
3. Description of heart rhythm
4. Respirations
   Rate and depth
   Character
   Presence of Cheyne-Stokes respirations
   Position assumed by patient
5. Blood pressure
   Both arms
   Both legs (at initial evaluation)
6. Presence of pain
   Location
   Radiation
   Quality
   Duration
   Intensity
   Circumstances precipitating pain
7. Presence of cough and sputum
8. Emotional reaction of the patient to his symptoms
9. Response of patient to the treatment

EVALUATION OF CARDIAC FUNCTION

In order to determine accurately the nature and the exact location of cardiovascular defects, many studies are done. To begin with, a complete history of the patient is taken from his birth to the present. The physical examination should be complete and include fluoroscopy (often with barium swallow) and x-ray study of the chest to determine heart size and chamber enlargement. Tests for the evaluation of cardiac function include measurements of peripheral and central venous pressure, circulation time (p. 364), vital capacity (p. 230), electrocardiography, roentgenographic examination of the chest, serum enzyme tests (SGOT, LDH, CPK), ballistocardiogram, cardiac catheterization and angiocardiography.

Electrocardiography

The electrocardiogram is a visual representation of the electrical activity of the heart, as reflected by changes in electrical potential at the skin surface, these changes being detected and recorded graphically by an electrocardiograph. Impulses generated within the heart, traveling via the conduction pathways and spreading throughout the myocardium are depicted in the form of waves that have characteristic patterns and correspond in frequency to specific events in the cardiac cycle. Based on the direction, contour and relative location of 5, or occasionally 6, peaks in each cycle, precise information is obtainable with respect to the origin of the initial impulse, or "pacemaker," the manner of its spread and the nature of the response throughout the heart. Therefore, precise diagnoses are possible in patients with arrhythmia, conduction defects, myocardial damage of various types, including old and recent coronary occlusions, and a number of other disorders as well. Electrocardiography is discussed in detail on pages 408-410.

Cardiac Catheterization

Right heart cardiac catheterization involves the passing of a small-lumen tube into the right atrium by way of the median basilic and subclavian veins and the superior vena cava (Fig. 19-2). This is carried out under direct visualization with a fluoroscope. Pressures within the right atrium are measured and recorded, and blood samples are removed for measurements of the hematocrit and oxygen saturation. The catheter is then passed through the tricuspid valve, and similar tests are performed on the blood within the right ventricle. Finally, the tube is introduced into the pulmonary artery, i.e., through the pulmonic valve, and as far as possible beyond that point, where "capillary" samples are obtained and "capillary" pressures (also known as wedge pressures) are recorded. Then the catheter is withdrawn.

Right heart catheterization is a relatively safe and usually comfortable procedure. It usually takes 2 to 3 hours and is done in a room that can be darkened to permit use of the fluoroscope.

Left heart catheterization involves the passage of a small catheter into the left atrium or ventricle either by puncture of the atrial septum with a specially designed needle, the retrograde passage of a catheter through the aortic valve from a peripheral artery, or direct puncture of the left ventricle through the skin of the anterior chest. It is most often performed to

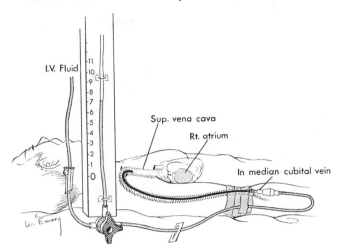

FIG. 19-3. Central venous pressure via median cubital vein. (From Gilbo, D.: Nursing assessment of circulatory function. Nurs. Clin. N. Amer., 3:53-63, 1968)

evaluate the mitral or aortic valve or the coronary arteries. Almost always pressure measurements are combined with x-ray studies (angiography), requiring the injection of radiographic contrast material.

After having made a continuous recording of the arterial pressure and of the pressures within the right atrium, the right ventricle and the pulmonary capillary bed, and intermittent recordings of the total oxygen consumption, along with measurements of the hematocrit and oxygen capacity of blood specimens as specified, it is possible to compute with accuracy the cardiac output; to estimate the pulmonary blood flow in terms of rate and resistance; to evaluate valve function with respect to all valves; and to evaluate the efficiency of pulmonary ventilation, based on the degree of equilibrium established between pulmonary capillary blood and the air in the alveoli. Most important, an accurate and precise diagnosis is possible with respect to the existence and the location of any shunt between systemic venous and arterial channels permitting the bypassing of the pulmonary circulation.

Following the catheterization, the catheter is slowly withdrawn and a dressing is placed over the cutdown site. The patient is usually permitted to resume his normal activities. In the period following cardiac catheterization, the puncture (or cutdown) sites should be watched for hematoma formation, the peripheral pulses checked, and any complaint of pain, numbness, or tingling in the extremities should be reported. Transient arrhythmias during or shortly after the procedure are expected and need not cause the patient concern.

Angiocardiography

This is a technique of injecting dye through an arterial catheter into the heart or selected artery; this procedure is useful in outlining structural abnormalities such as occlusions, defects or fistulas, and it may show abnormal heart valve function. The coronary arteries can be catheterized to show narrowed sclerotic coronary arteries.

The *aortogram* is a form of angiography to outline the lumen of the aorta and the major arteries arising from it. Renal artery stenosis as a cause of hypertension can be diagnosed by this method.

X-ray films and fluoroscopy of the heart and chest show size, shape and position of the heart and indicate which areas may be enlarged or otherwise abnormal.

Central Venous Pressure

This is monitored in such acute states as shock by passing a catheter into the vena cava and attaching it to a pressure recording device, so that continuous variations may be noted as a guide to use of parenteral fluids and anti-shock drugs (Fig. 19-3) (See also Fig. 15-10).

At times it is important to record the *blood pressure in all four extremities*—especially in the initial evaluation of a patient. Normally, blood pressure is higher in the legs than in the arms, but in the presence of coarctation of the aorta, the blood pressure in the legs is low.

Circulation Time

The technique of performing the circulation time test is to inject Decholin intravenously and to time the interval from the injection to when the patient reports a bitter taste on the tongue. This is known as the arm-to-tongue circulation time, and is 12 to 15 seconds in duration.

Enzyme Tests

SGOT (serum glutamic oxaloacetic transaminase), the LDH (lactic dehydrogenase) and CPK (creatine phosphokinase) are enzymes contained within the heart muscle cells. In injury to myocardial cells, these enzymes are released in the bloodstream and elevated levels are found in the serum. LDH is very nonspecific for the heart, being found in many body cells. SGOT is present in liver and muscle as well as in heart cells, and to be evaluated as a test of heart function, one must know that there is no liver or skeletal muscle damage. CPK is more specific, being present only in heart and muscle. With a clinical picture of myocardial infarction and in the absence of skeletal muscle disease, SGOT and CPK are very good confirmatory tests, because many times the electrocardiogram is not diagnostic.

CARDIAC ARRHYTHMIAS

The rate and the rhythm of the heartbeat depend on the speed and the regularity with which electrical impulses are generated by the pacemaker—normally the SA node—and on the functional integrity of the conduction system that distributes these impulses through the myocardium. The activity of this node, as previously pointed out, is subject to the influence of the autonomic nervous system. Moreover, it responds to chemical changes in the blood and is highly susceptible to the action of several drugs. Its normal activity may be altered and its conduction pathways interrupted as a result of local disease. And its function as a pacemaker can be usurped by the AV node or by some other "hyperirritable" focus elsewhere in the conduction system. Moreover, heart muscle has the ability to contract on its own, without benefit of nervous control; this property becomes important in patients with complete heart-block, whose ventricles beat at a slow, unvarying pace, approximately 28 beats per minute, or the so-called idioventricular rate. Factors such as these, affecting the production or the distribution of pacemaking impulses, may speed or slow the heart rate, producing tachycardia or bradycardia respectively, or disrupt its rhythm, i.e., cause an arrhythmia. (The term *arrhythmia*, as it commonly is applied, refers to abnormalities of heart rate, as well as to irregularities of rhythm.)

The existence of an arrhythmia may or may not be responsible for symptoms; it may or may not represent a manifestation of serious underlying heart disease; and it may or may not jeopardize, per se, the health and the safety of the patient. How various arrhythmias differ with respect to clinical features, complications and clinical significance is the topic of the following sections, in which certain of the more common and important types are described.

Ectopic Beats

The most common cardiac irregularity is that caused by ectopic beats that occur ahead of schedule (called *premature beats*). While the heart is contracting regularly and all of its beats are originating in the sinoatrial node, some overly irritable portion of the wall of the atrium or the ventricle suddenly starts an abnormal impulse to contract. Each premature beat follows very soon, but not immediately, after one of the regular beats. (It cannot follow immediately. No stimulus can arouse the ventricle then, for each contraction momentarily uses up all the available energy of the myocardium. This brief period is called the *refractory phase* of the beat.) The premature beat itself may not be noted by the patient; he is more apt to detect the next normal beat, which tends to be unusually forceful because of the usual post-ectopic pause that allows the heart to overstuff itself with venous blood. The patient may say that the heart "jumped," "turned over," or "jarred the whole body."

Premature beats occur in many types of heart disease, but the patient often is unconscious of them. On the other hand, the premature beats of which patients complain may arise in hearts that are organically normal; ectopic beats sometimes merely signify that the patient is nervous, smokes too much, drinks too much coffee, etc.

Paroxysmal Atrial Tachycardia

In the condition called *paroxysmal atrial tachycardia,* the heart suddenly doubles or trebles the number of its systoles per minute, continues at this rate for a while and then, just as suddenly, resumes its normal speed. Such attacks of regular, rapid heart action, during which the heart is not under the control of the sino-atrial node, may last for minutes, hours or even days in otherwise healthy persons. Similar attacks of tachycardia occur in patients with valvular and other types of heart disease, and these are often of more serious consequence. How much patients suffer from such attacks depends on the personality of the individual. Most patients feel exhausted and have shortness of breath while the attacks last, often a sense of fluttering under the sternum and possibly a peculiar feeling of apprehension; but the majority suffer no serious distress. A few, however, have pronounced cardiac palpitation and even severe anginal pains.

The cause of paroxysmal tachycardia in people without organic heart disease is not known, but the chances are that some spot in the wall of the atrium, less often in that of the ventricle, is hyperirritable from birth and occasionally usurps for a while the function of the sino-atrial node as the heart's pacemaker. This condition usually has little or no serious importance unless the heart rate is very fast or the attack is prolonged.

Treatment. Sedation with barbiturates or tranquilizers may be tried. The patient should stop smoking and cut out coffee and other stimulants such as amphetamines, which are often used in weight-reduction programs. A search for thyrotoxicosis should be carried out. If these measures are unsuccessful, a variety of drugs may be tried, of which a digitalis preparation is probably one of the safest.

Atrial Fibrillation

Atrial fibrillation, indicated by a pulse that is totally irregular in force and rhythm, develops in the following conditions: in about one half of all patients with severe cardiac disease, in hyperthyroidism, in acute fevers, sometimes in digitalis intoxication and in patients with atherosclerotic and hypertensive heart disease. The condition may be continuous or it may occur for limited periods of time only (paroxysmal fibrillation).

The presence of atrial fibrillation means that the sino-atrial node has entirely lost control of the heart rhythm and that numerous parts of the atrial wall are being stimulated to contract simultaneously and with great rapidity, with the result that the atrium merely quivers, that is, fibrillates. An atrium beating in this manner sends a confused medley of stimuli to the ventricles, which respond as strongly and to as many impulses as possible.

In atrial fibrillation, all grades of irregularity in force and rhythm are seen. Sometimes the tumultuous beating is so severe that the condition is called *delirium cordis.* In other patients the symptoms are absent or so mild that the condition is detected only after a routine physical examination or electrocardiogram. Physical activity does not regularize a fibrillating heart. This is an important point in diagnosis, since it excludes the somewhat similar irregularity due to the presence of numerous premature beats, because these are sometimes abolished by exercise in the patient without heart disease.

The ventricle may receive as many as 500 stimuli per minute. Although the refractory period allows it to respond to fewer than half that many impulses, nonetheless the ventricle is likely to beat at an excessive speed—so rapidly that it does not have time to fill adequately between successive beats. This inadequacy leads to a reduction in cardiac output. The heart rate at the apex may range from 150 to 220 beats per minute, but because of gross variations in stroke volume, there usually is a pulse deficit at the wrist compared to the apex beat (radial pulse slower than apical rate).

Treatment. The object of treatment is to protect the ventricles and improve their efficiency by reducing the rate of their contractions. This is accomplished by digitalis, a drug that stimulates the vagus nerve and retards the rate of atrioventricular conduction, thus blocking most of the stimuli originating in the quivering atria. An attempt may be made to restore the cardiac rhythm to normal by cardioversion, that is, by administering a brief electrical shock; thereafter, digitalis is often continued prophylactically, together with drugs like Pronestyl (procaine amide) or quinidine, which reduce the electrical excitability of the myocardium. It is important to bear in mind that the fibrillating atrium is a favored site for the formation of a thrombus; should it harbor such a thrombus, restoration of its rhythm to normal may cause the clot to be dislodged and then propelled into the pulmonary or systemic circulation with consequences, such as pulmonary or cerebral infarction, that potentially are fatal. Atrial thrombus formation is favored by prolonged fibrillation.

Atrial Flutter

This disturbance of heart action is characterized by a tachycardia of the atrium, this chamber beating regularly at a rate around 300 times a minute, while the ventricle, protected by a greater or lesser degree of heart-block, responds to each second, third, or fourth atrial contraction. The result is a pulse rate that is seldom over 150 per minute. Before treatment the ventricular rate is usually regular at about 140 to 150 beats per minute because it is responding to every other atrial beat (2:1 AV block). After digitalis has been given to slow the ventricular rate, the pulse is usually irregular or only semi-regular, often doubling or halving its rate. This condition may resemble fibrillation, which possibly is due to a related mechanism; moreover the 2 conditions often alternate. Atrial flutter is seen commonly in elderly persons, in whom it may persist for months or years with few or no symptoms other than palpitation. Fainting spells occur in a few patients.

Treatment. The best treatment of flutter is cardioversion, or digitalis in sufficiently large doses to cause a higher degree of heart-block. Following digitalization, the flutter may persist or atrial fibrillation may ensue; however, restoration of normal sinus rhythm occurs in a significant number of instances.

Heart-Block

Heart-block results from disturbances of the atrioventricular bundle that keep some (*partial block*) or all (*complete block*) of the stimuli from the atria from reaching the ventricles. In cases of *partial block,* if each second stimulus is blocked, the pulse is regular but slow; if each third or each fourth stimulus fails to pass, a bigeminal or trigeminal pulse is observed. However, as a rule, the result of partial heart-block is an irregular pulse. The diagnosis is made best from electrocardiograph records, which show that some atrial beats meet with no response from the ventricles.

Complete heart-block implies complete independence of the atrial and ventricular contractions, the bundle of His having become impassable for stimuli. The block may be temporary or permanent; if permanent, the ventricles may initiate and control their own contractions for many years, beating at a regular pace but slowly, about 28 beats per minute, which is characteristic of the idioventricular rhythm. However, such stability is the exception rather than the rule, because the majority of patients with lesions involving the bundle exhibit a variety of ventricular arrhythmias and tend to shift from one to another. Associated with each shift may be a temporary cessation of cardiac output, followed at once by a precipitous fall of the arterial pressure nearly to zero. *When cardiac output is reduced suddenly, the most sensitive area to react to*

a lessened oxygen supply is the cerebrum. With halting of the cerebral blood flow, the brain rapidly becomes hypoxic, the patient loses consciousness and may have a convulsive seizure. Without prompt resumption of effective ventricular contractions, death is inevitable. Such an episode is termed a "Stokes-Adams attack" and its recurrence is the hallmark of "Stokes-Adams disease" (or syndrome).

Transient complete heart-block may be induced with large doses of digitalis and its analogues, quinidine and certain poisons. In patients with "carotid sinus sensitivity" it may be produced by overstimulation of the vagus. Moreover, it may develop in the course of acute rheumatic fever. Complete block, which may be permanent, can result from damage to the bundle of His by an impinging, invasive or ulcerative lesion in the septum, such as a gumma or a tumor. However, it most often follows an occlusion of the posterior coronary artery, which provides this bundle with its principle blood supply.

The treatment of heart-block is to remove the cause, if possible. When complete or partial block is attended by episodic arrhythmias and Stokes-Adams attacks, treatment is decidedly indicated and is available. Long-range definitive therapy involves installation of an electrical pacemaker, i.e., transvenous electrode, within the lumen of the right ventricle or the implantation of an electrode directly on the wall of the left ventricle (see p. 367). In either case, the contraction stimulus is supplied by a miniaturized and subcutaneously implanted electronic pacemaker. The medical, surgical and nursing implications of Stokes-Adams disease (syndrome) will now be considered.

Stokes-Adams Disease

As a result of arteriosclerotic coronary artery disease or after myocardial infarction, tissue necrosis may occur and scars form in a location that coincides with the pathways of the electrical impulses through or below the AV node, interrupting their conduction and producing atrioventricular block. The conduction defect produces unpredictable disturbances of ventricular rhythm that are manifested by either a slow idioventricular rhythm, ventricular standstill, and less commonly, even ventricular tachycardia or ventricular fibrillation. The block may be transient or permanent, partial or complete. The resultant reduction in cardiac output produces cerebral ischemia and presents as dizziness, syncope, convulsions, or death. Once the conduction defect has taken place these patients must be treated vigorously to increase the ventricular rate. Such drugs as Isuprel, which is sympathomimetic, and atropine, which is parasympatholytic, are sometimes helpful stop-gap measures for increasing the rate for adequate cardiac output. However, even with vigorous

Fig. 19-4. The Chardack-Great-batch Cardiac Pacemaker as it fits into a subcutaneous pocket below the shoulder. The electrode is threaded through the jugular vein for its descent through the superior vena cava, atrium and into the ventricle where it is attached to the myocardium. (Medtronic, Inc.)

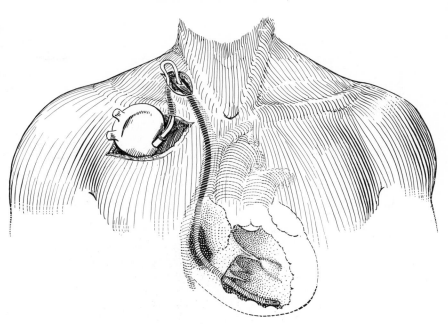

medical management, life expectancy is probably less than 2 years.

Because the life-endangering defect is the disturbance in ventricular rhythm, some other source of stimuli must be used to sustain an adequate ventricular rate. This has become possible through direct electrical stimulation of the myocardium, utilizing an external source of electricity and transmitting the impulses through intracardiac electrodes, or electrodes implanted directly on the ventricular muscle. Stokes-Adams disease is the major indication for external pacing of the heart. Another is a somewhat similar conduction defect that sometimes occurs as a complication of open-heart surgery of the interventricular septum; depending on whether the conduction tissue is destroyed or merely injured, the heart will require permanent or temporary pacing.

Temporary Cardiac Pacing

The cardiac arrest that occurs in Stokes-Adams attacks can be reversed quickly by pounding on the sternum or by external cardiac massage (see p. 425). Here, perhaps more than in any other field, nursing care makes the difference between life and death. Therefore, nurses must learn to administer external cardiac massage to sustain the patient until the external pacemaker can be applied.

Patients with Stokes-Adams attacks are admitted to the hospital immediately and placed on a medical program. Electrodes are attached to the chest wall overlying the heart and connected to a monitoring system. The monitoring system contains an oscilloscope, an external pacemaker, and a defibrillator. The oscilloscope allows constant observation of the electrocardiograph pattern, the pacemaker can be started quickly when the impulses from the heart cease, and the defibrillator is used to stop ventricular fibrillation. Since a high voltage is necessary to pace the heart through the chest wall, it is very painful and distressing, and a low voltage system of which the patient is not conscious must be put in place as soon as possible.

Another method of temporary pacing is done in the fluoroscopy room. After preparing the patient, a cardiac electrode is passed into the right ventricle of the heart by way of the anterior jugular vein in the right side of the neck, the subclavian, or through the basilic vein of the arm (Fig. 19-4). This electrode is similar to a cardiac catheter, but it has 2 electrodes within and 2 connections remaining on the outside. The 2 connections are attached to a low voltage (10 to 12 v.), external transistorized battery-powered pacemaker. This pacemaker produces a current of about 2 milliamperes and is capable of pacing the heart without sensation to the patient.

Although this electrode may be used for extended periods of time, even up to several weeks, the disadvantages are that sepsis may occur where the electrode enters the skin, and it is cumbersome for the patient to manage. However, it allows adequate time for studying the patient, for the heart to recover from its insult, or for obtaining an implantable pacemaker.

The safest pacemakers are those that sense any spontaneous ventricular beats and are thereby inhibited from firing in competition with any occasional, nor-

POSTOPERATIVE MANAGEMENT FOLLOWING PACEMAKER IMPLANTATION*

THERAPEUTIC PLAN	RATIONALE	NURSING RESPONSIBILITY
Meperidine hydrochloride 25-35 mg. q. 3 h., p.r.n. for pain.	Following thoracic surgery, respirations are depressed. A small amount of a less depressing narcotic is ordered at more frequent intervals. Care must be taken not to depress cough reflex.	Traumatized tissue, apprehension, need to cough and take deep breaths do not lessen pain. Observe for pain and pain-filled non-verbal expressions; administer medication and/or provide other comfort measures— mere presence, understanding, positioning, planning care about rest periods.
B.P. & pulse q. 15 min. until stable; q. ½ h.; q. 1 h.	Prime indicators of adequate heart function. Constant monitoring to ascertain effectiveness of pacemaker.	Accurate and alert readings and recordings to prevent complications. Apical beat, radial pulse and oscilloscope must synchronize.
Aqueous penicillin 1,000,000 U. q. 6 h. and chloramphenicol 500 mg. IM q. 6 h.	There is natural intolerance of foreign object by the body; this area becomes subject to infection.	Administration of intramuscular medications at proper intervals to maintain antibiotic titer.
First urine specimen to laboratory.	To determine possible presence of hemoglobin in urine, secondary to transfusion reaction. Presence of acidosis.	Collection of specimen and immediate delivery to laboratory.
1000 cc. 5% Dextrose/ water IV to run for 8 h.	For nutritional needs. No saline because of retention possibility. Slowly, not to overload cardiovascular system.	Start IV in site where rigid positioning is not necessary. Observe frequently for infiltration and regulation.
Sips of water.	Begin fluid replacement to limit IV needs into the cardiovascular system.	Offer frequent and small amounts. Explain why necessary.
Chest suction —25 cm./H$_2$O	To drain pleural space and enhance return of subatmospheric intrapleural pressure; re-expansion of lung. To determine drainage and blood loss.	Explanation. Observe and record accurate hourly amount and character of fluid (a calibrated adhesive strip on collection). Avoid kinks or loops in tube. Provide comfort in positioning.
Abdominal tube (from pouch) to suction.	Small amount of suction prevents accumulation at site and hastens healing.	Same as above.
Cough and deep breaths, q. 2 h.	To increase pulmonary volume and prevent retention of mucus, leading to atelectasis.	Explanation, reminders, ecouragement. Assistance splinting operated area.
Bland diet.	To avoid excessive stimulation and fatigue of regular diet.	Provide small amounts, appetizing foods.
Portable upright chest x-ray. (Shield abdomen with lead apron.)	To ascertain re-expansion of lung and freedom from atelectasis. Shield is precaution for pacemaker.	Careful explanation to allay fears. Assist in positioning patient.
Phenobarbital 15 mg. q. 4 h.	To allay or decrease apprehension.	Proper administration, observation and recording.
Ambulation (second day)	Prevent postoperative vascular and pulmonary complications.	Assistance. Avoid time immediately after meals. Watch tubes.
Thoracentesis (not always routine)	To remove retained fluids. (Eighth operative day 150 ml. removed.)	Explanation and support for patient. Assist physician. Stop if patient coughs.

* Sr. M. C. Moore: Nursing care of a patient with an implanted artificial pacemaker. Cardio-Vascular Nursing, Vol. 2, Winter, 1969, American Heart Assoc. Inc.

mally-conducted or ectopic beats. Such instruments are called "demand" pacemakers, in that they fire only when the heart rate falls below a certain limit (usually around 70 beats per minute). The batteries that power the instruments presently available last about 3 years, after which the power pack must be replaced. A vigorous search for a more lasting power source is under way. (See Chap. 20 for pacing in the Cardiac Care Unit.)

Surgical Implantation of the Myocardial Pacer

Preoperative Preparation of the Patient. The discussion thus far has dealt with the stabilization of the patient in preparation for surgical implantation of a pacemaker. This represents part of the preoperative preparation of the patient. Concern, understanding of the patient's needs and the offering of explanations constitute the support offered by the nurse.

Before the open operation these patients need tremendous reassurance. They realize that their hearts are diseased and therefore are frightened by the thought of a heart operation. However, this fear is managed best by acquainting the patients with the fact that the risk of surgery is less than the risk of their disease.

The most common surgical procedure is the transvenous approach; it consists of implanting a power-pack into a subcutaneous pocket in the axillary region and connecting it to a second transvenous electrode catheter, this one so arranged that no part of it traverses the skin. The temporary catheter electrode and battery-operated external pacer may then be removed. This procedure is the most common one because it does not involve major thoracic surgery, and the average Stokes-Adams patient is quite elderly and hence a relatively poor risk. However, the transvenous electrode sometimes slips out of the right ventricle into the pulmonary artery, and is subject to still other vicissitudes that interrupt pacing. When these episodes occur more than a very few times in a given patient, open chest surgery (thoracotomy) is performed and 2 electrodes are attached to the surface of the left ventricle.

Postoperative Nursing Management. Complications that may occur following the thoracotomy approach are similar to those following this kind of surgery in the elderly patient (p. 268). Occasionally, the newly-paced heart may go into congestive heart failure and pleural effusion may develop. The nurse should be informed of these possibilities, be able to recognize symptoms, and confer with the physician; digitalis and diuretics are then given.

After installation of the intracardiac electrode, the patient's pulse must be watched very carefully until the optimal voltage is determined. Because the impulse is transmitted through a column of blood rather than directly to the myocardium, the heart does not respond to every impulse until the voltage controls are optimally adjusted and readjusted as necessary. Following installation of the pacemaker the patient is relatively out of danger, but close attention again must be given to vital signs.

The major complication following pacemaker implantation is, of course, a faulty unit that ceases to function. Under these circumstances the patient is treated as in a Stokes-Adams attack with external massage, external pacemaker, a medical program, and then a temporary transvenous pacemaker until the defect is corrected or a new pacemaker can be implanted.

Rehabilitation. Because the patient begins to feel so much better, he often develops a false sense of security. The conduction defect is corrected and his disability is relieved, but the underlying problem is still present. Without the pacemaker his former symptoms would return. Because of this, the patient and/or his family should take time to count the pulse for a full minute at least twice daily. A rate increase may indicate the weakening of the battery and should be reported. The patient also should know of energy-saving activities (literature available from the local Heart Association) and reminded that periodic check-ups with his physician are essential.

Cardiac Arrest and Resuscitation

Cardiac arrest is defined as the sudden, unexpected cessation of the heartbeat. All heart action may stop, or asynchronized muscular twitchings (ventricular fibrillation) may occur. The incidence of cardiac arrest in the operating room varies, but is thought to approximate 1 in 1,200 operations. The factors that play a major role in the etiology of arrest are the following: anoxia caused by airway obstruction; inadequate ventilation; anesthetic depression; hypotension; retention of CO_2 (hypercapnia); coronary occlusion and myocardial infarction; and neurogenic reflexes. Outside of the operating room, cardiac arrest may result from drowning, electric shock, carbon monoxide and other types of poisoning, drug reactions, and suffocation, and coronary artery disease or occlusion.

There is a 4-minute interval between the cessation of circulation and the appearance of irreversible brain damage. During this period, the diagnosis of arrest must be made and the circulation must be restored. *The most reliable sign of arrest is the absence of a carotid pulsation.* Valuable time should not be wasted taking the blood pressure, or listening for the heartbeat. *Details of the resuscitation procedure may be found on pages 425-426.*

Postresuscitation Measures

After cardiac resuscitation, close observation of the vital signs is important because of the high incidence of recurrent arrest. Adequate pulmonary ventilation must be maintained. Oxygen therapy is administered. Tracheal aspiration may be helpful. When bronchial secretions cannot be cleared by coughing or aspiration, a tracheotomy is performed. Pneumothorax is a common complication, due to rib fracture during massage. If cardiac massage is performed incorrectly the sternal xiphoid process may puncture the liver producing hemorrhage. The patient may be restless and noisy following resuscitation from cerebral hypoxia. Seizures are relatively common from metabolic acidosis.

The patient's temperature is taken hourly; a rapid rise usually indicates cerebral damage and cerebral edema. The latter may be treated by hypothermia or agents to lower intracerebral pressure (mannitol infusions or the like).

Nursing of Patients
With Cardiac Arrhythmias

The medical and nursing management of patients with arrhythmias has been radically changed by the use of monitoring devices, electrical defibrillation, cardiac pacing and drugs. The concept of monitoring patients with an arrhythmia is one of *prevention* of a subsequent cardiac catastrophe. Armed with comprehensive knowledge about the action of the heart, the nurse seeks to make meaningful patient observations. There is a need to recognize the symptoms that can be noted before a death-producing arrhythmia occurs. By readily recognizing a problem, nursing judgments are made and a plan of action instituted *before* the monitoring alarm sounds.

Not infrequently the nurse is the first to recognize the existence of an arrhythmia, based on her examination of a patient's pulse. Examination of a pulse never should become "routine." The nurse invariably should seek to correlate its rate, rhythm and character with other facets of her patient's condition. In so doing, she cannot fail to improve her acuity as a clinical observer and thus add continuously and materially to her accumulating stores of knowledge.

Nurses should be diarists, recording everything of significance that they observe. Of all members of the health team they are the ones who spend the most time with the patient and, as a result, are in the best position to acquire significant data. For example, their recorded description of a patient's appearance and behavior during an episode of arrhythmia very often proves invaluable and, in many instances, this information otherwise is unobtainable.

The pulse should be counted carefully for at least one full minute. Variations in force and frequency, as well as general characteristics and overall rate, should be noted. If an abnormality is detected, it should be reported without delay. The carotid pulse should be counted in addition to the radial pulse, and, if an arrhythmia is suspected, the apical pulse rate should be measured by auscultation as well. It must be borne in mind that abnormal beats may not be detectable at the wrist, since a very weak pulse wave often fails to reach the periphery and, in this event, the apical and radial rates will not correspond. Both must be counted simultaneously but independently by 2 observers for no less than one minute, in order to determine the degree to which they differ quantitatively, i.e., the pulse deficit. The greater the deficit, the less efficient the ventricular contractions are assumed to be, and the less favorable the clinical evaluation of cardiac function.

The electrocardiogram is of great value in establishing the type of rhythmic disturbance that is present. This recording is most informative during the course of an arrhythmic episode. Arrhythmias are prone to be transient and elusive. Should the nurse discover evidence of such a disorder in a patient previously free of cardiac arrhythmia, or in whom a diagnosis of arrhythmia has not been established with certainty, she should see that an electrocardiogram (ECG) is recorded. It is quite helpful in reducing patient anxiety if the nurse explains to the patient the basic principles of the electrocardiogram and its application in his particular case. The patient should not drink ice water or, for that matter, any cold drinks. The ingestion of cold fluids may trigger premature beats or atrial fibrillation.

If the patient is constipated (from medications, reduction of activity and food intake), straining at the stool can cause reduction of cardiac output, increased venous pressure and a fall in blood pressure that may lead to an arrhythmia, myocardial rupture or pulmonary embolism. Constipation and straining are avoided by giving laxatives, suppositories and stool softeners according to the individual patient's needs.

Many patients with an arrhythmia complain of palpitation, shortness of breath, dizziness and precordial pain, and they are prone to be anxious. Anxiety tends to beget more symptoms, which promote increased anxiety with further aggravation of symptoms, etc., until fear and anxiety far outweigh the actual gravity of the organic disorder. From the standpoint of this patient's cardiac status, as well as his comfort, it is important that this vicious cycle be broken. Broken it can be, and readily, by a display on the part of the nurse of an attitude that at once expresses confidence and composure, that evinces understanding and implies capability; an attitude that is founded securely on clinical experience, sound education and detailed knowledge of the problem, and an attitude to which this knowledge lends the necessary conviction.

Electrocardiography and the interpretation of cardiac arrhythmias is discussed in further detail in chapter 20.

PATIENTS WITH
CORONARY ARTERY DISEASE

Underlying Pathophysiology of
Coronary Arteriosclerosis

Commonest of all the disorders of the heart is coronary arteriosclerosis or, more specifically, atherosclerosis. This disease produces degeneration and fibrosis of the myocardium and eventual cardiac failure. Or it may cause more acute episodes of myocardial hypoxia that are manifested by attacks of angina pectoris and that lead eventually to acute myocardial infarction. Atherosclerosis, the prevailing type of arteriosclerosis, begins with fatty degeneration of the vascular intima, a process that subsequently extends to involve also the media. Waxy cholesterol plaques become deposited on the inner lining of the arteries, interfering with the absorption of nutrients by the endothelial cells that compose the lining, and obstructing the blood flow by their protrusion into the lumen of the vessel. The vascular endothelium in involved areas becomes necrotic, then scarred, further compromising the lumen and impeding the flow of blood. At sites such as these, where the lumen is narrow and the walls rough, there is a great tendency for clots to form, which explains the fact that intravascular coagulation, followed by thromboembolic disease, is among the most important complications of atherosclerosis (and among the more important of all the diseases to which man is heir!).

A second form of arteriosclerosis is characterized by thickening and calcification of the arterial media, converting the vessel into a relatively inflexible tube with a very narrow lumen. Patients with hypertension exhibit such changes with some regularity and with consequences that are usually benign. Unfortunately, hypertension promotes ordinary atherosclerosis as well with a vengeance, which is responsible for most of its major dangers and complications (see p. 353).

Coronary atherosclerosis produces symptoms and complications through narrowing of the arterial lumena, and obstruction of blood flow therein. This impediment to blood flow persists and progresses, to the extreme detriment of all tissue cells that depend for their survival on the native components of blood and on various other constituents that it transports. In greatest jeopardy are the cells that require more than the average amount of oxygen, dextrose, amino acids, or other nutrients—such as the brain, the kidneys and the heart muscle. Myocardial cells, deprived of their customary and normal supply of nutrients and oxygen, undergo degeneration and eventually are replaced by fibrocytes, the harbingers of scarring. Altered in structure, its functional efficiency forever impaired, the heart eventually must fail.

The cardinal symptom of relative myocardial hypoxia is pain of cardiac origin. This is also the outstanding feature of the angina pectoris syndrome, as well as an early, prominent manifestation of myocardial infarction.

Angina Pectoris

Angina pectoris is a syndrome that is featured by paroxysms of pain in the anterior chest, produced as a result of insufficient coronary blood flow and myocardial hypoxia. This may be a purely relative matter: i.e., in the face of constant coronary flow in an indi-

vidual previously without symptoms, acute myocardial hypoxia, with the classic symptoms of angina pectoris and with characteristic changes on electrocardiogram, may occur at any time as a result of any number of factors, especially the following: physical exertion, especially exertion of an unaccustomed type; strong emotion; exposure to cold; or a heavy meal. The majority of patients with angina pectoris are males over 45, who ostensibly had been in excellent health and considered themselves to be perfectly fit.

The pain varies greatly in severity, from a sense of mere upper substernal pressure to pain that is agonizing. Typically it comes on with exertion and disappears with rest. In advanced cases it may come on during bed rest. If severe and typical, it starts over the precordium and the upper sternum, radiates to the left shoulder and sometimes down the inner surface of the arm to the elbow, the wrist, and even to the fifth and ulnar aspect of the fourth fingers. Occasionally it seems to start in the throat, hence the name *angina*. In some cases it is reflected to the right shoulder or arm; in others, to the upper abdomen, in which case it may simulate gallstones. When it is at all severe, the patient at once immobilizes himself. He cannot do otherwise; he cannot speak, his face is ashen, and he is covered with clammy sweat. With rest, the attack passes off completely, leaving him comfortable. Along with the physical pain, the patient also suffers a mental agony, a sense of impending death. This apprehension is so characteristic that when it occurs alone, as it sometimes does, it is sufficient for diagnosis.

Management

The basic program of care for the patient with angina pectoris embodies 3 aspects: (1) the amelioration of symptoms during attacks; (2) the abortion of attacks, or curtailment of their duration; and, (3) prevention of recurrences. Each patient must be evaluated and treated on an individual basis.

During an anginal attack the presence of a capable, knowledgable and understanding nurse is definitely beneficial from the therapeutic standpoint, tending, as it does, to allay apprehension, therefore helping to reduce a tachycardia or an elevation of cardiac work that, if present, might promote or prolong myocardial hypoxia.

The pain of an acute anginal attack usually is controlled with 1 or 2 tablets of nitroglycerin (glyceryl trinitrate), containing from 0.3 to 0.4 mg. and placed under the tongue or in the buccal pouch. Instruct the patient to keep the tongue still and avoid swallowing saliva until the tablet is dissolved. Its action is rapid and, in most patients, very effective. The patient should be reassured as to the nonhabituating qualities of the drug and cautioned to carry it with him at all times. For some patients the inhalation of amyl nitrite is equally effective. This agent, a liquid, is stored and distributed in tiny sealed glass tubes, which may be broken in a handkerchief and inhaled, as needed. Various longer acting nitrate derivates may be prescribed for prophylaxis Propranolol (a beta-adrenergic receptor blocking agent), in varying dosages, has been found to decrease the number of anginal attacks. It reduces the oxygen requirements of the myocardium and is useful in patients who have limited exercise capacity.

If a patient senses that an attack is imminent he should cease all unnecessary movement, the objective being to reduce to a minimum the oxygen requirements of his ischemic myocardium, hoping that its needs can be met by the limited supply presently available and the impending attack thereby averted.

There are patients whose attacks occur predominantly in the morning. This peculiar predilection obviously calls for a change in the schedule of daily activities. As a first step, the patient should plan to rise earlier each morning so that he may complete his shaving, washing and dressing in a more leisurely fashion and, hopefully, may maintain this unhurried pace throughout the entire day—performing his scheduled tasks and meeting whatever commitments he has without haste or a sense of pressure. Sound teaching for any patient with angina pectoris would be to initiate all movements with deliberation; avoid exposure to cold; avoid tobacco; eat regularly but lightly; and, if overweight, correct obesity.

Nursing Assessment of the Patient with Anginal Pain

If the patient is in the hospital, the nurse can observe with care and record all facets of his activity, with particular regard for the activities that have been found to precede and may precipitate attacks of anginal pain. When do attacks tend to occur? Shortly following a meal? After engaging in certain activities? After physical activity in general? After visits from members of the family, or others? Where is the pain located? How does the patient describe the pain? Was the onset of pain gradual or sudden? How long did it last—seconds? minutes? hours? Was the pain steady and unwavering in quality? How many minutes after taking nitroglycerine did the pain last? What was the mode of abatement? The answers to these questions, ascertained from observation, can provide valuable clues to the conduct of an effective convalescent program and a basis for designing a logical program of prevention.

As a group, patients with angina pectoris are inclined to be tense and fearful, especially if they have lived with their diagnosis for a short time only and as

PATIENT EDUCATION

A patient with heart disease should learn to regulate his activity according to his individual response. The goal is always to prevent progression of disease and the development of congestive heart failure.

THE PATIENT WITH ANGINA PECTORIS

I. To prevent an episode of anginal pain:
  A. Use moderation in all activities of life.
    1. Participate in a normal daily program, the activities of which do not produce chest discomfort, shortness of breath and undue fatigue.
    2. Avoid overeating.
      (a) Refrain from engaging in physical activity one hour after meals.
      (b) Attempt to keep weight slightly below normal.
    3. Shun situations that are emotionally stressful.
    4. Stop smoking.
    5. Try to avoid cold weather if possible.
      (a) Dress warmly in winter.
      (b) Walk more slowly in cold weather.
    6. Avoid activities that require *heavy* effort (carrying heavy objects).
  B. Follow general principles of good hygienic living.

II. To cope with an attack of anginal pain:
  A. Carry nitroglycerine at all times.
    1. Renew nitroglycerine supply every three months.
    2. Take nitroglycerine before emotionally stressful situations if possible.
  B. Place nitroglycerine under tongue at first sign of chest discomfort.
    1. Do not swallow saliva until the tablet is dissolved.
    2. Stop and rest until all pain subsides.

yet do not comprehend or are unwilling to accept its implications. There are favorable aspects to every situation—including this patient's—however bleak it may appear. Of these, he needs to be made aware and reminded constantly. Moreover, he should be encouraged to participate actively, and as soon as possible, in a systematic program of convalescence and prevention—a program that is calculated to bolster and sustain his morale, restore self-confidence and foster independence. Its major objective and its principal effort, to which the nurse is a most important contributor, is his education (see above). Education of the cardiac patient, conducted on a fairly sophisticated level, is designed to acquaint him with the basic nature of his illness and to furnish him with the facts he needs if he is to reorganize his living habits in a way that is effecitve, i.e., that will reduce the frequency and the severity of the anginal attacks, delay the progress of the underlying disease and help to protect him from other complications. Moreover, teaching the patient to live by good hygienic prin-

Fig. 19-5. The arrow points out a myocardial infarction. (Armed Forces Institute of Pathology, Neg. No. 55-19447)

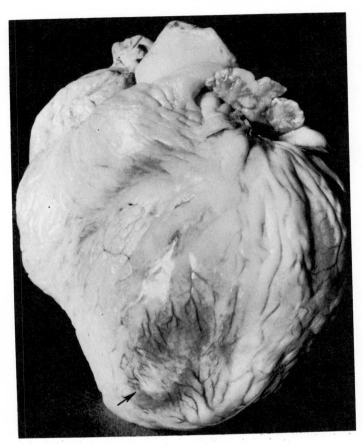

ciples and offering him empathetic reassurance is part of the therapy for the patient with angina.

Myocardial Infarction

This term refers to the process by which myocardial tissue is destroyed in regions of the heart that are deprived of their blood supply after closure of the coronary artery or one of its branches, either by a thrombus or through obstruction of the vessel lumen by atherosclerosis.

Symptoms

The majority of patients with myocardial infarction are men over 40 with arteriosclerosis of the coronary vessels and often with arterial hypertension. In a typical patient, the pain starts suddenly, usually over the lower sternal region and the upper abdomen, and is continuous; but it may increase steadily in severity until it becomes almost unendurable. It is a heavy viselike pain, which may radiate to the shoulders and down the arms, usually the left. Unlike the pain of true angina, it begins spontaneously (not following effort, emotional upset, etc.), persists for hours or days and is relieved neither by rest nor by nitrites. The pulse

may become very rapid, irregular and feeble, even imperceptible, and the heart may dilate. Gallop rhythm (accentuated third heart sound making the three heart sounds similar to those of a galloping horse) often develops. It is important to note that about 15 per cent of the patients with acute myocardial infarction, diagnosed on the basis of subsequent electrocardiograms, deny having experienced any pain or discomfort whatever. These are the so-called "silent coronaries."

From the first, the patient with a severe occlusion may be in shock; his color is ashen, he breaks out in a clammy sweat and in a few minutes is confined to bed. Vomiting is common. In a few hours his temperature rises, his blood pressure falls to an unusually low point, the leukocyte count rises to 15,000 or 20,000. Changes are seen with great regularity in the electrocardiogram; changes testifying not only to the presence, but also to the location, of the infarct. The SGOT rises in 6 to 12 hours and reverts to normal in 3 to 4 days (see p. 364).

Prognosis

The possibility of recovery depends on the size of the infarct. Some patients die instantly, others in a few minutes or hours. Other patients live a few days, often from 4 to 10, and then die either from softening and rupture of the infarcted area or from myocardial failure. Others suffer from embolus during the following week. (The inner surface of the infarcted area of the heart wall is covered by a blood clot, fragments of which may break loose.) About 50 per cent of all infarct patients recover from the acute attack. Of those who live long enough to get to a hospital, a much higher percentage survive, especially if an intensive coronary care unit is available. A small infarct may heal with scar formation, leaving the patient fairly well, but a second occlusion often occurs later, or the patient develops heart failure. Of those who recover, about 80 per cent can return to normal duties.

Medical and Nursing Management

The most critical period for the patient with a myocardial infarction is during the first 48 hours following the attack. Ventricular fibrillation and cardiac arrest are common causes of sudden death. Ideally, all patients with myocardial infarctions should be admitted to a cardiac care unit for four to five days (see pp. 406, 421-423). It is believed that this action would prevent most of the deaths from arrhythmias.

Medical management and nursing care of the patient with myocardial infarction are designed to: (1) alleviate shock; (2) relieve pain; (3) rest the myocardium; (4) prevent complications; (5) achieve physiologic and functional rehabilitation; and (6) halt the progression of arteriosclerosis, the lesion that is basically responsible for the myocardial infarct. If a cardiac care unit is available, the patient is immediately taken to this unit.

Shock. The patient is admitted to the unit as an emergency, probably on a stretcher and in a state of shock. The same principles of nursing care that are applicable in other shock states are likewise appropriate in the care of this patient. The sitting position may further depress the arterial pressure; therefore, he should not be permitted to adopt it. Unnecessary movements on his part should be discouraged; he should be lifted from the stretcher to the bed.

The patient's pulse and respiratory rates should be measured at frequent intervals, as a guide to the progress of his vascular collapse. Shock must be treated with vigor; the longer it persists, the greater the peril to the patient.

If the patient is severely hypotensive and his skin is cold and clammy, an intravenous infusion of dextrose solution may be started. This serves as a vehicle for the injection of a vasopressor drug, such as Levophed or Aramine and a route of administration that permits the most precise regulation of dosage. The administration of vasopressor agents assists in restoring aortic blood pressure and ensures adequate coronary perfusion. The nurse, under the direction of the physician, can readjust the flow rate as often as necessary in accordance with fluctuations in the blood pressure until such time as the pressure has become stabilized at a normotensive level.

Management of Pain and Hypoxia. Narcotics are given to alleviate pain and apprehension. If pain is only moderately intense, it should respond to intramuscular Demerol; if severe, its control may require intravenous morphine. The wise nurse takes the precaution of measuring the patient's blood pressure and counting the pulse and the respiratory rates before administering these narcotics, because they may depress further the arterial pressure of a patient who already is hypotensive. If pain persists despite analgesic medication, or if the patient appears to become increasingly restless, complains of headache or exhibits pronounced tachycardia, it may be assumed that he is suffering from hypoxia and is a candidate for oxygen inhalation therapy.

Although most patients with acute myocardial infarctions have tachycardia, a number of patients have been found to exhibit a slowing of the pulse (bradycardia) and falling of the blood pressure. A falling heart rate associated with falling arterial pressure indicates deterioration of the patient's condition. If this occurs, atropine may be injected slowly intravenously (0.3 to 2.0 mg.) to raise the heart rate and arterial pressure.

Promotion of Rest. The key element in the treatment and the nursing care of patients with myocardial infarction is rest—physical and emotional—which should be as nearly complete as can be arranged and should be continued until the circulatory status has been restored to normal and the area of infarction has healed, i.e., no less than 3 to 6 weeks.

Oxygen requirements are greater during pressure loads than during volume loads. *Any sudden physical effort is to be avoided.* Over-reaching and straining at the stool should be cautioned against. Exciting television programs are also contraindicated. Proper temperature of the room is most important as restlessness arising from a warm and humid environment increases cardiac output.

The patient should be spared every unnecessary physical exertion. This may create difficulties in the case of a patient who insists on taking care of himself. During the acute stage the patient should be disturbed as little as possible during the hours of sleep, so that maximal rest is received each day. Visits from casual acquaintances and business associates should be deferred, and close friends and relatives, who *are* admitted, should be instructed to avoid lengthy and controversial discussions.

Contrary to prevailing concepts, the recumbent position is not necessarily the posture of choice from the standpoint of cardiac rest. On the contrary, the work of the heart appears to be at a minimum when the patient—especially the elderly patient—is sitting in a chair. This observation is the basis for the "armchair" treatment of heart failure. ("Armchair treatment" does not mean ambulation; it means *rest in an armchair!*).

Ambulation usually is not permitted until 3 or 4 weeks have elapsed after an episode of infarction. The precise time when a particular patient may ambulate is dictated by many considerations and is determined on the basis of the total clinical picture. Moreover, physical exertion is not the sole factor that increases the work of the heart. Others, quite as important from the standpoint of the myocardial burden, include obesity, which should be brought under control, speedily and permanently; arterial hypertension, which, if severe and persistent, should be accorded topmost priority in treatment; anemia, which should be corrected without delay, by whatever means are appropriate; and tobacco smoking, which stimulates peripheral and coronary vasoconstriction and tachycardia and, therefore, should be avoided.

Diet. The diet may be liquid, soft or regular, depending on the patient's circulatory status and comfort. In general, high residue and fermentative foods should be avoided and small feedings supplied at frequent intervals during this acute stage. Sodium is restricted. Ice water and cold fluids are to be avoided, as the ingestion of cold drinks may trigger an arrhythmia.

Nursing Surveillance and Prevention of Complications. The patient's prognosis may be jeopardized by the advent, during the initial 2 weeks, of any one of several complications, including arrhythmias, thromboembolism, congestive failure, and myocardial rupture. To be on the alert for any such development is an important nursing responsibility.

Cardiac Arrhythmias. Arrhythmias are the major cause of death following an acute myocardial infarction. This kind of complication is especially common following posterior myocardial infarcts, inasmuch as the posterior coronary artery furnishes the principal blood supply to the conduction system of the heart.

Experience in cardiac monitoring units has shown a high proportion of patients with myocardial infarctions develop or have arrhythmias. By the use of electronic monitoring equipment the heart beat may be observed constantly. If a beginning arrhythmia can be detected early and treated vigorously, the more serious derangements of cardiac rhythm may be avoided (see chap. 20).

When monitoring equipment is not available and to ensure that an arrhythmia will not fail to be detected, at the earliest possible moment, the pulse should be counted at frequent intervals, preferably by auscultation at the apex and for no less than one full minute. The occurrence of extrasystoles and dropped beats, ordinarily considered of minor import, should be viewed with concern in a patient with a fresh myocardial infarct, for it may signal the onset of a more serious arrhythmia. Any change in the rate, the rhythm, the volume or the character of the patient's pulse should be reported in detail and without delay.

Thromboembolism. Clots tend to form on the interior wall of an infarcted ventricle. From these so-called "mural thrombi" embolic material is likely to separate and find its way into the pulmonary or systemic circulation. Other and more common sources of emboli in patients with myocardial infarction are the leg veins, where blood flow, owing to muscular inactivity and reduced cardiac output, is likely to be sluggish. Phlebothrombosis in the legs may be prevented by the application of elastic stockings and by the performance of leg exercises, including frequent and repeated flexion of the feet and the toes. Deep breathing exercises should be done hourly. Another prophylactic measure of value is the administration of an anticoagulant drug, such as Dicumarol, which inhibits clot formation by reducing the production of factors responsible for the evolution of thrombin. The responsible nurse will see to it that the anticoagulant medication is withheld on each occasion until the daily prothrombin clotting time has been reported by the laboratory, and will inform the physician at once if the results of the test are not within the desired range.

Congestive Failure. This complicaton ensues if myocardial damage is so extensive that cardiac efficiency is impaired, i.e., to the point that ventricular emptying is incomplete and cardiac output is inadequate. The nurse must be on the outlook for the premonitory symptoms of dyspnea and edema—symptoms that may presage the rapid onset of serious pulmonary edema. In an effort to avoid excessive fluid retention, the physician is likely to restrict routinely the sodium intake of all of his patients with a myocardial infarction. (The treatment of congestive heart failure is discussed on page 385.)

Myocardial Rupture. Another complication, likewise a hazard during the first 2 weeks after an infarct, is myocardial rupture, which is almost always fatal. This is most apt to occur in patients with severe hypertension. Of course, the risk is increased by factors or circumstances that tend to elevate the systolic arterial pressure—some of which can be avoided or at least moderated. Among these factors are vigorous coughing and straining at stool which, from the standpoint of arterial pressure, are as stressful as weight lifting or even more so.

THE NURSE AS A CASE FINDER
Prevention of Coronary Heart Disease

Epidemiological studies and observations by cardiologists reveal that there are coronary risk factors that tend to make an individual more prone to develop coronary heart disease. This information is important in the *prevention* of premature coronary heart disease as well as forestalling recurring episodes in patients with known atherosclerotic disease. These factors include:

Hypercholesterolemia
Hypertension
Diabetes Mellitus
Obesity
Habitual dietary intake of excessive calories, total fats, saturated fats, cholesterol, carbohydrates and salt.
Physical inactivity
Cigarette smoking
Positive family history

Patient Education

Certain general rules for living are usually prescribed at this stage, the character of which must vary widely from patient to patient, owing to marked differences in practicalities and individual personalities. The nature of these instructions are decided by the physician, ideally after joint discussion with the nurse whose familiarity with the patient as a person lends great significance to her views of his long-term management. Questions that will pertain may concern such matters as requirements for rest, criteria for controlling activities, recommendations as to diet and the use of tobacco. In relation to smoking, it may be pointed out that most sudden deaths that occur in individuals with a past history of a myocardial infarction are due to cardiac arrhythmia, notably ventricular fibrillation, and that most of the individuals so afflicted are habitually heavy smokers. Logically, any individual who has sustained a myocardial infarct is well advised to eliminate the use of tobacco.

The patient's progress is followed with the aid of repeated electrocardiograms and determinations of the erythrocyte-sedimentation rate. His cardiac function is estimated on the basis of his symptoms and physical signs. Gradually his self-confidence should be built up and a mode of living established, with respect to work, recreation and hobbies, that will enable him to live a useful, happy and active life within the limits of his health. (See patient education summary, p. 377.)

Control of Arteriosclerosis. Obviously, since myocardial infarcts are the result of coronary artery obstruction and since the cause of the latter is usually atherosclerosis, every possible effort should be made to arrest the progress of this vascular lesion. To be sure, atherosclerosis is a multifactorial disease with its occurrence and course dependent on a hereditary predisposition and influenced greatly by the existence of uncontrolled diabetes, obesity or arterial hypertension. Persistent elevation of the blood cholesterol with excessive proportions of saturated, relative to unsaturated, fats in the diet also may be implicated in its pathogenesis. Some of these factors are amenable to control. For example, either diabetes or arterial hypertension, if present, should be managed under constant medical supervision.

The obese patient should lose weight until an optimal nutritional status is attained, a goal that is unlikely to be achieved and, ideally, should not be attempted without the advice and the guidance of a physician. The role of saturated versus unsaturated fatty acids in the diet and of the blood cholesterol level is another area amenable to dietary (and drug) control.

Rehabilitation. The nurse can assist the patient toward his goal of independence even when he is on strict bed rest. This assistance is given by asking the patient's preference in small matters and by directing his thinking toward the time when he will be active again. The objective here is not to change the patient's life pattern but to make necessary modifications. During the recovery phase, find out the fears and hopes of the patient and help him to mobilize his own resources to make these modifications. His questions must be answered truthfully and his confidence built in those who are responsible for his care. These are positive approaches in preventing the patient from becoming a cardiac cripple.

It has been shown that with narrowing of the coronary arteries there is an associated growth of collateral vessels. It takes time for the patient to develop an adequate collateral (secondary) circulation after a myocardial infarction. As the collateral vessels develop, the oxygen supply to the myocardium is increased, and the patient is gradually permitted to return to normal activities. It is desirable to train the patient for each added activity. If the patient has to climb stairs, he should start with a few steps at a time and each day gradually increase the number until he can tolerate a full flight of steps.

The same principle applies to any activity that the patient must attempt in his job. The work situation is analyzed, and the patient is trained and conditioned for each new activity, such as walking the distance to the bus, lifting objects and so forth. The patient is cautioned to stop before he becomes fatigued. The amount of work that he is usually able to assume depends on his occupation as well as the severity of the attack. Most patients can return to a full work status if they can learn to live within their cardiac reserve. Achieving this means stopping activities before becoming fatigued. On the other hand, a regular program of vigorous exercise may be prescribed if the heart has not been so badly damaged that congestive failure is present. There is considerable evidence to indicate that regular exercise to the point of producing a light sweat is a valuable prophylactic measure for the postconvalescent patient. The nurse has a role in restoring the patient's confidence and helping him to adopt his new physical activity status.

PATIENTS WITH ENDOCARDIAL DISEASE

Underlying Pathophysiology

The endocardium is the endothelial layer of tissue that lines the heart's cavities and covers the flaps of its valves. Of the diseases that affect it, the majority represent various types and stages of inflammation, i.e., *endocarditis*, or its aftermath. They include: (1) rheumatic endocarditis, one of the many complications of acute rheumatic fever; (2) bacterial endocarditis, produced by direct bacterial invasion of the endocardium, particularly that portion covering the valve leaflets; and, (3) chronic valvular heart disease, based on structural deformities of the heart valves, either of congenital origin or acquired as a result of either rheumatic or bacterial endocarditis in the past. Whenever an area of endocardium becomes inflamed, for whatever reason, there forms at that site a fibrin clot, called a *vegetation*. In time this clot becomes converted into a mass of scar tissue. The scarred endocardium becomes thickened, stiffened, contracted and deformed. A fringe of vegetations ranging along the free margins of the valve flaps, marking the site of earlier erosions, represents the basic lesion of endocarditis and is the forerunner of chronic valvular heart disease.

Rheumatic Endocarditis

Rheumatic fever is a disease—a preventable disease—that usually has its onset in childhood following a hemolytic streptococcus infection. Whereas the most prominent symptom of rheumatic fever is polyarthritis, the most serious damage occurs in the heart, where every structural component is likely to be the site of an inflammatory reaction. The heart damage and the joint lesions as well, are not infectious in origin, in the sense that these tissues are invaded and directly damaged by destructive organisms; rather, they represent a sensitivity phenomenon, occurring in response to prior contact with a bacterium: specifically, the *beta*

PATIENT EDUCATION

A patient with heart disease should learn to regulate his activity according to his individual response. The goal is always to prevent progression of disease and the development of congestive heart failure.

THE PATIENT WITH MYOCARDIAL INFARCTION

I. To modify activities during convalescence so that complete recovery is realized:
   A. Avoid physiologic and psychogenic stresses.
      1. Do not engage in strenuous activities the first six months following myocardial infarction.
      2. Avoid air travel for 2 to 3 months.
      3. Avoid any activity that produces dyspnea or undue fatigue.
      4. Keep away from extremes of heat and cold.
      5. Take off weight (if directed) and avoid smoking.
      6. Shorten work hours when first returning to work.
      7. Have a daily rest period.
   B. Pursue a pleasurable hobby that affords release of tension.

II. To undertake an orderly program of increasing exercise and activity for long term rehabilitation:
   A. Engage in a regimen of physical conditioning with a gradual increasing of activity levels.
   B. Plan and participate in a *daily* program of exercise that develops into a program of *regular* exercise for a lifetime.

---

hemolytic streptococcus. Blood leukocytes accumulate in the affected tissues to form nodules, which eventually are replaced by scars. The myocardium is certain to be involved in this inflammatory process, i.e., *rheumatic myocarditis* develops, which temporarily weakens the contractile power of the heart. The pericardium likewise is affected, i.e., *rheumatic pericarditis* also occurs during the acute illness. These myocardial and pericardial complications usually are without serious sequelae; on the other hand, the effects of *rheumatic endocarditis* are permanent and often crippling.

Rheumatic endocarditis anatomically manifests itself first by tiny translucent vegetations, which resemble beads about the size of the head of a pin, arranged in a row along the free margins of the valve flaps. These tiny beads look harmless enough and may disappear without injuring the valve flaps, but more often their results are serious. They are the starting point of a process that gradually thickens the flaps after years, rendering them just a little shorter, just a little thicker than normal, just a little shriveled along their edges—not much, but enough to prevent them from closing the orifice of the valve perfectly. Hence a leak develops; the valve is said to be "regurgitant." In other patients the inflamed margins of the valve flaps become adherent, with the result that the valve orifice is narrowed, or "stenotic."

A very small percentage of patients die as the immediate result of acute rheumatic fever; when death does occur at this stage, usually it is due to acute myocarditis. Most patients recover with gratifying speed and their recovery ostensibly is complete. However, although free of symptoms, the patient is left with certain permanent residuals that often gradually lead to progressive valvular deformities. The extent of cardiac damage, or even its existence, may not have been apparent on clinical examinations during the acute phase of the disease. Eventually, however, the heart murmurs that are characteristic of valvular stenosis, regurgitation, or both, become audible on auscultation and, in some patients, even detectable as "thrills" on palpation. The myocardium usually can compensate for these valvular defects very well for a time, despite its increased burden. As long as it can do so, the patient remains in apparent good health. However, sooner or later it fails to compensate—and decompensation, when it occurs, is signaled by the manifestations of congestive heart failure, described on pages 384-385.

Treatment

The patient with rheumatic endocarditis should be confined to bed as long as he is febrile and remain quiet thereafter until the erythrocyte sedimentation rate (a fair though nonspecific index of rheumatic activity) returns to normal. Salicylates customarily are prescribed in large doses, and invariably to good effect, so far as the elimination of fever and arthritis are concerned. However, neither these nor any other drugs appear to affect the development or the progress of rheumatic endocarditis.

The patient with rheumatic endocarditis, whose valve function is faulty but whose disease is quiescent, does not require therapy as long as his heart pumps effectively. Nevertheless, he faces the threat of recurrent attacks· of acute rheumatic fever, of bacterial endocarditis, of embolism from vegetations or mural thrombi in the heart, and of eventual cardiac failure. The relation between valvular disease and congestive heart failure is discussed on page 379; the treatment of heart failure, on page 385.

Prevention

Unfortunately, rheumatic fever is prone to recur unless forestalled by prophylactic antimicrobial therapy, and each attack renders the patient more susceptible to a subsequent recurrence. Furthermore, each attack adds to the valvular damage already present, further impairing cardiac function and hastening the advent of eventual decompensation. Obviously, it is in the area of prevention that the medical team can make its most significant contribution to the welfare of the patient with rheumatic endocarditis.

THE NURSE AS A CASE FINDER
Prevention of Rheumatic Heart Disease

Rhematic fever is a preventable disease. By eradication of rheumatic fever, the great cardiac crippler—*rheumatic heart disease*—would be virtually eliminated. Through the use of penicillin therapy in patients with streptococcal infections, almost all primary attacks of rheumatic fever could be prevented. The symptoms of streptococcal pharyngitis are:

Fever (38.9° to 40° C., or 102° to 104° F.)
Chilliness
Sore throat (sudden in onset)
Diffuse redness of throat with exudate on oropharynx
Enlarged and tender lymph nodes

The nurse should be familiar with the symptoms of streptococcal pharyngitis and aware of its role in relation to rheumatic fever, so that she may be convincingly emphatic in her instructions to individuals so afflicted—especially individuals with a past history of rheumatic fever. Early and effective treatment of streptococcal infections, including streptococcal pharyngitis, has been shown to prevent the onset as well as the recurrence of acute rheumatic fever. Rheumatic fever subjects must be especially wary of contact with persons with symptoms suggesting bacterial pharyngitis, or who are known to have contracted a streptococcal infection within a period of 3 months. Any patient with evidence of bacterial pharyngitis should be regarded as a candidate for antibiotic therapy, pending the results of a throat culture. Moreover, almost every patient with a history of rheumatic fever should receive monthly prophylactic injections of penicillin therapy, in order to avoid another streptococcal infection. The patient must recognize and should accept the fact that he is a "rheumatic fever patient," and as such can lead a normal life only if he is willing to submit to certain limitations and inconveniences. In relation to this facet of his education, the nurse is in a position to play a very important role.

Bacterial Endocarditis

Subacute bacterial endocarditis is a febrile disease usually resulting from infection of a heart valve that has been damaged by rheumatic fever, or one that is abnormal by virtue of a congenital defect. However, bacterial endocarditis does attack normal valves of the aged. The incidence of this disease is highest among individuals between the ages of 20 and 40.

Fortunately the incidence of bacterial endocarditis is now declining due to the lower incidence of rheumatic fever.

Pathophysiology

Subacute bacterial endocarditis is caused by streptococci of the *viridans* group, organisms of low virulence that normally inhabit the mouth and the gastrointestinal tract. Characteristically, 1 to 3 weeks before the onset of his illness the patient has had a bacterial pharyngitis or has been subjected to a dental extraction, or to oral, genitourinary or rectal surgery—procedures that almost invariably are attended by transient bacteremia. Such bacteremias are extremely common, and ordinarily are harmless, thanks to the protective activities of the reticuloendothelial system. However, on heart valves that are abnormally vascularized or otherwise altered by prior disease, blood-borne bacteria are prone to lodge—and there they thrive. As they multiply they cause the valve leaflets to become eroded; on these erosions, fibrin is deposited and vegetations form, in accordance with the sequence described above. The bacteria themselves become enmeshed in a network of fibrin that, in turn, forms a barricade against the phagocytic cells and immune antibodies in the circulating blood, thereby protecting the bacteria from destruction and ensuring their continuing growth.

The onset of subacute bacterial endocarditis usually is insidious and seldom can be dated with precision. Typical symptoms include weakness, malaise and intermittent fever, with alternating chills and sweats. A unique feature of the disease is the appearance of small painful swellings, called "Osler's nodes," on the tips or lateral borders of the fingers and toes. Petechial hemorrhages are to be found on the skin and the conjunctivae. Clubbing of the fingers is common. If the disease runs a protracted course the patient loses a substantial amount of weight and becomes very anemic. His complexion acquires a "cafe-au-lait" hue as a result of the anemia. The pulse rate is accelerated. A mild leukocytosis is present, and a bacteremia usually can be demonstrated by means of a blood culture.

As the blood courses through his heart, vegetations may separate from the diseased valve and be carried to distant sites in the body. Embolic fragments from this source, or from a mural thrombus in the heart, may lodge in the kidneys, the brain or elsewhere, including myocardium, often with serious and occasionally lethal consequences.

Acute bacterial endocarditis differs from the subacute variety only with respect to the infecting organism, which is relatively virulent (e.g., the hemolytic streptococcus, *Staphylococcus aureus*, the pneumococcus or the gonococcus), and the clinical course, which progresses more rapidly and is relatively stormy. The most conspicuous symptoms are those of sepsis: high fever, chills, prostration and marked leukocytosis.

Treatment

The basic objective of therapy is to eradicate the invading organisms. This is accomplished by the administration of an antimicrobial drug, one selected on the basis of blood cultures and the sensitivity tests that are applied to the organism isolated from these cultures. Penicillin, given in massive doses (e.g., 2 million units or more intramuscularly or intravenously each day for 4 to 6 weeks) sufficiently early in the course of the infection, is curative in most patients.

Whereas eradication of the infection usually can be achieved, thanks to modern antibacterial chemotherapy, the valvular damage produced is irreparable, except by valve replacement surgery (if the patient is a good enough risk). The ultimate prognosis of the patient who has been "cured" of bacterial endocarditis often depends to a large extent on the degree to which his cardiac efficiency has been impaired.

Chronic Valvular Heart Disease

If the heart muscle remains strong, the circulatory apparatus can adjust itself efficiently even though a valve is injured badly. The details of such adjustment, called *compensatory changes,* include modifications in the rate and the character of the heartbeat, changes in the blood pressure, hypertrophy of the myocardium, a redistribution of the blood in the body, etc., all changes that lessen the untoward results of the valve defect.

Aortic Stenosis

Pathophysiology. Narrowing of the orifice between the left ventricle and the aorta is a lesion found most frequently in elderly men. Often it is the result of arteriosclerosis or rheumatic fever. The flaps of the aortic valve fuse and partially close the opening between the heart and the aorta. The left ventricle overcomes this obstruction to circulation by contracting more slowly, but with greater energy than normal, forcibly squeezing the blood through the very small hole.

Symptoms and Diagnosis. The first heart sound is a long-drawn rough and vibrating *r-r-r-r-rub-dub.* If one rests the hand over the aortic area, he feels a vibration that is the most intense of all cardiac thrills and that resembles the purring of a cat.

The pulse is slow in rate and small in volume; the pulse pressure is low. Because the blood is squeezed slowly into the aorta, the ascent of each pulse wave is gradual and its apex is rounded.

To compensate for this condition, the left ventricle shows the strain by a thickening of the muscle wall. Other signs and symptoms are dizziness and fainting

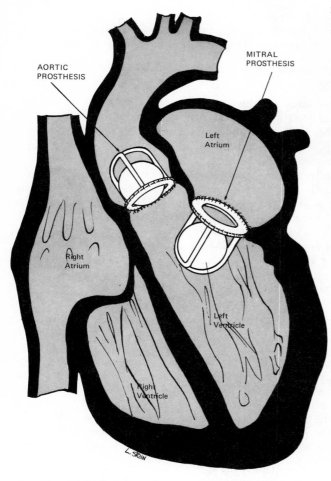

FIG. 19-6. Position of aortic and mitral Starr-valve prostheses in the heart.

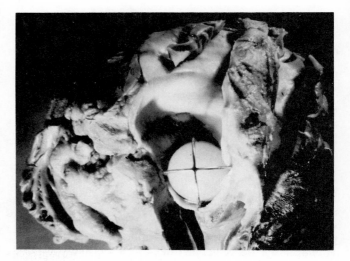

FIG. 19-7. Starr-valve shown in place in the aortic valve of the heart. The aorta has been cut open, to show the valve (post mortem specimen).

because of reduced blood volume to the brain, anginal-type pain in the chest because of lessened blood supply to the heart, and a low blood-pulse pressure because of diminished blood flow. Left heart catheterization is the most accurate diagnostic procedure. Pressure tracings are taken from the left ventricle and base of aorta. The systolic pressure in the left ventricle is considerably higher than in the aorta during systole.

Treatment. Because the aortic valve cusps fuse and the leaflets become rigid, scarred and, in advanced disease, calcified, it is necessary to repair and restore function through surgery. Otherwise, the uncorrected condition will lead to congestive heart failure. By direct vision, utilizing cardiopulmonary bypass, the calcified portions may be removed and the commissures opened, the valves and cusps may be reconstructed, or the cusps may be replaced with artificial cusps. Most commonly, the valve is replaced by a ball-valve. In over half of the patients, the mitral valve is also diseased,

and both valves may have to be replaced. Research is still going on to find artificial materials for ball-valves that are tolerated by the body and that do not promote local thrombosis and embolism. Chronic anticoagulant therapy is now required following valve replacement. Nursing management is similar to that of other patients having heart surgery (see pp. 399-404).

Aortic Insufficiency (Regurgitation)

Aortic regurgitation is caused by inflammatory lesions that deform the flaps so that they fail to seal perfectly the aortic orifice during diastole. This valvular defect is usually the result of endocarditis of the rheumatic type or the bacterial type, but occasionally is due to syphilis.

Because of the leak in the aortic valve during diastole, some of the blood in the aorta, always under high pressure, hisses back into the left ventricle, which must handle both the blood that the left atrium normally delivers into it through the mitral orifice and that returning from the aorta. The left ventricle dilates to accommodate this increased volume, hypertrophies in order to expel it, and does so with more than normal force, thus raising the systolic blood pressure. By another reflex the cardiovascular system tends to become accommodated: the peripheral arterioles become relaxed, so that the peripheral resistance is lessened and the diastolic pressure greatly lowered. The pulse pressure is considerably increased in these cases, and one of the characteristic signs of the disease is the pulse which strikes the palpating finger with quick sharp strokes followed by sudden collapse (Corrigan's or water hammer pulse). The nature of

FIG. 19-8. (*Top*) The mitral valve. The valve on the left is a normal valve. The other two show fusion of the commissures in various locations. (*Bottom*) Commissurotomy of a stenotic mitral valve. (*Left*) The posterior commissure is being opened by finger fracture, utilizing the fingernail to help tear open the posterior commissure. (*Right*) The anterior commissure is being opened by a special knife, designed to fit into the surgeon's glove. (Johnson, J., and Kirby, C.: Surgery of the Chest, Chicago, Year Book Pub.)

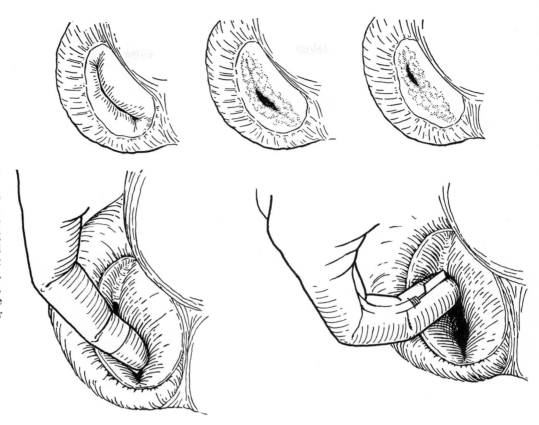

the pulse wave is quite unmistakable, and the capillary pulse is pronounced. The diagnosis often can be made when shaking hands because of the throb of the entire hand. Using cineangiography, an opaque dye can be injected into the root of the aorta, usually by way of a catheter passed from the femoral artery. In aortic regurgitation, the opaque liquid can be seen passing into the left ventricle.

Compensation may remain excellent for a long time, but when the left ventricle dilates because of weakness, a relative mitral insufficiency arises and a train of events leading to cardiac failure is initiated.

Treatment. The damaged valve is replaced by a ball-valve prosthesis, using cardiopulmonary bypass.

Mitral Stenosis

Mitral stenosis is by far the most common of the cardiac lesions produced by acute rheumatic fever and is considered the typical lesion. It has been estimated that nearly 1,000,000 persons in the United States have mitral stenosis.

Pathophysiology. In this disorder, acute rheumatic endocarditis has glued the mitral valve flaps (commissures) together and, by shortening the chordae tendineae, has pulled the flap edges almost down to the tips of the papillary muscles, thus greatly narrowing the mitral orifice. Normally, one should be able to put three fingers through this orifice with ease, but in well-marked cases of stenosis one can hardly pass a lead pencil through it. The left ventricle is not affected, but the left atrium has great difficulty in emptying itself through the narrow orifice into the ventricle. Therefore it dilates and hypertrophies. Since no valve protects the pulmonary veins from a backward flow from this atrium, the pulmonary circulation becomes markedly congested. As a result of the abnormally high pulmonary arterial pressure that must be maintained by the right ventricle, it is subjected to an unfunctional strain and eventually fails.

Symptoms and Diagnosis. Patients with mitral stenosis are prone to be cyanotic, short of breath, to cough and to suffer from "bronchitis." Hemoptysis is a common symptom. The pulse is small in volume and often irregular because of fibrillation. The apex beat is in about normal position and not conspicuous on inspection; but on palpation, the shock of the first sound is felt as a characteristically brief, sudden tap. At this point also, over an area or not more than an inch in diameter, is felt and heard a characteristic purring crescendo thrill, due to the atrial systole. This, steadily increasing in intensity, ends in the above-mentioned brief tap. In many patients this thrill appears only after exercise. At the pulmonary area one feels a similar tap, but this is the shock of the second sound. Diagnostic aids that assist the cardiologist in making an accurate diagnosis are angiography, cineangiography, left heart catheterization and ultrasound technique to determine the mobility of the mitral valve.

Commissurotomy for Mitral Stenosis. When left atrial enlargement develops in a patient with mitral stenosis, as shown by roentgenograms, and the patient experiences fatigue and dyspnea on exertion, early operation usually is indicated. In selected patients, it is possible for the surgeon to free the thickened and fused valve flaps by fracturing them with his index finger (finger-fracture method), by cutting them with a special knife, or using a ventricular dilator. (Fig. 19-8)

In this closed surgical technique, it is necessary for the pleura and the pericardium to be opened after making an incision through the third or the fourth interspace. Procaine is infiltrated around the base of the left atrial (auricular) appendage, and a purse-string suture is applied. When the tip of the appendage is excised, the surgeon is able to insert his finger; by tightening the purse-string suture there is little blood loss while the surgeon fractures or cuts the commissures. When the surgeon withdraws his finger, immediately the purse-string suture is closed tightly.

This procedure ("closed valve" surgery, as opposed to open heart surgery with a pump oxygenator) carries a relatively low mortality rate but is often followed by recurrent stenosis in a few months or years. Replacement with an artificial valve is now commonly performed, especially when conditions are not favorable for finger fracture, e.g., when the valve is densely fibrotic or calcified.

Postoperatively, there should be a gradual improvement in the patient, such as reduction of the pulmonary pressure, less dyspnea on exertion and increased energy to lead a more normal life. If deterioration of the valve does occur, it is likely that calcium is again being deposited; there also is a possibility of peripheral emboli. Although the closed surgical procedure continues to be the one of choice, deterioration and other circumstances may influence the surgeon to relieve mitral stenosis by open heart surgery, at which time the valve is replaced by a ball-type prosthetic valve. Management of such a patient is similar to that described on pp. 399-404.

Mitral Regurgitation

The typical mitral lesion of rheumatic origin produces not only stenosis but also regurgitation of that valve. Shortening or tearing of one or both of the mitral valve flaps prevents the perfect closure of the mitral orifice, while the powerful left ventricle is forcing the blood into the aorta. Then at each beat, the left ventricle forces some of the blood back into its atrium; this blood is added to the blood then beginning to flow into this chamber from the lungs. The left atrium must dilate and hypertrophy. This backward flow of blood from the ventricle also checks the current of blood flowing under low pressure from the lungs, which, therefore, become congested, and this, in turn, throws an extra strain on the right ventricle. Therefore, the result of even a slight mitral leak always involves both lungs and the right ventricle.

Patients with mitral insufficiency are sometimes just a trifle cyanotic; after exertion they may actually become blue. Even while compensation is good, palpitation of the heart, shortness of breath on exertion and cough due to chronic passive pulmonary congestion are common symptoms. The pulse may be regular and of good volume, but not infrequently it becomes irregular, either as a result of extrasystoles or fibrillation, which may persist indefinitely.

For severe regurgitation, surgical replacement with an artificial valve is indicated.

Tricuspid Lesions

Tricuspid regurgitation, the result of disease of the tricuspid valve flaps, occurs rarely, though more often in children than in adults. The usual cause is severe rheumatic endocarditis.

Symptoms. The symptoms of tricuspid regurgitation are marked. At each beat the right ventricle forces blood in two directions: through the pulmonary valve, the normal direction, and back through the leaking tricuspid valve into the right atrium. The flow of venous blood from the systemic circulation is impeded, causing signs of general cyanosis and overfilling of all the veins of the body. A pulse wave similar to that sent by the left ventricle throughout the arterial tree may be transmitted into the larger veins. Therefore, the liver, now swollen to perhaps 2 or 3 times its normal size, pulsates. The walls of the stomach and the intestines, the kidneys and other abdominal organs, since they are turgid with venous blood, cannot function well and give rise to symptoms of chronic passive congestion. The skin of the legs and the dependent portions of the body becomes edematous. Fluid collects in the abdominal cavity (ascites) and in the pleural cavities (hydrothorax). If the heart can compensate again, circulation improves at once, the congestion of the various organs is relieved, and all symptoms due to it disappear.

Tricuspid stenosis may also follow acute rheumatic fever, but is rare. Neither regurgitation nor stenosis of the rheumatic tricuspid valve occur as isolated lesions except very rarely; in almost every case they are not the major cause of the patient's disability, but merely add to the cardiac burden and worsen the prognosis a bit more. Surgery of the aortic or mitral valve is usually all that is required.

Lesions of the Pulmonary Valve

Pulmonary valve disease with either regurgitation or stenosis is due to congenital malformations. The reader is referred to a textbook of pediatric nursing.

PATIENTS WITH MYOCARDITIS

The heart is a muscle, hence its efficiency depends on the health of its individual muscle fibers. When this is good, the heart can function well in spite of severe valvular injuries; when it is poor, life is in jeopardy.

Acute myocarditis, or acute inflammation of the cardiac muscle tissue, occasionally resembles other inflammations in that an inflammatory exudate is present, as in cases secondary to an acute endocarditis or pericarditis. But usually myocarditis appears as an acute degeneration of the heart muscle fibers, which are replaced later by fibrous tissue cells.

Etiology

Acute myocarditis may develop as a complication of many acute infections, or it may be caused by a virus of the Coxsackie group. By far the commonest cause, however, is *beta hemolytic streptococcus* Lancefield type A infection, following which myocarditis may occur as a late complication 2 to 3 weeks after the acute febrile phase. This is the so-called "rheumatic myocarditis," a constant feature of acute rheumatic fever. Another type, a toxic form of myocarditis, eventually occurs in severe hyperthyroidism. Other rarer types and several idiopathic varieties are also known.

The symptoms of acute myocarditis usually are indefinite. Often the first evidence of its presence is suddenly developing cardiac dilatation with heart failure, which may rapidly lead to death. In other cases, its presence is suggested by breathlessness, a low blood pressure, disturbances of rate and rhythm and evidences of cardiac enlargement.

Management

The main requirement is complete rest in bed, for sudden death may follow the slightest exertion of the body. Every attempt is made to anticipate the patient's needs and wishes. He is fed, bathed, lifted and turned so that his strength may be conserved. The necessity for such assistance is explained to the patient, with emphasis on the fact that it is but a temporary need that will be eliminated as soon as the inflammatory process subsides. Digitalis is a mainstay of management.

Convalescence

The convalescence should be prolonged and carefully guarded, because heart failure often occurs after the patient seems to be practically well, and relapses or a relentless progressive downhill course are not uncommon.

PATIENTS WITH PERICARDITIS

Pericarditis, as its name implies, refers to an inflammation of the pericardium, the membranous sac enveloping the heart. This inflammation may be due to infection by organisms brought to it by way of the bloodstream in the course of a bacteremia or by extension of an infectious process involving an adjacent organ, such as a tuberculous lymph node, an infected pleura or a mediastinal abscess. It appears often in the course of acute rheumatic heart disease that is the result of infection. Noninfectious pericardial inflammation occurs in uremia and occasionally in coronary thrombosis over the area of myocardial infarction. Acute benign pericarditis is an inflammatory lesion caused by any of several viruses and, rarely, by immune reactions.

The patient may complain of chest pain and dyspnea. Pain, if present, varies from mild to severe. Usually it is felt in the central substernal region, radiating to the shoulder and the neck. It is likely to be aggravated by respiration, thus demonstrating its pleural origin. (Infectious pericarditis nearly always is accompanied by acute pleuritis.)

Nursing Assessment

In the course of her observations the nurse should attempt to discover whether or not the pain is influenced by respiratory movements, with or without the actual passage of air; by flexion, extension or rotation of the spine, including the neck; by movements of the shoulders and the arms; by coughing; or by swallowing. Notation of these relationships may be very helpful in establishing a diagnosis. Typically in acute pericarditis the pain is increased by respiration (with passage of air), by coughing and, occasionally, by swallowing; it is uninfluenced by posture or other movements.

Dyspnea occurs as a result of compression of the bronchi or the parenchyma of the lung by the distended pericardium. The patient obviously is ill, in distress, restless and anxious; his complexion is pale. He prefers to adopt a forward-leaning or a sitting posture. Pericarditis per se often gives rise to no signs other than fever and the production of a friction rub that is audible on auscultation and is synchronous with the heartbeat.

Pericardial Effusion

This may accompany the general anasarca of nephrosis, pericarditis or advanced congestive heart failure. In this type of case, the fluid is noninfected and is of low specific gravity and protein content. However, in pericarditis due to infections other than tuberculosis, the fluid is likely to be purulent, and from it the organism can be cultured. Blood occasionally finds its way into the sac (hemopericardium) as a result of traumatic injury, tumor of the pericardium or dissecting aneurysm. When caring for a patient who has sustained an automobile accident, ascertain whether his chest impinged on the steering wheel, and report this information. It should be borne in mind that hemopericardium may follow any chest injury, even in the absence of external laceration or rib cage fracture.

Whatever the character of the fluid, if it accumulates in sufficient amount, the heart action is embarrassed. The blood pressure drops and fluctuates with respiration (pulsus paradoxicus), being lowest on inspiration, at which phase the pulse may be imperceptible. The venous pressure tends to rise, as is evident by the development of engorged neck veins and generalized edema. The heart sounds become feeble in intensity, there are signs of cardiac enlargement and compression of the left lung posteriorly. This is a life-threatening situation, demanding close and constant observation. This should include hourly measurements of the arterial pressure and pulse rate, for on the course of these vital signs hinges the decision regarding the need for pericardial paracentesis.

To improve the cardiac function, if it becomes impaired seriously, a pericardial tap is performed, all the available fluid being aspirated through a needle inserted usually near the apex. Tapping may have to be performed repeatedly and at frequent intervals, depending on the speed of fluid reaccumulation. The type of pericarditis most apt to require frequent tapping and eventual surgical removal of the pericardium is the tuberculous variety. Purulent exudates may require open drainage through a surgical chest wall incision.

Treatment. The principal element of medical and nursing management is to ensure that the patient is kept on bed rest until the fever has disappeared and the patient's clinical signs are normal. Analgesia (usually in the form of acetylsalicylic acid, which also has an anti-inflammatory effect) is given for the patient's distressing chest pain. Morphine may be needed for severe pain. If congestive heart failure develops, digitalization is carried out.

Patients with bacterial infections of the pericardium are treated with the antimicrobial agent of choice for each particular patient, based on identification and sensitivity tests.

Chronic Constrictive Pericarditis

Usually of tuberculous origin, this disease is a chronic inflammatory thickening of the pericardium with an obliteration of the pericardial space. Often the adherent pericardium becomes calcified. The heart action is much embarrassed by this tough, unyielding enclosure, and edema, ascites and hepatic enlargement result. The fixation of the heart to the pericardium often produces a retraction of the chest wall with every heartbeat. Surgical removal of the constricting diseased pericardium (pericardectomy) is the only treatment of any benefit. This is done by excising carefully the thickened covering of the heart.

THE PATIENT IN CONGESTIVE HEART FAILURE
Underlying Pathophysiology

The majority of patients with heart disease sooner or later display the combination of symptoms and signs that we recognize as the syndrome of congestive heart failure. The manner of its onset, its predominant features and its course vary considerably from one individual to another, depending on the nature of the cardiac disorder, the clinical status of the patient and the factors that have led to its occurrence. There are many possible predisposing factors: for example, the myocardium may have been subjected to severe and prolonged strain as a result of systemic or pulmonary arterial hypertension or due to the presence of valvular disease. On the other hand, the myocardium may have been weakened by the advent of an acute myocarditis, an arrhythmia, a myocardial infarct, or prolonged dietary deficiency.

The clinical manifestations of congestive heart failure stem primarily from three major alterations of circulatory dynamics, derangements that are common to most of these patients: (1) the cardiac output is diminished to the extent that vital organs no longer are profused adequately with arterial blood, their oxygen and nutritional requirements fail to be met and they suffer from deprivation; (2) the pulmonary vascular bed no longer is emptied efficiently by the left atrium and ventricle, with the result that the pulmonary vessels become engorged, pulmonary hypertension develops, and pulmonary edema may supervene; (3) blood returning to the heart from the periphery is not dispatched onward into the pulmonary vessels rapidly enough to avoid congestion in the systemic veins and venules; the venous pressure rises, the liver and other organs become congested and fluid escapes through the walls of engorged capillaries to form dependent edema and ascites.

When the blood supply to the kidneys is reduced, glomerular filtration is decreased, and tubular reabsorption increased, with the result that excessive amounts of sodium and water are retained in the body. This is the situation in congestive heart failure, renal blood flow becoming diminished in these patients as a consequence of a reduction in cardiac output. Moreover, the abnormal tendency to retain water is exaggerated through the action of aldosterone, an adrenal hormone that enhances tubular reabsorption of sodium and therefore promotes the formation of edema. Production of this hormone is increased in patients with congestive heart failure. Impairment of renal blood flow eventually leads to other and more serious abnormalities of kidney function, as evidenced by albuminuria and azotemia (nitrogen retention, or uremia).

Pulmonary engorgement impairs respiratory efficiency and is responsible for dyspnea in these patients. In the ambulatory patient, breathlessness is most severe at night after he has retired. It is at this time that his blood volume, already somewhat excessive, is further augmented by edema fluid reabsorbed from the legs, and is at its maximum. His venous pressure is maximal and pulmonary congestion is most extreme. This sequence of events is responsible for attacks of so-called "paroxysmal nocturnal dyspnea." In addition to dyspnea, the patient in failure is likely to cough a good deal, and may even experience hemoptysis. He may be short of breath even at bed rest (orthopnea). However, the most dramatic and most dangerous complication of pulmonary congestion is pulmonary edema, discussed on page 390.

Failure of the systemic venous blood to be propelled with normal rapidity into and through the pulmonary circulation results in an increase in the systemic venous pressure and venous stasis. Peripheral edema forms, owing to the escape of fluid from engorged capillaries and venules. The liver and other splanchnic organs become congested, and ascitic fluid may accumulate, following venous hypertension and vascular engorgement. Splanchnic congestion impairs the appetite and promotes gaseous abdominal distention. Consequently, nutrition suffers and tissue substance is lost, although weight loss may be obscured by the edema.

Impairment of cerebral blood flow and reduced oxygenation of the arterial blood together explain some of the neurologic complications of congestive heart failure, including symptoms of physical exhaustion and undue fatigue, difficulty in mental activity, impairment of memory, excessive drowsiness (or insomnia), and even hallucinations and delirium.

Heart failure does not necessarily involve both ventricles simultaneously, or equally. For a time one of these may perform far below its normal level of efficiency, while the other remains relatively unaffected. Whether the right or the left ventricle is affected earlier depends on the nature of the circumstances responsible for the failure. For example, with the advent of congestive heart failure in a patient with arterial hypertension, whose left ventricle has been subjected to undue strain for many years, the left ventricle loses its efficiency earlier and to a greater extent than does the right. As long as this disparity exists, an increased proportion of the blood volume tends to accumulate in the lungs behind the failing left ventricle, with the result that the patient experiences symptoms of pulmonary congestion and is a candidate for the development of pulmonary edema. This is the situation in so-called left ventricular failure.

When the strain is imposed predominantly on the right ventricle, as in patients with long-standing pulmonary disease and pulmonary hypertension, the power of the right ventricle is reduced before that of the left, and to a more marked degree. The manifestations of failure under these circumstances are most prominent in the splanchnic area and the distal extremities, appearing in the form of dependent edema, hepatic engorgement and ascites, i.e., the picture of "right-sided failure." Failure of either ventricle is followed inevitably, and within a brief period of time, by equal impairment of the other.

An estimated two million persons are being treated each year in this country for congestive heart failure. Approximately 10 to 15 per cent of all medical hospital admissions are for congestive failure. This is becoming an increasingly serious problem in older patients.

Management of Congestive Failure

The basic objectives in the treatment of patients with congestive failure are (1) to reduce the cardiac load by lessening the tissue demand for blood and by eliminating factors that tend to stimulate cardiac activity unnecessarily; (2) to reinforce the action of the heart, improving its effectiveness as a pump and thereby delivering more blood to the tissues; and (3) to eliminate the excessive accumulation of body water.

Rest

If the cardiac load is to be decreased, it is essential that the patient have both physical and emotional

Nursing Care Plan

LONG RANGE GOAL To re-establish self confidence & self esteem taking into consideration the limitations of pt's illness.

IMMEDIATE GOAL(S) To prevent the frequent occurrence of chest pain.

To relieve apprehension concerning her shortness of breath.

PROBLEMS	NURSING APPROACH	EVALUATION	OUTCOME
Intermittent chest pain c̄ apprehension. (Pain apparently from impending occlusion of coronary artery with subsequent ischemia.)	1. Medicate c̄ analgesic prescribed by physician 2. Oxygen by oropharyngeal catheter constantly. 3. Restrict activity to reduce physical stress.	Sleeping quietly most of the day Nasal catheter is annoying & irritating to nares.	Appears rested & free from pain after receiving medication. Nasal catheter changed to nasal cannula.
Loneliness (recently widowed; no children, says her close friends "are all dead!")	Introduce & build nurse-patient rapport on a one-to-one basis.	Seems to feel free to discuss her feelings c̄ members of the nursing staff.	Told her minister that the nurses are "real nice & treat me as a person — not just another old lady."
Premature Ventricular Contraction (has had many P.V.C.'s which have been multi-focal)	Note occurrence & frequency of P.V.C.'s. Determine if P.V.C.'s are associated c̄ clinical symptoms Administer antiarrhythmic drugs as ordered.	P.V.C.'s occurring infrequently and falling free of the vulnerable period (away from the T wave) Free of symptoms — Drug therapy apparently successful.	Free of signs of ht. failure. No acute episodes noted.
Prevention of acute episodes of failure.	Limit intake (oral & I.V.) according to order. Measure output; administer diuretic when ordered. Restrict sodium intake. Observe for mood changes, anorexia, nausea & vomiting. Observe respiratory exchange — Observe for venous distention & peripheral dependent edema.	Free of symptoms Diuretics given.	

Fig. 19-9. Mrs. C. C., a 78-year-old retired seamstress was admitted to the Cardiac Care Unit with a diagnosis of congestive heart failure with an impending myocardial infarction. She assumed the orthopneic position and had marked peripheral edema. The above care plan was written on the third day following admission to the hospital.

rest. Rest lessens the tissue demand for oxygen, and for the supply and the removal of metabolites in general. The patient may be impressed by the importance of this therapeutic approach when he hears that each day of complete rest spares the heart approximately 25,000 contractions.

Body Alignment. In order to secure proper rest, the body should be in proper alignment. A semirecumbent position, with a pillow placed longitudinally under the back, is restful. Moreover, in this position the venous return to the heart and the lungs is reduced, pulmonary congestion is alleviated, and impingement of the liver on the diaphragm is minimized. A footboard should support the feet in order to avoid footdrop. The lower arms should be sup-

ported with pillows to eliminate the constant pull of their weight on the shoulder muscles, which is very tiring. The orthopneic patient may sit on the side of his bed with his feet propped up on a chair, his head and arms resting on an over-the-bed table, and his lumbosacral spine supported by a pillow. The patient with pulmonary congestion rests comfortably in an armchair, a position that is especially advantageous because it tends, more than any other, to reduce the shift of fluid from the periphery to the lungs. The patient who spends the entire day in an armchair finds that lying in bed with his head elevated provides a welcome change at night.

Hygienic Care. Although, during the acute stage of congestive failure, a partial bath may suffice and may be the extent of bathing permissible, a full bath each day is to be preferred as a source of relaxation and as a circulatory stimulant.

The nurse must be ever conscious of the fact that prolonged immobility, combined with the presence of tissue edema, favors the development of decubiti. Nursing measures to forestall this complication include frequent massaging of the skin with emollient lotions, the placing of small sheepskin pads under bony prominences, and areas of tenderness, letting the patient lie on a sheepskin, or by placing the patient on an alternating pressure pad mattress.

Promoting Sleep. Patients in congestive failure are unusually prone to be restless and anxious at night. A quiet, well-ventilated room predisposes to sound sleep. To some patients, the presence of a member of the family provides the necessary reassurance. Others are relieved of their anxiety and insomnia by illumination of the bedroom throughout the night. They should be observed repeatedly for possible respiratory arrhythmia, such as Cheyne-Stokes respirations, indicating a disturbance in the function of the respiratory center. If such an arrhythmia is discovered, it may be worthwhile to test the effect of oxygen inhalations, administered briefly each night just before retirement.

Soporific drugs have a definite place in the care of the patient with congestive heart failure and insomnia. Paraldehyde and chloral hydrate are among the safest of the soporific agents, and are as likely as any to be effective. It should be recalled that the patient with hepatic congestion is unable to detoxify drugs with normal rapidity, and should be medicated with unusual caution. As a result of cerebral hypoxia, with superimposed nitrogen retention, he may react unfavorably to soporific drugs, becoming confused and increasingly anxious in response to medication. Such a patient should not be restrained; restraints are likely to be resisted, and resistance inevitably increases the cardiac load. If he insists on getting out of bed he should be installed comfortably in an armchair. As his cerebral and systemic circulation improve, the quality of his sleep will improve.

Rest is not possible without relaxation. Emotional stress produces vasoconstriction, elevates the arterial pressure and speeds the heart. Relaxation may be secured by avoiding situations that tend to promote anxiety and agitation. Patients who are particularly prone to be tense should be maintained in a less reactive, even drowsy state, in order to eliminate any emotional stimuli that would exact unnecessary and undesirable demands on the heart.

Pain of cardiac origin is relieved effectively by one or more tablets of nitroglycerine placed under the tongue, or by inhalations of amyl nitrite. Oxygen therapy is very helpful.

Digitalis Therapy

Digitalis leaf and its glycosides slow and strengthen the heart beat and exert a diuretic effect in congestive heart failure. The dose is quite variable from person to person and only averages can be given as examples. Digitalis leaf is given as 100-mg. tablets at the rate of 3 to 6 tablets daily, depending on the rapidity of digitalization desired by the physician, until the optimal effect is obtained. The closer one comes to ingesting 1 gm. of digitalis leaf in 24 hours, the more likely toxic effects are to occur. These include nausea, vomiting, arrhythmias (especially premature ventricular contractions [PVC's] and bigeminy—double beat), yellow vision and too slow a pulse rate. The usual dose of digitalis leaf required for full digitalization is around 1 gm.; this dose may be somewhat less if the drug is rapidly administered, and somewhat greater if it is slowly administered, because about 100 mg. of the drug are excreted daily. The usual maintenance dose is 100 mg. daily, again with rather wide individual variations.

The purified cardiac glycosides have become popular in recent years. Digitoxin, 0.1 or 0.2 mg. tablets, usually digitalizes a patient in a dose of 1.2 mg. over 24 to 72 hours, and the daily maintenance dosage is 0.1 or 0.2 mg. This is a very slowly excreted drug, so that the toxic effects of overdosage may be prolonged for weeks, and doses that seem to be adequate for maintenance may be slowly cumulative, so that digitalis toxicity insidiously appears.

Digoxin, 0.25 or 0.5 mg. tablets, usually digitalizes a patient in a total dose of 3 to 3.5 mg. over a 24- to 72-hour period, with a daily maintenance dose in the range of 0.25 to 0.5 mg. Digoxin also comes as an intravenous preparation and this form is usually given as 1 mg. initially and 0.25 mg. every 4 to 6 hours to a total dose of about 1.75 mg. Digoxin parenterally may be used for the immediate postoperative period, when patients are unable to take digitalis by mouth and it is decided that their daily maintenance dose not be omitted.

For rapid or emergency digitalization, Cedilanid may be used, 0.8 mg. IV, followed by increments of 0.4 mg. every four to six hours and a maximum of 1.6 mg. in 24 hours. This drug has rapid onset and rapid excretion and is not used for daily maintenance therapy.

Remember that clinical hypokalemia, or the total body deficit of potassium, is attended by a higher than usual risk of digitalis toxicity at lower than ordinary digitalis dosage levels. Also, remember that hypokalemia may exist even in the face of normal serum potassium, as often occurs in patients on prolonged thiazide diuretic therapy. With the advent of potent diuretics, digitalis intoxication has become increasingly common. The appearance of such intoxication may be subtle, with the patient simply losing his appetite, or it may be dramatic, with the sudden onset of arrhythmia, nausea, and vomiting.

Diet

The optimal diet for most patients with congestive heart failure is low in bulk, caloric value, fat and sodium. The average patient in this group, being somewhat overweight and relatively inactive, can subsist quite satisfactorily on a low-energy diet. Since abdominal distention elevates the diaphragm and interferes with respiration, gas-forming foods should be avoided. Small, frequent feedings are preferable to large bulky meals for the same reason. However, the most important consideration with respect to the diet is its sodium content, for the amount of sodium in the body determines the degree of its hydration; restriction of sodium intake is the key to success in the prevention and treatment of overhydration, or edema. The failing heart retains salt in the body, and in turn, water is retained.

The diet prescription should specify the precise weight of sodium that may be ingested each day, usually 200 to 600 mg., in contrast with the 2 to 4 gm. that is the average daily intake of a normal individual on an unrestricted diet.

The patient must be taught the purposes and the principles of sodium restriction, equipped with food tables listing items of low sodium and high sodium content and given specific instructions regarding the use of these tables. Merely to supply vague generalizations on the subject of meal planning only serves to de-emphasize its importance. Obviously, before the nurse can consider herself in a position to impart this instruction to her patients, she herself must possess a reasonable knowledge of the subject.

Diuretic Therapy

If edema is not controlled adequately by sodium restriction and digitalization alone, one or more diuretic drugs may be prescribed. Widely used for this purpose is chlorothiazide (Diuril). The organic mercurial drugs promote the urinary excretion of sodium, and therefore water. They must be given intramuscularly, subcutaneously or intravenously. As much as 3,000 to 5,000 ml. of urine may be excreted in response to a single mercurial injection. Ethacrynic acid and furosemide, 2 relatively new diuretics, are even more potent—so much so that they must be given with caution in order to prevent electrolyte

depletion and vascular collapse. As a basis for evaluating the effectiveness of therapy, patients receiving diuretic drugs should be weighed daily at the same hour, and these measurements should be entered in the permanent hospital record.

A voluminous diuresis entails many voidings in rapid succession, which may prove quite taxing for the sick patient. In order to minimize fatigue and conserve his energy the patient who is debilitated or very ill should be assisted on and off the bedpan or, better, the bedside commode.

Before diuretic therapy is commenced, the possibility of a urinary tract obstruction must be excluded. The elderly male patient should be treated with special vigilance, inasmuch as the incidence of urethral obstruction due to prostatic hypertrophy is high among such individuals. Signs of bladder distention should be sought routinely by palpation of the abdomen in the midline, just above the symphysis pubis.

Large and repeated diureses can lead to potassium depletion. This poses new problems for the cardiac patient, for among the complications of hypokalemia are marked weakening of cardiac contractions and the precipitation of digitalis toxicity in individuals receiving digitalis, thereby increasing the likelihood of a dangerous arrhythmia (see p. 364). To lessen the risk of hypokalemia and its attendant complications, patients receiving diuretic drugs should also be supplied with potassium salts as a supplement.

Regulation of Fluid Intake. The total amount of fluids should be limited, since an excess of water, unless the sodium intake is restricted carefully, is retained in the body, increasing the edema and adding to the burden of the heart. The daily total volume of all fluids ingested, which should be measured and charted, in general should be from 1,500 to 2,000 ml. in 24 hours. The patient may become interested in recording the amounts of fluids ingested. This may help him to restrict liquids and permit adequate spacing of fluid intake during the course of 24 hours. The fluid intake is regulated best to correspond to the urine output, fluids for each day being calculated on the basis of the total urinary excretion for the previous 24 hours. Charting of the fluid balance daily, together with daily weighing of the patient (at the same time), is an excellent and simple way of determining the progress of cardiac and renal function. In this way, the tendency to water retention, which indicates increased cardiac insufficiency or renal failure, is recognized early, and, similarly, diuresis, indicating improvement in the function of these systems, is estimated quantitatively.

Promotion of Bowel Elimination. The bowels are kept as nearly empty as possible of gas as well as solids by the use of such cathartics as compound licorice powder, cascara and mineral oil. The importance of this is twofold; it aids in the elimination of water from the intestine and facilitates the passage of stools. Straining at stool involves considerable muscular effort which, for these patients, may prove to be very dangerous.

It often happens that patients with lesser grades of cardiac decompensation are kept in bed too long and kept much too quiet. Also, after a prolonged stay in bed, the severe cases are not re-educated carefully and deliberately enough to physical activity. The patient with fever, of course, should remain quietly in bed until his temperature remains normal, but for those without fever, there are definite advantages in allowing mild exercise. This exercise, however, should be planned carefully. At first it is ideal for the patient, lying flat on his back or propped up in bed, systematically to engage in free-arm and free-leg movements. Later, he is allowed to sit in a chair and then to walk for increasing distances. Mild exercise improves muscle tone and aids in venous return. The pulse response to sitting up and walking is observed carefully and recorded in the nurse's notes.

Psychological Considerations

This aspect of treatment is especially important in patients who have experienced a complete reversal in their mode of life: from normal activity to almost complete inactivity for an appreciable period of time. The patient's interests must be distracted from his own fears and symptoms, which are apt to be alarming enough, and projected into the surrounding environment. As his strength improves and more activity is permitted, he should be encouraged to become increasingly self-reliant and to perform whatever functions, such as eating, bathing and reading, as seem possible and desirable. These activities in themselves usually are diverting enough, at least for a time. Other and more pleasurable pursuits also should be made possible, such as access to a radio or television set, a library and equipment for some creative project; and new interests should be cultivated, the possibilities for which are endless.

Prevention of Recurrent Episodes of Congestive Heart Failure

All too frequently patients keep returning to the clinic and hospital for recurring episodes of congestive heart failure. Not only does this create psychological, sociological and financial problems, but the physiological burden on the patient can be serious. Previously normal organs of the body may be ultimately damaged. Repeated attacks can lead to pulmonary fibrosis, liver cirrhosis, enlargement of the spleen and kidneys and even brain damage due to

PATIENT EDUCATION

A patient with heart disease should learn to regulate his activity according to his individual response. The goal is always to prevent progression of disease and the development of congestive heart failure.

THE PATIENT WITH CONGESTIVE HEART FAILURE

I. To live within the limits of the cardiac reserve:
 A. Obtain adequate rest.
  1. Have a regular daily rest period.
  2. Shorten working hours if possible.
  3. Avoid emotional upsets.
 B. Accept the fact that taking digitalis and restricting sodium intake will be a permanent way of life.
  1. Take digitalis daily exactly as prescribed.
  2. Restrict sodium as directed.
   (a) Become familiar with permitted and forbidden food and drink.
   (b) Avoid laxatives, antacids or any preparation that may contain sodium.
   (c) Ascertain the amount of sodium in local drinking water through inquiry of local department of health.
  3. Take diuretic as prescribed.
  4. Weigh at the same time daily to detect any tendency toward fluid retention.
 C. Avoid excesses in eating and drinking.
  1. Go on a weight reduction program until optimal weight is reached.
  2. Rest after lunch.
 D. Control chronic cough and report symptoms of respiratory infection to physician.
 E. Engage in prescribed exercise program to improve circulation and muscle tone.
 F. Keep *regular* appointment with physician or clinic.
II. To be alert for symptoms that may indicate recurring congestive heart failure:
 A. Gain in weight.
 B. Loss of appetite.
 C. Shortness of breath upon activity.
 D. Swelling of ankles, feet or abdomen.
 E. Persistent cough.
 F. Frequent urination at night.

insufficient oxygen during acute episodes. *To keep the patient on his therapy requires patient education, involvement and cooperation.* Many of the recurrences of congestive heart failure appear to be preventable. These include failure to follow the drug therapy *properly*, dietary indiscretions, inadequate medical follow-up, excessive physical activity and failure to recognize recurring symptoms. A summary of what the patient should know about his condition is given above.

It must be emphasized that cough medicines, alkalizers, pain remedies, etc., contain fairly large amounts of sodium. The patient must be warned against their use as well as be advised to rinse his mouth with clear water when using toothpaste and mouthwashes. In some areas the drinking water has a high sodium content and the patient should contact his local health department to find the sodium content of his drinking water. Congestive heart failure can be controlled. The patient must never become lax in following his therapeutic program. Careful follow-up of patients with heart lesions, maintenance of correct weight, sodium restriction, prevention of infection, avoidance of noxious agents such as coffee and tobacco, avoidance of unregulated or excessive exercise—all aid in preventing the onset of congestive heart failure. In patients with valvular heart disease, surgical correction of the defect at the appropriate time may spare the heart and prevent failure.

Acute Pulmonary Edema

Pathophysiology

Pulmonary edema represents the ultimate stage of pulmonary congestion, in which fluid has leaked through the capillary walls and is permeating the airways, giving rise to dyspnea of dramatic severity. Pulmonary congestion, it will be recalled, comes about when the pulmonary vascular bed has received more blood from the right ventricle than the left can accommodate and remove. The slightest imbalance between inflow on the right and outflow on the left side of the heart may have drastic consequences: for example, if with each heart beat the right ventricle pumps out just one more drop of blood than the left, within the space of only 3 hours the pulmonary blood volume will have expanded 500 ml.!

Most patients with pulmonary edema have chronic heart disease of a type that imposes a strain preponderantly on the left ventricle, such as arterial hypertension or aortic valvular disease. The development of this complication signifies that cardiac function has become grossly inadequate. Terminally the pulmonary capillaries, engorged with an excess of blood that the left ventricle has been incompetent to disgorge, no longer are able to retain their contents. Fluid, first serous and later bloody, escapes into the adjacent alveoli, through the communicating bronchioles and bronchi and thence, mixed with air and churned by respiratory agitation, out of the mouth and the nostrils, producing the ominous "death rattle."

But death from pulmonary edema is by no means inevitable. If appropriate measures are taken, and taken promptly, many attacks can be aborted and many patients can survive this complication to benefit from measures directed against its return. Fortunately, pulmonary edema usually does not develop precipitously, but is preceded by the premonitory symptoms of pulmonary congestion. Moreover, even after it has become well-established, it usually does not progress to a fatal termination with lightning rapidity; its course may occupy a period of many minutes, even hours, during which time treatment may prove to be effective.

Symptoms

The typical attack of pulmonary edema occurs at night after the patient has been recumbent for a few hours. Recumbency increases the venous return to the heart and favors the resorption of edema fluid from the legs. The circulating blood becomes diluted, and its volume expands. The venous pressure mounts and the right atrium fills with increasing rapidity. There is a corresponding increase in the right ventricular output, which eventually surpasses the output from the left ventricle. The pulmonary vessels become engorged with blood, and proceed to leak. Meanwhile the patient has been increasingly restless, oppressed with anxiety and unable to sleep. His complexion is grey; his hands are cold and moist; his nail beds become cyanotic. He has been coughing incessantly and producing increasing quantities of mucoid sputum. As his pulmonary edema progresses his anxiety becomes more acute. He is confused, then stuporous. He breathes noisily and moistly, nearly suffocated by the blood-tinged frothy fluid that now is pouring into his bronchi and trachea. He literally is drowning in his own secretions. The situation is precarious and demands immediate action.

Management

The prime objectives of therapy, simply stated, are the following: (1) to reduce the right atrial inflow of systemic venous blood; and (2) to increase the left ventricular outflow.

To retard the venous return to the heart, i.e., the right atrial inflow, the patient is placed in the near-upright orthopneic position, head and shoulders up, feet and legs down, thus favoring the pooling of blood in dependent portions of the body. As long as, and to the extent that, blood accumulates in the periphery, correspondingly less blood returns to the heart. An attempt is made to reduce the blood volume and increase the oncotic pressure of the blood (hence render it less susceptible to leakage) through dehydration and, to this end, diuretics are administered in the form of Mercuhydrin or Diuril injections, or both.

Phlebotomy. One of the most effective means available for lowering the venous pressure, hence reducing the venous return to the heart, is the rapid withdrawal of from 500 to 700 ml. of blood from a peripheral vein

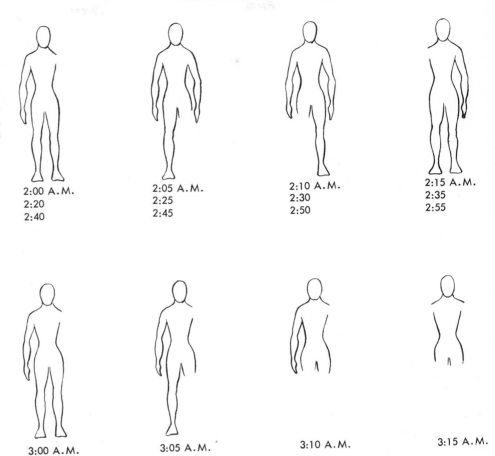

FIG. 19-10. Rotating tourniquet technic. Timing of compression and release of extremities and the sequence of rotation and sequence of removal of tourniquets during a course of tourniquet therapy which was prescribed for 1 hour starting at 2 A.M. Anatomy shown in figures indicates extent of circulation.

2:00 A.M.
2:20
2:40

2:05 A.M.
2:25
2:45

2:10 A.M.
2:30
2:50

2:15 A.M.
2:35
2:55

3:00 A.M.

3:05 A.M.

3:10 A.M.

3:15 A.M.

(i.e., a phlebotomy, or venesection). The resulting decrease in venous return is accompanied by a corresponding decline in the right ventricular. output. Accordingly, the pulmonary artery pressure drops, the pulmonary vessels become less congested and the lung capillaries, no longer congested, reabsorb the fluid that has escaped. The edema clears; the immediate danger has passed. The efficacy and technical simplicity of phlebotomy commend its use in the management of pulmonary edema of all types. All that is required is a standard blood donor set, a supply of which should always be readily available to the clinical staff, plus a reasonable familiarity with its use. The only important contraindication to this procedure is the presence of marked anemia.

Rotating Tourniquets. Another therapeutic measure that achieves essentially the same objectives as does phlebotomy consists in the production of venous stasis in the extremities by either applying tourniquets or inflating pneumatic cuffs around the upper arms and legs, the immediate effect of which is equivalent to removing about 1,000 ml. of circulating blood. Ideally, 4 sphygmomanometer cuffs are employed for this purpose, since these permit the regulation of compression precisely as desired: i.e., to a point slightly above the level of diastolic pressure. In lieu of cuffs, 4 rubber tubes (2 feet long, with an outside diameter of $\frac{5}{16}$ to 1½ inches) may be used; these are tightened sufficiently to cause venous congestion without obliterating the arterial pulse. If this procedure is to be accomplished safely and with maximal benefit, the tourniquet tension on every extremity and on every application must be correct. Moreover, the timing of their application and release must adhere rigidly to a schedule that ensures that 3 of the 4 extremities are compressed and one is free at all times throughout the procedure; that no extremity is compressed continuously for periods of longer than 15 minutes; and that no less than 5 minutes shall intervene between consecutive periods of compression applied to the same extremity. The proper routine is depicted in Figure 19-10. The 15-minute limitation on continuous stasis, and the specification regarding periods of release, are intended to reduce the risks of phlebothrombosis and fatal pulmonary embolism, to which patients in congestive heart failure are uniquely predisposed and which are increased decidedly as a result of the injudicious application of tourniquets. Patients who are to receive this treatment should be reassured as to its nature and purpose; otherwise, they are certain to be disturbed by the attending discomforts and alarmed by the cyanotic discoloration of their congested extremities. The multiplicity of duties and activities involved in tourniquet therapy is sufficient to engage the full attention of one individual, and the importance of the procedure is such as to warrant its assignment as the sole responsibility for the time being of one member of the team.

Oxygen. Oxygen may be administered by intermittant positive pressure, tent, or mask. Oxygen concentration must be high enough to provide blood oxygenation and to overcome the pressure barrier of the edema fluid. Because of their relatively low density and viscosity, helium-oxygen mixtures are breathed with less effort than 100 per cent oxygen or oxygen diluted with atmospheric air; hence, they may be employed to advantage in the treatment of pulmonary edema. If the respiratory passages are obstructed by foamy edema fluid, the oxygen may be bubbled through 95 per cent ethyl alcohol or 2-ethylhexanol, which exert an antifoaming action.

Drugs. In order to improve the contractile force and increase the output of the left ventricle the patient is digitalized, as described on page 387. In addition to strengthening the heart action, steps are taken to reduce to a minimum those factors that tend to stimulate cardiac output. Morphine is given subcutaneously, intramuscularly or intravenously in 15- to 30-mg. doses to relieve anxiety, pain and dyspnea. It must be realized that dyspnea per se involves a great deal of muscular effort, and from the standpoint of pulmonary ventilation is a most unrewarding activity. Thus, the more rapid and shallow the respirations become, the more oxygen is consumed by the respiratory muscles, whereas this type of breathing contributes very little more, if any, to the oxygenation of the blood than does the slower, quieter and deeper type of respiration. A reduction of the respiratory rate is one of the important objectives behind the administration of morphine. Excessive respiratory depression, on the other hand, is a complication to be guarded against and watched for carefully in patients receiving that drug.

Diuretics such as Mercuhydrin, Thiomerin, ethacrynic acid intravenously quickly start the excretion of excess salt and water. Aminophylline given slowly intravenously acts as a bronchodilator and mild diuretic and is often used in conjunction with the above drugs.

Allaying Anxiety. This is a most important consideration in treating patients with pulmonary edema, a cardinal feature of which is basic, primitive fear—fear that is self-intensifying and that tends in itself to intensify the severity of the condition. Apropos of the patient's apprehension and need for reassurance, the nurse must never forget that her patient, however oblivious to his surroundings he may appear, nevertheless may be capable of perceiving and responding to actions, words and appearances that to him represent either a favorable omen or are of ominous significance, to which many a recovered patient can testify. She must not be too quick to assume that he no longer is eligible for, or capable of benefiting from, her reassuring words and acts.

Prevention

As is the case with most medical and surgical complications, pulmonary edema is easier to prevent than to treat. Thus, if recognized in its early stages when the presenting symptoms and signs are solely those of pulmonary congestion, the situation may be corrected by relatively simple measures. These include: (1) vertical positioning of the patient to restore ventricular balance; (2) digitalization to improve myocardial efficiency, and, (3) the elimination of exertional and emotional stress to reduce the left ventricular load. The long-range approach to the prevention of pulmonary edema must be directed at its precursor, namely, pulmonary congestion, the prevention of which depends on the lightening of this load by a variety of means which have already been discussed—including the prevention of overhydration and elimination of edema, the curtailment of physical activity, the correction of obesity and the control of pulmonary infections and of arterial hypertension, if present. Surgical treatment may be performed to eliminate or to minimize valvular defects that limit the flow of blood into or out of the left ventricle, thereby impairing the cardiac output and predisposing the patient to the development of pulmonary congestion and edema.

A final point, and one that is especially important in relation to the role of the nurse in this prophylaxis, concerns the problem of iatrogenic (physician-produced, or therapeutically-induced) pulmonary edema precipitated by the administration of parenteral fluids too rapidly or in too great a volume. Intravenous infusions tend to elevate the venous pressure and increase the venous return. Given injudiciously to patients with little or no cardiac reserve, such injections readily initiate pulmonary edema. Accordingly, when intravenous fluids are given to elderly patients, or to patients with known cardiac disability, they should be administered at a slow, measured rate, the recipient having been placed and supported in the orthopneic position and kept under close observation throughout the procedure.

Fig. 19-11. Diagram showing heart and large vessels and the various defects which might be treated surgically. The defects which require surgical therapy are described in the text. The heart has as a prime objective the propulsion of an adequate volume of blood through two systems, the pulmonic and the systemic. The flow through these two systems must be balanced exactly, since any disequilibrium results in the accumulation of fluid on one side or the other.

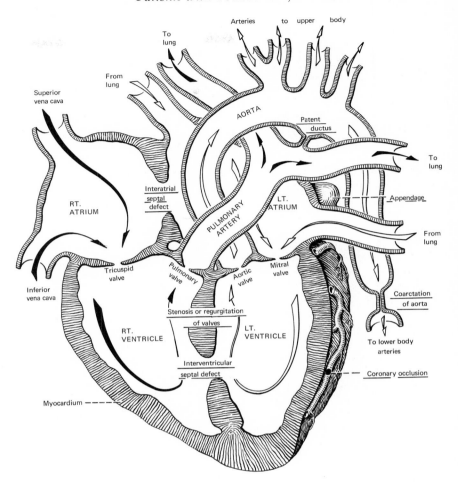

CARDIOVASCULAR SURGERY

Historical Survey

Surgery of the heart has made rapid strides in the last decade; however, experimental work was reported at the beginning of the 20th century. In 1896 Rehn reported the first successful repair of a lacerated right ventricle. In 1923 Cutler, Levine and Beck performed the first surgery for mitral stenosis, and in 1938 Dr. Robert Gross did the first ligation of a patent ductus arteriosus. The excision of a coarctation of the aorta and reconstruction by primary anastomosis was performed successfully by Dr. Gross in Boston and Dr. Crafoord in Stockholm in 1945. Dr. Charles P. Bailey did a successful mitral commissurotomy in June, 1946. Dr. Alfred Blalock and Dr. Helen Taussig of Baltimore improved the circulation of "blue babies" (the problem of tetralogy of Fallot) by shunting the blood into the pulmonary circulation after anastomosing the right subclavian artery to the right pulmonary artery. Dr. Willis Potts modified this technique by anastomosing the left pulmonary artery to the aorta.

Operations were being performed around the heart,

but intracardiac surgery was impeded because there was no means for working within the heart in a dry field. Finally, in 1952, Floyd John Lewis, in Minneapolis, used hypothermia to close the first atrial septal defect by direct approach. Among other effects, the length of time that the oxygen supply to such vital organs as the brain and the spinal cord can be interrupted is increased from 4 minutes to 8 minutes at subnormal body temperatures.

However, what was still needed was a pumping device to take over the functions of both heart and lungs for as long as was necessary to operate. After many years of work, John Gibbon of Philadelphia used a "heart-lung" machine in 1953 during an operation to repair an atrial septal defect; the pump oxygenator worked for 26 minutes during surgery. Open-heart surgery can now be done successfully, employing the "heart-lung" machine. An impressive variety of defects can be corrected, including patent ducts, coarctation of the aorta, aortic aneurysms, atrial and ventricular defects and scarred, leaking and stenosed heart valves. The "heart-lung" machine has been refined, simplified and popularized. Meanwhile, C.

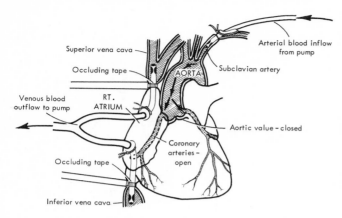

FIG. 19-12. Extracorporeal circulation, illustrating flow of blood from the body and return. The coronary arteries are filled, but no blood enters the cardiac chambers (except coronary venous return). (From Storer, Pate, and Sherman: The Science of Surgery. New York, McGraw-Hill, 1964)

Walton Lillehei, of Minnesota, developed the ingenious idea of using a donor, especially the father of a child, to perform as a heart and lungs to do the work of the patient during the operation. However, this technique risks two lives instead of one. Various heart valve replacements are now commonplace in repairing defective valves.

Presently, artificial hearts or heart-assist devices are being designed and studied experimentally. Moreover, in December of 1967 the first heart transplantation operations were performed by Dr. Christiaan Barnard in Capetown, South Africa, and by Dr. Adrian Kantrowitz in New York. In 1968 approximately 100 heart transplants were done in various parts of the world. Physicians agree that the procedure has passed the initial experimental stage and shows promise of helping carefully selected patients.

The most common of all heart defects continues to defy the surgeon's efforts: stenosis or blockage of the coronary arteries. However, several recently developed procedures are under extensive clinical investigation. Unfortunately, the merits of some of these have not been established with certainty, while the operative mortality of the more definitely beneficial procedures remains formidably high.

Special Techniques in Cardiovascular Surgery

The scope of intracardiac surgery has been limited in the past by the inability to visualize lesions inside the chambers of the heart. The use of hypothermia, the pump oxygenator and a variety of available grafts has made this kind of surgery possible. Hyperbaric oxygenation (performed in a pressure chamber) is a new technique used in surgery of certain forms of congenital heart disease.

Hypothermia

With the use of techniques that lower body temperature, the amount of anesthetic agent can be reduced and the danger of surgical shock lessened. Blood base is reduced. Moreover, it is known that if the heart stops for about 4 minutes and oxygenated blood is not pumped to the brain at normal temperatures, the patient will suffer irreparable brain damage. If the patient's general temperature is lowered, the length of time during which the brain and the spinal cord can be deprived of oxygenated blood can be prolonged to about 8 minutes without such damage. However, the difficulty with hypothermia is that when the patient's temperature gets down to about 26.4° C. (80° F.), the likelihood of ventricular fibrillation or cardiac standstill is great. The correction of this is relatively easy in the warm heart, which has no abnormalities, but in abnormal cooled hearts, restoration may be very difficult. For this reason cardiac hypothermia is used less frequently since the advent of the pump oxygenator.

Extracorporeal Circulation (Pump Oxygenator "Heart-Lung" Machine)

The pump oxygenator takes over the functions of the heart and the lung during surgical intervention on the heart. By diverting venous blood (coming into the right atrium by way of the superior and the inferior venae cavae) into the oxygenator, providing the means of oxygenation of the blood and pumping it back into the arterial system by way of the femoral or the subclavian artery, the heart-lung machine achieves the functions of these major organs of the body (Fig. 19-12).

An interior thoracotomy incision is made by entering the third or the fourth intercostal spaces, and the pericardium is incised. Tape tourniquets are passed about the superior and the inferior venae cavae, and plastic catheters are inserted, through which blood is drawn into the pump oxygenator. Into the right or the left femoral artery in the groin, a catheter is passed upward into the iliac artery for the return of oxygenated blood from the machine into the circulatory system.

Three types of pumps are in use and several kinds of oxygenators. Whereas early "heart-lung" machines oxygenated the blood by a process known as "filming" (letting it run thin over a flat surface), De Wall suggested bubbling oxygen through the blood and defoaming it to get rid of excess bubbles. Another method of oxygenation is by a membrane interphase. Most methods provide satisfactory oxygenation and carbon dioxide elimination. The heart may be open for periods up to 60 minutes; however, most defects can be repaired in less than 15 or 20 minutes.

Grafts

By grafts, one usually means blood-vessel or synthetic grafts. At the turn of the century, a femoral artery was replaced by the femoral artery of another person. Viability of a graft was thought to be important, but this is no longer true. A blood vessel may be obtained for use as a graft under sterile or unsterile conditions. If unsterile, it may be sterilized by radiation, ethylene oxide or a chemical disinfectant.

A graft may be preserved by freezing it very rapidly to avoid damaging it and then drying it by drawing out all the moisture in a vacuum. A freeze-dried graft may be kept in a sealed container for several years. When it is needed, the graft is dropped into a saline solution, where it soon becomes flexible, pliable and similar to its original state.

Today grafts are available as flexible, "accordion-pleated" tubes of Dacron and Teflon. Weaveknit, a non-texturized Dacron yarn, is more pliable, lighter in weight and less likely to fray or run when cut than other commonly used materials.

Artificial Heart or Heart-Assist Devices

Single-chambered pumps to serve as auxiliary or "booster" hearts designed to assist rather than replace a failing heart are being investigated. Likewise, complete prosthetic hearts have been designed and tried under experimental laboratory conditions. Although over 20 different kinds of pumps have undergone trials in animals, to date artificial hearts are still unavailable for more than isolated use, but they hold interesting promise for the future.

The most difficult problem in constructing an artificial heart or heart-assist device lies in discovering a suitable material. To qualify, the material must not damage blood cells or plasma proteins, promote clotting, harm tissue or cause toxic reactions. Tremendous wear and tear must be endured for many years. Another problem is to develop a satisfactory source of power. External power sources are not as desirable as an implantable source. Various possibilities are being investigated. Of course, the heat generated by a power source must be controlled, or at least a method devised whereby the body can tolerate and dissipate such energy.

The following are some devices now being developed:

(1) The DeBakey left ventricular bypass device—an air-driven, diaphragm pump that takes blood from the heart's left atrium and discharges it into the axillary artery, then to the subclavian artery and into the aorta.

(2) The Kantrowitz left-ventricular assist pump is also an air-driven, diaphragm pump that takes up blood from the ascending aorta while the natural left ventricle contracts and discharges blood into the descending aorta as the left ventricle refills. This device increases the efficiency of the left ventricle.

(3) The Kolff total heart replacement is an air-driven device consisting of two separate diaphragm-type blood pumps; one supplies blood to the lungs and the other to the body. The pumps have receiving as well as pumping chambers and the device can vary both its rate and stroke volume.

Heart Transplantation

The major physical problem in heart transplants, as in all other transplant operations, is immunologic rejection, the process whereby the body sets up a reaction to destroy the new organ. Antilymphocytic globulin (ALG) appears to prevent organ rejection, but after a few months some patients develop a resistance to the drug. Tissue matching appears more effective in predicting good matches between relatives (as is done in kidney transplants), but this technique is inadequate for heart transplants from unrelated cadavers. An additional problem being worked on is the need to find a satisfactory way of storing organs for at least one week (Fig. 19-13).

Ethical, moral and economic problems are also significant in heart transplantation. When is a person physically and legally dead? How much is a life worth? When is it permissible to let a patient die? Who decides which person should benefit from a life-saving procedure? How must our ideas regarding the sanctity of the body be changed? Criteria to assist in answering these questions need to be set up to provide guidelines for medical action.

Nursing Considerations

At present, transplantation of a heart is a life-saving procedure; because of this, the patient and his family are made aware of the problems and risks. Numerous laboratory tests are done to assess the patient's clinical condition and to aid in the selection of a donor. Postoperatively the patient requires cardiac monitoring, assisted ventilation, and hemodynamic studies. His preoperative condition will determine the extent of instruction that will be possible or necessary. He may be too ill to receive any instruction, however, his immediate family will appreciate knowing what to expect. The psychological support of the patient and the family is extremely important. This is a time when crucial decisions must be made relative to the cost of

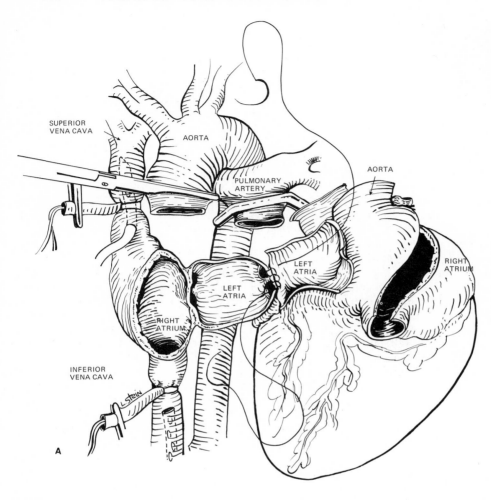

SUPERIOR
VENA CAVA

AORTA

PULMONARY
ARTERY

AORTA

LEFT
ATRIA

RIGHT
ATRIUM

LEFT
ATRIA

RIGHT
ATRIUM

INFERIOR
VENA CAVA

A

Fig. 19-13A. The Cooley method of transplanting a donor heart. The donor's left atrium is being sutured to the remnant of the recipient's left atrium. (Continued with 19-13B on p. 397.)

the surgery, medical and nursing care, family concerns and obligations, emotional involvement, and moral, religious and ethical considerations.

The immediate preoperative preparation of the heart transplant patient is similar to that of other open-heart surgical patients. Timing is a significant factor, because the time of surgery is determined by the immediate availability of a donor heart. Postoperative readiness is undertaken at least a half hour before the patient leaves the operating room. Nurses assigned to care for this patient wear caps, surgical foot coverings, and masks. Every attempt to prevent infection is undertaken. Details of care are similar to that of postoperative open-heart surgical patients. Monitoring devices, respiratory and circulatory aids, as well as observation of the patient as a whole, are evaluated continually to detect arrhythmias, fluid accumulation, respiratory or circulatory distress.

After the immediate postoperative period, the effect of immunosuppressive therapy is ascertained; this in-

cludes signs of infection such as fever, leukocytosis, and bone marrow depression. Lesser obvious signs may be indicative of the onset of rejection; therefore, any change in behavior or clinical signs should be noted, followed, and reported.

Surgery for Congenital Heart Disease

Anomalies due to defective development of the heart are numerous in variety. Some affect its position only. In some persons, the heart lies in the right instead of the left half of the chest (dextrocardia). Such abnormalities in position may affect the heart and the large blood vessels only, or all the viscera of the abdomen also may be inverted (situs inversus). Such persons may be quite healthy.

Defects in the development of the heart itself are much more serious. In general, each of these represents the persistence of some feature normal to this organ at some stage of its development. The most common of these defects is a patent ductus arteriosus.

FIG. 19-13B. The donor's right atrium is sutured to the recipient's right atrium. Then the aorta and the pulmonary artery of the donor heart is approximated to the patient's aorta and pulmonary artery. Sometimes the heart begins to beat automatically when the blood is directed through it; at times, an electric shock is necessary to initiate a beat in the heart.

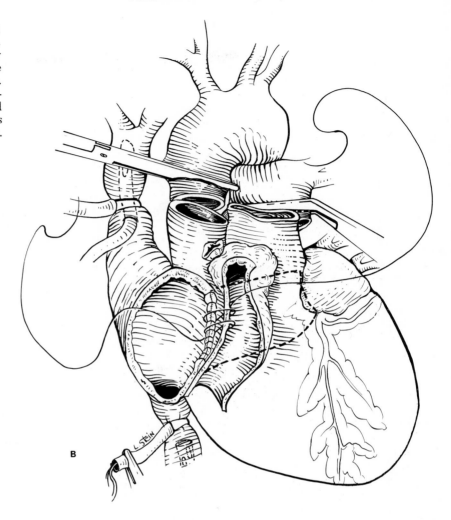

Patent Ductus Arteriosus

Normally in fetal life the ductus arteriosus is open between the pulmonary artery and the arch of the aorta, such being essential to life in utero. This should close soon after birth but, if closure does not occur, the patient usually shows signs of its abnormal existence in the form of retarded or seriously restricted growth, hypertrophic heart, a subsequent streptococcic endocarditis and, at times, aneurysmal dilatation, embolus and so forth. To prevent these occurrences, the duct is preferably doubly ligated and divided. The best time for such a ligation is between the ages of 4 and 12 (Fig. 19-14).

Pulmonary Stenosis

This is a congenital narrowing of the pulmonary artery at its exit from the heart. It leads to an inadequate flow of blood through the lungs. The treatment is to enlarge the opening so that there is an adequate blood flow from the right heart to the lungs.

Tetralogy of Fallot

When pulmonary stenosis is accompanied by a defect of the interventricular septum, a shift of the aorta to the right side and a hypertrophy of the right ventricle, the condition is called *tetralogy of Fallot*. Children so affected are spoken of as *blue babies*.

Clinical signs of tetralogy of Fallot are cyanosis and "clubbing" of fingers, a heart of normal size, a murmur at the base, and no pulmonic second sound. Exercise tolerance of the individual shows marked variation. Operation is indicated when the primary difficulties are lack of circulation to the lungs and cyanosis.

Three methods now are used in the treatment of tetralogy of Fallot. The Blalock and Taussig method of directing blood to the lungs is by an anastomosis between the pulmonary artery and one of the aortic branches, such as the left subclavian, the left common carotid or the innominate. The Potts method is a direct anastomosis between the aorta itself and the pulmonary artery. This increases the flow of blood through the lungs and relieves the cyanosis. Results of this type of surgery are generally satisfactory. The color becomes pinker, the blood becomes thinner, the "clubbing" of fingers and toes begins to disappear, and the patient becomes stronger and more active. A definite attack on the pulmonic stenosis and ventricular septal defect is also possible, using the heart-lung machine, but the risk is higher.

Septal Defects

The walls (septa) separating the atria and the ventricles of the heart also are subject to congenital defects that can be corrected often by surgery.

Atrial Defects. The clinical picture presented by the patient with an atrial septal defect is variable. Inhibition of growth, dyspnea, limitation of activity and systolic murmur may be apparent in large septal defects. Cardiac catheterization is the most reliable technique for making a final diagnosis. A large defect usually leads to progressive cardiac enlargement, increased pulmonary flow and eventual right heart failure.

The repair of atrial septal defects is to close the opening extending between the right (venous) and the left (arterial) sides of the heart. This may be done in various ways. At times, it may be done by suturing a part of the heart wall into the hole; in other instances, by entering the heart and directly closing the opening by suture or by the use of a patch of plastic material sutured into place to close the hole.

Ventricular Defect. In the patient with this defect, the flow of blood is from left to right because of higher pressure in the left ventricle; hence, the patient is not cyanotic. The chief sign is a loud systolic murmur over the base of the heart. Cardiac catheterization is the most conclusive diagnostic procedure. The treatment obviously is to close the defect; however, this has been far from satisfactory by the closed method. With open-heart technique, the technical problems still lead to a rather high operative mortality.

Coarctation of the Aorta

About one fourth of all patients with congenital narrowing of the aorta (see Fig. 19-15) live relatively normal lives; however, most patients begin to show symptoms as they approach adolescence. Hypertension is noted in the upper extremities and lower pressure in the lower extremities, often so low that a pulse is not palpable in the vessels. The chief difficulty is that as such an individual grows older, extreme hypertension can occur in the upper part of the body, causing headache, cerebrovascular accidents, rupture of the aorta and death. The life expectancy at birth of a patient with coarctation of the aorta is estimated at 32 years or less.

This condition, which occurs twice as often in males as in females, can be corrected surgically in one of two ways. The coarctation can be removed, and the 2 ends of the vessel can be anastomosed. At times, this is impossible because of an inelastic aorta or because the defect may involve a long section of the aorta. In these patients, it is necessary to use a graft. The ideal time for surgery is from ages 8 to 16. Before the age of 8 the vessel is too small, and after 16, degenerative changes begin to take place in the arterial walls.

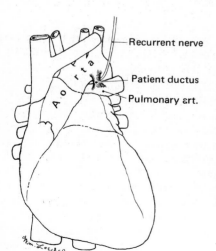

FIG. 19-14. Diagram of the heart and the great vessels, showing patent ductus arteriosus. This is a congenital communication between the aorta and the pulmonary artery. It closes as a rule. However, when it remains open, often it is necessary to close it surgically.

Recurrent nerve
Patient ductus
Pulmonary art.

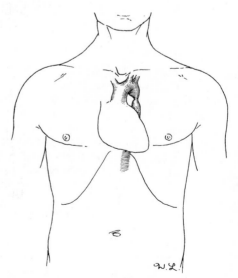

FIG. 19-15. Diagram showing the narrowing of the aorta in the usual position found in coarctation of the aorta.

Cardiovascular Surgical Nursing

Cardiovascular surgical nursing is challenging, dramatic and demanding; progress in recent years has been great. Whereas many patients will be remarkably improved by an operation, many other patients, for one reason or another, will not be eligible for surgery. It is important for the nurse to recognize that, as in any other kind of surgery, the patient is evaluated and treated on an individual basis. Many of these patients know much about heart disease and their own history; therefore, it is necessary for the nurse to be well-informed in order to interpret, teach and care for her patient in keeping with his needs.

Observation of the patient is perhaps even more important in cardiovascular nursing than in other clinical areas. By knowing the patient preoperatively, she will know his habits, his preoccupations and interests, his activity limitations, his worries and the place he assumes in his family. She will recognize changes in mood and personality shifts. Circulatory and respiratory changes often occur rapidly; therefore, the nature and the effect of such signs and symptoms must be reported accurately and intelligently.

Auditory as well as visual signs may be significant. A change in the character of breathing may be heard, or a "different" sound may be detected as the nurse listens with a stethoscope against the patient's chest. In this kind of nursing, it is essential that she become familiar with heart-and-lung sounds; any opportunity that presents itself for her to "listen" with a stethoscope should be seized. The sense of feeling is another important avenue of perception. The rhythm and the nature of the pulse elicited in places other than the wrist have clinical value.

Psychological Support. Since it has been established that the incidence of psychological complications and postoperative psychoses is higher in cardiac surgery patients than in other major surgical patients, the nurse needs to recognize that these patients have greater fears, conscious and subconscious, than other patients. Just the thought of his heart not beating during part of surgery may worry a patient as he tries to determine what the chances are of his heart resuming its beating. The nurse can assist in alleviating the patient's fears by explaining the purpose of each experience that he will have, the persons involved and the effects of the procedure. This explanation is determined on an individual basis, since some patients wish to know more than others. Behavior or verbal reaction that might indicate over-concern can be reported to the physician, who would decide on preventive therapy or the need for psychiatric consultation. Familiarity with the environment, staff, near-by patients and hospital routine is very important to this patient. Opportunity to talk to a recovering patient often is more effective in estab-lishing his confidence than any other means. The spiritual adviser serves to support and sustain the religious faith of this patient and his family rather than dwelling on the possibility of death.

Socioeconomic aspects are major considerations that are reflected in the care and the treatment of the cardiac surgical patient. Usually, he has had a long medical history leading up to the decision to undergo surgery. He may have had consultations, distance to travel to a cardiac surgical clinic, and preliminary checkups prior to his admission to a hospital, where at least 2 weeks are spent undergoing various diagnostic tests. This is costly. Then the decision is reached regarding the treatment of choice. Aside from the usual charges, the surgical patient may need at least a dozen pints of blood for the "heart-lung" machine, special medications that are varied and expensive, intensive nursing care for at least the first 5 postoperative days and many roentgenograms and laboratory studies. Upon discharge from the hospital, it is not uncommon for the patient to be asked to stay at a nearby hotel within walking distance of the cardiac clinic for about a week, during which time additional evaluation is done and more concrete individual advice is given regarding his future activity. Health insurance may cover a part of the financial burden; however, much must be assumed by the patient and his family.

The concern, the support and the value of the family must never be minimized in the early or long-range plans for the individual patient. The nurse is in a strong position to assist the patient-family relationship as she teaches, interprets, encourages and understands their many problems.

Preoperative Care

Only those aspects of nursing care that are unique to the cardiovascular surgical patient are mentioned here. (The principles of surgical care outlined in Chap. 9 would be applicable throughout.)

Regardless of the publicity and the frequency with which heart surgery is being performed today, the individual about to face such an operation is worried and concerned. He needs to know that he is in competent hands. Meeting his emotional and spiritual needs is a vital part of his preparation; his postoperative progress depends on it.

In addition to diagnostic tests, the preoperative cardiovascular patient has complete blood studies and chest roentgenograms. He has his blood pressure taken and the apical-radial pulse rate noted every 4 hours; he is also weighed daily. This is done in order to establish a base line or guide as to the level at which these indices are normal for each particular patient. As for the dietary regimen, he may be on a restricted sodium diet, depending upon the degree of congestive failure.

His diet is planned to achieve optimal nutritional levels. The need for diuretics and digitalis are evaluated at this time.

Preoperative Instruction of the Patient. A planned "talk" about what to expect preoperatively and postoperatively, such as the reason for chest tubes, oxygen therapy, fluid, blood and replacement therapy, drug therapy, turning and so forth, is given informally and individually to each patient. This will help greatly in the postoperative period. At this time, any questions the patient might have are answered or referred to the physician, the social worker or the person who can supply the answer. The individual nature of such instruction must be emphasized. Some patients desire or require more than others.

Coughing and deep breathing activities are extremely important for proper aeration of the lungs postoperatively. The patient should be encouraged to practice coughing effectively by (1) taking a deep breath, (2) tightening the stomach muscles and (3) exploding the cough.

This may be the ideal time to acquaint the patient with the treatment methods used in respiratory therapy and those used for artificial ventilation (see Chap. 15).

Immediate Preoperative Nursing Care. Over and above the routine immediate preparation, the wrists and the ankles may be shaved in anticipation of a "cut-down." This is performed early on the day of surgery; a plastic catheter is used to cannulate the vein, and a blunted 15-gauge or 18-gauge needle is used to connect the plastic tube to the intravenous set. A "cut-down" is done so that easy access to a vein may be always present.

A nasogastric tube may be inserted before surgery to prevent abdominal distention and nausea postoperatively. Before administering the preoperative medication, a record should be made of the patient's blood pressure, temperature, pulse and respiration. Any unusual change in these signs should be reported. An indwelling catheter may be ordered for insertion into the urinary bladder; this may be done after the patient is anesthetized.

Postoperative Nursing Management

Proficiency in nursing care is essential for the recovery of the patient. The nurse must be skilled in the use of ventilatory equipment, monitoring devices, resuscitative aids and fluid therapy equipment. Meaningful observation, intelligent interpretation, and accurate recording are the components of essential nursing care. By being informed about the operative course of her patient, the nurse is in a better position to anticipate possible problems.

In general, all postoperative patients who have had heart and great vessel surgery are cared for in the same manner as chest surgical patients, with the possible exception of the coronary artery surgical patient. When it is realized that death resulting from heart surgery occurs more frequently in the first 48 hours postoperatively and not on the operating table, the nurse will be impressed by the necessity for expert and effective care.

Vital Signs. These are significant because complications can be anticipated very early when the signs begin to deviate. For example, low systolic and pulse pressures may indicate reduced blood volume; lowered systolic, diastolic, and pulse pressures may suggest a developing metabolic acidosis. It is important to keep the blood pressure at desirable levels to prevent irreversible shock and damage to the heart, the brain, the kidneys and the liver. Postoperative care of patients with mitral or aortic commissurotomy tolerate lowered blood pressures such as 80 or 90 without ill effects. However, should the systolic pressure fall below 80, it may be necessary to administer neosynephrine or some other vasopressor drug.

If hypotension persists, a thrombus may be blocking a graft or anastomosis site. Other problems that may result from hypotension are cerebral ischemia, myocardial infarction and renal shutdown.

The blood pressure of patients who have had coronary artery surgery (revascularization surgery) must be watched more closely. Their blood pressure ought to be maintained not lower than 10 points below the preoperative level.

With an increase in blood pressure, the anastomosis or graft may disrupt. Pain or activity may cause an increase in pressure and should be controlled by medication. A safe range in blood pressure is from 20 mm. above to 20 mm. below the normal systolic reading.

Volume and rhythm of pulse should be noted as well as the rate. Pulse irregularity must be reported, since it may be indicative of fibrillation and subsequent cardiac arrest. An increased pulse rate may be the first sign of shock, hemorrhage or heart failure.

It is important in the immediate postoperative period to check the peripheral pulse because of the hazard of peripheral emboli, particularly in patients who have had mitral valve surgery. However, there are patients whose peripheral pulses are not discernable immediately postoperatively, and this information should be made known to the nurse by the surgeon. Peripheral pulses need not be counted but simply verified as to their presence. Check points are the temporal artery, the radial artery, the posterior tibial artery and the dorsalis pedis artery. If these pulses are not detected, check the next proximal pulse.

The physician should be notified of any temperature over 38.9° C. (102.2° F.), inasmuch as this causes extra work for the heart. Lower temperatures ranging from 34.4° C. (94° F.) to 36° C. (96.8° F.) ought to be reported also, since this may indicate shock or cardiac decompensation. In raising the body temperature, an electric blanket may be used at the request of the surgeon; hot water bottles should *not* be used.

General Observation. Cyanosis must be watched for and corrected. The lighting in the unit should allow optimal observation of nail beds, lips and skin. Blanching or mottling in the extremities may indicate embolic phenomenon, especially when accompanied by numbness, tingling, loss of motion and/or pain. Report the least suspicious sign at once.

Venous distention of the neck may be noted as the patient regains consciousness. This results from straining due to chest pain, discomfort and even the presence of the endotracheal tube; eventually, it will disappear.

Check surgical dressings, especially posteriorly, for signs of hemorrhage or constriction.

Maintaining Patency and Function of Equipment. This includes the intravenous infusion, nasogastric tube connected to its suction machine, ECG leads, assisted breathing apparatus, indwelling catheter attached to a drainage tube and bottle, and proper function of the water-sealed chest drainage. Two Kelly clamps should be available near the water-seal drainage equipment to be used in the event of accidental disconnection. (These are discussed in more detail on p. 260.)

Maintaining a Patent Airway. *Retained Secretions.* This is a common problem in thoracic and cardiac postoperative surgical patients. Signs include apprehension, perspiration, rapid pulse, dyspnea, cyanosis, a "wet" cough, if any, and wet noisy respirations. A steady rise in temperature and pulse is often a sign of retained secretions and, possibly, of atelectasis. If secretions are not removed, atelectasis and cardiac failure result; this is inexcusable.

Coughing must be done in such a way that secretions down deep are brought up and expelled. The nurse can assist the patient by splinting the chest with her hands or arms. It has been found helpful to support the upper abdomen when encouraging the patient to cough. If secretions cannot be brought out in this way, endotracheal suctioning must be done. At times it may be necessary to perform a bronchoscopy or a tracheotomy.

Aerosol therapy using a mucolytic agent also aids in the removal of secretions. Through surface action wetting characteristics and thinning action, mucolytic agents aid in the control and elimination of secretions. With supersaturation the secretions are maintained in liquid form and the cilia can function more efficiently with less viscid secretions; therefore, secretions may be brought to the area where they can stimulate the cough reflex and be eliminated. The cough reflex is more effective on these thinned and watery secretions and the pain and trauma of the paroxysmal bouts of coughing are reduced.

Positioning and Turning. Usually, the patient is kept flat in bed until the systolic blood pressure is over 100 mm. Hg. Before the head of the bed is raised, the blood pressure should be noted and repeated 5 minutes after the new position is assumed. If the blood pressure has dropped, lower the patient and wait for at least 30 minutes before elevating again.

Patients who have had mitral, aortic or congenital heart surgery usually may be turned from side to side every 2 hours and placed in a semisitting position; however, check the individual patient's specific orders and nursing care plan. Postoperative coronary artery surgical patients are usually kept quiet on their backs for 48 hours. Turning these patients even 15° may cause a marked drop in blood pressure. After 48 hours, they may turn from the back to the right side every 2 hours. Patients who have had mammary artery implants are never turned to the left side, because of interference with lung expansion and the possibility of herniation of the heart from its pericardial sac.

The bed never should be elevated at the knees without a written order from the surgeon. Such a position after surgery on the descending aorta or vessels of the legs may produce thrombosis by inhibiting the flow of blood through the lower extremities.

Inhalation Therapy. For ease of ventilation of the lungs, oxygen is given by face mask at 8 L. per minute until the patient has fully reacted. Then oxygen by oropharyngeal catheter is administered at approximately 6 L. per minute. Proper positioning of the tube is important as well as frequent cleaning of the tube.

Drainage Systems. *Water-sealed Drainage.* A catheter is introduced through a stab wound in the lower part of the chest. An extension of this catheter with its distal end placed under a fluid level permits excess air and fluid to drain from the pleural space but allows nothing to re-enter. Another reason for chest drainage is to maintain subatmospheric pressure in the pleural cavity. The drainage bottle must be secured at the side of the bed, and a clamp must be available at all times to close the tube near the chest wall in the event of accidental disconnection of the tubing or suction bottle (see also p. 260).

Watch for excessive drainage of blood. It is usual to expect 400 to 500 ml. of serosanguineous drainage in 24 hours following mitral commissurotomy, and up to 1,200 ml. in 24 hours for a mammary artery implant. If there is no drainage, fluid may be accumulating in the thorax, with ultimate cardiac embarrassment.

For valvular surgical patients, drainage tubes usually

are removed in 24 hours. Patients with mammary implants retain their drainage tubes longer.

To prevent clots from forming in the tubes, they are milked or stripped as necessary. This may be done by hand or with a specially designed chest-tube stripper (Mueller).

A suggested method of noting the amount of drainage in a given period of time is to place an inch-wide strip of adhesive tape vertically on the drainage bottle. A line is drawn on the tape at hourly intervals to indicate the level of drainage at that time.

Nasogastric Suction. A common occurrence with postoperative cardiac surgical patients is paralytic ileus. Often as a result of trauma to the vagus nerve during surgery, there is a temporary inability of the stomach to empty properly, and gastric dilatation results. For patients who have had surgery for coronary artery insufficiency, the stomach must be kept deflated to relieve pressure on the heart and help to prevent angulation of the implanted artery; this may occur when the heart is pushed upward by a distended stomach. For these reasons, nasogastric suction is used.

General Postoperative Management. Pain. Patients may have a considerable amount of chest pain postoperatively, due mostly to rib retraction during surgery. Demerol Hydrochloride (50-100 mgm. every 3 to 4 hours) is given during the first 24 to 48 hours after surgery. The patient must be evaluated carefully so that enough medication is given to keep him fairly comfortable and yet not more than necessary, which would depress him generally and his cough reflex specifically.

The nurse is challenged to keep the patient as comfortable as possible by changing his position, supporting dependent parts, splinting his chest as he coughs, etc., before resorting to narcotics. When such medications are used, less than the average dose is given; the patient is observed for undue depressant effects. Narcotic antagonist drugs are available should this occur.

Thereafter, it is advisable to decrease the amount and the frequency of sedation and attempt to determine the cause of restlessness if possible, such as oxygen want, fear, position discomfort and so forth.

Nutrition and Fluids. Fluids are given as soon as tolerated; they should not be too hot or too cold, for this may set up cardiac irregularities. Since fruit juices may cause nausea, they are omitted in the beginning. A return to soft and normal diet is done as soon as the patient wishes, except for those patients who have had coronary artery surgery. Food should be postponed until abdominal cramps and the passage of flatus have passed.

The nurse should be aware that cardiac patients may exhibit unusual thirst and drink large quantities of fluids. In instances of fluid retention, it may be necessary to restrict fluid intake. Because fluid balance in the cardiac patient is of extreme importance, all fluid intake and output must be recorded. Also, it may be necessary to weigh the patient daily.

Physical Rehabilitation. Deep breathing is encouraged to ventilate and expand the lungs. It is carried out deliberately, slowly and quietly through the nose. The patient must not become overtired.

After the first 24 hours, patients are encouraged to move. A "pull" can be made from a double thickness of muslin (approx. 3 yds. long and 4-inches wide). By doubling this to form a loop that is placed around the foot end (center) of the bed, the ends can be drawn through the loop, thereby securing it. The ends serve as a "pull" for the patient; these can be tied together in a knot to facilitate grasping.

Patients have a tendency toward left shoulder pain, which results in "a frozen left shoulder" unless combated vigorously throughout the postoperative period. These patients must be urged to move their left shoulder freely, starting soon after operation. This does not mean passive motion by moving their left arm with their right arm. It means active motion of left hand—combing hair, reaching for various objects, buttoning neck buttons and so forth.

When surgery has not involved the lower extremities, leg exercises (flexion and extension) should be performed every 2 hours postoperatively.

Medications. Antibiotics are given routinely postoperatively to help prevent infections. Such therapy is usually maintained for 10 to 12 days in order to minimize any tendency for reactivation of rheumatic fever. Vitamin supplements are added as soon as solid food is tolerated. Digitalis may or may not be ordered, as determined by the cardiologist. Quinidine is usually given to convert atrial fibrillation to normal sinus rhythm.

First Postoperative Day. A portable upright chest plate is taken to determine the rate of lung expansion and to detect fluid collection, pneumothorax or emphysema.

A hematocrit, a red blood count and a hemoglobin test are done to indicate the degree of blood loss during surgery. Also, a routine urinalysis is done.

Complications. Although the first 48 hours are most critical, it is several days before the patient has really passed the danger point. Possible complications are: (1) *respiratory:* hypoxia, respiratory failure, pneumothorax, atelectasis; (2) *circulatory:* hemorrhage, arterial insufficiency, metabolic acidosis, over-oxygenation, distention of the left side of the heart, heart block; (3) *renal shutdown.* In addition, there may be problems of fluid imbalance, muscle spasm, hiccup, pain, worry and apprehension. The nurse caring for a patient who has had heart surgery needs to be aware that these problems can occur; she is in a position to detect early symptoms and to ward off major difficulties by prompt attention and action.

Psychological Aspects. On the whole, patients who have had explanations preoperatively and an opportunity to talk out their fears, anxieties and concerns seem to make a better adjustment to the postoperative phase of their treatment.

States of depression in the postoperative cardiac patient have ranged from mild, transient depression to a full-blown depression with suicidal tendencies. Those patients with transient personality changes resulting from their reluctance to leave the shelter of a "cardiac life" require special understanding and support. For varying lengths of time, these people have been sick and have held the center of attention in the family circle. After surgery, a weaning process must start.†

Convalescence

From the fifth to the eighth days, the patient may be allowed to dangle his feet, then gradually be allowed out of bed until full mobilization is reached by the twelfth to the fourteenth day. This is determined on an individual basis.

Tests are done on the day prior to discharge for comparison with the preoperative studies and with future studies. Changes can be noted that are indicative of the success of the operative procedure. These tests are also useful in determining future medical treatment, the nature of activities and the type of diet.

Instructions for Convalescence After Operation.* Patients, regardless of the ease with which they tolerate surgery, should set aside a minimum of 8 weeks for convalescence. This period should be devoted to the recovery of strength depleted by the previous illness and the rigors of hospitalization.

During the first week exercise is limited to walking for short periods in the morning and the afternoon.

† Bolton and Bailey studied 1,500 patients in an attempt to determine if there were some particularly characteristic preoperative elements that would be of significant help in predicting the likelihood of patients' developing postoperative psychoses. Results: There seems to be no relationship to sex, age, severity of heart disease, duration of failure, or complications of surgery that would lead to cerebral ischemia. However, postoperative psychoses occurred more frequently in cases of acquired heart disease that had a dynamically significant mitral insufficiency. (Bolton, H. E., and Bailey, C. P.: Psychosomatic Aspects of Cardiovascular Surgery *in* Cantor, A. J., and Foxe, A. N.: Psychosomatic Aspects of Surgery. p. 40. New York, Grune, 1956.)

* Bailey Thoracic Clinic: *Your New Way to Health,* a brochure for patient instruction.

This should be done on level ground in the home or outside for 15 or 20 minutes. Shorter periods are advised if fatigue develops. Stair-climbing is permitted, but since this requires a greater output of energy, it should be done slowly and only when necessary.

The remainder of the waking day is spent out of bed and in relaxing activities such as reading, painting, knitting, writing or speaking with visitors. A nap after the noon meal is beneficial. Showers or tub baths may be taken from the start. It is necessary to avoid drafts and to keep warm in order to prevent respiratory infections; 10 hours of sleep is the minimal requirement, and it is wise to retire before 11 o'clock.

After the first week, exercise is more liberal. Walking can be continued for longer periods. Regular rest will prevent unusual fatigue. Patients may enjoy a leisurely drive, although they should refrain from doing their own driving for several weeks.

Usually, an unrestricted diet is prescribed. Meals are to be ample, eaten with leisure and followed by a half hour of relaxation. In instances where partial improvement rather than complete cure has been accomplished, continued sodium restriction may be necessary for 3 months, sometimes indefinitely.

At the conclusion of the first 2 weeks of home care, the patient should be able to attend to all his duties without unusual fatigue or difficulty. Shortness of breath and ankle swelling should not be present. Persistence of these complaints requires medical care.

Pain in the area of the incision is common for a varying length of time. Occasionally, the discomfort is a bandlike tightness or numbness. Although an annoying complaint, it is not a serious one and is readily controlled with such simple drugs as aspirin. A gradual subsidence of this distress will be noted after the first several weeks, although damp weather and other climatic changes occasionally cause its return.

It is most important to guard against infection of any type. A common cold may develop into a serious illness if ignored. To prevent upper respiratory infections, avoid fatigue, exposure and direct contact with persons already infected. If, despite these precautions, respiratory infection should occur, bed rest, warmth and prompt medical care must be instituted immediately in a patient with rheumatic heart disease.

A suitable antibiotic must be taken before and after any dental extraction. It is necessary to consult one's physician for the drug of choice before such dental work is undertaken.

A decision to return to a full working status must await a complete evaluation of the patient's cardiac condition. This is generally scheduled at the end of the 8-week period following operation.

Women with household responsibilities have generally undertaken light duties, such as dusting and cooking, prior to the 8-week examination. However, approval for full household duty should await the result of this medical review.

In re-establishing a routine of life, sound habits must be formed. Health cannot be bought with a single stroke of the surgeon's knife. Exhausting routines may wipe out the benefits already won. Sensible adjustments have been made by people of all temperaments and walks of life. Cardiac surgery cannot erase all the consequences of years of illness. It remains for the patient to regulate his life sensibly in order to protect the gains this modern miracle of treatment has made possible.

BIBLIOGRAPHY

Books

Andreoli, K. G., *et al.*: Comprehensive Cardiac Care. St. Louis, C. V. Mosby, 1968.

Bailey, C. P. (ed.): Rheumatic and Coronary Heart Disease. Philadelphia, J. B. Lippincott, 1967.

Benack, R. T.: Congestive Heart Failure. Springfield, Ill., Charles C Thomas, 1966.

Blake, T. M.: An Introduction to Electrocardiography. New York, Appleton-Century-Crofts, 1968.

Friedberg, C.: Diseases of the Heart. Philadelphia, W. B. Saunders, 1966.

Gefter, W. I., *et al.*: Synopsis of Cardiology. St. Louis, C. V. Mosby, 1965.

Karvonen, M., and Barry, A. (eds.): Physical Activity and the Heart. Springfield, Ill., Charles C Thomas, 1967.

Metheney, N., and Snively, W.: Fluid balance in the patient with cardiac disease. *In* Nurses' Handbook of Fluid Balance, pp. 195-211. Philadelphia, J. B. Lippincott, 1967.

Myerson, R. M., and Pastor, B. H.: Congestive Heart Failure. St. Louis, C. V. Mosby, 1967.

Stamler, J.: Lectures on Preventive Cardiology. New York, Grune and Stratton, 1967.

The President's Commission on Heart Disease, Cancer, and Stroke: A National Program to Conquer Heart Disease, Cancer and Stroke. Washington, D.C., U.S. Government Printing Office, 1964.

Articles

Braunwald, E. (ed.): Symposium on beta adrenergic receptor blockade. Amer. J. Cardiology, *18*:303-475, Sept., 1966.

Burke, G.: The treatment of angina pectoris. Geriatrics, *22*:168-174, May, 1967.

Cortes, F. M.: Treatment of pericardial diseases. Mod. Treatment, *4*:123-225, Jan., 1967.

DeGraff, A. C., and Fisch, S. (eds.): Treatment of arteriosclerotic heart disease. Mod. Treatment, *3*:563-657, May, 1966.

Dolan, J. A. (ed.): Symposium on nursing problems of persons with cardiovascular disorders. Nurs. Clin. N. Amer., *1*:1-72, March, 1966.

Gibson, T. C., *et al.*: Community nursing visits to patients with cardiovascular disease. Amer. J. Pub. Health, *57*:1004-1008, June, 1967.

Griep, H., and DePaul, Sister: Angina pectoris. Amer. J. Nurs., *65*:72-75, June, 1965.

Grossman, B. J.: Chemoprevention of rheumatic fever. Med. Clin. N. Amer., *50*:279-283, Jan., 1966.

Gunnar, R. M., *et al.*: The physiologic basis for treatment of shock associated with myocardial infarction. Med. Clin. N. Amer., *51*:69-81, Jan., 1967.

Hunn, V. K.: "Cardiac pacemakers," Amer. J. Nurs., *69*:749-754, April, 1969.

Kelly, A.: Current cardiovascular diagnostic measures and associated nursing care. J. Nurs. Educ., *5*:13-17, Nov., 1966.

Larson, E. D.: The patient with acute pulmonary edema. Amer. J. Nurs., *68*:1019-1021, May, 1968.

Luisada, A. A.: The signs and symptoms of valvular disease and heart failure. Clinical Symposia *20*:3-29, Jan.-Feb.-March, 1968.

Malmude, A.: Coronary heart disease. Nurs. Sci., *3*:414-428, Dec., 1965.

Mattingly, T.: Symposium: primary myocardial disease. Circulation, *32*:845-851, Nov., 1965.

McIntyre, H.: Clinical nursing and the congestive heart failure patient. Cardio-Vascular Nurs., *3*:19-22, Sept.-Oct., 1967.

Merkel, R., and Sovie, M. D.: Electrocution hazards with transvenous pacemaker electrodes. Amer. J. Nurs., *68*:2560-2563, Dec., 1968.

Motock, E. C.: A patient with sarcoma of the pericardium. Nurs. Clin. N. Amer., *1*:15-22, March, 1966.

Olson, E. (ed.): The hazards of immobility. Effects on cardiovascular function. Amer. J. Nurs., *67*:781-782, April, 1967.

Poole, P. E.: Implementing behavior in male patients with coronary artery disease. Nurs. Res., *15*:172-175, Spring, 1966.

Rawlings, M. S.: Heart disease today. Amer. J. Nurs., *66*:303-307, Feb., 1966.

Semler, H. J.: Management of acute myocardial infarction. ANA Conference Group on Medical-Surgical Nursing and American Heart Association, ANA, 1965.

Smith, B. C.: Congestive heart failure. Amer. J. Nurs., *69*:278-282, Feb., 1969.

Sobel, D. E.: Personalization on the coronary care unit. Amer. J. Nurs., *69*:1439-1442, July, 1969.

Symposium on Care of the Cardiac Patient. Nurs. Clin. N. Amer., *4*:563-649, Dec., 1969.

Torrens, P., and Hanchett, E.: Public health nursing and the congestive heart failure patient. CardioVascular Nurs., *3*:15-18, July-Aug., 1967.

Turrell, D.: The cardiac patient returns to work. Amer. J. Nurs., *65*:115-117, Aug., 1965.

U. S. National Heart Institute: Fact Sheet: Artificial parts for the heart and blood vessels. Dept. of Health, Education and Welfare, 1967.

————: The Framingham heart study: habits and coronary heart disease. 1966.

Warren, J. V.: Acute myocardial infarction. Postgrad. Med., *38*:101-104, Aug., 1965.

Welch, W.: Medical aspects of congestive heart failure. Cardio-Vascular Nurs., 3:9-13, May-June, 1967.

Whitehouse, F. A. (ed.): The coronary spectrum. J. Rehab., 32, March-April, 1966.

Yokes, J. A.: The clinical specialist in cardiovascular nursing. Amer. J. Nurs., 66:2667-2670, Dec., 1966.

Zoll, P. M., and Lilienthal, A. J.: Control of heart action by electrical means. Disease-A-Month, Sept., 1966.

Cardiovascular Surgery

Artificial Parts for the Heart and Blood Vessels, Fact Sheet: National Heart Institute, U. S. Dept. of Health, Education & Welfare, 1967.

Brambilla, M. A.: A teaching plan for cardiac surgical patients. Cardio-Vascular Nurs., 5:1-4, Jan.-Feb., 1969.

Cardiovascular Surgery, Heart Information Center, National Heart Institute, National Institute of Health, 1968.

Druss, R. J., and Kornfeld, D. S.: The survivors of cardiac arrest. A psychiatric study. JAMA, 201:291-296, 1967.

Effler, D. B.: "The surgical treatment of myocardial ischemia," Clinical Symposia 21:1, Jan.-Feb.-March, 1969.

James, E. E.: The nursing care of the open heart patient. Nurs. Clin. N. Amer., 2:543-558, Sept., 1967.

Kantrowitz, A.: Frontiers in heart surgery. Rhode Island Med. J., 50:470-479, July, 1967.

Kennedy, M. J.: Coping with emotional stress in the patient awaiting heart surgery. Nurs. Clin. N. Amer., 1:3-13, Mar., 1966.

Kimball, C. P.: Psychological responses to the experience of open heart surgery, The Amer. J. of Psychiatry, 126:348-359, Sept., 1969.

Lunde, D. T.: Psychiatric complications of heart transplants, The Amer. J. of Psychiatry, 126:369-373, Sept., 1969.

Maclean, D. M., and Fowler, E. A.: Heart transplant. Amer. J. Nurs., 68:2124-2127, Oct., 1968.

Pitorak, E. F.: Open-ended care for the open heart patient. Amer. J. Nurs., 67:1452-1457, July, 1967.

Powers, M.: Emotional aspects of cardiovascular surgery. Cardio-Vascular Nurs., 4:7-10, Mar.-Apr., 1968.

Rubenstein, D., and Thomas, J. K.: Psychiatric findings in cardiotomy patients, The Amer. J. of Psychiatry, 126:360-369, Sept., 1969.

PATIENT EDUCATION

Brams, W. A.: Managing Your Coronary. ed. 3. Philadelphia, J. B. Lippincott, 1966.

American Heart Association
44 E. 23rd Street
New York, New York 10010
  Many booklets, slides and teaching materials are available.
  Booklets available by prescription:
  Your Mild Sodium Restricted Diet
  Your 1000 Milligram Sodium Diet—Moderate
  Your 500 Milligram Sodium Diet—Strict
  Special Foods for Sodium Restricted Diets
  Anticoagulants, Your Physician and You
  Anticoagulant Emergency Identification Card
  If Your Child Has a Congenital Heart Defect
  After a Coronary
  If You Have Angina
  Heart Attack
  Heart Disease Caused by Coronary Atherosclerosis
  After a Coronary
  If You Have Angina
  Heart Attack
  Heart Disease Caused by Coronary Atherosclerosis
  Planning Fat-Controlled Meals for 1200 and 1800 Calories
  Planning Fat-Controlled Meals for Approximately
    2000-2600 Calories
  Reduce Your Risk of Heart Attack
  What We Know About Diet and Heart Disease
  Physical Activity and Your Heart
  High Blood Pressure
  What Everyone Should Know About Smoking and
    Heart Disease

United States Department of Health, Education and Welfare
  Heart Information Center
  National Heart Institute
  Bethesda, Maryland 20402
    A Handbook of Heart Terms
    Congestive Heart Failure—A Guide for the Patient
    Rheumatic Fever
    Hardening of the Arteries
    Inborn Heart Defects

CHAPTER **20**

The Patient in The Cardiac Care Unit

- *The Concept of Intensive Coronary Care*
- *The Primary Role of the Cardiac Care Nurse-Clinician*
- *Electrocardiography and the Interpretation of Cardiac Arrhythmias*
- *Clinical Pharmacology of Anti-Arrhythmic Drugs*
- *Arrhythmias of Major Importance in the CCU*
- *Nursing Management of the Patient with Acute Myocardial Infarction*
- *Nursing Management of Complications other than Cardiac Arrhythmias*
- *Special CCU Nursing Techniques*
- *The System of Intensive Cardiac Care*

THE CONCEPT OF INTENSIVE CORONARY CARE

Acute myocardial infarction from coronary artery occlusion is a frequent, dangerous, and treacherous illness. Over half a million persons die of this illness annually in the United States. The victim may die with little or no advance warning, especially in the first few minutes, hours or days after the onset of the attack. A leading cause of mortality is the development of serious cardiac arrhythmias. These dangerous cardiac arrhythmias involve abnormally fast or slow rates of beating, abnormal origin of the dominant pacemaker, abnormal distribution over the ventricles of the electrical impulse that triggers contraction, uncoordinated or disorganized beating, or no beating at all. The appearance of these complications either alone or in various combinations grimly foreshadows impending death.

Over the course of the past decade, 3 new techniques have become available that have greatly improved the prospects for survival from the serious or otherwise lethal cardiac arrhythmias. These 3 techniques (closed-chest cardiac massage, cardioversion, and cardiac pacemaking) are defined on pp. 419, 425-426. When they are applied quickly and appropriately in conjunction with arrhythmia-suppressing drug therapy, myo-

cardial infarction mortality in hospitalized patients can be reduced by about one third—that is, from roughly 30 per cent to 20 per cent.

Shortly after these techniques became available, it was realized that the tendency of many myocardial infarction patients to die suddenly often made it impossible to apply the necessary life-saving technique quickly enough. Unless the cerebral circulation is restored within 4 minutes after cardiac arrest, the brain of an adult patient progressively sustains irreversible and ultimately lethal damage; if acute myocardial infarction patients are housed all over the hospital on different wards, the required equipment and specially-trained personnel often cannot reach the bedside in sufficient time to prevent this damage. Because of this need for rapid application of resuscitative measures, the development of a special area in the general hospital for the care of all myocardial infarction patients was a logical step, so logical that 3 coronary care units were started independently and nearly simultaneously in 1962, one in Canada and 2 in the United States. More recently, the concept has quite properly been generalized to include special intensive care of other types of heart disease as well. As a result, the term *cardiac care unit* is now often used in place of *coronary care unit;* the common abbreviation, CCU, is appropriate for both.

Fig. 20A. Nursing in the cardiac care unit requires special skills. The nurse is counting the patient's apical pulse rate. Behind her is a cardiac monitor. A calibrated chamber has been placed in the line for intravenous fluid administration to insure accurate fluid intake. The ventilator is attached to the tracheostomy tube with sufficient slack to minimize strain on the tube and discomfort to the patient.

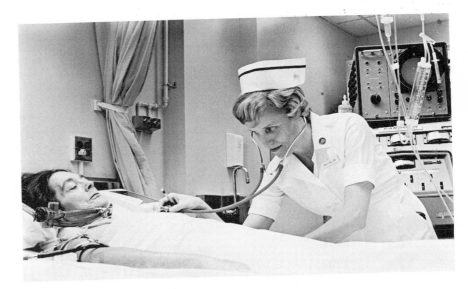

Although the initial impetus to the establishment of coronary care units was the need for rapid resuscitation of patients who were about to die, another benefit was recognized early. This concerned the desirability of preventing potentially lethal arrhythmias in the first place by means of constant surveillance of the patient's electrocardiogram and the administration of appropriate arrhythmia-suppressant drugs whenever early warning signs of a serious arrhythmia appeared. Experience has shown that the death rate is higher if one waits until serious arrhythmias are already present and only then plunges ahead under suboptimal, emergency conditions to attempt resuscitation of an already severely compromised patient.

The basic principles of a CCU are listed in Table 20-1. The first 3 elements are functions that follow obviously from the preceding discussion; the last 2 are organizational considerations that are of at least equal importance if a CCU is to function with maximal effectiveness.

TABLE 20-1. Basic elements of a cardiac care unit

1. Gathering into one location in the hospital.
   (a) All patients with recent myocardial infarctions.
   (b) Special equipment for coronary care.
   (c) Specially trained coronary care personnel.
2. Careful and continuous monitoring and observation of the myocardial infarction patient.
3. Delegation of responsibility so that urgently necessary preventive or therapeutic measures may be carried out quickly by trained personnel.
4. Proper organization to develop and continue high standards of patient care.
5. An ongoing educational program to maintain and enhance CCU staff skills.

THE PRIMARY ROLE OF THE CARDIAC CARE NURSE-CLINICIAN

Traditional hospital organization calls for a professional nurse to be continuously available to each patient throughout every moment of hospitalization, whereas the physician is ordinarily only intermittently present at the bedside of the patient. As a result of this, the coronary care nurse-clinician is a central figure on the CCU team, where a specially trained person must be constantly available for continuous monitoring, preventive therapy, and emergency resuscitation. Here the traditional role of the nurse must be enlarged to include medical diagnosis and authorization for emergency treatment in the absence of a physician. The factor of over-riding importance that has led to this enlargement of nursing responsibility has again been the 4-minute post-arrest time limit after which the brain begins to deteriorate irreversibly. Because experienced physicians can be stationed at the CCU around the clock in only a few hospitals, it has become essential that many coronary care nurses be specially educated to assume these new responsibilities.

The Impact of the CCU on the Nursing Profession

The cumulative impact of the delegation to nurses of increased responsibility and scope of activity in the thousands of CCU's now operating in the United States alone has introduced a new dimension of professionalism into nursing. By and large, the professional nursing organizations have responded favorably to the challenge, with the result that no significant legal problems have arisen in terms of state nursing practice regulations, nor is there any reason to anticipate such difficulties in the future.

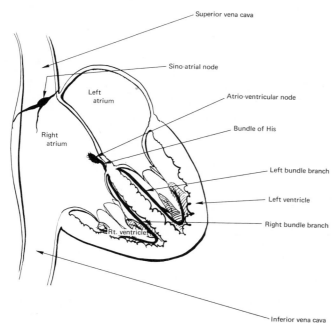

FIG. 20-1. Drawing of the pacemaker and conduction system of the heart.

Another major effect of the widespread development of CCU's has been to increase greatly the prestige of bedside nursing because a good CCU nurse has special skills and responsibilities that are unusually complex and demanding.

The reader should not conclude that the CCU nurse is repeatedly thrown back on her own resources, without any professional support to draw upon in making important diagnostic and therapeutic decisions. In a properly run CCU, a physician experienced in the management of myocardial infarction and other aspects of cardiology must be available daily. As CCU medical director, this individual must be willing to devote several hours a day to the CCU if it is to function properly. Because of the enhanced professionalism that is promoted by the CCU nurse-physician team's collaborative approach to vital bedside decision-making, a properly run CCU can be a highly rewarding source of increased career satisfaction to its participating nurses.

ELECTROCARDIOGRAPHY AND THE INTERPRETATION OF CARDIAC ARRHYTHMIAS

Ability to make correct electrocardiographic interpretations of cardiac arrhythmias is a basic tool of the CCU nurse. Without this diagnostic skill, she cannot carry out her most important function—prompt pro-

phylactic or therapeutic intervention. Electrocardiographic interpretation is not a traditional nursing function, but it is a skill that can be readily learned with proper education.

Electrophysiology

The beating heart is an electromechanical system in which an electrical event—depolarization of the heart muscle cells—serves as a preliminary stimulus to mechanical contraction. Resting (repolarized) heart muscle cells are charged electrically so that the inside of each cell is negative with respect to the outside, with the cell membrane serving as the interface. When a cell is depolarized, these charge relationships between inside and outside are reversed as sodium ions pour into the cell and potassium ions flow out, due to an alteration in cell membrane permeability that is characteristic of the depolarization process. The charge-reversal process starts at one part of a cell, from which it spreads to envelop the entire cell. While this activation wave is spreading, the surface of the depolarized part of the cell has a negative electrical charge with respect to the surface of the resting, polarized part. As a result of this imbalance, an electrical current flows in the body, most intensely in the electrically conductive body fluids immediately surrounding the depolarizing cell, but also in the body at large, with tiny currents even reaching the body surface. Following contraction, the expenditure of metabolic energy repolarizes the cells electrically (by redistributing potassium and sodium ions), so that the cycle may repeat itself to produce a sustained sequence of beats.

As currents flow in the body, the responsible electrons steadily drop in electrical potential energy as they travel along their particular current paths from the positive back to the negative part of the cell membrane. Therefore, different regions of the body show variations in electrical potential (voltage), depending on the particular point (early or late) they happen to occupy in the current path of the electrons that traverse a particular part of the body. The clinical electrocardiogram (ECG) is a graphic record (on a time base) of voltage differences between 2 parts of the body's skin surface as the waves of electrical depolarization and repolarization sweep over the heart.

The depolarization wave starts in a single cell, the pacemaker. Even normal pacemaker cells are seemingly defective, i.e., they are unable to maintain the repolarized state indefinitely. Instead, the transmembrane difference drops steadily following repolarization, due to a steady, slow leakage of sodium ions into the cell. When this process goes far enough, it becomes regenerative: the cell membrane suddenly becomes quite permeable to sodium, and rapid depolarization begins. The latter causes an intense flow of electrical current in the vicinity of the pacemaker cell—strong enough to initiate depolarization in nearby cells. The result is a wave of depolarization that sweeps like a prairie fire over the heart until all cells are depolarized.

Pacemaker cells may normally be found in many parts of the heart, but usually the only ones that initiate beating are found in the sino-atrial (SA) node. These cells are usually in control because they leak sodium faster, and consequently depolarize themselves more rapidly, than other "latent" pacemaker cells. However, when the heart is injured, as by an acute myocardial infarction, some of the injured cells may begin to leak sodium even faster than the SA node cells, with the result that impulse formation begins in an abnormal site, thereby producing a cardiac arrhythmia. At other times, injured cells may no longer be able to depolarize or repolarize as rapidly as before, or even at all, so that the conduction path of the activation wave follows an abnormal course. The result again is a cardiac arrhythmia.

Normal beating is called sinus rhythm because it originates in the sino-atrial node, located high on the right atrium near the entrance of the superior vena cava (see Fig. 20-1). From that point, the wave of depolarization spreads over the atria; the currents resulting from sinus depolarization are too minute to be detected at the body surface, but atrial depolarization produces the P wave of the clinical electrocardiogram (see Fig. 20-2). The P wave lasts about 0.10 second.

After the electrical impulse reaches the atrioventricular (AV) node (or "nodal junction"), it passes through that area of tiny muscle fibers with much reduced amplitude and speed. The amplitude is again too small to be detected at the body surface; the resulting period of apparent electrical quiescence is called the P-R interval. The P-R interval is measured from the beginning of the P wave to the onset of ventricular activation; it normally lasts from 0.12 to 0.21 second, averaging about 0.16 second.

When the P-R interval exceeds 0.21 second, first degree AV block is diagnosed; second degree AV block occurs when some, but not all, P waves fail to reach (activate) the ventricles, which produces an irregular ventricular rate. Third degree or complete heart block is present when no P waves reach the ventricle at all; the ventricles beat regularly but very slowly (perhaps 28 beats per minute) under the control of a pacemaker in the AV node or in the wall of the ventricle itself— a so-called idioventricular pacemaker. The latter is particularly apt to be unreliable, especially when complete heart block develops during the course of an acute myocardial infarction. Unless special measures are taken, the patient is in constant danger of ventricular standstill and death.

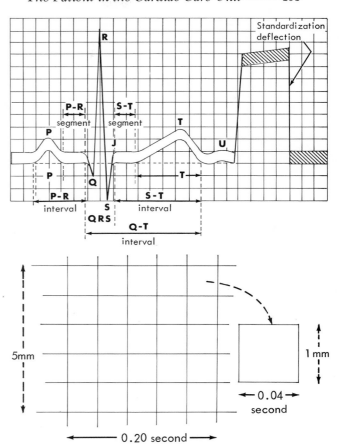

FIG. 20-2. *(Top)* Electrocardiographic wave form nomenclature. The J-point indicates a junction between the end of the QRS and the beginning of the ST-T complex. *(Bottom)* The fine lines of the grid markings of electrocardiographic paper are one millimeter apart both horizontally and vertically; the heavy lines are spaced at 5 millimeter intervals in both directions. At the conventional electrocardiographic paper speed of 25 millimeters per second, each fine line represents 0.04 seconds, and each heavy vertical line represents 0.20 seconds. At the conventional amplifier gain setting, a deflection which is one millivolt (1/1000th of a volt) will produce a deflection of one centimeter (the distance between two heavy horizontal lines) on the electrocardiograph paper.

When a depolarization wave is not blocked and reaches the far side of the AV junction, it enters specialized, rapidly-conducting fibers in the bundle of His and the right and left bundle branches. These serve almost as electric wires to bring the depolarization impulse to many parts of the ventricle at more or less the same time. The result is the nearly simultaneous contraction of many ventricular muscle cells, producing the high intravascular pressures characteristic of ventricular contraction. The electrical expression of ventricular depolarization is called the QRS complex (see Fig. 20-2). It normally lasts 0.07 to 0.10 second.

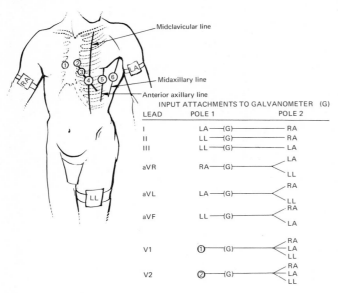

FIG. 20-3. Schematic illustration of the electrode locations and wiring arrangements for attaching a patient to an electrocardiograph machine when recording a conventional twelve lead electrocardiogram.

Any electrocardiograph has two basic input terminals (poles) so that the machine can compare the voltage prevailing at one location on the body surface with that prevailing at a second point. The last nine leads of the conventional twelve are composite leads in which the voltage prevailing at one location is compared to the average prevailing two or three other locations; hence, the right hand column of the schematic diagram shows more than one limb connection to the second input terminal for the lowest nine leads.

Electrocardiograph machines are conventionally wired such that an upward deflection is recorded whenever pole one is positive with respect to pole two. Pole one is sometimes referred to as the "exploring electrode."

The first and second precordial (V) leads are located to the right and left of the sternum in the fourth intercostal space. V4 is located on a line drawn vertically down from the middle of the clavicle, at the level of the fifth intercostal space. V3 is located half-way between V2 and V4, regardless of the rib interspace over which it might or might not lie. Similarly, leads V5 and V6 are located without regard to rib position on a line perpendicular to the long axis of the body, where that line intersects the anterior axillary line and the mid-axillary line, respectively.

The electrical manifestation of cardiac repolarization at the body surface is normally absent or negligible in amplitude except in the case of the ventricles. The latter have a sufficiently large mass of cells to cause significant currents to flow, even though the time course of ventricular repolarization is spread out over about 0.3 to 0.4 second. This repolarization wave is called the T wave. The duration of the T wave is usually measured quantitatively in conjunction with the QRS complex, the overall measurement being called the QT interval.

Leads

As indicated previously, an electrocardiographic tracing records the voltage difference prevailing between 2 points on the body surface. In practice, 12 different pairs of points are used in clinical electrocardiography, with each pair called a *lead*. Actually, only the 3 "standard" limb leads (using the right and left arms and the left leg) are such straightforward, 2-site ("bipolar") leads; the other 9 leads are called unipolar, in that the potential prevailing at one point is compared to the average prevailing between 2 (in leads aVR, aVL, and aVF, the so-called unipolar limb leads) or 3 other sites (in leads V1 through V6, the precordial leads) (see Fig. 20-3).

For arrhythmia monitoring purposes in the CCU, a single special lead is usually used; the full set of twelve leads is recorded less often—usually at daily intervals but sometimes more frequently, especially in the early postinfarction period. The special monitoring leads are chosen to permit greater comfort or freedom of

TABLE 20-2. QRS Nomenclature

Certain QRS nomenclature conventions exist which must be memorized if the CCU nurse is to be able to read the literature and communicate. They are as follows:

1. A downward deflection that initiates a QRS complex is called a Q wave.
2. An upward deflection (it must rise above the baseline) is always an R wave, whether or not it is preceded by a Q wave.
3. A downward deflection (provided it drops below the baseline—otherwise it is merely a notch) that follows an R wave is an S wave.
4. A second R wave after an S wave is an R' (called "R prime"), the third an R", etc.; a second S wave is an S', etc.
5. A completely downward QRS complex (no R waves at all) is called a QS complex.
6. When a QRS complex is being described in writing, capital letters are used for relatively big deflections and small letters for relatively small deflections. Thus, one might have a qRs, or a QRs, or a Qr, or a qRsr', etc. A QS deflection is always capitalized, regardless of its overall size.

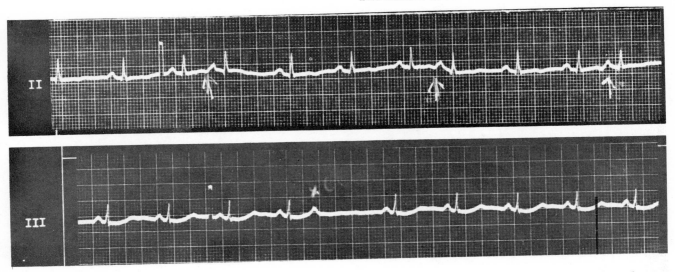

Fig. 20-4. The top strip shows atrial premature beats (marked by arrows) which were conducted to the ventricles, producing an associated QRS complex which is normal in configuration. The lower strip shows an atrial premature beat which occurred so early that it is superimposed on the T wave of the fourth beat. In consequence, the fourth T wave is unusually tall.

motion in bed for the patient, to reduce artifacts in the tracing attributable to muscle tremor, to maximize QRS voltage so that electronic monitoring equipment will not falsely record "cardiac arrest," and to keep the precordial area uncluttered in case cardioversion should suddenly become necessary. Too many different monitoring lead schemes are in use to enumerate them all here. Suffice it to say that for accuracy and helpfulness in the diagnosis of difficult arrhythmias, leads II and V1 are usually most rewarding. However, these are not usually used for long-term monitoring because they do not satisfy all of the essentials enumerated earlier in this paragraph; they should be recorded on a short-term basis (along with the other 10 conventional leads) whenever a difficult arrhythmia is encountered.

The gain (sensitivity) of the ECG amplifying circuit is conventionally adjusted so that when a 0.001 volt (one millivolt) signal is introduced in series with the lead by a calibration circuit, the galvanometer is deflected 1.0 centimeter, producing a distinctive square wave deflection like that in Fig. 20-2.

Arrhythmia Considerations

A strip of normal sinus rhythm, interrupted by a premature beat originating in the atrium as the third, seventh, and tenth P waves, is shown in Figure 20-4. The normal-looking QRS complex is typical of atrial premature beats, as is the atypical P wave. The P

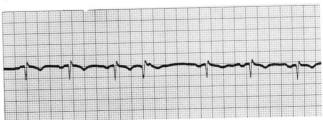

Fig. 20-6. The strip shows a nodal (junctional) premature beat. The impulse originated in the AV junction and was conducted downward into the ventricles, producing a normal QRS; the impulse also was conducted upward into the atria, producing an abnormal (in this case upright) P wave. The normal P waves in this example are inverted because the electrocardiographic lead in question is aVR. Not all nodal premature beats are conducted successfully back into the atria; in consequence, associated abnormal P waves need not always be seen.

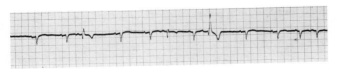

Fig. 20-5. The third, sixth, and eighth QRS complexes are aberrant conducted ventricular responses to atrial premature beats. Note that each of the three aberrant conducted QRS complexes are preceded by a premature P wave, or by a T wave which is deformed by a premature P wave. None of the three abnormal QRS complexes resembles the other two because the aberrant ventricular conduction has expressed itself to different degrees in each beat.

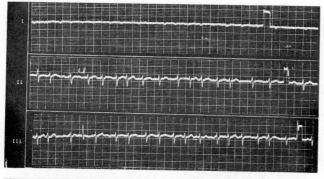

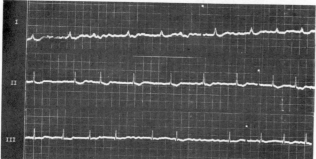

Fig. 20-7. *(Top)* Atrial fibrillation with rapid ventricular response. The fourth QRS complex in lead 3 is aberrantly conducted. The average ventricular rate is about 150. *(Bottom)* Atrial fibrillation after the administration of digitalis. The ventricular rate has now slowed to about 65. The characteristically rapid, irregular ("snake-track") base line representing chaotic atrial activity may now be seen clearly between each QRS-T complex.

wave is abnormal because the atria were depolarized from an abnormal initial site; the QRS is normal because the premature impulse entered the ventricles at the normal location (the distal end of the AV junction).

Infrequently, the QRS complex of true atrial premature beat is broad and slurred (like that of a ventricular premature beat) if it occurs so soon after the preceding beat that some but not all of the ventricular muscle has repolarized and is ready to conduct an impulse again. When this phenomenon is seen, the most common part of the ventricle to have experienced delayed recovery is the right bundle branch. Whatever the last part to recover, the phenomenon is called aberrant ventricular conduction; as suggested above, however, it is usually due to right bundle branch block (see Fig. 20-5). The phenomenon is of great importance diagnostically, because ventricular premature beats (VPBs) have a more serious significance than do atrial premature beats in the presence of an acute myocardial infarction. Ventricular premature beats

may be seen in Fig. 20-9.

Premature beats originating in the AV node resemble atrial premature beats except that the P-R interval is less than 0.12 second in duration, or may even be negative, with the P wave occurring after the QRS complex. The latter case indicates some difficulty of retrograde conduction into the atria from the node compared to the time required for forward conduction into the ventricles. About half the time, retrograde conduction fails altogether, producing a normal QRS complex (unless there is aberrant ventricular conduction) with no P wave at all (see Fig. 20-6).

Sequences of premature beats without intervening normal beats produce paroxysmal or sustained tachycardias: atrial, nodal, or ventricular. Still faster beating produces atrial or ventricular flutter. The faster the ventricular rate, the more serious the hemodynamic consequences for the patient, and the more likely is the occurrence of the ultimate in disorganized beating— fibrillation. When a heart chamber fibrillates, it ceases to propel blood. Atrial fibrillation produces a rapid, irregular ventricular rate. This is tolerable if the ventricular rate is sufficiently slowed by reducing the number of impulses transmitted through the AV node, which can be accomplished by administering digitalis (see Fig. 20-7). However, when the ventricles fibrillate, the patient dies almost immediately unless prompt action is taken to restore the circulation.

CLINICAL PHARMACOLOGY OF ANTI-ARRHYTHMIC DRUGS

A. *Autonomic Drugs*

The autonomic nervous system plays the most important role in setting the rate of the normal heart at the usual adult resting normal sinus rhythm rate of about 70 to 80 beats per minute. If all nerve connections to the adult heart are severed, the rate rises to 120 or 125 beats per minute. This new, higher value reflects the fact that the parasympathetic division of the autonomic nervous system exercises preponderant control over the normal resting heart, keeping it slower than its "natural" rate by means of tonic impulses transmitted over the vagus nerve to the SA node. With exercise, excitement, or other stimuli to the sympathetic division, vagal tone decreases in favor of sympathetic tone preponderance, and the heart rate may rise well above even the "natural" rate. The acceleration is achieved by the release of catecholamines, levarterenol (norepinephrine) and epinephrine, from storage sites in the nerve endings in the heart. Vagal slowing, on the other hand, results from the release of acetylcholine.

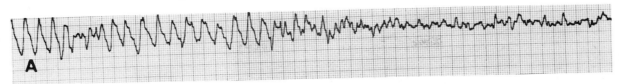

Fig. 20-8A. Ventricular fibrillation. Notice how rapidly the originally coarse deflections become smaller and finer (higher in frequency). The first four deflections could be called ventricular flutter (see Fig. 20-8D).

The autonomic heart rate control system can be manipulated, if necessary, by giving appropriate drugs, as in the following examples:

(1) To slow the heart, one might give:

    (a) Reserpine, to deplete the heart of catecholamines;

    (b) An acetylcholine-like drug, such as methacholine;

    (c) Digitalis, for its well-known vagotonic and direct depressant effects on the SA node;

    (d) Neostigmine, which inhibits the blood enzyme (choline esterase) that destroys acetylcholine;

    (e) Sympathetic blocking agents like propranolol or bretylium tosylate.

In clinical practice, vagomimetic agents are seldom either used or necessary to control a rapid sinus rhythm (sinus tachycardia), but are helpful at other times; digitalis and neostigmine, for example, may be used to promote reversion to normal sinus rhythm of a paroxysmal atrial tachycardia (a rapid, sustained ectopic rhythm originating in one of the atria).

(2) To accelerate the heart, or to stimulate a flagging pacemaker, one might give:

    (a) Epinephrine itself;

    (b) An epinephrine analog like isoproterenol;

    (c) A vagolytic agent like atropine.

B. Digitalis

This drug has direct and vagotonic depressant effects on the AV node, too. These properties are quite useful for producing partial AV block, to reduce the unduly large number of depolarizing impulses that would otherwise reach and excessively accelerate the ventricle in instances of very rapid atrial fibrillation. Moreover, digitalis is often useful for reducing mild degrees of atrial irritability (as in atrial premature beats or paroxysmal atrial tachycardia); in higher degrees of atrial irritability (flutter and fibrillation); the existing irritability may be enhanced, but such a result is by no means uniform.

It used to be taught that acute myocardial infarction was a contraindication to digitalis administration. However, it is now known that the drug may clearly be life-saving for many of the complications of myocardial infarction, both for arrhythmia control and to increase the force of beating, but the agent must be used more carefully and more skillfully than in the non-infarct patient. Overdosage can produce a wide variety of cardiac arrhythmias.

C. Quinidine and Related Drugs

These agents all tend to depress myocardial irritability and conductivity. The one now used most commonly in CCU's proper is lidocaine. It has less of a depressant effect on blood pressure than its relatives (quinidine, procainamide), but can only be given intravenously because it is inactivated when taken by mouth. When given to excess, these agents may cause complete heart block, cardiac standstill, or even marked ventricular irritability (ventricular tachycardia or ventricular fibrillation). When the patient is again up and about, an orally active agent such as quinidine may be used if irritability persists.

A variety of less potent anti-arrhythmic agents may be somewhat loosely considered in this general category: diphenylhydantoin, antihistaminics and, to a certain degree, most sedatives, analgesics, local anesthetics, and hypnotics. All of them tend to stabilize cell membranes, making it harder for them to depolarize. The sedatives and hypnotics, etc., naturally display this property more strongly on nerve than heart cell membranes.

ARRHYTHMIAS OF MAJOR IMPORTANCE IN THE CCU

There are 6 life-threatening arrhythmias that call for immediate action on the part of the cardiac care unit nurse. These arrhythmias and the principal therapeutic steps that they make necessary as soon as they are diagnosed are outlined on p. 421. An example of each arrhythmia may be seen in Figure 20-8A-F.

The need for immediate action is obvious in the case of ventricular fibrillation and cardiac standstill, since the cardiac output drops to zero and the blood pressure nearly to zero in the presence of either arrhythmia.

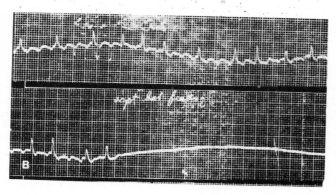

FIG. 20-8B. Cardiac standstill. The upper strip shows atrial flutter, as manifested by the sawtooth-like appearance of the base line which is characteristic of the atrial electrical activity in atrial flutter. The atrial rate is about 300 beats per minute; because of the very rapid atrial rate, the ventricles are able to respond only irregularly to every second or third beat. In the bottom strip, both atrial and ventricular activity cease suddenly, producing total cardiac standstill of all heart chambers.

Ventricular tachycardia requires urgent management because the sequence of ventricular muscular contraction is abnormal by definition—the pacemaker is located in an abnormal site in the ventricular wall. The electrical impulse that triggers contraction therefore spreads over the ventricles in an abnormal fashion. The cardiac output is almost always depressed, both because of the abnormal contraction sequence and because of the rapid heart rates that are usually seen. If the output falls far enough, the result is a drop in systemic arterial blood pressure and a consequent reduction in coronary artery perfusion. The latter is usually disastrous in the presence of the already impaired coronary blood flow—the hallmark of acute myocardial infarction. In fact, ventricular tachycardia may start a vicious circle in which the initial drop in coronary perfusion causes further impairment of myocardial contractility—the latter resulting in a still lower systemic blood pressure, further impairment of coronary perfusion and so forth until death rapidly follows.

Sinus bradycardia is dangerous because the more marked degrees of heart rate slowing are associated

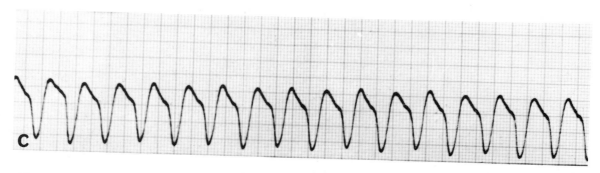

FIG. 20-8C. Ventricular tachycardia. Observe the very broad and rapid QRS complexes at a rate of about 145 beats per minute. Atrial activity (P waves) cannot be clearly seen.

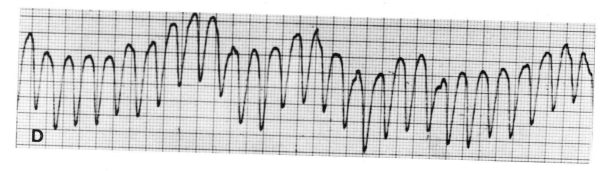

FIG. 20-8D. Ventricular flutter. Ventricle flutter resembles ventricular tachycardia except that it is extremely rapid. In this instance, the heart rate is over 240 beats per minute. Atrial activity at a different (dissociated) rate can nonetheless be made out: A particularly clear P wave can be seen to follow just after the tenth QRS deflection and again following the thirteenth, fourteenth, sixteenth and twentieth QRS deflections.

with a drop in cardiac output, with results that are similar to those just listed for ventricular tachycardia; furthermore, sinus bradycardia may be the forerunner of cardiac standstill.

Like the more severe degrees of sinus bradycardia, complete AV heart block due to acute myocardial infarction is associated with a reduced cardiac output because of the invariably slow ventricular rate. Moreover, the so-called idioventricular pacemaker that keeps the ventricles beating (the normal pacemaker impulse from the sino-atrial node is no longer available due to the AV block) is notoriously less reliable and stable than the normal sinus pacemaker, and is often associated with an abnormal heart muscle contraction sequence as well. As a result, cardiac standstill often follows the development of complete AV heart block unless pacemaker electrodes are inserted to maintain normal rates of beating.

There are several other arrhythmias that are not in themselves deleterious to cardiac function but which

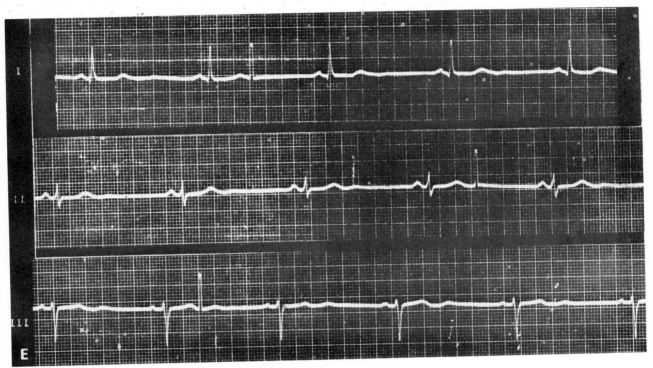

FIG. 20-8E. Sinus bradycardia. Observe the very slow atrial and ventricular rate, with a P wave preceding each QRS complex. The ventricular rate is slightly irregular (sinus **arrhythmia**), which is characteristic of sinus bradycardia.

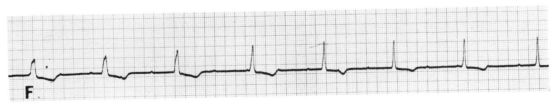

FIG. 20-8F. Complete atrioventricular (A-V) heart block. Observe that the atrial rate (about 97 beats per minute) is more than twice as fast as the ventricular rate (about 42 beats per minute). Consequently, there is no fixed relationship between P waves and QRS complexes. Note that the shape of the QRS complex changes gradually from morphology prevailing during the first two ventricular beats to that prevailing during the last four QRS complexes. This reflects a change in the pacemaker location. The ventricles were being driven by a focus in the ventricular wall during the first two beats but was under the control of the A-V node during the last four beats, with sharing of the ventricle between both foci during the third and fourth beats which consequently are fusion beats (see Figure 20-9).

nonetheless indicate the need for prompt preventive treatment (see Fig. 20-9). These are the various types of ventricular premature beats that indicate a high degree of ventricular irritability: ventricular premature beats with a very short coupling interval (the QRS complex of the ventricular premature beat falls on the T wave of the preceding beat); multiform ventricular premature beats (the abnormal QRS complexes show more than one shape, suggesting that multiple foci of irritability are present); and runs of more than one ventricular premature beat in sequence. The last is obviously a significant harbinger of future difficulty, since ventricular tachycardia is merely a sustained run of ventricular premature beats (a common definition being that 5 or more ventricular premature beats in sequence constitute ventricular tachycardia). In any event, each of these different types of increased ventricular irritability may be followed at any time by either ventricular tachycardia or ventricular fibrillation.

Indeed, it is the rule in most CCU's that the mere occurrence of 5 or more ventricular premature beats per minute calls for the administration of an anti-arrhythmic drug. However, it must be kept in mind that ventricular irritability at times may be the result of excessive prior administration of an anti-arrhythmic drug!

NURSING MANAGEMENT OF THE PATIENT WITH ACUTE MYOCARDIAL INFARCTION*

When a patient is brought to the CCU, the nursing admission procedure must be carried out with deliberate haste so that basic information will be available as soon as possible for use in the event of a sudden emergency. Sudden emergencies are extremely common in acute myocardial infarction. Furthermore, the

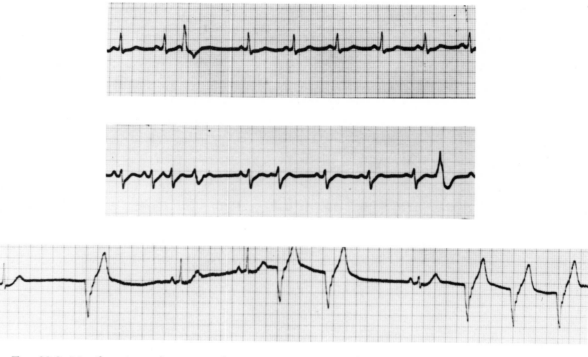

Fig. 20-9. Manifestations of serious and potentially dangerous ventricular irritability. The third beat of the top strip shows the R wave of a ventricular premature beat occurring so early that it coincides with the latter portion of the T wave of the preceding normal beat. The middle strip shows multiform ventricular premature beats; observe that the fourth and tenth beats are both unusually broad and deformed, but that the QRS complex assumes different shapes in each of these two beats. The bottom strip shows runs of ventricular premature beats, increasing in frequency. The seventh beat is intermediate in configuration between the normal beats (beats number 1, 3, and 4) and the abnormally broad and deformed beats originating in the ventricles. This intermediate beat is probably a fusion beat in which the ventricles were partially activated through the normal pathway and partially by the abnormal focus in the ventricles.

* See also pp. 373-377.

earlier in the course the patient is seen, the more likely is an emergency to be encountered. Many patients die within a few seconds or minutes after coronary artery occlusion, and a number of others develop ventricular fibrillation within minutes of admission to the CCU, sometimes even when they originally seem to be in no significant distress.

Guidelines for admission and nursing management of a patient with an acute myocardial infarction appear on pages 421-423. It is obvious from inspecting the table that much physiological data on the patient must be gathered, many nursing activities carried out, and various solutions and drugs administered. It is of critical importance that all of this information be recorded in a neat, systematic fashion that provides easy subsequent summary and access. The more sick the patient, the more urgent the need to see the patient's minute to minute progress in order to evaluate the effectiveness of the medical and nursing interventions in use; moreover, the sicker the patient, the greater will be the rate and volume of data collection. Consequently, it is important that all of the information on each patient be recorded on specially designed forms. An admission form should be filled out first. A general form would then be started on uncomplicated patients, with special additional forms being used to record the course of patients in shock and/or congestive heart failure.

The admission form should have designated entry spaces for such things as: name, date, time, responsible physician, admission diagnosis, age; name, address, and telephone number of the next of kin; known diseases, medications to the time of entry, drug sensitivities, diet, general appearance, vital signs, emotional state and state of consciousness, severity and frequency of pain, initial electrocardiographic findings, initial nursing actions, and comments. On forms used subsequently, 4 columns should be set up for filling out in parallel, with headings as follows:

(1) Date and time
(2) Physiologic data reflecting the patient's condition and progress
(3) Medication given, and other nursing measures
(4) Comments

All of this tabulated information not only greatly facilitates proper management of the patient; it is also very helpful when periodic reports are to be made of overall experience in the unit. Such reports have some interest for administrative purposes, but are absolutely essential for evaluating the effectiveness of therapeutic measures being used and for detecting the need for improvement in certain areas or analyzing the reason for unusual successes.

NURSING MANAGEMENT OF COMPLICATIONS OTHER THAN CARDIAC ARRHYTHMIAS

As indicated previously, coronary care units at present are most effective in reducing the mortality of acute myocardial infarction by preventing the development of otherwise lethal cardiac arrhythmias, and effective to a lesser degree by successfully resuscitating patients who have developed such arrhythmias. The other principal cause of death is heart failure, broadly defined. After an infarct cuts off the blood supply to a significant percentage of the ventricular muscle mass, the resulting impaired contractility may cause an acute drop in blood pressure (cardiogenic shock), and/or may set in motion a series of endocrine defenses against loss of blood pressure or blood volume that result in excessive retention of salt and water by the kidney. The consequences of this accumulation depend upon its location: if it occurs in the lungs, the result is pulmonary edema; occurrence in the abdomen results in the swelling of ascites, and in the extremities, the familiar leg edema of congestive heart failure. (The nursing management of congestive heart failure is summarized on pp. 423-424.) See also pp. 384-390.

The prompt management of pulmonary edema and the lesser degrees of congestive heart failure exerts a favorable influence on mortality, but two thirds of all patients with sustained drops in systemic blood pressure and the concomitant shock syndrome continue to die despite intensive treatment.

There are a few recent but as yet incompletely verified claims of much better results in the treatment of cardiogenic shock in CCU's that are organized to provide extensive physiologic monitoring over and above the universally monitored electrocardiogram and occasionally monitored central venous pressure. The new measurements may include serial determinations of cardiac output; blood pH, blood oxygen, carbon dioxide and lactic acid content, and continuously monitored arterial blood pressure. These measurements are generally made by medical technicians assigned to the CCU around the clock; in a few units, however, they are made by members of the nursing staff assigned in rotation to this function. The educational impact of the latter practice is profoundly rewarding to the nurse, since it gives her direct and immediate data for physiologically evaluating the effect of nursing measures. The patients concerned are in such critical and rapidly-changing states that this sort of evaluation and nursing awareness is of course immensely beneficial to them as well. It does require the employment of more nurses (or technicians) in CCU's, and the acquisition of expensive equipment, but nonetheless the trend to physiologic monitoring is spreading.

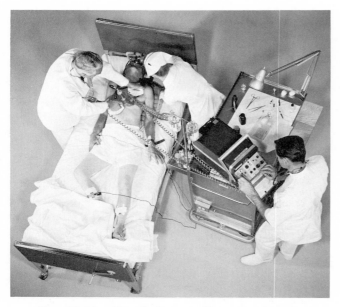

Fig. 20-10. Closed-chest cardiac resuscitation is attempted by a skilled team. The nurse is often the one who detects initial changes in the patient and immediately alerts the team. (Travenol Laboratories)

Cardiogenic shock occurs in about 12 per cent of hospitalized patients. It is initiated by failure of the injured heart to function adequately as a pump because of impaired contractility. Thus both shock as well as acute congestive heart failure with pulmonary edema are often considered together under the heading of "pump failure" or "power failure." The nursing management of shock is summarized on pp. 424-425.

If one excludes deaths due to such complications as rupture of the infarcted ventricular wall and pulmonary embolism (about 10% and 7% of the total hospitalized patient mortality, respectively), almost all of the myocardial infarction deaths in a properly-run CCU occur in patients with pump failure. The CCU techniques of continuous preventive surveillance and preventive drug management, as well as the immediate availability of cardioversion, pacemaking, and closed-chest resuscitation now make deaths from primary cardiac arrhythmias a relative rarity. Patients still die from refractory arrhythmias, but these deaths usually occur only in patients who also have power failure.

SPECIAL CCU NURSING TECHNIQUES

The above observations make it clear that the cardiac care unit nurse must receive special training in many areas. She must be able to make rather sophisticated electrocardiographic arrhythmia diagnoses. She must also be carefully trained in the relevant clinical pharmacology of anti-arrhythmic and circulation-supporting drugs. At times she must start treatment with certain

drugs, on her own initiative, and at other times must be able to adjust properly the rate of administration of a drug that has already been started. As an example of the former type of drug administration one may cite the immediate need for the administration of sodium bicarbonate solution intravenously as a part of the resuscitation process in cardiac arrest (ventricular fibrillation or cardiac standstill). A common example of the second type of drug administration by the CCU nurse is the need for continuous adjustment in the rate of intravenous administration of lidocaine to the patient with marked ventricular irritability. By adjusting the rate of administration, a nurse is in effect controlling the total amount of drug given.

The emergency procedures that the CCU nurse must be able to carry out when the heart suddenly stops beating are the most dramatic parts of her repertoire of expertise. She is the first line of defense when these emergencies occur when the medical staff is not available. To be effective, she must be well-trained, confident, and duly authorized to act in the absence of a physician. The details of these procedures are discussed below.

Resuscitation

In the absence of a physician, the cardiac care unit nurse must be prepared to carry out all of the steps required for closed-chest cardiac resuscitation. These steps are outlined on p. 425. In practice, at least 2 trained individuals are required to carry out the resuscitation measures listed. This is the basis for the oft-stated requirement that there be at least 2 trained individuals on each nursing tour of duty in a CCU.

The first column on p. 425 gives those steps that are directly related to the resuscitation procedure *per se* regardless of the setting—either inside or outside of a CCU. The second column lists steps that the nurse would also take in the actual CCU setting or indicates the implications of differences in procedure. Still other variations may be advisable, depending on the actual administrative organization and facilities available in the individual CCU. The reasons behind the various steps are largely self-evident, and the underlying principles would apply in almost any CCU.

Cardioversion

When ventricular fibrillation occurs in the CCU and a physician is not present, the CCU nurse must be prepared to administer an electric shock of several thousand volts to the patient's chest wall to bring about defibrillation. This procedure (cardioversion) should ideally be carried out within seconds of the onset of ventricular fibrillation to minimize cerebral and circulatory deterioration. However, the patient who cannot be immediately defibrillated may sometimes be tided over the danger period by closed-chest cardiac massage until defibrillation can be performed. Indeed, this constitutes the main indication for cardiac massage outside the CCU. Since electrical defibrillation equipment must always be readily available in a CCU, closed-chest resuscitation is not as often needed in the CCU as elsewhere in the hospital when a sudden or unexpected death occurs.

The CCU nurse must realize that the amount of blood flow that can be sustained by closed-chest cardiac massage is always subnormal, inevitably resulting in some circulatory deterioration. Consequently, if ventricular fibrillation is present, cardioversion should be carried out as quickly as possible. The necessary steps are outlined on p. 426.

Although the administered shock usually has an amplitude of several thousand volts, the intensity is never thus calibrated in voltage units. The cardioversion shock is actually measured in *joules* (sometimes called watt-seconds, although this term is now being eliminated in keeping with a nomenclature convention reached by international engineering agreement). Four hundred joules is the highest setting available on most commercial cardioversion equipment, and this is the setting that should be used for ventricular defibrillation. Time is not available for a "titration" procedure with repeated tries at gradually increasing voltage settings until reversion occurs, because of the rapidity with which the unperfused brain (and infarcted heart) deteriorates. In the absence of a physician, the trained CCU nurse will also find it necessary at times to revert a sustained ventricular tachycardia by means of cardioversion, because when this arrhythmia occurs in an acute myocardial infarction patient, it often deteriorates into ventricular fibrillation due to its adverse effects on the circulation, as mentioned previously. Lower joule settings may be tried at first, starting with 150 to 200 joules, for reversion of ventricular tachycardia.

Cardiac Pacemaking in the CCU

Electrical shocks of much lower intensity than those required to defibrillate the heart will cause cardiac contraction in many hearts that have recently gone into ventricular standstill. Each shock is followed by a cardiac beat; if the normal cardiac pacemaker does not start to function again, the heart rate can be adjusted to any desired figure merely by adjusting the rate of the artificial electrical pacemaker.

The electrodes for artificially pacing the heart were originally applied to the surface of the chest wall, but this is no longer done except under special emergency circumstances because it is quite painful to the patient.

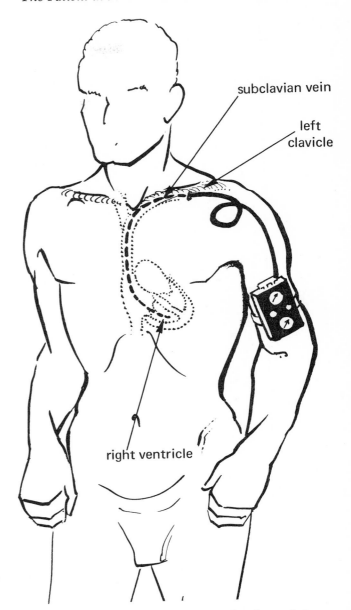

FIG. 20-11. In this illustration, a bipolar catheter electrode has been inserted transvenously to the apex of the right ventricle. The vascular system was entered by means of a needle puncture of the right subclavian vein. The pacemaker power-pack and control unit has been attached to the patient's right arm, leaving plenty of slack so that motion of the arm will not dislodge the catheter. The nurse caring for a patient with a temporary transvenous pacemaker should make certain that no metal parts of the output terminal or pacemaker's wires are exposed. All such bare metal should be scrupulously covered with non-conductive tape in order to prevent accidental ventricular fibrillation from stray currents which might reach the heart if exposed metal parts were to come in contact with a metal conductor such as a bed rail.

TABLE 20-3. Principal elements of CCU equipment

A. Mobile or cart-mounted equipment.
   1. Electrocardiograph.
   2. Capacitor-discharge type cardioversion apparatus, optionally capable of being synchronized to fire only during a QRS complex.
   3. Electronic pacemaker equipment.
   4. Rotating tourniquet equipment (automatic or manual).
   5. Endotracheal intubation equipment.
   6. Intermittent positive pressure breathing (IPPB) equipment (a volume-controlled ventilator should also be available, if possible).
   7. Gas-driven closed-chest automatic cardiac massage equipment, which can move with a patient on a stretcher if necessary.
   8. Crash cart with emergency drugs and intravenous fluids. Several preceding items on this list are often incorporated into the crash cart; also cutdown trays, sterile drapes and gloves, antiseptic solutions, etc.
   9. A mobile image-intensifier fluoroscope is of great aid for passing transvenous catheter electrodes, etc., at the bedside at odd hours.

B. Equipment at the central nursing station.
   1. Oscilloscopic display of the patient's ECG; other monitored physiologic signals may also be displayed on various gauges. It is very helpful to have a paper-writing electrocardiograph that can optionally record any displayed ECG in more permanent form for detailed analysis. Unless this can be done quickly and remotely at the nursing station, much valuable information will be lost.
   2. Intercommunication master set.
   3. Alarm indicators.
   4. Records storage and processing equipment, bulletin board, telephone, and so forth as in a conventional nursing station.
   5. A library of recent textbooks on cardiology, electrocardiography, coronary artery disease, etc., with reprints of key articles from the periodical literature.

C. Equipment installed at each bedside.
   1. Compressed oxygen (and medically-clean compressed air, if possible).
   2. Suction outlets.
   3. Individual, simple (not synchronized to fire only on a QRS complex) cardioversion apparatus for ventricular defibrillation at each bedside.
   4. Elapsed time clock to record duration of cardiac arrest.
   5. Alarm button or switch.
   6. Ceiling-mounted "sky-hooks" or their equivalent for administering intravenous fluids.
   7. A call switch for the patient's use.
   8. An intercommunication outlet, arranged so that a conversation can be initiated from the nursing station only.
   9. Numerous electrical wall plug-in sockets; some should be in the head-panel (for electric razors, etc.) and others wall-mounted to either side of the bed and arranged so that they are not all blocked by ordinary, non-emergency bedside equipment (bedside stands, etc.).
   10. A small monitor-display oscilloscope; heart rate or blood pressure channels and other devices may be included or displayed on other gauges.

There are other disadvantages as well, the most important for CCU purposes being that external pacing (that is, with the electrodes on the skin surface of the chest wall) is rarely successful in cardiac standstill due to acute myocardial infarction.

The preferred method for temporary electrical pacing of the heart is the transvenous introduction of an electrode catheter into the right ventricle by way of a superficial vein. Two electrodes are necessary to complete the electrical circuit. The second electrode may be attached to the skin surface, but better results are obtained if a bipolar electrode catheter is used—that is, a catheter that puts both electrodes within the right ventricle. Some monopolar catheters are flexible enough to be "floated" into the right heart by the bloodstream when they are introduced while the heart is still beating normally. However, the rate of successful initial placement is only 60 to 70 per cent, and these very flexible catheters often subsequently wash out into the pulmonary artery, with consequent cessation of pacing. Better results are obtained when a somewhat stiffer, bipolar transvenous catheter electrode is placed into the right ventricle under fluoroscopic control. This can be done quickly even under emergency circumstances, without the need for transporting a seriously ill patient, if a fluoroscope unit is an integral part of the CCU. The general arrangement may be seen in Figure 20-11.

The CCU nurse is not expected to pass pacemaker electrode catheters, but she must be familiar with the indications and complications of the procedure and with the operating instructions for the pacemaker equipment being used. She will often find it necessary to change the amplitude of the stimulation impulse, and she will sometimes be called upon to adjust the rate of stimulation. To help prevent infection, careful nursing attention must also be directed daily to the site where the transvenous catheter electrode penetrates the patient's skin.

In addition to cardiac standstill, complete AV heart block following acute myocardial infarction is another indication for transvenous electrical pacing of the heart. The heart block that results from an acute infarction is usually not permanent, so that the transvenous electrodes can usually be removed in a few days or week. When the heart block is permanent, a second electrode is introduced and attached beneath the skin to a surgically-implanted miniaturized power supply. The procedures and equipment are identical to those used in the case of patients with Stokes-Adams syncopal attacks due to AV block not associated with acute myocardial infarction.

GUIDELINES FOR NURSING IN THE CARDIAC CARE UNIT

A. Techniques for Controlling Lethal Cardiac Arrhythmias

1. *Closed chest cardiac massage:* The lower portion of the sternum of the pulseless supine patient is rhythmically pressed downward against the vertebral column, squeezing the intervening heart and causing blood circulation to a limited degree.

2. *Cardioversion:* A brief but intense electric shock is applied to the chest wall to coordinate the disorganized electrical activity of a heart in ventricular fibrillation.

3. *Cardiac pacemaking:* Brief but relatively weak electric shocks are applied periodically to induce beating in the presence of cardiac standstill or to accelerate a heart in which the spontaneous rate of beating is too slow to meet circulatory needs.

B. Six Arrhythmias Requiring Immediate Treatment

Arrhythmia	*Principal Management Procedures*
1. Ventricular fibrillation	Cardioversion. Closed-chest cardiac massage may also be required if cardioversion is delayed, is not immediately effective, or if an anti-arrhythmic drug like lidocaine has to be given first before cardioversion is successful.
2. Cardiac standstill (ventricular arrest)	Pacemaking by means of transvenous intracardiac electrodes, preceded by isoproterenol infusion if the electrode catheter has not previously been placed in anticipation of standstill. Closed-chest cardiac massage is sometimes required initially.
3. Ventricular tachycardia	Cardioversion if the tachycardia is not rapidly controlled by intravenous administration of an anti-arrhythmic drug such as lidocaine.
4. Ventricular flutter (Very rapid ventricular tachycardia, often progressing directly to ventricular fibrillation)	Cardioversion
5. Sinus bradycardia (unduly slow heart rate with normal cardiac electrical impulse formation and conduction)	Pacemaking by means of transvenous intracardiac electrodes if satisfactory heart rates cannot be maintained by tolerable doses of atropine.
6. Complete atrioventricular heart block	Pacemaking by means of transvenous intracardiac electrodes.

C. Immediate Nursing Management of the Uncomplicated Acute Myocardial Infarction Patient[*]

Nursing Measures	*Rationale and Implications*
Admission procedures	
1. Measure and record vital signs, including both radial and apical pulse rates.	Tachycardia may signify congestive heart failure, shock, or cardiac arrhythmia. Bradycardia, an irregular rate, or a discrepancy between the apical and radial pulse rates, also indicates arrhythmia. Tachypnea may indicate congestive failure or pulmonary embolism. Marked arterial hypotension is the prime indicator of shock. Low arterial blood pressure is especially dangerous in acute myocardial infarction because it lowers perfusion pressure in an already compromised coronary artery circulation.

[*] The order of procedure will vary somewhat according to the patient's condition.

GUIDELINES FOR NURSING IN THE CARDIAC CARE UNIT (*Continued*)

2. Relieve suffering. Supply analgesic medication within prescribed limits.

Pain associated with myocardial infarction is apt to be agonizing and difficult to relieve. The pain is often attended by fear of impending death, emotional agitation, and physical restlessness, which tend to elevate arterial blood pressure and increase cardiac work. However, overadministration of narcotics and sedatives may contribute to the development of shock.

3. Provide rest. Strict, continuous bed rest is required initially. Later the patient may be assigned to an armchair, as the therapeutic regimen selected and the patient's condition permit; hypotension is one contra-indication.

The objective is to reduce the frequency and vigor of cardiac contractions, lowering oxygen requirements of the damaged and ischemic myocardium, thus:
  (a) relieving anginal pain;
  (b) minimizing further ischemic damage;
  (c) minimizing incidence of cardiac failure;
  (d) reducing likelihood of heart rupture.

4. Attach ECG monitoring electrodes.

This provides the constant information needed for optimal arrhythmia prevention and treatment.

5. Start humidified oxygen inhalation.

This brings more oxygen to the hypoxic heart muscle; chest pain may be relieved and serious complications diminished in frequency or extent.

6. Start a slow intravenous infusion of 5 per cent glucose in water.

A means for rapid injection of intravenous medication should be provided for early, against the possibility of later emergency need.

7. Record a full 12-lead ECG.

This is necessary to provide a permanent record for subsequent comparison to assess the clinical course and as a baseline for interpretation of any subsequent complex arrhythmia.

8. Reassure the patient by maintaining a cheerful and encouraging attitude, by explaining the meaning of CCU procedures and equipment, and by displaying quiet competence. The patient's family will profit greatly from similar explanations, which may be made in part by distributing a previously prepared brochure. This approach makes more time available for patient care.

Emotional disturbance increases cardiac work and the likelihood of serious cardiac arrhythmias because of resulting neuroendocrine discharges. As a consequence of the well-publicized dangers of an acute "heart attack," even the initially uncomplicated patient as well as his family are apt to be highly anxious. After receiving appropriate reassurance and explanations, the patient's family will interact in a more supportive and understanding way with both the patient and the CCU staff.

9. If not already done, notify attending physician, CCU director or his representative on call, according to hospital policy.

Self-explanatory.

10. Place patient on the danger list.

Self-explanatory.

11. Apply elastic stockings from toes to groin, when not contraindicated.

Pulmonary emboli from leg veins are a frequent complication of myocardial infarction; application of elastic stockings is designed to minimize the incidence. Anticoagulant drugs are also often prescribed for the same reason, when contra-indications to their use are not present.

12. Instruct the patient in calf- and foot-flexing exercises. These must be repeated hourly during waking hours each day as long as the patient is bedfast.

This measure also improves leg vein circulation by minimizing blood stasis and subsequent clotting, thereby reducing the frequency of pulmonary embolism.

GUIDELINES FOR NURSING IN THE CARDIAC CARE UNIT (*Continued*)

Postadmission nursing activities

1. Record urinary output.

A depressed urine flow is a sensitive indicator of impending shock, and provides a rough guide to the state of water balance and kidney function.

2. Listen to the patient's chest with a stethoscope daily primarily to seek evidence of congestive heart failure, or lung complications.

Nurses in the CCU should become skilled in chest auscultation to help assure early detection of congestive heart failure (and other complications associated with auscultatory lung findings). Auscultation can best be learned at the bedside.

3. Explain dietary restrictions, prohibitions against smoking, and urination/defecation procedures to the patient.

To reduce cardiac work, a low caloric, low sodium diet is usually prescribed, sometimes consisting only of skimmed milk for the first 48 hours. Because of the frequency of post-infarction stress peptic ulcer, antacid medication is sometimes routinely prescribed. The early skimmed milk diet is also recommended for this reason as well. Explanation of dietary restrictions enhances patient cooperation and improves patient morale. The same is true when the no-smoking rule is explained. Smoking not only has short- and long-term noxious effects on the heart, but is contraindicated in areas where oxygen is usually administered because of the fire hazard.

Stool softeners are usually prescribed to minimize the stress of defecation; straining at stool may even induce rupture of the infarcted heart.

4. Instruct and assist the patient in the use of the bedside commode.

The effort associated with use of a bedpan is considerably greater than that expended by the patient who is assisted to a bedside commode *by 2 persons.*

5. Assist patient to bedside chair, if chair is prescribed.

Complete bed rest, except for the use of a commode, is indicated for the first 2 or 3 days for all patients. Thereafter, some patients are allowed to sit in a chair for gradually increasing periods, especially those with congestive heart failure. This position inhibits fluid accumulation in the lungs. The cardiac output and work are also lower in the sitting position than in the supine. Unless a mechanical hoist is used, or the patient is in a special electric bed that can be folded to the seated position, the patient should again be assisted to and from the chair by 2 persons.

D. Nursing Management of the Patient With Congestive Heart Failure with Pulmonary Edema*

Nursing Measures

Rationale and Implications

1. Place patient in semi-Fowler's or seated position.

This improves ventilatory efficiency and reduces fluid accumulation in the lungs.

2. Give morphine unless advanced primary lung disease with carbon dioxide retention is present.

This reduces the increased cardiac work load induced by dyspnea and anxiety; morphine has remarkable additional beneficial effects over and above sedation, for reasons that are not clearly understood. When carbon dioxide retention due to advanced chronic lung disease is present, the respiratory reflex depression caused by morphine is dangerous.

* See also pp. 384 to 392.

GUIDELINES FOR NURSING IN THE CARDIAC CARE UNIT (*Continued*)

3. Give vasopressor agents if low blood pressure is present (systolic pressure below 85 or 90).

A seated position is detrimental to blood pressure maintenance, although the danger can be reduced by the simultaneous use of vasopressors.

4. Administer oxygen by intermittent positive pressure breathing (IPPB).

The increasing resulting intrathoracic pressure reduces fluid extravasation into the lungs and reduces venous return to the overburdened heart (the induction of shock must therefore be guarded against). Antifoaming agents are sometimes added to the humidifying solution to reduce the deleterious effects on intrapulmonary gas exchange caused by bubbling and foaming of extravasated fluid.

5. Apply and continue the use of rotating tourniquets.

Either automatic or manual methods trap blood in extremities, which act as peripheral blood reservoirs; the result resembles a phlebotomy to lower effective blood volume (which is almost invariably elevated in congestive heart failure).

6. Administer a rapidly-acting digitalis preparation.

Ouabain is commonly prescribed for intravenous injection because of the rapidity with which this cardiotonic agent acts.

7. Administer a diuretic agent.

Furosemide or ethacrynic acid are often prescribed because of their potency and rapid action to reduce excessive blood and extracellular fluid volume.

8. Attend the patient constantly.

This helps reduce the cardiac workload attributable to the characteristic anxiety displayed by these critically ill, suffocating patients.

E. Nursing Management of the Patient with Cardiogenic Shock

Nursing Measures

Rationale and Implications

1. Place patient in supine or Trendelenburg position, unless pulmonary edema is present.

The filling pressure of the heart is characteristically lowered in shock, unless acute congestive heart failure is also present. Lowering the head and thorax increases venous return and increases filling pressure.

2. Administer oxygen.

The lowered coronary artery perfusion pressure resulting from the hypotension of shock can be rapidly lethal in the presence of heart damage already inflicted by recent coronary artery occlusion.

3. Monitor pulse and blood pressure frequently.

The patient's condition in cardiogenic shock is very fragile and subject to rapid change, requiring frequent adjustments in management. In particular, an intravenous vasopressor agent (see below) can induce undesirable, marked increases in both pulse and blood pressure when given to excess; careful adjustment of its rate of administration, based on pulse and blood pressure responses, is mandatory.

4. Monitor central pressure.

This is a useful guide to the therapeutic repletion of lowered blood volume, when present.

5. Administer cardiotonic, vasopressor and acidosis-combatting agents, as prescribed.

The weakened heart may respond favorably to digitalis administration, or to vasopressors to improve coronary artery perfusion pressure. An increase in blood pressure is also often needed to prevent deterioration of other vital organs. Vaso-

GUIDELINES FOR NURSING IN THE CARDIAC CARE UNIT (*Continued*)

6. Carefully observe and record the volume and dose of intravenously administered fluids and drugs; special attention should also be given to the patency of intravenous lines and to urinary output.

dilator drugs are sometimes helpful for the latter purpose in noncardiogenic shock but are risky in postmyocardial-infarction shock because of the danger of lowering coronary artery perfusion pressure.

Sodium bicarbonate or other antacids are usually given intravenously to combat the lactic acidosis of shock, because acidosis impairs the effectiveness of endogenous or administered vasopressor agents.

Extravasation of a vasopressor-like levarterenol causes tissue necrosis and sloughing. Fluid balance and the response to carefully administered drugs is of vital importance in shock therapy because of the fragile state of the patient. The preservation or resumption of urinary output is a good prognostic sign, indicating that the perfusion of body tissues is reasonably good.

F. Closed-chest Cardiac Massage and Resuscitation

Basic Steps

A. Immediate steps with only one rescuer present:

Additional CCU Measures or Considerations

1. Call for help but don't wait for it; note time.

Press alarm button at patient's bedside and start elapsed time clock.

2. Punch chest over the precordium once or twice; cardiac standstill may sometimes be terminated by a sharp blow, or a patient who has merely fainted may respond to it.

The differential diagnosis between cardiac standstill, ventricular fibrillation, or syncope should be obvious in a patient whose ECG is already being monitored. Ventricular fibrillation should be defibrillated (cardioverted) as soon as diagnosed.

3. Hyperextend the patient's neck and hold jaw forward to open the air passages.

A second person will make ready to apply a self-inflating respiratory bag-and-mask device (such as an Ambu bag).

4. Inflate the patient's lungs 3 or 4 times with mouth-to-mouth or S-tube ventilation; repeat every 20 to 30 seconds.

Endotracheal intubation should be carried out if the resuscitation effort is not immediately successful, when skilled personnel and sufficient help are present to prevent disruption of other resuscitative steps during intubation. Without an endotracheal tube in place, prolonged lung insufflation of the unconscious patient will produce gastric dilatation with air, with subsequent regurgitation and aspiration of gastric contents.

5. Place patient on his back on a firm surface, preferably in a Trendelenburg position if possible, to minimize the danger of aspiration and to increase cerebral blood flow.

When a mechanical external cardiac compression device is used, a firm backing for counter-pressure is an intrinsic part of the apparatus. Two people are necessary to place the patient in the apparatus expeditiously.

6. Intermittently and rapidly depress the lower half of the sternum with the heel of one hand, aligned with the long axis of the patient's sternum. Both hands should be used to provide sufficient power, but only the heel of one hand should touch the patient's chest, to minimize rib fractures and other trauma. The depression stroke should be 4 to 5 cm. (1½ to 2 inches) in length, repeated at a rate of about 70 strokes per minute.

GUIDELINES FOR NURSING IN THE CARDIAC CARE UNIT (*Continued*)

B. Additional steps when 2 or more rescuers are present:

1. One person should take over responsibility for ventilation, and another for chest compression.

2. An intravenous line or cutdown should be instituted, and 2 ampules (88 mEq.) of sodium bicarbonate solution should be given intravenously as soon as practicable; repeat doses of 44 mEq. should be given every 5 minutes until recovery has taken place or the resuscitation effort abandoned.

3. An ECG should be recorded.

4. Defibrillate (cardiovert) the patient immediately if ventricular fibrillation is found.

5. In the presence of ventricular standstill, pacemaking by means of electrodes placed on the surface of the chest may be tried, although it will rarely be effective in the presence of acute myocardial infarction. A physician should plunge a needle electrode directly into the heart instead as soon as possible.

   Drugs such as isoproterenol or epinephrine should be prescribed for intravenous administration in an attempt to restart spontaneous beating and to support it, if successful, until a transvenous pacemaker electrode can be inserted.

The same is true in the CCU; however, the crash cart should first be brought to the bedside if only 2 rescuers are present.

A transvenous pacemaker electrode may already be in place—and should be used in the presence of standstill, with a considerable chance of a successful myocardial response even in the presence of acute infarction.

G. The Cardioversion Procedure for Ventricular Defibrillation

1. Expose the patient's anterior chest.

2. Turn on the electric power and charge the cardioversion circuit to the 400-joule setting (the machine's dial should always be left in this position).

3. If the machine has a synchronization circuit for atrial arryhthmia reversion, make sure that it is not activated; otherwise, the apparatus fruitlessly seeks a non-existent QRS complex before firing the electrical discharge, regardless of how often the manual discharge button is pressed.

4. Apply electrode paste to the paddle electrodes if they are not routinely kept in tubs of paste at all times.

5. Place the paddle electrodes on the chest along the longitudinal axis of the heart—that is, with one paddle centered over the right second intercostal space parasternally, and the other centered over the presumed location of the cardiac apex.

6. Administer the electrical shock by pressing the discharge button.

7. Re-examine the monitored electrocardiogram to see if further shocks are necessary, either immediately or after appropriate drug therapy.

THE SYSTEM OF INTENSIVE CARDIAC CARE

A CCU must be equipped with a number of special devices which, unfortunately, are rather costly, particularly when considered in the aggregate. However, almost all of the items listed in Table 20-3 must be on hand if a CCU is to function effectively at anything near its potential for saving lives. The need for most of the items is either implicit or explicit in the preceding discussion.

For details concerning administration of a CCU, staffing requirements, and physical facilities needed, see the Bibliography at the end of this chapter.

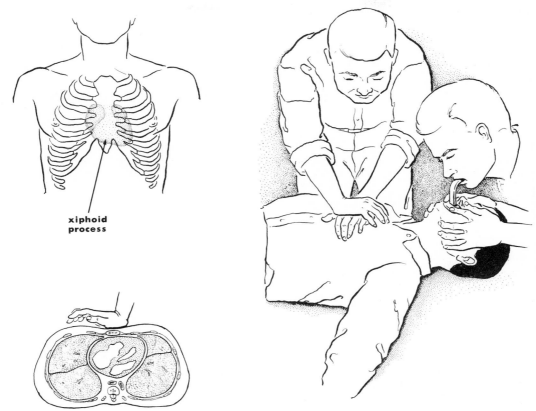

xiphoid process

Fig. 20-12. Closed-chest cardiac massage.

BIBLIOGRAPHY

Books

Dreifus, L. S. (ed.): Mechanisms and Therapy of Cardiac Arrhythmias. New York, Grune and Stratton, 1966.

Hurst, J. W.: Introduction to Electrocardiography. New York, McGraw-Hill, 1968.

Meltzer, L. W., *et al.*: Intensive Coronary Care: A Manual for Nurses. CCU Fund, Philadelphia Presbyterian Hospital, 1965.

Nite, G., and Willias, F. N.: The Coronary Patient: Hospital Care and Rehabilitation. New York, Macmillan, 1964.

Whipple, G. H., *et al.*: Acute Coronary Care. Boston, Little, Brown, 1970.

Articles

Andreoli, K. G.: The cardiac monitor, Amer. J. Nurs., 69:1238-1243, June, 1969.

Cahill, D.: The nurse's role in closed chest cardiac resuscitation. Amer. J. Nurs., 65:84-88, March, 1965.

Chater, S. S.: Research critique: the coronary patient. Nurs. Res., 15:246-251, Summer, 1966.

Doyle, J.: Etiology of coronary disease: risk factors influencing coronary disease. Mod. Concepts of Cardiovascular Dis., 35:81-88, April, 1966.

George, J.: Monitoring the myocardial infarction patient. Nurs. Clin. N. Amer., 1:549-557, Dec., 1966.

Gordon, T., and Garst, C. C.: Coronary heart disease in adults. Vital Health Statistics, 11:1-46, Sept., 1965.

Graham, L. E.: Patients' perceptions in the C.C.U. Amer. J. Nurs., 69:1921-1922, Sept., 1966.

Jenkins, A. C.: Successful cardiac monitoring. Nurs. Clin. N. Amer., 1:537-547, Dec., 1966.

Kinlein, M. L.: Nursing the coronary patient. J. Rehab., 32:39-41, March-April, 1966.

Langhorne, U.: The coronary care unit. JAMA, 201:92-95, 1967.

Lown, B. (ed.): Symposium on coronary care units. Amer. J. Cardiol., 20:449-508, Oct., 1967.

Meltzer, L. E.: Coronary care, electrocardiography and the nurse. Amer. J. Nurs., 65:63-67, Dec., 1965.

Pinneo, R.: Nursing in a coronary care unit. Cardio-Vascular Nursing, 3:1-4, Jan.-Feb., 1967.

Ritota, M. C.: Diagnostic Electrocardiography, Phila., J. B. Lippincott, 1969.

Special report on cardiac care units. Mod. Hosp., 108:104-124, March, 1967.

CHAPTER **21**

Patients with Conditions of the Mouth, Neck and Esophagus

- *Dental Conditions and Care of the Teeth*
- *Conditions of the Lips, Mouth and Neck*
- *Conditions of the Esophagus*

It has been said that one's general appearance reveals much about an individual, and that the facial expression discloses much about the personality. A pleasant smile is an asset, and as is the appearance of healthy, even, white teeth.

The mouth with its lips, teeth and tongue is a vital facial structure related not only to a person's appearance and nutritional well-being, but also is a means of communication and personal contact. Any disturbance in appearance or function affects the physical and emotional reaction of the individual. Understanding, patience and explanations are required of those who care for persons who have problems involving the mouth and face, whether the difficulty is a toothache, ill-fitting dentures, mouth cancer or a traumatic disfigurement.

DENTAL CONDITIONS AND CARE OF THE TEETH

Care of the Teeth

Healthy teeth require conscientious and effective cleaning. To achieve maximal benefit from toothbrushing, the latter should be performed immediately after eating. The purpose is to remove food particles that lodge in crevices, around and between the teeth, and to prevent tartar formation.

Proper hand brushing of the teeth requires a firm-bristled brush of a size that permits easy access to all surfaces. The upper teeth are brushed downward and the bottom teeth upward so that the gum is not pushed away from the tooth. Horizontal scrubbing is reserved for lateral molar surfaces. Ten strokes is recommended for each surface. The normal movements of muscles used in eating and the normal flow of saliva aid greatly in keeping the teeth clean. Even so, it is necessary to brush the teeth in the morning and evening and after each meal to keep the mouth healthy.*

Many ill patients do not eat and salivate normally, which reduces the natural cleaning process. If the patient is unable to clean his teeth adequately, he must be taught to do so, perhaps being aided by the nurse. If a patient cannot brush his teeth, such as someone disabled by cerebrovascular disease or trauma, an oral lavage (half water and half hydrogen peroxide) can be sprayed into the mouth around the teeth using a squeeze plastic bottle with a fine hole tip. Gly-Oxide† also can be used. When this solution comes into contact with tissue, oxygen is released and exerts a me-

---

* Detailed discussion of general preventive measures, the nurse's role in health education, use of dentifrices and mouthwashes, mouth care, importance of proper nutrition, and so forth are found in fundamentals of nursing texts.

† International Pharmaceutical Corp. 10 per cent carbamide peroxide in a vehicle of anhydrous glycerol.

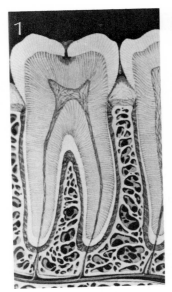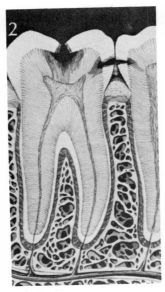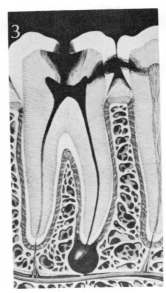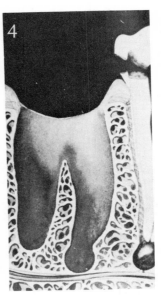

FIG. 21-1. Progress of decay. Left to right: (1) Early stages of dental decay. The enamel has been pentetrated. (2) The softer dentin has been attacked. (3) The pulp has been killed and an abscess formed. (4) The molar is extracted. The bicuspid is abscessed. (American Dental Association)

chanical cleansing action. The patient can be asked to alternate blowing and sucking the solution for half a minute before emitting it into the emesis basin. For those who can bite but cannot brush, a sponge rubber device is available that allows the teeth to compress and release alternately the fluid-filled cells of a sponge. The foaming action and massage of gums helps prevent gingivitis.

The electric brush is more effective in cleansing someone else's teeth than the conventional hand toothbrush. While the left hand of the nurse retracts the lips and cheeks, the right hand can direct the electric brush to all surfaces of the patient's teeth. Even the tongue may receive a beneficial light brushing. Following use of any toothbrush, it should be cleaned thoroughly with soap and water and allowed to dry.

Dental Caries

At least 95 per cent of Americans sooner or later experience tooth decay. This is an erosive process that results from the action of bacteria on fermentable carbohydrates in the mouth, which in turn produces acids that dissolve tooth enamel. The extent of damage to the teeth depends on several factors, the most significant of which are (1) the presence of dental plaques; (2) the strength of the acids and the ability of the saliva to neutralize them; (3) the length of time the acids are in contact with the teeth; and (4) susceptibility of the teeth to decay. Dental plaques are gluey, gelatin-like substances that adhere to the teeth

and afford protection for the bacteria. The initial action that causes damage to a tooth occurs under a dental plaque.*

Dental decay begins with a small hole, usually in a fissure or flaw of the enamel, or in an area that is hard to clean. Left unchecked, it penetrates the enamel into the dentin. Because the dentin is not as hard as the enamel, decay progresses somewhat more rapidly and in time reaches the pulp. When the blood, lymph vessels and nerves are exposed, they become infected, and an abscess may form either within the tooth or at the tip of the root (Fig. 21-1). Soreness and pain usually accompany the abscess. As the infection increases, the face may become swollen and there may be pulsating pain. The dentist can determine by x-ray pictures the extent of damage and the type of treatment needed. It may be necessary to extract the tooth.†

Measures used in the prevention and control of dental caries are reducing the intake of sugars, practicing effective mouth care as described, and fluoride applications to the teeth or drinking fluoridated water.

Fluoridation. By adjusting the fluoride level in the drinking water to an optimal healthful level of one part per million, up to two thirds of tooth decay can be prevented. Such a concentration of fluoride makes tooth enamel more resistant to the acids that are formed in the mouth. When ingested from birth to

* The American Dental Association: Dental Health Facts for Teachers. p. 11. 1966.
† *Ibid.*, p. 12.

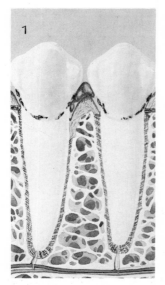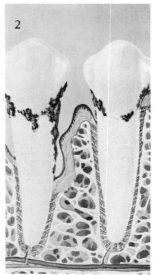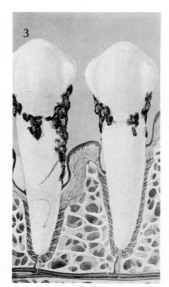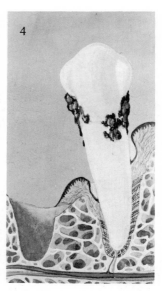

Fig. 21-2. Progress of periodontal disease. Left to right: (1) Irritations cause gums to withdraw from teeth. (2) Further destruction. (3) Most of the tissues have been destroyed. (4) One tooth is lost—the other weakened. (American Dental Association)

about 10 years of age, fluoridated water can give permanent protection. Some sections of the western United States have natural fluoridation; other areas of the country have enacted legislation for controlled fluoridation of public water supplies. In these areas, studies have demonstrated a reduction in dental decay. Fluoridation also seems to lessen the possibility of malocclusion and gingival disease.*

Most areas of this country, however, do not have fluoridated water and people must find other ways of receiving the benefits of fluoride. Four other methods are possible. (1) Vitamin preparations can include fluoride. Treatment must start early in life and continue until the age of 10. (2) A concentrated solution can be applied directly to the teeth. This is done by the dentist and has the advantage of professional control while encouraging regular check-ups. (3) Sodium fluoride can be added to the water in the home; however, home fluoridators that operate automatically are expensive and may do little good since children drink most of their daily water supply in school. (4) Sodium fluoride can be provided in tablet or liquid drops as a dietary additive; this, too, is expensive and often impractical.

* The addition of stannous fluoride to dentifrices helps to prevent tooth decay if used regularly. Acid phosphate fluoride and mon-fluoride phosphate give evidence that they may equal or surpass the results obtained with stannous fluoride dentifrices. (Horowitz, H. S., and Heifetz, S. B.: Individual fluoridation and fluorides for the individual. Clin. Ped., 5:103-108, Feb., 1966.)

Dentoalveolar Abscess or Periapical Abscess

This is a suppurative process involving the apical dental periosteum and the alveolar process in the periapical region. It may appear in 2 forms. The acute form is usually secondary to a suppurative pulpitis that arises from an infection that extended from dental caries. The infection of the dental pulp extends through the apical foramen of the tooth to form an abscess about the apex at its site of implantation in the alevolar bone. The abscess produces a dull gnawing continuous pain, often with a surrounding cellulitis and edema of the adjacent facial structures. The gum opposite the apex of the tooth is usually swollen on the cheek side where the abscess is prone to point. The swelling and cellulitis of the facial structures may make it difficult to open the mouth. In well developed abscesses there may be a systemic reaction, fever and malaise.

Medical and Nursing Management. In the early stages of the infection, a drill opening into the pulp chamber may relieve tension and so relieve pain and provide drainage. Most often the infection has progressed to periapical abscess and drainage must be provided by an incision through the gingivae down to the jaw bone. A foul pus escapes under pressure. The postoperative care consists of hot saline mouthwashes given at least every 2 hours except when the patient is asleep. He should be encouraged to expectorate the foul pus that escapes and a basin should be within easy reach. External heat in the form of hot compresses or a heating pad hasten the subsidence of the inflammatory swelling and soreness. In patients with a high fever, an antibiotic (penicillin) is usually administered. It goes without saying that bed rest and a soft diet are necessary during the acute stage. Analgesic drugs are used as necessary to relieve pain. The nurse must recognize that the pain and swelling may interfere with an adequate fluid intake, and a special effort must be made to overcome any deficit. After the inflammatory reaction has subsided, the tooth may have to be extracted or appropriate root canal therapy given.

Chronic dentoalveolar abscess is a slowly progressive infection with the same mode as the acute form. It differs from the acute form in that the process may progress to a fully formed abscess without the patient knowing it. The infection eventually leads to a "blind dental abscess" that is really a periapical granuloma. It may enlarge to as much as 1 cm. in diameter. It is often discovered in x-ray examination and is treated by tooth extraction or by root canal therapy, often with apicoectomy.

Periodontal Disease

Periodontal disease is a condition affecting the gums (gingivae) and other supporting structures (bone, cementum and periodontal membrane). At the onset, there is little discomfort and few other signs of the condition. Later there may be bleeding, infection, gum recession and loosening of the teeth. This may cause teeth to fall out or require extraction. It is estimated that 1 in 4 persons have the disease at some stage of its development, and up to 90 per cent of all persons in their 40's are affected. Dental authorities suggest that the principal reason most people after age 50 require dentures is the effect of this increasingly prevalent disease (Fig. 21-2).

Malocclusion, poor fillings and inadequate diet are suspected causes of periodontal disease; in addition, improper cleaning and poor mouth hygiene contribute to the problem. Tartar or calculus that cannot be brushed from the teeth tends to build up and requires professional removal twice a year. If this is not done, gums become swollen and tender, infection progresses and pockets collecting pus and bacteria are formed between the gums and teeth. The bone supporting the teeth is destroyed and the tooth becomes loose.

Some authorities believe that this condition is frequently associated with other systemic diseases, such as diabetes and certain skin and blood disorders; however, conclusive evidence is lacking. At present the best advice is to brush the teeth carefully at least twice a day (after breakfast and dinner), and to have them cleaned professionally twice a year. Such a cleaning should include the area below the gum line. Poor occlusion should be corrected, crooked teeth straightened and missing teeth replaced with bridgework or another form of splinting. Not too long ago such work by an orthodontist was considered a luxury and done only for cosmetic reasons. Today the value of such treatment is seen in the prevention of periodontal disease and other mouth problems. In the near future, perhaps 3-dimensional photography will assist periodontists in measuring the changes in the shape or elevation of the gum, signs that allow early detection of periodontal disease.

Orthodontal Correction for Malocclusion

Malocclusion is the faulty relationship between the teeth when the jaws are closed. Correction of malocclusion requires three factors: an orthodontist who has special training, a patient who cooperates, and adequate time. Most treatments begin when the patient has shed his last primary tooth and the last permanent successor has erupted, usually around 12 or 13 years of age.

In order to realign the teeth, the orthodontist gradually forces the teeth into a new location by the use of wires or bands. This therapy is commonly known as teeth-straightening. The patient may object to the effect of these devices on his appearance, and this is a psychological burden that must be overcome if good results are to be achieved in the future. During this time, it is essential that the patient keep his mouth meticulously clean. In the final phase of treatment, a retaining device is worn for several hours each day to support the tissues as they adjust to the new location of the teeth. Encouragement is often necessary for the individual to persist in this most important part of the treatment. When an adolescent is admitted to the hospital for some other problem while undergoing orthodontal correction, it may be necessary to remind him to continue wearing the retainer, if it does not interfere with the problem requiring hospitalization.

Dental Implants and Transplantation

Successful research is being done involving the transplant of teeth. Experimenting continues with "tooth" banks. Some researchers have restricted their transplants to undeveloped or "bud" teeth while others are trying to transplant teeth at many stages of development. However, at present, homotransplants (person-to-person) will have to await additional research to combat the rejection process. Successful autotransplants (using the patient's own teeth) have been reported. For example, a defective first molar has been replaced successfully by the patient's own third molar. Several successful implants of teeth have been made from acrylic and other plastics.

Dental Extraction

A tooth is extracted because it is defective, damaged or in the path of future orthodontal correction.

Extraction wounds usually heal quickly and without complications if simple precautions are taken. Lessened activity reduces the likelihood of bleeding. Cold applications soon after extraction, such as an ice bag or cold moist cloth to the side of the face for about 15 minutes of every hour for several hours, relieve discomfort and swelling. Rinsing the mouth is not done the first day so that the clot is not disturbed. Thereafter rinsing and cleansing of the teeth is resumed.

Oozing of blood may be apparent the first day, but if more occurs than just oozing, place clean folded gauze pad directly on the bleeding spot. Instruct the patient to close his teeth tightly over the pad to apply pressure for about 30 minutes. Repeat if necessary. If there is prolonged or severe pain, swelling or bleeding, the dentist should be notified. (See Chap. 17 for special precautions to be taken with patients having hematologic problems.)

Impacted Third Molars. It is desirable to have the patient hospitalized when all 4 molars are to be extracted at one time. Using endotracheal general anesthesia, the oral surgeon inserts a mouth retractor to provide exposure. Incisions are made laterally in the mandible to approach the impacted tooth. Bone that is removed from the jaw eventually regenerates. Closure of the mucous membrane is accomplished with black silk sutures. Soreness and edema are noticeable, but can be relieved by analgesics and ice packs. Liquids may be offered from a spouted container if the facial muscles are too sensitive to allow the patient to suck from a straw. After the fifth day, stitches are removed and mouthwashes can proceed from saline to sodium peroxyborate monohydrate (Amosan). Brushing of the teeth is resumed when the gums have healed. Any pain or swelling after one week should be reported; infection is common but can be easily treated with drainage, packing and antibiotics.

Artificial Dentures

It is common practice for people to postpone indefinitely the final decision to obtain artificial dentures, even though there is no possibility of having the few remaining teeth repaired. The improved appearance, better nutrition and reduced likelihood of infection are positive aspects of obtaining dentures that can be presented by the nurse to the hesitant patient. When dentures have been obtained, patience is required in learning to use them effectively.

Dentures require careful scrubbing, using a good denture brush, mild soap and water, salt and sodium bicarbonate. The addition of a drop of household chlorine acts as a deodorant and gives a fresher taste. Most dentists recommend that dentures be removed at night, scrubbed and allowed to soak in a proprietary cleaner.

Pressure or irritation caused by dentures should be reported to the dentist, who can make the proper adjustment. Uncorrected pressure areas may cause lesions that in turn may become malignant.

Many persons now prefer to have "immediate dentures." Usually the back teeth are extracted first, which allows the tissues time to heal. Meanwhile, the artificial teeth are made and ready for placement immediately after the front teeth are extracted.

Partial dentures should not be left in place for prolonged periods without removing for a good cleaning. They are held in place with metal clasps that encircle the teeth. These clasps can be spread using gentle force with two index fingers. One side can be loosened and then the other. When reapplying, the cleaned partial dentures usually can be pressed into place.

CONDITIONS OF THE LIPS, MOUTH AND NECK

Trauma of Lips

Wounds of the face and the lips rarely become infected because of the rich blood supply of that region. If an accidental wound is cleaned and sutured early, healing is rapid. This is the case also in the event of an intentional wound of the surgeon's making. Dressings are both unnecessary and conspicuous. The wounds are sutured best with silk or nylon and painted with Whitehead's varnish. Primary healing occurs without much scarring.

Stomatitis

This is an inflammatory condition of the mouth. It may occur as a primary disease or as a symptom of a systemic disease. As a primary disease it may arise from local pathogens such as Vincent's fusospirochete and the viruses of *Herpes simplex* and of measles; from local trauma such as cheek-biting, jagged teeth, ill-fitting dentures; from excessive use of irritants such as alcohol, tobacco, hot foods, etc.; or from sensitization to substances such as toothpastes and mouthwashes. The systemic diseases causing stomatitis may be avitaminosis, blood disorders such as pernicious anemia, infectious mononucleosis or leukemia, systemic infections such as syphilis, and various drugs such as iodides, mercury, barbiturates and lead.

The clinical signs and symptoms of stomatitis vary widely, from painful ulcers of the mucous membrane often covered with a pseudomembrane, to widespread gangrene (noma) of the mouth. Smears and cultures of the lesions and a careful examination of the patient help to make the diagnosis. When systemic disease, anemia, vitamin deficiencies and systemic infections are thought to be the cause of the stomatitis, appropriate treatment is given. Local infections are treated with specific antibiotic therapy, usually penicillin. When the painful mouth ulcers prevent eating, temporary relief may be obtained by rinsing the mouth with a local anesthetic solution before eating. Antiseptic mouthwashes are given at least every 2 hours. In caring for these patients, the nurse should use sterile precautions, and the dishes and utensils should be treated as for a patient on infectious precautions.

Herpes Simplex Infection

The herpes simplex virus most commonly produces the familiar *herpes labialis* (cold sore, fever blister or canker). The infection may take the form of an acute herpetic gingivostomatitis. Small vesicles, single or clustered, may erupt on the lips, the tongue, the cheeks and the pharynx. These soon rupture, forming sore, shallow ulcers that are covered with a gray membrane. Herpes infections appear often in association with other febrile infections, such as pneumococcus pneumonia, meningococcic meningitis and malaria. The herpes virus does not yield in the slightest to any of the chemotherapeutic agents that have become available to date. However, some relief is experienced with supportive medications containing *Lactobacillus acidophilus* (e.g., Lactinex).

Canker Sores (Aphthous Ulcers)

One of the most common lesions of the mouth are recurrent aphthous ulcers (canker sores). Because of the local discomfort they produce, the difficulty experienced in getting rid of them and their possible resemblance (to the untrained eye) to other more serious conditions, they are also one of the most distressing lesions to the person so afflicted. Aphthous ulcers are shallow ulcers found in the mucous membrane of the mouth, most often on the innerside of the lips, cheeks and in the sulcus between the lips and gums. However, they may appear anywhere in the mouth—including on the tongue. They begin with a burning, tingling sensation and slight swelling of the mucous membrane, which soon becomes a shallow ulcer with a whitish center surrounded by a red border. These ulcers are especially painful when eating, and acid or spicy foods particularly aggravate them. Since these ulcers are tender to pressure, any abrasion of or movement of the skin around the ulcer tends to make activities such as speaking and facial movements painful. The ulcers may be single or multiple, and they often tend to heal at one site and recur elsewhere. The sores may appear at anytime in life; most often they begin in childhood or adolescence, and may appear as frequently as once a month. In most cases, however, they do not occur more than once a year or so. These ulcers last only a short time—from 4 to 20 days—and eventually heal spontaneously, leaving no scar.

In spite of intense studies, no definite cause can be found for canker sores. Despite what you may have heard to the contrary, they are not caused by too much or too little "acid" in the system, "bad" teeth, poor oral hygiene, or nutritional deficiency. These studies have apparently ruled out a virus as a causative agent. The latest information available appears to point to psychosomatic factors as the cause. There seem to be definite predisposing factors—such as emotional or mental stress—to their occurrence. In females, they seem to appear at the time of menstrual periods, and they occur much more frequently among women than men. Fatigue, change in a life situation, and anxiety are other predisposing factors.

Because these studies have uncovered no specific cause, there is no specific treatment for canker sores. Where anxiety is an obvious etiologic factor, tranquilizing drugs may be beneficial. Mouthwashes of various types have not proved particularly helpful in ridding the patient of his sores, although some oxygen-liberating agents (such as hydrogen peroxide), as well as some mouthwashes containing antibiotics have been used to alleviate symptoms with variable results. Solutions of corticosteroids have been found to relieve the pain and discomfort of the ulcers when applied locally. Fortunately these ulcers eventually heal spontaneously in a relatively short time.

Vincent's Angina

This is commonly called "trench mouth" or Vincent's infection, and is a pseudomembranous ulceration affecting the edges of the gums, the mucosa of the mouth, the tonsils and pharynx. It is caused by a combination of 2 organisms, a spirochete and a fusiform bacillus. Smears made from the ulcerations are found teeming with the characteristic organisms and establishes the diagnosis.

The chief symptoms are painful bleeding gums. Swallowing and talking are painful, especially when infection has spread to the tonsils and pharynx. There may be a mild fever and swelling of the lymph nodes in the neck.

Treatment and Nursing Management. Objectives of medical and nursing care are directed toward controlling and treating the infection, reducing fetid breath, making the patient comfortable and maintaining his nutrition. The plan of care includes hourly mouth washes or irrigations consisting of fluids rich in free oxygen (to combat the anaerobic spirochete), such as dilute hydrogen peroxide or sodium perborate in a 2 per cent solution. Antibiotics given parenterally are effective. Food should be of liquid or soft consistency to reduce trauma to the gums. Highly seasoned or strongly acid foods should not be served; it is also desirable to avoid smoking and alcohol. Patient education is stressed so that recurrence does not occur due to uncorrected mouth problems and poor hygiene. Methods of preventing transmission to others also must be emphasized, such as sterilizing dishes and eating utensils before they are used again.

Ludwig's Angina

This is an acute septic inflammation of the tissues of the floor and the submaxillary region of the mouth and neck. Its onset is sudden: the patient has difficulty in talking and swallowing, he has pain and neck swelling and, finally, dyspnea. The patient is profoundly toxic, but does not exhibit the high temperature and the leukocytosis that might be expected. Death may occur suddenly due to edema of the glottis that produces asphyxia or to intense toxemia.

Medical and Nursing Management. Fortunately for these individuals, antibiotic therapy often is able to abort the infection and to ward off serious complications. The treatment is early incision with drainage, then the application of hot wet dressings to the neck and the use of hot mouthwashes. If dyspnea develops, a tracheostomy must be performed. The nurse must watch these patients closely for respiratory difficulty, stertorous (noisy) breathing, cyanosis or rapid increase in swelling. These symptoms are the early signs of beginning respiratory obstruction.

Patients with Disorders of the Salivary Glands

Acute Inflammation—Parotitis

The most common inflammation of the salivary glands is *parotitis* (inflammation of the parotid gland); however, infection can occur in the other glands as well. The essential lesion of mumps (infectious parotitis) is an inflammation of the salivary gland, usually the parotid. A form of parotitis is sometimes seen in sarcoidosis; the uveo-parotid syndrome or uveo-parotid fever characterized by fever, uveitis, lacrimal and salivary gland enlargement. Parotitis also can occur as a serious complication of other infectious diseases such as pneumonia. Elderly, acutely ill and debilitated individuals whose salivary glands fail to secrete sufficiently because of general dehydration often acquire parotitis. The infecting organisms travel from the mouth through the salivary duct. Because of parched mouths and not chewing solid food, older people offer poor defense against invasion of the parotid ducts by pathogenic organisms.

In all the above-mentioned conditions, except mumps, the offending organism usually is the staphylococcus. The onset of this complication is sudden, with an exacerbation of the fever and of the symptoms of the primary condition. The gland swells, becomes tense and tender, pain is felt in the ear, and there is interference with swallowing. The swelling rapidly increases and the overlying skin soon becomes red and shiny. Occasionally, facial nerve palsy may occur with parotid gland disease.

Prevention Postoperatively. In order to prevent parotitis in the postoperative patient, any necessary dental work should be done before surgery. In addition, optimal patient preparation includes maintaining an adequate nutritional and fluid intake plus good mouth hygiene. After surgery, having the patient chew gum or suck hard candy may prevent obstruction of the salivary gland ducts.

Treatment and Nursing Care. At the onset of the swelling, an icebag may be applied over the affected gland, and chemotherapy may be instituted with penicillin or one of the sulfonamides. A suppurating gland may require incision and drainage.

Syphilis causes both acute and gummatous parotitis. In all cases of these 2 luetic conditions the gland swells gradually and there is salivation. However, there is seldom any pain, and there is little tendency to suppuration. All patients respond readily to antiluetic therapy.

Salivary Calculus (Sialolithiasis)

Salivary stones may develop in the submaxillary gland following glandular infection or ductal stricture due to trauma or inflammation. Sialograms (x-ray pictures taken with a radiopaque substance injected into duct) may be required to show obstruction of the duct by stenosis. Salivary stones are composed mainly of calcium oxalate. If located within the gland, they are irregularly lobulated and vary in diameter from 3 to 30 mm. Stones in the duct are small and oval.

Calculi within the salivary gland cause no symptoms unless infection arises; but a calculus that obstructs the gland's duct causes sudden, local and often colicky pain, which is suddenly relieved by a gush of saliva. Where this condition exists, the gland is swollen and quite tender, the stone itself often is palpable and its shadow may be seen on roentgenograms. The calculus can be extracted fairly easily from the duct in the mouth; sometimes enlarging the orifice permits the stone to pass spontaneously. It may be necessary to remove the gland if there are repeated recurrences of symptoms and calculi in the gland itself.

Tumors of the Salivary Glands

Neoplasms of almost any type, but the great majority of them malignant, develop in salivary glands, and in 75 per cent of all patients these develop in one parotid. They may remain small and quiescent for years, then suddenly begin to increase in size. Neoplasms are diagnosed on the basis of history and physical examination; tests such as needle biopsy are contraindicated. Recently, encouraging results in detection of neoplasms have been reported with radiosialography (scanning with Te99m).

The best treatment of parotid tumor is the early and complete excision of the mass. Fortunately, most of these growths occur superficially rather than in the deep retromandibular lobe. Partial excision of the gland, along with all of the tumor combined with careful dissection to preserve the vulnerable facial (7th) nerve is the common procedure. For more involved tumors, it may be necessary to sacrifice the nerve (see p. 785) when a parotidectomy is done. If the tumor is malignant or mixed, irradiation therapy follows surgery. Local recurrences are common; the recurrent growth usually is more malignant than the original one. Postoperatively, the nurse should be aware that the patient may have some facial paralysis (if the nerve was not excised) due to tissue trauma and edema. This will gradually subside.

Fracture of the Mandible, Jaw Repositioning or Reconstruction

These fractures may be simple fractures without displacement, resulting from a blow on the chin, or they may be very complicated, involving loss of tissue and bone from a severe accident. Mandibular fractures are always compound. In simple fractures, without loss of teeth, the jaw is immobilized by fixing it to the upper jaw with wires. The wires are placed around the teeth in both the upper and lower jaw, on each side of the fracture line. The lower jaw is held tight against the upper jaw by cross-wires or rubber bands placed around the wires about the teeth (Fig. 21-3). This simple form of fixation is used when there are teeth that can be used in the wire fixation. In other cases, in which teeth are missing or bone displacement has occurred, various other forms of fixation can be used. Some of these are applied in the mouth, such as metal arch bars; other methods are more involved, requiring pins inserted into the bone with fixation to a plaster head piece. The nursing problem then is one of treating a fracture compounded in the mouth in a patient who cannot open his jaws.

Nursing Responsibility

Immediately following surgery, the patient should be placed on his side with his head slightly elevated. The nasogastric suction tube inserted during surgery is connected to low pressure suction; this removes stomach contents and lessens the danger of their aspiration. Antiemetic drugs are also administered. Prevention of vomiting is most desirable. If the patient

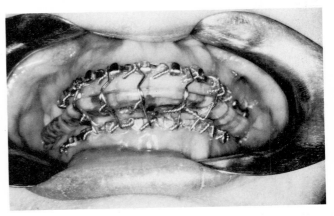

FIG. 21-3. For this patient's intermaxillary fixation, arch bars were placed about the maxillary and mandibular arches of teeth. The intermaxillary wires are the vertical ones between the arch bars. It is these wires that must be cut in an emergency. (Marsh Robinson, D.D.S., M.D.)

does vomit, and the wires are cut, surgery and rewiring have to be repeated later. A plier-type of wire cutter (or scissors, if rubber bands are used) should be taped to the head of the bed for emergency use.

Clearing of the nasopharyngeal area can be done with a small catheter inserted through the nasal orifice. The oral cavity can be aspirated by first inserting a tongue blade to move the cheek away from the teeth; insert the catheter where teeth are not in close position, where a tooth is missing or in the space behind the third molar.

Constant attention by the nurse in the postsurgery recovery time is necessary. As the patient regains consciousness, he needs to be reminded again that his jaw is wired but that he can breathe and swallow. As he emerges from anesthesia, his head may be elevated. If an extraoral appliance is used to immobilize the mandible, the patient needs instruction on positioning so that he does not roll onto the device. To prevent dry and cracking lips, a lubricant is applied.

Careful attention to the hygiene of the mouth must be insisted upon, using warm alkaline mouthwashes or oxygenating rinses at least every 2 hours and after each feeding. In addition, the mouth should be inspected at least once or twice daily to ensure thorough cleansing. A flashlight and a tongue blade to retract the cheeks are essential equipment. If permissible, a small soft toothbrush can be used carefully.

The diet must necessarily be liquid, but sufficient caloric and fluid intake can be given easily to these patients. They can be fed through a straw without much difficulty and occasionally soft foods may be given with a spoon. Water should be given after each liquid feeding, followed by a mouthwash.

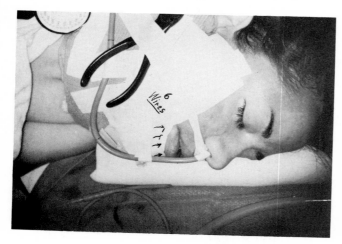

Fig. 21-4. This patient shown in the lateral position in the recovery room had surgery for mandibular prognathism, necessitating intermaxillary fixation. Note the wire cutter attached to the collar bandage, the bandage marked with the location and number of intermaxillary wires, the Levin tube in place, and a nasopharyngeal tube and suction catheter readily available. Also note the manometer available to ascertain blood pressure. (Marsh Robinson, D.D.S., M.D.)

Usually the patient is out of bed the first postoperative day, and the length of time for ambulation is gradually increased each day.

Patient Education and Convalescent Care

Depending on conditions, including age and the patient's stability, most patients are able to leave the hospital before the wiring is removed. Of prime importance is the proper functioning of the fixation appliance, and to ensure this, the patient has to see his physician at certain intervals. At these examinations,

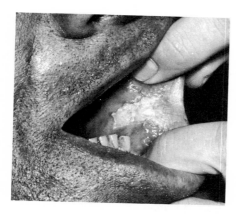

Fig. 21-5. Leukoplakia. Note the white patches above and to the right of the teeth.

he also is checked for cleanliness of the mouth and the device as well as his general nutritional condition. This means that he needs to know how to give himself mouth care, how to feed himself and what kinds of foods to take. If there are any sites of irritation, these need to be reported. This instruction is given to the patient before he is discharged.

Precancerous Lesions

Leukoplakia buccalis (also called "smoker's patch") and the related *keratosis labialis* are seen in middle-aged adults, more than 80 per cent of them men. These conditions are characterized early by the appearance of one or two small, thin, often crinkled, pearly patches on the mucous membrane of the tongue, the mouth, or both, due to keratinization of the mucosa and sclerosis of its underlying tissue (Fig. 21-5). In time, most of the tongue and the mouth may become covered by a creamy white, thick, fissured or papillomatous mucous membrane that desquamates occasionally, leaving a beefy-red base. This condition results from chronic irritation by carious, infected or poorly repaired teeth, by tobacco and by highly spiced foods. It will disappear in time after cessation of smoking. Occasionally it is due to lues. Not infrequently, cancers start in the keratinized patches.

Carcinoma may arise in any part of the mouth and cancer in this area (including cancer of the pharynx) accounts for 3 per cent of all cancer deaths in this country. Males are afflicted 3½ times more than females. Of the 7,000 oral cancer deaths annually, the distribution by site[*] is estimated as follows:

Lip	27%
Tongue	22%
Other oral mucosa	16%
Salivary gland	14%
Floor of mouth	11%
Other mesopharynx incl. tonsil	10%

Because the mouth is such an accessible and observable site, more intensive professional and patient educational programs are needed for early detection of mouth lesions. The nurse should urge the patient with a white patchy area, sore spot, or ulceration of lips, gums or mouth that fails to heal after 2 weeks to see a physician. Often the individual feels a roughened area with his tongue. Since pain is often one of the last symptoms to appear, a painless condition should not prevent further professional examination; this includes swelling, numbness or loss of feeling in any part of the mouth.

Squamous cell (epidermoid) carcinoma constitutes

[*] Oral Cancer Control. U. S. Dept. H.E.W., PHS Publication No 1542, August, 1966.

over 90 per cent of all mouth cancer. The next most common type arises from the submucous glands, adenocarcinoma. The third grouping includes malignancy of the jaw bone. The year cure rate is below 30 per cent. Most oral cancers can be prevented by good dental care and no smoking. In tobacco chewers, the mucous membrane of the cheek is the commonest site. A jagged tooth and poor dental hygiene may be the cause. Betel and areca nut, used widely for chewing in South India, is believed to be related to that country's high incidence (40 per cent of all cancers) of oral cancer.

Cancer of the Lip

This tumor, usually called an epithelioma, occurs most frequently on the lower lip in men as a chronic ulcer. Predisposing factors may be chronic irritation of a warm pipe stem, or prolonged exposure to the sun and wind. More significantly, however, is the tendency for leukoplakia to progress to an epidermoid lip cancer. A typical lesion is a painless indurated ulcer with raised edges. Any wart or ulcer of the lip that does not heal in 3 weeks should be biopsied.

Small lesions usually are excised liberally; larger lesions involving more than one third of the lip may be treated best by radiotherapy because of superior cosmetic results. The choice depends upon the extent of the lesion, the skill of the surgeon or radiologist, and what is necessary to cure the patient while preserving the best appearance. Fortunately only about 10 to 15 per cent of lip cancers metastasize. When lymph nodes appear to be involved, a neck dissection is indicated.

Cancer of the Tongue

The early stage of cancer of the anterior undersurface of lateral aspects of the tongue usually is detected as a small ulcer that has not healed in 3 weeks, or it may be an area of thickening. After several months, the cancer invades the underlying muscle body of the tongue. Pain or soreness of the tongue on eating hot or highly seasoned foods and limitation of motion is noticeable. As the growth spreads to neighboring structures, symptoms such as excessive salivation, slurred speech, blood-tinged sputum, trismus and pain on swallowing liquids develop. If untreated, the patient is unable to swallow and earache, faceache and toothache become almost constant. Unable to eat or sleep, he finally succumbs to hemorrhage (lingual artery), cervical lymph node metastasis, or general debilitation.

The only cure is surgery following early recognition of the condition. The enlargement of lymph nodes indicates metastases. This may necessitate more extensive surgical dissection combined with radium and x-ray therapy. When the tongue is involved, it is

necessary often to perform a *hemiglossectomy* or a *glossectomy*.

Malignancy at the base of the tongue produces less obvious symptoms: slight dysphagia, sore throat, salivation and some blood-tinged sputum. This is a difficult site for effective radiation and because of the mutilating effects of total glossectomy and the likelihood of metastasis, the cure rate of posterior tongue cancer is very low.

Nursing Management of the Patient with Oral Cancer

Psychosocial and Environmental Considerations. The patient with a mouth or facial problem requires patience and understanding. Quite naturally he tends to withdraw from people, is self-conscious about mouth odors and is sensitive about his appearance. The nurse is challenged to get through to him, encourage his expression of fears and concerns, and offer him support and explanations as necessary. The immediate family need to be aware of their supporting role and in turn, should be informed of the plan of therapy for the patient.

Particular areas of patient concern are fear of pain, ability to communicate, drooling, feeding and swallowing. In addition, he may express a strong desire for solitude and be self-conscious of his appearance. (The need to remove, temporarily, any large mirrors in the room should be considered by the nurse.) The results of surgery or radiation concern him, especially the fear of disfigurement; if the resection is extensive, the possibility of prosthetics (fitting an artificial part) may be explained.

A therapeutic environment must be maintained by good room ventilation, particularly with the patient who has a malodorous cancer lesion. A room deodorant may be advisable.

Mouth Hygiene and Adequate Nutrition. To reduce the number of bacteria and to keep the mouth clean are important objectives before as well as after surgery or radiation. If the patient is conscious and able to help himself, the nurse can teach him effective mouth care. He may need reminding and proper supplies. These may include an effective toothbrush or gauze-padded applicator stick as well as oxygen-releasing and antimicrobial mouth-rinsing solutions. Essence of caroid is a good agent for cleansing a dry, crusted, foul tongue in the debilitated, dehydrated patient. (See care of teeth, p. 428; also, fundamentals of nursing texts.) If the patient is a mouth-breather, he needs more mouth attention than the average person. The use of swabs of mineral oil with lemon juice or milk of magnesia and mineral oil is refreshing. Lanolin applied to dry and cracking lips is soothing.

Dentures must be removed frequently and cleaned. Before they are replaced, the mouth also should be cleaned. Often care is given to the teeth, but the "furred" or coated tongue is neglected and bad breath continues. In the unconscious patient, the nurse is wholly responsible for maintaining good mouth hygiene. The use of a special mouth tray with all necessary applicator sticks, padded tongue depressors, mouthwashes, lubricants and so forth encourages frequent mouth attention.

The general physical condition of a person often is reflected in his mouth. Therefore, good nutritional levels must be maintained. If the breath has a foul odor, the nurse must encourage and assist the patient with his oral hygiene before and after each feeding. Often a bad taste in the mouth spoils the taste of food and limits the intake of nourishment.

Individuals with mouth lesions may have feeding problems. The use of a plastic straw or a teaspoon may be effective. Feeders employed with children may be of use. Food should be soft or liquid and nonirritating; i.e., not too hot or too cold and not highly seasoned. It should be served attractively to tempt the patient to take it. Small, frequent feedings are more desirable than large, less frequent ones. The desires as well as the nutritional needs of the patient should be taken into consideration. If he is not able to take anything by mouth, it may be necessary to feed him by means of a nasogastric tube. Before feedings are given, the position of the tube must be checked by injecting slowly, drop by drop, 1 or 2 ml. of saline. If the tube is in the esophagus, as it should be, the patient should have no reaction. If it is in the trachea, he coughs violently. The care of this tube is similar to that of a gastrostomy tube (see p. 469). As the patient progresses to the point where he can insert his own feeding catheter, he should be given time, privacy, assistance and encouragement. Perhaps a mirror will help.

Salivation and Mouth Odors. If the lesion is such that the patient salivates constantly, this may be relieved somewhat by inserting a gauze wick in the corner of the mouth. The saliva that drops from the end of the wick may be caught in a small basin. Another way of removing mouth secretions is by the use of a small rubber catheter attached to a suction apparatus. Mouth wipes, as well as a paper bag attached to the bed or the bedside stand to receive soiled tissues, always should be on hand. An effective way of holding dressings of the mouth or the lower jaw in place is by the use of a face mask. The strings can be tied at the top of the head.

To combat odors, the doctor may order such oxidizing agents for a mouthwash as potassium permanganate 1:10,000, hydrogen peroxide in half strength, sodium perborate and so forth. In extensive mouth sores, a power spray can clean wounds effectively and necrotic tissue can be removed more easily.

Surgical Intervention. General preparation for surgery is similar to that described on p. 101. Depending upon the nature of the operation, the anesthesia may be local or general. The surgery may be confined to the lip, involve only the tongue, or include resection of facial tissue and the mandible with possible dental extraction. If there is metastasis to the lymph nodes of the neck, neck dissection may be necessary. Postoperatively, the chief objective is to maintain a patent airway. The patient is placed in the prone position, in the supine position with the head turned to the side, or the lateral position with special emphasis on facilitating drainage from the mouth. Suctioning may be required; precautions are necessary to avoid injury to the suture line and sensitive tissues such as exist in a hemiglossectomy. Perhaps a dental suction tip may be required until such time as the patient is able to take care of his own secretions.

Mouth irrigations are given to keep the mouth clean, provide comfort and assist in the healing process. The prescribed solutions may be normal saline, diluted hydrogen peroxide, sodium bicarbonate solution, alkaline mouthwash or others. Gentle lavaging using a catheter inserted between the cheek and teeth loosens mucus and is refreshing. A power spray has the advantage of getting the solution into inaccessible areas.

Speech Rehabilitation. Speech often is interfered with or is difficult. Simply to supply the patient with a pad of paper and a pencil or "magic slate" will supply the means whereby he can express his needs and thoughts and may make a tremendous difference in his depressed condition. Often these patients are reluctant to associate with other patients; they prefer to be alone. If there are 2 or more patients with a similar condition, they can help each other. It is easier for them, and for others, if they have their meals apart from other patients.

The patient's family and friends should be encouraged to visit so that he is aware that others care about and for him. He can be helped to care for his appearance. With speech training and adjustment to a prosthesis, he will become increasingly aware that the future holds promise for him.

Radium. If radium implants are used, the usual radium precautions are observed. When radium needles are implanted, each needle has a thread attached to it. The patient should know upon waking that these are present and that they are not to be removed. The power spray is effective in cleansing the mouth when these are in place. Radium may be implanted in a moulage (molded dental compound), and this may be applied to some part of the mouth for a specific length of time. It is usually permissible to remove the mold for meals and at night. When it is reinserted, it is important for the nurse to note that it is in its proper position. (For care of radium, see p. 610.)

Convalescent and Extended Care in the Home

The post-hospital objectives of patient care are similar to those in the hospital. The individual who is recovering from treatment for a mouth condition needs to breathe, to secure nourishment, to avoid infection, and to be alert for adverse signs. The patient, his family or person responsible for his home care, the nurse and whoever else may be involved such as a speech therapist, dietition, psychologist, and so forth, need to prepare an individualized plan. If suctioning the mouth or tracheostomy tube is required, what equipment and how to use it as well as where it can be obtained must be determined. Consideration is given to the humidification and aeration of the room as well as measures to control odors. How to prepare foods that are nutritious, properly seasoned and of the right temperature can be explained. Perhaps it may be more feasible to use commercial baby food than to prepare liquid and soft diets in a blender. The use and care of prostheses must be understood. The importance of cleanliness with dressings and mouth care is reviewed. The person caring for the patient needs to know the signs of obstruction, hemorrhage, infection, depression, and withdrawal as well as what to do about these problems. Follow-up visits to the clinic or physician are important to determine progression or regression and to receive any modifications in medication or general care.

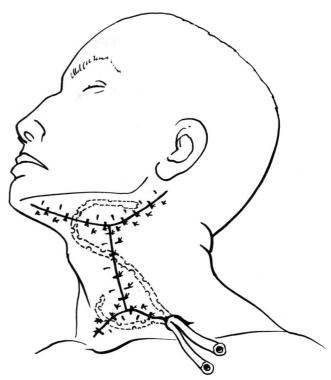

Fig. 21-6. Diagram showing extent of radical neck dissection and the position of the drainage tubes.

Palliative Patient Care

Because of further extension of a malignancy by metastasis and necrosis, it may not be possible medically to halt the spread of disease. All efforts are then directed toward comfort measures, including those physical, psychological and spiritual. With the family's help this may be continued in the hospital, nursing home or the patient's own home.

The Patient with Radical Neck Dissection

Malignancies of the head and neck, including cancers of the lips, tongue, gums, palate, tonsils and of the mucosa of the mouth, pharynx and larynx, may be treated early by surgery or irradiation with good results. These cancers are in an area that can be easily seen and early diagnosis and treatment given. Most observers agree that such patients do not die from recurrence at the site of the primary growth, but rather from metastasis to the cervical lymph nodes in the neck, which often takes place by way of the lymphatics before the primary lesion has been treated. The nodes involved are only on one side of the neck, unless the tumor is located at or near the midline, in which case the nodes of both sides of the neck may contain metastic tumor.

Because radiation does not give good results in controlling the metastic cancer in the lymph nodes in the neck, an operation called a "radical neck dissection" is performed. This operation attempts to remove all of the lymph-node bearing tissue of one side of the neck. It may be done at the time of the treatment of the primary tumor, or carried out independently at a later date.

The operation is radical, as the name implies, and involves removal of all the tissue under the skin from the ramus of the jaw down to the clavicle, and from the midline back to the angle of the jaw in one mass. This includes removing the sternomastoid muscle and other smaller muscles as well as the jugular vein in the neck, because the lymphatic nodes are found widely distributed throughout these tissues.

During or after the procedure a tracheostomy is often performed. Because there may be profuse drainage of serum and lymph after such an extensive procedure, drainage tubes or Hemovac suction are often used in the wound.

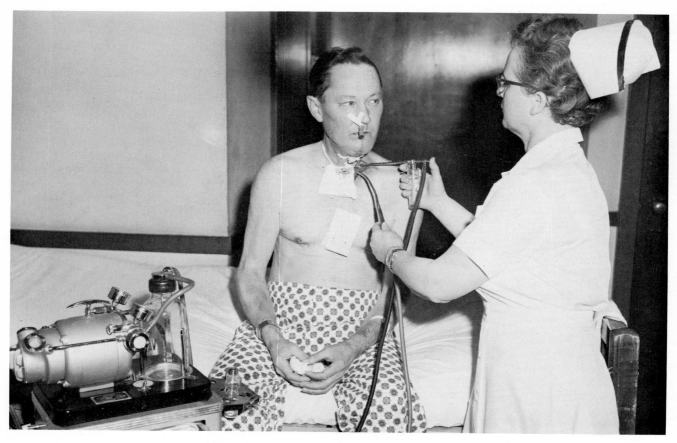

Fig. 21-7. With a radical neck dissection, this patient has a tracheostomy tube inserted. To keep a drainage area clean, the nurse is using a power spray with antiseptic solution in her right hand while holding a suction tip in the left hand. Note the hanging end of a Montgomery strap on the anterior chest; after sterile dressings are applied, the strap will be laced over the dressing as it meets the strap from the left posterior shoulder. (William R. Nelson, M.D.)

Postoperative Nursing Management

The principles of nursing care described on pp. 129 and 145 can be applied to the patient who has extensive neck surgery. In addition, the nurse should recognize specific needs of this patient, which can suggest appropriate action. Paralleling his physical needs are the patient's needs for emotional support stemming from his concern about (1) his being able to breathe normally, (2) his ability to swallow, (3) his ability to speak, (4) his appearance, and (5) the prognosis.

After the endotracheal tube or airway has been removed and he has recovered from anesthesia, the Fowler position will help the patient to breathe more easily and he will be more comfortable. Signs of respiratory embarrassment, such as dyspnea, cyanosis, and changes in vital signs must be watched for, since they may suggest edema, throat irritation from the endotracheal tube, hemorrhage, or inadequate drainage. In this situation, the physician should be summoned.

Coughing is encouraged to remove secretions. In the sitting position, with the nurse supporting the neck with her hands, the patient may be able to bring up bothersome secretions; if this technique fails, he may have to be suctioned.

If drainage tubes are used in the wound, the surgeon may have applied pressure dressings to obliterate dead spaces and to provide immobilization. These may need to be reinforced from time to time. Dressings are observed for evidence of hemorrhage and constriction, which may affect respiration. Drains may be removed before the massive dressings are changed in about 5 days. Lighter dressings permit greater freedom of movement (Fig. 21-7).

With suction drainage (Hemovac), there is no need for pressure dressings because the skin flaps are drawn down tightly; approximately 80 to 120 ml. of serosanguineous secretions are drawn off by a portable suction unit the first day (Fig. 21-8). This amount diminishes thereafter. Aeroplast or other antiseptic plastic sprays protect the wound. The patient usually

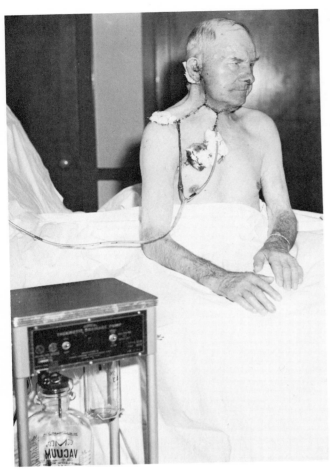

FIG. 21-8. This patient had a radical neck dissection as well as a parotidectomy for extensive parotid malignancy. To close the parotid incision, it was necessary to graft skin. The portable suction is drawing off sero-sanguineous secretions. The pressure dressings are covering skin grafts. (William R. Nelson, M.D.)

is allowed out of bed the first postoperative day.

Lower facial paralysis may occur due to injury of the facial nerve during the dissection, so this should be watched for and reported if noted. Likewise, if the superior laryngeal nerve is damaged, the patient may have difficulty with aspirating liquids and food because of the partial aesthesia of the glottis.

The person with extensive neck surgery often is sensitive about his appearance, when either the operative area is covered by bulky dressings or when an incision line is exposed as with Hemovac drainage. If the nurse accepts the patient and his appearance as he is and expresses a positive, optimistic attitude, the patient is more likely to be encouraged. In spite of the wide

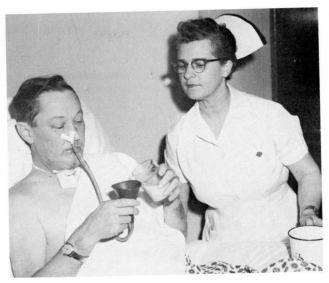

FIG. 21-9. Nasogastric tube feeding is being done by the patient who has had a radical neck dissection and tracheostomy. (William R. Nelson, M.D.)

removal of tissue, the cosmetic and functional defects are less than might be expected. The patient also needs an opportunity to voice his concerns regarding the success of the surgery and his prognosis. Most of these individuals are able to maintain and gain weight and are soon restored to economic independence. (When palliative care is necessary, the principles presented on p. 192 can be followed.)

CONDITIONS OF THE ESOPHAGUS

The esophagus is the mucus-lined tube that leads from the pharynx through the chest to the stomach.

Trauma

The esophagus is not an uncommon site of injury. Stab or bullet wounds of the neck and chest often produce such injury. Swallowed foreign bodies—dentures; fish bones, and so forth—may injure the esophagus as well as obstruct its lumen. Usually, foreign bodies can be removed with the aid of the esophagoscope. When the foreign body is made of metal, such as bobby and safety pins, needles, jacks, nails and tacks, it may not be safe to allow the object to make its slow way through the stomach and intestinal tract. Now available is a bar magnet that is fastened to a cable; the operator may turn the magnet ON or OFF as he directs it with the aid of fluoroscopy.* Consequently, it is possible to

* Luborsky, F. E., Drummon, B. J., and Pinta, A. Q.: Recent advances in the removal of magnetic foreign bodies from the esophagus, stomach, and duodenum with controllable permanent magnets. General Electric Research Laboratory. No. 64-RL-3595M, Feb. 1964.

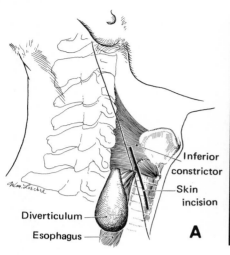

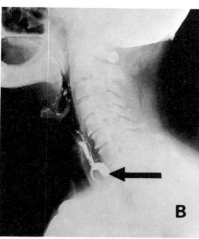

FIG. 21-10 (A). Diagram showing how diverticulum projects through the muscles of the upper portion of the pharynx. (B) Roentgenogram showing the appearance of an esophageal diverticulum. Note the retention of barium in the diverticulum.

maneuver the magnet and the object, e.g., a safety pin can be maneuvered so that the pin is withdrawn with the coiled section coming first rather than the sharp pin point. A skilled esophagoscopist can remove open safety pins through the esophagoscope. The injuries to the esophagus are the more serious part of the problem, because they may lead to deep cervical or mediastinal abscess or to stricture formations. Drainage of such abscesses requires a thoracic exposure.

Chemical Burns

The patient who accidentally or intentionally swallows a strong acid or base (such as lye) is emotionally

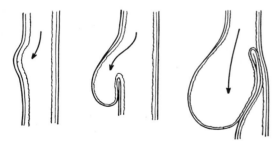

FIG. 21-11. Early, intermediate and late phases in the development of pharyngoesophageal diverticulum. When fully developed, the diverticulum is in a completely dependent position, and its orifice appears on esophagoscopy to be the continuation of the esophagus. At the same time, compression of the esophagus by the sac containing food and fluid compromises the distal esophageal orifice. It can be understood that the blind passage of a nasal tube or esophagoscopy, unless expertly performed, may result in perforation of the diverticulum. (Rhoads et al: Surgery, 4th ed., Phila., J. B. Lippincott, 1970.)

distraught as well as in acute physical pain. (Emergency treatment is discussed on p. 965.) Neutralization should be attempted and the patient treated immediately for shock and pain.

The acute chemical burn of the esophagus has associated severe burns of the lips, the mouth and the pharynx with pain on swallowing and, sometimes, difficulty in respiration due either to edema of the throat or a collection of mucus in the pharynx. The patient may be profoundly toxic. If he is able to swallow, fluids should be given in small quantities at a time. Secretions should be aspirated from the pharynx if respiration is embarrassed. The necessity for high fluid intake may require administration by parenteral means.

When the acute stage subsides, the patient may swallow normally for a time, but usually multiple stricture levels form in the esophagus. These may be dilated by the retrograde bouginage method of Tucker. A gastrostomy opening is made and a braided silk string is swallowed. One end is brought out through the gastrostomy opening and the other end through the nose. The 2 ends are tied together and form a complete loop. Dilatation is obtained by pulling larger and larger bougies upward through the esophagus by means of the string. It is important that this string be left in place at all times. The gastrostomy is kept open by means of a gastrostomy tube, through which feedings may be given if necessary. Dressings around this tube should be changed whenever soiled. The tube should be changed daily to prevent irritation about the wound. (See Gastrostomy, p. 610.)

The Patient with an Esophageal Diverticulum

A *diverticulum* of the esophagus is an outpouching of the wall of this structure, usually in the cervical region and on the posterior aspect (Figs. 21-10, 21-11).

FIG. 21-12. *(Top)* Minor surgical approach. Dilatation of the lower esophagus with rubber balloon technic in cases of cardiospasm (achalasia). The dilator is passed, guided by a previously swallowed thread, into the upper stomach. When the balloon is in proper position it is distended by pressure sufficient to dilate the narrowed area of the esophagus. (Olsen, Ellis and Creamer: Achalasia of the cardia, Am. J. Surg. 93:299-307)

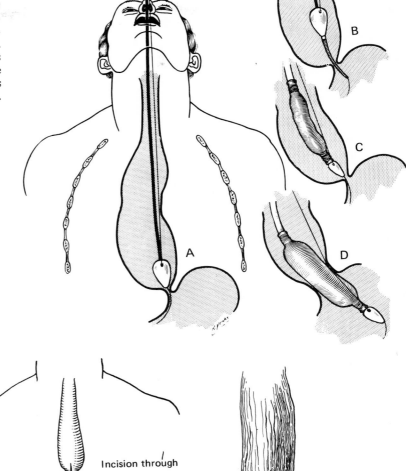

(Bottom) Major surgical approach. Treatment of achalasia. The esophagus is approached from in front on the left side. An incision is made through the muscularis of the esophagus sufficiently to allow a pouting of the esophageal mucosa. Separation of the muscular fibers relieves the narrowing at the lower end of the esophagus and permits the patient again to swallow normally.

Incision through muscle of constricted area

Esophageal mucosa pouting through incision in muscular wall

Esophageal hiatus

The patient first notices difficulty in swallowing, with fullness in the neck, and often he states that it feels as though his food stops before it reaches the stomach. He may complain of belching and gurgling. The diverticulum or pouch becomes filled with food or liquid; this is later regurgitated and may cause coughing by irritating the trachea. The food retained in the diverticulum tends to decompose, causing the breath to have a foul odor. Since the disease is progressive, the only means of cure is surgical removal of the diverticulum.

Medical and Nursing Management. To determine the exact nature and location of a diverticulum, roentgenograms using barium are done (Fig. 21-10). Esophagoscopy usually is contraindicated because of the danger of perforation of the diverticulum with resulting mediastinitis. Even the blind passing of a nasal tube should be avoided, and only guided into the stomach under direct vision of a lighted scope. Because this patient is often a victim of unbalanced diet and fluid levels, an evaluation of his nutritional state is done to determine dietary needs.

When a patient has difficulty in swallowing, it is usual to limit his diet to those foods that pass more easily. Blenderized meals supplemented with vitamins are usually ordered.

Some surgeons prefer to make a transverse cervical

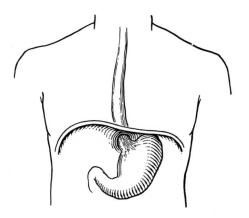

Normal position of
esophagus and stomach

Fig. 21-13. Anatomy of hiatal hernia of the two types. The sliding type of hernia with the short esophagus passes directly through the esophageal hiatus. In the para-esophageal type, the cardio-esophageal junction is in approximately its normal position, but a mass of the cardiac end of the stomach passes through the hiatal hernia beside the esophagus.

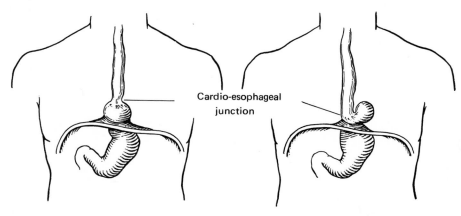

Cardio-esophageal
junction

Sliding hiatal hernia   Paraesophageal hiatal hernia

incision, but most commonly a vertical incision extending along the anterior border of the sternocleidomastoid muscle is made (Fig. 21-11). Care is taken to avoid undue trauma to the common carotid artery and internal jugular vein. The sac is dissected free and amputated flush with the esophageal wall. When the diverticulum occurs lower in the esophagus, it may be necessary to use a transthoracic approach, in which case the nursing management is similar to that described for chest operations (p. 258).

After operation, the nurse must feed the patient through a nasogastric tube that usually is inserted at the time of operation. The feedings may include any liquid, but a careful record of their kind, amount and character must be kept. After each feeding, the tube should be irrigated carefully with water. The wound also must be observed for evidences of leakage from the esophagus and a developing fistula.

Cardiospasm (Achalasia of the Cardia)

Cardiospasm or *achalasia* is a term used to denote benign stenosis of the lower end of the esophagus. This is usually associated with a lack of peristaltic activity in the esophagus itself and often with a failure of the cardiac sphincter of the stomach to open. Narrowing of the esophagus just above the stomach results in a gradually increasing dilatation of the esophagus in the upper chest, and the symptoms produced are those of difficulty in swallowing. The patient has a sensation of food sticking in the lower portion of the esophagus; as the condition progresses, regurgitation of the food is common, sometimes spontaneously and other times brought on by the patient because of the discomfort that is produced by the prolonged distention of the esophagus with food that will not pass into the stomach. The cause of this condition is believed to be a degeneration of the nerves that go to the involuntary muscles of the esophagus. Emotional upsets aggravate the problem. Cardiospasm is diagnosed by roentgenograms (Fig. 21-12) which show the marked dilatation of the upper esophagus and the narrowing of its lower end.

Medical and Nursing Management. The treatment of achalasia is divided into 2 parts: minor and major surgery. The minor surgical therapy, stretching of the narrowed area of the esophagus, is accomplished by the distension of a bag placed in this area through the mouth (Fig. 21-12). This bag (Plummer) is passed along a previously swallowed thread that leads into the stomach. Other dilating agents (bouginage) may be the use of French bougies or mercury-weighted dilators. Hydrostatic dilatation usually gives good results, but the dilatation required may result in a rupture of the esophagus in a small number of cases.

Major surgical treatment (Fig. 21-12) consists in a division of the muscular fibers that enclose the narrowed area of the esophagus, allowing the mucosa to pouch out through the divided area in the muscle layers. This permits food to be swallowed without obstruction, and the operation is used with very good results. The operation is spoken of as *esophagomyotomy* and is reserved usually for the later and more resistant lesions, whereas dilatation is more often practiced in early lesions. When the above operation is extended to include the cardiac end of the stomach, it is referred to as a *cardiomyotomy*. The incisional approach determines the nature of postoperative nursing care through the chest; the care is similar to the patient who has had a thoracotomy.

The Patient with Hiatus Hernia

The esophagus enters the abdomen through an opening in the diaphragm to empty, at its lower end, into the upper part of the stomach. The opening in the diaphragm normally encircles the esophagus tightly; therefore, the stomach lies within the abdomen completely. In a condition known as *hiatus* (or *hiatal*) *hernia*, the opening in the diaphragm through which the esophagus passes becomes enlarged, and part of the upper stomach tends to come up into the lower portion of the thorax. This complication may be present in many patients without giving any symptoms, but there is often a feeling of fullness in the lower chest and a splashing sound noted in the substernal area in patients in whom the hiatal hernia is large. In addition, the gastric juice produced by the stomach mucosa tends to be loculated in the portion of the stomach above the diaphragm, and for this reason ulcerations and bleeding occur in this group of patients. Finally, the erosive action of the gastric juice on the stomach and the lower esophagus may produce a condition known as esophagitis, with

the production of pain and discomfort in the substernal area.

All of these symptoms produce an uncomfortable and often very ill patient if bleeding is a factor.

Medical and Nursing Management. In those hernias that are found incidentally in the x-ray examination (Fig. 21-13) and that do not produce symptoms, no treatment is necessary. Many of these hernias are of the sliding type in which the stomach tends to extend into the chest when the patient is lying down, but it goes back into the abdomen when the patient is erect (Fig. 21-13). In those patients in whom the hernia is present constantly, and even in the sliding type of hernia in patients who are symptomatic, surgical correction of the abnormality is necessary. The stomach is replaced into the abdomen and the enlarged esophageal opening is made smaller so that the stomach cannot extend above the diaphragm. This operation may be performed from the abdomen, in which case the stomach is pulled down and the crura of the diaphragm are brought together behind the esophagus. Otherwise, the operation may be performed through the left chest, separating the ribs. The esophagus is identified and the herniated portion of the stomach is pulled down into the abdomen, and again the esophageal opening in the diaphragm narrowed by sutures from above.

The immediate postoperative care of these patients is that used for any thoracotomy or laparotomy. In patients with thoracotomy a chest tube is often introduced, which is placed in underwater drainage or suction. The drain is usually taken out in a day or two, after the lung has completely expanded. The patient is given fluids and food on the second or third day after operation, and gradually increasing amounts of food are given as tolerated by the patient. In some individuals, edema at the site where the esophagus passes through the diaphragmatic hiatus may cause some delay in food intake for a time, but usually this subsides without incidence in 2 or 3 days.

The Patient with Esophageal Varices

Varices of the lower esophagus are really a secondary manifestation of cirrhosis of the liver. This subject is discussed on p. 523.

The Patient with Cancer of the Esophagus

Recognition and Diagnosis. Two per cent of all cancer deaths in the United States are due to cancer of the esophagus; approximately 80 per cent occur in men and most involve the middle third of the esophagus. Chronic trauma such as produced by the frequent use of alcohol, tobacco, spicy food and poor mouth hygiene appear to be underlying factors. In the Orient, the drinking of large quantities of very hot tea is suspected

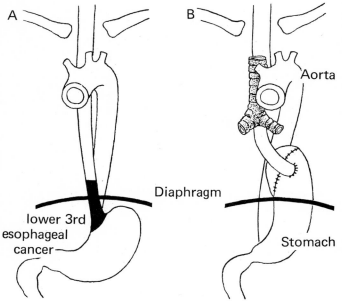

FIG. 21-14. (A) Black portion of esophagus indicates carcinoma. (B) Relations of the viscera after resection of a carcinoma of the lower fourth of the thoracic segment and the abdominal segment of the esophagus. The proximal esophagus is relatively long and a large segment of the stomach, including the lesser curvature, the cardia and the fundus, has been resected. The anastomosis lies in the lower portion of the mediastinum.

of contributing to the high incidence of esophageal malignancy.

The patient is first aware of intermittent and increasing difficulty in swallowing. At first only solid food gives trouble but, as the growth progresses and the obstruction becomes more complete, even liquids cannot pass into the stomach. Regurgitation of food and saliva occur, hemorrhage may take place and there is a progressive loss of weight and strength due to starvation. Later symptoms include substernal pain, hiccough, respiratory difficulty and foul breath.

The diagnosis is confirmed by x-ray examination and by esophagoscopy. Bronchoscopy usually is performed also, especially in tumors of the middle and the upper third of the esophagus, to determine whether the trachea has been involved by the tumor and to help in determining whether the lesion can be removed.

Surgical Management. Surgical removal of the growth is the only hope of cure. This can be accomplished by an approach through the thorax or through the abdomen and the thorax for lower esophageal lesions. The portion of the esophagus containing the growth is removed, and the continuity of the gastrointestinal tract is reformed by bringing the stomach into the chest and implanting the proximal end of the

esophagus into it (Fig. 21-14). The chest is closed after insertion in the pleural cavity of a drain that is led under water or is attached to a suction apparatus.

Lesions in the middle and the upper thirds of the esophagus, particularly, are often not suitable for surgical excision. However, in some clinics success has been reported in which a tunnel is created beneath the sternum and a resected segment of either jejunum or colon replaces the diseased esophagus. A palliative procedure in which a plastic tube is introduced through a cervical incision has been done with resultant symptomatic relief, improvement in nutrition and amelioration of psychological symptoms.

Radiation is used in some clinics before surgery; in others, it is used after surgery. The ideal method of treating this problem has not yet been found; each patient is approached in a way that appears best for him. If the growth is found to be inoperable either before or at operation, a gastrostomy often is performed as a palliative procedure to permit the administration of food and fluids (see p. 469).

The high mortality rate among patients with cancer of the esophagus is due to 3 factors. (1) Usually this is an older patient in whom the incidence of pulmonary and cardiovascular disorders is high. (2) Before significant symptoms occur the tumor has already invaded surrounding structures. It is impossible to excise a liberal area of tissue because of the proximity of vital structures. (3) The malignancy tends to spread to nearby lymph nodes, and the unique relation of the esophagus to the heart and lungs makes these organs easily accessible to the extension of the tumor. In several series of operative cases 45 to 80 per cent showed evidence of metastasis when examined in the operating room.

Nursing. The principles of nursing management are similar to those given the patient having a radical neck dissection. (p. 439).

BIBLIOGRAPHY

Dental

American Dental Association: Dental Health Facts for Teachers. 1966.

American Dental Association: Fluoridation Facts. Answers to Criticisms of Fluoridation. 1967.

Haas, R. L.: The case for fluoridation. Amer. J. Nurs., 66:328-331, Feb., 1966.

Ramfjord, S. P.: Epidemiological studies of periodontal diseases, Amer. J. Pub. Health, 58:1713-1722, Sept., 1968.

Screiber, F. C.: Dental care for long-term patient. Amer. J. Nurs., 64:84-86, Feb., 1964.

Stanley, M. K., and Bader, P.: Adult teeth can be straightened. Amer. J. Nurs., 62:94-97, Feb., 1962.

Tank, G., and Storvick, C. A.: Caries experience of children. II. Relation of fluorides to hypoplasia, malocclusion and gingivitis. J. Amer. Dent. Assoc., 70:100-104, Jan., 1965.

Parotid Gland

Frazell, E. L., Strong, E. W., and Newcombe, B.: Tumors of the parotid. Amer. J. Nurs., *66*:2702-2708, Dec., 1966.

Martin, H.: Surgical removal of parotid tumors. Ciba Clin. Symposia, *13*:121-131, Oct.-Nov.-Dec., 1961.

Work, W. P.: Therapy of salivary gland tumors. Arch. Otolaryng., *83*:89-91, Feb., 1966.

Facial Injury

Robinson, M., and Van Volkenburgh, S. T.: Intermaxillary fixation: immediate postoperative care. Amer. J. Nurs., *63*:71-72, Jan., 1963.

Weiss, L., and Weiss, E.: Facial injuries and nursing care. Amer. J. Nurs., *65*:96-100, Feb., 1965.

Mouth

Andrews, M. S.: Mr. F—His face and his family. Nursing in Relation to the Impact of Illness Upon the Family. Amer. Nurses Assn., *2*:34-42, 1962.

Cahn, L. R., and Slaughter, D. P.: Oral cancer, a monograph for the dentist. New York, American Cancer Society, 1962.

Farr, H. W., and Hislop, R.: Cancer of the tongue and nursing care of patients with mouth or throat cancer. Amer. J. Nurs., *57*:1314-1319, Oct., 1957.

Guyton, A. C.: The sense of taste. *In* Textbook of Medical Physiology, ed. 3, pp. 760-765. Philadelphia, W. B. Saunders, 1966.

Nicholl, M.: A patient with cancer of the tongue. Amer. J. Nurs., *63*:132-133, Sept., 1963.

Redman, B. K., and Redman, R. S.: Oral care of the critically ill patient. *In* Bergersen: Current Concepts in Clinical Nursing. pp. 107-118. St. Louis, C. V. Mosby, 1967.

Taritano, J. J., Wooten, J. W., and Taritano, P. N.: Nursing care after oral surgery. Amer. J. Nurs., *69*:1493-1496, July, 1969.

Neck Surgery

Hamm, W. G.: Nursing care in surgery of the head and neck. Nurs. Clin. N. Amer., *2*:475-481, Sept., 1967.

MacComb, W. S., and Fletcher, G. H.: Cancer of the head and neck. Baltimore, Williams & Wilkins, 1967.

Martin, H.: Radical neck dissection. Ciba Clin. Symposia, Oct.-Nov.-Dec., 1961.

Newcombe, B.: Care of the patient with head and neck cancer. Nurs. Clin. N. Amer., *2*:599-607, Dec., 1967.

Zavertnik, J. J.: Emotional support of patients with head and neck surgery. Nurs. Clin. N. Amer., *2*:503-510, Sept., 1967.

Esophagus

Burge, J. P., and Ochsner, J. L.: Management of esophageal tumors. Surg. Clin. N. Amer., *46*:1457-1467, Dec., 1966.

Passos, J. Y.: Esophageal perforation, a case study. Amer. J. Nurs., *65*:73-76, May, 1965.

PATIENT EDUCATION

American Dental Association
211 East Chicago Ave.
Chicago, Illinois 60611
>Your New Dentures. 1965.
>Immediate Dentures. 1963.
>Toothbrushing. (Folder) 1965.

Dept. of Health, Education, and Welfare
U.S. Government Printing Office
Superintendent of Documents
Washington, D.C. 20402
>Pyorrhea and Other Gum Diseases. 1967.
>Oral Cancer Control. 1966.

American Cancer Society
219 East 42nd Street
New York, New York 10017
>Oral Cancer Examination Procedure

CHAPTER **22**

Patients with Gastric and Intestinal Problems

- *General Considerations and Patient Evaluation*
- *Problems Related to the Stomach and Duodenum*
- *Problems Involving the Small and the Large Bowel*

GENERAL CONSIDERATIONS AND PATIENT EVALUATION

Scope of Nursing Patients with Gastrointestinal Disorders

Abnormalities of the gastrointestinal tract are numerous and exemplify every type of major pathology that has been described in connection with other organ systems. Congenital, inflammatory, infectious, traumatic and neoplastic lesions have been encountered in every portion and at every site along its 25-foot length. In common with many other organ systems, it is subject to circulatory disturbances, faulty nervous control and senescence.

Quite apart from the multiplicity of organic diseases to which the gastrointestinal tract is heir, there are many extrinsic factors—some related to disease, others not—which can interfere with its normal functions and produce symptoms duplicating those of intrinsic gastrointestinal disease. An anxiety state, for example, often finds its chief expression in the syndrome of functional indigestion or motor disturbance of the intestine. Moreover, certain organic diseases have been ascribed to emotional imbalances. Peptic ulcer and chronic ulcerative colitis, for example, have been explained on a psychogenic basis by many observers. Such diseases are commonly referred to as "psychosomatic" disorders,

a term that underlines, so to speak, the importance of the mind-body relationship in the pathogenesis. Regarding the importance of this relationship there can be no doubt, because regardless of the fundamental etiology, the severity, course and outcome of these conditions are influenced greatly by the mental health of the patient.

The nurse should be thoroughly cognizant of the relation between the level of her patient's mood and his appetite and bowel function, and between his sensory awareness and the manner in which he interprets sensations. She must also recognize the importance of her own attitude toward the patient and his complaints as an influential factor capable of modifying his symptoms in either direction. Her display of genuine tolerance and sympathetic interest toward the patient is often the key to his cooperation, and if that is obtained the major obstacle to therapeutic success has been removed.

The Function of the Gastrointestinal Tract

The gastrointestinal canal is a tube, about 25 feet in length, through which the food passes and is subjected to the action of various digestive fluids and enzymes. All solid food, to get within the body, must first be liquefied, because only liquids can be absorbed into the blood vessels and the lymphatics in the stomach and the intestine.

Constituents of food, even though in liquid form, in most cases must first be modified chemically before they can be absorbed.

Carbohydrates. Although our daily diet contains many different sugars and starches, practically the only carbohydrate that the tissue cells utilize as fuel is glucose (dextrose), of which there is little in our food. Therefore, all ingested carbohydrates, if they are to be used, first must be changed into glucose. The bulk of the carbohydrate in fruits and vegetables is in the form of starch, although the riper, the softer and the sweeter these foods are, the more of their carbohydrates are in sugar form—because the plants store their carbohydrates in the form of starches and, like the human body, transform them into sugar before they metabolize them. All starches, which are relatively insoluble, must be changed into sugars before they are absorbed. All the complex sugars first must be broken down to simple sugars, like glucose, levulose and galactose, and all of these must be converted or "inverted" into glucose.

Fats. Most of the fats in our food are liquid at body temperature but are insoluble in water. All fats are combinations of glycerin and various fatty acids. This combination is split up by digestion. The glycerin thus set free is easily absorbed as such, while the fatty acids promptly unite with alkalies to form true soaps, which likewise are absorbed easily. Most of our food fat, however, is not split thus, but instead is divided by the action of the bile salts into microscopic globules. In other words, it is emulsified, and emulsions as well as solutions are able to pass through the intestinal mucous membrane into the lymphatic vessels.

Proteins. These are complex materials that are not absorbed until they have been split into single fatty acids, glucose and amino acids, all of which are absorbed readily. Having passed through the mucous membrane of the intestinal wall, many are resynthesized into complex compounds. The glycerin and fatty acids may be reunited to form fats of a different character, and the amino acid products of protein digestion, circulating in the blood, are resynthesized into the particular proteins of which the body cells are composed.

Oral Digestion

All foods are prepared for digestion in the mouth, and starch digestion actually begins there. The solid foods are ground into pulp by the teeth, which makes gastric digestion easier; and in the mouth food is mixed with saliva containing ptyalin, an enzyme that initiates starch digestion. The food may be in the mouth for but a few seconds, but this salivary digestion continues until the acid of the gastric juice has destroyed the ptyalin. Foods should be well masticated. There is much truth in the old proverb that "food well chewed is half digested," for the smaller the particles of meat and vegetables that are swallowed, the more accessible is the food to the digestive juices. Moreover, thorough mastication is desirable because it stimulates the secretion of gastric juice.

Swallowing. A complex motor act involving highly coordinated contractions of the tongue and the pharynx, swallowing propels the food from the mouth into the esophagus.

The Esophagus

The esophagus is a muscular tube about 9 inches long, equipped with both circular and longitudinal muscle fibers. It conducts the ingested material into the stomach, wavelike contractions of its wall expressing its contents into the gastric reservoir.

The Stomach

The stomach is a distensible pouch situated between the esophagus and the duodenum. During a meal it distends to become a large hollow receptacle capable of holding about 1,500 ml. The organ is situated in the upper abdomen, almost entirely on the left side of the body, for the most part tucked away beneath the ribs. The lesser curvature, or upper margin, of the stomach is 7.6-15.2 cm. (3 to 6 inches) long. The greater curvature is considerably longer, its length depending on the degree of gastric distention. At its widest point the stomach, when full, measures 10.2-12.7 cm. (4 to 5 inches). There are two orifices to the stomach: the cardiac orifice (inlet), and the pylorus (outlet). Both orifices are ringed with muscle tissue by which they can be closed.

Gastric Juice. The gastric mucosa secretes each day several hundred milliliters of a clear, colorless liquid, the function of which is to start the digestion of the food proteins. Gastric juice contains *pepsin,* an enzyme that splits and dissolves proteins; *hydrochloric acid,* necessary for this peptic digestion; and *rennin,* the effect of which is to clot milk and thereby prevent its absorption before it has been digested properly by the intestinal enzymes.

Gastric secretion normally is stimulated in 1 of 2 ways: (1) through the nervous system, and (2) by chemical substances from the food that are absorbed into the gastrointestinal mucosa. The earlier stimulus of secretion is psychic; it is a response to the odor, the appearance and the taste of appetizing food. When we do not enjoy our food, or when we are under some mental stress, the secretion of gastric juice is inhibited and digestion gets a bad start. Equally important in the secretion of gastric juice is stimulation by a hormone, *gastrin.* This hormone is produced by the mucosa of the antrum, and is carried by the bloodstream to the acid-pepsin producing cells of the body of the stomach. Gastrin is produced when the antrum is distended with food and by certain products of protein digestion.

Practically no food is absorbed in the stomach; all is passed on into the duodenum, there to become exposed and acted on by the pancreatic juice and the bile.

The Duodenum

The duodenum is a muscular tube about 30.48 cm. (12 inches) long and forms the upper end of the small intestine. The stomach communicates with the duodenum through the pylorus. The common bile duct and the pancreatic duct enter the duodenum at a point 8 to 10 cm. below the pylorus.

The first food swallowed enters an empty stomach. At once the pylorus closes tightly. If the proper stimulus is present, the walls of the stomach soon begin to pour out gastric juice, and a gentle churning movement (gastric peristalsis) begins, the effect of which is to mix the food thoroughly with the juice. As the mass of food is pressed toward the pylorus, the liquid portion (chyle) is allowed to enter the duodenum, but the food that is still solid is retained in the stomach until it is liquefied by the mechanical action of peristalsis and the chemical effects of the gastric juice. This process normally requires 1 to 6 hours. If, at the end of a few hours, any solid masses of food remain, they are forced on, through the pylorus, by powerful expulsive stomach contractions.

Pancreatic Juice. The pancreatic duct opens into the duodenum approximately 10 cm. distal to the pylorus. Through this duct is secreted a digestive juice containing three enzymes: *trypsin, lipase* (steapsin) and *amylase* (amylopsin). Trypsin is a powerful proteolytic enzyme that digests proteins more rapidly and completely than pepsin. In contrast with pepsin, trypsin acts, not in an acid, but in an alkaline medium. It is manufactured in the pancreas as *trypsinogen,* which has no digestive power—otherwise, the pancreas and its duct would themselves be digested. It acquires its potency in contact with the mucous membrane of the duodenum, owing to another enzyme, *enterokinase. Amylase* is practically the same as the ptyalin of saliva. Its function is to break down starches and complicated sugars in food to the simple sugars: glucose, levulose, etc. *Lipase* is an enzyme that splits fat into its 2 components, glycerin and fatty acids. In childhood, the pancreatic juice also contains lactase, important in the digestion of milk sugar.

Bile. This liquid, which is secreted by the liver, also enters the duodenum at this point. Many of its constituents are waste products, no longer of use to the body, but bile also contains alkalies, which help to neutralize the acid from the stomach and to form soluble soaps from the fatty acids that are liberated from food fats as a result of the action of lipase. The bile salts are important in the emulsification and absorption of fats and fat-soluble vitamins from the intestine. Bile is formed almost continuously, but most of it is formed during digestion. Some of it is stored in concentrated form in the gallbladder, which serves as a reserve tank. It probably is this stored bile that enters the duodenum first when intestinal digestion begins.

The Intestine

The intestine is a muscular tube, approximately 6 m. (20 ft.) long, extending from the pylorus to the anus. The first 30.48 cm. (12 in.) beyond the pylorus comprise the duodenum, which has been discussed. The proximal two fifths of the small intestine beyond the duodenum is called the *jejunum,* the lower three fifths, the *ileum.* The ileum opens into the colon or large bowel, and just below this juncture of ileum and colon, at a point that is protected by the ileocecal valve, the *vermiform appendix* is connected.

Enzyme Action. Along the whole length of the small intestine is secreted a fluid containing several enzymes, the function of which is to complete the chemical process of digestion. These include *enterokinase,* already mentioned as the activator of trypsinogen; *secretin,* the substance that stimulates the pancreas to secrete its digestive juice; *erepsin,* which completes the enzymatic breakdown of proteins that was initiated by pepsin and trypsin; and a carbohydrate-splitting enzyme for each simple sugar: *maltase,* to invert maltose into dextrose; *invertase* for the inversion of cane sugar into dextrose and levulose; and *lactase* to convert milk sugar into dextrose.

Thorough mixing of the chyle—the liquefied food masses—with the digestive fluid is accomplished by rhythmic peristaltic contractions of the muscular intestinal wall that split up the masses and churn them repeatedly for several minutes in small segments of the bowel. At intervals during this process, the chyle is propelled onward through the intestine by peristaltic waves running longitudinally along its entire length. One layer of muscle fibers of the intestinal wall is arranged as a ring around the bowel lumen; when this contracts, the lumen is constricted. Another layer of fibers runs parallel with the lumen; when this contracts, the intestinal loop is shortened. These 2 movements, passing in orderly succession down the bowel and coordinated so that they push its contents along, are called *peristaltic waves.*

As the digested material courses through the small intestine, the utilizable portion is absorbed through its lining and enters the lymph vessels and the blood vessels in the wall of the intestine. The mucous membrane lining the bowel wall is thrown into folds and has a surface much like velvet, being covered completely with fingerlike processes known as *villi,* which

TERMINOLOGY AND TOPOGRAPHY

Before studying about patients with specific gastrointestinal problems and operations, the nurse should be familiar with the prefixes denoting abdominal organs and the suffixes used to denote the diseases of or operations on these organs.

Suffixes used to denote the names of diseases and operations are:

itis—inflammation of—as *appendicitis*, an inflammation of the appendix.

otomy—to make a cut into—as *gastrotomy*, to make an opening into the stomach.

ostomy—to make a mouth or opening into—as *cystostomy*, to insert a tube into the urinary bladder.

ectomy—to cut or remove—as *salpingectomy*, to remove the fallopian tube.

pexy—to sew up in position—as *nephropexy*, to sew the kidney up in position.

orrhaphy—to repair a defect—as *herniorrhaphy*, to repair a hernial defect.

plasty—to improve by changing the position of the tissue—as *pyloroplasty*, an operation to enlarge the pyloric opening of the stomach.

(See also the appendix.)

Organs	Prefix	
Stomach	Gastr	*Gastritis*—inflammation of stomach
Pylorus	Pylor	*Pylorectomy*—removal of pyloric end of stomach
Liver	Hepa	*Hepatitis*—inflammation of liver
Gallbladder	Cholecyst	*Cholecystitis*—inflammation of gallbladder
Common bile duct	Choledoch	*Choledochitis*—inflammation of common bile duct
Small intestine	Enter	*Enteritis*—inflammation of intestine
Colon	Col	*Colitis*—inflammation of large colon
Appendix	Appendic	*Appendicitis*—inflammation of appendix
Urinary bladder	Cyst	*Cystitis*—inflammation of urinary bladder
Fallopian tube	Salping	*Salpingitis*—inflammation of fallopian tube
Ovary	Oophor	*Oophoritis*—inflammation of ovary
Pelvis of kidney	Pyel	*Pyelitis*—inflammation of pelvis of kidney
Kidney	Nephr	*Nephritis*—inflammation of kidney
Rupture	Herni	*Herniorrhaphy*—repair of hernia
Loin or abdomen	Lapar	*Laparotomy*—incision in the abdomen

Abdominal Topography. For purposes of convenience in description, the abdomen has been divided into nine regions by imaginary lines, as illustrated in Figure 22-1A.

The abdominal cavity normally contains a small amount of fluid that lubricates the peritoneal surfaces. This cavity is lined with a thin, glistening membrane called the *peritoneum*. This structure covers all the abdominal organs, forming folds between which the coils of intestine are located. Some organs (such as the liver, the pancreas, the kidney and the urinary bladder) are not covered completely by peritoneum; hence inflammations of these structures may not always involve the general abdominal cavity but may develop into retroperitoneal extensions or abscesses.

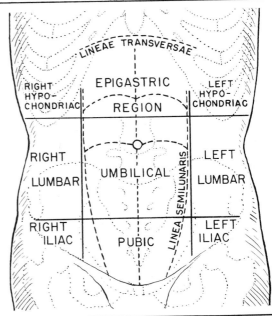

FIG. 22-1A. Regions of the abdomen.

vastly increase its absorbing surface. By the time the chyle reaches the ileocecal valve, practically all that is of value has been absorbed. That which is left is the indigestible part of the food, consisting largely of cellulose, some of the constituents of the bile and the intestinal fluids, many epithelial cells thrown off from the intestinal wall and, finally, vast numbers of the bacteria that grow in the intestine, eventually comprising at least one fifth of the solid feces.

The colon is about 1.5 m. (5 feet) long. It starts as a pouch, called the *cecum,* into the side of which the ileum and the appendix open. It then ascends upward toward the liver as the *ascending colon,* crosses the abdomen as the *transverse colon,* descends into the left flank as the *descending colon* and terminates in a short curve, called the *sigmoid flexure,* which leads into the rectum.

The colon receives the liquid residue of intestinal digestion at the ileocecal valve. Its chief function is the absorption of fluid from the residue. Thus, as the fecal contents of the colon pass from the right to the left colon and thence to the sigmoid and rectum, they become at first a soft mushy mass, and finally a formed stool.

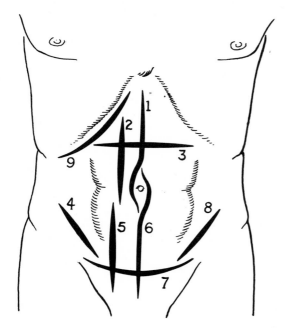

Fig. 22-1B. Diagram to show the various abdominal incisions which are used. (1) Upper midline incision. (2) Upper right rectus incision. (3) Transverse incision in the upper abdomen. (4) Gridiron incision on the right. (5) Lower right rectus incision. (6) Lower midline incision. (7) Pfannenstiel incision. (8) Left gridiron incision. (9) Subcostal incision.

Abdominal Incisions and Operative Procedures

Incisions

Laparotomy or *abdominal section* are terms used to describe any operation that involves opening the abdominal cavity. The gridiron or the McBurney incision (Fig. 22-1B) is the simplest. It opens the abdomen through a small wound made by spreading the fibers of the muscles through which it passes. This incision is suitable especially for operations upon the appendix, and, as it has the advantage of being closed without tension, it makes a firm wound in which hernias rarely form.

More widely useful, however, are the vertical incisions made in the midline or to either side of it. These are made to pass between or through the rectus muscles. Many other types of incisions may be made, depending on the preference of the surgeon.

Operative Procedures

In making abdominal incisions, the wound always is protected from skin contamination by the fastening of towels, gauze sponges or plastic material to its edge. Bleeding points are caught and ligated as they appear, and the tissues are divided layer by layer as they are encountered.

In all operations on the gastrointestinal tract, the surgeon makes an opening into a tube filled with many kinds of bacterial life. Because of the highly acid juices of the stomach, the upper intestine and the stomach are believed to contain less bacteria than the lower. Nevertheless, whenever the intestinal tract is opened, there is danger of the spread of infection from it into the peritoneal cavity unless strict precautions are taken. Moist sponges are placed round the portion through which the incision is to be made, and all tissues not directly implicated in the operation are covered as completely as possible. Rubber- or plastic-covered clamps may be placed on the intestine in order to prevent the escape of its contents. When the incision in the intestine has been made, the contents of the opened loop are sponged out and the sponges are discarded.

When the openings in the intestines have been closed, all instruments, needles, sutures, scissors and so forth that have been used are removed from the operating table. Soiled sponges are discarded after the suture line has been mopped off with moist gauze, and fresh sterile towels or covers are placed about the operative field. The surgeon's gloves and those of his assistants should be changed before the operation is continued.

These precautions are taken in every gastrointestinal operation and are observed rigidly in operations on the large intestine, where infection is found most commonly. Closure is made in the reverse order, and each layer is united accurately until the wound has been closed. As a general rule, sutures are not placed in fat or muscles, but only in the firm aponeurotic layers, which are able to hold the wound closed until healing has taken place. Reinforcing, "stay" or tension sutures of heavy silk or wire often are employed to give added strength and to prevent the formation of dead space in the wound.

The Role of the Nurse in Gastrointestinal Diagnosis

One of the most interesting aspects of gastroenterology is the problem of clinical diagnosis in patients with digestive complaints. Part of the diagnostic difficulty arises from the fact that, despite the large array of etiologic possibilities, the number of symptoms referable to the digestive system that are distinctive and of diagnostic value is surprisingly limited; dysphagia, anorexia, nausea, vomiting, hematemesis, melena, constipation, diarrhea and abdominal pain comprise practically the entire list. Therefore, unusual importance attaches to the precise quality of each symptom presented, its mode of onset, its duration, the timing of its recurrences, its relation to meals and other events and the character of associated symptoms.

The observant, well-informed nurse can contribute materially to the diagnosis in many cases of digestive-tract disease and in most cases with functional disturbances of the gastrointestinal tract, for she is in an admirable position to observe and discuss with the patient those symptoms that are potentially so informative.

Given the proper tools, the correct diagnostic approach and the expert collaboration of the nurse, the physician usually can establish a diagnosis. Correct gastroenterologic diagnoses are rewarding indeed, for in no other category of disease is correct treatment more urgently required, and in none are opportunities for benefit or cure so numerous.

Because of the elusive nature of many gastrointestinal disorders, the patient under investigation is likely to be subjected to a battery of complicated tests. Of course a complete history and physical examination are carried out. The tests may include repeated roentgenographic studies after the ingestion and the rectal instillation of barium, the collection and the examination of numerous stool specimens, intubation of the stomach or the small bowel and aspiration of their contents, and usually one or more endoscopic procedures as well.

Preparation of the patient for each gastrointestinal roentgenologic study involves fasting, catharsis, retention enemas and colonic irrigations. His muscles sore from lying on many hard, narrow examining tables, with "gas pains" from hunger, tired and probably anxious, the patient may have a few new complaints to impart after his rigorous work-up, and small wonder!

Each examination should be explained carefully to the patient in advance. During the procedure he expects and deserves the full attention of the attending doctor and nurse, whose conversation should be calculated to alleviate his anxiety and elicit his full cooperation.

Roentgenography of the Upper Gastrointestinal Tract

The entire gastrointestinal tract can be delineated by x-rays following the introduction of barium sulfate as the contrast medium. This material, a tasteless, odorless, nongranular and completely insoluble (hence, not absorbable) powder, is ingested in the form of a thick or thin aqueous suspension for purposes of upper gastrointestinal tract study ("upper G.I. series") and is instilled rectally for visualization of the colon ("barium enema"). For purposes of examining the upper gastrointestinal tract, the fasting patient is required to swallow barium under direct fluoroscopic examination. As the contrast medium descends into the stomach, the position, patency and caliber of the esophagus are visualized, enabling the examiner to detect or exclude any anatomic or functional derangement of that organ. He is able to make an important observation relating to the heart, namely, the presence or the absence of right atrial involvement. An enlarged right atrium invariably impinges on the esophagus, revealed by the resulting pressure defect in the esophagus.

The roentgenographic appearance of the lower esophagus after a swallow of thick barium suspension enables detection of esophageal varices, a manifestation of liver cirrhosis. Fluoroscopic examination extends next to the stomach, as its lumen fills with barium. The motility and the thickness of the gastric wall and the mucosal pattern are observed for evidence of spasms, ulcerations, malignant infiltrates and other anatomic abnormalities, including pressure defects from without. The patency of the pyloric valve and the anatomy of the duodenum are also observed under the fluoroscope, with particular reference to possible ulceration of the mucosa, spasm of the wall or displacement of the structure as a whole by a tumor in the adjacent area.

During the fluoroscopic examination, roentgenograms are exposed in order to obtain a permanent record of the findings. Additional roentgenograms are taken at intervals, for as long as 24 hours thereafter, as a means of estimating the rate of gastric emptying and the degree of small bowel motility. A truly detailed study of the small intestine involves the continuous infusion, through a duodenal tube, of 500 to 1,000 ml. of a thin barium sulfate suspension. This is carried out as a separate procedure. The barium column fills the intestinal loops and is observed continuously by fluoroscope and filmed at frequent intervals as it progresses through the jejunum and the ilium.

The following are the nursing specifications that are applicable in connection with the G.I. series:

(1) The patient is to receive nothing by mouth after 12 o'clock midnight prior to the test.

(2) During this interim, the patient is to receive no purgative, however mild, and no other medication unless specifically ordered.

(3) Breakfast and the noonday meal are to be omitted on the day of the test.

(4) The evening meal may be offered and nourishment provided until midnight.

(5) After midnight the patient is to resume fasting. Nothing is permitted by mouth after midnight on the second day of the test until the final roentgenogram is taken.

(6) Breakfast is again held on the second day of the test and the patient remains in the fasting state until the last roentgenogram is taken.

Roentgenography of the Colon (Barium Enema)

As the first step in an x-ray study of the colon, the fasting patient receives a rectal instillation of a barium sulfate suspension, which is viewed in the fluoroscope and then filmed. If the patient has been prepared satisfactorily, with the colonic contents having been evacuated completely by enemas, the contour of the entire colon, including cecum and appendix (if patent), is clearly visible and the motility of each portion readily observed.

The following orders may be specified for the patient who is to be prepared for barium enema:

(1) A saline enema is administered early in the preceding evening.

(2) Saline enemas are repeated until returns are clear.

(3) The patient is to receive nothing by mouth after midnight.

(4) Two hours after completion of the x-ray study, the patient is to receive an oil retention enema.

(5) This is followed 2 hours later by saline clearing enemas.

(6) On the following day, the oil retention enemas are again administered to assure adequate evacuation of the barium suspension.

Barium Double Contrast Enema. Examination of the colonic mucosa for detailed inspection of small lesions may be carried out by insufflating the lower gastrointestinal tract with air immediately following spontaneous evacuation of the barium enema.

Barium predisposes to constipation and eventually fecal impaction, the prevention of which is a very important consideration in the care of any patient who is undergoing these studies.

Stool Examination and Gastric Analysis

Examination of the Stool. The basic examination of the stool includes an inspection of the specimen for its amount, consistency and color, and a screening test for melena. Special tests indicated in specific cases may include tests for fecal urobilinogen, fat, nitrogen, parasites, food residues and other substances.

The color of stools varies from light to dark brown, depending largely on the urobilin content. (Milk-fed infants pass stools that are golden-yellow in color, due to unchanged bilirubin.) Various foods and medications affect stool color as follows: meat protein produces a dark brown coloration; spinach, a green hue; carrots and beets, red; cocoa, dark red or brown; senna and santonin, a yellowish hue; calomel, green; bismuth, iron and charcoal, black; and barium, a milky-white appearance. Blood in sufficient quantities, if shed into the upper gastrointestinal tract, produces a tarry black color; blood entering the lower portion, or passing rapidly through the gastrointestinal tract, will appear bright or dark red. Even considerable quantities of hemoglobin may fail to produce a distinctive color, in which event it is termed "occult blood."

The stools in cases of steatorrhea are generally bulky, greasy, foamy, foul in odor and gray in color with a silvery sheen. The "acholic" stool of the patient with biliary obstruction is light gray or "clay-colored," due to the absence of urobilin.

Mucus or pus may be visible on gross inspection of the stool in cases of chronic ulcerative colitis (p. 483) or other ulcerative lesions of the lower bowel. Patients with constipation, obstipation or fecal impaction may pass small, dry, rocky-hard masses called "scybala." Their passage may traumatize the rectal mucosa sufficiently to cause hemorrhage, in which case these masses are streaked with red blood.

Tests for Melena. The most common stool tests are based on the benzidine, gum guaiac or the orthotolidin reaction. A recent form of the guaiac test is the Hemoccult test. A dry paper slide is used on which the stool specimen is smeared. The slide comes in an envelope that can be mailed if needed and examined later.

Gastric Analysis. Examination of the gastric juice offers means of estimating the secretory activity of the gastric mucosa and of ascertaining the presence or the degree of gastric retention in cases of patients suspected of having pyloric or duodenal obstruction. A diagnosis of pernicious anemia (p. 307) is excluded by the finding of acid, and a diagnosis of gastric carcinoma may be established by the discovery of cancer cells in the gastric juice.

The fasting patient is intubated through a nostril with a Levin duodenal tube, a small rubber tube with catheter tip marked at points 45, 55, 65 and 75 cm.

FIG. 22-2. Patient having gastroscopy. Note the extreme flexibility of the tube with the patient in the sitting position. (Adapted from McNeer, G., and Pack, G. T.: Neoplasms of the Stomach. Philadelphia, Lippincott, 1967)

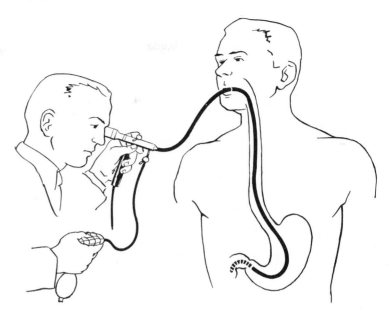

from the distal end. The fasting patient is placed in a sitting position, suitably draped, and given an adequate explanation of the character and the purpose of the procedure that is contemplated. Participation of the patient through active swallowing and control of gagging is essential to the success of intubation. If the tube inadvertently enters the trachea instead of the esophagus, vigorous coughing will ensue and air currents coinciding with inspiration and expiration will be felt at the proximal orifice, the signal for prompt withdrawal and reinsertion of the tube. Passage through the esophagus may be facilitated by having the patient sip small quantities of water. If neither nostril is patent, the Levin tube or the Rehfuss duodenal tube, which is equipped with a small perforated metal bulb at the tip, may be introduced through the mouth. However, the nasal route, unless barred mechanically, is preferred, since it is far less prone to stimulate gagging.

When the second marker of the Levin tube is at the point of entering the nares, the tip of the tube, 55 cm. distant, should be within the stomach. Once in place, the tube is secured to the patient's cheek by means of a small strip of adhesive tape, and the patient is placed in a semireclining position. If he exhibits any tendency to gag, he is instructed to pant gently with his mouth wide open, the effect of which is to minimize contact between the tube and the soft palate. The entire stomach contents are aspirated by gentle suction into a syringe. The color of the specimen is recorded as an indication regarding presence or absence of bile or blood. The presence or the absence of mucus and of food particles is noted. The acidity of the specimen is determined by means of an indicator dye, such as Töpfer's reagent, by indicator paper or by means of a

pH meter. Other examinations in special instances may include cytologic study by the Papanicolaou technique for the presence or the absence of carcinoma cells. Tubercle bacilli may be sought by culture techniques for guinea pig inoculation. Enzyme analysis of the gastric juice is sometimes indicated.

One of the most important items of information to be gained from gastric analysis relates to the ability of the mucosa to secrete hydrochloric acid. Patients with pernicious anemia secrete no acid, and patients with severe chronic gastritis or gastric cancer secrete little or no acid, whereas patients with peptic ulcer invariably secrete some acid and usually an excess amount of it. If the first sample aspirated from the stomach is found to be neutral or alkaline, 3 additional samples are obtained at 20-minute intervals and tested in similar fashion following the subcutaneous injection of histamine (0.1 ml. of a 0.5% solution of histamine base) or after the intravenous injection of 10 to 20 units of regular insulin. Either of these agents is likely to stimulate maximal production of hydrochloric acid by the gastric mucosa. If, for any reason, the use of these stimulants is contraindicated, a "test meal" may be substituted in the form of 50 ml. of 7 per cent alcohol by mouth.

Tubeless Gastric Analysis. A relatively simple, convenient and reliable method for determining gastric acidity, and one that dispenses with the necessity for gastric intubation, involves the feeding of a blue dye (azure A) and subsequent examination of the urine for the presence or the absence of that dye. The dye, when ingested, is bound to an insoluble resin from which it is released only in the presence of acid. Com-

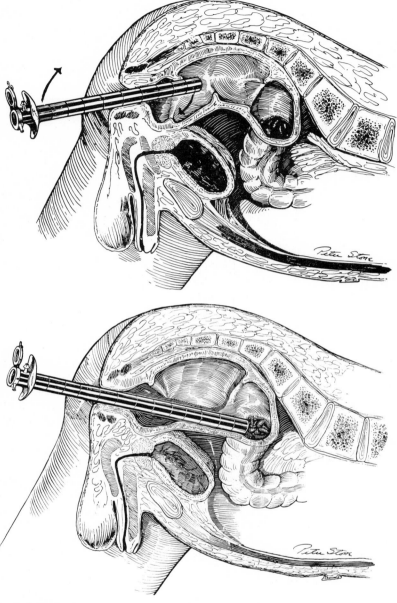

Fig. 22-3. Sigmoidoscopic examination. (*Top*) Direction of motion as the sigmoidoscope enters the rectum. (*Bottom*) The sigmoidoscope reaches the rectosigmoid junction.

bined with the resin, it cannot be absorbed from the gastrointestinal tract; freed from this combination, it is absorbed and is excreted promptly in the urine. Its appearance in the urine therefore serves to indicate that the resin-dye complex has been exposed to acid. Explicit instructions are given in each test unit. Of course, this test provides no information except as regards the presence or absence of gastric acidity. Furthermore, its results, if they appear to show no acid, are not necessarily valid in the presence of liver disease or in patients with obstructive lesions of the gastrointestinal or the urinary tract.

Esophagoscopy is discussed on page 441.

The *gastroscopic examination* affords direct visualization of the gastric mucosa. It is especially valuable when a gastric neoplasm is suspected. The patient is placed in a fasting state for 6 to 8 hours before the examination. One half hour before the procedure he is premedicated with Demerol. The patient's lips, oral cavity and pharynx are sprayed with pontocaine and the passage of the gastroscope is done smoothly and slowly. This fiber gastroscope is almost completely flexible and gives the physician an opportunity to view a large part of the gastric wall. Experienced gastroscopists may recognize a cancer and remove a piece of the tumor for microscopic examination.

The Rectal Examination

Visual inspection and digital examination of the anus and the rectum are indispensable for detection and identification of lesions involving these structures. Moreover, rectal examination is extremely useful in the diagnosis, or for the exclusion, of many intra-abdominal and pelvic conditions, including appendicitis, diverticulitis, salpingitis, tumors of the ovary, the uterus and the colon, and prostatic lesions of various types.

As the first step, the buttocks are spread apart with gauze pads or tissue wipes, and the anus and the perianal area are surveyed for fistulas, hemorrhoids, abscesses, fissures and other abnormalities. Next, with his examining index finger covered with a glove or a finger cot, the physician procedes to palpate the anal orifice and the rectum. The nurse should ensure that the requisite items are at hand, including a nonsterile glove or finger cot, lubricant, tissue wipes and a light source. During the procedure she should station herself at the patient's side to lend support and reassurance and to help him to assume the positions necessary for this examination.

Rectal examinations frequently are carried out in the lateral (Sims's) position. The patient, draped with a sheet, lies on his left side (if the physician is right-handed), lower leg extended and upper leg flexed on the abdomen.

Anoscopy, Proctoscopy and Sigmoidoscopy. By means of tubular instruments that incorporate small electric lights, the lumen of the lower bowel may be viewed directly. The anoscope is employed to examine the anal canal; proctoscopes and sigmoidoscopes, to inspect the rectum and the sigmoid respectively for evidence of ulceration, tumors, polyps or other pathology. It goes without saying that such an examination requires that the lower bowel be empty of feces; to this end, a cleansing soapsuds enema should be given at least 2 hours before endoscopy. Commercially prepared enemas may be used. Nevertheless, fecal material may remain to obstruct the examiner's view; to wipe it away, long swabs with generous cotton tips must be available.

The patient to be endoscoped assumes the knee-chest position, resting on his knees, feet extending over the edge of the bed or the examining table. Knees spread apart to give steady support, the patient leans over, and rests the side of his face on the bed or the table, with his forearms on either side of the head and his hands placed one on top of the other above the head. His back is now inclined at about a 45-degree angle and he is in proper position for the introduction of an anoscope, proctoscope or sigmoidoscope. Maximal convenience and comfort are afforded by a table that has been especially designed for rectal endoscopy —the so-called "proctoscopic table," which tilts the patient into the optimal position. (Fig. 22-3).

The patient undergoing a proctosigmoidoscopic examination should be kept informed as to the progress of the examination and praised for his cooperation. Let him know that he will experience the feeling of pressure and will feel like he is going to have a bowel movement. Explain that this is from the pressure of the proctoscope and will last only a brief period of time.

Many offices and hospitals are equipped with special rooms that are designed and outfitted primarily for proctoscopy. These include facilities for applying suction through long tubes that are introduced through the scope to remove any secretion, exudate, blood or excreta that might be obstructing the area of observation. After each use these tubes must be cleansed thoroughly by aspirating water through them, and the collecting bottles should be emptied and cleaned likewise. Disposable sigmoidoscopes are now available that eliminate the need for cleaning.

As part of the endoscopic examination, one or more small pieces of tissue may be removed for histologic study, a procedure referred to as a biopsy. This is done with small biting forceps introduced through the proctoscope. If present, rectal and sigmoidal polyps may be removed through the proctoscope by means of a wire snare with which to grasp the pedicle or stalk, and an electrocoagulating current to sever it and to prevent bleeding. It is extremely important that all tissue that is excised by the endoscopist be placed immediately in moist gauze or in an appropriate receptacle, labeled correctly and legibly, then delivered without delay to the pathology laboratory.

Gastric and Intestinal Intubation

Tubes inserted into the stomach and the intestine are used to aspirate the contents of these organs in the active and prophylactic treatment of many intra-abdominal lesions. The nasogastric catheter or so-called short tube is introduced through the nose or the mouth into the stomach. By aspiration, the gas and the fluids that collect in the stomach may be removed. It is especially valuable in the postoperative care of many patients after abdominal operations and especially in the treatment of vomiting postoperatively.

The long tubes or double lumen tubes are made of rubber or plastic that are introduced through the stomach into the intestinal tract. They are used to aspirate the intestinal content and so to prevent gas and fluid distention of the coils of intestine. The long tubes are the Miller-Abbott, the Harris and the Cantor and Devine tubes. These are used in the active treatment of intestinal obstruction, especially that of the small intestine. They also are used prophylactically, being inserted the night before the operation to prevent obstruction after abdominal operation. By their use the intestine is threaded on the tube and so shortened and held together compactly, making it relatively easier to pack off the intestine at the time of operation on the colon. Usually, the tubes are allowed to remain in place after operation until peristalsis is resumed, as shown by the passage of gas by rectum. Intubation usually is practiced in the treatment of all forms of intestinal obstruction, but it is especially effective in paralytic ileus and in postoperative obstruction. These patients can be given liquid nourishment by mouth with the tube in place but clamped off.

Types and Use of Gastrointestinal Tubes

Miller-Abbott Tube. This is a double lumen, No. 16 Fr. 10-foot tube: one lumen of the tube is used to inflate the balloon at the end of the tube; the other, entirely independent, is used for aspiration. Before inserting the tube, the balloon should be tested, its capacity measured and then deflated completely. The tube should be lubricated sparingly and chilled well before the doctor inserts the tip through the patient's nose. Markings on the tube indicate the distance it has been passed.

Harris Tube. This is a single-lumen mercury-weighted tube of about 6 feet, and a lumen of 14 on the French scale. This tube has a metal tip that is introduced first into the nostril after having been lubricated. The mercury-weighted bag follows. The weight

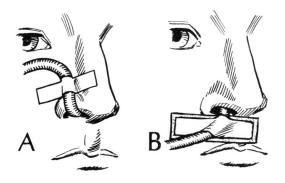

Fig. 22-4. (A) Excessive pressure by the tube on the ala nasi should be avoided. (B) Satisfactory method for securing the tube which will prevent injury to the nasopharyngeal passages. Method of tube fixation: Apply a thin coat of tincture of benzoin to the area under the nose and place a strip of non-allergic tape on the prepared area. The nasogastric tube is fixed in position by anchoring it on top of the tape. By using this method, the nares may be cleaned frequently and the tube reanchored without causing undue discomfort to the patient. (Adapted from Artz, C. P., and Hardy, J. P.: Complications in Surgery and their Management, Saunders, 1967)

of the mercury carries the bag by gravity. As this is a single lumen tube that is used wholly for suction and irrigating, there is no difficulty in irrigating it. Usually a Y tube is attached to the end of the tube, so that the suction apparatus is attached to one side, and an outlet with a clamp is available on the other side for irrigating purposes.

Cantor Tube. The Cantor tube is 10 feet long and No. 18 Fr. Its distinguishing feature is that it is larger and has the mercury-filled bag at the extreme end of the rubber tubing.

Devine Tube. The Devine tube is a double lumen tube that has an air vent. One lumen is used to suction out intestinal contents while the other simultaneously draws air into the intestine to prevent collapsing of the intestinal mucosa around the tube.

To Introduce Nasogastric Tube and Attachment of Suction Apparatus: 1. The nasogastric tube is prepared for use by sterilizing and placing it in a basin containing cracked ice for at least 5 minutes. After lubricating the end of the tube with water-soluble jelly, the nurse assists the patient to hyperextend his head while the surgeon introduces the tube through the nostril. The nurse should provide the tape fixation for use when the tube has been inserted the required distance.

2. The nasogastric catheter is attached to the tube leading to the trap bottle, usually by a Y tube. The other end of the Y tube is attached to a small piece of rubber tubing closed by a clamp. Through this tube irrigations of the nasogastric catheter may be accomplished.

3. The tube line from the nose to the trap bottle is fixed in position on the bed so that there will be no pulling upon it. This may be accomplished by a safety pin through the bed sheet or by adhesive-tape loops that may be tied or pinned to the bed.

To Irrigate Nasogastric Catheter: Keep the nasogastric catheter open by the injection of a measured amount of saline or isotonic electrolyte solution through the Y tube connection, using a Luer-tip or Asepto syringe. The physician directs the amount of solution to be used. When fluid is injected, the tubing on the other side of the Y connection leading to the trap bottle should be clamped. Suction should not be made with a syringe unless ordered.

To Maintain Adequate Intake: While gastric-suction drainage is in use, an adequate parenteral intake should be maintained. The amount and the type of fluids are prescribed by the physician.

Keep Accurate Records of: (1) Drainage, amount, color and type, every 12 hours.

(2) Amount of fluid instilled by irrigation of the nasogastric catheter and the amount of water taken by mouth.

(3) Amount and character of vomitus, if any.

(4) Duration of any period in which the suction apparatus did not appear to function.

(5) Effects produced by the treatment.

Nursing Management of Intubated Patients

Before the patient is intubated, it is wise for the nurse or the doctor to explain the treatment and its purpose. A cooperative patient adds much to the success of the procedure. He may be allowed to sit up, and a towel can be spread bib-fashion over his chest. Tissue wipes should be available. The patient ought to be screened from other patients, and the doctor should have adequate light. Often the physician will swab the nostril and spray the oropharynx with pontocaine to dull the nasal passage and the gag reflex and make the procedure more tolerable. Holding ice chips in the mouth for a few minutes will have the same effect. Encouraging the patient to breathe through his mouth or pant often helps, as does swallowing of water if permitted.

When the tube is passed to the desired distance, the nurse should fasten the catheter to the nose with tape (Fig. 22-4). A minimal amount of adhesive for the maximal effect should be used. The tube then is connected to the suction apparatus. Enough leeway should be allowed to permit the patient to turn without risk of dislodging the tube. Rigid mouth and nostril hygiene must be followed in caring for these patients, as these tubes may be in place for several days. Applicator sticks dipped in water can be used to clean the nose. This can be followed by mineral oil. Frequent mouth attention is comforting. If the nasal and pharyngeal mucosa is excessively dry, steam or cool vapor inhalations may be beneficial. Throat lozenges, an ice collar, chewing gum (if permitted) and frequent movement also assist in relieving discomfort.

Patients undergoing suction decompression are susceptible to water and electrolyte problems. Symptoms indicating a fluid volume deficit include dryness of skin and mucous membranes, decreasing urinary output, lethargy and exhaustion and a drop in body temperature. The nurse should assess the intubated patient for these signs as well as measure and record the amount of fluid lost by suction.

When it is desirable to remove the tube, it is necessary to deflate the balloon and withdraw it gently and slowly for about 6 to 8 inches at intervals of 10 minutes until the tip reaches the esophagus, when the remainder is withdrawn rapidly out of the nostril. Should the tube not come out easily, force should not be used—the physician should be notified. As it is withdrawn, the tube should be concealed in a towel, because it is not a pleasant spectacle and may cause the patient to vomit. After its removal the patient will be grateful for good mouth care.

PROBLEMS RELATED TO THE STOMACH AND THE DUODENUM

Functional Gastric Disturbances

Indigestion

As a result of disturbed nervous control of the stomach or of disease elsewhere in the body, many individuals suffer intensely from "indigestion," although their stomachs are without a trace of disease. Abdominal pain is the most common complaint of these individuals. This pain is usually in the upper abdomen and it usually is associated with eating, occurring during or immediately after a meal. Its character may be described as crampy, it may be a feeling of fullness, distention or burning. The types of food that cause the most discomfort are apt to be fatty foods, probably because they remain in the stomach longest and because these patients commonly have an abnormal aversion to fatty foods. Coarse vegetables and highly seasoned foods likewise cause considerable distress. Alkalies, such as sodium bicarbonate, afford only partial relief or perhaps none at all. The basis for the abdominal distress is obviously the patient's own normal gastric peristaltic movements. These anxious and hypersensitive individuals gradually have become acutely conscious of sensations that normally are not noticed, and that are interpreted as pain.

Psychic Vomiting

This is a common symptom in persons with an anxiety neurosis and may be exhibited by any normal individual in a tense situation. Such vomiting may be only occasional or it may be frequent—after every meal. Usually the amount vomited is very small, so small that the nutrition is not in the least disturbed, which is an important diagnostic point; but some severely neurotic individuals develop persistent vomiting to such a degree that they eventually starve to death. The usual neurotic vomiting is not preceded by nausea; the patient simply regurgitates his food and expectorates. Children sometimes learn the trick and are proud of it.

Aerophagia (Air Swallowing)

This is not an unusual symptom of tense persons. It may appear in attacks lasting for hours. Some individuals eructate large amounts of air. One may wonder at the source of the air, but by watching observes that unconsciously they are continually swallowing it.

In most psychoneurotic individuals the gastric symptoms form only a part of the total picture, but, in some patients, severe stomach symptoms overshadow all others and require careful study to rule out organic gastrointestinal disease. The fact that the patient is manifestly neurotic or hysterical, however, does not prove that his gastric symptoms are functional, because a neurotic individual has the same chance of contracting gallbladder disease or carcinoma of the stomach as have other individuals. All possible diagnostic methods should be employed before a definite diagnosis of functional indigestion has been decided upon. Nervous dyspepsia is diagnosed incorrectly in many cases, not only of organic gastrointestinal disease, but also of unsuspected tuberculosis, cardiac decompensation, uremia, pernicious anemia and atypical migraine. Too much care cannot be taken.

Organic Gastric Disturbances

Pylorospasm

In this disturbance, the muscle closing the orifice between the stomach and the duodenum, instead of relaxing, contracts vigorously and painfully at the time that the stomach wall is contracting. The result is upper abdominal pain, occasionally very severe. This usually is due to the presence of a small peptic ulcer near the pylorus.

Hyperacidity

The so-called *heartburn, acid eructation,* etc., are due to reverse peristalsis. Because of spasm of the pylorus, reverse peristalsis churns the gastric juice to the cardiac end of the stomach, whence it is forced up the esophagus and into the pharynx where it can be tasted.

Gastritis

Acute Gastritis

Inflammation of the stomach is a complaint so common that its symptoms need not be described in detail. Often it is due to some dietary indiscretion. The individual eats too much or too rapidly or eats food that is noxious because it is too highly seasoned or is infected. Acute gastritis also may be the first sign of an acute systemic infection. However, the best examples of acute gastritis are those due to alcohol, to overindulgence in salicylates and to uremia.

The gastric mucous membrane of a stomach that is the seat of acute gastritis is red and swollen and secretes a paucity of gastric juice containing very little acid but much mucus. The patient has uncomfortable feelings in his abdomen, with headache, lassitude, nausea, often vomiting and hiccuping. The vomiting relieves him considerably, because it removes the irritating substances. The tongue is coated, and the flow of saliva is increased. If the irritating food is not vomited but reaches the bowel, colic and diarrhea may result. As a rule, the patient is well in about one day, although he may not have much appetite for the next 2 or 3 days.

Treatment consists in the parenteral administration of glucose and saline as long as the vomiting persists. When the patient is able to take nourishment by mouth, a bland diet, perhaps supplemented by alkalies, is offered.

Chronic Gastritis

In early cases of chronic gastritis, the mucous membrane of the stomach is thickened and its rugae are prominent. As time passes, both its lining and its walls become thinned and its secretion lessens in quantity and in quality, eventually consisting almost entirely of mucus and water.

One of the important causes of chronic gastritis is chronic uremia. Among the local causes of gastritis are benign and malignant ulcers of the stomach and cirrhosis of the liver complicated by portal hypertension, the latter causing the chronic congestion of the stomach wall.

The diagnosis is established on upper gastrointestinal x-ray series and by gastric analysis.

Symptoms of chronic gastritis vary greatly. The appetite may be poor (anorexia) or too good (bulimia); there is usually some distress ("heartburn") after eating, and often there are eructations of gas. The taste in the mouth is bad; there is usually considerable nausea and perhaps some vomiting, especially early in the morning.

Treatment consists of having the patient eat only easily digested, properly prepared food and chew it well. Because the muscles of the stomach are weakened, he should eat only small amounts at a time and, therefore, eat more frequently.

The diet may consist entirely of milk for a few days, subsequently replaced by a soft diet. Whatever special treatment might be indicated depends on the basic cause of the gastritis in each individual patient.

The Patient with Peptic Ulcer

A peptic ulcer is an excavation formed in the mucosal wall of the stomach, in the pylorus or in the duodenum, and is due to the erosion of a circumscribed area of its mucous membrane. This erosion may extend as deeply as the muscle layers or through the muscle to the peritoneum. Peptic ulcers are more apt to be in the duodenum than in the stomach, but, whether on the gastric or on the duodenal side, most of them occur near the pylorus, a few being situated in the pylorus itself. As a rule, they occur singly, but there may be a number of them present at once.

The etiology of peptic ulcer is poorly understood. It is known that peptic ulcers occur only in the areas of the gastrointestinal tract that are exposed to hydrochloric acid and pepsin. The disease occurs with the greatest frequency between the ages of 20 and 40, but it has been observed in childhood, even in infancy. It seems to develop in persons who are emotionally tense, but whether this is the cause or the effect of the condition is uncertain. Important predisposing factors associated with recurrence of activity in peptic ulcer include emotional stress, eating hurried and irregular meals, excessive smoking and the season of the year, because this disease tends to appear and recur most commonly in the spring and the fall.

Certain drugs predispose to peptic ulceration. These include the salicylates, Reserpine, phenylbutazone (Butazolidine) and the steroids. Susceptible patients who must take these drugs should be instructed to ingest milk and crackers between meals and at bedtime. By a buffering action the intake of food tends to protect the mucous lining of the stomach.

Symptoms

Pain. As a rule, the patient with peptic ulcer complains of pain, or a gnawing sensation, sharply localized in the midepigastrium or in the back. It is believed that the pain occurs when the increased acid content of the stomach and duodenum erode the lesion and stimulate the exposed nerve endings.

The pain recurs from 1 to 3 hours after meals and becomes progressively more severe toward the end of the day. This pain typically is relieved quite promptly by food or alkalies, either of which neutralizes the free acid in contact with the ulcer. If the patient takes neither food nor alkali, the pain gradually wears off as the secretion of acid stops and it empties into the intestine. The character of the pain may be described as a dull, burning sensation, a feeling of emptiness or gnawing pain so severe that the patient is in agony. Some relief is obtained by local pressure on the epigastrium. Sharply localized tenderness can be ·elicited by gentle pressure in the epigastrium at or slightly to the right of the midline. In assessing the patient's pain the nurse observes and records the following factors: Where is the pain located? Does it radiate? How long does it last? Is it relieved by food or alkalies? How does the patient describe the pain?

Vomiting is the second classic symptom of peptic ulcer. It is due to pyloric obstruction caused by either muscular spasm of the pylorus or of mechanical obstruction. The latter may be due to scarring or to acute swelling of the inflamed mucous membrane adjacent to the acute ulcer. The vomiting may or may not be preceded by nausea; usually it follows a bout of severe pain, which is relieved by ejection of the acid gastric contents.

Complications

There are 3 major complications of a peptic ulcer: hemorrhage, perforation and pyloric obstruction.

Hemorrhage. Manifested by hematemesis, melena, or both, hemorrhage is the common complication of peptic ulcer. Occasionally this appears without any antecedent history of dyspepsia. Early symptoms may be giddiness and faintness; nausea may precede or accompany bleeding. A large amount of blood, even 2,000 to 3,000 ml., may be vomited. The patient may become almost exsanguinated, and rapid blood replacement may be required to save his life. When the hemorrhage is of large proportions, most of the blood is vomited; when small, much or all of the blood may be passed in the stools, which, due to the digested hemoglobin, appear tarry black. Chemical tests (benzidine, guaiac or orthotolidine) are necessary to detect occult blood that does not alter the gross appearance of the stools, since this type of melena is decidedly more common than gross hemorrhages from the bowel.

Hemorrhage, which can be massive and fatal, requires the speedy application of measures designed to halt the bleeding and then to replace the lost blood. Small, frequent, bland feedings are provided to prevent hunger contractions. Demerol hydrochloride may be indicated if the patient is extremely restless or in pain. Whole-blood and/or plasma transfusions are employed to keep the circulating blood volume at a safe level. One does not wait for a drop of blood pressure before embarking on transfusion therapy if there are signs of tachycardia, sweating and coldness of the extremities. The blood pressure and pulse rates should be taken at half-hourly intervals when bleeding is suspected. It is important to observe the color, consistency and the volume of stools and vomitus.

The nurse plays an important role in observing and reporting these symptoms immediately, then carrying out the procedures indicated in cases of oligemic shock, as outlined on page 146.

Gastric Cooling. This procedure is used in the treatment of many types of upper gastrointestinal bleeding, such as bleeding from gastric and duodenal ulcers. The method involves the insertion of a balloon into·the upper stomach and lower esophagus through which is circulated a water-alcohol mixture cooled to a temperature of 0° to +2° C. The coolant solution is delivered into the balloon through a small plastic tube and withdrawn through another plastic tube, so that the mixture in the balloon is maintained at a cooling temperature. The solution is cooled and circulated with a specially designed cooling and pump apparatus, which is also fitted with an air monitor that removes any air from the circulating fluid. The coolant solution is used in amounts of 400 to 600 ml. initially if the patient is an adult and has had no previous gastric surgery. The balloon is sausage-shaped; with a distendable section resting in the upper stomach and a longer narrower portion resting in the esophagus.

The result of gastric cooling is to depress the flow of gastric secretion by about 90 per cent, thus reducing gastric digestion, and to decrease gastric blood flow by about 70 per cent. In addition, pressure of the distended balloon in the upper stomach and esophagus has an effect. These measures usually stop the bleeding within 2 hours. Usually the temperature of the coolant is maintained at the low temperature for 6 to 8 hours, then the balloon volume is slowly decreased to about 200 ml., and the temperature of the circulating fluid is raised slowly to about 18° to 20° C.

NURSING OF THE PATIENT WITH GASTRIC COOLING. The cooling effect of the relatively prolonged treatment is often found to produce systemic hypothermia unless counteracted by external heating. The heat is best provided by an "electric blanket," which should be installed on the bed before the gastric cooling is started. The nurse should remember that many of these patients with bleeding ulcers are in the older age group of patients (over 60 years) and are in the "poor risk" group, not only because of the bleeding, but also because of the effects of cooling.

After cooling, the stomach reacts by a temporary hypersecretion of acid gastric juice. To counteract the effects of this hypersecretion, chilled milk or antacids are introduced by drip into the stomach through a nasogastric tube. The tube should be ready and the prescribed solution for the drip, so that the drip can be started as soon as the balloon is removed.

In some cases of massive bleeding, a nasogastric tube is inserted first to lavage the stomach. Normal saline is used for the lavage to remove blood and clots. Often the No. 18 French tube is too small, and a No. 22 French size is used. The normal saline solution may be taken by mouth and the fluid withdrawn through the tube by suction. Often the nasogastric tube is left in place during the cooling procedure. The character of the fluid aspirated from it serves as an indicator of the status of the hemorrhage.

The procedure of gastric cooling falls in the province of the attending physician, but the observation of the patient and the fluid aspirated from the stomach are among the important responsibilities of the nurse. Gastric cooling is probably the most effective method of controlling hemorrhage from ulcers, but it should be understood that the control may be only temporary and may necessitate more definitive treatment—usually surgical.

Perforation. Perforation of a peptic ulcer may occur unexpectedly, without much evidence of preceding indigestion. Perforation into the free peritoneal cavity is one of the abdominal catastrophes, and the symptoms and signs are those of an acute surgical abdomen. The typical history is that of sudden severe upper abdominal pain, persisting and increasing in intensity, accompanied by vomiting and collapse.

The pain may be referred to the shoulders due to irritation of the phrenic nerve in the diaphragm. The abdomen is extremely tender and board-like in rigidity, and signs of shock develop. Immediate surgical intervention is indicated because chemical peritonitis develops within a few hours following perforation and is followed by a bacterial peritonitis. Therefore, the perforation must be closed as quickly as possible.

Pyloric Obstruction. Pyloric obstruction occurs when the area surrounding the pyloric sphincter becomes scarred and stenosed from spasm, edema or from scar tissue that is formed when the ulcer alternately heals and breaks down. The patient has symptoms of nausea and vomiting, constipation and weight loss. In treating the patient, the first consideration is the relief of the obstruction by gastric decompression. When the patient's clinical course has been prolonged and there is evidence of much inflammation and scarring and spasticity, surgery is usually performed.

Study of Patients with Peptic Ulcer

The nurse plays a large role in the study of patients with peptic ulcer. Since an ulcer usually bleeds, at least in small amounts, the appearance of blood in the stools is an important diagnostic finding. The stools should be collected as requested by the physician. Frequently, it is important to avoid food containing meats for a period of time before stool collection for occult blood.

A great deal of information of value both to the internist and to the surgeon concerns the secretion of gastric acid. In ulcer of the duodenum especially, this secretion is more than normal, and its acid content is very high. For this reason, an analysis of the gastric juice obtained by aspiration of the juice through a tube is an important diagnostic procedure (p. 454). Often, stimulation of the acid is carried out by using injections of histamine.

There are many techniques for gastric analysis. The type that is preferred by the physician in charge is the one that the nurse should follow. Careful collection and marking of the aspirates at intervals are necessary.

Therapeutic Regimen for the Patient with an Ulcer

The major objective of therapy is to control gastric acidity. This is accomplished by appropriate sedation and neutralization of the gastric juice at frequent and regular intervals with milk drinks and antacids. Sometimes antispasmodics are given to reduce pylorospasm and intestinal motility. Anticholinergic agents may be prescribed to inhibit gastric secretion.

Ideally the patient should be on bed rest until he is free of pain and eating normally. Sedatives and tranquilizers are given according to the individual patient's needs. These may be prescribed on a regular schedule. The surroundings of the patient should provide an optimal milieu for healing.

The patient may become quite drowsy, in which event he will require close supervision when ambulatory, as well as protective rails on his bed, in order to avoid injury. Heavily sedated patients should be turned frequently and should be required to wear elastic stockings constantly as a prophylactic measure for the prevention of thrombophlebitis.

The diet and the medication schedule require the closest cooperation on the part of patient and nurse, for it is extremely important that they be followed carefully. Ulcer pain, as has been stated, can be agonizing, and the responsibility for its relief necessarily devolves on the nurse, who must see that the patient receives his feedings on time. Since the main objective of treatment at this stage is to protect the ulcer from exposure to acid gastric juice, the patient is given calcium carbonate or aluminum hydroxide at regular intervals throughout the day and night. These agents do not produce alkalosis and their constipating effect is relieved by an occasional dose of magnesium carbonate. The consistency of the patient's stools and his symptomatic reaction to the antacid compounds should be noted.

In addition to the antacid compounds, one of the many anticholinergic drugs usually is given to suppress gastric secretion or to delay gastric emptying and, thereby, increase the effectiveness of the antacid compound. Among the antisecretory drugs are atropine or belladonna, Pro-Banthine and Prantal Methylsulfate. Pro-Banthine, in a dose of 0.2 mg. per Kg., is similar in effectiveness and toxicity to Prantal, given I.M. in doses of 0.1 mg. per Kg. of body weight. Both are preferable to atropine and belladonna from the standpoint of toxic side-effects, but the latter are similar in quality, regardless of which particular agent is used. Symptoms of toxicity for which the nurse should be alert include dryness of the mouth and the throat, excessive thirst, difficulty in swallowing, flushed dry skin, rapid pulse and respiration, dilated pupils and emotional excitement.

The purpose of the dietary treatment is to neutralize the free hydrochloric acid in the stomach. *Frequent and regular* feedings are most successful in achieving these goals and keeping the patient's symptoms relieved. Skim milk, milk or milk and cream given regularly at 1-hour or 2-hour intervals may comprise the entire diet for the first few days. For milk-allergic ulcer patients, a soya bean formula such as Sobee can be used along with bland foods to avoid the milk products.

During this period the nurse is responsible for giving the patient his feedings. If the patient proves to be reliable, the ingredients of his diet may be left at his bedside in a receptacle that keeps the milk at a desirable temperature. The responsibility for seeing to it that the patient takes these feedings still rests with the nurse. A patient on such a regimen may become uncooperative because of dissatisfaction with his diet. If so, the diet may be modified.

The patient and his family should be educated in the reasons for, as well as details of, his ulcer regimen to assure their maximal cooperation. The present trend in ulcer therapy is toward greater latitude in the choice of the dietary constituents, the emphasis being placed on regular feedings rather than on antacid and antispasmodic agents.

Therapy during the night is scheduled in such a manner that sleep will not be curtailed, but at the same time periods of fasting do not exceed 2 or 3 hours, for many of these patients secrete gastric juice continuously day and night. Observe the patient to see when his pain begins. Milk should be given *before* pain starts.

In a few days, after the pain has been controlled, a regular schedule of frequent bland feedings is inaugurated, supplemented by powders or other neutralizing substances as needed. Ideally, the stomach at no time is overloaded; at no time is free acid present in excess or peristalsis vigorous. Dilute orange juice supplies vitamin C (ascorbic acid), which is otherwise lacking in the diet. As progress is made from the simple milk diet, trays must be served attractively and with attention to specific preferences so that the patient will eat with enthusiasm all that is given him. The food should be of bland character, containing all the essential constituents in proper balance, and it should not provoke the secretion of gastric juice or be monotonous. This diet usually is continued for several weeks after discharge, even after all symptoms have disappeared.

Peptic ulcer patients with intractable pain despite hourly milk, antacid and anticholinergic drug therapy often benefit from a continuous intragastric Sustagen drip through a nasogastric tube for 24 to 72 hours.

Psychological Support

Peptic ulcer patients often may be irritable and demanding and take offense easily. The patient may be preoccupied with some concrete problems as a conscious basis for his anxiety. Usually he is eager to discuss them with the nurse during her unhurried contacts with him, and such discussions afford him satisfaction and relief. Indeed, her very presence, as she responds to his many calls, brings relief. If the nurse is aware of her therapeutic role in relation to her patient she will understand the real significance of his repeated signals.

Nursing measures should be carried out punctiliously and in a manner calculated to make them acceptable to the patient. This is usually accomplished by a show of confidence and understanding, by making every effort to accommodate his likes and dislikes within the limits prescribed, and by means of rational detailed explanations when indicated. His day-to-day response to treatment should be observed with care and recorded for the medical and nursing care plans.

Many patients with acute ulcer symptoms, due to proved ulcer, derive complete temporary relief from nothing more than severance of all connections with environmental anxiety-producing factors—unfavorable diet and hygienic conditions notwithstanding. Such a solution is rarely practicable, however, for environ-

ments, particularly internal emotional environments, are not easily shed. Freedom from ulcer recurrences is favored by adherence to a sound hygienic routine of living, which implies regularity of habits in general, moderation in all pursuits, adequate rest daily, ample relaxation, good diet discipline and, at least in this instance, abstinence from caffeine and alcohol, which have acid-producing potential. Smoking likewise is contraindicated for ulcer patients. Nicotine increases gastric motility and the flow of gastric acid.

Beneficial alterations of stress situations frequently are possible through wise counseling by the physician (in some cases aided by a psychiatrist) of the patient and the patient's family. The basis of such counsel may be established by the observation of a nurse who

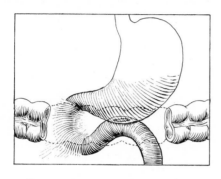

Posterior gastrojejunostomy. The jejunum is sutured to the stomach behind the colon, which has been cut away to show the anastomosis.

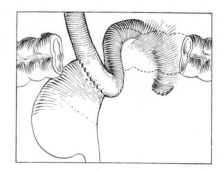

Subtotal gastric resection with posterior gastrojejunostomy. The resected portion includes the first part of the duodenum, the pylorus and from two thirds to three quarters of the stomach. The stump of the duodenum is closed by suture, and the side of the jejunum is anastomosed to the end of the stomach (Polya) posterior to the colon.

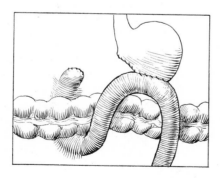

Subtotal gastric resection with anterior gastrojejunostomy (Hofmeister type). The resection is as in B. The anastomosis is made anterior to the colon, the side of the jejunum is anastomosed to part of the cut end of the stomach, and the rest is closed by sutures.

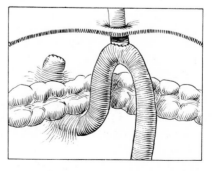

Total gastrectomy. The entire stomach is removed and the esophagus is anastomosed to a loop of jejunum under the diaphragm.

FIG. 22-5. Types of gastric operations.

has been able to elicit pertinent information in this connection. An increased food budget may be required to provide an adequate bland diet for the patient. (Extra food expense can be eliminated, or held to a minimum, by providing standard family items that have been processed with a sieve or a "blender," or by using commercial baby foods, flavored to taste and served warm.) Ulcers are prone to recur, despite medical and surgical measures, if the patient must return to the same environment to face the same problems that earlier had played a contributory role in their production.

Surgical Treatment of Peptic Ulcer

Most patients with peptic ulcer respond to medical treatment. Surgery is required in only about 15 per cent of ulcer patients. Complications, however, may develop that demand surgical therapy. These complications are perforation, hemorrhage, obstruction to the pylorus, or inability to control the ulcer pain by medical means—a complication most often described as "intractability." The purpose of operation is to relieve complications and treat the tendency to ulcer formation.

Since the ulcers are believed to result from the acid pepsin of the stomach, the operations are designed to lower the production of acid by the stomach to a point at which further ulcerations will not occur. This may be done either by removing a large part of the acid-forming cells of the stomach, usually the distal two thirds or three quarters, or by removing the acid-stimulating mechanism of the stomach, i.e., dividing the vagus nerves and removing the antral portion of the stomach. The excessive gastric acid is produced in duodenal ulcer largely by stimulation that arrives over the vagus nerves. The antral portion of the stomach also stimulates acid production by way of the hormone *gastrin* produced in its mucosal layer and absorbed into the bloodstream and carried to the acid-producing cells of the stomach. By removing these 2 stimulating factors, acid secretion is reduced to a minimum.

Another method of treating the patient with a peptic ulcer is by cutting the vagus nerves and performing an operation for drainage of the stomach. The drainage operation is performed because vagotomy is often followed by gastric retention, since the vagus nerves provide the motor impulses to the gastric musculature and their division is often followed by gastric atony. The drainage operations may be gastroenterostomy or pyloroplasty. The vagotomy divides the nerves that are known to stimulate gastric acid hypersecretion in most cases of duodenal ulcer. The gastric drainage operation not only drains the atonic stomach produced by the vagotomy but also reduces the stimulation of gastric acid by reducing the formation of gastrin produced in the antral area of the stomach. In other patients a vagotomy and pyloroplasty may be performed, ligating the bleeding vessel in the base of the ulcer through the incision made for the pyloroplasty.

An almost immediate operation must be performed on those patients who reach the hospital with ulcers that are perforated and draining gastric or intestinal contents into the abdominal cavity. The abdomen is opened and the perforation through the ulcer is sutured and overlaid with omentum. In a few patients it may be necessary also to perform an anastomosis between the stomach and the jejunum. Ulcers complicated by a gradually increasing closure of the pyloric opening of the stomach occur usually in older people. In these individuals, a conservative type of operation—posterior gastrojejunostomy—may be used (Fig. 22-5).

It is difficult to distinguish benign ulcers of the stomach from cancer of the stomach. Therefore, many surgeons are of the opinion that most large gastric ulcers should be treated by operation.

In patients whose bleeding is the outstanding symptom, there usually is a period of transfusion in preparation for the operative procedure. This is especially important in older patients in whom recurrence of hemorrhage often ends fatally. In these patients, the ulcer-bearing area is removed or the bleeding vessel is ligated.

As much as three fourths of the stomach proper often is removed with the ulcer. The end of the duodenum is closed. The opening in the stomach then is sutured partially and the remaining opening is sutured to the side of the jejunum (Fig. 22-5).

In the case of intractable ulcer not amenable to any type of medicinal or other conservative treatment, the foregoing operation is often advised. In this type of operation it is hoped, in both gastric and duodenal ulcers, not only to remove the ulcer-bearing areas in both the duodenum and the stomach but to reduce the acid pepsin secretion of the stomach to a level that will prevent the appearance later of ulcers on the margin of the stoma or even in the jejunum.

Preoperative Nursing Care. Often the cause of the ulcer is not removed by surgical intervention alone. Constant fear or worry may be disturbing the individual. Only when this factor is eliminated can the best results be looked for. The surgeon and the nurse must realize that the "psyche" has much influence over the "soma," and all efforts to allay the apprehension and the fears of the patient should be employed. Perhaps an immediate preoperative worry is fear of the anesthesia or of malignancy. Because these patients have a long illness, they are discouraged frequently and often are helped by spiritual therapy.

PRINCIPLES OF MEDICAL AND NURSING MANAGEMENT OF THE PATIENT WITH A PEPTIC ULCER

Major Problems
- A. Pain and dyspepsia
- B. Anxiety and emotional distress
- C. Promotion of physical and emotional rest
- D. Prevention of complications

Objectives
- I. To assure mental and physical rest:
  - A. Bed rest to remove patient from stressful environment
  - B. Written nursing-care plan to provide for optimal coordinated care
  - C. Sedatives and soporific medications to promote relaxation and sleep
  - D. Medications and dietary feedings given on time
- II. To rest the motor and secretory activities of the stomach through a therapeutic diet:
  - A. Bland protein and fat foods to neutralize acidity
  - B. Small feedings to rest the gastrointestinal tract
  - C. Frequent feedings to absorb excess acid
  - D. Nonstimulating foods to avoid irritation of the gastric mucosa
  - E. Progression to nutritionally adequate diet as rapidly as possible
- III. To relieve pain and discomfort and promote healing:
  - A. Antacid drugs given to neutralize gastric secretions and afford symptomatic relief
  - B. Anticholinergic drugs given to decrease gastric motility and reduce volume of gastric secretions
  - C. Adequate hydration to relieve side-effects of anticholinergic drugs
  - D. Therapeutic diet as ordered
- IV. To assist the patient to accept and follow his therapeutic program:
  - A. Demonstrate interest in patient and eliminate factors producing anxiety.
  - B. Teach importance of taking prescribed medication and diet on time.
  - C. Assist patient to develop insight into causes of his tension and frustration.
  - D. Implement and reinforce instructions issued by the doctor.
  - E. Teach the importance of moderation in all activities.
  - F. Encourage the elimination of smoking.
  - G. Stress the value of psychiatric interviews if prescribed.
- V. To recognize the complications of peptic ulcer:
  - A. Perforation
    1. Assist with transfusion to treat shock.
    2. Prepare to institute nasogastric suction to remove gastrointestinal secretions.
    3. Give drugs to control pain.
    4. Prepare patient for immediate surgery.
  - B. Hemorrhage
    1. Prepare for prompt and rapid transfusion for blood replacement.
    2. Administer sedation to allay anxiety and keep patient at rest.
    3. Assist with gastric intubation for aspiration of stomach contents.
    4. Evaluate clinical response to blood replacement.
    5. Observe continuously to maintain blood pressure at physiologic level.
    6. Observe urinary volume.
    7. Observe stools for melena.
    8. Prepare for surgical intervention if indicated.

Economic and social factors may have influenced the patient to such an extent that long hours of work, no recreation, tension, fatigue, etc., have contributed in good measure to his illness. The nurse might seek these factors tactfully in an effort to aid the physician as he directs treatment so that a recurrence of the patient's ulcer might be eliminated.

The patient has laboratory analyses, roentgenologic series and a general physical examination before surgery is attempted. The function of the nurse is to prepare the patient for each of these diagnostic measures by explaining their nature and significance to him. Specific physical preparation is prescribed by the physician.

Before operation is begun on the upper intestinal tract, attention should be given to the hygiene of the mouth. The teeth of these patients usually are bad, and the nurse should urge frequent mouthwashes and a thorough brushing of the teeth at least 3 times daily.

The nutritional and fluid needs of the patient are of major importance. In those patients with pyloric obstruction, there usually is prolonged vomiting with resultant weight and fluid loss. Every effort must be made to restore an adequate nutritional level and to maintain an optimal fluid and electrolyte balance. Again, the nurse plays a key role in helping her patient to achieve a satisfactory preoperative status so that postoperative hazards are kept at a minimum.

Gastric suction through a nasogastric tube is used often to empty the stomach, especially in patients with pyloric obstruction, and a Levin tube often is inserted before the patient goes to the operating room; this is left in place for operative and postoperative use. It is important that the colon be empty when the patient comes to surgery. Usually this is ensured by an enema the day before operation. If gastrointestinal roentgenograms have been made shortly before the day of operation, it is most important that the patient have enemas to remove completely the barium that may remain in the colon. The nurse should report it when the enema returns still show the whitish color of barium in the fecal material. The patient usually is limited to full fluids during the 24-hour period preceding surgery. The abdomen should be prepared from the nipple line to the symphysis, although the incision usually is made in the upper right quadrant or the midline.

Patient Education

Patients who have been operated on for peptic ulcer often need instruction as to their diet for months after operation, because, even though the ulcer has been removed, secondary ulcers sometimes occur. The best way to prevent these is to reduce the amount of the acidity of the gastric juice and to avoid coarse foods. Therefore, patients are instructed to avoid foods that tend to stimulate acid secretion in the stomach. Such foods are as follows:

All acids, e.g., vinegar, pickles, sour foods.
Raw fruits, e.g., apples, grapes, lemons, oranges.
Meat-stock soups, e.g., bouillon, consommé.
Condiments and spices, e.g., excess of chili and black pepper, mustard, horseradish, cloves, nutmeg.
Concentrated sweets, e.g., honey, molasses, candy.
Coarse foods, e.g., nuts, corn, cabbage.

For the first 6 months, the patient may require 6 small meals a day because of his reduced gastric capacity. He must avoid overeating.

Merely to hand a patient awaiting discharge from the hospital a diet list is not sufficient preparation. He should be helped to realize that emotional factors have a definite effect on food digestion. The need for peace of mind is important; both he and his family should know this. If some of his problems remain unsolved, perhaps the medical social worker can help. The patient must realize that he is a responsible partner in his own treatment.

The patient should resume normal activities and responsibilities gradually. Time should be allowed daily for rest periods; these should follow each meal to promote good digestion. Good habits of sleeping and relaxing should be formed. Finally, moderation in all activities must be practiced. Follow-up visits to the physician are an important part of convalescent care.

Gastric Cancer

Cancer of the stomach, a disease that still accounts for more than 20,000 annual deaths in the United States, is typically a disease of middle age. It occurs chiefly in persons over 40, but is seen occasionally in younger people. The most common type of neoplasm of the stomach is carcinoma; sarcomata and lymphomata are relatively rare.

Symptoms and Diagnosis

The early symptoms of this disease are often indefinite, since most of these tumors start on the lesser curvature, where they cause little disturbance to the gastric functions. Later, after they have spread to the cardiac orifice, or especially to the pylorus, the suffering may be distressing; this is due not to the cancer as such, but to disturbance in gastric motility. Weight loss, weakness, anemia and sometimes icterus appear late in the disease. Pain in gastric cancer, as in cancer in almost all other parts of the body, is a late symptom. Whereas pain is, to the average layman, a sensitive indicator of disturbed physiology or disease, it is ironic that pain rarely warns the individual who has cancer while there is still an opportunity of curing it.

The most important early symptoms are: a progressive loss of appetite; the appearance of, or change in, gastrointestinal symptoms that have been increasingly apparent for a matter of weeks or months only; and the appearance of blood in the stools. If the tumor causes obstruction at the cardiac orifice, vomiting or a feeling of fullness will immediately follow the meal. If it is near the pylorus it eventually obstructs this channel, and vomiting becomes a prominent symptom. A certain number of patients apparently have experienced no symptoms attributable to gastric disease, but, having died for some other reason, are found at necropsy to have cancer of the stomach.

The dyspepsia mentioned is by far the most important of all early symptoms. If two persons were to describe their dyspepsia in much the same words, but one were to say his trouble began when he was a young man and had been present more or less ever since, while the other were to declare that he had had a normal digestion until he was 40 years old or more, it would be reasonable to postulate, tentatively, that the former has no cancer, while the latter may have one. If, in addition to this unprecedented development of dyspepsia, he has lost weight and strength and has become rather pale, we may be more confident of the suspected diagnosis.

Another important symptom occasionally present is the vomiting of coffee-ground vomitus. The blood that leaks slowly from the cancer (large hemorrhages are rare in patients with gastric cancer) is altered chemically and forms small clots or precipitates; there-

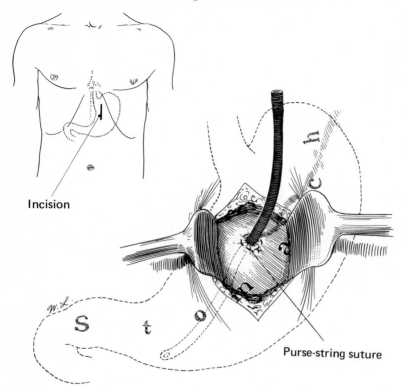

Incision

Purse-string suture

FIG. 22-6. The patient with a gastrostomy. Inset shows site of incision. A tube is inserted into the anterior gastric wall and held in place with several purse-string sutures.

fore, the vomitus acquires that appearance. The patient may not vomit, but one may constantly find traces of blood in the stools if these are examined chemically by the guaiac or benzidine test. This is a very early valuable sign of cancer anywhere along the gastrointestinal canal, but it is by no means confined to patients with malignancy, bleeding being a common complication of benign peptic ulcer as well.

If we examine the gastric juice, we find quite early that there is no free hydrochloric acid present. Often we do find some lactic acid formed from the gastric contents within one hour after the meal. Cytologic examination of the sediment from a centrifuged specimen of gastric juice examined by the Papanicolaou technique may show the presence of carcinoma cells; if so, the diagnosis is established. Sometimes the cancer is palpable, especially if it is located near the pylorus. We may find also in the abdomen other tumors, metastases of this gastric malignancy. The metastases are most apt to be located on the surface of the liver, in the skin at the umbilicus, in the left supraclavicular node, etc. In the early diagnosis of gastric cancer, roentgenologic, fluoroscopic and gastroscopic examinations are most valuable, as they often demonstrate the trouble before other signs appear. Dyspepsia of more than 4 weeks duration in any person over 40 calls for complete roentgenographic examination of the gastrointestinal tract, for no other single method offers a comparable means of diagnosing gastric cancer at a curable stage.

Treatment

At this writing there is no successful treatment of gastric carcinoma except removal of the tumor. This type of tumor does not respond to x-ray therapy or to any chemotherapeutic agents. Since surgery is the only method of therapy and since it is impossible to determine before operation the extent of the tumor and whether it can be cured, all patients with carcinoma of the stomach, with few exceptions, must be operated on. If the tumor can be removed while it is still localized to the stomach, many patients can be cured. If the tumor has spread beyond the area that can be excised surgically, cure cannot be effected. However, in many of these patients, effective palliation may be obtained by resection of the tumor. Although a radical operation is necessary to remove gastric cancer and the area to which it may have spread, as a rule some part of the stomach can be preserved. However, in some patients the entire tumor can be removed only by total gastrectomy. If a radical subtotal gastrectomy has been performed, the stump of the stomach is anastomosed to the jejunum, as in the gastrectomy for ulcer. When total gastrectomy is performed, gastrointestinal continuity is restored by an anastomosis between the ends of the esophagus and the jejunum, or sometimes a part of the colon may be interposed between the esophagus and the small intestine to act as a substitute stomach.

These patients should receive preparation similar to that for operation on peptic ulcers. Blood transfusions often are needed before, during and after operation. Gastric suction drainage usually is employed to empty the stomach both preoperatively and postoperatively.

Some of the complications that may follow gastrectomy are shock, hemorrhage, vomiting, peritonitis, obstruction, hiccup, parotitis, pulmonary embolus and phlebitis. For a full description, see pages 470-471.

Gastrostomy. This operation, in which a permanent opening is made into the stomach, is performed for the purpose of administering food and fluids when an impermeable stricture of the esophagus exists. The esophageal stricture may be due to scar-tissue contracture. In children, it occurs often as a result of lye burns, and in older people it is due most frequently to a carcinomatous growth.

Preoperative Preparation. The purpose of the operative procedure should be explained to the patient so that he will have a better understanding of his postoperative course. Fluids are administered by vein; the nature of the solution is determined by the fluid, the electrolyte and the nutritional needs of the patient.

Operation. The anterior gastric wall is grasped through the left rectus incision and a tube is inserted into the stomach. A plastic siliconized tube is used. The proximal end is flanged to fit snugly against the skin so that it will not pull out. (A purse-string suture is sometimes used for fixation.) The end of the tube is brought through the wound to the anterior abdominal wall and clamped. (Fig. 22-6.)

Postoperative Nursing Care. The psychological care of this patient is as important as his physical and nutritional care. The observing nurse will note his reactions and handle the situation accordingly.

The patient may be given fluids (10% glucose solution is best) through the tube at once if he is much dehydrated. At first only an ounce or 2 at a time is given, but the amount is increased gradually until, by the end of the second day, from 6 to 8 ounces may be given at one time provided this quantity is tolerated.

Tube Feedings. There have been several recent innovations in the preparation of tube feedings. Powdered feedings that are easily liquefied are commercially available. Since the advent of the food blender, a normal diet can be liquefied and fed through a tube. Blenderized tube feedings allow the patient to follow his usual diet pattern and thus are psychologically more acceptable. Good bowel function is promoted, since the fiber and residue content are similar to that of a normal diet.

Warm milk, cream, eggs, sugar, olive oil, broths and so forth may be given through the tube. The nurse may prepare a tray containing a funnel to which a tubing and a glass adapter are attached. This would be attached to the gastrostomy tube at the time of feeding. Water at room temperature should be available and used to precede and follow the feeding. The feeding should be warmed by placing it in a basin of water. Feedings never should be given directly from the refrigerator.

The feeding should be allowed to flow into the stomach by gravity. The flow can be regulated by raising or lowering the receptacle. Force never should be used. If there seems to be an obstruction, stop the feeding and report the condition to the surgeon.

The diet mixture may be divided into 4 feedings for the day and 3 for the night. They must be given very slowly. If the patient becomes nauseated, the fats must be decreased in amount and then increased gradually until the caloric requirement again is met. Water should be given as ordered through the tube.

Feedings should be recorded carefully as to amount of fluid and contents, in order that the surgeon may know whether the patient is obtaining enough to satisfy his caloric, nutritional and fluid requirements. After each feeding, the tube should be irrigated with warm water and clamped. Neglect of this procedure may cause the catheter to become clogged. The nurse in charge of a patient with a gastrostomy always should have a duplicate tube sterilized and ready for use. After 5 or 6 days, the tube may be removed if loose, and a fresh one, lubricated with petrolatum, inserted. The tube is held in place by a thin strip of adhesive that first is twisted about the tube and then firmly attached to the abdomen. A small dressing is applied over the tube and the whole is held in place by a firm abdominal binder. Thereafter the tube should be changed every 2 or 3 days, and adults should be taught how to do this for themselves. Once the opening into the stomach has been established, there is no possibility or necessity for a sterile technique in changing and introducing a gastrostomy tube. The tube should be clean but not necessarily sterile. The patient should learn also how to feed himself and should know what foods may be taken.

The skin about a gastrostomy opening requires special care. Sooner or later it may become irritated due to the action of gastric juices that leak out around the tube. If uncared for, the skin becomes macerated, red, raw and painful. Daily dressing of the wound averts this in large measure. However, it is well to apply some bland ointment, such as zinc oxide or petrolatum, to the area about the tube.

After several weeks, the tube may be removed and inserted only for feedings. Between times, the gastrostomy opening may be protected by a small gauze pad that is held in place by adhesive.

Nursing Surveillance for Complications After Gastric Resection. *Shock* has been mentioned as a complication, especially in very ill patients. The restoration of normal temperature and the administration of fluids are the prophylactic measures necessary in every case. For symptoms and treatment of shock, see pages 146-149.

Vomiting may occur once or twice after operations on the stomach. The vomitus usually is composed of a dark, bloody fluid. Usually, nausea and vomiting disappear after 8 or 10 hours. If vomiting continues after the first 24 hours, it is due probably to blood retained in the stomach. A change of position or a glass of warm water or sodium bicarbonate solution may aid in draining the stomach or inducing vomiting. The nasogastric tube often is inserted to provide continuous gastric drainage by suction.

Hemorrhage is occasionally a complication after gastric operations. The patient exhibits the usual signs (p. 149) and usually continues to vomit bright blood in considerable amounts. Emergency treatment is the administration of morphine and the placing of an icebag on the abdomen. Adrenalin hydrochloride solution may be given in water or saline by mouth for its effect in producing vasoconstriction. The nurse should be prepared for the administration of blood and intravenous fluids.

Pulmonary Complications frequently follow upper abdominal incisions because of the tendency to shallow respiration. Therefore, the nurse should urge the patient to breathe deeply several times each hour when awake in order to obtain full aeration of the lungs. A change in position, turning the patient from side to side, also is an aid in preventing these complications.

The dumping syndrome is a label loosely applied to postoperative symptoms that come on after eating. It is probable that it results from a rapid emptying of gastric contents into the small intestine, which has been anastomosed to the gastric stump. Symptoms are varied and may consist of palpitation, sweating, a feeling of faintness and weakness which may last only a few minutes or for as long as 30 minutes, even forcing the patient to lie down for a time.

There may be several causes for these symptoms, including a small gastric remnant remaining after the operation, the large opening from the gastric stump into the jejunum and the ingestion of food high in carbohydrates and electrolytes that have to be diluted in the jejunum before absorption can take place. The ingestion of fluid at mealtime is another factor in the rapid emptying of the stomach into the jejunum. The symptoms that occur are probably brought about by rapid distention of the jejunal loop anastomosed to the stomach and a withdrawal of water from the circulating blood volume into the jejunum to dilute the high concentration of electrolytes and sugars. Most patients with "dumping syndrome" recognize that meals high in sugars and salt produce these symptoms; consequently, they avoid these foods. They also have found that a dry meal (without liquids) reduces the appearance of "dumping" symptoms. Surgeons are attempting to reduce "dumping" by formation of smaller stomas and larger gastric stumps. On rare occasions, reoperation may be necessary to correct this syndrome.

Diarrhea is a troublesome complication in the occasional patient who has had a vagotomy. This symptom usually disappears in the first few weeks after operation, but when it is present it demands symptomatic therapy, usually by ingesting Kaopectate and at times, paregoric in small doses.

Vitamin B_{12} Deficiency. Total gastrectomy brings to an abrupt, complete and final halt the production of "intrinsic factor," the gastric secretion that is required for the absorption of vitamin B_{12} from the gastrointestinal tract (see page 307). Therefore, unless this vitamin is supplied by parenteral injection and continues to be supplied by that route throughout his life, the patient inevitably suffers from vitamin B_{12} deficiency, his status in time becoming identical to that of a patient with pernicious anemia in relapse. All of the manifestations of pernicious anemia, including macrocytic anemia and combined system disease, may be expected to develop within a period of 5 years or less, to progress in severity thereafter and, in the absence of therapy, to prove fatal. This complication is avoided by the regular monthly intramuscular injection of 100 to 200 micrograms of B_{12}, a regimen that should be started without delay after gastrectomy.

General Nursing Care After Gastric Surgery

In the operating room the administration of fluids is begun by transfusion and infusion, as much as from 2,500 to 3,000 ml. being given daily for the first 2 or 3 days. This is one of the best methods of warding off postoperative shock, a condition especially prone to develop in patients who have undergone operation for bleeding, perforated ulcer or cancer.

When recovery from anesthesia is complete, the patient is placed in the Fowler position, as this favors drainage of the stomach. Change of position from one side to the other at frequent intervals tends to prevent postoperative pulmonary and vascular complications. Nothing is given these patients by mouth for at least 24 hours. This precaution is taken to allow the suture line to seal off thoroughly and thus minimize the danger of leakage and peritonitis. Antibiotic and vitamin therapy are instituted parenterally. To relieve dryness of the mouth during this period, mouthwashes should be given at frequent intervals. To allow the patient to moisten his lips with ice that is enclosed in a piece

PRINCIPLES OF NURSING MANAGEMENT OF A PATIENT
FOLLOWING A GASTRIC RESECTION

Major Problems

1. Postoperative pain and discomfort
2. Maintenance of adequate nutrition
3. Prevention of complications

Objectives

I. To relieve the patient of pain and discomfort:

  A. Frequent turning for comfort and the prevention of pulmonary and vascular complications.

  B. Meticulous oral hygiene to counteract mouth dryness.

  C. Analgesics or narcotics for pain control.

  D. Parenteral antibiotics for prevention of infection.

  E. Oral fluids withheld until ordered (to allow sealing of suture line).

  F. Gastric suction to remove liquids, blood and gas in stomach.

II. To promote adequate nutrition:

  A. Intravenous fluids to prevent shock and maintain optimal fluid and electrolyte balance.

  B. Oral fluids when audible bowel sounds are present.

  C. Fluids to be increased according to patient's tolerance.

  D. Bland diet with vitamin supplements as indicated by patient's condition.

  E. Supplementary iron-vitamin therapy to ensure adequate intake.

  F. Avoidance of foods that may initiate development of "dumping syndrome."

III. To develop an awareness of complications that may follow gastric surgery:

  A. Shock

    1. Evaluate drainage from dressing and drainage bottle.

    2. Evaluate blood pressure, pulse and respiratory rates.

    3. Give blood and fluid replacement at time ordered.

  B. Hemorrhage

    1. Watch drainage for presence of blood.

    2. Evaluate blood pressure, pulse and respiratory rates.

    3. Start blood replacement if indicated.

  C. Pulmonary complications

    1. Encourage deep breathing and coughing to counteract voluntary diaphragm splinting.

    2. Promote frequent turning and moving to mobilize bronchial secretions.

    3. Ambulate when ordered to increase respiratory exchange.

  D. Thrombosis and embolism

    1. Encourage participation in self-care activities to increase circulation.

    2. Encourage early ambulation to minimize stasis of venous blood.

    3. Use elastic stockings as indicated to prevent venous stasis.

    4. Check dressing and binders for tightness that impairs circulation.

  E. Wound evisceration

    1. Use abdominal binders if ordered for support.

    2. Prevent distention and wound infection.

    3. Support incision when coughing.

    4. Promote good nutrition.

    5. Inspect dressing frequently.

  F. "Dumping syndrome"

    1. Teach patient to avoid eating large meals.

    2. Avoid salty, or highly concentrated carbohydrate foods.

    3. Take fluids between meals.

    4. Avoid liquids with meals.

    5. Eliminate sweets from the diet.

    6. Eat regularly, slowly and in a relaxed environment.

    7. Lie down after meals.

    8. Take anticholinergic drugs before meals (as directed) to lessen gastrointestinal activity.

IV. To promote the rehabilitation of the patient:

  A. Help him to modify his environmental stresses.

  B. Encourage him to remain under medical supervision.

  C. Advise adequate caloric intake after discharge from the hospital.

  D. Weigh regularly.

  E. Have yearly hematologic study and medical evaluation for evidences of pernicious anemia.

of gauze often is refreshing. The nurse also can use an applicator stick dipped in mineral oil and lemon juice to swab dry lips. Very often a nasogastric tube attached to a suction apparatus is used to remove mucus, liquids, blood, gas and materials that accumulate in the stomach during the first 24 to 48 hours after operation. Repeated irrigation of the tube with syringe and physiologic saline or Ringer's solution may be needed to keep the tube open. The amount of solution used should be charted. With the nasogastric tube it is important for the nurse to give care to the nostrils. An applicator stick moistened with water and followed by an applicator stick dipped in mineral oil can be used to clean the nostril.

When fluids are ordered, they should be given warm and sparingly at first. Beginning with 4 or 8 ml. every half hour, the amount is increased gradually until 90 or 120 ml. are being taken. Warm weak tea with sugar and lemon is very acceptable. Cold fluids usually cause distress. If the patient does not vomit, more fluid may be given by mouth. On the third or fourth day, milk and other bland liquids may be added to the diet, and on the fifth day a routine diet should be instituted. Should the patient vomit, eruct or hiccup at any time, the intake should be stopped and instructions requested.

After radical resections of the stomach in the treatment of carcinoma, the remaining gastric stump may be extremely small; after total gastrectomy, there is no gastric reservoir at all. The nutrition of these patients is the important postoperative therapy. Since they cannot eat large meals, frequent smaller ones are necessary. These should be high in caloric value, with foods that do not require much churning for digestion. This means a diet rather high in eggs, milk, butter and cream. If vegetables are taken, they should be pureed or soft. Fruits should be stewed or finely chewed.

PROBLEMS INVOLVING THE SMALL AND THE LARGE BOWEL

Constipation

Chronic Constipation

Constipation is a term which describes an abnormal infrequency of defecation, and also abnormal dryness of the stools. Most normal persons have one bowel movement a day. Some, however, go 2, 3 or 4 days without a movement; their stools are normally moist, and they suffer no discomfort. On the other hand, some constipated persons at times have a diarrhea of liquid stools, due to the irritation caused by the presence in the colon of hard, dry fecal masses. Such stools contain a good deal of mucus, secreted by glands in the colon in response to these irritating masses. In severe constipation, the rectum may become impacted, that is, filled with masses of hard feces that must be removed by the fingers or first softened by instillations of oil before they can be washed out by an enema.

There are few organic causes of chronic constipation. The most important of these are morphine addiction, lead poisoning and cancer of the large bowel, a condition in which constipation usually alternates with diarrhea. Painful hemorrhoids and anal fissures, by inducing rectal spasm, also may lead to temporary constipation. Other factors that predispose to its development include limitation of muscular exercise, unfamiliar diet, weakness, debility and fatigue.

By far the most common type of constipation has a functional, rather than organic, basis. Many patients develop a habit constipation because of the careless or neurotic habit of delaying each bowel movement as long as possible. The rectal mucous membrane and musculature become insensitive to the presence of fecal masses, and consequently the stimulus required to produce the necessary peristaltic rush for defecation becomes increasingly greater. The initial effect of this fecal retention, or hoarding, is to produce irritability of the colon, which at this stage goes frequently into spasm, especially after meals, giving rise to colicky mid abdominal or low abdominal pains. Eventually, after several years, perhaps, the colon loses muscular tone; it is essentially unresponsive to normal stimuli. The patient may be said to have *atonic constipation,* whereas in the earlier stage the condition is sometimes referred to as *spastic constipation,* although they should not be regarded as separate entities.

Teaching the Patient. In simple or functional constipation, the role of the nurse is that of assisting with the re-education of the patient. The physiology of defecation should be explained carefully, with particular emphasis on the importance of heeding promptly the urge to defecate. Instruct the patient to have a regular time for defecation, preferably after a meal. Thinking about the act of defecation, i.e., "auto-suggestion," may be an aid in initiating the reflex. A small footstool to promote flexion of the thighs ensures an optimal posture during defecation.

Patients who worry about having a *daily* bowel movement need reassurance. Carefully explain that some healthy persons have a bowel movement 3 times daily while others do so only 2 or 3 times a week. Knowing that some of the food eaten may normally remain in the intestinal tract 48 hours after ingestion will help the patient to understand and accept the fact that a daily bowel evacuation is not always necessary. The use of laxatives should be discontinued. If the feces remain too long in the rectum and become dehydrated, and hardened, the patient may be instructed to take 2 or 3 oz. of warm oil in the form of a rectal instillation at bed time. A small enema of physiologic saline the next morning should help to alleviate this condition.

Measures helpful in breaking the constipation habit include:

(1) Regular time to go to stool each day.

(2) A large glass of prune juice, or lemon juice in warm water each morning.

(3) Bulk-forming laxative that does not irritate the bowel, such as Metamucil, one heaping teaspoonful in a glass of water followed by a second glass of water, once or twice daily.

(4) Plentiful daily fluid intake.

The patient must know what constitutes a normal diet. When teaching the patient, emphasize the similarities between his prescribed diet and the normal diet. In general, a high-residue, high-fiber diet is prescribed for atonic constipation; a bland or low residue diet is indicated for the patient with an irritable colon. Approximately the same amount of foods should be eaten at each meal, and the patient should ingest 2 liters of fluid daily (or more if he perspires freely).

It takes time to break bad habits and form new ones. It takes time to teach the patient. Remember that repetition is one of the laws of learning. The wise use of every patient contact to help the patient to adjust to his new regimen of treatment will do much to help to develop a nurse who is worthy of the patient's confidence.

Acute Constipation

Obstipation (no bowel movements) is indicative of bowel obstruction or adynamic ileus.

Acute constipation, in contrast with the chronic variety, always indicates an acute and, frequently, a serious disorder. The symptom may prompt one to order a laxative, but it must be remembered that acute constipation may be an early symptom of acute appendicitis, and that a purge given in this condition may well produce perforation of the inflamed appendix. In general, one should not prescribe a cathartic for fever, nausea or pain merely because the bowels fail to move; and, before such medication is offered, it must be quite clear that no inflammatory disease of the intestinal tract is present.

Enemas are relatively safe as regards the possible perforation of an inflammatory lesion of the bowel, provided that they are administered with extreme caution. Saline solutions, or water alone, may be instilled, but nothing more irritating than these, and the nurse should be prepared to halt the irrigation at once if pain is induced or increased in the slightest degree.

Complications and Nursing Implications of Constipation

The maintenance of elimination is basic to the care of every patient. The mechanical difficulties and the physical discomforts associated with defecation and micturition that harass the bed patient are widely known. It is doubtful, however, whether this aspect of medical and nursing care is generally recognized as a problem of considerable magnitude, the implications of which, in some instances, are far from trivial. The effort entailed in defecation is considerable. With the use of a bedpan the muscular strain is inevitably greater, and when constipation is imposed in addition, the performance of this function can be extremely fatiguing, if not altogether exhausting. This is a serious consideration in the management of patients with congestive heart failure, which may be dangerously aggravated in patients with recent myocardial infarction and susceptibility to cardiac rupture, and in those with arterial hypertension.

Straining at stool has a striking effect on the arterial blood pressure. During the period of active straining, the flow of venous blood in the chest is temporarily impeded due to an increase in intrathoracic pressure that tends to collapse the large veins in the chest. The atria and the ventricles receive less blood, and consequently less is delivered by the systolic contractions of the left ventricle; the cardiac output is decreased, and there is a transient drop in arterial pressure. Almost immediately after this period of hypotension, a rise in arterial pressure occurs; the pressure is elevated momentarily to a point far exceeding the original level (the "rebound" phenomenon). In patients, with arterial hypertension, this compensatory reaction may be exaggerated greatly, and the peaks of pressure attained may be dangerously high—sufficient, indeed, to rupture a major artery in the brain or elsewhere. It is not possible to make other than a rough estimate of the frequency with which the act of defecation is the terminal event and brings on death due to vascular accidents that result from straining at stool. The danger is not sufficiently appreciated, however, particularly in patients with vascular diseases of the type described. Inasmuch as straining is promoted by constipation, the latter cannot be dismissed as altogether inconsequential; on the contrary, it must be concluded that the regularity and the consistency of the stools, as well as the mechanical aspects of defecation, are matters of prime concern.

To facilitate elimination, the patient should assume the normal position for defecation. In most instances there is less strain to the patient if he can be assisted to a bedside commode. A bedpan placed on a chair will suffice if a commode is not available. Or the patient may be seated on the bedpan at the side of the bed with his feet supported on a chair. If he cannot sit up, a small support should be placed under the lumbosacral curve to minimize strain and increase his comfort while using the bedpan.

The Primary Malabsorption States

The above term is applied to 3 closely related conditions: namely, tropical sprue, idiopathic steatorrhea (nontropical sprue) and celiac disease. Tropical and nontropical sprue are diseases of adults; in clinical manifestations and pathologic changes, the 2 conditions are very similar. However, their geographic incidence and their causes differ and they respond to different treatments. Celiac disease is limited to childhood but resembles idiopathic steatorrhea in all other respects, and probably represents the juvenile phase of that disease. Other causes are extensive resection of the small bowel and tumor infiltration of the small bowel wall.

The pathologic defect is similar in all 3 conditions. The principal lesion involves the mucosa of the small intestine especially the intestinal villae, which become severely blunted or are lost altogether. As a result, the absorptive surface within the small bowel is substantially reduced in area and food absorption is correspondingly impaired. The hallmarks of the malabsorption syndrome of whatever cause are diarrhea or frequent loose, bulky, foul stools with increased fat content and often greyish in color; associated weakness, weight loss and lack of well-being.

Patients with the malabsorption syndrome, if neglected, become weak and emaciated due to starvation. Failing to absorb the fat-soluble vitamins A, D and K, they develop the corresponding avitaminoses. Manifestations of abnormal bleeding are likely to appear as a result of K deficiency and hypoprothrombinemia (p. 324). Anemia develops, which is of the macrocytic type characteristic of folic-acid deficiency (p. 309). Impaired absorption of calcium may be responsible for gradual demineralization of the skeleton and, in the case of children with celiac disease, for the stunting of growth. Moreover, calcium deficiency may lead to extreme neuromuscular hyperirritability, including attacks of hypocalcemic tetany.

The basic factor in the pathogenesis of idiopathic steatorrhea and celiac disease is a specific and profound intolerance to a protein substance (gluten) contained in wheat, rye and barley. A constituent of gluten, *gliadin,* for reasons that are not clear, exerts toxic effects on the mucosa of the small intestine, damaging or destroying its villi and crippling its function. The increased familial incidence of these disorders suggests that a hereditary factor, i.e., an inborn error of metabolism, may be involved, and that enzymatic activities governing the digestion of gliadin may be affected. In any case, the elimination of gluten from the patient's diet is followed by striking clinical improvement. His diarrhea ceases and his nutritional status is restored to normal. This gratifying remission may be expected to last as long as the patient remains on a gluten-free diet, and no longer. Unfortunately, the total exclusion of gluten is difficult to accomplish, since this substance is incorporated into many foods as a binder and filler. It is contained in almost every bakery product, "wheat-free" or otherwise, and is an ingredient of other foodstuffs as well, including some brands of ice cream.

The factors primarily responsible for the onset and the progression of tropical sprue have not as yet been clarified. Its clinical course appears to be unaffected by the presence or the absence of gliadin in the diet; hence gliadin intolerance seemingly plays no role in its pathogenesis. Of greatest benefit in this condition is the administration of folic acid, which usually is prescribed in 5-mg. doses by mouth, 3 times each day until a remission is established, and once daily thereafter for a period of 4 to 6 months. The beneficial effects of folic acid in patients with tropical sprue appear with such regularity and on occasion are so striking as to suggest that this particular malabsorption syndrome may be attributable to, as well as productive of, folic-acid deficiency.

Diarrhea

Diarrhea is one of the cardinal symptoms of small-bowel disease. It is a condition in which there is unusual frequency of bowel movements, as well as changes in the amount, the character and the consistency of the stools. In acute cases the stools are grayish-brown, foul smelling and filled with undigested particles of food and mucus. The patient complains of abdominal cramps, distention, intestinal rumbling (borborygmus), anorexia and thirst. Painful spasms (tenesmus) of the anus may attend each defecation.

Diarrhea and its associated symptoms occur in a variety of disorders. The efficient nurse will facilitate the diagnosis in each case by recording her discerning observations, including the patient's symptoms, behavior and remarks. Accurate description of abnormal stools is of great importance in diagnosis. For example, watery stools are characteristic of small-bowel disease, whereas loose, semisolid stools are associated more often with disorders of the colon. Voluminous, greasy stools suggest intestinal malabsorption, and the presence of mucus and pus in the stools denotes inflammatory enteritis or colitis.

Nocturnal diarrhea may be a manifestation of diabetic neuropathy.

Acute Diarrhea

Most acute diarrheas are due to the stimulating effect of some irritant on intestinal peristalsis. The irritant stimulating the diarrhea may arise from a localized infection or ulceration in the intestinal wall, due, for example, to a carcinoma, a diverticulitis or a tuberculous lesion. The irritant may be chemical. Castor oil, after it has been acted upon by the digestive juice, is an example of a mild intestinal irritant, as are most of the vegetable cathartics. Certain unripe fruits, which cause crampy diarrhea, likewise belong in this category.

The inflammatory response to these mild irritants is slight; little or no mucous membrane lining is destroyed on exposure to them unless their concentration in the intestinal fluid is excessive. Their chief effect is to produce hyperemia (vascular dilatation, with local increase in blood flow, in other words, blushing) of the intestinal mucosa and increase in mucous secretion. There also occurs a motor response of hyperperistalsis, which persists until the irritant is excreted. This explains the symptoms of crampy diarrhea. Some chemicals, such as mercuric chloride, are extremely caustic. They cause intense circulatory congestion of the intestinal walls and necrosis of its lining membrane, which separates away in shreds. The unfortunate individual who ingests such a caustic experiences severe crampy diarrhea with persistent passage of liquid bloody stools. The eventual outcome, usually, is death.

Infectious. By far the most common intestinal irritants are the products of certain bacteria, whether their growth occurred in the intestine or in the food before it was eaten. In the case of the enteric pathogens, the organisms causing bacillary dysentery, bacterial growth with release of the irritating toxins takes place in the intestine. On the other hand, practically all cases of food poisoning, or ptomaine poisoning, are due to the ingestion of food heavily contaminated and already containing the toxin. *Staphylococcus aureus*, for example, if given an opportunity to grow in food, produces an exotoxin that is extremely irritating to the intestinal tract.

Whether the gastrointestinal tract is exposed to toxins introduced in food or produced by bacteria growing within the intestine, an infectious enterocolitis is produced. The inflammatory response may vary from mild hyperemia and hypermotility of the gastrointestinal tract to severe inflammation of the intestine, depending on the virulence of the infecting organism and the amount of toxin liberated. Clinically, except for the presence of diarrhea, there is little similarity between a case of food poisoning due to the ingestion of food containing bacterial toxins and a case of bacillary dysentery. The diarrhea in food poisoning is explosive in onset, develops within a very few hours following the toxic meal and, except in severe cases, subsides within 1 or 2 days—as soon as the toxin is excreted and the inflammatory response subsides. There is little or no fever, and usually the only associated symptoms are those directly attributable to the diarrhea, namely, dehydration and weakness. Dysentery due to the growth of gastrointestinal pathogens within the gastrointestinal tract, on the other hand, develops with a more gradual onset, persists for several days or weeks, and there are striking constitutional symptoms in addition to the diarrhea. These clinical differences are quite understandable when it is realized that in the infectious diarrheas a bacterial invasion of the intestinal mucosa is involved. Then, not only must the bacterial toxins be excreted or destroyed, but also the bacteria themselves must be eradicated, and this takes considerably longer.

Diagnostic Evaluation. The diagnosis of an acute diarrhea is based on the course of the disease: the type of onset and progression, the presence or absence of fever and a study of the stools, which are examined for bacteria as well as for blood and pus. In cases of possible infection, the suspected food is tested by bacteriologic cultures. It is very important to remember that diarrhea often is present in various systemic infections. It may be the initial misleading complaint in certain of the exanthemata before the appearance of the rash, or appear as an early symptom of hepatitis. It may complicate or mask such conditions as mastoiditis, pneumonia and pyelitis.

Treatment. Patients with acute diarrhea are placed at bed rest until the episode has terminated. They may be treated with a sedative drug, such as a barbiturate, or with a more powerful opiate, for example, paregoric or opium tincture. Fluid and electrolyte replacement, orally or parenterally, is an extremely important measure, symptomatically as well as supportively. During the acute stages very little is prescribed by mouth other than water, bouillon (for its salt content) and milk, the last furnishing water, electrolytes and also calories. Potassium replacement, accomplished by the parenteral injections of an appropriate electrolyte solution (pp. 84-87), is necessary in very severe diarrheal disorders, particularly in infants and young children. Sulfonamide chemotherapy, with sulfadiazine or Gantrisin, may be indicated in infectious cases.

Prevention. All cases of acute diarrhea should be treated as potentially infective until they are proved otherwise. If the diarrhea is of infectious origin, those caring for the patient should determine whether there is any diarrhea among his family and neighbors. Ask him about his recent sources of food and water. Every nurse is a case finder. By reporting a larger than usual number of cases of diarrhea, she assists the local health officer to discover whether an epidemic is starting in the community.

Proper precautions to avoid the spread of the disease through contamination of the hands, the clothing, the bed linen, etc., with feces or vomitus must be taken.

Diarrhea always should be regarded as a potential risk under conditions of crowding; outbreaks occur with particular frequency in institutions such as prisons, boarding schools and army camps, in trailer camps and even in hospitals, unless sanitary precautions are observed rigidly and constantly. Precautions include ensuring that proper storage and refrigeration facilities are available and are used for the handling of all fresh fruits and meats. Meat products should be cooked thoroughly, and all cooked meats should be refrigerated immediately unless they are consumed promptly. Milk and milk products should be refrigerated constantly and protected against exposure. Food items that are particularly prone to infection and provide the best environment for bacterial growth include custards and cream fillings, such as are prepared in éclairs, cream pies, layer cakes, cream puffs, etc. Such materials should be cooked thoroughly and then be brought to refrigerator temperature immediately unless they are to be eaten within a very few hours after cooking.

Isolation Technique and Precautions. The following precautions should be observed meticulously, not only in this, but also in other communicable enteric infections, including enteritis due to *Salmonella* infection and dysentery of all types.

SCREENING. The patient's room should be completely screened against the entry of flies and other insects; if the patient is treated in an open ward, the area adjacent to his bed should be framed and screened.

LINENS. All nurses, doctors, and other hospital personnel in contact with the patient should wear gowns and scrub their hands with soap and running water after each contact. All bed linen and clothing should be collected in an individual precaution bag and sterilized by autoclaving, by boiling or by soaking for 1 hour in a 5 per cent formalin or 2 per cent cresol solution.

DISHES. All dishes, trays and eating utensils should be sterilized after use by boiling for 15 minutes. Uneaten food is collected in a paper bag and burned in the incinerator.

DEJECTA. Depending on the nature of the equipment for sterilizing bedpans and their contents, the following procedures may be adopted.

All feces should be sterilized in the bedpan by completely covering them with 5 per cent cresol or 10 per cent formalin solution for 30 to 60 minutes. Formed feces should be broken up with a stick to facilitate

adequate exposure to the antiseptic. Urine and bath water similarly should be exposed to these antiseptic solutions. Dejecta never should be discarded into toilets without previous sterilization, because flies may have access to the material itself or to the water in the bowl, which has become contaminated and is infective. (These measures are unnecessary if automatic bedpan washing equipment of the type delivering water sprayed at high temperature and city sewage disposal facilities are available.)

MISCELLANEOUS ITEMS. Each patient should be equipped with his own individual thermometer, bedpan, basin, urinal and toilet articles. Wastes, wipes, etc., are collected in paper bags and disposed of by burning in an incinerator.

VISITORS. Nonprofessional visits should be kept to a minimum, and all persons admitted should be obliged to wear gowns and observe precautions as instructed, i.e., refrain from touching the patient, his bed, bedside table or any object that the patient has handled or is within his reach.

Home Nursing. Precautions to be observed in caring for patients with infectious enteritis in the home include the following:

Linens should be boiled for 30 minutes or soaked for 1 hour in a 2 per cent Lysol solution.

Liquid waste and excreta should be collected in a special container, allowed to stand for 1 hour with equal parts of 5 per cent chlorinated lime solution and then emptied. Bedpans and urinals may be soaked for 1 hour in a 2 per cent Lysol or a 5 per cent chlorinated lime solution.

Public Health Teaching. Proper housekeeping, especially in kitchen maintenance, is obviously very important in the prevention of epidemic diarrhea. All materials used in the preparation and the serving of food must be cleansed rigorously and kept in immaculate condition. All food handlers should receive detailed instructions in hygienic principles and practices and, on the development of any illness that is potentially infectious, should be relieved of their duties immediately.

Appendicitis

The appendix is a small tube about 4 inches long and as large around as the little finger. Its structure is similar to the ileum. One end of the appendix is closed and the other opens into the cecum just below the ileocecal valve. No definite function can be assigned to it in man. It fills with food and empties as regularly as does the cecum, of which it is a part. It empties inefficiently, however, and its lumen is very small, so that it is prone to become obstructed and is particularly vulnerable to infection, or appendicitis.

Symptoms

Acute appendicitis starts typically with a progressively severe generalized or upper abdominal pain, which, within a few hours, becomes localized in the right lower quadrant of the abdomen. This pain usually is accompanied by a low-grade fever and often by vomiting. At McBurney's point, located halfway between the umbilicus and the anterior spine, one expects to find local tenderness on pressure and some rigidity of the lower portion of the right rectus muscle. A moderate leukocytosis is often present. Loss of appetite is common.

Just how much tenderness there will be, how much muscle spasm, whether or not there is constipation or diarrhea, etc., depend not so much on the severity of the appendical infection as on the location of the appendix. If the appendix curls around behind the cecum (retrocecal appendix), pain and tenderness may be felt in the lumbar region; if its tip is in the pelvis, these signs may be elicited only on rectal examination. Pain on defecation suggests that its tip is against the rectum; pain on micturition, that it is near the bladder or impinges on the ureter. Eventually, the inflamed appendix fills with pus and then is apt to perforate. Once it has ruptured, the pain is relieved temporarily, and for a short time the patient feels much better. However, the symptoms soon recur and increase in severity as a local abscess forms or general peritonitis develops (Fig. 22-7).

Complications

If the appendix can be removed before inflammation has progressed to the point of perforation, there is no further trouble. The abdomen can be closed at once, and the patient can be out of the hospital in a few days. However, if perforation has occurred, the patient may develop generalized peritonitis (p. 478), or an appendiceal abscess may result, in which case the surrounding loops of bowel become adherent and wall off the spreading peritonitis. A certain number of patients having appendicitis, on whom operation was performed too late or not at all, develop the dangerous complication of pylephlebitis, that is, a spread of the infection into the portal venous system, thence to the liver, where abscesses develop. This complication is to be suspected in a patient with chills, fever and jaundice following an attack of abdominal pain suggestive of appendicitis.

Nonoperative Treatment

Operation is always indicated if acute appendicitis is suspected, unless there is good evidence that perforation has occurred recently and a generalized peritonitis has developed. In this case the patient is treated

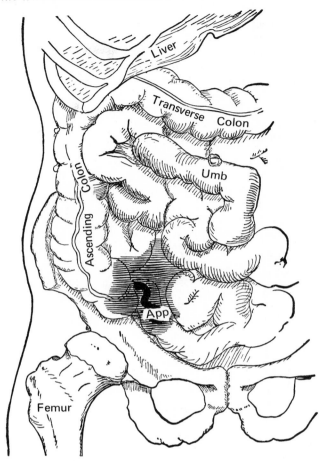

Fig. 22-7. Acute appendicitis, gangrene of the appendix, perforation and spreading peritonitis. In this case, the appendix was not removed, and the inflammation spreads to the surrounding loops of bowel. An abscess will form in the shaded area, or the inflammation may spread through the entire peritoneal cavity.

conservatively with parenteral electrolyte and amino acid solutions, gastric suction, drainage and antibiotics, in the expectation that the infection will localize and be susceptible to surgical drainage. As long as the question of operation is undecided, morphine is withheld, even in the face of moderate suffering, because it may mask the patient's symptoms. After the decision has been made, he may be sedated comfortably.

Preparation for Operation

This depends entirely on the length of time spent in the hospital before operation. If an emergency operation is necessary, shaving of the abdomen, voiding by the patient and the administration of the prescribed hypodermic injection are required. Usually an enema is not given but, if one is ordered, it is given low and slowly. Chemotherapy and/or antibiotics are administered before and after surgery.

If the patient has been suffering from acute abdominal pain, he accepts the operation as a means of relief. This acceptance of surgery makes his anesthetic and postanesthetic course a relatively easy one. The operation may be performed under general or spinal anesthesia. The usual incisions are the McBurney, the muscle-splitting or the gridiron and the lower right rectus incision. After the peritoneum has been opened, the appendix is brought into the wound and its mesentery is ligated with a surgical gut ligature. The appendix is freed and a purse-string suture is inserted round its base. After cutting through the organ at its base between clamps or ligatures, using the electrocautery or a knife followed by pure phenol and alcohol, the stump is inverted and the purse-string is tied. The appendix, the knife, the hemostats and the forceps used when the appendix was severed no longer are sterile, and they should be discarded. Sponges used to protect the wound and intestine also should be removed from the table. If the appendix has perforated and caused an abscess or a peritonitis, drainage tubes must be inserted.

Postoperative Nursing Care

Appendectomy Without Drainage. As soon as the patient recovers from the anesthesia he should be placed in the Fowler position. Morphine, from 0.016 gm. to 0.011 gm. (gr. ¼-⅛), may be given at intervals of 3 or 4 hours. Fluids are usually given as soon as the patient can tolerate them unless the patient has been dehydrated. In this case they are given intravenously. Food may be given as desired the day of operation if the patient's condition permits. An enema may be given on the morning of the third day. The stitches are removed from the incision between the fifth and the seventh days, usually in the physician's office.

After removal of the appendix a complication that at times is annoying is the inability to void. The patient may be allowed to stand with support or to sit on the edge of the bed with the feet on a chair. In this manner, the necessity for catheterization may be averted.

Appendectomy With Drainage. The treatment of patients after an appendectomy requiring drainage is complicated by local or general peritonitis. They should be placed in strict Fowler position as soon as they recover from the anesthetic and treatment for peritonitis should be instituted as described on page 479. These patients should be watched carefully for many days for signs of intestinal obstruction and secondary hemorrhage. Secondary abscesses may form

in the pelvis, under the diaphragm or in the liver. These cause an elevation of temperature and pulse rate with an increase in the leukocyte count. A fecal fistula, with the discharge of feces through the drainage tract, develops at times. The complication arises most often after the drainage of an appendiceal abscess. The attention of the surgeon should be drawn to feces on the dressings.

Meckel's Diverticulum

Meckel's diverticulum is a congenital abnormality consisting of a blind tube, comparable with the appendix, that usually opens into the distal ileum near the ileocecal valve. It represents a remnant of a fetal structure, the omphalomesenteric duct, which in fetal life connects the embryonic yolk sac with the digestive tract. A portion of this duct persists as a diverticulum in approximately 2 per cent of the population. It is more common in men than in women. It usually opens into the ileum at a point 1 to 3 feet proximal to the ileocecal valve. Most diverticula are less than 4 inches long, although on rare occasions they may even exceed 3 feet in length.

The importance of Meckel's diverticulum lies in the fact that its mucosal lining not infrequently is composed in part of aberrant, or misplaced, tissue—tissue characteristic of another portion of the gastrointestinal tract. It may, for example, contain gastric or jejunal mucosa, or even pancreatic tissue. Such aberrant tissues tend to ulcerate. Thus, the diverticulum may give rise to gastrointestinal hemorrhage—its most common manifestation in childhood; it may become inflamed and lead to intestinal obstruction, or it may perforate, causing peritonitis.

The most common symptoms of a diseased Meckel's diverticulum are abdominal pain, typically umbilical in location, or the passage of stools containing blood. This blood is not apt to be tarry black, as in the case of a slowly bleeding gastric or upper intestinal lesion, nor yet bright red, as would be expected from a colonic hemorrhage, but, rather it is a dark crimson color. The treatment is surgical excision of the diverticulum.

Peritonitis

Peritonitis is inflammation of the peritoneal cavity. Usually it is due to bacterial infection, the organisms coming from disease of the gastrointestinal tract, the internal genital organs of the female and, less often, from outside by injury or by extension of inflammation from an extraperitoneal organ such as the kidney.

Symptoms depend, of course, on the location and the extent of the inflammation, and these in turn are determined by the disease causing the peritonitis. At first a diffuse type of pain is felt. This tends to become constant, localized and more intense near the site of the process. The area of the abdomen affected becomes extremely tender and the muscles become rigid. Rebound tenderness and ileus may be present. Usually, nausea and vomiting occur and peristalsis is diminished. The temperature and the pulse rate increase, and almost always there is an elevation of the leukocyte count. These early signs and symptoms of peritonitis also are the symptoms of the disease causing the condition.

Treatment and Nursing Care

Treatment is directed toward removing the cause: if this is an acutely inflamed appendix, an appendectomy is performed; if it is a ruptured duodenal ulcer, the opening in the duodenum is closed; and so on.

If the cause of the peritonitis is removed at an early stage, the inflammation subsides and the patient recovers. Frequently, however, the inflammation is not localized and the whole abdominal cavity becomes involved. The patient is acutely ill. He has severe pain and must be treated gently. Treatment and nursing care are concerned with combating the infection, establishing and eliminating the cause of the peritonitis, and making the patient as comfortable as possible.

Nothing is given by mouth; therefore, good mouth hygiene must be carried out by the nurse. Fluids of saline and glucose are administered by vein in an attempt to establish an adequate fluid level and to ensure an adequate urinary output both before and after operation. This is important, for many toxins are thrown off in this way. The effectiveness of this regimen can be attained only by the accurate recording of fluid intake and output by the nurse. This includes the measuring and the recording of vomitus. The antibiotics, especially penicillin and streptomycin or chlortetracycline or oxytetracycline, may be given parenterally.

It is essential that the nurse observe and record symptoms accurately. Her description of the nature, the location and the shifts of pain in the abdomen is very important. She may do much in establishing confidence and hope in the patient, who realizes very often the seriousness of his condition.

When he has recovered from the anesthetic after operation, the patient is placed in the Fowler position to facilitate drainage. Nothing is given by mouth and he continues to receive fluids by vein. To prevent vomiting and distention, a gastrointestinal tube is passed through the nose into the stomach and/or the intestine. This tube is connected to a suction source and must be checked by the nurse to see that it works properly. Obviously, it will be necessary to give care to the nose and the mouth to keep the patient com-

fortable. Cotton applicators dipped in water or mineral oil are effective in cleaning the nose. The use of a toothbrush and a mouthwash by the patient is refreshing. Mineral oil with lemon juice is pleasant as a lubricant for dry lips.

Drains are inserted frequently during the operation, and it is essential that the nurse observe and record the character of the drainage. Care must be taken in moving and in turning the patient to prevent dislodging or removing the drains accidentally. When the temperature and the pulse rate fall, the abdomen becomes soft, peristaltic sounds return and the patient begins to pass gas and have bowel movements, the peritonitis is subsiding. Food and fluids can be given by mouth in increasing amounts and parenteral fluids are reduced.

Two of the most common complications that must be watched for are wound evisceration and abscess formation. Any suggestion from the patient that an area of the abdomen is tender or painful or "feels as if something just gave way" should be reported to the surgeon.

Intestinal Tuberculosis

Primary tuberculous infections of the bowel wall are rare; the majority of cases develop as a complication of pulmonary tuberculosis. The disease spreads in the lymph channels of the intestinal wall, forming a ring of tubercles, which, coalescing, form an encircling ulcer in its mucous membrane. Tuberculous intestinal ulcers give few informative symptoms: merely chronic indigestion, with more or less flatulence, and diarrhea, but little pain. X-ray examination of the small and the large bowel is of great aid in the diagnosis of this disease. The treatment is that of tuberculosis in general. (See Chap. 16.)

Tuberculous Peritonitis

This infection presumably reaches the peritoneal cavity from caseous mesenteric lymph nodes. There are three forms of the disease: acute tuberculous peritonitis, peritonitis with effusion and adhesive peritonitis. Usually, however, one speaks merely of a "wet" and a "dry" form.

Symptoms

Acute tuberculous peritonitis rarely develops as abruptly as the acute pyogenic types described above. The pain usually is less severe, local tenderness and muscle spasm are more vague, the patient is less ill, and he tends to improve progressively. Indeed, in most patients, the local symptoms and signs are few or absent altogether; often the only physical sign elicited is immobility of the abdominal wall during respiration, a sign that is quite suggestive of this disease. On pal-

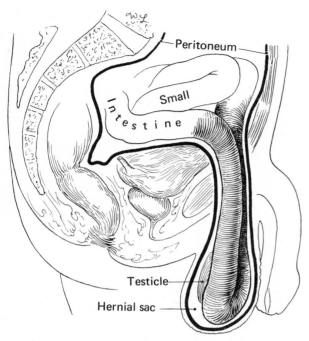

FIG. 22-8. *Inguinal* hernia. Note that the sac of the hernia is a continuation of the peritoneum of the abdomen and that the hernial contents are intestine, omentum or other abdominal contents that pass through the hernial opening into the hernial sac.

pation, the abdomen feels doughy rather than rigid. An irregular fever is characteristic, and either diarrhea or constipation may be present.

The "wet" form of the disease, in addition to the symptoms just described, is characterized by a striking distention of the abdomen, caused by a large amount of free fluid in the peritoneal cavity, and also by tympanites (gaseous distention of the intestines).

In the adhesive form of tuberculous peritonitis, the peritoneal cavity largely becomes obliterated by adhesions. There may be present large masses consisting of caseous tuberculous exudate walled in between the viscera, all of the bowel bound together into one mass, the omentum thickened and rolled up into a mass, visceral organs encased in a thick shell of tuberculous tissue or collections of clear fluid exudate encapsulated in various parts of the abdominal cavity. While these lesions are developing, patients may have varying degrees of malaise, loss of weight and strength, fever and anemia.

Treatment

Tuberculous peritonitis of all types improves following a regimen of chemotherapy and rest such as has been described for tuberculous infections in general.

Mesenteric Thrombosis

If one of the larger arteries supplying the intestine becomes plugged, that segment of the bowel supplied by this artery soon will become gangrenous; in other words, intestinal infarction occurs. Mesenteric thrombosis is most common in individuals past middle age who are suffering from generalized arteriosclerosis. Sclerosis of the mesenteric arteries, as in the case of the coronary or the cerebral arteries, predisposes to thrombosis of these vessels. Another cause of their sudden occlusion is embolism, for example, from a mural thrombus in the heart or from an endocarditis.

The symptoms of mesenteric thrombosis are sudden severe diffuse abdominal pain, distention, shock, which is often profound, and passage of blood in the stools.

Treatment

Treatment of the condition is a surgical emergency. Unless the infarcted portion of the bowel is removed promptly, intestinal perforation surely will occur through the gangrenous wall, with fatal peritonitis as the end result.

Abdominal Angina

"*Abdominal angina*" or arterial insufficiency of a chronic, low-grade nature may appear in arteriosclerotic patients. It is characterized by crampy abdominal pain after eating, especially if the patient exercises, because of an inability to increase the blood supply to the intestine as needed for digestion. This condition is often a forerunner of mesenteric thrombosis or bowel infarction. It is treated surgically by revascularization procedures.

Abdominal Hernia

A *hernia* (spoken of by the laity as "rupture") is a protrusion of a viscus through the wall of the cavity in which it is naturally contained. This definition may apply to any part of the body; for instance, the protrusion of the brain after a subtemporal decompression is called *cerebral hernia*. However, in general, the term is applied to the protrusion of an abdominal viscus through an opening in the abdominal wall.

Based on National Health Survey findings, it is estimated that approximately 2,900,000 people in the United States—about 15 per 1,000—have a hernia. Hernia is a major cause of hospitalization, especially among men, in whom it occurs 3 times more frequently than in women.

Most hernias result from congenital or acquired weakness of the abdominal wall, coupled with sustained increased intra-abdominal pressure from coughing, straining or from an enlarging lesion within the abdomen. Once the hernia occurs it has a tendency to increase in size.

The hernial sac is formed by an out-pouching of the peritoneum and may contain the large or small intestine, omentum and, occasionally, the bladder. When the hernia first is formed, the sac is filled only when the patient is on his feet, the contents returning to the abdominal cavity as soon as he lies down.

Types

There are 4 types of abdominal hernia. The most common type is the *inguinal*. This hernia is due to a weakness of the abdominal wall at the point through which the spermatic cord emerges in the male and the round ligament in the female. Through this opening the hernia extends down the inguinal canal and often into the scrotum or the labia. It is common in the male, and it may appear at any age (Fig. 22-8).

Femoral hernia appears below Poupart's ligament (i.e., below the groin) as a round bulge. It is more frequent in women.

Umbilical hernia results from failure of the umbilical orifice to close. It is most common in obese women and in children as a protrusion at the umbilicus.

Ventral or *incisional* hernias occur due to a weakness of the abdominal wall. They are due most frequently to previous operations in which drainage was necessary, complete closure of the tissues being impossible. Weakened by infection, only a slight bulge results at first, but this increases gradually in size until a definite hernial sac is produced.

There are many other forms of hernia, some of which occur inside the abdominal cavity. Such a hernia is spoken of as *internal* hernia.

Complications

As time goes on, adhesions form between the sac and its contents, so that the hernia becomes *irreducible*. Any hernia, whether previously reducible or not, may at any time become incarcerated or strangulated. An *incarcerated* hernia is one in which the intestinal flow is obstructed completely. In a *strangulated* hernia the contents not only are irreducible, but the blood and the intestinal flow through the intestine in the hernia are stopped completely. This condition obtains when the loop of intestine in the sac becomes twisted or swelling occurs and a constriction is produced at the neck of the sac. The result then is an acute intestinal obstruction, plus the added danger of gangrene of the bowel. The symptoms are pain at the site of strangulation, followed by colicky abdominal pain, vomiting, and swelling of the hernial sac.

Treatment

Surgical. In most cases the hernia should be repaired by operation; otherwise, it is in continual danger of strangulation. When this occurs, operation becomes imperative, and it is attended invariably by considerable increased risk.

The operation comprises removal of the hernial sac after dissecting it free from surrounding structures, replacing its contents in the abdominal cavity and ligating it at the neck. The muscle and the fascial layers then are sewed together firmly over the hernial orifice to prevent a recurrence. When the tissues are not sufficiently strong, reinforcement can be obtained by overlaying the suture line with synthetic mesh, which is also sutured in place. The presence of the mesh stimulates more than the usual amount of fibroblastic activity and thereby enhances the strength of the repair. When a strangulation has occurred, the operation is complicated by an intestinal obstruction and injury to the bowel.

Mechanical. In infants, a hernia may at times be helped by the application of a truss, an appliance having a pad that is held snugly in the hernial orifice and should keep a reducible hernia reduced. A truss also may be used in the treatment of a hernia in adults when, because of age, or disease, it seems inadvisable to subject the patient to the risk of an operation. *A truss does not cure a hernia;* it simply prevents the abdominal contents from entering the hernial sac.

Preoperative Nursing Management. In emergency conditions of strangulated or incarcerated hernia, the nurse prepares her patient as in any other acute surgical problem. However, most patients are individuals who are in good physical condition and are having a herniorrhaphy as elective surgery. The patient may be prompted by the knowledge that an unrepaired hernia may become a serious emergency, or he may have difficulty securing employment because of this condition.

The suprapubic region and the anterior surface of the upper thigh should be shaved carefully. It is important for the patient not to have a cold or a cough. Such a strain may break the sutures and defeat the purpose of surgery. When he goes to the operating room, his bladder must be empty.

Postoperative Nursing Management. Prolonged bed rest is not necessary after such operations, and in most cases patients are allowed out of bed a day or 2 after operation. In the event of edema and swelling of the scrotum, bed rest may be prolonged somewhat, and a suspensory bandage or a jock strap may be necessary to give support and to provide pressure.

The chief complication to be watched for in connection with the repair of a hernia is the retention of urine. The patient may have problems in voiding after spinal anesthesia. When these patients may not stand or sit up and, if conservative measures fail to give relief, catheterization must be performed.

Infection, or at least an imperfect healing, is all too

NAME MRS. JOAN BOSWICK   AGE 27   MARITAL STATUS S Ⓜ W D   DOCTOR ROBERT WALLACE

DATE OF ADMISSION 4/24   OCCUPATION ELEMENTARY   RELIGION UNITARIAN   HOSPITAL INSURANCE BLUE CROSS

ROOM 618   SCHOOL TEACHER

MAJOR NURSING AND THERAPEUTIC OBJECTIVE(S) TO KEEP PATIENT AT PHYSICAL AND EMOTIONAL REST.

PROBLEM	NURSING APPROACH	RESULTS AND EVALUATION
CRAMPING ABDOMINAL PAIN. STATES PAIN IS MORE SEVERE AFTER EATING (ON BLAND HIGH CALORIC, HIGH PROTEIN DIET).	TR. OF BELLADONNA STARTED BEFORE MEALS PER ORDER (4-25). APPLY WARM HOT WATER BOTTLE TO ABDOMEN AFTER MEALS. DO NOT GIVE ICED LIQUIDS (WARD AIDES ADVISED) (SIGN POSTED ABOVE ICE CHEST).	STATES WARMTH ON ABDOMEN "HELPS PAIN".
HAVING 10-14 BLOODY STOOLS DAILY. 4/26 COMPLAINING OF SEVERE RECTAL TENESMUS FOLLOWING BOWEL MOVEMENT.	4/26 DR. WALLACE HAS GIVEN PERMISSION FOR PT. TO HAVE DIOTHANE UNG. AT BEDSIDE FOR USE AFTER BOWEL MOVEMENTS. HAS BEEN TAUGHT HOW TO INSERT.	DIOTHANE UNG. SEEMS TO GIVE MRS. BOSWICK SOME RELIEF BUT SHE NEEDS TO BE REMINDED TO USE IT.
4/27 Becomes quite tense around mealtime, states that "eating just makes my diarrhea worse".	Try soft radio music while eating. "Pink lady volunteer" will visit c̄ pt. during mealtime. Give Butobarbital 30 min. after meals. Employ short interaction c̄ pt. regarding purpose of medication. Let pt. know that the medication meets a need expressed by her.	Radio music "makes me nervous & jumpy." Appears to enjoy companionship of older volunteers, uncommunicative c̄ younger volunteer workers.
4/28 CRIES AT INTERVALS THROUGHOUT DAY BUT REACTS WITH HOSTILITY WHEN SOMEONE ENTERS ROOM AND FINDS HER CRYING.	DO NOT IGNORE CRYING. RECOGNIZE HER NEED TO CRY AND ACCEPT THE ANGER THAT ACCOMPANIES IT.	SEEMED LESS HOSTILE AFTER NURSE SAID, "YOU HAVE A RIGHT TO CRY."

FIG. 22-9. Sample nursing care plan for the patient with ulcerative colitis.

frequent in these wounds. The elevation of temperature several days after operation or soreness in the operative region should lead to the discovery of the trouble. If early remedial measures are taken, the patient's convalescence is not delayed.

The patient should be instructed specifically as to his activity after leaving the hospital. As a rule, athletics and extremes of exertion are not permitted for at least 6 or 8 weeks after the operation.

Regional Ileitis

Pathophysiology

Regional ileitis is an inflammatory disease of the small intestine. Its cause is unknown. It has numerous names (terminal ileitis, cicatrizing enteritis, etc.) indicating that the disease usually affects a local area of the small intestine—usually the area of the terminal ileum, just before the ileum joins the large bowel. The disease is characterized by inflammation of the intestinal wall with swelling (edema). As it progresses, it tends to thicken the intestinal wall, at first by edema, and later by the formation of scar tissue and granulomas. This interferes with the function of the intestine because the lumen of the intestine is constricted. The result is that the intestine has to work harder to push the products of upper intestinal digestion through its narrowed lumen. This causes crampy abdominal pains, and since intestinal peristalsis is stimulated by the eating of food, the crampy pains occur after meals. To avoid these bouts of crampy pain, the patient avoids food or takes it only in amounts and types inadequate for normal nutritional requirements, so that weight loss, malnutrition and secondary or macrocytic anemia occur. In addition, ulcers form in the lining membrane of the intestine and other inflammatory changes take place, resulting in a constant irritating discharge that is emptied into the colon from the weeping, swollen intestine. This causes a chronic diarrhea. The end result is a very uncomfortable person, thin and emaciated from inadequate food intake and constant fluid loss. In some cases, the inflamed intestine may perforate and form intra-abdominal abscesses and abscesses about the anus. Melena may occur and also the malabsorption syndrome (see p.

474). Fever is not a prominent symptom, except when abscesses are present.

This disease affects both sexes equally and appears more often in those of Jewish origin. There is a definite familial occurrence. Regional enteritis may occur in any decade of life, but it reaches its highest incidence between the ages of 15 and 35.

Treatment

In mild cases, conservative treatment is employed, consisting of a dietary regimen low in roughage to improve nutrition. Sedative drugs and the corticosteroids are used as anti-inflammatory measures. When the symptoms do not respond to these conservative measures, or when massive bleeding occurs, surgical treatment is necessary.

Ulcerative Colitis

Ulcerative colitis is an ulcerative and inflammatory disease of the colon and rectum. It is characterized by multiple ulcerations, diffuse inflammation and desquamation of the colonic epithelium. Most commonly the disease begins in the rectum and sigmoid and spreads upward, ultimately involving the entire colon. The complications of ulcerative colitis are: skin ulcers, arthritis, malnutrition, anemia, abscess formations, stricture, erythema nodosum and amyloidosis.

The cause of the disease is unknown. In some patients, an autoimmune mechanism may be responsible for the development of ulcerative colitis. Some authorities consider ulcerative colitis to represent an example of psychosomatic disease. There may be several precipitating factors, the net effect of which is a self-perpetuating destructive infection of the mucosal lining of the large intestine. It is a serious disease accompanied by systemic complications, and the mortality rate is high. Eventually, 10 to 15 per cent of the patients develop carcinoma of the colon.

The following is a sample case history of a patient with ulcerative colitis. (See p. 482 for a sample nursing care plan for this patient.)

> Mrs. Joan Boswick, a school teacher, began having recurring bouts of diarrhea soon after the death of her mother. She continued teaching until she was having 12 to 14 bloody stools daily containing mucus and pus. She experienced increasing discomfort from abdominal cramps and began to lose weight. When she finally "gave up" and went to her physician, he immediately hospitalized her for diagnostic evaluation and treatment.

Diagnostic Evaluation

In the diagnosis of chronic ulcerative colitis, dysentery due to the common intestinal organisms and especially *Endameba histolytica* infection, must be ruled out by careful stool examination. Sigmoidoscopy and barium enema x-ray examination are of value in distinguishing this condition from other diseases of the colon with similar symptoms.

Therapeutic Regimen

The medical treatment of ulcerative colitis is summarized as follows:

(1) Well-balanced, bland, low residue, high protein diet;
(2) Psychological support of the patient and psychiatric evaluation when indicated;
(3) Education of the patient to accept and learn to live with a chronic disease;
(4) Administration of nonabsorbable sulfas such as salicylazo-sulfapyridine (Azulfidine), 1 gm. 4 times a day, orally;
(5) Administration of sedatives;
(6) Corticosteroid therapy orally, parenterally or by enema in patients with severe symptoms;
(7) Supplemental vitamin therapy;
(8) Iron replacement;
(9) Anticholinergics.

Nursing Support

The patient with acute ulcerative colitis is placed at bed rest and given sedative drugs, i.e., barbiturates in sufficient dosage to ensure constant drowsiness for several days. The purpose of this sedation is to reduce to a minimum the colonic peristalsis in order to rest the infected bowel. Tincture of belladonna or atropine may also be given to lessen gastric motility. Sedation is continued until the patient's stools approach normal frequency and consistency. Meanwhile, the patient is watched carefully for signs of colonic perforation and hemorrhage, a calamitous complication of this disease.

Antibiotics and sulfonamides may be given to combat secondary infections. While the patient is acutely ill he is maintained on parenteral replacement of vitamins, fluids and electrolytes. When he is able to tolerate food, he is placed on a highly nutritious, low residue diet that is liberalized as his symptoms are brought under control. Cold fluids increase gastric motility and are to be avoided. Since this disorder may cause inadequate absorption of vitamin K from the intestinal tract, parenteral vitamin K therapy is usually given. Blood transfusions are administered to correct existing anemia. Anodyne suppositories relieve painful rectal spasms produced by frequent diarrheal stools. ACTH and adrenal steroid hormones are important adjuncts in the therapeutic regimen of some patients, because they promote a feeling of well-being and decrease the patient's toxic symptoms. If there is severe proctitis, nightly rectal instillations of prednisolone acetate (30 mg.) dissolved in 50 ml. of tapwater may improve the appearance of the bowel and produce a remission of symptoms. The nurse should remember that these patients may develop intestinal perforation and peritonitis without warning and their symptoms may be masked while taking systemic corticosteroid therapy. Therefore all complaints as well as the behavior of the patient should be assessed carefully.

Surgical Treatment for Ulcerative Colitis

Approximately 20 per cent of patients with ulcerative colitis require surgical intervention. Indications for surgery include: no improvement and continued deterioration in the patient's condition, profuse bleeding, perforation, stricture formation, and indications of carcinoma development. The operation of choice is usually a total colectomy (removal of the colon) and ileostomy; any procedure more limited will prove to be of only temporary benefit in most cases.

Preoperative Care. A prolonged period of preparation with intensive fluid, blood and protein replacement is necessary before operation is attempted. Chemotherapy and antibiotics are useful adjuncts.

Usually, the patient is on a low residue diet offered frequently in small feedings. All other preoperative measures are similar to general abdominal surgery.

Psychological Support. For a patient with ulcerative colitis the preoperative care should include an understanding of the problems faced by the patient. These may be social and emotional, as well as physical; they may have resulted from or contributed to the diseased condition. His personality may be affected by innumerable factors. Let him know that his complaints are understood. Fear and anxiety accompanies diarrhea. Any patient who is suffering from the discomforts of frequent bowel movements and rectal soreness is anxious, discouraged, and depressed. The patient with this condition is often a hypersensitive individual. Encourage him to talk and ventilate his feelings. This is an outlet for emotional tension. Listen to the matters that may be disturbing him. Direct attention to the individual patient, not to his bowel condition. The nurse's evident interest in the patient will aid in gaining his confidence, which is an important part of his preoperative treatment.

Postoperative Care. If it is known before operation that a patient is to have an ileostomy, it is well to begin psychological preparation at that time. The acceptance of an ileostomy is often difficult, and the patient deserves all the support that can be given to him. It is necessary to develop in him a point of view that an ileostomy is a challenge; if accepted with courage he can master it and proceed to live normally and effectively. This is difficult to bring about in many individuals, and the task of developing a proper attitude in the patient becomes a challenge for the nurse. Other patients who have had ileostomies are an excellent source of help to this patient.

The opening of the small intestine on the abdomen discharges continuously the liquid contents of the small intestine. Because these discharges contain digestive enzymes, they are highly irritating to the skin of the abdomen. As soon as operation is completed, a temporary plastic bag with an adhesive facing is placed over the ileostomy and firmly pressed onto surrounding skin. The contents draining from the ileostomy are thus kept from coming in contact with skin and are collected and measured as the bag becomes full. After the ileostomy has had a chance to heal, a permanent appliance is obtained and held in place on the skin with a special cement.

Because these patients lose much fluid and food in the early postoperative period, an accurate record of fluid intake, urinary output and rectal discharges is necessary to help the surgeon to gauge the fluid needs of the patient. Fluids, blood and a low-residue, high-calorie diet are given in large amounts until the patient becomes accustomed to the new digestive arrangement.

Such patients probably are the most challenging of all to nurse. Their prolonged illness makes them irritable, anxious and depressed. The nurse must recognize that the patient's behavior often is a result of complex socioeconomic pressures. She must be consistent in expressing sincere friendliness and exhibiting a non-judgmental attitude. Operation often results in an almost immediate change in the patient's mental outlook and, as soon as he learns to care for his ileostomy, he becomes a normal, affable and attractive person. A patient, empathetic and tolerant nurse is most important in the recovery of these patients.

Rehabilitation and Patient Education Following an Ileostomy

There are certain rehabilitation problems unique to the ileostomy patient. One is irregularity of bowel evacuation. The patient with an ileostomy cannot establish regular bowel habits because the contents of the ileum are fluid and are discharging continuously. Therefore the patient must wear an appliance day and night for the rest of his life. The appliance should be regarded as an intestinal prosthesis, and as important to this patient as the artificial leg is to the amputee. It is sealed to the skin with a special cement and permits the patient to carry on normal activities without fear of leakage or odor.

Another major problem is that of skin excoriation around the stoma. Not only does the ileostomy drainage contain enzymes that rapidly excoriate the skin, but the skin may also be irritated by the cement used in putting the appliance on and by the trauma of removing the appliance. Small ulcers, reddened areas and skin blemishes may develop near the stoma. Some patients report success in healing excoriated areas by swabbing them with milk of magnesia; others use calamine lotion on the skin. Plain tincture of benzoin may be helpful to some patients. (However, compound tincture of benzoin is irritating to the skin.) The skin should be thoroughly clean and dry before the appliance is cemented on. If an exudative dermatitis persists, karaya gum washers are available to unite the appliance and the skin that do not have to be cemented in place.

A regular schedule for changing the appliance should be established before leakage occurs. In teaching the patient to use and care for his appliance, the following points are essential:

To remove the appliance:
(1) Sit or stand in a comfortable position.
(2) Fill a medicine glass with the prescribed cement solvent. Apply a few drops of solvent with a medicine dropper between the disc of the appliance and the skin. *Do not pull off the appliance.*

To remove cement from the skin:
(1) Use a cotton ball soaked in cement solvent. Wet the skin around the stoma until the cement is softened. Avoid rubbing the skin, because solvents are irritating.
(2) Wash the skin with a soft cloth moistened with *tepid* water and mild soap.

To put on the appliance: (See Fig. 22-10)
(1) Dust the prescribed gum karaya powder on the moist reddened skin around the stoma. Remove excess powder.
(2) Put a few drops of cement on the index finger and apply the cement as thinly as possible on the skin around the stoma.
(3) Place the appliance on a flat surface with the disc-side up. Apply a thin coat of cement to the disc, making sure that the entire area near the hole in the disc is covered. Apply a second thin coat of cement to the skin and to the appliance. The cement on the skin and disc must be dry before the pouch is put in place. Apply the pouch *firmly* to the skin and hold the disc tightly for a few minutes until it firmly adheres to the skin.

The amount of time that the individual can keep the appliance sealed to his body depends on the location of the stoma and the person's body structure. Usually the normal wearing time is 2 to 4 days. The appliance is emptied every 4 to 6 hours. The pouch has an emptying spout at the bottom that is closed with a rubber band or special clip made for this purpose.

The appliance is cleaned and aired according to the manufacturer's directions. There are many deodorizers and cleaning aids available that the patient can

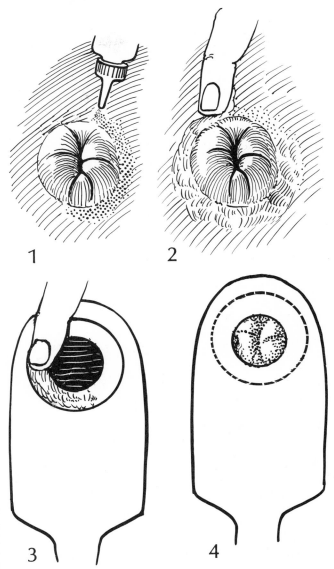

FIG. 22-10. A method of putting on an ileostomy appliance. (1) Dusting the gum karaya powder on the reddened moist skin immediately around the stoma. (2) Applying the cement around the stoma. (3) Applying the cement on the disc of the pouch. (appliance.) (4) Centering the pouch over the stoma and holding it firmly until it adheres to the skin. (Redrawn from Merck Sharp and Dohme)

use. There are also ostomy appliances available that do not have to be cemented to the skin. An ostomy appliance is fitted to the individual patient and the patient's needs determine the type of appliance to be worn.

The United Ostomy Association, Inc.,* is a nonprofit

* 1111 Wilshire Blvd., Los Angeles, California 90017.

TABLE 22-1. Comparison of colostomy and ileostomy

Categories	Colostomy	Ileostomy
Definition	A portion of the colon is brought through the abdominal wall, thereby creating a temporary or permanent opening.	A portion of the ileum is brought through the abdominal wall, thereby creating a permanent opening.
Indications	(1) Obstructive processes of the lower intestinal tract.	Ulcerative colitis in the vast majority of cases.
	(2) Congenital or traumatic disruption of the intestinal tract.	
	(3) Cancer of the rectum or sigmoid flexure where anastomosis is not possible.	
Purpose	To provide an outlet for intestinal waste products.	To serve as an exit for waste products when the colon has been removed.
Location in bowel	Colon	Ileum
Reservoir	Limited	None
Incidence of evacuation	24 to 48 hours with control measures	Constant
Consistency of discharge	Semi-formed, nonirritant	Liquid, irritant
Means of control	Diet, dressings, irrigations, dilation of the stoma	Cement-on bag
Return to normal activity	All	All

From American Cancer Society: Colostomy and Ileostomy Care. A Guide of Practical Information for Nurses.

health service agency dedicated to the rehabilitation of ostomates. This organization gives patients useful knowledge of living with an ostomy through an educational program of literature, lectures, and exhibits. Local associations provide visiting services by qualified members and give hope and rehabilitation services to new ostomy patients.

Diverticulosis and Diverticulitis

A *diverticulum* is a saccular dilatation, a blind passage, so to speak, leading from the lumen of the bowel. (An abnormal example is Meckel's diverticulum, an outpocketing of the ileum.) Diverticula, in fact, may occur anywhere along the course of the gastrointestinal tract, from the esophagus to the rectum. These defects may be congenital. They may be the result of local degeneration and weakening of the muscular wall, or they may be due to mechanical factors, such as a constant pulling on the intestinal wall from without or pressure from within its lumen. An individual who possesses diverticula is said to have *diverticulosis*.

Diverticula of the large bowel occur in from 5 to 10 per cent of adults. When present, they are usually multiple and tend rather to involve the distal portions of the colon. In contrast with Meckel's diverticulum, the colonic diverticula are rarely congenital defects, but are acquired, usually during adulthood. The cause of the diverticula is thought to be herniation of the lining mucous membrane through defects in the muscular layer of the colon, this herniation arising as a result of chronic overdistention of the bowel. Whatever their cause, large bowel diverticula are more apt to cause trouble than those situated in the small intestine. Whereas the contents of the latter are fluid in consistency, the material passing through the colon becomes increasingly firm and viscid, and diverticula located in the region where the fecal matter is most dehydrated, namely, in the sigmoid and the descending colon, are most apt to become obstructed. Obstruction of a diverticulum, as in the case of the appendix, leads to infection and inflammation. This is referred to as *diverticulitis*.

Diverticulitis usually occurs in patients over 40 years of age. It is by no means rare. It has been estimated that approximately a third of the patients with diverticulosis at one time or another experience diverticulitis. The condition may occur in acute attacks or it may persist as a long-continued, smoldering infection. Inflammation of a diverticulum, if its obstruction continues, tends to spread to the surrounding bowel wall, giving rise to irritability and spasticity of the colon. If the infection is unusually severe, perforation of the colon can occur, with resultant peritonitis. If the inflammation is less acute and more slowly progressive, the result may be extensive scarring and abscess formation involving the bowel wall and eventually producing some degree of lower intestinal obstruction. Complications of this severity fortunately are rarely seen.

The most common symptom of a moderately severe acute diverticulitis is crampy pain in the left lower quadrant of the abdomen, with associated flatulence, slight nausea and a low-grade fever. Milder grades of the condition may give rise only to bouts of soreness, mild cramps in the lower abdomen and irregularity of bowel habit. Hemorrhage occurs in 10 to 20 per cent of the cases. The bleeding is not persistent but may be massive. The diagnosis is made on the basis of fluoroscopic and x-ray findings with a barium enema. Direct visualization by means of sigmoidoscopy occasionally is helpful.

Guidelines for Therapeutic Management

The treatment of the patient with acute diverticulitis consists of the elimination of roughage from the diet, hot applications to the lower abdomen and repeated warm-saline enemas. Systemic and, more especially, the surface-acting antimicrobials are of great value. Those most commonly used are the so-called bowel antiseptics, such as sulfathalidine and neomycin. These drugs reduce the bacterial flora of the bowel, diminish the bulk of the stool and soften the fecal mass so that it traverses more easily the area of inflammatory obstruction. Surgery is reserved for patients whose conditions are complicated by colonic perforation, obstruction, abscesses or fistulae.

Patient Education

A very important aspect of the treatment is prevention of recurrences. To this end, patients who have experienced diverticulitis should, henceforth, restrict themselves to a low-residue diet, eliminating particularly the coarser cereals and vegetables. It is especially important that they establish a regular bowel habit. To promote regular and complete evacuation, an adequate fluid intake should be maintained, and mild laxatives should be employed whenever necessary. (See bowel training, p. 176.)

Although there is no conclusive evidence that diverticulosis or diverticulitis predisposes the patient to develop carcinoma of the colon, these diseases frequently coexist. The patient should be reminded to stay under continuing medical supervision and follow up.

Surgical Treatment of Diverticulitis

Surgical care of patients with diverticulitis is required in the treatment of the complications of this disease; perforations with peritonitis, abscess, profuse hemorrhage, colonic obstruction and the formation of fistulas. Many of these indications require emergency operations, but when time permits bowel preparation, low-residue diet, bowel antiseptics and cleansing enemas are given. The operation performed varies with the operative findings. When possible, the area of diverticulitis is resected and the remaining

bowel joined end to end (primary resection and end-to-end anastomosis). In some cases such an operation may appear impossible or inadvisable, in which case a colostomy is performed in the right transverse colon. By so diverting the fecal flow from the area of diverticulitis, the inflammatory process is permitted to subside and a later operation on the colon containing the diverticulitis is removed and an anastomosis performed. When this method of treatment is chosen, the colostomy is only temporary, and after the area of diverticulitis has been removed and the intestinal continuity established by the anastomosis, the colostomy is closed. Thus, this is a 3-staged procedure, requiring the care for a colostomy during part of the treatment (see p. 489). This colostomy, on the right side of the transverse colon, drains liquid or mushy feces and requires that a bag be worn constantly. Irrigations are rarely of value in this type of colostomy, but ordinary cleanliness is obtained by baths or showers, using soap and water to cleanse the skin about the colostomy stoma. It is best to have 2 colostomy bags so that one may be emptied, cleansed and deodorized while the other is worn. Such a colostomy, although requiring daily care, should permit the patient to be up and active, eating a regular diet. (The nursing management of the patient with a colostomy is discussed on pp. 489-493.)

Tumors of the Intestine

Tumors of the small intestine, as in the case of duodenal tumors, are rare. Lipomata (fatty tumors), fibromata (connective tissue tumors), and angiomata (blood vessel tumors) are all benign in character. Some of these may take the form of polyps projecting into the intestinal lumen. Their chief importance lies in the fact that they may give rise to intussusception (p. 493). Sarcoma and lymphosarcoma—malignant tumors of connective tissue and lymphoid tissue, respectively—may arise in the small bowel, producing intestinal hemorrhage or obstruction.

Tumors of the colon, on the other hand, are relatively common. In fact, cancer of the colon and rectum is now the most common type of internal cancer in the United States. Benign polyps are much more common in the large than in the small intestine. They may be very numerous. When multiple, the condition is referred to as polyposis—often, apparently, a congenital abnormality. These polyps not infrequently become cancerous.

The Patient with Cancer of the Colon

Cancer of the colon (Fig. 22-11) and the rectum always arises from the epithelium lining the intestine. The effects produced depend largely on its location. As in the case of cancer elsewhere in the gastrointestinal tract, the chief symptoms are the passage of blood in the stools, anemia, obstruction and perforation. A suddenly developing obstruction may be the first symptom of cancer involving the colon anywhere between the cecum and the sigmoid, for in this region, where the bowel contents are liquid, a slowly developing obstruction will not become evident until the lumen is practically closed. Cancer of the sigmoid and the rectum causes earlier symptoms of partial obstruction, with constipation alternating with diarrhea, lower abdominal crampy pains and distention. Any patient with a history of inexplicable change in bowel habit and the passage of blood in the stools should be studied carefully to rule out cancer of the large bowel. The possibility that a rectal carcinoma exists, detectable but still asymptomatic and still operable, is one important reason for the inclusion of a rectal examination as part of every routine physical examination. Helpful additional symptoms, often present, are those of progressive weakness, anorexia, weight loss, anemia and lower abdominal pain. The most important diagnostic procedures are the abdominal and rectal examinations, sigmoidoscopy, repeated examination of the stools for the presence of

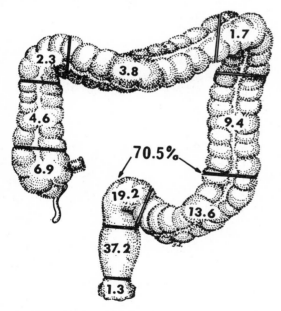

Fig. 22-11. Distribution of cancer of the colon. Half of the cancers of the colon or rectum can be felt by the examining finger or be seen by visualizing the rectum. Over 70 per cent can be visualized by a sigmoidoscopic examination. Therefore these procedures should be a part of the annual physical examination and the nurse should encourage the patient to have them. (Rhoads *et al*: Surgery. J. B. Lippincott, 1970)

blood, determination of the blood-hemoglobin concentration for anemia and, usually the most conclusive of all, the barium roentgenologic examination.

Nursing Aspects

Preparation for Operation. This includes the shaving of the abdomen and the perineum, and rectal irrigation that is continued until the fluid returns clear. Usually a high-caloric, low-residue diet is given for several days before operation if time and the patient's condition permit. If an emergency does not exist, these patients are prepared for several days by being given intestinal antiseptics of the sulfa group (sulfasuxidine or sulfathalidine) and neomycin. These are given by mouth to reduce the bacterial content of the colon and to soften and decrease the bulk of the contents of the colon. The nurse should pay attention to any mention of pain and its location. She also should record fluid losses, such as would occur by vomiting and diarrhea. This will aid in regulating the fluid intake and maintaining proper balance. Preoperative intestinal intubation with a Miller-Abbott or Cantor tube facilitates the performance of intestinal surgery and minimizes postoperative distention. In the event that there is any possibility of a permanent colostomy, the patient should be informed of it by the surgeon, and he should be assured that it can be handled effectively and need not interfere with his usual social and business life. He should be assured also that he need not develop into a dependent person. This mental preparation of the patient is an extremely important part of his preoperative care.

The patient is sent to the operating room with an indwelling catheter in place.

Operative Treatment. This will depend on the position and the extent of the cancer. When the tumor can be removed, the involved colon is excised for some distance on each side of the growth to remove the tumor and the area of its lymphatic spread. If distant (liver) metastasis has occurred, the tumor may be excised for palliation but without hope of cure. The intestine may be reunited by an *enterocolostomy* or by an end-to-end anastomosis of the colon. When the growth is situated low in the sigmoid or the rectum, the colon is cut above the growth and brought out through the abdominal wall, forming thus an abdominal anus, called a *colostomy*. The growth then is removed from below by a perineal incision. (*Abdominoperineal resection*, Fig. 22-12.)

In the event that the tumor has spread and involves surrounding vital structures, it is considered to be inoperable. When the growth in the rectum or the sigmoid is inoperable, and especially when symptoms of partial or complete obstruction are present, a colostomy may be performed. A loop of the colon, near the

FIG. 22-12. Abdominoperineal resection for carcinoma of rectum. (*Top, left*) Tumor in rectum. (*Top, right*) At operation, the sigmoid first is delivered and a colostomy is established. The distal bowel has been dissected free to a point below the pelvic peritoneum. The pelvic peritoneum is sutured over the closed end of the distal sigmoid and rectum. The perineal resection includes removal of the rectum and free portion of the sigmoid from below. (*Bottom, left*) The perineum is closed loosely about drains placed beneath the peritoneum in the hollow of the sacrum. (*Bottom, right*) The final result after healing.

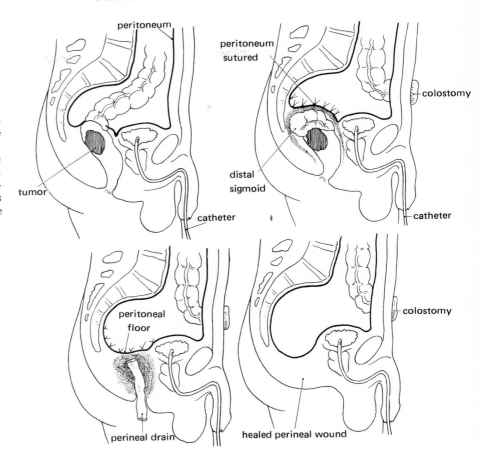

Care and Teaching of the Patient with a Colostomy

junction of the descending colon and the sigmoid, is brought out of the abdomen through a lower left rectus incision and maintained in place by a plastic rod or rubber tube inserted underneath the loop. If the obstruction is complete, the loop may be drained by the insertion of a rubber tube or by the use of a right-angled tube called a Paul's tube, which is held in the intestine by a purse-string suture. When the obstruction is incomplete, the colostomy loop is allowed to remain unopened for several days to permit the peritoneal cavity to become thoroughly sealed off. During this time the patient is given a liquid diet. The intestine is opened by electrocautery, as hemorrhage is slight after its use.

Care and Teaching of the Patient with a Colostomy

From the point of view of safety, the permanent colostomy, as we know it today, is a lifesaving procedure that is compatible with active participation in social and business life, and as such its drawbacks pale into insignificance. A philosophical acceptance of this and readjustment of one's daily habits are not achieved in one day, but getting used to this, as to any other handicap, can be accomplished by being put on the right track

and facing each day with courage, optimism, and determination.*

Nursing Emphasis. A *colostomy* (a temporary or permanent opening of the colon through the abdominal wall) is, as we have seen, used often in the treatment of ulcerative colitis, tumors of the colon, and some intestinal obstructions. The nurse cannot teach effectively if all facets of the problem facing a patient with a colostomy are not known; if, on the other hand, she has a broad understanding of colostomy care but does not know her patient, again she will fail. To give adequate support, care and instruction to this patient, the nurse must know not only basic information, but also she must know her patient. What does he think, feel, express, suppress, desire, fear and so forth? In her daily contacts with the patient who has a colostomy, valuable rapport can be established to facilitate his adjustment. The nurse must understand and practice the psychology and the principles of learning as they apply to each particular individual.

* Dubois, E. C.: Hints on the management of a colostomy. Amer. J. Nurs., 55:72, 1955.

Psychological Preparation. Thousands of people who have colostomies are engaged actively in business today. With the improvement of surgical and nursing procedures, and the assistance of patients who have "lived" with their colostomies, it is now possible to give intelligent assistance to the person about to have a colostomy or an ileostomy.

The support and the teaching of a patient must be individualized. Therefore, the same approach may not be appropriate for all patients. Before operation, some may find that a simple line drawing illustrating the nature and the function of the lower intestinal tract is helpful. By this means the deviations necessary for his particular situation can be explained. For others, having another patient who has had a colostomy talk to them presents a comfortable opportunity for the expressions of fears and doubts. In still other situations, some surgeons believe that a minimal amount of explanation should be given the patient preoperatively; simply telling a patient that he will have major surgery in order to correct his problem is sufficient. In other words, the extent of psychological preparation must be approached on a personal basis.

The patient needs to know what a colostomy is and how it functions; he should know that it need not hamper his way of living and that with patience, as well as some trial-and-error methods, he will be able to manage, control and master it.

As in the care of any other surgical patient, the nurse must know the plan of care to be followed, and she must know her patient. During the interval of preoperative care she should encourage the patient to talk out his concerns and fears; in this way the nurse will be able to direct and help him.

Postoperatively, many surgeons are getting the patient out of bed on the first postoperative day, and he is encouraged to care for his colostomy from the very first irrigation. The return to normal diet is more rapid, and every effort is made to encourage him to live as he did before his operation. Psychologically, this appears to de-emphasize the abnormality of the situation.

It is well to remember that this is a strange and new experience for the patient. Most likely he has never seen an incision under surgical dressings and, less likely, a colostomy. The shock of this first sight may be minimized if he has seen drawings and perhaps a picture or two of the anatomy involved. The nurse should have all her equipment organized before removing the dressing.

The colostomy is opened on the second or the third postoperative day by the surgeon, and often there is an evacuation of loose stools. In anticipation of this the nurse will have protected the bedding with a plastic sheet covered with a towel, and she will have an emesis basin positioned at the side of the patient.

Regulating the Colostomy. *Colostomy Irrigations.* The stoma on the abdomen does not have voluntary muscular control and may empty at irregular intervals. The purpose of irrigating a colostomy is to empty the colon of gas, mucus and feces so that the patient can go about his social and business activities without fear of fecal drainage. By irrigating the stoma at a *regular* time there is less gas and retention of irrigating fluids. It is best to irrigate after a meal as ingestion of food stimulates peristalsis and defecation.

The initial irrigation is usually done on the fourth or fifth postoperative day. There are 2 methods of irrigating a colostomy: the conventional one using an enema irrigation procedure, and the other utilizing a bulb syringe method.

IRRIGATION BY ENEMA. The following equipment is used:

Irrigating set (2-quart can or bag, tubing, adapter)
Catheter, clamp, colostomy irrigator
Solution at 40.5° C. (105° F.)
Petrolatum to lubricate catheter
Toilet tissue to clean around colostomy before and after irrigation
Newspaper or paper bag to receive soiled dressings
A place to set or hang the irrigating container
Dressings for colostomy following irrigation

The patient may sit up in bed or preferably in a chair before the toilet in the bathroom. A rubber or plastic sheet can be used as a trough leading to the toilet bowl. Encourage the patient to watch the procedure and explain each step as it is performed. The catheter, lubricated with petrolatum to reduce friction, is inserted 2 to 3 inches at first and the solution is allowed to run into the colon.

The catheter then can be inserted gently up to 6 to 8 inches. At first, only about 500 ml. of solution is given, and this may be increased gradually every day up to 1,500 ml. The temperature of the solution is about 40.5° C. (105° F.), and the irrigating can is placed about 18 to 24 inches above the level of the colostomy opening. The purpose of the irrigation is to empty the distal bowel of fecal material. As distention of the colon is an effective stimulus for bowel evacuation, the irrigating solution should be introduced in such amount and with such pressure as to distend the bowel and give the patient a feeling of fullness. If the patient complains of cramps, the level of the can may be lowered to lessen the force of the flow. The patient should be taught that the rate of flow of solution varies with the pressure and the caliber of tube. Pressure depends on height; therefore, when increased pressure is desired, the container of solution may be raised and vice versa. Solutions may be soapy solution, plain water or saline. The irrigation may be given daily, every other day or every 3 days according to the experience of the patient. Some patients prefer

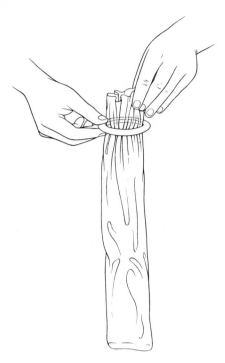

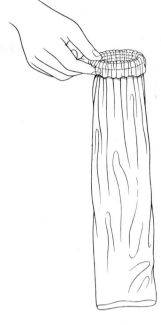

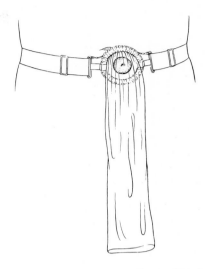

Insert one end of drainage sheath through the plastic ring.

Fold over the edges of the sheath and roll around ring securely and evenly.

The ring with sheath is placed over the stoma, and the belt clips hooked onto the ring. This holds the appliance securely over the opening.

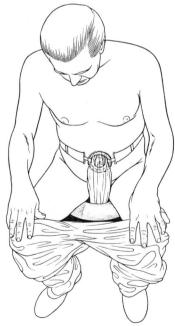

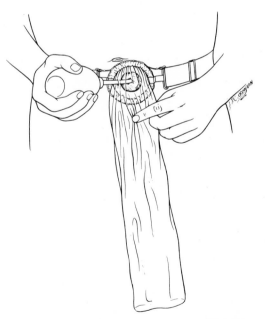

After cutting a small hole in the sheath above and to one side of the stoma, it is tucked between the legs so that it leads directly into the toilet.

Moisten the tip of the syringe with a standard lubricating jelly. Insert the lubricated syringe tip through the hole of the drainage sheath and gently into the stoma about 3 to 5 inches.

Fig. 22-13. The bulb syringe method of colostomy irrigation. (Postel, A. H., Grier, W. R. N., and Localio, S. A.: Training the Patient in the Bulb Syringe Method of Colostomy Irrigation. New York, New York University Medical Center, 1965)

to take a warm bath after an irrigation. This promotes a feeling of cleanliness and relaxation. During the irrigation, when done at home, it may be pleasant and diverting to have a radio nearby. While waiting for the return flow, it may be an opportune time to read. (The entire procedure usually takes between 45 minutes and 1 hour.) Nothing but flatus and a slight amount of mucus should escape from the colostomy between irrigations.

IRRIGATION BY BULB SYRINGE. The second method of colostomy irrigation is the *bulb syringe* method. This type of irrigation stimulates fecal return rather than washing it out. There is no prolonged trapping of water in the colon and no spillage or accidents during the day.

The patient is seated on the toilet. An 8-ounce soft rubber bulb syringe is used. The hard nozzle is cut off and a No. 24 French catheter is attached to the end of the bulb syringe. *No more than 24 ounces of water is used.* The bulb syringe method is shown in Fig. 22-13.

The patient may massage the lower part of the abdomen to ensure adequate return. The bag is left in place for 15 minutes, after which the stoma is covered with a piece of gauze and held in place by a girdle, elasticized shorts or an elastic belt. The patient washes the pitcher and bulb syringe with soapy water, and the procedure is complete.

Other Types of Colostomies. "Wet" colostomies are those through which both urine and feces are excreted because of transplantation of ureters into the colon. These colostomies are never irrigated, because of the danger that contaminated material will be forced into the ureters and produce infection.

In a double-barrel colostomy, there are 2 openings, the proximal and distal segments of colon. The proximal portion is the functioning colon, whereas the distal end is irrigated only to keep it clean and free of mucus. If there is an obstruction in this section, it may be necessary to siphon the fluid. In case the cancer has not been removed, it is well to irrigate the lower loop, from anus to colostomy, every 2 or 3 days, to remove the irritating mucus that collects. If the growth has been removed by the perineal route, the wound should be watched carefully for signs of hemorrhage. The close proximity of the wound to the sacrum necessitates a frequent change of dressings in order to keep the area clean and dry.

Care of Perineal Wound

The perineal wound usually contains a drain or packing that is removed gradually so that on about the seventh day all drains are out. There usually are sloughing bits of tissue that must come away for the following week or 10 days. This process is hastened by mechanical irrigation of the wound. An irrigating can with 1:5,000 potassium permanganate solution and a soft rubber catheter at the tip facilitates this procedure, which should be carried out at least once daily until the wound is clean. The nurse often gives these irrigations. During the procedure it is important to protect the bed with an extra waterproof sheet and absorbent pads, and it may be well to time the irrigation so that it can be performed before the patient receives morning care.

Choice and Care of Suitable Equipment

Early in the postoperative care of the colostomy or ileostomy patient, the use of a plastic stoma bag is effective in preventing skin irritation and reducing offensive odors. Such protection is relatively inexpensive, since the bags are disposable. Various types of irrigating sets are available from surgical supply houses.

Colostomy bags may be worn immediately after irrigation; then a change to a simple dressing may be effective. Patients are instructed in the care and the cleaning of equipment to prolong its life and keep it free of odors. Cleaning by soap or a detergent and water and exposing it to fresh air usually is sufficient; however, it may still be necessary to deodorize the appliance; liquid deodorizers are available to use in washing and soaking equipment. The other aspect of the problem is the control of odors arising from the body excreta as they collect in the appliance. Readily soluble deodorizing tablets may be inserted in plastic or rubber bags, or putting a few drops of chlorphyll solution into the bag will help in the control of odors. Powdered charcoal also may be sprinkled into the bag to absorb odors.

As a rule, colostomy bags are not necessary. As soon as the patient has learned a routine for his irrigation, bags may be dispensed with, and a simple dressing of disposable tissue often covered with Saran wrap is held in place by an elastic belt of girdle. Except for the escape of gas and a slight amount of mucus, nothing comes from the colostomy opening between irrigations; therefore, the inconvenience of a colostomy bag is unnecessary.

Hygienic Measures

In general, the patient needs to be reminded that good health practices will aid materially his feeling of well-being and his positive adjustment to his colostomy. His diet should be adequate and well-balanced; laxatives are never used. Lastly, it is valuable to observe a habit time for doing certain activities, e.g., mealtime, irrigation time, bedtime, and so forth.

Soap and water should be used to clean the skin. Dry thoroughly. Consult the physician before trying skin medications.

Selection of Appropriate Diet

After a liquid diet, the physician usually orders a low-residue diet. It is necessary to begin with a strict diet, but later it can be more liberal as indicated below.

Colostomy Diet No. 1. Used in the hospital while first gaining control and at any time later when loose movements occur.

Breakfast: Large portion of cream of wheat with boiled milk, and sugar if desired; 2 hardboiled eggs; dry toast; 1 glass of boiled milk

Lunch: Creamed soups (creamed lettuce soup 3 or 4 times a week); creamed fish or meat; baked or mashed potato; boiled rice or custard

Dinner: Meat or fish, creamed whenever possible; escalloped vegetable—no spinach or carrots; soft pudding, custard or junket

Colostomy Diet No. 2. Used after gaining control in the hospital (2 weeks) and continued for 2 months at home.

Cereals—cream of wheat, farina, strained oatmeal, puffed wheat or rice

Eggs—any way except fried

Breads—white, plain or toasted; soda crackers

Soups of all kinds except tomato or corn, not highly seasoned

Potato and Substitutes—baked, mashed, creamed or boiled potato; macaroni; spaghetti; noodles; boiled rice

Meats and Substitutes—roast beef or lamb; broiled steak or lamb chop; oven-baked bacon
   Stewed, creamed, boiled or baked chicken
   Cheese, cottage and cream (white)
   Fish, broiled, baked or creamed

Desserts—Jello, junket, custard, tapioca and cornstarch pudding, plain ice cream, plain cake, sponge and angel cake, plain cookies

Colostomy Diet No. 3. Added to No. 2 after 2 months if control is still effective.

Raw lettuce and celery

Fruits—bananas, canned pears, peaches, apricots, applesauce, baked apple (no skin)

Vegetables—asparagus, beets, green beans, carrots, squash, peas, spinach

Orange juice

AVOID: spices, highly seasoned foods, fried foods, raw fruits and vegetables, gas-forming foods such as onions, turnips, cabbage family, beans, nuts, melons, carbonated drinks, iced-drinks. Also avoid overeating and eating at odd times.

The patient will be able to tell that certain foods interfere with control and these should be eliminated. It becomes an individual matter.

Intestinal Obstruction

An intestinal obstruction is inability of the intestinal contents to flow normally along the intestinal tract. There are two types of intestinal obstruction: (1) mechanical and (2) adynamic or paralytic. In the *mechanical* type there may be an intraluminal obstruction or a mural obstruction from pressure on the intestinal walls. In *adynamic* or *paralytic ileus* the intestinal musculature is unable to propel the contents along the bowel due to toxic or traumatic affection of the autonomic nervous system.

An obstruction may be partial or complete. Its seriousness depends on the region of bowel that is affected, the degree to which the lumen is occluded and, especially, the degree to which the blood circulation in the bowel wall is disturbed. Small bowel obstruction is always serious, because, as a consequence of persistent vomiting, it leads to profound disturbances in the electrolyte balance of the body: first, to alkalosis, from the loss of the gastric hydrochloric acid; then, to profound dehydration and acidosis, due to the loss of water and sodium from the small intestine. If the obstruction is only partial and develops slowly, the symptoms are relatively mild. Large bowel obstruction, even if complete, is also comparatively undramatic, provided that the blood supply to the colon is not disturbed.

Causes

One of every three cases of acute intestinal obstruction is due to cancer of the large bowel (see p. 488). Intestinal obstruction very occasionally results from a foreign body lodged in the bowel. This may be false teeth, jewelry, a large fruit stone, a gallstone, a mass of parasitic worms, etc. In other cases, a stricture of the bowel is the result of the contracting scar of an ulcer in its wall, due, for example, to tuberculosis. The intestine may become pinched in a peritoneal pocket (hernia) or linked by peritoneal adhesions. A loop of intestine may become twisted about itself (volvulus). Hernia (pp. 480-482) is one of the most common and important causes of intestinal obstruction.

Intussusception is another cause of intestinal obstruction. In this condition, the bowel, above a certain point, pushes itself into the bowel below that point, much as a telescope is shortened by pushing one section into the next. This likewise occurs through peristalsis. The point at which intussusception most commonly develops is at or near the ileocecal valve. The telescoping, or invagination, also may start at the point of attachment of a tumor in the colon—particularly a pedunculated tumor—as a result of its becoming engaged by a peristaltic wave and propelled along the colon, dragging into the lumen that portion of the

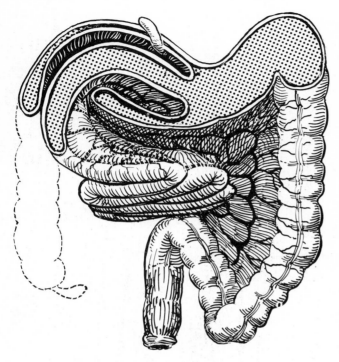

Fig. 22-14. Intussusception. The ileocecal type in which the ileocecal valve and cecum invaginate into the colon.

wall to which its pedicle is attached (see Fig. 22-14). When intussusception starts at the ileocecal valve, the terminal portion of the small bowel may invaginate its way down the whole length of the large bowel and protrude at the anus. Any child who has been seized with pain in the abdomen and then passes blood and mucus in the stools should be examined with the possibility of intussusception in mind.

Postoperative Adhesions. After abdominal operation, there are many areas produced within the abdomen that are not completely healed, and to these areas loops of intestine may become adherent. The attachment of these loops of small intestine through inflammatory adhesions usually is only temporary and of no particular moment. However, occasionally these inflammatory adhesions may produce a kinking of an intestinal loop, which causes obstruction of the intestinal flow. This intestinal obstruction usually appears on the third or fourth day after operation, when peristalsis normally is resumed and when food and fluids are being given to the patient for the first time. The symptoms are typical of any intestinal obstruction—crampy abdominal pain, distention, vomiting, etc.

In most cases of postoperative inflammatory obstruction, the difficulty may be relieved by intestinal intubation. By decompressing the bowel above the site of the obstruction, the inflammation is permitted to subside, and the obstruction is relieved. When the obstruction cannot be relieved by this conservative means, a reoperation may be necessary to free the adherent intestine and to permit the intestinal flow to be resumed.

Paralytic Ileus

A paralytic ileus occurs when peristaltic movement becomes paralyzed due to the effect of trauma or toxins on the nerves that regulate intestinal movement. This may happen after back injuries, after operation on the kidney and frequently with peritonitis.

The result is a distention of the intestine with gas produced by decomposition of the intestinal contents or by the swallowing of air. The lack of peristalsis results in an accumulation of this gas in the intestine, causing distention. Few or no peristaltic sounds can be heard, and the patient may be extremely uncomfortable, if not in marked pain. This condition is spoken of as *paralytic ileus* to distinguish it from *organic ileus,* which is caused by an organic obstruction of the intestine. Relief of the distention associated with paralytic ileus often is obtained by intestinal intubation (see p. 457).

Symptoms of Intestinal Obstruction

The symptoms of intestinal obstruction depend on what part of the bowel is obstructed.

The initial symptom of *small bowel* obstruction is usually pain, wavelike in character. Constipation ensues. The patient may pass blood and mucus, but no fecal matter and no flatus. Vomiting occurs. This is often characteristic. If the obstruction is complete, the peristaltic waves become extremely vigorous and assume a reverse direction, the intestinal contents being propelled toward the mouth instead of toward the rectum. If the obstruction is in the ileum, fecal vomiting takes place. First, the patient vomits the stomach contents, then the bile-stained contents of the duodenum and the jejunum and, finally, with each paroxysm of pain the darker, fecal-like contents of the ileum are ejected. Soon, due to the loss of water, sodium and chlorides in the vomitus, the unmistakable signs of dehydration become evident. The patient complains of intense thirst, drowsiness, generalized malaise and aching. The tongue and the mucous membranes become parched; the face acquires a pinched appearance. The abdomen becomes distended, and the lower the obstruction in the gastrointestinal tract, the more marked is the distention. If the situation is allowed to continue uncorrected, shock appears due to dehydration and loss of plasma volume. The patient is prostrated; the pulse becomes increasingly weak and rapid; the temperature and the blood pressure are lowered;

the skin is pale, cold and clammy. At this point, death may supervene rapidly.

Large bowel intestinal obstruction differs clinically from the small bowel type in that the symptoms develop and progress relatively slowly. This difference is due to the fact that the colon is able to absorb its fluid contents and it can distend to a considerable degree beyond its normal full capacity. In patients with an obstruction in the sigmoid or the rectum, constipation may be the only symptom for days. Eventually the abdomen becomes markedly distended; loops of large bowel become visibly outlined through the abdominal wall, and the patient suffers from crampy lower abdominal pain. Finally, fecal vomiting develops, and the terminal features are essentially those of ileum obstruction. In patients with fecal impaction there is no shock.

Nursing Assessment and Care

Most cases of intestinal obstruction are surgical problems. From the medical standpoint, it is essential that the conditions be recognized. They must not be confused with other, more benign causes of constipation, vomiting, abdominal pain and distention. A purgative never is given to a patient suspected of having obstruction, for this will seriously aggravate the situation.

The most important criteria by which obstruction is distinguished, as such, include the existence, location and character of pain, the presence of distention and the absence of flatus or defecation. The eliciting of this type of evidence is within the scope of the nurse's responsibility. In addition, the nurse must measure, record and chart 4-hour temperatures, pulse rates and blood pressure readings as well as fluid intake and output. Any stool that might be passed, or a portion thereof, is to be saved for direct inspection by the physician as well as to be tested for the presence of occult blood. Arrangements for that test as well as for urinalysis, hemoglobin measurements and blood cell counts should be made promptly on request by the physician or automatically on the nurse's own initiative if circumstances warrant it in this type of emergency.

If the disorder is an incarcerated external hernia, an attempt may be made to reduce it, not by applying pressure to the extruded mass, but simply by having the patient lie flat on his back with knees flexed and with an ice compress placed continuously over the mass. This position and the cold may cause the edema and swelling of the incarcerated bowel to subside, allowing the loop to escape back through the ring or opening into which it has worked itself. If reduction does not occur, prompt surgical intervention is necessary.

Preoperative Care

Before attempting surgery on an ill patient with intestinal obstruction, steps are taken to correct the dehydration and to decompress the dilated bowel. Adequate amounts of physiologic saline solution with dextrose are given intravenously to replace the sodium, chloride and water lost in the vomitus and to supply nourishment. Decompression is accomplished by intubating the small intestine with a Miller-Abbott tube, for example, and constantly aspirating the fluid and gaseous contents, employing constant suction siphonage.

Preoperative preparation is the giving of a small enema and, if the patient's condition permits, the shaving of the entire abdomen. These measures often are supplemented by decompression of the intestine by the use of suction attached to a Miller-Abbott, a Cantor or a Harris tube. The tubes frequently become clogged and must be irrigated with normal saline by the nurse at frequent intervals. Extreme care must be exercised in irrigating the Miller-Abbott tube, in that the irrigating solution must be introduced into the portion marked "Suction." The other lumen leads to the distensible rubber bag and serious accidents have occurred (rupture of the intestine) when, by mistake, nurses have introduced fluid into the bag meant for irrigation.

Surgical Intervention

The surgical treatment of intestinal obstruction depends largely on the cause of the obstruction. In the most common causes of obstruction, such as strangulated hernia, obstruction by adhesions, and so forth, the operation consists of repair of the hernia or division of the adhesion to which the intestine is attached. In some hernias, it may be necessary to remove the strangulated portion of bowel and perform an anastomosis. Operation for intestinal obstruction may be simple or complicated, depending on the duration of the obstruction and the condition of the intestine found at operation. In occasional patients, intestinal intubation may not be sufficient to decompress the bowel. In these cases, it is not uncommon to introduce a catheter into the distended intestine. This catheter is brought out through the abdominal wall, usually through a separate incision, to decompress the intestine and is spoken of as a *tube enterostomy*.

When the large intestine becomes obstructed, usually by cancer, it is frequently necessary to relieve the colonic obstruction before it is possible to resect the cancer itself. This is done by inserting a large tube into the cecum (cecostomy) or by making an opening in the colon above the site of the obstruction by bringing a loop of colon up to the skin surface. When this is opened, the obstruction is relieved and the tumor

SUMMARY OF THE PRINCIPLES AND OBJECTIVES OF MEDICAL, SURGICAL AND NURSING MANAGEMENT OF THE PATIENT UNDERGOING INTESTINAL SURGERY

Preoperative Objectives:

I. To ensure optimal patient condition for surgery:

A. Give whole blood or packed red cells as ordered to patient debilitated by bleeding, infection or a malignant neoplasm.

B. Correct fluid and electrolyte deficiencies preoperatively.

1. Give intravenous infusions of lactated Ringer's solution, etc. as ordered prior to surgery to prevent electrolyte imbalance and diminished renal function during surgery.

C. Promote the nutrition of the patient.

1. Correct existing protein deficiencies before operation.

2. Encourage between-meal feedings.

3. Give intravenous protein hydrolysates or albumin if indicated.

D. Assist in diagnostic examinations to evaluate the patient's pulmonary, cardiac, hepatic and renal functions.

1. Evaluate T.P.R. and B.P. at prescribed intervals.

2. Give medications and treatments indicated when heart failure is present.

3. Support the patient undergoing diagnostic bowel studies.

E. Insert indwelling catheter immediately before surgery to prevent manipulation and trauma to the bladder.

II. To eliminate bacteria from the intestinal tract to prevent postoperative infection:

A. Employ effective measures to empty the colon.

1. Give laxatives as directed to cleanse the bowel by catharsis.

2. Administer enemas and colonic irrigations to rid the bowel of feces and gas.

3. Offer a low-residue diet to reduce feces content in lower bowel.

4. Place patient on liquid diet at the prescribed interval before surgery.

B. Give antibacterial agents (intestinal antiseptics) to control the bacterial flora of the gastrointestinal tract.

1. Give drug combinations (usually sulfathalidine and neomycin) as ordered.

2. Observe patient for symptoms of pseudomembranous enterocolitis.
   (a) tender distended abdomen
   (b) vomiting, diarrhea
   (c) fever

III. To decompress gastrointestinal tract through an indwelling tube to minimize vomiting and distention:

A. Use a Levine tube for stomach and upper small bowel decompression.

B. Use a Miller-Abbott tube for intestinal decompression.

Postoperative Objectives:

IV. To supply fluids and electrolytes and body nutrients to the patient in the immediate postoperative period:

A. Use an intravenous catheter if I.V. therapy is to be carried out for more than a few days.

1. Use arm for placement of intravenous catheter to permit greater patient mobility.

2. Examine needle site for evidences of thrombophlebitis or chemical phlebitis.

3. Elevate patient's head and back (after he regains consciousness) while he is receiving intravenous infusions.

B. Record type of intravenous fluid, starting time, finishing time, amount absorbed and any untoward reactions.

C. Employ meticulous oral hygiene measures when patient is not taking fluids by the oral route.

V. To ensure continuing function of the nasogastric tube so that postoperative aspiration, distention and ileus are minimized:

A. Record amount and type of gastrointestinal aspirate.

B. Watch for symptoms of fluid volume deficit.
   1. Skin dryness
   2. Lethargy, etc.

C. Promote comfort of intubated patient.

1. Lubricate nares with water-soluble ointment.

2. Turn the patient frequently.

3. Humidify the room to decrease dryness of mucous membranes.

4. Apply cold compresses to neck periodically if patient complains of sore throat.

D. Remove tube when peristalsis is re-established (indicated by auscultation, the passage of flatus by rectum, and the clinical symptoms of the patient). (This is done on order of the physician.)

VI. To promote the comfort and safety of the patient:

A. Give analgesic agent according to clinical symptoms and needs of the individual patient.

1. Assess the patient for hypotension and restlessness.

2. Use special caution in giving narcotics to elderly patients.

SUMMARY OF THE PRINCIPLES AND OBJECTIVES OF MEDICAL, SURGICAL AND NURSING MANAGEMENT OF THE PATIENT UNDERGOING INTESTINAL SURGERY (*Continued*)

B. Combat sleeplessness with appropriate nursing measures and prescribed sedatives and hypnotics.

C. Encourage the patient to turn, breathe deeply and cough at specified intervals.

D. Change the dressing when indicated if patient has a draining wound, ileostomy or colostomy.

E. Encourage the patient to ventilate his feelings and anxieties about his condition.

VII. To observe the patient for complications:

A. Intra-abdominal infections (peritonitis, intra-abdominal abscesses, retroperitoneal abscesses)

B. Intracolonic infections

C. Wound infections

VIII. To encourage the patient to have follow-up examinations following surgery:

A. Inform the patient to expect periodic x-ray examinations of the colon, chest, lumbar spine (especially if patient has cancer)

B. Reinforce the physician's instructions concerning regular follow-up examinations.

C. Advise the patient to report any unexplained symptoms or recurring symptoms immediately to his physician.

---

can be treated at a later time. This operation is called a *loop colostomy* (see p. 488).

Postoperative Care

After operation, fluids must be given to these patients in large amounts. An accurately kept intake and output record is essential, since it is information that is needed if the nutritional needs of the patient are to be met. If an enterostomy has been performed, a bottle is attached to the side of the bed and a tube connected with the enterostomy tube, inserted in it. If peristalsis is active and the tube has been placed properly in the bowel, a considerable amount (from 500 to 1,000 ml.) of fecal fluid should drain away in the first 12 to 15 hours after operation. Frequently the fenestra of the enterostomy tube becomes clogged by fecal masses and, obviously, the drainage ceases until the tube is cleared. The nurse should observe the amount of drainage accumulating in the collection bottle and, if there is no increase in the quantity of fluid for several hours, she should regard it as an indication that the tube has clogged. Many surgeons make sure that the fenestra remains open by having the nurse inject a half ounce of warm saline solution into the enterostomy or colostomy tube at intervals of 2 to 4 hours. The skin about the enterostomy is protected by strips of petrolatum gauze, aluminum paint or zinc ointment. Again, it is emphasized that an accurate record must be kept on these patients.

The Patient with Anorectal Conditions

Patients with anorectal disorders seek medical help primarily because of pain and rectal bleeding. Other frequent complaints are protrusion of hemorrhoids, anal discharge, itching and swelling.

Bleeding is frequently seen in anorectal disease. (The commonest cause of rectal bleeding is hemor-

rhoids.) The patient's description of the bleeding as well as the nurse's assessment assists the physician in making the diagnosis. The bleeding may be bright red but occasionally it is a darker color due to its remaining in the rectal ampulla before expulsion and also from admixture with feces. Bleeding from the anal canal usually has a bright red appearance.

Nursing Assessment

In assessing the patient's signs and symptoms, the following should be investigated:

(1) Is there blood coating the stool or is it mixed with the feces?

(2) Is there pain during evacuation? Is there associated abdominal pain?

(3) How long does the pain last after evacuation?

(4) How does the *patient* describe the pain?

(5) Is any protrusion noted from the anus?

(6) Is a discharge evident? Mucoid? Purulent? Bloody?

Anal Conditions

Ischiorectal abscess is located in the fatty tissue beside the anus. Usually it is caused by infection from the rectum. Treatment consists of incision and drainage. Packing is inserted, and this demands daily changing. The first dressing of these wounds may be extremely painful; therefore, it is well to protect the edges of wounds with petrolatum gauze and to loosen the packing before removing it, by soaking it with peroxide of hydrogen. These wounds are allowed to heal by granulation. Bowel movements should be formed rather than liquid or soft. Cathartics or mineral oil are not usually used.

Fistula in ano is a tiny tubular tract that has its skin opening beside the anus and goes from there by a

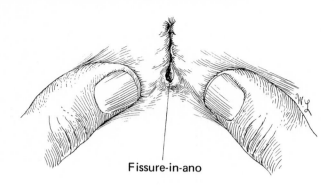

Fig. 22-15. Various types of anal lesions.

Fissure-in-ano

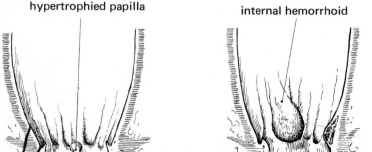

hypertrophied papilla   internal hemorrhoid

fistula   external hemorrhoid

tortuous route into the anal canal. Pus is leaking constantly from the cutaneous opening, making it necessary for the patient to wear a protective pad. (Fig. 22-15.)

Three or 4 hours before operation, the perineum should be shaved and the lower bowel evacuated thoroughly, several warm soapsuds enemas being used. The patient should be allowed to evacuate the enemas on a commode. The last enema should return clear and should be evacuated entirely.

For operation, the patient usually is placed in the lithotomy position, and the sinus tract is identified by inserting a probe into it or by injecting the tract with methylene blue solution. The fistula then may be dissected out or laid open by an incision from its rectal opening to its outlet. The wound is packed with gauze.

Postoperative treatment and complications are the same as those described under "Nursing Management of Patients Having Rectal Surgery" (pp. 499-501).

Fissure in ano is a longitudinal ulcer in the anal canal. It is associated frequently with constipation,

and its most pronounced symptom is excruciating pain when the bowels move. The same preoperative preparation as for fistula in ano is indicated. Several types of operations may be performed: in some cases the anal sphincter is dilated and the fissure is excised; in others, a part of the external sphincter is divided. This gives a paralysis of the external sphincter with consequent relief of spasm and permits the ulcer to heal. When there is a large overhanging sentinel hemorrhoid, excision of the ulcer and of the hemorrhoid is performed. (Fig. 22-15.)

Hemorrhoids are simply varicose veins in the anal canal. They may come and go and almost everyone has them at some time. They are very common in pregnancy. When they fade away they may leave a telltale skin tag. They occur in 2 locations. Those occurring above the internal sphincter are called *internal hemorrhoids* and those appearing outside the external sphincter *external hemorrhoids*. They cause itching, bleeding at stool and pain. Internal hemorrhoids prolapse frequently through the sphincter and cause considerable discomfort. If the blood within them clots and becomes infected, they grow painful and are said to be *thrombosed.* (Fig. 22-15.)

The medical treatment consists in keeping the stools soft and using witch hazel compresses and sitz baths.

The preoperative treatment is that described for fistula in ano (pp. 497-498).

The operation usually is digital dilatation of the rectal sphincter and removal of the hemorrhoids by the use of a clamp and cautery or by ligation and excision. After completion of the operative procedures, a small tube, often covered with petrolatum gauze, may be inserted through the sphincter to permit the escape of flatus, and also of blood if there should be any hemorrhage. Instead of the tube, some surgeons place pieces of Gelfoam or Oxycel gauze over the anal wounds. Dressings in such cases are held in place by a T-binder.

A pilonidal cyst is found in the intergluteal cleft on the posterior surface of the lower sacrum. It is thought by some to be formed by an infolding of epithelial tissue beneath the skin, which may communicate with the skin surface through one or several small sinus openings. Hair frequently is seen protruding from these openings, and this gives the cyst its name—*pilonidal*—a nest of hair. The cysts rarely give symptoms until adolescence or early adult life, when infection produces an irritating drainage or an abscess. This area is easily irritated by perspiration and friction.

Trauma appears to play a part in producing the inflammatory reaction in these cysts.

In the early stages of the inflammation, the infection may be controlled by antibiotic therapy. Once an abscess has formed, as in cases of a hair-containing sinus, surgery is indicated. When an abscess is present, incision and drainage are performed. Usually, however, because the abscesses tend to recur or form secondary sinuses that cause irritating drainage, radical excision of the cyst is necessary. In patients with hair-containing sinuses without marked inflammatory reaction, operation is necessary for the same reason. The entire cyst and the secondary sinus tracts are excised. In many cases the resulting defect may be sutured, but in some the defect may be so large that it cannot be closed entirely, and it is allowed to heal by granulation.

The nursing care of these patients is relatively simple. In those with abscess, hot moist applications are used frequently. After excision of the cyst, the care is that of any superficial wound. For the first few days, this patient often is more comfortable lying on his abdomen or side with a pillow between his legs. Most patients may be allowed out of bed soon after operation, and their postoperative care is carried out in the doctor's office.

Preoperative Nursing Management of Patients Having Rectal Surgery

Patients facing rectal surgery are usually nervous and irritable. The nursing approach should focus on the special psychological problems involved. This patient has a special need for privacy. The perineum is shaved carefully before surgery. This may vary with the nature of the operation. Usually a lower bowel irrigation is ordered, which should be given at least 2 hours prior to surgery. The skin area should be cleaned as thoroughly as possible.

Postoperative Nursing Management

The first 24 hours after rectal surgery there may be painful spasms of the sphincter and muscles. Therefore control of pain is of prime consideration. Liberal use of analgesics during this time may be necessary. After 24 hours have elapsed, topical anesthetic agents may be beneficial for relief of local irritation and soreness.

Voiding may be a problem due to a reflex spasm of the sphincter at the outlet of the bladder and a certain amount of muscle guarding from apprehension and pain. All methods to encourage voluntary micturition should be tried before resorting to catheterization. After rectal operations patients are usually allowed out of bed to void.

After hemorrhoidectomy, hemorrhage may occur from the veins that were cut. If a tube has been inserted through the sphincter after operation, evidence of bleeding should be apparent on the dressings. If, however, the patient feels faint, restless, and anxious and the pulse rate increases, the nurse should recognize internal or concealed hemorrhage and give appropriate treatment until the surgeon can be obtained.

Hygiene of the perianal area is important for patient comfort. This is accomplished by gentle cleansing with warm water and *drying* with absorbent cotton wipes. The patient should be instructed to avoid rubbing the area with toilet tissue after he leaves the hospital.

To relieve soreness and pain, moist heat is employed in the form of warm compresses and sitz baths 3 or 4 times daily and especially after each bowel movement. Moist heat is soothing and relaxes sphincter spasm. An icecap to the head or over the heart helps to prevent the faint feeling experienced by many patients during sitz baths. Wet dressings saturated with equal parts of cold water and witch hazel help relieve edema. Petrolatum should be applied around the anal area when wet compresses are being used continuously to prevent skin maceration. Instruct the patient to assume a prone position at intervals as this position promotes dependent drainage of edema fluid.

The patient may be so fearful of pain that he fails

TABLE 22-2. Summary of immediate complications following gastric and intestinal surgery

Anticipation and vigilance for complications have first priority in caring for postoperative patients. Prompt recognition and management of these complications can prevent prolonged disability and, in some instances, death.

Operative Procedure	Complication	Nursing Assessment and Action
Gastric resection	Hemorrhage	Observe gastric aspirate in drainage bottle for evidence of bleeding. Observe the suture line for bleeding. Prepare patient for blood transfusion. Obtain aspiration equipment and cold saline solution. If bleeding continues, prepare patient for surgical intervention.

	Leakage from duodenal stump
	Duodenal disruption
		Evaluate for pain, elevation of temperature, accelerated pulse rate, abdominal rigidity, and deteriorating clinical course.
		Observe for appearance of bile-stained drainage.
		Prepare for surgical drainage.
		  Obtain drainage equipment.
		  Prepare for intravenous infusions and blood transfusions.
		  Institute nasogastric suction.
		  Protect skin from irritating drainage.

	Pancreatitis	Assess for abdominal pain, rapid pulse and elevation of temperature.
		  Establish continuous gastric suction.
		  Maintain fluid and blood volume and electrolyte balance.
		  Control pain.
		  Give medications and antibiotics as ordered.

Surgery of small intestine	Paralytic ileus	Continue constant nasogastric suction. Ensure adequate parenteral therapy.
	Mechanical obstruction	Evaluate patient for intermittent colicky pain, nausea and vomiting. Prepare for intestinal intubation, electrolyte replacement and re-operation if patient does not respond to conservative treatment.

	Infection:
	  Intraperitoneal infections
	  Abdominal wound infection
		Assess for evidences of constant or generalized abdominal pain, rapid pulse and elevation of temperature.
		Prepare for tube decompression of bowel.
		Restore fluid and electrolytes by I.V. route.
		Give antibiotics as directed.

Surgery of large intestine	Wound complications: Infection	Watch temperature graph for evidences of spiking fever. Observe for redness, tenderness and pain around wound. Assist in establishing local drainage. Obtain culture of drainage material for culture and sensitivity studies.

	Wound disruption	Watch for sudden appearance of profuse serous drainage from wound.
		  Cover wound area with sterile towels held in place with binder.
		  Prepare patient immediately for surgery.

	Anastomotic complications: Dehiscence of anastomosis	Prepare patient for surgery.
	Fistulas	Employ bowel decompression. Give parenteral fluids to correct fluid and electrolyte defects.

TABLE 22-2. Summary of immediate complications following gastric and intestinal surgery (*continued*)

Operative Procedure	Complication	Nursing Assessment and Action
	Intra-abdominal septic conditions: Peritonitis	Evaluate patient for nausea, hiccuping, chills, spiking fever, tachycardia. Give antibiotics as ordered. Prepare patient for drainage procedure. Institute intravenous fluid and electrolyte therapy. Prepare patient for re-operation if his condition deteriorates.
	Abscess formation	Administer antibiotics as directed. Apply hot compresses as ordered. Prepare for surgical drainage.
	Paralytic ileus	Initiate nasogastric intubation. Prepare patient for x-ray study. Ensure adequate fluid and electrolyte replacement. Give antibiotics if patient has symptoms of peritonitis.
Appendectomy	Peritonitis	Observe for abdominal tenderness, fever, vomiting, abdominal rigidity and tachycardia. Employ constant nasogastric suction. Correct dehydration. Give antibiotic agents.
	Pelvic or lumbar abscess	Evaluate for anorexia, chills, fever, and diaphoresis. Watch for "diarrhea," which may indicate pelvic abscess. Prepare patient for rectal examination. Prepare patient for operative drainage procedure.
	Subphrenic abscess	Assess patient for chills, fever and sweats. Prepare for x-ray examination. Prepare for surgical drainage of abscess.
	Ileus: Paralytic ileus	Employ nasogastric intubation and suction. Replace fluids and electrolytes by intravenous route.
	Mechanical ileus	Prepare for operation if diagnosis of mechanical ileus is established.

to respond to the signal for defecation and thus develops constipation. Usually cathartics are avoided. It is better to have a formed stool rather than many liquid or soft ones. The painful sphincter spasm can be relieved at once by a hot sitz bath or hot compresses. Mineral oil may be ordered. Some surgeons prefer that a warm oil retention enema be given when the patient feels a desire to defecate; a soapsuds enema given through a well-lubricated catheter may be prescribed if there has been no bowel movement by the third day after operation. The food preferred by the patient is given usually.

The patient may assume any position that is comfortable. The prone position or side lying position with a pillow between the knees are quite comfortable for these patients. A foam rubber ring will increase greatly the patient's sitting comfort. Early ambulation is generally encouraged.

Patient Education

When it is time for the patient to be discharged from the hospital, he should know how to take sitz baths and how to test the temperature of the water. Sitz baths may be given in a bathtub, which necessitates the application of very warm water 3 or 4 times a day. If this tends to make some postoperative patients weak, sitz baths may be given by employing a dish pan or some large container with enough water to cover the perineum. The patient should be informed about his diet and made aware of the significance of proper eating habits. Also, he ought to know what laxatives he can take safely and why exercise is important. The surgeon usually outlines a schedule in detail to cover the daily routine. This can be reviewed with the patient by the nurse.

BIBLIOGRAPHY

Books

Artz, C. P., and Hardy, J. D.: Complications in Surgery and Their Management. Philadelphia, W. B. Saunders, 1967.

Calman, C. H.: Atlas of Hernia Repair. St. Louis, C. V. Mosby, 1966.

Gius, J. A.: Fundamentals of General Surgery. Chicago, Yearbook Medical Publishers, 1966.

Guyton, A. C.: Textbook of Medical Physiology. Parts IX and X. Philadelphia, W. B. Saunders, 1966.

Happenie, S. D.: Colostomy: A Second Chance. Springfield, Charles C Thomas, 1968.

Harrison, T. R.: Principles of Internal Medicine. Section 7. New York, McGraw-Hill, 1966.

McHardy, G.: Current Gastroenterology. New York, Harper and Brothers, 1963.

McNeer, G., and Pack, G. T.: Neoplasms of the Stomach. Philadelphia, J. B. Lippincott, 1967.

Metheny and Snively: Nurses' Handbook of Fluid Balance. Philadelphia, J. B. Lippincott, 1967.

Nyhus, L. M., and Harkins, H. N.: Hernia. Philadelphia, J. B. Lippincott, 1965.

Randall, H. T., *et al.:* Manual of Preoperative and Postoperative Care. Philadelphia, W. B. Saunders, 1967.

Rhoads, Allen, Harkins and Moyer: Surgery, ed. 4. Philadelphia, J. B. Lippincott, 1970.

Stomach and Small Intestines

Allen, J. G.: Acute appendicitis. Hosp. Med., *3*:61, June, 1967.

Beranbaum, E. R., *et al.:* Barium studies with visceral angiography. Amer. J. Gastroenterology, *46*:21-27, July, 1966.

Butler, F. S.: The permanent gastrostomy: A modern revised feeding technique involving the precision diet. J. Amer. Geriatrics Soc., *15*:174-182, Feb., 1967.

Case, T. C.: Acute abdominal problems in the aged. Geriatrics, *21*:180-188, Aug., 1966.

Donaldson, R. N.: Diet and gastrointestinal disorders. Gastroenterology, *52*:897-900, May, 1967.

Fason, M. F.: Controlling bacterial growth in tube feedings. Amer. J. Nurs., *67*:1246-1247, June, 1967.

Foster, F. P.: Peritonitis: a plan when treatment fails. Med. Clin. N. Amer., *50*:551-563, March, 1966.

Ingelfinger, F. J., and Ochsner, A.: Medical and surgical aspects of duodenal ulcer. Postgrad. Med., *40*:429-438, Oct., 1966.

Judd, E. S. (ed.): Gastrointestinal surgery. Surg. Clin. N. Amer., *47*, August, 1967.

Olson, E. (ed.): The hazards of immobility. Effects on gastrointestinal function. Amer. J. Nurs., *67*:785-787, April, 1967.

Postlethwait, R. W.: Peritonitis. Hosp. Med., *3*:12-25, Sept., 1967.

Steigmann, F., and Hyman, S.: Acute gastrointestinal hemorrhage. Postgrad. Med., *41*:252-259, March, 1967.

Colon

Agarwal, S. L.: A review of intestinal obstruction. Internat. Surg., *46*:113-117, Aug., 1966.

Amdrup, C.: Colostomy care: Natural evacuation or irrigation? Amer. J. Digest. Dis., *12*:747-748, July, 1967.

Atik, M.: Intestinal obstruction. G.P., *35*:128-137, Feb., 1967.

Cihlar, J., *et al.:* Courage with a colostomy (a care study). Amer. J. Nurs., *67*:1050-1051, May, 1967.

Colcock, B. P.: Carcinoma of the colon. Surg. Clin. N. Amer., *47*:647-655, June, 1967.

Dlin, B. M., Perlman, A., and Ringold, E.: Psycho-sexual response to ileostomy and colostomy, Amer. J. Psychiat. *126*:374-381, Sept., 1969.

Fry, W. A., and Daicoff, G. R.: Principles in the selection of colostomy. Hosp. Med., *3*:12-16, July, 1967.

Katona, E. A.: Learning colostomy control. Amer. J. Nurs., *67*:534-541, March, 1967.

Kirsner, J. B.: Possible immune mechanisms in ulcerative colitis. Postgrad. Med., *40*:387-390, Oct., 1966.

Moore, F. T., *et al.:* A protocol for ileostomy management. Amer. J. Surg., *3*:687-690, 1966.

Paine, J. R.: Cancer of the colon. Postgrad. Med., *39*:596-600, June, 1966.

Postel, A. H., *et al.:* A simplified method of irrigation of colonic stoma. Surg. Gynec. Obstet., *121*:595-598, Sept., 1965.

Rider, J. A.: Management of ulcerative colitis. Hosp. Med. *2*:85-91, Oct., 1966.

Turnbull, R. B.: Construction and care of the ileostomy. Hosp. Med., *2*:38-43, March, 1966.

Wilson, J. P.: Cancer of the rectum and colon. Nurs. Forum, *4*:59-66, No. 2, 1965.

Hernia

Inguinal and femoral hernias. Ciba Clin. Symposia, *18*, April-May-June, 1966.

Anorectal Conditions

Castro, A. F.: Diagnosis and management of common rectal and anal disorders. G.P., *34*:78-92, Dec., 1966.

Hopping, R. A.: Common disorders of anus, rectum and sigmoid. Ciba Clin. Symposia, *16*, Oct.-Nov.-Dec., 1964.

Howard, G. T.: Surgical management of hemorrhoids. Amer. J. Proctol., *17*:213-220, June, 1966.

Montague, J.: Better care for patients with rectal ailments. Amer. J. Nurs., *65*:83, Nov., 1965.

Nesselrod, J. P.: Anatomy, pathogenesis and treatment of hemorrhoids and related anorectal conditions. Rev. Surg., *23*:229-253, July-Aug., 1966.

Thomas, B.: Nursing in rectal disorder. Canad. Nurse, *62*:38-39, March, 1966.

Turell, R. (ed.): New perspectives in colorectoanal surgery. Surg. Clin. N. Amer., *45*, Oct., 1965.

PATIENT EDUCATION

Serino, J. S.: Your Ulcer. Philadelphia, J. B. Lippincott, 1966.

United States Public Health Service
U.S. Government Printing Office
Superintendent of Documents
Washington, D.C. 20402
    Cancer of the Stomach. (HIS) Publication No. 120
    Peptic Ulcer. (HIS) Publication No. 71
    Cancer of the Colon and Rectum. (HIS) Publication No. 124

Trask Laboratories
Box 72
Newton, Mass. 02158
Booklet of General Information and Instruction for Persons With Colostomies. $.25

American Cancer Society
(Local Chapter)
Care of Your Colostomy.

John F. Greer Co.
5335 College Ave.
P.O. Box 2898
Oakland, California 94618
General Information about the Colostomy.

Institute of Physical Medicine and Rehabilitation
New York University Medical Center
New York, New York 10016
Postel, A. H., Grier, W. R. N., and Localio, S. A.: Training the Patient in the Bulb Syringe Method of Colostomy Irrigation. A Manual for Nurses. 1965. $.50

QT Inc.
227 Commonwealth Avenue
Boston, Mass. 02116
Manual for Ileostomy Patients. (Sections written by physicians.) $2.20
Your Ileostomy. $.10

Ileostomy Association of Los Angeles, Inc.
1710 N. LaBrea Avenue
Los Angeles, California 90046
Pearce, V.: Ileostomy Information. $.50

United Surgical Supplies Co.
Port Chester, New York 10574
Brubaker, W.: A Message to All New Ileostomy, Colostomy, and Ileal Bladder Patients. $.35

Merck Sharpe and Dohme
West Point, Pennsylvania 19486
Helpful Notes for Colostomy and Ileostomy Patients. 1967.

American Medical Association
535 N. Dearborn Street
Chicago, Illinois 60610
Montague, J. F.: Living with an ostomy. (Reprinted from Today's Health, April, 1967)

United Ostomy Association Inc.
1111 Wilshire Blvd.
Los Angeles, California 90017
Ostomy Quarterly. Official world publication; paramedical journal. $2.00 per year for 4 issues.

CHAPTER 23

Patients with Disorders of the Liver and the Biliary Tract

- *Physiologic and Pathologic Perspectives*
- *Conditions of the Liver*
- *Conditions of the Biliary System*

PHYSIOLOGIC AND PATHOLOGIC PERSPECTIVES

Structural Components

The liver is a large organ, weighing about 1,500 gm., or 3 lbs. Most of it is located behind the ribs in the upper right-hand portion of the abdominal cavity (Fig. 23-1). It is made up of myriad small units called *lobules*, each just large enough to be visible with the naked eye and all similar in size, shape and function. Each lobule has somewhat the shape of a thimble. It is composed of liver cells and vessels.

Through its center runs a tiny tributary to the hepatic vein, which carries the blood to the heart. Along the periphery of each lobule course 3 or 4 tiny branches of the portal vein, which conducts the blood from the digestive organs to the liver. These portal and hepatic veins are connected by a multitude of small capillaries, and around these the liver cells are arranged. The liver thus is composed of multitudes of cells, and on one side or several sides of each of these a capillary is situated. Through these capillaries flows practically all the blood from the stomach, the intestines, the pancreas and the spleen, so that every bit of nourishment that is absorbed from the gastrointestinal tract into the blood has to come into close contact with these liver cells.

There is another type of cell in the liver, likewise situated close beside the capillaries, namely, Kupffer's cells. These are phagocytic cells and belong to the reticuloendothelial tissue, distributed also in other organs throughout the body, especially in the spleen, the bone marrow and the lymph nodes. The function of these Kupffer cells appears to be in part the engulfing of particulate matter in the blood, including defective or old red blood cells ready to be retired from circulation. The hemoglobin from the red cells is split chemically; its iron-containing fraction is conserved for the formation of more hemoglobin, and the rest is converted into bile pigment.

Within the liver cells start tiny bile ducts, or canaliculi, which unite between the rows of liver cells to form larger ducts comparable in size with blood capillaries. These in turn unite and course along between the liver lobules, forming still larger ducts which eventually lead into the large *hepatic duct*, a tube about 2 inches in length and ¼ inch in diameter. Beneath the liver is the gallbladder, a pouch that can hold from 30 to 50 ml. of bile. Connected to the gallbladder is a duct, called the *cystic duct*, which is about ½ inch in length and ⅛ inch in diameter. The hepatic duct and the cystic duct unite to form the *common bile duct*, a tube about 3 inches long and about ¼ inch in diameter, which terminates in the duodenum at the Ampulla of

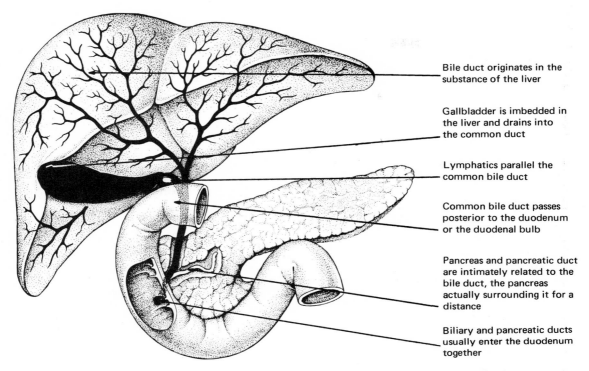

Bile duct originates in the substance of the liver

Gallbladder is imbedded in the liver and drains into the common duct

Lymphatics parallel the common bile duct

Common bile duct passes posterior to the duodenum or the duodenal bulb

Pancreas and pancreatic duct are intimately related to the bile duct, the pancreas actually surrounding it for a distance

Biliary and pancreatic ducts usually enter the duodenum together

FIG. 23-1. Anatomic relationships of the biliary tract. (Iber, F. L.: Hospital Medicine *4*:No. 6, June, 1968)

Vater. The hepatic duct; its continuation, the common bile duct; its offshoot, the cystic duct; and the gallbladder all together comprise what is referred to as the *biliary tract* (Fig. 23-1).

Biochemical Activities

The functions of the liver are numerous and varied. This organ receives by way of the portal vein all the blood returning from the gastrointestinal tract—blood that carries all the products of carbohydrate and protein digestion. The digested carbohydrate arrives in the liver in the form of glucose. Here it is converted into glycogen (glycogenesis) or animal starch, and is stored as such. From this storage depot of glycogen a constant supply of carbohydrate is released into the bloodstream (glycogenolysis)—again in the form of glucose—the rate of its release varying according to the changing body requirements. Most of it eventually serves as body fuel, being metabolized in the tissues to provide heat and energy; some is transformed again into glycogen and stored in the muscle tissues; the rest is converted into fat and stored by special cells (fat cells) located chiefly in the subcutaneous tissues and within the abdominal cavity. The liver also is capable of manufacturing glucose from non-carbohydrate sources, such as proteins, fats and lactates

(glucogenesis), so that the body is not solely dependent on food as a source of this substance.

The parenchymal cells of the liver likewise play an important role in *protein metabolism*. Here the amino acids derived from foods lose their amine groups and are incorporated into new proteins. Among these are many of the plasma proteins, including fibrinogen, prothrombin, the prothrombin accelerators and albumin. Just as in the case of carbohydrate, a certain amount of protein is stored in utilizable form in the liver, to be available as required. Moreover, it is in these cells that certain poisonous nitrogenous byproducts of protein digestion and metabolism are converted into nontoxic substances. For example, ammonia bodies are returned to the blood from the liver as urea, which is not poisonous; the urea is cleared from the bloodstream by the kidneys, which excrete it into the urine.

Liver cells play a key role in the metabolism of fatty acids and ketone bodies; and they prepare for the body, store for it and supply it with numerous other essential substances. One such material is necessary for the normal development of the immature red blood cell in the bone marrow. This substance is vitamin B_{12} (cyanocobalamine), and its deficiency leads to the development of pernicious anemia (p. 307). These cells are concerned in the manufacture and the storage of other vitamins, including vitamins A and D, as well as many components of the B complex. Certain metals, such as iron and copper likewise are stored here.

All of the aforementioned metabolites and synthetic products are secreted by the parenchymal liver cells into adjacent blood capillaries, which, in the center of each liver lobule, connect with a branch of the hepatic vein. The latter drains into the inferior vena cava, which conducts the blood directly to the heart. This mode of secretion by an organ—namely, into the blood —is termed *internal secretion*.

Bile Formation and Excretion

In addition to being an organ of internal secretion, the liver is also an excretory organ, its excretory product being the bile. Bile formation by the liver is taking place constantly. Its excretion into the gastrointestinal tract is not continuous, however, but intermittent. Between meals most of the bile produced by the liver is diverted into the gallbladder, where a large proportion of its water is absorbed, the final solution being 5 to 10 times more concentrated than that originally secreted by the liver. Following a period of fasting, as soon as fatty food passes through the pylorus from the stomach, the gallbladder empties this reserve of concentrated bile through the cystic duct, by way of the common bile duct, into the duodenum (Fig. 23-1).

The function of bile in intestinal digestion is to aid in the enzymatic transformation of fats into soluble soaps by causing them to emulsify, that is, break up into a suspension of very small globules that are more readily attacked by the fat-splitting enzymes in the intestinal fluid. Bile also serves as a vehicle for the removal of various substances that the liver cells clear from the blood, including bilirubin and urobilinogen.

Bilirubin is a pigment derived from hemoglobin. A by-product of hemolysis, this pigment constantly is being formed and introduced into the bloodstream by histiocytic cells engaged in the phagocytosis of outworn or defective erythrocytes. Attached to albumin, bilirubin circulates in the plasma until it comes in contact with a liver cell, which promptly absorbs it, separates it from its albumin attachment, conjugates it with glycuronic acid and secretes it, along with other bile constituents, into the adjacent bile canaliculus. Thence, by way of a succession of communicating channels within the liver and the hepatic ducts outside the liver, the bilirubin glucuronide escapes through the common bile duct into the duodenum. Subsequently, while in transit through the intestines, this pigment becomes converted into urobilinogen and most of it makes a direct exit from the body as fecal urobilinogen. However, some urobilinogen is absorbed through the intestinal mucosa into the blood; of this, a portion is excreted by the kidneys as urine urobilinogen, while the remainder is secreted by the liver cells into the bile and returns once again to the gastrointestinal tract.

Pathologic Perspectives

The most common circulatory problems involving the liver are based on increased venous blood pressure in the vena cava, causing liver vascular congestion or portal venous obstruction within the liver itself as a result of liver disease. Hepatic congestion, due to high systemic venous pressure, as in patients with right-sided heart failure, results in a large, tense liver that may pulsate. If the process is prolonged, lack of oxygen causes death of the parenchymal cells with replacement of fibrous tissue, resulting in a large, firm (cirrhotic) liver with a reduced functional capacity. Obstructed portal blood flow within a cirrhotic liver is the commonest cause of an abnormally high pressure in the venous system of the gastrointestinal tract, or portal hypertension. This leads to edema of the tract, the accumulation of fluid in the abdominal cavity, abnormalities of absorption, and to the increase of the collateral venous drainage with enlarged tortuous veins in the esophagus (varices), rectum (hemorrhoids) and abdominal wall.

The parenchymatous cells of the liver have many functions in connection with carbohydrate, protein, fat, vitamin and hormone metabolism. The liver is involved in the formation of plasma proteins, including several blood clotting components; in carbohydrate metabolism (control of blood sugar), in fat metabolism (oxidation of fatty acids), in lipid metabolism (synthesis of cholesterol), in detoxification and conjugation of drugs and hormones, in the degradation of red blood cell pigments (porphyrins) and many other activities. Of particular importance is the conversion of ammonia derived from the enzymatic removal of nitrogen from amino acids (deamination) into urea, the principal end product of nitrogen metabolism.

Disease of the liver parenchyma is caused by infectious agents as bacteria and viruses, anoxia, metabolic disorders, toxins and drugs, nutritional deficiencies and states of hypersensitivity. Probably the most common causes of parenchymatous damage are viral hepatitis and malnutrition, especially in alcoholism. The response of the parenchymal cells is much the same for most noxious agents: replacement of glycogen by lipids and fats (fatty infiltration), with or without cell death (necrosis) associated with inflammatory cell infiltration and growth of fibrous tissue. Cell regeneration can occur if the disease process is not too toxic to the cells. The end result of severe parenchymatous disease is a firm (cirrhotic) normal to small-sized liver, smooth or irregular (hobnail), and perhaps portal hypertension due to intrahepatic obstruction to

LIVER BIOPSY AND THE ROLE OF THE NURSE

A procedure that facilitates greatly the diagnosis of most hepatic disorders is the liver biopsy, i.e., the sampling of liver tissue by needle aspiration for purposes of histologic study. The responsibilities of the nurse in relation to liver biopsy and the rationale of her participation in this procedure are summarized below:

Nursing Activities

Ascertain in advance that hemostasis tests have been requisitioned, completed and reported, and that compatible donor blood is available.

Measure and record the patient's pulse, respirations and arterial pressure immediately prior to biopsy.

Describe to the patient in advance:
1. Steps contemplated
2. Sensations expected
3. After-effects anticipated
4. Restrictions of activity to be imposed afterward

Give support to the patient during the procedure

Expose the right side of the patient's abdomen.

Instruct the patient to inhale and exhale deeply several times, finally to exhale and to hold his breath at the end of expiration.

 The physician promptly introduces the biopsy needle by way of the transthoracic (intercostal) or transabdominal (subcostal) route, penetrates the liver, aspirates and withdraws. The entire procedure is completed within 5 to 10 seconds.

Inform the patient to resume breathing.

Immediately following the biopsy, assist the patient to turn on his right side, place a pillow under his costal margin and caution him to remain in this position, recumbent and immobile, for several hours.

Measure and record the patient's pulse and respiratory rates and his arterial pressure at 10- to 20-minute intervals for the prescribed period of time, or until his status proves to be stable, and his condition has been pronounced to be satisfactory. Be alert to detect and to report promptly any increase in pulse rate or any decrease in arterial pressure, any complaint of pain or manifestations of apprehension.

Rationale

Many patients with liver disease have clotting defects and are abnormally prone to bleed.

Prebiopsy values provide a basis on which to compare his vital signs and evaluate his status following the procedure.

Explanations serve to allay his fears, to ensure his cooperation and to reinforce his instruction.

The proximity of an understanding nurse enhances comfort and promotes a sense of security.

The skin at the site of penetration will be disinfected and infiltrated with local anesthetic.

Holding the breath immobilizes the chest wall and the diaphragm; penetration of the diaphragm thereby is avoided, and the risk of lacerating the liver is minimized.

In this position the liver capsule at the site of penetration is compressed against the chest wall, and the escape of blood or bile through the perforation is impeded.

These signs may indicate the presence and the progress of hepatic bleeding or bile peritonitis, the most frequent complications of liver biopsy.

---

portal blood flow or jaundice due to intrahepatic obstruction of bile channels.

Biliary disease generally is associated with obstruction of biliary channels, either of the small bile canaliculi (cholangioles) inside the liver (intrahepatic) or the bile ducts outside the liver (extrahepatic). The end result is accumulation of bile pigments in the liver and blood to produce jaundice. Cholangiolitic hepatitis is found principally in viral hepatitis and in drug reactions (methyltestosterone, chlorpromazine). These conditions are associated with obstruction and often proliferation of the cholangioles, cellular infiltration, and fibrosis of the periphery of the liver lobules. Chronic cholangiolitis can result in primary biliary cirrhosis. Generally, the liver architecture is relatively normal. Extrahepatic biliary obstruction is due to neoplasm (progressive and uninfected) or to benign causes such as gallstones or strictures (intermittent with chronic secondary infection). Here the bile regurgitates from the fine biliary canaliculi by leakage or rupture into the liver sinusoids, causing bile staining of the liver. Generally, parenchymal cells are not

ALKALINE PHOSPHATASE

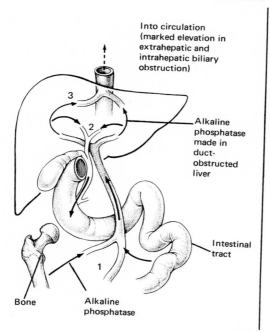

Into circulation (marked elevation in extrahepatic and intrahepatic biliary obstruction)

Alkaline phosphatase made in duct-obstructed liver

Intestinal tract

Bone

Alkaline phosphatase

RATIONALE

Alkaline phosphatase delivered to the liver (1) is excreted in the bile, as indicated by solid arrows (2). In the event of biliary obstruction, serum alkaline phosphatase increases by virtue of impaired bile flow pathways and increased hepatic manufacture, as indicated by dotted arrow (3).

QUESTIONS ANSWERED

Is the biliary tract blocked? Has it been blocked recently?

SERUM BILIRUBIN

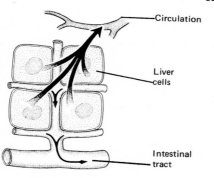

Circulation

Liver cells

Intestinal tract

RATIONALE

Interruption of the normal bile pathways to the intestinal tract (arrow) results in increased serum bilirubin levels.

QUESTION ANSWERED

Is there jaundice?

SERUM AMYLASE

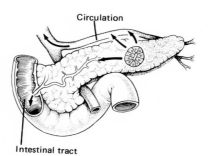

Circulation

Intestinal tract

RATIONALE

Obstruction and inflammatory disease of the pancreas interfere with the normal flow of amylase into the intestinal tract and result in increased serum levels.
Serum amylase levels are markedly elevated in acute pancreatitis.

QUESTION ANSWERED

Is the pancreas inflamed or the duct obstructed?

Fɪɢ. 23-2. Rationale underlying some laboratory tests. (Iber, F. L.: Hospital Medicine 4:No. 6 June, 1968)

| **TEST** | **QUESTIONS ANSWERED OR INFORMATION GAINED** |

DUODENAL INTUBATION

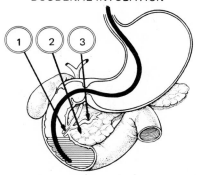

1 Is the bile duct patent? Is there pus (from examination of bile and biliary sediment)?

2 Is there carcinoma of pancreas or duodenum (from cytologic examination)?

3 Is there obstruction of the pancreatic duct (from examination of pancreatic juice for bicarbonate and enzyme)?

SELECTIVE CELIAC AXIS ARTERIOGRAPHY

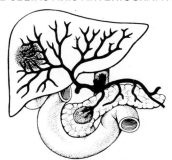

Demonstrates the arterial supply of the pancreas to show tumors

SPLENIC PORTAL VENOGRAPHY

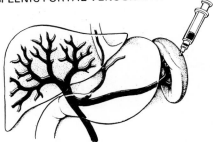

Demonstrates the splenic portal vein and collaterals to show venous invasion and portal collateral circulation

PERITONEOSCOPY

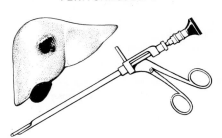

Visualizes the anterior surface of the liver, the gallbladder, and occasionally the mesentery

Fig. 23-3. Test requiring special techniques. (Iber, F. L.: Hospital Medicine *4*:No. 6:61 June, 1968)

damaged but fibrosis and cellular infiltration occurs, and if the process is prolonged cirrhosis can occur. Disease of any of the 4 systems, if sufficiently extensive or prolonged, gradually involves the others; and the end result is cirrhosis with obstruction of bile channels and of portal blood flow.

The liver has remarkable powers of recovery and over 70 per cent of the parenchyma may be damaged before function tests are abnormal. Function is generally measured in terms of enzyme activity, alkaline phosphatase, transaminase, detoxification of Bromsulphalein, abnormal protein concentration formation or thymol turbidity, cephalin flocculation, or the presence of abnormal constituents in the blood (blood ammonia).

If the liver is sufficiently damaged, the capacity of the liver to maintain metabolic stability of the body is insufficient for the metabolic requirements, and the liver is said to fail. The events leading to cirrhosis may proceed over a period of years, but liver failure may occur rapidly when more than 70 per cent of the functional capacity is gone.

Liver Function Tests

In order to differentiate among the many possibilities of liver disturbances, it is necessary to perform a number of tests. There are many tests because the liver has many functions. (Table 23-1 follows; Figs. 23-2, 23-3 illustrate tests frequently done to ascertain presence of biliary tract disease.)

TABLE 23-1. Liver function studies

Test	Normal	Clinical functions
I. *Pigment Studies*		
A. Serum bilirubin, direct	0.-0.3 mg. %	These are measures of ability of liver to conjugate and excrete bilirubin. They are abnormal in liver and biliary tract disease, causing jaundice clinically.
B. Serum bilirubin, total	0.-0.9 mg. %	
C. Urine bilirubin	0	
D. Urine urobilinogen	0-1.16 mg./24 hrs.	
E. Fecal urobilinogen (infrequently used)	40-280 mg./24 hrs.	
II. *Dye Clearances*		
A. Bromosulphalein excretion (BSP test)	< 5% retention in 45 minutes	BSP binds to albumin in blood. Liver cells unbind BSP, conjugate it and excrete it in bile. Normal clearance depends on hepatic blood flow, functioning liver cell mass and lack of obstruction. Retention is increased in liver cell damage or decreased liver blood flow.
B. Indocyanine Green	500-800 ml./sq. m. body surface/min.	Extracted from blood and excreted by liver. Depends on hepatic blood flow, functioning liver cells and lack of obstruction.
III. *Protein Studies*		
A. Total serum protein	7.0-7.5 gm. %	Proteins are manufactured by the liver. Their levels may be depressed in a variety of liver impairments.
B. Serum albumin	3.5-5.5 gm. %	
C. Serum globulin	1.5-3.0 gm. %	
D. Serum protein electrophoresis	Albumin 63-69% of total	
	Alpha 1 Glob. 3.9-7.3%	
	Alpha 2 Glob. 3.9-7.3%	
	Alpha 2 Glob. 6.9-11.8%	
	Beta Glob. 6.9-11.8%	
	Gamma Glob. 9.8-20%	
IV. *Prothrombin Time*		
Response of prothrombin time to vitamin K	100% return to normal.	Prothrombin time may be prolonged in liver disease. It will not return to normal with vitamin K in severe liver cell damage.
V. *Serum Alkaline Phosphatase*	Varies with method. 2-5 Bodansky units.	Manufactured in bones, liver, kidneys, intestine. Excreted through biliary tract. In absence of bone disease, it is a sensitive measure of biliary tract obstruction.

TABLE 23-1. Liver function studies (*continued*)

Test	Normal	Clinical functions
VI. *Serum Transaminase Studies* A. SGOT B. SGPT C. LDH	40 units 35 units 400 units	Based on release of enzymes from damaged liver cells. These enzymes are elevated in liver cell damage.
VII. *Blood Ammonia* (Arterial)	20-50 mgm./ml.	Liver converts ammonia to urea. Ammonia level rises in liver failure.
VIII. *Flocculation Tests* A. Cephalin flocculation B. Thymol turbidity (These protein reactions are too nonspecific to be of great value.)	0-14 units 0-5 units	Depend on ability of serum proteins to stabilize colloidal suspension. Abnormal in liver and other diseases. Positive thymol turbidity also produced by elevated gamma globulin levels.
IX. *Cholesterol* Ester	150-250 mg. % 60% of total	Elevated in biliary obstruction (each of excretion). Decreased in parenchymal liver disease.
X. *Radiologic Studies* A. Splenoportogram B. Cholecystogram and cholangiogram C. Liver scan with radioiodine-tagged rose bengal D. Plain film of abdomen E. Barium study of esophagus		To determine adequacy of portal blood flow. For gallbladder and bile duct visualization. To show size, shape of liver. To show replacement of liver tissue with scars, cysts, or tumor. To determine gross liver size. For varices. Varices in esophagus indicate increased portal pressure.
XI. *Liver Biopsy*		To determine anatomic changes in liver tissue.
XII. *Measurement of Portal Pressure*		Elevated in cirrhosis of the liver.
XIII. *Esophagoscopy*		To search for esophageal varices.
XIV. *Electroencephalogram*		Abnormal in hepatic coma and impending hepatic coma.

CONDITIONS OF THE LIVER

Special Problems of Patients with Disorders of the Liver

The complications of liver disease are numerous and varied. In many instances their ultimate effects are incapacitating or lethal; their advent is ominous, and their treatment is notoriously difficult. Among the most important of these complications are severe gastrointestinal hemorrhages and excessive water retention with ascites and edema, the result of circulatory changes within the diseased liver leading to portal hypertension; impairment of the central and peripheral nervous systems and abnormal bleeding tendencies, attributable to the inability of malfunctioning liver cells to metabolize certain vitamins; and hepatic coma, reflecting the incomplete metabolism of protein fragments by the diseased liver (see Fig. 23-4).

The Jaundiced Patient

When for any reason the bilirubin concentration in the blood becomes abnormally increased, all the body tissues, including the sclerae and the skin, become tinged with a yellow or a greenish-yellow color. This condition is called *jaundice*. There are 3 types of jaundice: (1) hemolytic jaundice, which is attributable to an abnormally high concentration of bilirubin in the blood, the amount exceeding the capacity of normal liver cells to excrete it; (2) hepatocellular jaundice, due to the inability of diseased liver cells to clear normal amounts of bilirubin from the blood; and (3) obstructive jaundice, caused by an impeded or interrupted flow of bile through the external ducts draining the liver (extrahepatic obstruction) or through their radicles within the liver parenchyma (intrahepatic obstruction).

Hemolytic jaundice is the result of an abnormally great destruction of the red blood cells, the effect of which is to flood the plasma with bilirubin so rapidly that the liver, although functioning perfectly normally, cannot excrete this pigment as rapidly as it is formed. This is the type of jaundice that is encountered in patients with hereditary spherocytosis (p. 312), auto-immune hemolytic anemia (p. 313), erythroblastosis fetalis, hemolytic transfusion reactions (p. 95) and other hemolytic disorders. The bilirubin in the blood of these patients is of the unconjugated or "free" type. Fecal and urine urobilinogen are increased; on the other hand, the urine is free of bilirubin. Patients with this type of jaundice, unless their hyperbilirubinemia is extreme, do not experience symptoms or complications as a result of the jaundice *per se*. However, very prolonged jaundice, even if mild, predisposes to the

formation of "pigment stones" in the gallbladder, and extremely severe jaundice—e.g., in patients with levels of free bilirubin above 20 to 25 mg. per cent—is attended by a definite risk of possible brain-stem damage.

Hepatocellular Jaundice. This is jaundice due to liver cell damage or functional impairment. The cellular damage may be from infection such as in infectious hepatitis, homologous serum hepatitis (from virus infected blood transfusion) or yellow fever virus, drug or chemical toxicity (such as carbon tetrachloride, chloroform, phosphorus, arsenicals, certain psychotherapeutic drugs or ethanol). Cirrhosis of the liver is a form of hepatocellular disease that may produce jaundice; it is usually but not always associated

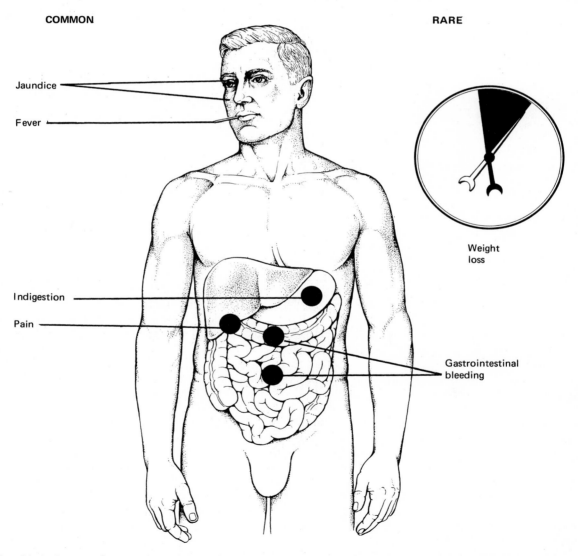

Fig. 23-4. Signs and symptoms of biliary tract disease. (Iber, F. L.: Hospital Medicine 4:No. 6 June, 1968)

with excessive alcoholic intake. It may be a late result of viral-caused liver cell necrosis. In prolonged obstructive jaundice there may eventuate cell damage so that both types appear together.

Patients with hepatocellular jaundice may be mildly or severely ill, with lack of appetite, nausea, loss of vigor and strength, and they may show weight loss. In some instances of hepatocellular disease there may be no jaundice clinically. The SGOT, serum glutamic oxaloacetic transaminase, and the SGPT, serum glutamic pyruvic transaminase, are two intracellular enzymes of the liver that are liberated with cellular necrosis and rise in the bloodstream. These are excellent tests for liver cell damage. In addition, the BSP, bilirubin alkaline phosphatase may be elevated, and the urine urobilinogen rises. In long-standing cases the serum proteins are abnormal, and the prothrombin time prolonged. At onset there may be complaints of headache, chills and fever if the cause is infectious. Depending on the cause and extent of the liver cell damage, hepatocellular jaundice may or may not be completely reversible.

Inborn Errors of Biliary Metabolism. Gilbert's syndrome consists of an increased unconjugated bilirubin that causes jaundice. Liver histology and liver function tests (other than elevated bilirubin) are normal. There is no hemolysis. Gilbert's syndrome is due to a diminution of glucuronyl transferase; it is a familial condition, and is asymptomatic. Other conditions that are caused by inborn errors of biliary metabolism include Dubin-Johnson syndrome (chronic idiopathic jaundice with pigment in the liver) and Rotor syndrome (chronic familial conjugated hyperbilirubinemia without pigment in the liver), and "benign" cholestatic jaundice of pregnancy with retention of conjugated bilirubin, probably secondary to unusual sensitivity to the hormones of pregnancy.

Obstructive jaundice of the extrahepatic type may be caused by plugging of the bile duct by a gallstone (Fig. 23-9), by an inflammatory process, by a tumor, or by an enlarged gland pressing on it. Or the obstruction may involve the small bile ducts within the liver substance (i.e., intrahepatic obstruction), caused, for example, by pressure on these channels from inflammatory swelling of the liver substance or by an inflammatory exudate within the ducts themselves. Intrahepatic obstruction due to stasis and inspissation of bile within the canaliculi is an occasional occurrence following the ingestion of certain drugs, which accordingly are referred to as "cholestatic" agents. These include phenothiazine (e.g., Sparine, Trilafon, etc.), phenothiazine derivatives (e.g., Thorazine), sulfonamide drugs, tolbutamide (Orinase) and other antidiabetic drugs, arsphenamine, thiouracil, and p-aminobenzoic acid (PAB). Whether the obstruction is

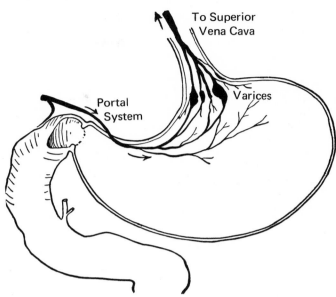

FIG. 23-5. Diagram of the stomach, showing the venous circulation of the lesser circulation of the lesser curvature in a severe case of cirrhosis of the liver. The current of blood now will flow toward the esophagus, and the fine anastomoses will be distended into varices. These have thin walls and rupture, causing profuse hemorrhages into the stomach.

intrahepatic or extrahepatic, and whatever its cause may be, if bile cannot flow normally into the intestine, but is dammed back in the liver substance, it is reabsorbed into the blood and there carried over the entire body, staining the skin and the sclerae. It is excreted in the urine, which becomes a deep orange color and foamy in appearance. Because of the decreased amount of bile in the intestinal tract, the stools become white or clay-colored. The skin may itch intensely, requiring repeated starch baths and oil inunctions. Dyspepsia and especially an intolerance to fatty foods may develop temporarily, due to impairment of fat digestion in the absence of intestinal bile. Here the SGOT and SGPT do not rise but the bilirubin and alkaline phosphatase are elevated.

Portal Hypertension

One set of problems, largely limited to patients with hepatic cirrhosis, arises as a result of obstruction to the flow of portal venous blood through the liver, the effect of which is to elevate the blood pressure throughout the entire portal venous system. Portal hypertension accounts for the formation of esophageal, gastric and hemorrhoidal varicosities, which are prone to rupture and often are the source of massive hemorrhages from the upper gastrointestinal tract and the rectum, as described on page 523. Portal hypertension accounts also for the large accumulations of fluid (ascites) in the abdominal cavity that are characteristic of patients with cirrhosis. As ascites forms, the volume of extracellular fluid throughout the body shrinks; in response to this shrinkage, the adrenal glands are stimulated to secrete increased quantities of the hormone aldosterone, which in turn causes the kidneys to retain sodium and water to excess and is responsible for the generalized edema of cirrhosis. The management of gastrointestinal hemorrhage, ascites and edema in patients with liver disease and portal hypertension are discussed on pp. 522-525.

Nutritional Deficiencies

A second group of complications that are common to patients with severe chronic liver disease of all types is caused by failure of damaged liver cells to make certain vitamins available in an active form to the body. Among the specific deficiency states that occur on this basis are vitamin A deficiency, beriberi, polyneuritis and Wernicke-Korsakoff psychosis, all attributable to a deficiency of thiamine; skin and mucous membrane lesions characteristic of riboflavin deficiency; "rum fits," which probably are due to pyridoxine deficiency; hypoprothrombinemia (p. 324), characterized by spontaneous bleeding and ecchymoses, due to vitamin K deficiency; the hemorrhagic lesions of scurvy, i.e., vitamin C deficiency; and the macrocytic anemia of folic acid deficiency. The threat of these avitaminoses provides the rationale for supplementing the diet of every patient with chronic liver disease with ample quantities of vitamins A, B complex, C and K. (The student is referred to a text on nutrition in disease.)

Hepatic Coma

Hepatic coma, one of the dreaded complications of liver disease and a manifestation of profound liver failure, in essence is ammonia intoxication. Its principal manifestations are those of brain dysfunction and damage. It may be caused by failure of the liver cells to detoxify (by converting to urea) the ammonia that constantly is entering the bloodstream as a result of its absorption from the gastrointestinal tract, its production by metabolizing kidney tissue, and its liberation from contracting muscle cells. Enzymatic and other functions are disrupted.

Clinical Features. The earliest symptoms of hepatic coma, i.e., the manifestations of impending coma, include minor mental aberrations and motor disturbances. The patient appears to be slightly confused; he becomes untidy; there is a faraway look in his eye; he tends to drowse during the day and to wander at night; and he may exhibit a coarse, or "flapping" tremor, especially of the hands. In a more advanced

stage there are gross disturbances of consciousness, and the patient is completely disoriented with respect to time and place. With further progression of the disorder he lapses into frank coma and is likely to succumb.

Aggravating and Precipitating Factors. As indicated above, a factor in the pathogenesis of liver coma is the accumulation of ammonia in the blood. The largest source of blood ammonia is the enzymatic and bacterial digestion of proteins (including dietary and blood proteins) in the gastrointestinal tract. Ammonia from this source is *increased* as a result of gastrointestinal bleeding, a high protein diet, the ingestion of ammonium salts (e.g., ammonium chloride, prescribed as a diuretic), bacterial growth in the small bowel, and uremia. On the other hand, gastrointestinal ammonia is *decreased* by elimination of protein from the diet and by the administration of bowel sterilizing antibiotics, such as neomycin sulfate, kanamycin sulfate and chlortetracycline.

Ammonia is supplied also by the kidneys as they carry out the deamination of various amino acids. Ammonia from the kidney is *increased* following the administration of diuretics (such as chlorothiazide, and steroid drugs), following the restriction of dietary sodium, and in patients with potassium depletion. Ammonia from muscle tissue is *increased* during exercise.

As might be anticipated in part from the foregoing comments, liver coma may be induced in susceptible patients as a consequence of any of the following: gastrointestinal bleeding; any infection, especially an enteric infection; a surgical procedure; any acute disturbance in water and electrolyte balance, especially hyponatremia (sodium depletion), hypokalemia (potassium depletion) and water intoxication; the administration of diuretic agents, such as acetazolamide (Diamox) or chlorothiazide (Diuril); the ingestion (or injection) of ammonium salts; and protein feedings.

Nursing Management. The patient with impending hepatic coma should be observed several times each day from the standpoint of his neurologic status. A daily record should be kept of his handwriting and his performance in arithmetic. His fluid intake and output and, if feasible, his body weight should be charted each day. His vital signs should be measured and recorded every 4 hours. Evidences suggesting pulmonary or other infection should be sought frequently and carefully, and reported promptly, if observed.

If it becomes apparent that liver coma is indeed impending, the patient's protein intake is reduced sharply, or eliminated altogether for the time being, and an antibiotic drug is prescribed for sterilization of the bowel (e.g., chlortetracycline, neomycin sulfate or kanamycin sulfate, 6 to 8 gm. orally on the first day and 4 gm. daily thereafter). Sedative and analgesic drugs, if prescribed at all, are administered to this patient in very conservative doses and under very close observation.

The Patient with Viral Hepatitis

Of increasing importance to those concerned with public health is the increasing incidence of viral hepatitis. Peaks of maximal incidence occurred in 1954 and 1961 in the United States, which leads some authorities to suggest a seven-year cycle. Although mortality rate is low, the importance of the disease is due to its ease of transmission, morbidity, and prolonged loss of time from school or employment. The nurse is especially concerned with the problem of viral hepatitis not only because of the care of the patient so afflicted, but because of the apparent health needs of the community required for its elimination: (1) proper public and home sanitation, (2) conscientious individual hygiene at all times, (3) safe practices of food preparation and dispensation, (4) effective health supervision in schools, dormitories, barracks and camps, and (5) repeated health educational programs.

Two major forms of viral hepatitis have been identified—both caused by evasive filtrable viruses: (1) infectious hepatitis, and (2) serum hepatitis. These have world-wide distribution, with outbreaks occurring in both epidemic and sporadic form. Extensive damage to the liver occurs as a result of the disease; lesions may be of considerable size and many weeks may be required for regeneration of the cells and recovery to take place.

Infectious Hepatitis (Epidemic Hepatitis, Catarrhal Jaundice, IH Virus or A Virus)

The mode of transmission of this disease is probably through the ingestion of foods or liquids infected by the virus, although a respiratory mode of transmission has not been excluded. Typically, a child acquires the infection at school and brings it home where haphazard sanitary habits spread it through the family. An infected person who handles food in a restaurant can spread the disease, or people drink sewage-contaminated water, or eat shellfish from sewage-polluted shoreland. As in the case of homologous serum jaundice (see below), the infection can be acquired as a result of an inoculation, e.g., a blood transfusion.

The incubation period is estimated to be from 2 to 7 weeks (usually 25 days) and the disease usually occurs in the fall and winter. The course of the illness may be prolonged (usually shorter in the young and much more serious in those after age 40), lasting from 4 to 8 weeks, and is characterized chiefly by jaundice, which at its peak may be intense. Symptoms of a mild

upper respiratory infection, with low-grade fever, may be present for a few days at the onset, even before the jaundice becomes apparent. Indigestion is present to a varying degree, marked by vague epigastric distress, anorexia, nausea, heartburn and flatulence. These symptoms tend to clear as soon as the jaundice reaches its peak—perhaps 10 days after its original appearance. The liver and the spleen are often moderately enlarged for a few days after the onset; otherwise, apart from the jaundice, there are few physical signs to be elicited.

Medical and Nursing Management. Bed rest during the acute stage and the provision of a diet that is both acceptable and nutritious are part of the treatment and nursing care. During the period of anorexia the patient should receive frequent small feedings, supplemented, as needed, by intravenous infusions of glucose. Since this patient would rather not look at food or eat, it requires gentle persistence and ingenuity to whet his appetite. Optimal food and fluid levels need to be maintained to counteract probable weight loss and unduly prolonged recovery. Even before the icteric phase, however, many patients recover their appetites and thereafter need no reminders to maintain a good diet.

Prognosis. Recovery from epidemic hepatitis is the rule; a rare case progresses to an acute liver necrosis (acute yellow atrophy), terminating in cirrhosis of the liver or even death. Infectious hepatitis confers immunity against itself; the person may acquire other forms of hepatitis, however.

Prevention, Control and Community Concern. Three ways to reduce the risk of contracting infectious hepatitis are:

1. Good personal hygiene stressing careful handwashing.

2. Community sanitation—safe food and water supply as well as effective sewage disposal.

3. Gamma globulin—infectious hepatitis can be prevented by the administration of gamma globulin given intramuscularly in a dose of 0.02 to 0.05 ml. per kg. of body weight during the period of incubation if this treatment is instituted within a period of a few days following exposure. This bolsters the person's own antibody production and provides about 6 to 8 weeks of immunity.

Homologous Serum Jaundice (Serum Hepatitis, SH virus, B virus)

This disease, the importance of which was recognized during World War II, occasionally follows the therapeutic or prophylactic injection of materials containing human serum, such as convalescent serum, certain vaccines and whole blood or plasma. It also may be transmitted by medical or dental instruments, or other skin-puncturing instruments such as tatooing

TABLE 23-2. A comparison of two forms of viral hepatitis

	Infectious hepatitis	Serum hepatitis
A. OTHER NAMES	Epidemic hepatitis, catarrhal jaundice, IH virus, A virus	Serum hepatitis, SH virus, B virus
B. EPIDEMIOLOGY		
1. Infectious Agent	Known: Filtrable virus	Unknown: Filtrable virus
2. Method of Transmission	Oral-anal route with respiratory spread possible	Parenteral route with infusion of blood or blood products from an infected person
	Blood transfusion, blood serum or plasma from infected person	Use of contaminated needles, syringes for parenteral infusion
	Contaminated syringes or needles	
	Contaminated food, milk, or water	
3. Incubation Period	2 to 7 weeks; usually 25 days	2 to 5 months; usually 2½ to 3 months
4. Occurrence	Worldwide, sporadic or in epidemic proportions	Worldwide
	Children and young adults usually. More recently, older persons afflicted	Recipients of blood and blood products
	Time of year: Fall and winter	
C. NATURE OF DISEASE		
1. Signs and Symptoms	*Pre-icteric phase:* Headache, fever, anorexia, nausea, vomiting, some abdominal tenderness, palpable pain over liver	Similar to infectious hepatitis but more severe
	Icteric phase: Dark urine, jaundice, liver enlarged Recovery within 4 months	Pre-icteric phase more prolonged Convalescence longer
2. Specific Treatment	Adequate rest, fluids and nutrition	Same
D. PREVENTION	Good sanitation	Reject donors who have had serum hepatitis
	Proper personal hygiene	Maintain 6-month interval of time since last serving as donor
	Proper safeguards to prevent use of blood and its components from infected donors	Transfuse only when justifiable
	Effective sterilization procedures	When feasible, use blood substitutes
	Careful screening of food handlers	Use effective heat sterilization for syringes and needles
	Safe preparation and serving of food	Use fresh sterile syringes and needles for each injection
E. CONTROL OF PATIENT AND ENVIRONMENT	Isolation of patient (explain reason to patient)	No isolation
	Disposal of nose and throat secretions in tissues, bags and then to incinerator	Equipment contaminated with blood needs immediate cleaning, disinfection and disposition.
	Careful bedpan handling	
	With good sewage disposal, feces disposal is no problem; without good disposable, use effective means of disinfection before disposal	
	Isolation of bedpan; terminal sterilization	
	Patient education in meticulous personal hygiene habits	
	Use disposable dishes or autoclave regular dishes (boiling at least 30 min.)	
	Discard thermometer at end of isolation period	

or ear-piercing needles. Drug addicts acquire the disease from hypodermic needles that have come in contact with blood or serum and have not been properly sterilized.

Clinically, the disease closely resembles epidemic hepatitis. However, the incubation period is relatively much longer: between 2 and 6 months. The mortality is appreciable, ranging from 0.1 to 10 per cent, depending on the infective dose and the condition of the patient.

Symptoms and signs of serum jaundice are not necessarily more severe than the IH type; actually they may be more insidious. The patient may just simply lose his appetite and turn yellow. In addition to jaundice, he may have dyspepsia, abdominal pain, generalized aching, malaise and weakness. The liver usually is enlarged, and splenomegaly is common. In contrast with epidemic hepatitis, respiratory symptoms are minimal or absent, and the occurrence of fever is rare.

Medical and Nursing Management. It is important that bed rest be continued until the progress of the hepatitis has definitely subsided, and, subsequently, the patient should be restricted in his activities until the hepatic enlargement and the elevation of serum bilirubin have disappeared. Adequate nutrition should be maintained and supplemental nutrients provided by the administration of ample quantities of vitamin B complex, carbohydrates and proteins. Other therapeutic measures employed to control the dyspeptic symptoms and general malaise include the use of salicylates, alkalies, belladonna and mild barbiturate soporifics.

Convalescence may be prolonged, complete symptomatic recovery sometimes requiring as long as 3 to 4 months. During this stage, gradual restoration of physical activity is permitted and encouraged following complete clearing of the jaundice.

Preventive Considerations. Individuals receiving infected blood or blood derivatives are protected from homologous serum jaundice by the concomitant injection of gamma globulin. However, infective blood donors cannot be identified with certainty, and supplies of gamma globulin are far from sufficient to permit its routine use in conjunction with every transfusion. The use of disposable syringes, needles and lancets reduces the risk of spreading this infection from one patient to another in the process of collecting blood samples or administering parenteral therapy.

Individual-dose ampules for medication administration is essential and is the prescribed policy of most hospitals. Among narcotic addicts where groups share the same needle, serious outbreaks of hepatitis have occurred. Persons known to have had serum or infectious hepatitis are asked not to donate blood to the Red Cross or other blood programs.

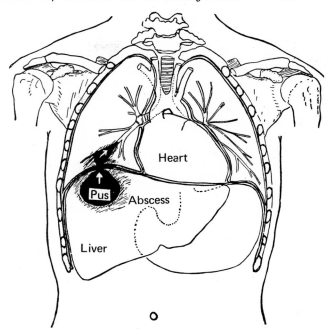

Fig. 23-6. Diagram of an abscess of the liver perforating through the lung into a bronchus. The preceding inflammation will have obliterated the peritoneal and the pleural cavities in the path of the abscess.

Toxic Hepatitis

Several chemicals are liver poisons, which, when taken by mouth or injected parenterally, produce acute liver cell necrosis or toxic hepatitis. The chemicals most commonly implicated in this disease are arsenic, chloroform, carbon tetrachloride, phosphorus and gold compounds.

The milder cases of toxic hepatitis closely resemble those of epidemic hepatitis, being quite comparable in symptoms, signs and course. However, a considerable proportion of patients unfortunately progress to the stage of acute liver necrosis or acute yellow atrophy. Within a few days the jaundice becomes extremely intense. The fever mounts; the patient becomes deeply toxic and prostrated. Vomiting may be persistent, the vomitus containing blood. Hemorrhages appear under the skin. Delirium, coma and convulsions develop, and within a few days the patient usually dies.

There is little to be done in the line of treatment, except to provide comfort, supply repeated blood transfusions and intravenous glucose and saline solutions. A few patients recover, only to develop cirrhosis.

Liver Abscesses

The liver is a sieve through which flows all the blood returning from the gastrointestinal tract. Whenever an abscess develops anywhere along this tract, there is danger that an infected embolus will be transported by way of the portal venous system to the liver, and that secondary abscess formation will take place in that organ. Moreover, in patients with bacteremia, organisms may be carried through the hepatic artery to the liver and lodge there. Most bacteria promptly are engulfed and destroyed, but occasionally some gain a foothold and multiply. The bacterial toxins destroy the neighboring liver cells, and the necrotic tissue produced serves as a protective wall for the organisms. Meanwhile, leukocytes migrate into the infected area. The result is an abscess cavity full of a liquid containing living and dead leukocytes, liquefied liver cells and bacteria (Fig. 23-6). Pyogenic abscesses of this type are usually multiple and small. The liver may be fairly honeycombed by them. The result is an extremely serious disease, manifested by high fever, chills alternating with sweats, jaundice, painful enlargement of the liver, anemia, toxemia and eventual death. Specific chemotherapy is given in such cases, depending on the identity of the infective agent. (The student is referred to a text on pharmacology.)

Liver abscesses may be due to several kinds of bacteria and to a fungus (actinomycosis). The commonest agent, however, is a protozoan, *Entamoeba histolytica*, one of the most important causes of dysentery.

Hepatic Cirrhosis

Cirrhosis of the liver means scarring of the liver. Three kinds are generally considered:

1. Laennec's portal cirrhosis, in which the scar tissue characteristically surrounds the portal areas. This is most commonly due to chronic alcoholism.

2. Postnecrotic cirrhosis in which there are broad bands of scar tissue as a late result of a previous acute viral hepatitis.

3. Biliary cirrhosis in which there is pericholangitic, perilobular scarring. This type usually is the result of chronic biliary obstruction and infection (cholangitis) and is much more rare than Laennec's and postnecrotic cirrhosis.

The differentiation among the three types is largely one for the pathologist. Laennec's cirrhosis is a disease characterized by episodes of necrosis involving the liver cells, sometimes occurring repeatedly throughout the course of the disease. The destroyed liver cells are replaced by scar tissue, the amount of which in time may exceed that of the functioning liver tissue. The disease usually has a particularly insidious onset and a very protracted course, occasionally proceeding over a period of 30 or more years.

The basic mechanism responsible for the development of cirrhosis is yet to be described. It occurs with greatest frequency among alcoholics. However, many explain the role of alcohol in the production of cirrhosis on the basis of nutritional deficiency with reduced protein intake rather than on alcohol toxicity, and certainly some cases are observed among the abstemious.

Some individuals appear to be more susceptible than others to this disease whether they are alcoholics, malnourished or not. Other factors may play a role such as exposure to certain chemicals (carbon tetrachloride, chlorinated naphthalene, arsenic or phosphorus) or infectious schistosomiasis. Twice as many men as women are affected and the majority of patients are between 40 and 60 years of age.

Pathophysiology Including Symptoms

The liver early in the disease is apt to be large, its cells loaded with fat; later, as the replacing scar tissue contracts, it becomes small. Also, its surface often becomes rough, because the scar tissue within it is disposed in coarse bundles, which by contracting pull in the capsule at certain points and cause the islands of residual normal tissue and of new regenerating liver tissue to project in little lumps. Hence arose the term *hobnail liver*.

The following illustrates a sample case history:

Jim Donnelly, 49, as sales engineer for a highly competitive aviation and missile corporation, traveled across the country frequently and had many luncheon and dinner business meetings. After a bout of acute hepatitis, he noticed that his appetite was affected (anorexia) and that he had occasional nausea and some vomiting. Then evidence of jaundice appeared with a low-grade fever. His symptoms subsided for a few days, then recurred. This pattern continued for weeks. He was hospitalized and diagnosed as having a posthepatic relapse.

The late symptoms are due partly to chronic failure of liver function and partly to obstruction of the portal circulation. Practically all the blood from the digestive organs is collected in the portal veins and carried to the liver. Since these cirrhotic livers do not allow it free passage, it is dammed back into the spleen and the gastrointestinal tract, with the result that these organs become the seat of chronic passive congestion; that is, they are stagnant with blood and so cannot function properly. Such patients are apt to have chronic dyspepsia and changes in bowel habit, with constipation or diarrhea. There is a gradual weight loss. The spleen becomes congested. Fluid may accumulate in the peritoneal cavity (ascites), in which event diuresis is induced.

At certain points in the abdomen the portal circulation anastomoses with the general circulation, and through these channels some portal blood can flow to the heart without first passing through the liver. One of the points of collateral circulation is at the cardiac orifice of the stomach. The blood from the esophagus flows directly to the heart; that from the stomach flows to the liver. Veins always anastomose, so that blood here can choose between these 2 routes. When there is obstruction to the portal circulation, as in cirrhosis, portal hypertension develops, and, because of its increased pressure, a portion of the blood in the gastric veins escapes through the esophageal veins. Unfortunately, however, these veins become distended, forming esophageal varices, the thin walls of which often rupture. Thus, about 25 per cent of patients with cirrhosis experience small hematemeses, while some have profuse hemorrhages from the stomach.

Within the lower rectum there is a point at which the portal and the general circulations meet. In cirrhosis of the liver, venous varices form here, also. These are known as hemorrhoids. These, too, may rupture and cause severe hemorrhages. Of course, hemorrhoids are common, but in the majority of cases they are due to simple constipation, and involve the external hemorrhoidal veins (external hemorrhoids), which usually thrombose before they bleed. However, in cirrhosis, the internal hemorrhoidal veins dilate. Blood is less apt to clot in them, so that when they rupture they bleed severely.

Other late symptoms of cirrhosis are attributable to chronic failure of liver function. The concentration of plasma albumin is lowered, predisposing to the formation of edema. Because of inadequate formation, utilization and storage of certain vitamins, notably vitamins A, C and K, signs of their deficiency frequently are encountered—particularly hemorrhagic phenomena associated with vitamin K deficiency. Chronic gastritis and poor gastrointestinal function, together with the factors of poor diet and impaired liver function, account for a deficiency type of anemia likewise often associated with this disease.

Therefore, the *chief signs of liver cirrhosis* are fever, jaundice, gastrointestinal disturbances and enlargement of the liver in the early stages. Later in the disease this organ becomes smaller and nodular, the spleen enlarges, ascites appears, jaundice recurs, distended veins develop at the anastomotic points described previously, and spider telangiectases (dilated superficial arterioles resembling little bluish-red spiders) appear in the skin of the face and the trunk. As the condition progresses, edema, anemia, purpura and signs of polyavitaminosis are likely to appear. The patient may die in liver failure, experiencing increasing weakness, wasting and depression and finally delirium, coma and convulsions.

Medical Management and Nursing Intervention

General Assessment and Action. The ill cirrhotic patient requires the careful attention of the nurse who can make sound judgments and initiate nursing action. His weight and his fluid intake and output volumes must be measured and recorded daily. His position in bed should be adjusted for maximal respiratory efficiency, which is especially important if ascites is marked. Skin care must be observed meticulously because of the presence of subcutaneous edema and the relative immobility of the patient.

Rest permits the liver to restore itself, limits the demands of the body on it and increases the blood supply to it. Since the patient is more susceptible to infection, efforts to prevent respiratory, circulatory, and vascular disturbances need to be initiated. By so doing, such problems as pneumonia, thrombophlebitis and decubiti can be prevented.

The extent of liver disease and the kind of treatment are determined after studying the laboratory findings. Because the liver is a complex functioning organ, the tests are many (see Table 23-1). The patient needs to know why they are done, their importance to him and how he can assist. His physical condition and mental alertness determine the nurse's individualized approach.

Parenchymal liver cell function can be evaluated with cephalin flocculation tests (2+ to 4*) and thymol turbidity (increased). Serum albumin tends to fall and serum globulin rises. Enzyme tests indicate liver cell damage; serum alkaline phosphate rises, serum cholinesterase may decrease and SGOT increases. Excretory function is tested by the liver's ability to eliminate Bromsulphalein. In cirrhosis, the BSP is retained. Bilirubin tests are done to measure bile excretion or bile retention. In some clinics, the use of photolaparoscopy permits direct visualization of the liver and is used in conjunction with biopsy; this is still in the investigative stages.

Dietary Needs. The cirrhotic patient who has no ascites or edema and exhibits no signs of impending coma should receive a nutritious, high-protein diet supplemented by vitamins of the B complex and others, as indicated (including vitamins A, C and K). Since proper nutrition is so important, every effort to encourage the patient to eat must be made. This is as important as any medication. Often small frequent meals can be accepted better than 3 larger meals. Patient preferences are to be considered. Patients with prolonged or severe anorexia, or those who are vomiting or eating poorly for any reason, can be fed by tube with milk and enough added starch hydrolysate (e.g., Dextri-Maltose, Dexin, etc.) to satisfy their caloric requirements. Powdered Sustagen and Protinal (low

THE PATIENT WITH LAENNEC'S CIRRHOSIS

Problems	Nursing Implications
Anorexia	Encourage patient to eat meals and supplementary feedings Offer frequent small feedings Give attention to esthetic factors and attractive trays at mealtime Eliminate alcohol
Nausea and vomiting	Oral hygiene before meals Ice collar for nausea Tube feedings, as required
Weight loss and fatigue	Continuous encouragement of intake of high-protein, high-calorie diet Give supplementary vitamins (A, B complex, C and K) Parenteral fluids as ordered Conserve patient's energy
Abdominal pain	Bed rest to protect liver Antispasmodics and mild sedatives Encourage patient to eat slowly and chew thoroughly Observe, record and report presence and character of pain
Hematemesis	Be alert for symptoms of anxiety, epigastric fullness, weakness and restlessness Observe for presence of bleeding and shock Record vital signs at frequent intervals Keep patient quiet and limit activity Observe during blood transfusions Assist physician in passage of tube for esophageal balloon tamponade Measure and record nature, time and amount of vomitus Give meticulous oral hygiene Maintain patient in fasting state if indicated Administer vitamin K as ordered Stay in constant attendance during episodes of bleeding Offer cold liquids by mouth when bleeding stops (if ordered)
Melena	Observe each stool for color, consistency and amount
Constipation	Ensure adequate fluid and food intake Encourage abdominal exercises
Diarrhea	Increase fluid intake Give medications as ordered
Jaundice	Note and record varying degrees of jaundice of the skin and the sclerae Relieve pruritus with good skin care, bathing without soap and massage with emollient lotions Keep patient's fingernails short to prevent skin excoriation from scratching Give empathetic attention to patient's complaints and problems
Edema of extremities	Restrict sodium Administer diuretics as ordered Give careful attention and care to skin Turn and change position frequently Elevate extremities at intervals Weigh patient daily Record intake and output Passive range-of-motion exercises Small foam rubber supports under heels, malleoli, etc. Careful control of rate of flow of intravenous infusions

THE PATIENT WITH LAENNEC'S CIRRHOSIS (*Continued*)

Problems	Nursing Implications

Ascites

Assist patient during paracentesis:
1. Have him void before procedure
2. Position correctly and use pillow support
3. Record both the amount and the character of fluid aspirated
4. Protect puncture site with dry dressings
5. Check dressing for fluid seepage and evidence of wound infection

Give diuretics, potassium and protein supplements as ordered
Restrict sodium
Record intake and output
Give careful attention to skin
Elevate head of bed to facilitate breathing
Give pillow support under costal margin when in side-lying positions
Observe for symptoms of impending coma

Hydrothorax and dyspnea

Elevate head of bed
Conserve patient's strength
Change position at intervals
Assist patient during thoracentesis:
1. Support and maintain position during procedure
2. Record both the amount and the character of fluid aspirated
3. Observe for evidence of coughing, increasing dyspnea and/or pulse rate

Fever

Record temperature regularly
Encourage fluid intake
Give cool sponges for elevated temperature
Supply icecap to head as ordered
Give antibiotics as ordered
Avoid exposure to infections
Keep patient at rest
Note urinary volume and concentration

Hemorrhagic manifestations: ecchymosis, epistaxis, petechiae, and bleeding gums

Avoid trauma
Maintain safe environment
Avoid forceful blowing of nose
Prevent trauma to gums from toothbrushing
Encourage intake of foods with high content of vitamin C
Apply cold compresses where indicated
Record location of bleeding sites
Avoid constrictive clothing
Use small gauge needles for injections

Increasing stupor: mental changes, lethargy, hallucinations, and hepatic coma

Restrict dietary protein
Give small frequent feeding of carbohydrates
Protect from infection
Keep environment warm and draft-free
Pad the side-rails of the bed
Limit visitors
Provide careful nursing surveillance to ensure patient's safety
Avoid narcotics and barbiturates
Arouse at intervals
Give sensitive nursing care during terminal phase

sodium) can be given as protein supplements. Patients with diarrhea and fatty stools (steatorrhea) should receive pancreatin as a dietary supplement, in which case they probably will tolerate and absorb a normal diet.

The cirrhotic patient with ascites and edema should restrict his sodium intake to 200 to 500 mg. daily but maintain a normal protein, caloric and vitamin intake. Table salt, salty foods, salted butter and margarine and all the ordinary canned and frozen foods should be avoided. The taste of unsalted foods can be improved by using salt substitutes such as lemon juice, oregano and thyme. Commercial substitutes need to be cleared with the physician; for example, those containing ammonia could precipitate hepatic coma. Liberal use should be made of powdered low-sodium milk and milk products. If water accumulation is not controlled on this regimen the salt restriction must be more stringent, i.e., the daily sodium allowance should be reduced to 200 mg. and diuretics administered.

The cirrhotic patient with signs of impending or advancing coma should receive temporarily a low-protein or protein-free diet, but a high caloric intake should be maintained, and supplementary vitamins and minerals should be supplied (e.g., liquid potassium, if the serum potassium is normal or low, and if renal function is normal). As soon as the situation permits, the protein intake should be restored to normal or above.

Edema and Ascites. One method of reducing edema and ascites is to induce diuresis. This involves the reduction of sodium intake to approximately 200 mg. daily; restriction of fluids, if the serum sodium is low; administration of an oral diuretic drug, such as Hydrodiuril, and possibly injections of a mercurial diuretic, such as Mercuhydrin. Spironolactone (Aldactone), an aldosterone-blocking agent, also may be supplied to reinforce the action of these diuretics. Ethacrynic acid (Edecrin) is a new and very potent diuretic agent for oral or intravenous use starting with doses of 50 mg. per day and increasing as needed. Furosemide (Lasix), in doses of 40 to 80 mg. per day is also a newer diuretic agent of great potency. The diuretics because of their ability to produce electrolyte imbalance (excessive loss of sodium, potassium and chloride) should be used with caution in cirrhotic patients.

Accumulations of ascitic fluid often lessen or disappear in response to the diuresis program outlined above. To conserve the patient's body proteins, abdominal paracentesis is avoided for as long as possible. However, if the abdomen of the patient is tightly distended with fluid, and if the ascites shows no evidence of becoming reduced as a result of a low sodium intake, diuretics and spironolactone, the mechanical removal of the fluid is justified, provided that each aspiration is limited to 3 to 5 liters.

The nurse prepares the patient for the treatment by supplying the necessary information, instructions and reassurance. *She must be sure to have the patient void as completely as possible just prior to paracentesis.* Sterile equipment and appropriate receptacles are made ready. Preparatory to that procedure the patient is placed in the upright position on the edge of the bed, fully supported, with his feet resting on a stool and one arm fitted with a sphygmomanometer cuff. The trocar is introduced with sterile precautions through a stab wound in the midline below the umbilicus, and the fluid is drained through an effluent tube into a container.

During the procedure itself the nurse helps the patient to maintain the proper posture and observes him closely for evidence of vascular collapse, such as the appearance of pallor, increase in pulse rate or a decline in blood pressure, the latter having been recorded at frequent intervals from the beginning of the procedure. When the procedure is concluded, the patient is restored to his original recumbent position. The amount collected should be measured and recorded, and samples of the fluid, properly labeled, should be sent to appropriate laboratories for examination of the cellular sediment, its specific gravity, protein concentration and bacterial content.

Patient Education and Post-Hospital Care. At the time of discharge the patient receives detailed instructions, in part from the nurse, principally relating to his dietary habits. Of utmost importance is the exclusion of alcohol completely and permanently from his diet, a fact of which he doubtless is well aware. However, if he is to succeed in abstaining completely and permanently, he will need all the help he can possibly muster, possibly including that of a skilled psychiatrist, an admired and trusted religious adviser and the most effective group in this therapeutic field, Alcoholics Anonymous. Sodium restriction will have to continue for a considerable period of time, if not permanently; if this diet is to be followed correctly, the patient will require written instructions.

The success of treatment depends upon convincing the patient of his need to adhere willingly and wholeheartedly to the therapeutic plan. This includes rest, a sensible way of life, an adequate well-balanced diet and the elimination of alcohol. Recovery is neither rapid nor easy; there are frequent setbacks and apparent lack of improvement. For many persons, the loss of support given by alcohol is discouraging. The understanding nurse can play a significant role in offering support and encouragement to this patient.

The Patient with Bleeding Esophageal Varices

Pathophysiology and Symptoms

Esophageal varices are dilated tortuous veins usually found in the submucosa of the lower esophagus; however, they may extend well up into the esophagus and into the stomach. Such a condition nearly always is caused by portal hypertension which, in turn, is due to obstruction of the portal venous circulation within the substance of a cirrhotic liver (see p. 513). As venous blood from the intestinal tract and spleen seeks new avenues of return to the right atrium because of increasing portal vein obstruction, the pathophysiological effect is increased strain, particularly on the esophageal veins. Other lesser causes of varices are abnormalities of the circulation in the splenic vein or superior vena cava.

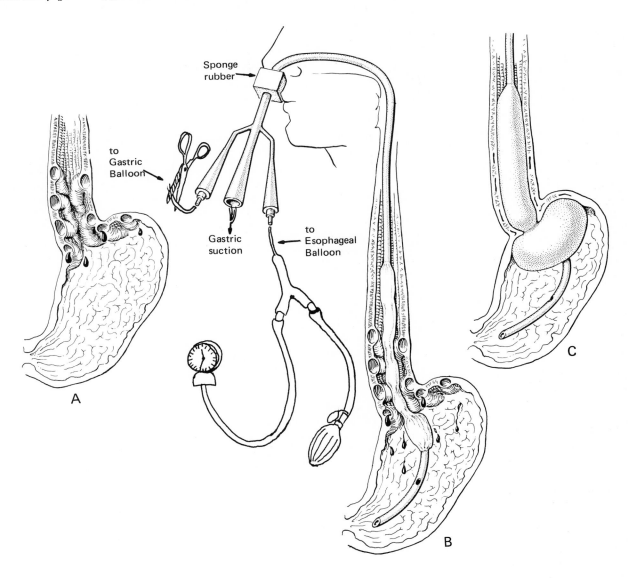

Sponge rubber

to Gastric Balloon

Gastric suction

to Esophageal Balloon

A

B

C

FIG. 23-7. Diagram showing esophageal varices and their treatment by a compressing balloon tube (Sengstaken-Blakemore). (A) Dilated veins of the lower esophagus. (B) The tube is in place in the stomach and the lower esophagus but is not inflated. (C) Inflation of the tube and the compression of the veins which can be obtained by inflation of the balloon.

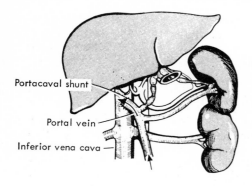

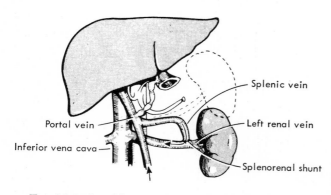

Fig. 23-8. Line drawing showing shunt procedures to relieve portal hypertension.

Esophageal varices should be suspected in the presence of hematemesis and melena, especially in the patient who has been addicted to alcohol. Usually these dilated veins cause no symptoms unless the mucosa over them becomes ulcerated. Then massive hemorrhage takes place, which if not controlled may result in death. Factors that contribute to rupture and hemorrhage are muscular strain from coughing or vomiting, esophagitis or irritation of vessels by poorly chewed foods or irritating fluids.

Assessment

In ascertaining the nature of the problem, the physician relies on various liver function tests, such as Bromsulphalein retention, serum transaminase, bilirubin, alkaline phosphatase and serum proteins (see Table 23-1). Esophagoscopy most clearly clinches the diagnosis, because even the site of hemorrhage may be seen; however, some physicians fear the risk of initiating hemorrhage or rupturing the esophagus, therefore, the decision to perform an endoscopic examination depends on the situation. Portal vein pressure can be measured in the operating room by introducing a needle into the spleen; a manometer reading above 250

mm. H_2O is abnormal. Splenoportography using Diodrast is studied in serial or segmental roentgenograms to detect extensive collateral circulation in esophageal vessels, which would be indicative of varices.

Nursing assessment includes an evaluation of the emotional concerns of the patient and any physical problems such as abnormal body discharges. Vital signs are taken and the nutritional needs are determined. If the patient was admitted for hemorrhage, the situation becomes an emergency.

Medical and Nursing Management

The patient with bleeding varices is seriously ill. The nurse remains in attendance and vital signs may be monitored. Before resorting to tamponade, some internists administer Pituitrin (S) because of its portal hypotensive action.

To control the hemorrhage, pressure is exerted on the cardiac portion of the stomach and against the bleeding varices by a double balloon tamponade (Sengstaken-Blakemore tube, Fig. 23-7). The carefully checked tube is chilled before the physician lubricates the tip and passes it through the mouth or nose of the patient into his stomach. The balloon in the stomach is inflated and the tube is pulled gently to exert a force against the cardia. The esophageal balloon is then inflated to the desired pressure (in both balloons this is 25 to 30 mm. Hg done under fluoroscopic control) as measured by the manometer. (After the balloon is inflated, there is a possibility of injury or rupture of the esophagus. There should be constant nursing surveillance at this time.) Traction is placed on the tube where it enters the patient. Gastric suction can be provided by connecting the proper catheter outlet to the suction machine. The tubing is irrigated hourly and drainage will indicate whether bleeding has been controlled. Some physicians circulate ice water in and out of the stomach balloon, which constricts gastric vessels. The pressures on the tubes and traction are released in 48 to 96 hours. If there is no bleeding, the tube is removed in 24 hours.

Although this method has been fairly successful, it is well to note some inherent dangers. If left in place too long, ulcers can develop in the stomach. If the tube suddenly ruptures, the result is disastrous, although using a brand new tested tube that is less than a year old may prevent this calamity. Another problem could result if the counterweight pulls the tube into the oropharynx, thereby causing asphyxiation. These potential dangers suggest the need for intensive and intelligent care. The balloon may be deflated at 8- to 12-hour intervals to prevent erosion and necrosis of the stomach and esophagus.

Bleeding also is treated by sedation and complete rest of the esophagus (parenteral feedings). Straining and vomiting must be prevented. Gastric suction usually is employed to keep the stomach as empty as possible. The patient complains of severe thirst, which may be relieved by frequent oral hygiene and ice chips if permitted. The nurse must keep close surveillance on the patient's blood pressure. Vitamin K therapy and multiple blood transfusions often are indicated. A quiet environment and calm reassurance by doctor and nurse will help to relieve the patient's anxiety.

Surgical procedures that may be employed are (1) injection of sclerosing drugs by way of the esophagoscope, (2) direct surgical ligation of varices, and (3) portacaval and splenorenal venous shunt operations.

Surgical By-Pass Procedures. In the present-day treatment of portal hypertension, certain by-pass procedures have been used to divert the blood from the portal system into the vena cava. The most common procedure is to create an anastomosis between the portal vein and the inferior vena cava, which is spoken of as a *portacaval anastomosis* (Fig. 23-8). As a result of shunting portal blood into the vena cava, the pressure in the portal system is decreased, and consequently the danger from hemorrhage from esophageal and gastric varices is reduced. When the portal vein cannot be used because of thrombosis or for other reasons, a shunt may be made between the splenic vein and the left renal vein (*splenorenal shunt*). Some surgeons prefer this shunt to the portacaval shunt, even though the portal vein could be used.

Both of these operations are rather extensive procedures and are not always successful because of secondary clotting in the veins used for the shunt. Nevertheless, this method is the only one by which a lowering of pressure in the portal system may be brought about, and since hemorrhages from the esophageal varices are often fatal, many of these relatively poor-risk patients must be subjected to these attempts to save their lives. The postoperative care of these patients is the care of patients with any abdominal operation, but care is complicated by the treatment of the cirrhotic liver, which is the main problem in the recovery of these patients.

Biliary Cirrhosis

A less common cause of cirrhosis is ascending infection of the biliary tract (cholangitis), with spread of the infection from the gallbladder by way of the hepatic duct to the small bile ducts in the liver substance. Prolonged obstructive jaundice may cause biliary cirrhosis. That portion of the liver chiefly involved, therefore, consists of the portal and the periportal spaces, where the bile canaliculi of each lobule communicate to form the liver bile ducts. These areas become the site of inflammation, and the bile ducts become occluded with inspissated bile and pus. An attempt is made by the liver to form new bile channels; hence, there is an overgrowth of tissue made up largely of disconnected, newly formed bile ducts and surrounded by scar tissue.

Symptoms and signs of this disease include intermittent jaundice and fever and the finding of an enlarged, hard, irregular liver, which eventually becomes atrophic. The treatment is the same as that described for portal cirrhosis, i.e., the treatment of any form of chronic liver insufficiency and, when indicated, surgical treatment designed to eradicate the biliary tract infection.

Postnecrotic Cirrhosis

Other types of cirrhosis include those of healed subacute yellow atrophy, syphilis of the liver and hemochromatosis, in which there occurs a pigment deposition with associated scarring not only of the liver but also of the pancreas and other organs.

Hepatic Tumors

Few cancers originate in the liver, and those that are primary in that organ usually start in the bile ducts. However, metastases are found in the liver in about one half of all late cancer cases. The primary growth may be almost anywhere, and since the bloodstream and the lymphatics from the body cavities nearly all reach the liver, malignant tumors anywhere in the trunk are likely to reach this organ eventually. Moreover, the liver apparently is an ideal place for these malignant cells to take root and to grow. Often the first evidence of a cancer in an abdominal organ is the appearance of one of its liver metastases, and, unless exploratory operation or necropsy is performed, the primary growth never may be discovered.

Diagnosis of malignant disease of the liver is made, regardless of the location of the primary tumor, when there is a recent loss of weight, loss of strength and anemia (the last being the commonest early symptoms of any cancer that interferes with nutrition), together with rapid enlargement of the liver, which on palpation presents an irregular surface. Jaundice is present only if the larger bile ducts are occluded by the pressure of malignant nodules in the hilum of the liver. Ascites occurs only if such nodules obstruct the portal veins, or if tumor tissue is seeded in the peritoneal cavity. The only treatment is palliative.

Surgical Management

Successful hepatic lobectomy for cancer can be done when the primary hepatic tumor is localized, or in the case of metastasis, when the primary site can be completely excised and the metastasis has not become too extensive. Capitalizing on the regenerative capacity of the liver cells, some surgeons have successfully removed 80 per cent of the liver.

Preoperative Evaluation and Preparation. As the patient is being prepared for surgery, his nutritional, fluid, emotional and physical needs are being evaluated and met. Meanwhile, he may be undergoing extensive laboratory and roentgen studies. The support, explanation and encouragement by the nurse will help him achieve the most desirable level for surgery. Optimism is automatically generated for this patient because not too long ago, liver surgery was unheard of. It may be necessary to prepare the intestinal tract by way of cathartic, colonic irrigation and intestinal antibiotics to minimize any possibility of ammonium intoxification and in case the intestine may have to be opened at surgery. Specific studies may include liver scanning, liver biopsy, pneumoperitoneal radiograph, splenoportal venography and blood tests, particularly serum alkaline phosphatase and serum glutamic oxaloacetic acid.

Surgical Intervention. If it is necessary to restrict blood flow from the hepatic artery and portal vein beyond 15 minutes (under normothermic conditions, 15-minute occlusion is permissible), it is likely that hypothermia will be used.

The nurse needs to be cognizant of the anatomy referred to by the surgeon in their care of these patients. The usual true (functional) division of the liver

is into 2 lobes, the larger (by 6 times) right lobe and the left lobe, with 2 smaller segments sandwiched between, the caudate and the quadrate.* Most surgeons prefer the anatomic (surgical) division of the lobes. Here the liver is divided into a right and a left lobe by a lobar fissure that is almost in line with the gallbladder bed and the inferior vena cava on the visceral surface. According to this division, the branching of hepatic vessels and the portal vein lend themselves to a more even segmentation. Obviously, a right liver lobectomy according to the surgical division is less extensive than it would be in the functional division.

For a right liver lobectomy or an extended right lobectomy (including medial left lobe), a thoracoabdominal incision is used. A generous abdominal incision is made for a left lobectomy. Basic principles that guide the surgeon are related to promoting adequate hemostasis, resecting all nonviable liver tissue, and promoting wide drainage that may include biliary decompression with a T-tube.

Postsurgical Nursing Management. By following the patient's experience in the operating room, the nurse is guided in the formulation of patient postoperative care objectives. There are potential problems related to cardiopulmonary involvement, portal

* Refer to your anatomy textbook.

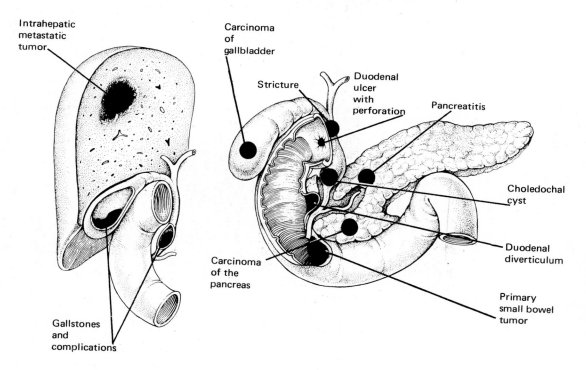

Fig. 23-9. Causes of biliary tract disease. (Iber, F. L.: Hospital Medicine 4:No. 6 June, 1968)

and general circulation, respiratory and metabolic function, as well as liver dysfunction. The patient requires constant attention for the first 2 or 3 days as described for abdominal and thoracic postsurgical nursing care (pp. 129 and 258).

Cortisone is often administered to facilitate liver cell regeneration. Early ambulation is encouraged under the knowledgeable supervision of the nurse who is able to translate untoward signs into desired action.

For more extensive malignancy of the liver, percutaneous infusions of antitumor drugs or radioactive gold (^{198}Au) may make the patient more comfortable. (Other measures are discussed on p. 192.)

CONDITIONS OF THE BILIARY SYSTEM

Estimates indicate that approximately 500,000 persons a year in the United States are hospitalized for gallbladder disease and that about two thirds of these are treated surgically. More women than men (4 to 1) acquire this disease; they are usually past 40, multiparous and overweight. By way of prevention, it is suggested that steps be taken to lose weight and to avoid fatty foods. Most (90 per cent) of the problems of patients with gallbladder disease are related to gallstones (cholelithiasis); infection is a common problem that may or may not be related to calculi; only 1 per cent of patients with biliary tract disease have neoplasms.

The Patient with Cholecystitis and Cholelithiasis

Calculi usually form in the gallbladder from the solid constituents of bile and vary greatly in size, shape and consistency. Upon analysis, they are found to be made of cholesterol, calcium combined with bilirubin, and inorganic salts. They are uncommon in children and young adults but become increasingly prevalent after age 40. The incidence of cholelithiasis increases thereafter to such an extent that one authority estimates that, by the age of 75, 1 of every 3 persons will have gallstones.

The presence of stones indicates some dysfunction of the gallbladder and the disease is spoken of as *chronic gallbladder disease*. The patient may notice 2 types of symptoms: those due to disease of the gallbladder itself—epigastric distress such as fullness and eructation after meals, heartburn and chronic pain in the upper right abdomen; and those due to obstruction of the bile passages (especially the cystic duct) by a gallstone—excruciating upper right abdominal pain that radiates to the back or right shoulder, usually associated with nausea and vomiting. These symptoms are more noticeable several hours after a heavy meal that included fried or fatty foods. Such a bout of *biliary colic* is caused by contracture of the gallbladder, which has been stimulated by fat; it is having difficulty releasing bile because of obstruction that in all likelihood is due to calculi. These symptoms generally are so severe as to require morphine or meperidine hydrochloride. (Some physicians believe these drugs may increase the spasm of the sphincter of Oddi; to give the patient relief, a nitroglycerin tablet is given under the tongue.)

The diet immediately after an attack is usually limited to low-fat liquids. Powdered supplements high in protein and carbohydrate can be stirred into skim milk. The following may then be added as tolerated: cooked fruits, rice or tapioca, lean meats, mashed potatoes, non-gas-forming vegetables, bread, coffee or tea. Avoid eggs, cream, pork, fried foods, cheese and rich dressings, gas-forming vegetables and alcohol. The patient needs to be reminded that fatty foods may bring on an attack. Rest is a vital part of recovery from an attack.

At times the gallbladder may be the seat of an acute infection that causes acute pain, tenderness and rigidity of the upper right abdomen, associated with nausea and vomiting and the usual signs of an acute inflammation. This condition is spoken of as *acute cholecystitis*. If the gallbladder is found to be filled with pus, there is said to be an *empyema* of the gallbladder.

Biliary Obstruction

Not infrequently a gallstone may pass from the gallbladder through the cystic duct and lodge in the common bile duct; or the head of the pancreas, through which the common duct passes, may be the seat of a carcinoma. Either condition may obstruct the flow of bile into the duodenum and result in the following characteristic symptoms.

The bile, no longer carried to the duodenum, is absorbed by the blood and gives the skin and the tissues a yellow color known as *jaundice*. The excretion of the bile pigments in some measure from the blood by the kidneys gives the urine a very dark color. The feces, no longer colored with bile pigments, are grayish, like putty, and usually are spoken of as clay-colored. There frequently is marked itching of the skin, and nausea occurs after eating fatty foods, because there is a marked disturbance of the digestion and absorption of fats when bile does not flow into the duodenum. Various laboratory tests of the blood (icteric index, van den Bergh, serum bilirubin, etc.) indicate the degree of pigment retention and therefore the depth of jaundice.

Operations on patients with obstructive jaundice are technically complex and the patients are usually quite sick because of extensive bile duct exploration. Therefore, these patients should receive special

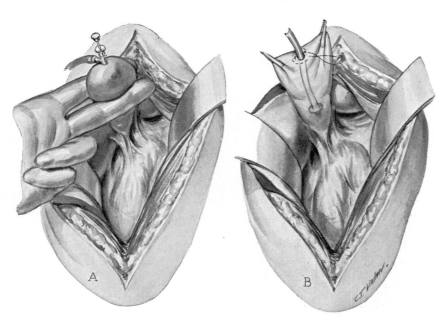

FIG. 23-10. Cholecystostomy. (A) The distended gallbladder is steadied by the hand of the surgeon as an aspirating trocar is placed into the lumen of the organ. (B) A Pezzer catheter is sutured into the gallbladder for purposes of drainage. (Thorek: Anatomy in Surgery, J. B. Lippincott, 1962)

preparation. The diet should be low in fats and high in protein and carbohydrate. Frequently it is wise to administer protein hydrolysates intravenously for a day or two before operation.

It is well known that the hemorrhagic tendency in jaundice is due to a deficient formation of the prothrombin. This is an important factor in the clotting of blood, which becomes deficient when the patient becomes jaundiced because of inadequate absorption of the fat-soluble vitamin K. Often the blood prothrombin may be raised adequately by administration of vitamin K, or a new supply may be added to the patient's blood by transfusion. Carbohydrates are given in large amounts by mouth and intravenously to build up the glycogen stores in the liver. The nurse should note the color of the urine and the stools and send specimens of these excreta to be examined for bile pigments. The operations performed depend on the cause of the biliary obstruction.

Roentgenography of the Biliary System

Cholecystography. Radiologic examination of the gallbladder is carried out for the detection of gallstones, and to estimate the ability of the gallbladder to fill, concentrate its contents, contract and empty in normal fashion. Very few gallstones are sufficiently radiopaque to be visualized by ordinary roentgenographic technique; they must be demonstrated as negative shadows in a gallbladder filled with a radiopaque substance. To this end an iodide-containing dye that is excreted into the bile by the liver and concentrated in the gallbladder is administered to the patient, either by mouth or by intravenous injection.

Drugs* given as contrast media include Telepaque, Cholografin, Oragrafin, and Priodax. These preparations are given in oral doses of 2 to 3 gm. 10 to 12 hours before x-ray study. Intravenous cholecystography involves the injection of an iodide approximately 10 minutes prior to roentgenography. During the interval between the administration of the iodide and the x-ray study, the patient is permitted nothing by mouth lest the gallbladder be stimulated to contract and thereby expel the contrast medium.

Nursing instructions to patients who are scheduled for x-ray studies of the gallbladder (cholecystogram; gallbladder series) are:

1. One hour or more after the evening meal, and approximately 10 hours before roentgenography, the patient receives six 0.5-gm. tablets or capsules of contrast medium by mouth.

2. These tablets are to be ingested 1 at a time, at intervals of from 2 to 5 minutes, together with a volume of water totaling at least 8 oz.

3. The patient then is to receive nothing by mouth, excepting water, until bedtime. Thereafter, until the roentgenogram is taken, not even water is permitted. If the patient vomits after the ingestion of the dye, the physician may suggest that the medication be given after nausea subsides or the test may be postponed.

4. Laxatives must not be given during this preparation period.

---

* Telepaque = iopanoic acid; Chlorografin methylglucamine = iodipamide methylglucamine; Oragrafin = sodium ipodate; Priodax = iodoalphionic acid.

Fig. 23-11. Choledochostomy. (A) An incision is made into the lesser omentum and the supraduodenal part of the common duct. (B) The stone is removed and a "T"-tube is inserted into the common duct. (C) The "T"-tube is in place, and the gallbladder is removed from below upward. (Thorek: Anatomy in Surgery, J. B. Lippincott, 1962)

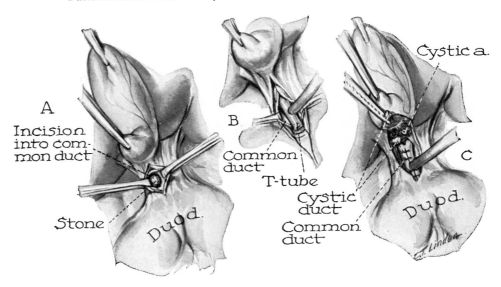

5. A saline enema is to be administered early in the morning of the test.

6. Breakfast is omitted.

The right upper abdominal quadrant then is photographed by x-ray. If the gallbladder has filled and concentrated the dye normally, it is seen as a pear-shaped shadow from 2 to 3 inches long under the right costal margin. If stones are present, there are mottled densities within this shadow corresponding to their outlines. Next, to test the contractility of the gallbladder, the patient is fed a fatty meal containing cream, butter or eggs, and the x-ray examination is repeated at intervals until the gallbladder has expelled the dye and becomes invisible (Graham-Cole test). If the gallbladder is found to fill and empty normally and to contain no stones, it is concluded that no gallbladder disease is present.

Percutaneous Transhepatic Cholangiography. The oral and the intravenous techniques just described permit the visualization of the gallbladder (and occasionally the larger ducts) only if the liver cells are functioning properly and are capable of excreting the radiopaque dye into the bile. Percutaneous transhepatic cholangiography, which involves the injection of dye directly into the biliary tree itself, is effective regardless of the state of liver function. Moreover, because of the relatively large concentration of dye that is introduced into the biliary system, all components of the latter, including the hepatic ducts within the liver, the common hepatic duct throughout its length, the cystic duct and the gallbladder, are delineated with clarity.

This procedure is useful in distinguishing jaundice caused by liver disease (hepatocellular jaundice) from that due to biliary obstruction; for investigating the gastrointestinal symptoms of patients whose gallbladders have been removed; for locating stones within the bile ducts; and in the diagnosis of cancer involving the biliary system.

The patient, fasting and well-sedated, lies prone on the x-ray table. The injection site, usually in the midclavicular line immediately beneath the right costal margin, is disinfected and anesthetized with Xylocaine. Through a small incision at this point is passed an 18-gauge spinal puncture needle, directed cephalad, posteriorly at a 45° angle and parallel to the midline. When the needle has penetrated to a depth of approximately 4 inches, the stylet is removed and replaced by a plastic connector tube with 50-ml. syringe attached. While gently applying suction, the operator slowly withdraws the needle until bile appears in the syringe. As much bile as possible is withdrawn, a radiopaque dye is injected (e.g., 20 ml. of 70 per cent Urokon Sodium) and an x-ray picture taken. Before removing the needle, the operator aspirates as much dye and bile as possible in order to forestall subsequent leakage into the needle tract into the peritoneal cavity and thus avoid the possibility of bile peritonitis.

Surgical Management and Nursing Responsibility

Surgical treatment is necessary for the relief of long-continued symptoms, for the removal of the cause of biliary colic and in patients who have acute cholecystitis.

Preoperative Care. In addition to x-ray studies of the gallbladder, the patient will have chest x-rays and examination of the urine and stools. Blood studies may include liver function tests (Table 23-1). Vitamin K preparations and perhaps blood transfusions may be given for a low prothrombin level. Nutritional requirements are respected; if the patient is not eating properly, it may be necessary to provide intravenous glucose with protein hydrolysate supplements. This will aid wound healing and help prevent liver damage. Some explanation regarding the patient's cooperation postoperatively in preventing complications can be most helpful, such as deep breathing and turning requirements.

Surgical Intervention. Preparation for a simple gallbladder operation is the same as for any upper abdominal laparotomy. Patients may be placed on the operating table with the upper abdomen raised somewhat by an air pillow or sandbag to make exposure easier.

Cholecystostomy. This is an operation performed for the relief of certain cases of acute cholecystitis and of chronic gallbladder disease (Fig. 23-10). The gallbladder is opened, the stones and the bile or the pus are removed, and a tube is sutured in the opening for drainage. As soon as the patient is returned to bed, the nurse should connect this tube to a drainage bottle placed at the side of the bed. Failure to perform this duty may result in the leakage of bile round the tube and its escape into the peritoneal cavity.

Cholecystectomy. This is the operation by which the gallbladder is removed after ligation of the cystic duct and artery. The operation is performed in most cases of acute and chronic cholecystitis.

Choledochostomy. In this operation an incision is made into the common duct for removal of stones (Fig. 23-1). After the stones have been evacuated, a tube usually is inserted into the duct for drainage. The gallbladder also contains stones as a rule. A cholecystectomy is performed.

When the common duct is obstructed because of the pressure of an inoperable carcinoma of the head of the pancreas, an operation is performed that leads the bile into the intestinal tract by a different route.

Nursing Intervention Postoperatively. As soon as recovery from anesthesia has occurred, the patient is placed in the low Fowler position. Fluids may be given by vein; nasogastric suction (tube probably inserted immediately prior to surgery) relieves the patient of distension. Water and other fluids may be given in 24 hours and an enema and a soft diet after 72 hours.

The location of the subcostal incision is likely to cause the patient subconsciously to splint the operative site by taking shallow breaths to prevent pain. Since full aeration of the lungs is necessary to prevent respiratory complications, analgesics should be given as ordered and the patient encouraged to turn and breathe deeply at frequent intervals.

As mentioned before, in patients with cholecystostomy or choledochostomy the drainage tubes must be connected immediately to a drainage bottle or bottles. In addition, tubing should be fastened to the dressings or to the bottom sheet with enough leeway for the patient to move without dislodging it. The nurse must exercise special care in turning or lifting these patients so as not to dislodge the tubes. The patient, in turn, must know why he cannot roll onto the tube and that at all times it must remain patent.

In order to prevent total loss of bile, the drainage tube or collecting bottle may be elevated above the level of the abdomen, so that bile drains through the apparatus only if pressure develops in the duct system. The bile collected should be measured and recorded every 24 hours, its color and character being charted. After 5 or 6 days of drainage, the tubes may be clamped for an hour before and after each meal, the purpose being to deliver bile to the duodenum to aid in digestion. Within 7 to 10 days the drainage tubes are removed from the gallbladder or common bile duct. Bile may continue to drain from the drainage tract in considerable quantities for a time and necessitate frequent change of the outer dressings and protection of the skin from irritation. Skin pastes of zinc oxide, aluminum or vaseline prevent the bile from literally digesting the skin. In chronic biliary drainage, it may be necessary to feed the patient his own bile. It may not be necessary to tell him this; instead, a simple statement to the effect that this is a special preparation to help his appetite may be sufficient. The bile should be chilled, strained and diluted with grape or apple juice.

In all patients with biliary drainage, the stools should be observed daily and their color recorded. At frequent intervals specimens of both urine and feces

TERMINOLOGY

Cholecystitis—Inflammation of the gallbladder

Cholelithiasis—Calculi in the gallbladder

Cholecystectomy—Removal of the gallbladder

Cholecystostomy—Opening and drainage of gallbladder

Choledochotomy—Opening into the common duct, usually to remove duct stones

Choledocholithiasis—Stones in the common duct

Choledocholithotomy—Removal of stones in common duct

Choledochoduodenostomy—Anastomosis of common duct to duodenum

Choledochojejunostomy—Anastomosis of common duct to jejunum

should be sent to the laboratory for examination for bile pigments. In this way the surgeon is able to tell that the bile pigment is disappearing from the blood and is draining again into the duodenum. A careful record of fluid intake and output should be kept and totaled for each 24 hours.

The diet of these patients should be low in fats and high in carbohydrates and proteins. The patients themselves usually refuse to eat fatty foods because of the nausea that follows. Vitamin K administration is continued after the operation.

These patients are especially prone to pulmonary complications, as are all patients with upper abdominal incisions. They should be taught to take 10 deep breaths every hour to aerate the lungs fully. Activating these individuals by getting them out of bed as early as permissible reduces the likelihood of thrombophlebitis and pulmonary atelectasis, complications to which the more obese patient is unusually susceptible. A scultetus binder may make the patient more comfortable when he first gets out of bed. Since he has a drainage bottle attached when ambulating, the bottle may be placed in a bathrobe pocket or fastened so that it is below the waist or common duct level.

Post-hospital Instructions. Ordinarily, barring complications, the patient may leave the hospital in 10 to 14 days. Usually there are no special dietary instructions other than to maintain a nutritious diet and avoid excessive fats. Follow-up visits to the family physician permit the patient's questions to be answered and give the physician an opportunity to observe his progress.

BIBLIOGRAPHY

Berkowitz, D.: Diagnosis of carcinoma of the pancreas. Hosp. Med., 3:14, March, 1967.

Bielski, M. T., and Molander, D. W.: Laennec's cirrhosis. Amer. J. Nurs., *65*:82-86, Aug., 1965.

Coodley, E..L.: Significance of serum enzymes. Amer. J. Nurs., 68:301, Feb., 1968.

Cunningham, L. M.: The patient with ruptured esophageal varices, components of nursing care. Amer. J. Nurs., 64:104-108, June, 1964.

Diseases of the liver. (Special issue) Postgrad. Med., *41*, Jan., 1967.

Glenn, F.: Surgical treatment of biliary tract disease. Amer. J. Nurs., *64*:88-92, May, 1964.

Gordon, J. E. (ed.): Control of Communicable Diseases in Man (Hepatitis). ed. 10. Amer. Pub. Health Assoc., 1965.

Hayter, J.: Impaired liver function and related nursing care. Amer. J. Nurs., 68:2374-2379, Nov., 1968.

Henderson, L. M.: Nursing care in acute cholecystitis. Amer. J. Nurs., *64*:93-96, May, 1964.

Iber, F. L.: Differential considerations in biliary tract disease. Hosp. Med., 4:61-80, June, 1968.

Kaplan, M. H., Bernheim, E. J., and Flunn, B. M.: Esophageal varices, components of nursing care. Amer. J. Nurs., *64*:104-108, June, 1964.

Koff, R. S., and Sear, H. S.: Internal temperature of steamed clams. New Eng. J. Med., 276:737-739, 1967.

Pack, G. T., and Islami, A. H.: Operative treatment of hepatic tumors. CIBA Clin. Symposia, *16*:2, Apr.-May-June, 1964.

Warren, K. W., McDonald, W. M., and Veidenheimer, M. C.: Trends in pancreatic surgery. Surg. Clin. N. Amer., 44:743-760, June, 1964.

Wilson, H., and Wolf, R. Y.: Hepatic lobectomy: indications, technique, and results. Surg., 59:472-480, March, 1966.

CHAPTER **24**

Patients with Disorders of the Pancreas

- *Physiology*
- *The Patient with Acute Pancreatitis*
- *The Patient with Chronic Pancreatitis*
- *The Patient with Pancreatic Cysts*
- *The Patient with Pancreatic Tumors*

PHYSIOLOGY

The pancreas is a very important gland that affects the digestion of food elements and the metabolism of sugar in the body. It lies across the upper abdomen behind the peritoneum and the stomach. Its external secretion, containing enzymes that are needed for the digestion of carbohydrates (amylase), proteins (trypsin) and fats (lipase), is delivered into the duodenum at the ampulla of Vater near the entrance of the common bile duct (Fig. 24-1). The stimulus for this enzyme production is the presence of food in the duodenum, in response to which a hormone (secretin) is liberated into the bloodstream and carried to the pancreas, causing the latter to secrete. Pancreatic secretion is stimulated also by nerve impulses transmitted by way of the vagus nerves.

In addition to this external secretion, the pancreas produces an internal secretion, or endocrine substance, *insulin*. This hormone is manufactured by small collections of cells scattered throughout the pancreas called the "islets of Langerhans," and is absorbed directly into the bloodstream. Insulin is required for the utilization of carbohydrate (sugar) by the body. (See p. 693.) Insulin is produced by the beta cells of the islets of Langerhans and glucagon, another hormone, is produced in the alpha cells of the islets. Glucagon has the property of increasing the blood glucose level, in contrast to insulin, which decreases blood glucose.

Both the internal and the external secretions of the pancreas are indispensable for normal body function. Any interruption of the production or interference in the delivery of the external secretion produces severe digestive and nutritional disturbances. Any shortage of insulin causes serious disturbance of carbohydrate metabolism.

THE PATIENT WITH ACUTE PANCREATITIS

Acute pancreatitis (inflammation of the pancreas) is brought about by the digestion of this organ by the very enzymes it produces, principally trypsin. Exactly how this autodigestion gets started is not known with certainty. However, in view of the frequent association of pancreatitis with gallbladder disease, it is believed that gallstones entering the common bile duct and lodging at the ampulla of Vater may obstruct the flow of pancreatic juice, or cause a reflux of bile from the common duct into the pancreatic duct, thus activating the powerful pancreatic enzymes within the gland. (Normally, these remain in an inactive form until the pancreatic juice reaches the lumen of the duodenum.) Spasm and edema of the ampulla of Vater, resulting from duodenitis, can probably produce pancreatitis. Infectious pancreatitis may occur as a complication of mumps or a bacterial disease. The excessive ingestion of alcohol appears to be another etiologic factor in this disease: a definite relationship can be established between alcoholic intake and the onset of symptoms in many patients with acute pancreatitis. Two forms of acute pancreatitis are encountered: acute edematous (or interstitial) pancreatitis, and acute hemorrhagic pancreatitis.

Acute Interstitial Pancreatitis

This condition is characterized by an edematous swelling of the gland and the escape of its enzymes into the surrounding tissues and the peritoneal cavity. Pancreatic lipase produces fat necrosis of the omentum, and the amount of peritoneal fluid increases because of the irritating effect of these digestive enzymes. Symptoms of the disease are caused by this irritation and to the edema and swelling of the inflamed gland. They include abdominal and back pain, nausea, vomiting and tenderness across the upper abdomen. Enzyme changes occur in the patient's blood, urine and peritoneal fluid. The more important diagnostic tests for acute pancreatitis include an estimation of blood amylase and blood lipase, which increase in amount early in the disease.

Since the pathologic process responsible for this disease is autodigestion of the pancreas, the objective of therapy is *to decrease the production of these enzymes.* Oral feedings are interrupted to control the formation of secretin; the patient is maintained on parenteral fluids. Anticholinergic drugs are administered to block the nerve impulses that stimulate pancreatic secretion. Gastric suction is employed. Demerol is given to relieve pain. Most attacks of acute interstitial pancreatitis are self-limited and may be expected to subside in 3 or 4 days.

Acute Hemorrhagic Pancreatitis

Acute hemorrhagic pancreatitis may represent a more advanced form of acute interstitial pancreatitis. Enzymatic digestion of the gland is more widespread and complete. The tissue becomes necrotic, and the damage extends to its vascular radicles, so that blood escapes into the substance of the pancreas and beyond into the retroperitoneal tissues. Symptoms are severe, consisting of pain in the upper abdomen and back, nausea, vomiting and the development of shock with hypotension, tachycardia, cold, clammy skin, and cyanosis. The serum amylase and the serum lipase evaluations are elevated.

Acute pancreatitis is classified into 3 types depending on the pathologic changes that occur. Mild acute

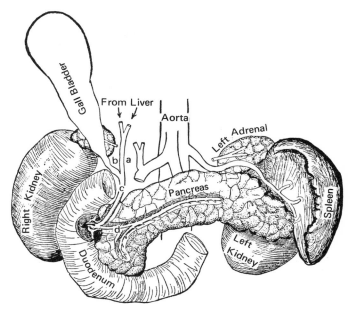

Fig. 24-1. Diagram of some of the abdominal organs. The stomach and the liver, which normally cover these organs, are not represented. (a) Hepatic duct. (b) Cystic duct. (c) Common duct; the arrow is in the ampulla of Vater. (d) Pancreatic duct, which is represented as exposed.

pancreatitis is not hemorrhagic. It is also known as acute pancreatic edema, an inflammatory reaction of relatively mild degree. More severe acute pancreatitis is hemorrhagic, and the most severe form is necrotic. Mild or moderate pancreatitis may subside completely and has a tendency to recur. Hemorrhagic necrosis has a 30 per cent mortality, and survivors may have chronic pancreatic insufficiency. Late complications consist of pancreatic cysts, or calculi. If the patient survives the initial shock, pancreatic necrosis often leads to the formation of secondary abscesses in the region of the gland, which are manifested clinically by mounting fever and leukocytosis. Such abscesses must be drained surgically during the later stages of the disease. Drainage is likely to be profuse and longstanding, so that these patients are certain to require close observation and constant care for a considerable period of time.

Treatment consists of the measures recommended for acute interstitial pancreatitis plus those indicated for shock (p. 146). They include intravenous fluid therapy, blood transfusion, antibiotics, drugs for the relief of pain and gastric suction. Careful nursing observation is extremely important, since this condition has a high mortality rate. A summary of the nursing management of patients with acute pancreatitis is found on p. 534.

THE PATIENT WITH ACUTE PANCREATITIS

Guidelines for Nursing and Medical Management

Major Goal of Therapy: To prevent recurrence and progression of the disease.

Nursing Actions	Rationale
Relieve pain and discomfort.	The agonizing pain is probably due to edema and distension of the capsule and peritoneal irritation.
Give Meperidine (Demerol) in fairly high dosages as indicated by the amount of pain present.	Meperidine acts by depressing the C.N.S. and thereby increasing the patient's pain threshold. Morphine is not usually given because it has a tendency to produce spasm of the sphincter of Oddi. Control of pain is important because restlessness increases body metabolism, which stimulates the secretion of pancreatic and gastric enzymes. The vagal stimulation to pancreatic secretion is stimulated by pain and anxiety.
Assist the patient to assume positions of comfort. Encourage the patient to turn at regularly scheduled intervals. Use pillow supports and foam rubber pads as necessary.	Frequent turning relieves pressure and aids in preventing pulmonary and vascular complications.
Minimize pancreatic secretion.	
Give antispasmodic and anticholinergic drugs as ordered.	Antispasmodic and anticholinergic drugs reduce gastric and pancreatic secretion.
Withhold oral intake.	The intestinal stimulus to pancreatic secretion is influenced by food and fluid intake.
Keep the patient on bedrest.	Bedrest decreases body metabolism and thus reduces pancreatic and gastric secretions.
Employ continuous nasogastric suction. 1. Measure gastric secretions at specified intervals. 2. Observe and chart color and viscosity of gastric secretions. 3. Ensure that the nasogastric tube is patent so free drainage occurs.	Nasogastric suction removes gastric contents and prevents gastric secretions from entering the duodenum and stimulating the secretin mechanism. Decompression of the intestines (if intestinal intubation is used) also assists in relieving respiratory distress.
Promote the comfort of the intubated patient. 1. Use water soluble lubricant around external nares to prevent irritation. 2. Turn patient at intervals to relieve pressure of tube on esophageal and gastric mucosa. 3. Give oral hygiene and gargling solutions to relieve dryness and irritation of oropharynx. 4. Utilize semi-Fowler's position frequently to decrease pressure on diaphragm and allow greater lung expansion.	
Give medications as directed.	
Give antibiotic drugs on ordered time schedule.	Edema, necrosis, hemorrhage and suppuration are present in varying degrees in acute pancreatitis. These conditions are the results of secondary infection. Pancreatic abscess and bacteremia may also be present.

THE PATIENT WITH ACUTE PANCREATITIS (*Continued*)

Nursing Actions	Rationale
Give insulin as directed if hyperglycemia is present.	
Replace the blood and fluid and electrolyte loss.	Electrolyte losses occur from nasogastric suctioning, severe diaphoresis, emesis and as a result of the patient being in a fasting state.
Give plasma and blood as directed.	During acute pancreatitis, plasma may be lost into the abdominal cavity, which diminishes the blood volume.
Give intravenous electrolytes (sodium, potassium, chlorides) as ordered.	The amount and type of fluid and electrolyte replacement is determined by the status of the blood pressure, the laboratory evaluations of serum electrolyte and blood urea nitrogen levels, the urinary volume and by the assessment of the patient's condition.
Combat shock if present.	Extensive acute pancreatitis may cause peripheral vascular collapse and shock. Blood and plasma may be lost into the abdominal cavity and therefore there is a decreased blood and plasma volume. The toxins from the bacteria of a necrotic pancreas may cause shock.
Evaluate the amount of urinary output.	Adrenocortical steroids may be used in the treatment of patients with shock who do not respond to conventional treatment.
Support patient's heart and lungs to prevent complications. Maintain blood volume with blood transfusions, plasma, albumin or dextran. Guard the patient's cardiopulmonary reserve. 1. Evaluate the pulse, respiratory rate and blood pressure at indicated intervals. 2. Give digitalis as ordered. 3. Give Intermittent Positive Pressure treatments as ordered.	Patients with hemorrhagic pancreatitis lose large amounts of blood and plasma which decreases effective circulation and blood volume. Replacement by blood, plasma, albumin or dextran assists in ensuring effective circulating blood volume. Acute pancreatitis produces retroperitoneal edema, elevation of the diaphragm, pleural effusion and inadequate lung ventilation. Intra-abdominal infection and labored breathing increases the body's metabolic demand, which further decreases pulmonary reserve and leads to respiratory failure.
Reduce the excessive metabolism of the body. 1. Give antibiotics as directed. 2. Place patient in an air-conditioned room. 3. Give oxygen if indicated. 4. Utilize a hypothermia blanket if necessary.	Pancreatitis produces a severe peritoneal and retroperitoneal reaction that causes fever, tachycardia and accelerated respirations. Placing the patient in an air-conditioned room and supporting him with oxygen therapy decreases the work load of the respiratory system and the tissue utilization of oxygen. Reduction of fever and pulse rate decrease the metabolic demands of the body.
Educate the patient to try to prevent further attacks of pancreatitis. Keep appointments with physician (or clinic) at specified times. Refrain from alcoholic beverages and avoid excessive use of coffee. Avoid heavy meals. Abstain from eating when nervous or tense.	Known causes of pancreatitis (gallbladder disease, gastric or duodenal ulcer, etc.) should be searched for and treated. Alcohol and coffee increase pancreatic secretion. Spicy foods and heavy meals are strong gastric stimulants.

THE PATIENT WITH CHRONIC PANCREATITIS

After repeated attacks of acute interstitial pancreatitis, or, in some instances, after the prolonged use of alcohol in large amounts, patients may develop a chronic fibrosis of the pancreatic gland itself, with obstruction of its ducts and destruction of its secreting cells. This type of pancreatitis is prone to appear in adult men and is characterized by recurring attacks of severe upper abdominal and back pain, accompanied by vomiting. Attacks often are so painful that morphine, even in large doses, does not provide relief. As the disease progresses, these patients may become addicted to opiates. Because of the destruction of the gland by fibrosis, the pancreatic secretions may be deficient in amount, or obstruction of the ducts by fibrosis may prevent the pancreatic juice from entering the duodenum and playing its role in digestion. As a result, the digestion of foodstuffs, especially proteins and fats, is disrupted. The stools become frequent, frothy (or soaplike) and foul-smelling due to the impairment of fat digestion, which results in a stool with a high fat content. This condition is referred to as "steatorrhea." As the disease progresses, calcifications of the gland may occur, and calcium stones may form within the ducts.

The treatment of chronic pancreatitis depends on its probable cause in each particular patient. When it develops in association with gallbladder disease, efforts are made to relieve the difficulty by operating on the biliary tract, exploring the common duct and removing the stones; usually, the gallbladder is removed at the same time. In addition, an attempt is made to improve the drainage of the common bile duct and the pancreatic duct by dividing the spincter of Oddi, a muscle that is located at the ampulla of Vater (this operation is known as a "sphincterotomy"). The nursing care after such an operation is the same as that indicated for all patients undergoing biliary tract surgery. A T-tube usually is placed in the common bile duct, which involves the necessity for a drainage bottle to collect the bile postoperatively.

In the absence of evidence indicating biliary tract disease, the most common cause of chronic pancreatitis is chronic alcoholism. In such patients, the pancreas becomes markedly fibrotic, to the extent that the pancreatic ducts may be obstructed. In some patients the obstruction may be relieved by sphincterotomy, but in others, the obstruction is located within the confines of the gland itself and therefore not amenable to this procedure. Other possible approaches include opening the pancreatic duct and placing the entire gland inside a loop of jejunum; or the tail of the pancreas may be removed and the remaining stump sutured into the end of a loop of jejunum. These somewhat complicated operations are performed with the object of draining the pancreatic juice by way of a route that by-passes the obstruction in the ductal system.

Despite these operative procedures the patient is likely to continue having pain and digestive difficulties from his pancreatitis unless he abstains completely from the use of alcohol. This point should be emphasized by the nurse in the course of her instruction of the patient and his family.

THE PATIENT WITH PANCREATIC CYSTS

As a result of the local necrosis that occurs at the time of acute pancreatitis, collections of fluid may form in the vicinity of the pancreas. These become walled off by fibrous tissue and are called pancreatic cysts. They are the commonest type of pancreatic cyst, most other types developing as a result of congenital anomalies.

Pancreatic cysts may attain considerable size. Because of their location behind the posterior peritoneum, when they enlarge they impinge on and displace the stomach or the colon, which are adjacent. Eventually, through pressure or secondary infection, they produce symptoms, in which event they must be drained. Drainage may be established into the gastrointestinal tract or through the skin surface. In the latter instance, the drainage is likely to be profuse and damaging to tissue because of its enzyme contents. Hence, steps must be taken to protect the skin in areas adjacent to the drainage site to prevent excoriation. Ointments protect the skin provided that they are applied before excoriation takes place. Another method involves the constant aspiration of juice from the drainage tract by means of a suction apparatus, so that enzyme contact is avoided. This method demands a great deal of nursing attention to be sure that the suction tube does not become dislodged from the drainage tract and that the entire apparatus functions properly without interruption.

THE PATIENT WITH PANCREATIC TUMORS

Carcinoma of the Pancreas

Cancer may arise in any portion of the pancreas: in the head, the body or the tail, producing symptoms and signs that vary depending on the location of the lesion and whether or not functioning, insulin-secreting pancreatic islet cells are involved. Tumors that originate in the head of the pancreas—decidedly the most common location—give rise to a distinctive clinical picture and will be discussed separately. Functioning islet cell tumors, whether benign (adenomata) or malignant (carcinomata) are responsible for the syndrome of hyperinsulinism, and are described on page 703. With these exceptions, carcinoma of the pancreas is notoriously lacking in clear-cut, characteristic symptomatology, and because of its rather nondescript features, patients with this form of cancer often are denied the advantages of an early diagnosis.

Patient Evaluation. Common to all types of pancreatic carcinoma are symptoms of rapid, profound, progressive and inexplicable weight loss; vague, ill-defined, upper or midabdominal discomfort totally unrelated to any gastrointestinal function and difficult to describe; and a boring pain in the midback that is unrelated to posture or activity. People with pancreatic carcinoma often find that they get some relief from pain by sitting bent forward. A full-length foam rubber pad placed under the patient has proven beneficial. Most likely to prove helpful in diagnosis is the gastrointestinal roentgenographic examination, which may demonstrate deformities in adjacent viscera caused by the impinging pancreatic mass. A very important clue, when present, is the development of signs that indicate insulin deficiency—glucosuria, hyperglycemia, and abnormal glucose tolerance.

Treatment. Therapy usually is limited to palliative measures. Definitive surgical treatment, i.e., total excision of the lesion, often is not applicable because of the extensive growth when the lesion is finally diagnosed, because by that time, widespread metastases—especially to the liver, the lungs, and the bones—are likely to have developed.

Tumors of the Head of the Pancreas

Tumors in this region are detected by the fact that they obstruct the common bile duct where it passes through the head of the pancreas to join the pancreatic duct and empty at the ampulla of Vater into the duodenum. Obstruction to the flow of bile produces jaundice, clay-colored stools and dark urine. This disease usually occurs in older, thin men. It must be differentiated from the jaundice due to a biliary obstruction caused by a gallstone in the common duct, which usually is intermittent and appears typically in obese individuals, most often women, who have had previous symptoms of gallbladder disease. The tumors producing the obstruction may arise from the pancreas, from the common bile duct or from the ampulla of Vater.

Operation is indicated in these patients, first to be sure that the jaundice is not due to an impacted gallstone, which can be removed with relative ease. If a

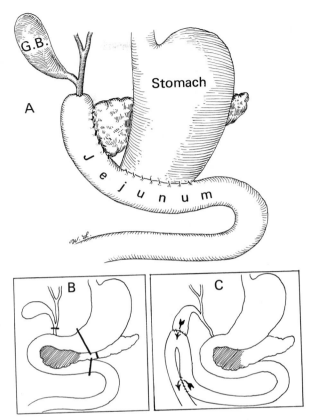

FIG. 24-2. Drawings which show types of operations for carcinoma of the pancreas. (A) Indicates the end-result for resection of the carcinoma of the head of the pancreas or the ampulla of Vater. The common duct is sutured to the end of the jejunum, and the remaining portion of the pancreas and the end of the stomach are sutured to the side of the jejunum. (B) Shows lines that indicate the amount of tissue removed. (C) An alternate method of treatment when an inoperable tumor of the head of the pancreas has been found. In such cases the bile may be permitted to flow again into the intestine by anastomosing the jejunum to the gallbladder. In addition, an accessory operation between the loops of jejunum has been performed.

tumor is found, it may be removed if it has not invaded many of the important structures adjacent to it (portal vein, superior mesenteric artery). The operation entails removal of the head of the pancreas, the duodenum and adjacent stomach and the distal part of the common bile duct. The stomach, the cut end of the pancreas and the common bile duct then are anastomosed to the jejunum. This operation, first suggested by Whipple, may be done in either 1 or 2 stages. It has resulted in the cure of many patients with cancer of the ampulla and the bile ducts, but unhappily it is only palliative in most cases of carcinoma of the head of the pancreas. When excision of the tumor cannot be performed, the jaundice may be relieved by diverting the bile flow into the jejunum. This is done by anastomosing the jejunum to the gallbladder (cholecystojejunostomy).

Nursing Management. When these patients come to the hospital, they are in such a poor nutritional and physical state that a fairly long period of preparation is necessary before operation can be attempted. Various liver and pancreatic function studies are carried out, vitamin K is given to restore the blood prothrombin activity, and diets high in protein often are given with pancreatic enzymes. Blood transfusions frequently are used as well.

Because of the extensive surgery performed, much depends on the nursing care after operation. This differs little from that after any upper abdominal operation, except that these patients are poor surgical risks, and therefore they need intensive nursing attention during the immediate postoperative period.

Pancreatic Islet Tumors

In the pancreas are located the islets (islands) of Langerhans—small nests of cells that secrete directly into the bloodstream and, therefore, part of the glands of internal secretion (endocrines). The secretion, insulin, is involved in the metabolism of sugar, and a deficient secretion produces diabetes mellitus. Tumors of these cells produce a hypersecretion of insulin, so that the body sugar is metabolized too rapidly. The fall of the blood sugar level (hypoglycemia) produces symptoms of weakness, mental confusion and even convulsions. These may be relieved almost immediately by taking sugar by mouth or by intravenous glucose. The 5-hour glucose tolerance test is helpful in diagnosing insulinoma and in distinguishing it from the more common functional hypoglycemia.

Once the diagnosis of a tumor of the islet cells has been made, surgical treatment with removal of the tumor usually is recommended. The tumors may be benign adenomas or they may be malignant. Complete removal usually results in a most dramatic cure. In some patients, such symptoms may not be produced by an actual tumor of the islet cells, but by a simple hypertrophy of this tissue. In such cases a partial *pancreatectomy*—removal of the tail and part of the body of the pancreas—is performed.

Nursing Emphasis. In preparing these patients for operation, the nurse must be alert for symptoms of hypoglycemia and be ready to give sugar, usually with orange juice, should they appear. After operation, the nursing care is the same as that following any upper abdominal operation.

Ulcerogenic (Zollinger-Ellison) Tumors

Some tumors of the islets of Langerhans are associated with a hypersecretion of gastric acid that produces ulcers in the stomach, the duodenum and even the jejunum. The hypersecretion is so great that even after partial gastric resection, enough acid to produce further ulceration may remain. When a marked tendency to develop gastric and duodenal ulcers is noted, an ulcerogenic tumor of the islets of Langerhans is suspected.

These tumors, which may be benign or malignant, are treated when possible by excision. Frequently, however, because of extension beyond the pancreas, removal is not possible. In many patients, a total gastrectomy may be necessary to reduce the secretion of gastric acid sufficiently to prevent further ulceration.

BIBLIOGRAPHY

Books

Guyton, A. C.: Textbook of Medical Physiology. pp. 922-926. Philadelphia, W. B. Saunders, 1966.

Harrison, E. T. (ed.): Principles of Internal Medicine. pp. 1096-1106. New York, McGraw-Hill, 1966.

Rhoads, J. E., et al.: Surgery, Principles and Practice. Philadelphia, J. B. Lippincott, 1970.

Articles

A ten year experience with carcinoma of the pancreas. Arch. Surg., 94:322-325, March, 1967.

Bartlett, M. K.: Might gallstones and recurrent pancreatitis have a common cause? Arch. Surg., 95:887-891, Dec., 1967.

Bauerlein, T. C., et al.: Carcinoma of body of pancreas: a diagnostic aid. Gastroenterology, 49:552-554, Nov., 1965.

Bufkin, W. J., et al.: Evaluation of palliative operations for carcinoma of the pancreas. Arch. Surg., 94:240-242, Feb., 1967.

Collins, J. J., Jr., et al.: Rationale for total pancreatectomy for carcinoma of the pancreatic head. New Eng. J. Med. 274:599-602, 1966.

Facey, F. L., et al.: Mechanism and treatment of shock associated with acute pancreatitis. Amer. J. Surg., 111:374-381, March, 1966.

Groziner, K. H.: Pancreatitis: progress in management. Surgery, 59:319-324, Feb., 1966.

Howard, J. M.: The natural course of pancreatitis: Its influence on results of therapy. Hosp. Med., 1:11-15, May, 1965.

Keddie, N. C., et al.: Acute pancreatitis: a clinical survey. Postgrad. Med. J., 42:234-239, April, 1966.

Klotz, A. P.: Laboratory tests for pancreatic function. Hosp. Med., 3:42-51, August, 1967.

Lowe, W. C., et al.: Carcinoma of the pancreas. An analysis of 100 patients. Amer. J. Gastroent., 47:412-420, May, 1967.

Marks, C.: Chronic relapsing pancreatitis. Amer. J. Surg., 113:340-345,. March, 1967.

Monge, J. J.: Survival of patients with small carcinomas of the head of the pancreas. Ann. Surg., 166:908-912, Dec., 1967.

Nardi, G. L.: Acute pancreatitis. Surg. Clin. N. Amer., 46:619-626, June, 1966.

Nugent, F. W., and Atendido, W.: Hemorrhagic pancreatitis. Postgrad. Med., *40*:87-94, July, 1966.

————, *et al.:* Treatment of acute pancreatitis. Surg. Clin. N. Amer., *48*:595-599, June, 1968.

Romer, J. F., *et al.:* Pancreatitis. A clinical review. Amer. J. Surg., *111*:795-798, June, 1966.

Rosen, R. G., *et al.:* Cytologic diagnosis of pancreatic cancer by ductal aspiration. Ann. Surg., *167*:427-432, March, 1968.

Sharma, T. C., *et al.:* Chronic relapsing pancreatitis. Amer. J. Gastroent., *48*:38-48, July, 1967.

Sodee, D. B.: Pancreatic scanning. Geriatrics, *22*:133-138, July, 1967.

Spencer, J. A., *et al.:* Management of chronic pancreatitis. Med. Clin. N. Amer., *48*:231-248, Jan., 1964.

Stefanini, P., *et al.:* Diagnosis and management of acute pancreatitis. Amer. J. Surg., *110*:866-875, Dec., 1965.

Tuzhilin, S. A.: Influence of high protein diet on chronic pancreatitis. Amer. J. Gastroent., *48*:103-109, Aug., 1967.

Walters, R. L., *et al.:* Traumatic pancreatitis. Amer. J. Surg., *111*:364-368, March, 1966.

Warren, K. W., *et al.:* Carcinoma of the pancreas. Surg. Clin. N. Amer., *48*:601-618, June, 1968.

————, *et al.:* Pancreatoduodenectomy for periampullary cancer. Surg. Clin. N. Amer., *47*:639-645, June, 1967.

CHAPTER **25**

Patients with Renal and Genitourinary Problems

- *Normal Structure and Function*
- *Examination of the Urine*
- *Examination of the Patient*
- *Nursing Problems Encountered in Patients with Urologic Conditions*
- *Problems Affecting the Kidneys*
- *Problems Affecting the Bladder*
- *Problems Affecting the Urethra*
- *Problems Related to the Male Reproductive System*

INTRODUCTION

Importance of Renal System to the Maintenance of Life

The kidneys and their drainage channels, the urinary tract, comprise the renal system. This organ assembly is mainly responsible for extracting the soluble metabolites from the blood and removing them from the body. Another and related aspect of its excretory function is the regulation of the water content and the electrolyte composition of the body fluids; the inorganic ions are excreted in the urine or retained in the body, depending on their individual concentrations in the plasma. Constant precision of operation on the part of the renal system is an absolute requirement for good health; in fact, if its functions are interrupted for more than a few days, death is inevitable. Details regarding the mechanisms of normal kidney function are poorly understood, and, insofar as diseases of the kidney are concerned, medical knowledge is quite as imperfect. The anatomic structure of this organ and its physiologic activities are discussed in the introductory paragraphs of this chapter; the remainder of which is concerned with problems associated with disorders of the renal system.

In common with other organs of the body, the kidneys are affected seriously by any factor that impedes the flow of blood through its substance. The slightest change in the renal circulation, however transient, is reflected at once by alterations in the volume and the composition of the urine. The nurse is well aware that an episode of oligemic shock lasting only 2 or 3 hours is sufficient to depress kidney function, and if shock is allowed to continue uncorrected or incompletely corrected a little longer, the patient may never survive the damage to his kidneys.

Close Relation of Renal and Cardiovascular Systems

Most of the diseases in which the kidneys are seriously and chronically involved are circulatory diseases, because of pathologic changes in the renal blood vessels causing a reduction of blood supply. Kidney failure, as might be expected, is common in patients with arteriosclerotic and hypertensive vascular disease, the renal situation in these patients being but one aspect of a generalized process. Glomerulonephritis (Bright's disease), in which renal insufficiency is most profound, also can be regarded as a vascular disease, one in which the pathologic process, in the early stages at least, is confined principally to the renal capillaries. In general, the tissue damage characteristically produced by vascular disease is extremely disruptive of organ function, and recovery, if it occurs at all, is seldom complete. Classic examples of its deleterious effects are to be found in patients with vascular disease of the kidney, who are notable for their susceptibility to renal failure, the duration of their ailment and the gravity of their prognosis.

Survey of Patient Problems

The clinical features of kidney disease depend chiefly on the presence or the absence of renal insufficiency, renal infection and arterial hypertension, one of its most important complications. Renal failure is reflected in the syndrome of uremia, a complicated situation clinically, with therapeutic problems as challenging for the nurse as any encountered in clinical practice. These problems are related to the failure of toxic metabolites to be excreted, the excess accumulation of certain materials in the blood, and the spillage of other materials that are essential to the body economy.

Infections of the kidney, causing diffuse inflammatory reactions or the formation of abscesses, are invariably serious because of their local destructiveness, their tendency to become widespread, and the occurrence of damaging complications. Stones and deforming scars that originate in an infection may interfere with urinary drainage. Moreover, permanent alterations of the renal blood vessels in pyelonephritis, a type of kidney infection, may be responsible for impairment of kidney function and also for chronic, incapacitating arterial hypertension. Fortunately, most urinary infections are responsive to modern antibacterial chemotherapy if treatment is selected appropriately and applied correctly.

NORMAL STRUCTURE AND FUNCTION

The kidneys are paired organs, each weighing approximately 125 gm., located in a position lateral to the bodies of the lower thoracic vertebrae a few centimeters to the right and the left of the midline. Anteriorly, they are separated from the abdominal cavity and its contents by layers of peritoneum; posteriorly, they are shielded by the lower thoracic wall. Each kidney, essentially a duplicate of the other, is composed of minute structural units that functionally may be regarded as little kidneys. To understand one of these renal units is to understand the whole kidney.

Nephron

Each renal unit, or *nephron*, is constructed of living cells arranged in the form of a tube, or *tubule*. Its wall is constructed with renal epithelial cells, on the outer side of which is a fine network of capillaries through which blood is constantly flowing.

At its upper end this tubule swells into a hollow ball called Bowman's capsule. At the pole of this ball, which is opposite the point where the tubule enters, the wall is pushed in, much as one can push one half of a rubber ball into the other half, by a knot of capillaries, the glomerulus. These glomeruli can be seen by the naked eye only as red dots about the size of a pinprick. The wall of this hollow ball is lined with flat epithelial cells quite unlike those lining the tubule. The tube, when it leaves the capsule, is quite tortuous and is called the *proximal convoluted tubule*. It then makes a long straight loop, the loop of Henle, which again becomes convoluted, after which it opens into a long straight tube, the *collecting tubule*, which grows larger and larger in its course.

The capillaries of the glomerulus, all of which branched from one vessel—a branch of the renal artery—unite again into one vessel which leaves the capsule, passes down the tubule and again is divided into the network of capillaries surrounding the tubule.

By a process similar to simple filtration, most of the constituents of the urine filter through the walls of the glomerular capillaries into the capsule, and this fluid passes down the tubule. Some of the substances filtered out into the glomeruli are of use to the body, and the convoluted tubules reabsorb these materials into the bloodstream. Much of the water is reabsorbed through the tubular walls. A portion of the tubule contributes to the formation of urine by secreting materials derived from the blood into the fluid passing through its lumen. The urine, as finally formed, flows down into the pelvis of the kidney.

The capillaries surrounding the tubules reunite to form the renal vein, the blood of which is now practically free of waste. A large amount of blood flows through the kidneys, nearly 10 times as much as through any other organ of the same weight. In this way the kidney continuously purifies the entire volume of blood.

Cortex

This is the most important part of the kidney because all the important structures of the kidney are here. It is a zone of about 4 to 6 mm. in thickness. In it the glomeruli are arranged on little vertical arteries, like bunches of grapes, and between these rows of glomeruli are the convoluted tubes. The loops of Henle and the collecting tubules together comprise pyramidal-shaped structures called *pyramids*, the apices of which project into the drainage portion of the kidney.

Pelvis

The pelvis is a sac with several fingerlike outpouchings extending into the substance of the kidney; these are called *calyces*, and into them the collecting tubules open. Distally, the pelvis becomes constricted to form the ureter, and this empties into the urinary bladder. The urine, therefore, flows down the tubes into the pelvis of the kidney, and then down the ureter to the bladder.

EXAMINATION OF THE URINE

Urinalysis provides a wealth of important clinical information and is regarded as an indispensable part of every clinical study. The more important urine tests are tabulated in the Appendix. Urine examination of every patient includes the observation and evaluation of urine color and clarity, measurement of urine acidity and specific gravity, tests for the presence of protein and sugar in the urine (proteinuria and glycosuria, respectively), and microscopic examination of the urine sediment after centrifuging for the detection of red blood cells (hematuria), white blood cells (pyuria), casts (cylindruria), crystals (crystalluria) and bacteria (bacteriuria). Numerous additional tests are applicable in special situations.

Collection and Preservation of Urine Samples

All urine tests are performed ideally on fresh specimens, preferably the first voiding of the day, since most urinary constituents are present in highest concentration at that time. Random specimens are satisfactory for most analyses, however, provided that they have been collected in clean containers and have been protected adequately against bacterial and chemical deterioration. Samples collected in the home should be voided into clean, dry, wide-mouth bottles of pint or quart size, equipped with screw-tops or clamp-tops, the mouth being sufficiently large to permit either the male or the female to void directly into them. All specimens should be refrigerated as soon as possible after they are voided and maintained at refrigerator temperatures until they are transported to the testing laboratory. If more than a few hours are to elapse between the times of collection and testing, the urine should be stabilized by the addition of a chemical preservative.

Collection bottles used in the hospital should be meticulously clean and dry. Moreover, they should be equipped with a tight-sealing closure of a type that is easily applied. Every urine sample must be labeled clearly with the patient's name and bed location; the label should also specify the date and the hour of the voiding and any other data that might pertain in an individual case, such as, for example, the occurrence of menstruation. Unless the urinalysis is to proceed at once, the specimen should be placed in a refrigerator immediately.

24-Hour Urine Collections

Many quantitative analytic tests are carried out on specimens that represent the entire urinary output of a patient over a 24-hour period. The reliability of such tests rests on the assumption that the sample is, in fact, representative of the 24-hour pool. This consideration applies in all electrolyte balance studies, measurements of protein and formed-element excretion, tests of radioactive vitamin B_{12} absorption, certain hormonal assays and other special tests. The receptacle accommodating the urine pool should be kept in a refrigerator or should contain a preservative. It should be labeled to identify the patient specifically, accurately and legibly and indicate the time that the collection was started. All voidings should be funneled promptly into this receptacle. Failure to transfer one specimen voided during the test period invalidates the test. The incidence of incomplete 24-hour collections is distressingly high. A successful collection requires the complete understanding and willing cooperation on the part of the patient and all unit personnel who happen to be concerned with the patient's care during the period in question. The organization and the supervision of these collections is the responsibility of the nurse in charge of the patient. Her instructions to her patient and her staff must be crystal clear.

"Sterile-Voided" ("Clean-Catch") Specimens

Urine samples voided in the usual way are practically useless for bacteriologic study because of inevitable contamination by organisms residing in the vicinity of the urethral meatus. Such contamination can be avoided by catheterizing the urinary bladder. However, since the dangers of catheterization have become recognized and its role in the production of chronic pyelonephritis has become understood, this procedure is no longer recommended except for specific indications. Reliable bacteriologic studies are possible without catheterization, utilizing the so called "sterile-voiding" technic of sampling.

The male patient is instructed to cleanse the penis thoroughly with soap and water, employing cotton pledgets or gauze squares. The first portion of the voiding is not collected but discarded. The next portion—the test sample—is voided into a sterile, wide-mouth bottle or large-caliber tube, which is protected by a sterile closure. The female patient, before voiding, must cleanse the vulva about the urethral meatus 3 or 4 times with soapy water, each time wiping the perineum backward toward the anus, then discarding the wipe. Following the lavage a midstream specimen is collected in a sterile receptacle.

Clinical Significance

Color and Clarity of Urine

The color of normal urine comes ultimately from the hemoglobin of hemolyzed red corpuscles. One part of the hemoglobin, containing iron, is split off and saved; the rest becomes bilirubin, the coloring matter of bile. In the intestine, bilirubin is slightly modified to form urobilinogen, and some of this is re-absorbed into the blood and excreted in the urine as urobilin. Usually, the higher the specific gravity of urine, the deeper is its color. Bile, which is excreted in the urine in patients with obstructive jaundice, darkens the urine. Its presence is best recognized not by the color of the urine but by its yellow foam when shaken. The presence of small amounts of blood lends a smoky appearance to the urine, that is, it is turbid and has a blackish-red tint.

Fresh acid urine is clear. Soon after standing there appears a feathery cloud, composed of mucus washed by the urine from the mucous membrane lining the urinary passages. If a person has not been drinking much water, but has ingested protein in large amounts, his urine forms a "brick dust" sediment in the presence of cold. This is merely a precipitate of the salts of uric acid that are present in every normal urine and are deposited whenever the urine is a little concentrated and cold.

If a urine is clear when voided, sediments that appear later have no importance. If a freshly voided urine is not clear, but contains a sediment that does not disappear on warming or on the addition of acetic acid, the sediment usually signifies the presence of bacteria, blood, pus or casts and is referred to as an "organized sediment."

Pigmenturia from Food, Drugs and Chemicals. The ingestion of beets may result in the transient appearance of pink or red urine. Certain cathartic agents, including aloes, cascara sagrada, rhubarb and senna, cause acid urine to turn yellow-brown and alkaline urine to turn red-violet in color. Antipyrine, one of the coal-tar analgesic drugs, in large doses produces deep red urine. Pyridium, a urinary antiseptic drug, colors the urine red. Thymol, an anthelminthic agent, produces a greenish tint. Santonin, another anthelminthic, colors acid urine deep yellow and alkaline urine pink. In cases of phenol (carbolic acid) poisoning, the urine becomes olive-green and blackens on exposure to air. Methylene blue, employed in the treatment of methemoglobinemia, confers a blue-green color. Phenolphthalein, contained in certain cathartic preparations, is colorless in acid urine but pink or red in alkaline urine. Phenolsulfonphthalein (PSP), used in a test of renal function (p. 547) and a procedure for measuring the residual urine volume, and Bromsulphalein (BSP), employed in a liver function test (p. 510), have the same effect as phenolphthalein on urine color.

Pigmenturia in Disease. Abnormal coloration of the urine has diagnostic importance. Tests for the identification and the quantitative estimation of urine pigments, and the nature of certain disorders that are responsible for pigmenturia follow.

Bilirubinuria. The presence of bilirubin in the urine (bilirubinuria or choluria) is abnormal. It signifies an obstruction to the excretion of that pigment by the liver into the intestine; that instead of escaping through the biliary tract into the intestinal lumen, it has been regurgitated by the liver cells directly into the circulating blood; and, finally, that the liver cells have succeeded in processing this pigment into the soluble glucuronide salt, the only form in which it can diffuse from the blood into the urine. Therefore, bilirubinuria is a sign of biliary obstruction, and jaundiced patients with bilirubin in their urine are presumed to have obstructive jaundice rather than jaundice due primarily to liver failure.

Urine containing bilirubin varies from deep yellow to light brown in color. A more specific indication of its presence in the urine is the appearance of yellow or brown foam when the sample is shaken in a glass container. In the absence of bilirubin, urine foam is white or straw-colored.

Hemoglobinuria. Minute traces of hemoglobin in the urine, as in microscopic hematuria, may escape visual detection. Oxyhemoglobin in more than trace amounts imparts a pink to dark red color to urine; reduced hemoglobin, a purple to black discoloration. Methemoglobin, an oxidation product of hemoglobin, may contribute a light- to dark-brown shade. The presence of hemoglobin or methemoglobin in the urine ordinarily reflects the presence of the corresponding pigment in the circulating plasma, i.e., hemoglobinemia or methemoglobinemia, which in turn signifies the rapid breakdown of red cells in the circulating blood, or "intravascular hemolysis." Hemoglobin liberated from red cells in this manner is rapidly oxidized to methemoglobin, which explains the methemoglobinemia and methemoglobinuria associated with certain hemolytic disorders. Intravascular hemolysis is a feature of paroxysmal nocturnal hemoglobinuria (p. 314), paroxysmal hemoglobinuria, hemolytic transfusion reactions (p. 95), hemolytic episodes following accidental injections of distilled water or other hypotonic fluids, and exposure to certain toxic agents.

The detection and the measurement of hemoglobin in the urine are possible by means of a test that depends on the appearance of a blue color when hemoglobin is mixed with benzidine and hydrogen peroxide in an acid solution. A more convenient method (Occultest) utilizes a reagent tablet containing orthotolidin and strontium peroxide.

Hemosiderinuria. The presence in the urine of hemosiderin, a breakdown product of hemoglobin, is expected in patients with hemoglobinuria and in hemochromatosis (p. 312). Hemosiderin is responsible for the appearance of a brown or black sediment in urine.

Myoglobinuria. Myoglobin, a pigment contained in muscle tissue exclusively, may appear in the urine following a severe crushing injury (crush syndrome); following the rupture, obstruction or prolonged spasm of a major artery in a traumatized limb; or as a complication of spontaneous femoral artery thrombosis. Myoglobin can be distinguished readily from hemoglobin by spectroscopy.

Porphyrinuria and Porphobilinuria. The porphyrins and porphobilin, precursors or degradation products of hemoglobin, are excreted in the urine in certain abnormal conditions, including 2 specific disease entities: intermittent acute porphyria and congenital light-sensitive porphyria.

The diagnosis of porphyrinuria and the specific identification of individual porphyrins in the urine depend on a combination of laboratory findings. Since some of these pigments are extremely unstable, their reliable identification requires samples of freshly voided urine.

Alkaptonuria. This term denotes an inborn metabolic defect, by which certain individuals fail to metabolize tyrosine and therefore excrete homogenistic acid in the urine. Alkaline samples containing this product turn black rapidly on standing.

Melaninuria. The pigment melanin and its colorless precursor, melanogen, are excreted in the urine of patients with melanosarcoma (Chap. 28). A freshly voided sample may be normal in color or only moderately tinged with brown. Eventually, however, it darkens and becomes entirely black as melanogen is oxidized to melanin.

Reaction (pH) of Urine

Urine acidity (pH) is estimated by immersing a strip of Nitrazine Paper in the sample and comparing the resultant color with those printed on a chart. The pH varies normally between 4.5 and 8.0 and is usually acid, i.e., less than 7. The concentration of hydrogen ions in the urine, or the urine pH, reflects the metabolic status of the patient. The urine reaction should be tested as soon as the sample is voided, because it becomes increasingly alkaline on standing. Bacterial contaminants multiply rapidly, decomposing the urea and liberating ammonia, which is a strong alkali. (Ammonia accounts for the disagreeable odor of stale urine.)

Acid urines are encountered in patients with metabolic acidosis and sodium depletion due to diarrhea or excessive sweating. Alkaline urines are voided after ingestion of alkalizing salts, following the vomiting of acid gastric juice and in patients with respiratory alkalosis. Transient alkalinization of the urine occurs after meals, which stimulate the production of hydrochloric acid in the stomach, a process involving the extraction of hydrogen ions from the blood. The resultant lowering of the hydrogen ion concentration in the plasma is reflected by a corresponding decrease in the urine. In cases of renal tract infection, urea-splitting organisms may alkalinize the urine before it is voided, as a product of their growth in the kidneys or the bladder. Constant alkalinity of freshly voided urine is important in such cases, not only as a diagnostic clue, but also as a factor that promotes the formation of renal and bladder stones. Renal tuberculosis represents one variety of urinary tract infection in which the urine reaction is characteristically acid; the tubercle bacillus does not split urea.

Urine Specific Gravity

By "specific gravity of urine" is meant the ratio of the weight of a given volume of urine to that of the same volume of distilled water when these are measured at the same temperature.

The specific gravity of urine is measured by the flotation of a hydrometer, or urinometer, a sealed glass bulb fitted at the upper end with a stem on which is mounted a calibrated scale and, at the bottom, with a small mercury bulb to provide ballast and to maintain the device in a vertical position when it is immersed. Urine is placed in a cylindrical receptacle and its temperature noted. The hydrometer is next introduced. The depth to which this sinks and at which its position becomes stabilized is determined by reading the scale at the junction of the stem and the fluid meniscus.

A specific gravity of 1.025 or more in the absence of albumin and sugar is fairly reliable evidence of normal renal function. On the other hand, if random samples from a patient consistently give specific gravity readings in the vicinity of 1.010, poor renal function is suspected.

Urine Concentration Tests. A simple, but not entirely reliable, test of renal function measures the capacity of the kidneys to concentrate the glomerular filtrate and consists in the determination of the specific gravity of urine voided 12 to 18 hours after all fluids and food have been withheld. Concentration below specific gravity 1.015 in these circumstances is regarded as being abnormal. Whereas this test is fairly reliable in an ambulatory patient, it is likely to yield misleading results in persons at bed rest, for they simply do not concentrate their urine to the maximal extent in less than 36 to 48 hours. Therefore, for reliable data, the dehydration period must be lengthened to a minimum of 36 hours. It would be highly undesirable to perform this test on any patient with high fever or with any feature predisposing to dehydration, and this would also apply to a patient in whom dehydration might be dangerous.

Abnormal Urine Constituents

Proteinuria (Albuminuria). Normal renal cells allow a trace of albumin to pass into the urine, but this trace is so minute that it cannot be detected by the ordinary tests. If any albumin can be recognized at all by these tests, albuminuria is present and indicates pathology. The cause of most long-standing albuminurias is nephritis. The amount of albumin in the urine of nephritic patients varies enormously. In the acute cases, a large quantity is present; the subacute cases have less, and the more chronic cases least.

Glycosuria. A large amount of sugar (glucose) in the urine is called glycosuria. Because glycosuria is an important symptom in diabetes mellitus, it is discussed under that disease, on page 694.

Ketonuria. The presence of ketone bodies (acetone, acetoacetic acid and beta-hydroxybutyric acid) in the urine is characteristic of diabetic ketoacidosis and individuals who are severely dehydrated or starved. The finding is indicative of incomplete fat metabolism (see Chap. 31).

Formed Elements in Urine

Hematuria. Red blood corpuscles may be found in the urine—either a few, or many, or in such quantity that the urine appears sanguineous. When their concentration is sufficient to color the urine red, the condition is called *gross hematuria*. One practically always finds red blood cells in the urine in acute nephritis and during the acute flare-ups of chronic nephritis. In these cases the urine is often not red, but more smoky in appearance.

The presence or absence of red blood cells is one of the important criteria for distinguishing a pure nephrosis, or the nephrotic stage of glomerulonephritis, from acute glomerulonephritis. Hematuria is seen in pyelonephritis, in pyonephrosis (different degrees of kidney bacterial infection) and in focal embolic nephritis such as occurs in bacterial endocarditis. It may appear as a manifestation of a hemorrhagic disease, such as thrombocytopenic purpura, or in Dicumarol toxicity. Red cells frequently are found in the urine in patients with renal stones, renal tuberculosis and carcinoma of the kidney.

Hematuria may also originate from sites in the genitourinary tract other than the kidney, such as the ureter, the bladder or the prostate. In all cases the source of the blood must be determined. The presence of red cells is usually detected on microscopic examination of the urine sediment. Sensitive hemoglobin tests based on the benzidine or orthotolidin reaction are useful for the screening of patients for hematuria, since the latter cannot escape detection even if the red cells are hemolyzed.

Pyuria. Small numbers of leukocytes are normally present in the urine. They are observed with regularity and in quantity in the urine of patients with nephritis and other inflammatory diseases involving the urinary tract. When present in sufficient number to give the fresh urine a cloudy appearance, the condition is called *pyuria*. Pyuria of marked degree occurs in pyelitis, pyelonephritis and pyonephrosis, in tuberculosis of the kidney and, most strikingly, in cystitis and urethritis.

Cylindruria. The term "cast" owes its origin to the manner in which these elements acquire their characteristic shape, molded as they are in the renal tubules. Thus, the tubular lumen becomes partially filled with a substance that hardens and forms a "cast" of their lumen. These casts are later washed out by the urine, where they can be found with a microscope.

Casts in the urine (cylindruria) have much the same clinical significance as proteinuria (albuminuria). As a rule, albumin and casts appear together, but for short periods either may be found alone.

It must be realized that casts deteriorate rapidly in unpreserved urine. Prolonged preservation may be accomplished, even in unrefrigerated specimens, by means of a chemical preservative. However, this may not be uniformly effective with respect to all the formed elements, and the morphology of those that persist may be altered beyond certain recognition. The fact remains that for examinaton of the urine sediment there is no substitute for fresh urine.

Crystalluria. Crystals are to be found in most concentrated urine specimens, their composition and morphology dictated by the pH of the specimen. In the majority of instances, their presence denotes no metabolic abnormality or other disorder. Their identification usually can be accomplished on the basis of their microscopic appearance alone.

Cystinuria. Definite pathologic significance attaches to the finding of cystine crystals in the urine, for they are indicative of a rare familial disorder known as "cystinuria." This is a life-long disease and represents one of the inborn errors of metabolism. Patients so affected are predisposed to the formation of renal and bladder stones composed of cystine.

Leucine and Tyrosine Crystals. If either of these varieties of crystal is encountered in the urine, the other is likely to be present. This form of crystalluria has ominous implications, indicating that massive tissue autolysis is in progress. It is associated most often with severe, diffuse and advanced liver necrosis destined to prove lethal.

Bacteriuria. The presence of bacteria in urine samples collected without special precautions or stored without adequate protection against contamination is of no significance. However, the demonstration, by microscopic examination or bacteriologic culture, of bacteriuria in catheterized specimens or in "sterile-voided" samples is potentially of great importance. In order to establish the significance of bacteriuria it is necessary to perform quantitative urine cultures. This involves the dilution of urine with sterile nutrient broth and the preparation of agar pour plates from this mixture. The number of organisms per ml. of urine can be estimated from the number of bacterial colonies that are visible on the plate after 24 to 48 hours of incubation at 37° C. Counts of 5,000 or more per ml. of urine are consistent with a diagnosis of urinary tract infection.

Urine Calcium

The concentration of calcium in the urine is important in the evaluation of bone disease. Associated with rapid decalcification of the skeleton, such as occurs in hyperparathyroidism (Chap. 31) and following the sudden cessation of normal physical activity, the urinary excretion of calcium is increased. A decrease in urine calcium may indicate an abnormal decrease in the blood calcium level, due, for example, to hypoparathyroidism or to vitamin D deficiency.

Urine Urobilinogen

Urobilinogen is a substance formed by the action of intestinal bacteria on the bilirubin in the bile. A portion of this urobilinogen is reabsorbed through the intestinal wall into the bloodstream and appears in the urine, the basis of the *urine urobilinogen* test. Normally there is always a certain amount present in the urine. If it is absent, it may be concluded that there is no bilirubin, hence no bile, reaching the intestine, due either to biliary tract obstruction or to failure of the liver to secrete bile. Blood containing urobilinogen is cleared of this substance as it passes through the liver, for the liver handles urobilinogen as it handles bilirubin, namely, by excreting it into the bile. If the liver cells are not functioning adequately, urobilinogen is retained in the blood, where its concentration becomes increasingly elevated. This high blood level of urobilinogen, in turn, is reflected by an abnormal increase in the urine urobilinogen. An increased urine urobilinogen is often one of the earliest signs of acute liver cell damage. Increased levels are also characteristic of patients with hemolytic anemia, whose bilirubin (hence urobilinogen) production is abnormally high as a result of rapid red cell destruction.

Hormone Assays in Urine

Chorionic Gonadotropin. Gonadotropic hormone, also called anterior pituitarylike substances (APL), is produced by placental tissue in the pregnant uterus. Its demonstration in the urine may provide the earliest indication of pregnancy, positive results being obtained in 98 per cent of pregnant women tested 10 days after the first amenorrhea. Urine tests for this substance may also be positive in patients with tumors containing chorionic tissue, such as testicular teratoma and chorioepithelioma, and in cases of retained placenta following obstetric delivery. Various procedures that are available for the detection of this hormone include the Friedman test, which employs a rabbit, the Aschheim-Zondek test, utilizing a mouse, and the African frog test. Each of the above tests is based on the observation of characteristic changes in ovarian structures following the injection of gonadotropic hormone. The procedure most widely used at present utilizes a male frog belonging to the species *Rana pipiens,* commonly known as the Leopard Frog, Grass Frog or Meadow Frog. One of these amphibians is injected with a sample of urine representing the first voiding of the day. One half to 1 hour after the injection, a drop of urine is secured from the frog. This specimen is examined for the presence or absence of spermatozoa, the former indicating a positive reaction. The validity of this procedure is enhanced by imposing a 24-hour period of fluid restriction prior to the voiding of the test sample, during which drugs of all types should be withheld, especially salicylates, barbiturates and hormones.

17-Ketosteroids. The concentration of 17-ketosteroids in the urine reflects the secretory activity of the adrenal cortex. Elevated levels are characteristic of patients with Cushing's disease and functioning adrenocortical tumors, whereas decreased levels are indicative of depressed adrenal function, as in Addison's disease or panhypopituitarism (see Chap. 31). Quantitative measurement of 17-ketosteroids requires the collection of a 24-hour urine sample. This is acidified throughout the collection period by the preliminary addition of 10 ml. of concentrated hydrochloric acid (or, if chlorides are also to be measured, of sulfuric acid). The urine should be refrigerated immediately after voiding and the analysis carried out as soon as possible following completion of the collection.

Catecholamines. Epinephrine and norepinephrine, representing the catecholamines, are hormones produced mainly by the adrenal medulla and serve as the chemical mediators of the sympathetic nervous system. Excessive quantities are produced by certain tumors, specifically pheochromocytoma (Chap. 31).

Urine tests in such patients demonstrate as much as a tenfold increase above normal. The catecholamines are measured by photofluorometric methods. Normal individuals excrete up to 200 micrograms of catecholamines per 24 hours, approximately one half of which is accounted for by derivatives of norepinephrine produced previously at sympathetic nerve endings. The excretion of more than 200 micrograms per day is indicative of pheochromocytoma.

Phenolsulfonphthalein (PSP) Excretion Test

For years, the easiest, quickest and, hence, most popular test of renal functional efficiency has been one that requires no blood chemistry but uses phenolsulfonphthalein, a harmless dye eliminated solely by the kidneys. After having emptied his bladder, the patient, in order to promote a free secretion of urine, drinks 400 ml. of water, cold but not iced, and 20 minutes later is given an intravenous injection of 1 ml. of a sterile solution containing 6 mg. of phenolsulfonphthalein. The patient is required to empty his bladder completely at intervals of 15 minutes, 30 minutes, 1 hour and 2 hours after the injection. Additional water is given to ensure an adequate output of urine. The amount of dye present in these specimens is then estimated by a simple colorimetric method. Normally, the first specimen will contain from 20 to 40 per cent, and the remainder enough so that the total amount of dye eliminated in 2 hours is 60 to 90 per cent of the amount injected. Interpretation of this test is not considered to be reliable unless the volume of each urine sample is 50 ml. or more.

EXAMINATION OF THE PATIENT

By direct palpation it is frequently possible to determine the size and the movability of the kidneys. Renal disease may produce tenderness over the costovertebral angle. By rectal examination in the male, the prostate gland may be palpated digitally as a part of the study of the urinary difficulty that occurs when it hypertrophies in older men.

Visualization (Roentgenograms)

Roentgenograms are used to study the urinary tract in many ways. The direct examination ("flat plate") is used to determine the size and the position of the kidneys and to visualize stones in the kidney, the ureter and the bladder. Various organic compounds of iodine, when given intravenously, are excreted rapidly by the kidney in the urine. The presence of these compounds makes the urine-producing parts of the urinary tract opaque to the x-rays, so that they can be delineated on the x-ray film; this is known as excretory urography (intravenous pyelogram, urogram) or occasionally mentioned as K.U.B. (kidney-ureter-bladder).

This is not only a method of outlining the urinary passages but also a test of kidney function. The position of the ureters is often marked by taking an x-ray film with ureteral catheters in place. Less frequently, the kidney pelvis and the ureters are studied by the injection of radiopaque solutions through ureteral catheters (*retrograde pyelogram*) or into the bladder through urethral catheters (*cystogram*).

Retrograde Pyelography. Retrograde pyelography is a procedure used to visualize the drainage structures during cystoscopy by introducing contrast material through catheters placed in each ureter. This procedure affords a clear and detailed image of the position and shape of the kidneys, the contour of the drainage structures, the position and caliber of the ureteral lumina and the contours of the bladder. Retrografin, which contains a topical antibiotic, is the most commonly used contrast material. A laxative is given the night before the examination. A low residue diet the day prior to the procedure is recommended so that a filled colon does not block visualization.

Excretory Urography (Intravenous Pyelogram or Intravenous Urogram). An excretory urogram (I.V.P.) visualizes the kidney and bladder by means of renal excretion of a radiopaque contrast material such as Hypaque (sodium diatrizoate) or Renografin-60 (meglumine diatrizoate). The contrast material is given intravenously in doses ranging from 20 ml. to 100 ml. or more. Multiple films are taken serially to visualize drainage structures. Preparation of the patient is desirable to avoid overhydration, which dilutes the contrast material causing inadequate visualization. The following preparation may be used: (1) a laxative is given the night before the scheduled examination; (2) a light evening meal is given. The patient is not permitted to eat or drink until after the examination is completed the next day.

Before the examination, the patient is carefully questioned to determine if he has a history of allergies. If he has a positive allergic history, a 0.2 ml. test dose of Hypaque or Renografin-60 is injected intradermally. If no skin reaction occurs in 15 minutes, the regular intravenous test dose of 1 ml. of contrast material is given. Although rare, as with the administration of any intravenous drug, an anaphylactoid reaction may occur. This reaction may occur even though the skin sensitivity test has been negative. All I.V. urogram rooms should have emergency drugs (epinephrine hydrochloride, vasopressors, etc.) as well as oxygen, tracheostomy equipment, and so forth ready for immediate symptomatic therapy in case such a medical emergency occurs.

Infusion Drip Pyelography. Intravenous drip pyelography is used when regular urographic techniques fail to show the drainage structures satisfactorily (e.g.,

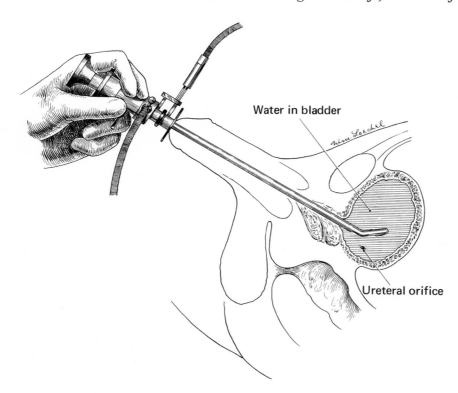

Water in bladder

Ureteral orifice

FIG. 25-1. A cystoscope being introduced into the bladder of the male. The upper cord is an electric line for the light at the distal end of the cystoscope. The lower tubing leads from a reservoir of sterile water that is used to inflate the bladder. Of course, the entire procedure of cystoscopy is a sterile one.

in a patient with an elevated blood urea nitrogen) or when prolonged opacification of the drainage structures is desired so that tomograms (body section radiography) can be made. The patient preparation is the same as for excretory urography. An infusion of a large volume of dilute solution of contrast material is rapidly administered intravenously. Films are obtained at specified intervals after the start of the infusion.

Radioisotope Studies of the Urinary Tract (Renogram)

Certain iodine-containing compounds, i.e., those employed in excretory pyelography, are concentrated and excreted in the kidneys after intravenous injection. After the administration of compounds labeled with radioiodine, the kidneys transiently contain radioactivity; the degree of radioactivity, determined by external counters, provides a measure of renal function. The most commonly used compound employed for this purpose is Hippuran [131]I. The patient is given an intravenous injection of [131]I. (The dose is 0.3 to 0.6 microcuries per kilogram of body weight.) Then the patient is placed in the sitting position before a pair of radiation counters, one directed toward the right and the other toward the left kidney. Both sites are counted simultaneously and continuously for 15 to 20 minutes by recording rate meters, to permit direct comparison of the two kidneys. A peak of radioactivity appearing within a few seconds reflects the renal blood flow; a second peak, approximately 5 minutes later, coincides with active tubular transport of the dye and filling of the renal tubules with concentrated dye. The excretion phase is also evaluated. In patients with unilateral renal disease, differences between the 2 kidneys with respect to blood flow, tubular function and excretion are clearly demonstrable by this technique.

Isotopic Localization of Renal Pathology (Renoscan)

Neohydrin is a diuretic compound that concentrates in the kidney tubules, but does not become concentrated in tumor tissue. After intravenous injection of Neohydrin labeled with radioactive mercury ([197]Hg), it is possible to delineate the kidneys by external scanning. If a lesion, such as a tumor or renal infarct, is contained within the kidney, it is readily detected by the absence of radioactivity in the involved area and the resultant defect in the scan.

Aortography

An outline of the kidney circulation is obtained by the injection of radiopaque material into the aorta near the renal arteries. This injection is made through a long needle that is introduced through the back while the patient is on the x-ray table; roentgenograms are made immediately. The kidney circulation thus visualized is often of great diagnostic value in searching for tumors, cysts and other renal disease.

The Cystoscopic Examination

A direct method of bladder study and visualization is by the cystoscopic examination. The cystoscope has a self-contained optical lens system and provides a magnified, illuminated view of the bladder. There is also a guide system that allows a ureteral catheter to be passed through the urethra and up into the kidneys. The cystoscope can be manipulated to allow complete visibility of the entire bladder.

There are 3 main pieces to this instrument. The *obturator* is designed to permit atraumatic passage of the cystoscope. After the cystoscope is passed into the bladder, the obturator is removed. Sterile distilled water is run in and out of the bladder to evacuate concentrated urine, pus and blood, thus allowing better visualization. A *telescope* with a very small lens is passed through the cystoscope, which enables the urologist to view the inside of the bladder (Fig. 25-1).

The cystoscope is an expensive and delicate instrument. It should be cleaned carefully and disinfected adequately. Ethylene oxide or glutaraldehydre is used to disinfect urological instruments. If a liquid disinfectant is used, the instrument should be placed vertically in a container so that air is not trapped within the cystoscope, thus preventing complete exposure of it to the disinfecting solution. After disinfection is completed, the cystoscope is rinsed with sterile distilled water to prevent burns from the glutaraldehyde solution.

Patient Preparation. Often the nurse is called upon to explain the meaning of a cystoscopic examination to her patient. This is a real part of preparation, because if he has no idea of the type of procedure that is to take place, his fears undoubtedly will make him tense. The preparation usually includes his drinking 1 or 2 glasses of water before going to the examining department. Often a sedative plus the instillation of a local anesthetic into the bladder is sufficient; however, depending on the patient, it may be necessary to use spinal or general anesthesia. Since this is a sterile procedure, complete aseptic technique is carried out.

Following such an examination, most patients prefer to remain in bed for the rest of the day. If there is any pain, a sedative may help. The application of a hot-water bottle to the lower abdomen is soothing. Fluids should be taken liberally. Occasionally following a cystoscopic examination the patient may have urinary retention. Hot sitz baths and relaxant medications are helpful.

Needle Biopsy of the Kidney

Technical advances have made needle biopsy of the kidney a relatively safe procedure. Renal biopsy is useful in evaluating patients with renal disease from both a diagnostic and prognostic viewpoint. A pyelogram is done before the biopsy and the kidney is specifically located in relation to the body's bony landmarks. These measurements are transferred and marked on the patient's back as a guide for biopsy needle insertion.

Before the biopsy, the hemogram, bleeding, clotting and prothrombin times as well as blood urea nitrogen levels are evaluated. The patient is typed and cross-matched and several units of blood are held in readiness. The sedated patient is placed in a prone position and a local anesthetic agent infiltrated into the skin of the biopsy site. The biopsy needle is introduced just inside the renal capsule of the outer quadrant of the kidney. The biopsy is performed while the patient holds his breath after a full inspiration. After the specimen is obtained, pressure is applied to the kidney and the patient lies flat for 24 hours.

The nurse must be watchful for hematuria, which may appear soon after biopsy. The kidney is a highly vascular organ and approximately one fourth of the entire cardiac output passes through it in about 1 minute. The passage of the biopsy needle lacerates the kidney capsule and bleeding can occur in the perirenal space. Usually the bleeding subsides on its own, but a large amount of blood can accumulate in this space in a short period of time without noticeable signs until cardiovascular collapse is evident. Therefore all urine voided by the patient is scrutinized for evidences of bleeding. Retroperitoneal hemorrhage acts as an irritant to the overlying posterior peritoneum, and produces abdominal pain, distention, nausea and vomiting. Continued perirenal bleeding necessitates blood transfusions. If the bleeding is life-threatening, a nephrectomy may have to be performed. The nurse should keep in mind that a delayed hemorrhage can occur a number of days after biopsy.

NURSING PROBLEMS ENCOUNTERED IN PATIENTS WITH UROLOGIC CONDITIONS

Emotional Problems

Conditions of the genitourinary tract may precipitate emotional stresses and problems. The patient may reveal feelings of guilt and shame when the external genitalia is examined and treated. Problems of incontinence may cause disgust and feelings of helplessness. Some patients are constantly uneasy over the possibility of an "accident," although others appear careless and indifferent. Operations on the male organs of reproduction are a threat to the masculinity of the patient—no matter what his age. He may react with anger and hostility to those caring for him, or his anger may turn inward and produce more than the usual amount of pain. Patients with urinary infections sometimes become depressed when they undergo prolonged periods of treatment. Anxiety in any stressful situation can produce urinary frequency and urgency. The urologic patient, as any other patient, needs to feel that he is respected as an individual and his problems are understood. He wants his questions answered, his fears allayed and his discomfort relieved. Reassurance is a part of nursing, and these patients may require more than the usual amount of reassurance, support and acceptance.

Retention

Retention is failure to expel the urine from the bladder. A person is said to have residual urine when urine remains in the bladder after voiding. The problem of retention may arise in any postoperative, acutely ill, elderly or bedridden patient. A patient may develop infection as a result of retention and may even have impairment of renal function. The nurse must be on guard for symptoms of retention, or they may be overlooked. The patient may not be able to void or may have urinary frequency, dribbling or straining when voiding. Also, he may have the sensation that he has not emptied his bladder. A patient with a long-standing prostatic obstruction may accommodate to this discomfort, and if it has had a gradual onset, he will not seek help until he is forced to do so by the problem of acute retention.

A mass in the suprapubic area that is either visible or palpable may be a sign of retention. The nurse should measure the volume of output in a given single voiding. Frequent voiding in small amounts may be indicative of urinary retention. Nursing measures, such as proper positioning to encourage micturition, offering fluids, placing the patient's hands in warm water, etc., should be used to assist the patient to void.

Frequency and Dysuria

The nurse often encounters the problems of frequency and dysuria (painful or difficult urination) in caring for patients with genitourinary conditions. Among the most common causes of frequency and dysuria are infections of the genitourinary tract. The patient complains of frequent urination accompanied by a burning sensation. To help the physician to find the cause and to eradicate the infection, the nurse must be specific in determining the time when the patient's discomfort occurs. When does the burning occur? Before voiding? During voiding? After voiding? Urethritis frequently causes burning during the act of voiding, whereas trigonitis may produce burning both before and after urination. Interstitial cystitis may cause urinary frequency and pain in the genital area. Dysuria associated with fever and chill usually is indicative of prostatitis or an infection in the upper urinary tract. Colicky pains suggest a stone or other obstruction of the urinary tract. Recording all available information associated with the patient's symptoms will help to assure a more accurate diagnosis.

Pigmenturia

Causes of urine of abnormal color or constituents have already been discussed (p. 543). The nurse should be alert for any abnormal appearance of the urine specimen.

Urinary Incontinence

Urinary incontinence presents many social and psychological problems. It may result from an inflammatory condition (cystitis) and be of a temporary nature, or it may result from a more serious neurologic condition (paraplegia) and be permanent. Usually, the patient's problems with incontinence lessen when he is making progress in other activities of daily living, such as walking. Most patients with urinary incontinence can be conditioned to gain urinary control through systematic habit-training or by the establishment of an automatic bladder. Such a program requires more nursing time than changing the patient's wet bed, but the rewards of seeing a patient lose his fear of embarrassment far outnumber the problems associated with his rehabilitation. The rehabilitation of a patient with urinary incontinence is discussed on pages 175 and 176.

Nursing Responsibilities

Observations

The nurse's role in the treatment of renal disease entails a number of difficult problems and responsibilities. To accomplish it properly, she must equip herself with a great many facts pertaining to clinical observation, pharmacology, therapeutics, medical technology, diet therapy, fluid balance and electrolyte metabolism, and she must, of course, be exceedingly well-versed in the practice of medical and surgical nursing. She must become familiar with the significance of a great many tests and with the methodology of these tests—at least to the extent of knowing what type of specimen is required in each instance, and how it should be collected, contained, preserved and stored. She must understand the significance and realize the importance of an accurate intake and output chart and daily record of the body weight as criteria for evaluating her patient's progress in response to therapy. She should understand the rationale behind each of several special diets. Drug therapy might involve the use of any one of several antibacterial agents, spasmolytic drugs, hypotensive drugs, anal-

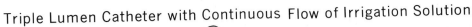

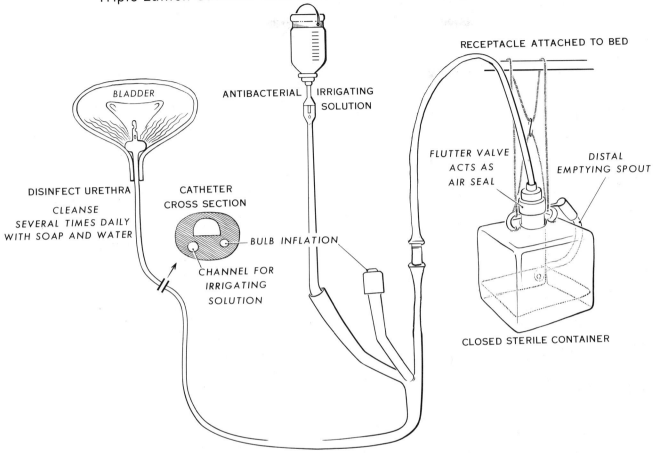

Fig. 25-2. Triple lumen catheter with continuous flow of irrigating solution.

gesic drugs, sedative drugs, opiates, digitalis, alkaloids and diuretics. Unusual psychological disturbances of organic, as well as emotional, origin will confront her very often, and her powers of clinical observation will be challenged by a great variety of symptoms and signs that reflect pathology in every organ system in the body.

Fluid and Electrolytic Balance

A major nursing problem in caring for patients with renal disorders is the maintenance of the fluid and electrolyte balance. The nurse must be astute in observing these patients and absolutely accurate in the recording of data. Every urologic patient has a fluid intake-output chart on which the nurse records all fluids ingested, regardless of their route, and the urine excreted. A 4-hour temperature chart and daily weight chart also are kept to assist the doctor in calculating the amount of fluid that the patient may receive. Other factors to be noted on the patient's record are complaints of thirst and signs of dehydration, e.g., excessive thirst, parched lips and tongue, dry and loose skin. Edema also should be reported if and when observed. Any directions regarding the intake of fluids or loss thereof must be understood thoroughly by the nurse and painstakingly explained in detail to other members of the team caring for the patient. In supervising intravenous therapy, the nurse is responsible for adjusting the flow rate in accordance with the physician's orders. In order to keep a check on the electrolyte balance, repeated blood examinations will be performed. The nurse must prepare the patient for this testing by explaining that these studies are necessary to help the doctor to plan the treatment of the condition and to be certain that the needed elements in the blood are maintained at a satisfactory level.

Maintaining Adequate Urinary Drainage

It is necessary for the patient with a disease of the urinary system to have proper drainage of waste products. A regulated diet and medications aid in establishing the desired chemical and electrolyte balance, whereas proper balance between intake and output aids in providing the necessary dilution and elimination of waste products.

Drainage of the urinary system is accomplished usually by the use of catheters, whether inserted directly into the kidney pelvis, the ureter or the bladder. The specific purpose for which a catheter is used, as well as the length of time it is left in place, establishes the criteria for selecting the proper catheter. The nurse should know where and why a catheter is used in each patient. Catheters come in an array of sizes and lengths and may have one or more openings placed in various positions near the tip. A catheter may be made of hard or soft rubber, woven fabric, silicone metal, glass or plastic. The tip may be opened or closed; its shape may be mushroom (Pezzer), winged (Malecot) or simply round and blunted.

Principles Underlying Catheter Management. No patient should be catheterized unless absolutely necessary. However, there are times when the catheter is a lifesaving instrument. Catheterization is indicated following certain genitourinary operations, in bladder obstruction, and when the patient is unable to void. Catheterization can lead to urinary tract infection. To safeguard the patient, the following points of care are essential in urethral catheter management:

(1) Strict surgical asepsis should be employed;

(2) The catheter should be smaller than the external urinary meatus to help to minimize trauma;

(3) The catheter should be lubricated well with an appropriate antimicrobial lubricant;

(4) The catheter should be passed gently and skillfully.

A bladder that has been overdistended has a weakened resistance and is easily invaded by bacteria.

When an indwelling catheter is necessary, a triple-lumen indwelling (3-way Foley) urethral catheter is preferred. This 3-way catheter allows urinary drainage through one channel, inflation of the bag with water or air through the second channel, and a continuous irrigation of the bladder, usually with neomycin-polymixin B solution, through the third channel. This antibacterial solution rinses the bladder and limits the multiplication of organisms; usually 30 to 60 drops per minute are sufficient. The catheter is attached to a *closed* sterile drainage system. If the drainage tube contains a drip chamber, this will serve as an airlock and prevent bacteria from ascending from the collection container. A drainage bag that can be emptied by a valve opening at the end of the bag is most desirable. If at all possible, no part of the drainage system should be disrupted or interrupted. It is most important that the area around the urethral orifice be cleansed with soap and water several times a day. Principles of physics having to do with gravity, fluid flow and pressure need to be reviewed in order to maintain adequate and safe outflow of drainage for the patient. Improper drainage occurs when (1) kinks or twists exist in the tubing, or (2) loops collect pools of drainage.

PROBLEMS AFFECTING THE KIDNEYS

Acute Renal Failure

Renal failure results from damage to the kidneys. It may develop slowly (chronic), or suddenly (acute). Acute renal failure, which is manifested by sudden oliguria or anuria, may be caused by acute glomerulonephritis; by shock, which produces tubular ischemia and impaired renal circulation; by chemical poisoning (carbon tetrachloride) or drug poisoning (salicylates). Following severe transfusion reactions, the hemoglobin filtering through the kidney glomeruli becomes concentrated in the kidney tubules to such a degree that precipitation occurs and may impair or halt the excretion of urine. Renal failure also follows burns, crushing injuries and infections, such as septic abortions. The kidneys become swollen and edematous, and the epithelial cells in the tubules may undergo necrosis.

The patient appears to be critically ill. He is lethargic with persistent nausea, vomiting, and diarrhea; his skin and mucous membranes are dry from dehydration; his breath may have the odor of urine. Drowsiness, headache, muscle twitching and convulsions are the central nervous system manifestations that are present in varying degrees. The urinary output is scanty and has a low specific gravity. All tests show depressed renal function; there is an elevation of the blood urea nitrogen, nonprotein nitrogen and serum potassium levels.

The kidney has a remarkable ability to recover from insult. Therefore, *the objectives of treatment are to remove the cause and then to maintain the patient in as normal a state as possible, so that the repair of renal tissue and the restoration of renal function can take place.* During the oliguric state the fluid intake is adjusted to provide *only* for the body needs. The nurse keeps a careful record of intake and output and the patient's daily weight. To maintain the fluid balance, the patient is given approximately 400 ml. of fluid daily, plus the amount lost from urine, vomitus, perspiration, etc. Since the patient is not excreting the end products of catabolism, there is an excessive accumulation of these products in the blood. Therefore, the diet given is low in protein and high in pure carbohydrates to aid in preventing ketosis and to minimize protein breakdown. Testosterone (25 to 50 mg. daily) also may be given to minimize protein catabolism. If the serum potassium reaches a dangerous level (6 mEq. per liter), cation-exchange resins are given orally or by retention enema to decrease the serum potassium.

Since sepsis is a serious complication, all measures to provide environmental asepsis are instituted. No one with a cold or an infection should be permitted in the patient's room. He should be turned frequently to help prevent pulmonary and skin complications. The nurse must watch for circulatory complications (pulmonary edema) that may develop from the excessive accumulation of body fluids. The elevation of serum potassium can produce cardiac arrhythmias and cardiac standstill. There may be a tendency to erythrocyte destruction, impaired red blood cell formation and platelet deficiencies. The patient should be watched for evidences of bleeding.

The oliguric phase of acute renal failure may last from 12 to 14 days and is followed by the diuretic phase. The patient begins to increase his urinary output until he is voiding 2,000 to 2,500 ml. daily. Blood chemistry evaluations are made to determine the amount of sodium, potassium and water needed for replacement. After the diuretic phase, the patient is placed on a high-protein and high-caloric diet. He is encouraged to resume his activities gradually, since he will have muscular weakness from excessive catabolism.

Dialysis. If the patient with renal failure does not respond to conservative methods of treatment, some method of dialysis may be performed to remove the waste products and to maintain the patient until renal recovery takes place. Methods of dialysis include *hemodialysis* and *peritoneal dialysis*. The main indication for dialysis is a high and rising level of serum potassium.

Hemodialysis. Several types of equipment are used, but the operating principle of each is a cellophane membrane placed between the patient's blood and a wash solution. The cellophane membrane has pores similar to those of the glomerular capillaries. Blood is

Peritoneal Dialysis Flow Sheet

DATE & TIME	SOLUTIONS & ADDITIVES	START	STOP	IN	OUT	BALANCE	CLINICAL EVALUATION
3/12 9 a.m.	2000 ml. Inpersol 1.5%	✓					B.P. 130/80. P. regular ⅌ of good
9²⁰	c̄ 8 mEq. KCl + 100 U Heparin		✓	2000 ml.			quality.
9⁴⁰		✓(drain)					
10	2000 ml. Inpersol 1.5%	✓	✓		2000 ml.	0	B.P. 140/90. M.S. 15 mg. I.M. for com-
10²⁰	c̄ 8 mEq. KCl + 100 U Heparin			2000 ml.			plaints of generalized abd. pain.
10⁴⁰		✓(drain)					Temp = 36.7 C
11 a.m.	2000 ml. Inpersol 1.5%	✓	✓		2000 ml.	0	Complaining of nausea. Medicated c̄
11²⁰	c̄ 8 mEq. KCl + 100 U Heparin		✓	2000 ml.			Compazine 10 mg. I.M. B.P. 132/90
11⁴⁰		✓(drain)					
12 noon	2000 ml. Inpersol 1.5%	✓	✓		1800 ml.	+200	Appears dyspneic. Resp. 26.—gasping.
	c̄ 8 mEq. KCl + 100 U Heparin						Dialysis stopped. Physician notified.
							Nasal O² @ 8 liters/min. started per
							order. Dialysis returns are sluggish.
							Pt. turned to Rt. ⅌ Lt sides c̄ sup-
							port to peritoneal catheter.
							Drainage facilitated. Color of returns
							appear pink-tinged. Specimen to
							bacteriology lab for culture ⅌ sensi-
							tivity.

Fig. 25-3. Peritoneal dialysis flow sheet. Heparin is added to maintain patency of peritoneal catheter. KCl is added to assist in maintaining electrolyte balance.

removed from the patient's radial or brachial artery and pumped through the cellophane tube, which is immersed in the rinsing fluid or bath of electrolyte solution. The nonprotein nitrogen retention products pass through the semipermeable membrane of the cellophane tube into the bath fluid. Thus the end products of protein catabolism, water and exogenous poisons are removed from the blood. The blood continuously recirculates from the patient through the dialyzing tube for a period of 4 to 7 hours. The temperature-controlled bath is changed intermittently to avoid the accumulation of toxins.

After this treatment the patient is watched for evidences of bleeding, as most patients are heparinized before and during dialysis to prevent the blood from clotting during the procedure. The cutdown site is observed for signs of phlebitis. The patient's vital signs as well as the volume and the appearance of his urine are recorded and reported.

Periodic hemodialysis for chronic kidney failure is discussed on page 558.

Peritoneal Dialysis. Peritoneal dialysis is based on the principle of diffusion of substances across a semipermeable membrane. In this technique, an appropriate sterile dialyzing fluid is introduced into the peritoneal cavity at intervals. The surface area of the peritoneum, which has a surface area of approximately 22,000 sq. cm., acts as the semipermeable membrane. With the development of nonirritating nylon catheters and improvements in commercial dialyzing solutions, peritoneal dialysis is fairly easy to perform. Peritoneal dialysis is used in renal failure to remove toxic substances and body wastes that are normally excreted by healthy kidneys. It is used in the management of patients with intractable edema, hepatic coma, hyperkalemia, azotemia, hypertension and uremia. The procedure can be intermittent or continuous. Although peritoneal dialysis can be carried out a few days after abdominal surgery, it is contraindicated in the presence of peritonitis.

Mr. John Callahan, a 45-year-old longshoreman, has been hospitalized for 30 hours with an obstructing staghorn calculus in his right kidney. Two years ago he had a left nephrectomy for a nonfunctioning kidney from multiple renal calculi. Since his urinary output was less than 300 ml. in a 24-hour period and his clinical condition was deteriorating, peritoneal dialysis was ordered to relieve the temporary kidney shutdown (Fig. 25-3).

Nursing Priorities for The Patient Undergoing Peritoneal Dialysis

A. RECORDING INTAKE AND OUTPUT VOLUMES INCLUDING:

1. URINE
2. VOMITUS
3. STOOL
4. DRAINAGE

B. KEEPING PERITONEAL DIALYSIS FLOW SHEET

C. WEIGHING PATIENT DAILY

E. TAKING VITAL SIGNS
1. LISTENING TO APICAL PULSE FOR EVIDENCES OF AN ARRHYTHMIA

2. EVALUATING FOR KUSSMAUL BREATHING

F. TURNING PATIENT WHILE SUPPORTING PERITONEAL CATHETER

G. ENCOURAGING DEEP BREATHING AND COUGHING

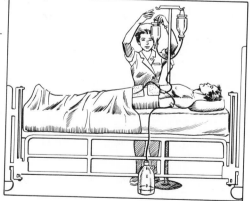

D. ENSURING INTAKE OF THERAPEUTIC DIET:

OFFERING SWEETENED FLUIDS AT PRESCRIBED INTERVALS

ASSISTING WITH ORAL HYGIENE MEASURES

H. ASSESSING PATIENTS SYMPTOMS AND BEHAVIOR:

WATCHING LEVEL OF CONSCIOUSNESS

EVALUATING FOR EVIDENCES OF UNTOWARD DRUG REACTIONS

FIG. 25-4. Nursing priorities for the patient undergoing peritoneal dialysis.

THE ROLE OF THE NURSE IN ASSISTING THE PATIENT UNDERGOING PERITONEAL DIALYSIS

Guidelines for Nursing Management

Peritoneal dialysis is a substitute for kidney function during renal failure. The peritoneum is used as a dialyzing membrane. The purposes of this therapy are to:

1. Aid in the removal of toxic substances and metabolic wastes;
2. Remove excessive body fluid;
3. Assist in regulating the fluid balance of the body.

Nursing Actions	Rationale
Prepare the patient emotionally and physically for the procedure.	Nursing support is offered by explaining procedural mechanics, providing opportunity for the patient to ask questions, allowing him to verbalize his feelings, and giving expert physical care.
Secure a signed operative permit.	
Weigh the patient before dialysis and every 24 hours thereafter, preferably on an in-bed scale.	The weight at the beginning of the procedure serves as a baseline of information. Daily weight is helpful in assessing the state of hydration.
Take temperature, pulse, respiration and blood pressure readings prior to dialysis.	A knowledge of the vital signs at the beginning of dialysis is necessary for comparing subsequent changes in vital signs.
Have the patient empty his bladder.	If the bladder is empty there is less likelihood of perforating it when the trocar is introduced into the peritoneum.
Make the patient comfortable in a supine position.	
The following is a brief resumé of insertion of the peritoneal catheter, which is done under strict asepsis.	
The abdomen is prepared surgically and the skin and subcutaneous tissues are infiltrated with a local anesthetic.	A surgical preparation of the skin minimizes or eliminates surface bacteria and decreases the possibility of wound contamination and infection.
A small midline stab wound is made 3 to 10 cm. below the umbilicus.	The midline area is relatively avascular.
The trocar is inserted through the incision with the stylet in place.	
The patient is requested to raise his head from the pillow after the trocar is introduced.	This maneuver puts the abdominal wall under tension and permits easier penetration of the trocar without danger of injury to intra-abdominal contents.
When the peritoneum is punctured, the trocar is directed toward the left side of the pelvis. The stylet is removed, and the catheter is inserted through the trocar and maneuvered into position. After removal of the trocar, the skin is closed with a purse string suture that is looped around the catheter. A sterile dressing is placed around the catheter.	
Take blood pressure and pulse every 15 minutes during the first exchange and every hour thereafter.	A drop in blood pressure may indicate excessive fluid loss from the glucose concentrations of the dialyzing solutions. The pulse is monitored for signs of arrhythmias. Changes in the vital signs may indicate impending shock or overhydration.
Take patient's temperature every 4 hours, especially after catheter removal.	An infection is more apt to become evident after dialysis has been discontinued.

THE ROLE OF THE NURSE IN ASSISTING THE PATIENT
UNDERGOING PERITONEAL DIALYSIS (*Continued*)

Nursing Actions	Rationale
Connect the catheter to the Y-tubing and allow 2 liters of warmed (40° C.) dialyzing solution to run in rapidly (10 to 20 minutes).	The solution is warmed to body temperature for patient comfort and to prevent abdominal pain. The inflow solution should flow in a steady stream. If this does not occur, it may indicate displacement of the catheter or occlusion by a blood clot.
Allow the fluid to remain in the peritoneal cavity for the prescribed time period (30 to 45 min.). Prepare the next exchange while the fluid is in the peritoneal cavity.	In order to remove potassium, urea, and other waste materials, the solution must be in the peritoneal cavity for the prescribed time period.
Unclamp the outflow tube. Drainage should take approximately 20 minutes, although the time varies with each patient.	The outflow drainage should run by gravity in a free-flowing stream. A closed sterile connecting system is desirable to prevent ascending infection.
If the fluid is not draining properly, apply firm pressure using both hands. Move the patient from side to side to facilitate removal of peritoneal drainage.	
When the outflow drainage ceases to run, clamp off the drainage tube, and infuse the next exchange.	The amount of drainage should closely approximate or be slightly more than the amount administered.
The process is repeated until the blood chemistry levels approach normal. The usual time is 24 to 36 hours, but patients with high urea blood levels may require much longer periods. The catheter may be left in situ and the dialysis done intermittently. (New administration sets are used every 4 to 6 exchanges.)	
Heparin and an antibiotic may be added to an exchange when ordered.	The addition of heparin prevents fibrin clots from occluding the catheter. An antibiotic is used as a prophylaxis against infection.
Promote patient comfort during dialysis: 1. Give frequent back care and massage pressure areas. 2. Change the dressing around the catheter, using *strict* asepsis.	The patient becomes fatigued during prolonged periods of dialysis.
Observe the patient for the following: 1. Respiratory difficulty	This is caused by pressure from the fluid in the peritoneal cavity. In severe respiratory difficulty, the fluid from the peritoneal cavity should be drained immediately and the physician notified.
2. Severe abdominal pain (usually occurs at end of inflow or outflow period)	Pain may be caused by the dialyzing solution not being at body temperature, incomplete drainage of solution, or as a forewarning of possible peritoneal infection. If severe pain persists, 10 ml. of 0.5 per cent procaine may be instilled through the dialysis tubing immediately before each exchange.
3. Bleeding	A small amount of bleeding around the catheter is not significant if it does not persist. During the first few exchanges, blood-tinged fluid from subcutaneous bleeding is not uncommon. The outflow drainage is usually straw-colored.

THE ROLE OF THE NURSE IN ASSISTING THE PATIENT
UNDERGOING PERITONEAL DIALYSIS (*Continued*)

Nursing Actions	Rationale
4. Shock	Symptoms of shock may occur due to excessive fluid loss. If a sudden drop in blood pressure occurs, drain the peritoneal cavity, clamp the tubing and notify the physician.
5. Protein loss	There may be a significant protein loss, because most serum proteins pass through the peritoneal membrane during dialysis. Serum albumin concentration determinations are done frequently throughout the dialysis.
6. Leakage	If leakage occurs around the catheter, change the dressing frequently, and use sterile plastic drapes to prevent contamination.

Keep accurate records (see Fig. 25-3):
1. Amount of solution infused and recovered
2. Exact time of beginning and ending of each infusion
3. Fluid balance
4. Number of exchanges
5. Medications added to dialyzing solution
6. Pre- and post-dialysis weight of patient
7. Assessment of patient's condition

Chronic Renal Failure (Uremia)

Every nurse should be acquainted with the characteristic signs of renal failure, including the early signs. Although sometimes its onset is sudden, in the majority of patients it begins with one or more of a group of symptoms—lethargy, headache, drowsiness, vomiting, restlessness, mental wandering, foul breath, etc.—which may persist for weeks. If active treatment is begun then, the renal failure may disappear. Otherwise, these symptoms become more marked, and others appear: the patient gradually or suddenly becomes increasingly more and more drowsy; the respiration becomes Cheyne-Stokes in character; a deep coma develops, often with convulsions, which may be mere muscle twitchings or severe spasms quite similar to those of epilepsy. A white powdery substance, composed chiefly of urates, appears on the skin, the "uremic frost." Unless treatment is successful, death soon follows.

Treatment and Nursing Care. The treatment and nursing care of renal failure should be prompt and vigorous; therefore, the nurse must report immediately any signs that she might observe. By the administration of sodium chloride intravenously (approximately 8 gm. daily by mouth or the equivalent in parenterally administered fluid), an attempt is made to maintain the alkaline reserve, which is rapidly depleted by the accumulated acids not being excreted normally; by

means of encouraging fluids and intravenous hypertonic glucose solution an attempt is made to stimulate diuresis. However, fluid and salt intake may be restricted to reduce the accumulation of fluid in the tissues. A careful record of intake and output must be maintained, and any change in the urinary output must be reported immediately. These patients should have very special protection from infections. No one should be allowed contact with a patient who has the slightest indication of an upper respiratory infection. This first sign of a cold, or even a suspicion on the part of the patient that he might be acquiring a cold, should be reported at once. All usual nursing measures should be carried out meticulously, especially those designed to protect him from chilling.

Early evidences of cerebral irritation should be reported. These may vary from slight twitching or headache to delirium. The patient must be protected from self-injury during involuntary movements, and it is advisable to pad side rails which should be in place whenever the patient is not under direct observation. The onset of convulsions should be recorded, as well as their duration, course, extent and general effect on the patient. The doctor should be notified at once, and suitable therapy should be initiated. Magnesium sulfate injected intramuscularly or intravenously has beneficial effects both as a sedative for the central nervous system and as a diuretic. Lumbar puncture

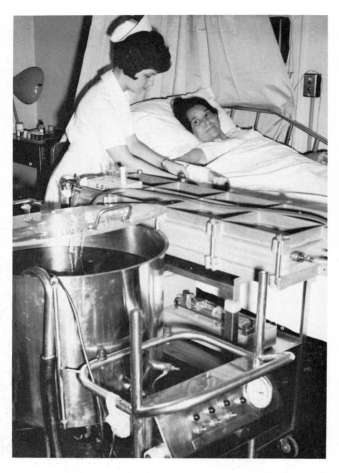

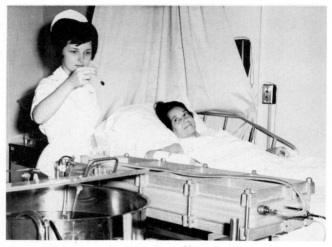

FIG. 25-6. The nurse checks the clotting time of the blood at hourly intervals. (Georgetown University School of Nursing)

FIG. 25-5. The nurse is caring for a patient with chronic renal failure who has periodic hemodialysis twice a week. The artificial kidney is the flat Kiil type. The round tank is the reservoir for the bath solution. Here the nurse is checking the tubing attached from the patient's cannula to the artificial kidney. The tubing must be exposed at all times so that the blood flow can be observed. (Georgetown University School of Nursing)

and draining the spinal fluid if it is under pressure will afford temporary relief. Such treatment may restore the patient to consciousness, and, if so, the immediate danger is past.

Periodic Hemodialysis for Chronic Kidney Failure. It is now recognized that patients with life-threatening chronic renal failure can be rehabilitated and live reasonably normal lives with repeated intermittent hemodialysis. Long-term dialysis is no longer considered experimental and dialysis centers are being established around the country as a result of recent Congressional appropriations. Patients are selected for the program who are free of irreversible complica-

tions, psychologically stable and well-motivated and who need dialysis therapy in order to live.

The technique of hemodialysis is the same as that described on page 553. However, a Silastic-Teflon arteriovenous cannula is permanently implanted in the radial artery and vein of the forearm; the leg is also sometimes used. The cannula is connected by a shunt that permits blood flow from one cannula to the other between treatments (see Fig. 25-7). This permits a ready access to the patient's circulation for intermittent hemodialysis. The patient, who usually lives at home, reports to the dialyzing center for his treatments. The shunt is removed and the cannulas are connected to tubes leading to the artificial kidney. The treatment may last for an 8- to 16-hour period once or twice a week, depending on individual needs. During periods of trauma or infection, the dialysis periods are increased. Although many patients work and live reasonably normal lives and remain surprisingly well, complications at the cannula shunt site can cause problems. Infection and clotting of blood in the shunt have been the principal causes of cannula failure, in which case the patient requires recannulization. The patient is taught to care for his own cannula. Using sterile technique, the area around the cannula is cleaned daily with an antiseptic solution and a dry sterile dressing is applied.

Since most uremic patients are anemic, blood transfusions are given regularly. The patient is maintained on a low-protein, sodium-restricted diet. The nurse in the dialysis unit has an important role in initiating treatment, monitoring dialysis, and supporting the patient during the procedure. Patients with virtually no renal function have been maintained for a number of years by periodic hemodialysis. Usually they hopefully anticipate a kidney transplantation operation in the future. Major problems with periodic hemodialysis programs yet to be solved include the heavy cost of securing enough trained personnel, facilities, blood and equipment. Estimates have been made that 5 to 20 million persons could benefit from periodic hemodialysis. Although this number staggers the imagination, one can appreciate the challenge involved in giving a person with chronic renal failure a chance to live. Recently, work has been progressing on developing a portable artificial kidney that would allow patients to be dialyzed in their own homes.

Renal Homotransplantation (Kidney Transplantation). Homotransplantation of the human kidney, although still in experimental form, holds great future promise in the treatment of kidney disease. Patients with irreversible chronic renal failure who are otherwise doomed to certain death may be considered for renal transplantation. This is a unique procedure, transplanting a kidney from either a living identical twin, sibling or parent or from a human cadaver donor to a recipient in terminal renal failure who requires support from dialysis in order to maintain life. Usually the patient's kidneys, which are nonfunctioning, are removed and he is maintained on a dialysis program until a kidney from a suitable donor is obtained. The donor kidney is transplanted retroperitoneally in either iliac fossa. The ureter of the newly transplanted kidney is transplanted into the bladder or anastomosed to the ureter of the recipient (Fig. 25-8).

The major limiting factor of this procedure is the body immunologic response that leads to rejection of the transplanted kidney. The recipient's body recognizes the new kidney as a foreign protein and attempts to destroy it. Rejection or threatened rejection of the kidney can occur several hours or several years after the transplant. The survival of a transplanted kidney depends upon the success of techniques that can suppress these immunologic reactions. In order to minimize or overcome the body's defense mechanism, immunosuppressive drugs [azathioprine (Imuran), prednisone, and actinomycin-C] are given. Because they suppress the immune response, i.e., the body's reaction to foreign protein, they also make the patient more susceptible to infection. Therefore, infection is a major complication encountered in a renal homotransplant program.

Postoperatively the patient is watched closely for signs of threatened rejection of the kidney. These include fever, swelling and tenderness at the site of transplant, decrease in urinary volume, rise in blood urea nitrogen and creatinine values and hypertension. Anorexia, malaise and a vague feeling of uneasiness may be noted by the patient. The nurse, of course,

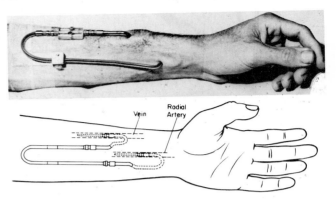

FIG. 25-7. (*Top*) The cannula, the semipermanent appliance in a patient's arm. The Silastic material is shown coming out of the patient's skin; one side is long and the other side short. The Silastic is connected to the Teflon joint, and the metal rings hold the Teflon inside the Silastic so that the cannula does not come apart. (*Bottom*) Schematic drawing showing the two Teflon tips within the vein and artery. The diameter of the beveled tips that are inserted in the vessels ranges from size 13 (⅛ inch) to size 18 (less than 1/16 in.). (Fellows, B. J.: The role of the nurse in a chronic dialysis unit. Nurs. Cl. N. Amer., 1:579, Dec. 1966)

records these signs and symptoms and reports them immediately.

The survival of a transplanted kidney remains a matter of concern to the patient, his family and his supporting medical team for many months. The psychological stresses to the patient are numerous as he copes with an uncertain outcome. This requires

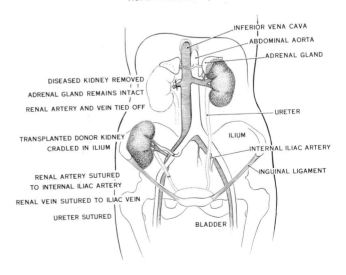

FIG. 25-8. Renal homotransplantation.

understanding and expert management of emotional crises by all concerned with his care.

Research is being devoted to solving the problem of rejection in kidney transplants. Tissue typing (identifying individuals with similar tissue characteristics) may provide a method of overcoming kidney rejection. The future goal is to overcome the body's natural defense mechanism by drugs or some other method.

The Patient with Acute Glomerulonephritis

Glomerulonephritis, or Bright's disease, refers to a disease in which the kidneys are seriously damaged and partially destroyed by an inflammatory process that originates as an immune response on the part of the kidneys. The stimulus of that reaction in most cases is a beta hemolytic streptococcus infection of the throat, which ordinarily precedes the onset of the nephritis by an interval of 2 to 3 weeks. It is assumed that the kidney receives its first exposure to the bacterial antigens in the form of toxins that are excreted into the urine. In glomerulonephritis, all of the renal tissues are badly injured, and they react to their injuries by progressive inflammatory, degenerative and healing processes. All the several renal tissues—glomeruli, tubules, blood vessels and stroma—are affected in every form of glomerulonephritis, but in each the tissues are involved in varying degrees.

All nephritic changes leave their scars. The process, once started, tends to progress, and the dangers of exacerbations are great. The striking clinical picture of late glomerulonephritis is less often the end-stage of one continuous process of long duration than it is the result of a series of repeated injuries extending over a period of years.

In acute glomerulonephritis the kidneys are large, swollen, fatty and congested. An exudate of blood plasma, red corpuscles and leukocytes escapes from the capillaries and infiltrates the kidney substance. The renal cells are so injured that they cannot do their work properly; many of them die.

Acute glomerulonephritis is predominantly a disease of youth. The cases that seem to have developed later are usually acute exacerbations of a quiescent glomerulonephritis already present. Acute glomerulonephritis in children usually develops in association with an acute upper respiratory infection, tonsillitis, scarlet fever or, indeed, any of the hemolytic streptococcal infections. It may appear also as a complication of infection caused by other organisms, particularly the hemolytic *Staphylococcus aureus*. The time relation is usually quite constant, that is, the infection precedes the first of the nephritic signs by approximately 2 weeks.

Symptoms. The symptoms of acute glomerulonephritis are extremely variable. Sometimes the disease begins suddenly, and even violently, with fever, occa-

sionally accompanied by a chill, headache, dizziness, nausea and vomiting, pains in the back, rapidly progressive swelling of the face and the feet—and such weakness that the patient cannot walk. The symptoms are seldom as definite as this, and acute glomerulonephritis is a good illustration of a dangerous disease that sometimes progresses to serious damage before the person suspects that he is sick. The child may feel merely tired, complain of headache and show only slight edema of the eyelids, while his urine shows every sign of a severe acute glomerulonephritis.

On the other hand, the acute exacerbations of unsuspected chronic glomerulonephritis may be mistaken for primary acute attacks. Although often uremic convulsions or sudden death may be the first indication of the chronic glomerulonephritis, yet the condition, which has been developing for years, may be manifested first by an acute attack that the patient believes to be his first. In the majority of cases, however, patients with acute exacerbations have from the first noticed that both ankles swell a little, that the face is pale, and that the eyelids are a little puffy. Otherwise, they may feel so well that they convince themselves that these signs are unimportant. Some of these patients have visual disturbances for a while, yet without evident lesions in the eyes; most develop a retinal hemorrhage or an albuminuric retinitis. In severe cases symptoms of psychosis, stupor, vomiting, convulsions and coma may develop. The arterial blood pressure usually is elevated.

The urine is scanty and bloody; there may even be none (anuria) for a day or two. Usually, however, the patient early in the disease passes from 50 to 200 ml. daily of a highly colored cloudy urine with a specific gravity between 1.020 and 1.025 (that is, low, considering the total amount) and with a thick sediment of red blood cells, leukocytes and all kinds of casts. This urine contains large amounts of albumin. A large percentage of patients have an increased antistreptolysin titre owing to a reaction to the streptococcal organism. There are usually rising blood urea nitrogen and serum creatinine levels. The patient may be anemic because of loss of the red blood cells into the urine and changes in the hemopoietic mechanism of the body.

As the patient improves, the amount of urine increases, whereas the albumin and the sediment diminish. Occasionally, perhaps oftener than we realize, the patient recovers entirely. Some patients become severely uremic and progress to a fatal termination within weeks or months, despite every form of therapy that can be offered; others, after a period of apparent recovery, insidiously develop chronic glomerulonephritis.

Medical and Nursing Management. The objectives of treatment are (1) to diminish the rate of nephron obstruction, (2) to decrease the metabolic demands on the kidneys, and (3) to improve kidney function. The treatment and nursing care of acute glomerulonephritis, or an acute flare-up of a more chronic condition, should begin with rest. This includes not only physical rest in bed but also the elimination of all worry and all causes of discomfort and restlessness. If residual streptococcal infection is suspected, penicillin is given. Evidences of cerebral edema indicate prompt spinal fluid drainage and dehydrating measures: parenteral magnesium sulfate acts as an excellent diuretic, as well as a sedative for the central nervous system, in patients with convulsions.

Pulmonary edema may occur as a result of fluid retention and cardiac failure, the basis for the latter in many patients being the rapid development of arterial hypertension, which subjects the left ventricle to a very real and unaccustomed strain. Its treatment varies in no essential respect from the routines applied in other types of cases, except for the use of mercurial diuretics, which are contraindicated in acute glomerulonephritis. The patient should be sedated, placed in an orthopneic position and digitalized, with oxygen inhalations supplied if necessary. The patient should be in a warm, well-ventilated room, protected from drafts. The sodium and the water intake should be reduced to a minimum.

Diet. In order to rest the kidney during the acute phase, the diet is low in protein. The amount of protein given depends upon the amount lost in the urine and the requirements of the individual patient. The intake of sodium is also limited, depending on the degree of edema present. The intake of fluids likewise should be restricted, with a maximal volume of 1,200 ml. per day permissible, depending on the degree of water retention, until signs of progressive recovery are evident. The chief source of nutrition in this early period may be foods composed largely of carbohydrates and fats. Thirst may be relieved by ice water, sipped in small amounts or furnished as a mouth rinse. With improvement in the patient's renal status, many of these restrictions may be relaxed, and his personal preferences and reactions may be heeded more closely in planning his diet with him.

Elements of Care. An accurate daily record of the patient's weight, fluid intake and urinary output is of value in estimating the renal function and as a basis for rational therapy. The total amount and the frequency of voided specimens are recorded faithfully by the nurse daily, and samples are saved for laboratory examination, which includes the determination of specific gravity, albumin and constituents of the sediment.

The condition of the skin and the surface membranes is important. Fresh air is desirable, but chilling definitely is to be avoided. Frequent massaging of the skin and changing of the patient's position in bed are recommended.

The edematous patient is given passive and active exercises to aid in increasing lymph and venous drainage, thereby decreasing the edema present. If there has been marked weight loss, debility or edema, skin care is of greater importance because of the susceptibility of such patients to decubitus ulcers. Oral hygiene never must be neglected. Regular elimination must be ensured.

An individualized therapeutic regimen is to be anticipated in these patients. The nurse must assist in securing the complete cooperation of the patient and ensure that treatments are carried out properly. She may be involved in special diagnostic procedures, including the P.S.P. urine excretion test, urine concentration, blood chemistry examinations, intravenous or retrograde pyelograms, cardiovascular function tests and others. She must also watch the patient for signs of complications such as cardiac failure, pulmonary edema or cerebral edema. These patients have their vital signs recorded every 4 hours and any significant change is reported immediately.

Convalescence. When the patient loses his edema, and the urine is free from albumin, casts and red blood cells, he is allowed to sit up, then to get out of bed (dressed warmly), and thenceforth to become increasingly active. However, he should avoid overexertion and exposure to cold for years. Should he contract a respiratory infection, he should go to bed and treat it seriously. A woman who has had glomerulonephritis requires special observation and attention during pregnancy.

Prevention. Prevention of glomerulonephritis may be a matter primarily of avoiding upper respiratory infections, as well as other acute and chronic infections, and of giving adequate treatment should they occur. It includes the control of the spread of these diseases by early reporting, isolation, use of prophylactic immunizations and antibiotic treatment, wherever indicated.

Social Aspects. The social significance devolves from the prolonged convalescence and continued ill health, which constitute economic problems. These patients have difficulty in securing insurance policies, for life expectancy in the nephritic group as a whole is materially shortened.

The Patient with Chronic Glomerulonephritis

Chronic glomerulonephritis is assumed to have its onset in the same manner as the acute form of the disease and to represent a milder type of antigen-antibody reaction, but one so mild that it can be overlooked easily. After repeated occurrences of these reactions, the kidneys are reduced to as little as one-fifth their normal size, consisting largely of fibrous tissue. Their cortex shrinks to a layer of 1 to 2 mm. in thickness, and in some areas it is gone entirely. The surface of the kidney is rough, because the renal tissue disappears in irregular patches, and bands of scar tissue distort the remaining cortex by contracting. The glomeruli suffer greatly. Many of them, and their convoluted tubes as well, disappear. The branches of the renal artery are thickened.

Symptoms. The symptoms of chronic glomerulonephritis are variable. Some patients with severe grades of this disease have no symptoms at all for a long time. They may discover their condition as the result of an application for life insurance, when the blood pressure is found to be elevated. Or it may be suggested during a routine eye examination, when vascular changes or hemorrhages are found. The first intimation others have is a sudden, severe nosebleed, a stroke, paralysis or uremic convulsion. Most patients merely notice that their feet are slightly swollen at night, but never markedly, unless an acute exacerbation of the nephritis is in progress. The majority of all patients have also such general symptoms as loss of weight and strength, increasing irritability and nocturia. Headaches, dizziness and digestive disturbances are common.

If these patients are examined carefully, it is likely that the heart will be found to be considerably enlarged, the arteries sclerotic and tortuous, the blood pressure high, and the radial artery resistant because of the arteriosclerosis. Epistaxis, hemorrhages from the lungs and the kidneys and into the retina and the cerebrum are common.

Later in the disease these patients do not "feel well"; they lose weight and strength; they have severe headaches, shortness of breath and dyspnea at night, suggesting bronchial asthma. Still later, Cheyne-Stokes respiration and the symptoms of chronic congestion of the gastrointestinal tract may appear. The heart dilates and fibrillates, and pulsus alternans and anginal pains appear, all of which indicate that the damaged heart cannot maintain an adequate output against such high arterial pressure. Various grades of edema develop, depending on the degree to which plasma albumin is decreased and on the severity of heart failure.

The examination of the eye grounds is most important. These patients complain of black spots before their eyes, flashes of light, dimness of vision and transitory blindness. On examination, thickening of the retinal arteries is seen, also retinal hemorrhages and exudates, and edema of the disks. The skin is dry, with a tendency to eczema and pruritus. Cachexia, with secondary anemia, is common. Later, cardiac edema, often confused with renal edema, and the symptoms of renal failure may appear.

Among the common symptoms of chronic glomerulonephritis are polyuria, frequent micturition, partic-

ularly at night, and a fixation of a specific gravity of the urine, that is, the urine does not show the normal variability of concentration due to what is eaten, drunk or done, but regardless of the patient's activities, it is all of practically the same composition. It never contains more than a trace of albumin, except during the occasional acute exacerbations, and this may be absent for weeks or be present only in the afternoon. Also, the urine contains so few casts that they may be difficult to find. Occasionally, red blood cells appear in the urine. Early in many patients the renal function tests indicate abnormal function. Eventually, there is evidence of marked renal decompensation by even the most gross tests.

In the so-called *nephrotic stage* of chronic glomerulonephritis the picture is striking. The skin has a pale, pasty color; often the whole body is swollen with edema, and almost always the face, the lower extremities and the dependent parts are so affected. The eyes are almost closed by the puffed lids, edema of the retina may interfere with vision, and the limbs appear to be twice their normal size. Often the finger can be pushed fully a quarter of an inch into the skin of the legs. This is referred to as *pitting edema*. Let an extremity hang down over the side of the bed, and more water accumulates, making it still larger. The fluid collects in the portion of the body that is in the lowest position. This is called *dependent edema*. These patients are truly "waterlogged." Fluid collects also in the abdominal cavity (ascites), which greatly distends the abdomen. It appears in one or both pleural cavities (hydrothorax, fluid in the chest); the patient is short of breath and must sit upright (orthopnea). Fluid may collect in the pericardial sac (pericarditis with effusion), and the patient is in consequence short of breath, cyanotic and has a weak pulse, especially during inspiration (paradoxical pulse). Repeated chest taps may be necessary to relieve the dyspnea (see p. 232).

Prognosis. The prognosis at this stage of the disease is poor. A few patients will improve, and they may enjoy fair health for many years. However, the great majority fail progressively and die in 1 or 2 years, often in a uremic condition.

Of importance in judging the progress of the disease is the weight, the red blood cell counts (there is danger of progressive anemia) and the blood pressure. One should watch also the blood urea nitrogen and phenolsulfonphthalein excretion curves.

Treatment and Nursing Care. The treatment of the ambulatory patient with chronic nephritis is entirely nonspecific and symptomatic, depending on the situation that presents itself at any given time. Thus, if hypertension is present, treatment is directed toward

Fig. 25-9. Commonly encountered male urogenital problems.

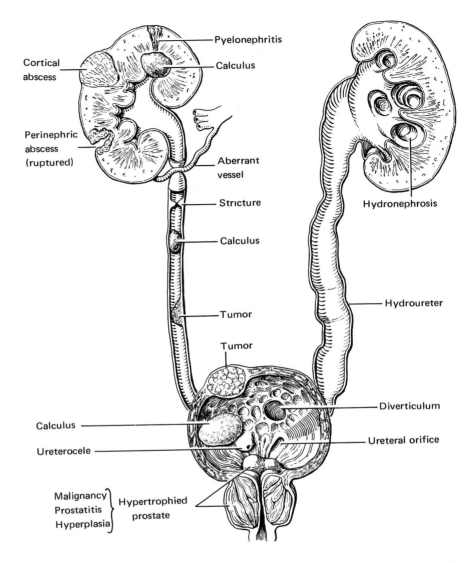

Pyelonephritis

Cortical abscess

Calculus

Perinephric abscess (ruptured)

Aberrant vessel

Stricture

Calculus

Hydronephrosis

Tumor

Hydroureter

Tumor

Calculus

Ureterocele

Diverticulum

Ureteral orifice

Malignancy
Prostatitis
Hyperplasia } Hypertrophied prostate

sparing the cardiovascular system; if chronic uremia is developing, treatment is directed toward readjustment of the diet and the fluid intake in an effort to maintain as normal a metabolic situation as possible. If there is apparent chronic renal tract infection, a possible factor in producing glomerulonephritis, steps should be taken to diagnose it and to treat it. This condition is apt to last from 10 to 15 years, and the patient naturally would insist on remaining active. Reasonable compromises must be made in the management of each patient; not only should the factors that are apt to precipitate acute exacerbations of his illness be borne in mind but also the total welfare of the individual.

Colds are to be avoided, and any infection of the nose, the throat or the mouth should be treated carefully. Climate is most important. A warm, agreeable

one may prolong life considerably. Moderate exercise in the open air is important. Hydrotherapy in the form of warm baths gives great comfort. The heart condition must be watched, and cardiac efficiency improved. Constipation should be avoided. The rule for this patient's life is "temperance in all things."

Treatment of patients with marked edema presents many difficulties. The patient is elevated in bed and made as comfortable as possible. He should be encouraged to drink as much fluid as he can eliminate, the weight being carefully followed for evidence of increasing fluid retention. Sodium restriction, however, is extremely important. The nurse should watch for all symptoms that suggest renal failure. Assistance should be secured in moving or lifting the patient so that he is protected from an accidental fall, and so that he may be relieved of any exertion in turning.

There should be no tugging or undue pressure on edematous areas.

If there is evidence of cardiac failure, digitalis is given to aid the heart. If anemia is present, the patient should receive iron, although little response will be forthcoming so long as renal failure continues.

If the nonprotein nitrogen blood level is normal, the diet should contain protein in excess of 80 gm. daily because of the theoretic value of a normal high-protein intake as a means of combating hypoproteinemia. Because of the proteinuria, the diet is high in protein to make up for this protein loss. The amount of protein intake depends on the degree of proteinuria present.

Nephrosclerosis

Nephrosclerosis is hardening or sclerosis of the kidney and usually is seen as a result of renal hypertension.

Malignant nephrosclerosis, as opposed to benign nephrosclerosis, though different in degree, merely represents the situation presented in the section on Chronic Glomerulonephritis. Patients with the malignant type progress rapidly to a fatal termination through the stages of albuminuria, increasing hypertension, failing renal function, and eye-ground changes and die usually within a few months. The factor responsible for this termination may be uremia, congestive heart failure due to hypertensive heart disease, or a cerebral accident. It occurs most commonly among people from the third to the fifth decade. So far as one can state at the present time, it is a generalized vascular disease that starts in the kidney and finally involves the entire vascular tree. It is always difficult to decide to what extent the vascular damage is responsible for, and to what extent it is a result of, the hypertension.

Patients that develop benign nephrosclerosis are most apt to be found in older age groups. These individuals rarely complain of renal symptoms, although for years the urine has a low and fixed specific gravity and contains a small amount of albumin and an occasional hyaline or granular cast. Only late in the disease does renal insufficiency appear. This type of renal disease is the result of a peculiar type of renal arteriosclerosis, which in a patchy manner produces wedge-shaped areas where glomeruli and tubules have largely disappeared, alternating with other areas where the renal units are practically intact—indeed, are able to function more actively than normal. The diffuse glomerular changes and the evidences of inflammation seen in glomerulonephritis are absent.

Hydronephrosis

Obstruction to the normal flow of urine produces a damming up of urine with a resultant back pressure on the kidney. If the obstruction is in the urethra or the bladder, the back pressure affects both kidneys, but if the obstruction is in the ureter, due to stone or kink, only one kidney is damaged.

The pelvis of the kidney (including the calyces) is the wide sac into which the urine is poured from the pyramids, and by narrowing to a small tube it becomes the ureter. The pelvis has thin walls whose inner surface is lined with the same type of mucous membrane as the ureter and the bladder.

The pelvis of the kidney and its calyces are distended by the partly dammed-up urine when the ureter is somewhat obstructed. If in such a case no inflammation is present and the fluid is clear, the condition is called *hydronephrosis* (Fig. 25-9). In order to cause dilatation of the pelvis of the kidney, the obstruction of urine must be gradual, partial or intermittent, but not sudden and total, for such would cause immediate anuria and therefore no distention at all of the pelvis.

Partial or intermittent obstruction may be caused by a renal stone that has formed in the renal pelvis but has dropped into the ureter and blocked it. The obstruction may be due to a tumor of some other abdominal or pelvic organ pressing on the ureter, or to bands of scar tissue resulting from an abscess or inflammation near the ureter that pinch it. The disorder may be due to an odd angle at which the ureter leaves the renal pelvis, or to an unusual position of the kidney, favoring a ureteral twist or kink. In elderly males the most common cause is urethral obstruction at the bladder outlet by an enlarged prostate.

Whatever the cause, if the fluid accumulates intermittently in the renal pelvis, it distends this and its calyces. If the obstructions are frequent, and the pressure that develops is high, in time atrophy of the kidney results, which causes the kidney to spread out into a thin cystlike shell. If, however, the pressure of the fluid is never very high, the kidney may not suffer much, although its dilated pelvis may almost fill the whole abdomen. In cases of hydronephrosis, the patient may scarcely know of his trouble, or he may have pains that are severe only when the fluid in the pelvis is under pressure.

Treatment. The treatment is to discover the cause of the obstruction and, if possible, to remove it. Sometimes the urine must be drained by catheter or by operation. If the cause is a tumor or bands of adhesions, removal is indicated. If the cause is benign prostatic hypertrophy, the prostate may have to be extirpated, partially or wholly, depending on the patient's condition and the degree of obstruction. When one kidney only is involved, and its function is nil, nephrectomy may be performed.

Nephroptosis

Nephroptosis, or movable kidney, is a condition found chiefly in thin, long-waisted women from 30 to 50 years of age. The pad of fat that normally surrounds the kidney is absent. The posture is usually poor and the abdominal muscles are relaxed, the result of which produces a weakness and a dragging pain in the loin. At times the kidney may sag so that it almost reaches the pelvis when the patient stands (floating kidney). This abnormal movability may produce torsion or kinks in the ureter. Acute pain, nausea and vomiting, and at times chills and fever may be produced by this obstruction to the ureter. These attacks are known as *Dietl's crises.* The attack often may be relieved by having the patient lie down with a pillow placed under the hips or by manipulating the kidney.

Treatment. The treatment of the condition is directed toward building up the general health. Belts often are applied to give abdominal support. One attack of Dietl's crisis warrants a complete urologic study (cystoscopy, pyelography, urography). If obstruction or infection is present from a ptotic kidney, surgical intervention may be necessary. The kidney is fixed in position by sutures in an operation called *nephropexy.*

Urinary Tract Infections and Pyelonephritis

It has been estimated that 3,300,000 Americans have infectious organisms in their urinary tract. Many of these persons will have no significant symptoms until they have far advanced kidney damage. There is some basis for every case of urinary tract infection. The majority are ascending infections, and the infection is favored by some mechanical defect, such as a congenital anomaly or a ureteral stone in the urinary tract, which produces stasis of urine. Permanent correction of this situation in many patients must entail more than mere temporary sterilization of the urine; it necessitates careful search for and, if possible, removal of the mechanical defect. Recurrent infection may destroy the nephrons, producing *uremia;* involve the renal arterial branches by fibrosis, producing *hypertension;* or cause bacterial invasion of the blood-stream, producing *sepsis* and death. Therefore, urinary tract infections are considered potentially serious.

Pyelitis signifies infection of the *kidney pelvis. Pyelonephritis is a bacterial infection of one or both kidneys that affects both the interstitial renal tissue and the renal pelvis.* The walls of the renal pelvis are lined internally with a mucous membrane that continues down the ureter to the bladder. When inflamed, this mucous membrane swells, its surface cells are discarded, its blood vessels become congested and may bleed, and pus pours out into the pelvis. When the disease is chronic, practically all this mucous membrane is destroyed, and then the pelvis is like any other abscess. Later, the ureter may become obstructed, and then the pus sac may become distended to large

size *(pyonephrosis).* Such an abscess may rupture, or the pus within it may thicken into a solid mass.

In kidney infections, the urine at first is cloudy because of the abundance of epithelial cells, mucus, pus and blood, and also, when its reaction is alkaline, because of the phosphate precipitate. When the infection is tuberculosis, however, the pyuria is acid. Some patients with pyelitis may on one day void a perfectly clear urine, since the ureter from the diseased pelvis is blocked; therefore, no kidney trouble is suspected. Then on the next day the urine may contain pus that has escaped from the diseased side. Should one kidney be entirely destroyed by disease, the other kidney, if normal, is quite able to do the work of both.

The causes of infection are many. They include infection by *E. coli* especially, or *M. tuberculosis* and other pyogenic bacteria. One must remember that bacteria (some of them quite virulent) frequently get into the body and are circulated by the bloodstream to the kidneys, which they sometimes, but not always, infect. However, the kidney's resistance to these organisms may be lowered by any condition that imposes an obstruction to its urinary drainage: a stone in the pelvis; a renal cancer; a twist in, or a tumor pressing on, the ureter; any congenital abnormality of the ureter or the bladder; or an enlarged prostate obstructing the urethra. Inflammation may start in the bladder and travel up the ureter to the pelvis. Pyelitis is most common in young girls and in pregnant women. Its greatest importance lies in the possible complication of this disease by pyelonephritis, wherein the infection spreads to the kidney, with occasionally serious results.

Symptoms. The symptoms of pyelitis and pyelonephritis vary greatly. In many patients they are spectacular, with high fever, a high leukocyte count and severe chills. Symptoms of frequency, slight dysuria, changes in urinary odor and appearance may indicate infection. Some patients experience pain in the back because of distention of the kidney pelvis, but this is rare. The large majority of patients are asymptomatic.

Diagnostic Evaluation. The diagnosis is made from repeated systematic examinations of the urine. The urine is collected by a midstream clean-catch technique. Bacterial counts of 100,000 organisms (colonies) per ml. of urine indicate a urinary infection. Successive urine cultures are also used to find bacterial species present. In all patients, the urine should be examined for tubercle bacilli. An intravenous urogram (IVP) detects abnormalities of function and shows any dilatations in the urinary system. Cystoscopic examination is also usually performed.

Treatment. The treatment depends on the cause of the infection. Any obstruction of the urinary system must be corrected, as these conditions will perpetuate the infection. If no obstruction is present, a high fluid intake is encouraged to prevent urinary stasis.

A urine culture is obtained to find the pathogens. The sensitivity test helps in the selection of an appropriate antibiotic. Throughout the course of treatment it is necessary to obtain repeated urine cultures and sensitivity tests, because a given antibiotic may lose its effectiveness.

Specific antibiotic therapy (Furadantin, penicillin, streptomycin, Chloromycetin) is continued until the infection is eliminated completely. The sulfonamides, with an unusually wide range of activity, ease of administration and ready availability, are employed extensively with this type of patient, the usual dosage being approximately equivalent to 1 gm. per liter of urine output per day.

Carbuncle of the Kidney

Carbuncle of the kidney is an infection of hematogenous origin that is caused usually by the staphylococcus. It usually follows a cutaneous boil or carbuncle and is characterized by fever, malaise, and dull pain in the region of the kidney. This type of infection, if recognized, usually subsides with chemotherapy and penicillin.

Perinephric Abscess

Perinephric abscess is an abscess in the fatty tissue about the kidney that may arise secondary to an infection of the kidney or as a hematogenous infection originating in foci elsewhere in the body. The symptoms often are acute in onset, with chills, fever, high leukocytosis and other signs of suppuration. Locally, there is tenderness posteriorly in the loin.

Treatment. The treatment consists of incision and drainage of the abscess by a lumbar incision. The use of suitable antibiotics is a standard procedure.

In the postoperative care the nurse should place the patient in the dorsal position. Because the drainage often is profuse, frequent changes of the outer dressings may be necessary.

Tuberculosis of the Kidney and the Genitourinary Tract

Clinically, tuberculosis of the kidney is uncommon, although microscopic lesions in the kidney are encountered not infrequently. However, such lesions cause few or no symptoms. The majority of cases with renal tuberculosis are due to extension of the infection to the kidney by way of the bloodstream. At first the symptoms are mild; there is usually a slight afternoon fever and a loss of weight and appetite. The process of tuberculosis generally starts in one of the renal pyramids; ulceration into the kidney pelvis follows; the germs are carried down with the urine into the bladder; the bladder is likely to become in-fected, with destruction of the ureterovesicle valve following, thereby presenting an opportunity for ascending infection of the previously healthy kidney.

Tuberculosis of the lower genitourinary tract is almost always secondary to renal tuberculosis, the infection having been propagated downward. Tuberculosis of the female genital tract is not necessarily a complication of urinary tract tuberculosis, but in the male, tuberculous epididymitis and prostatitis are almost invariably preceded by bladder involvement.

Tuberculosis of the urinary bladder is practically never a primary infection but an extension to the bladder of tuberculosis of a kidney or of the genital tract. This disease gives rise to several small ulcers, the majority of them near the trigone. The symptoms of bladder tuberculosis are those of cystitis in general but with an unusual degree of bladder irritability and frequent hematuria.

Symptoms. The clinical picture of renal tuberculosis is that of pyelitis: a urine containing pus, blood and also tubercle bacilli, which may be discovered only through guinea pig inoculation of the suspected urine. Suggestive early symptoms of this disease are an increased urinary output that contains considerable pus and yet is acid in reaction (in nearly all other pyurias the urine is alkaline), and early and frequent renal hemorrhage into the urine. The symptoms of pain, dysuria and urinary frequency, when they occur, are due to bladder infection. Symptoms of bladder irritability (viz., frequency of urination, nocturia) are a later manifestation of the disease.

Treatment. The current trend is toward medical treatment rather than surgical. The treatment of a patient having renal tuberculosis consists of the combined administration of streptomycin, 1 gm. biweekly, para-aminosalicylic acid, 12 gm. daily, or 0.15 to 0.30 gm. of isoniazid daily, together with the measures previously described as applicable to tuberculosis in general. For extensive unilateral renal tuberculosis, nephrectomy is the treatment of choice.

The Patient With Renal and Ureteral Calculi (Stones)

Stones are formed in the urinary tract by the deposit of the crystalline substances (uric acid, calcium phosphate and oxalate) excreted in the urine. They may be found anywhere from the kidney to the bladder and vary in size from mere granular deposits, called sand or gravel, to bladder stones the size of an orange. Certain conditions predispose to stone formation. These include renal infection, urinary stasis, periods of immobility and dehydration. Persons living in the "stone belt" (Southeastern, Southwestern and the Great Lakes region of the United States) have a higher incidence. Certain stones (e.g., cystine and uric acid stones) are genetic and familial

FIG. 25-10. Stone being removed from the bladder by crushing forceps (litholapaxy). Under direct vision through the cystoscope, a grasping forceps is introduced into the bladder to crush the stone and enable it to be removed or passed through the urethra.

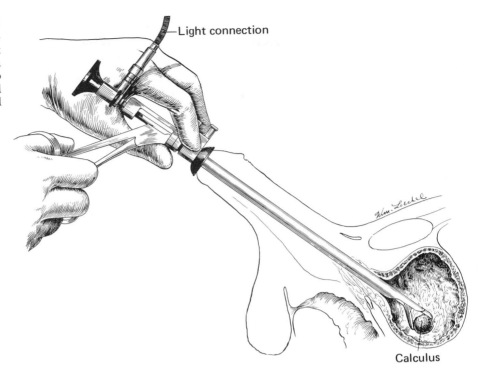

Light connection

Calculus

in etiology. Hyperparathyroidism is also responsible for renal stones in some patients. The majority of stones (90 per cent) are composed of calcium, with uric acid (5 to 8 per cent) and cystine (1 to 3 per cent) accounting for most of the rest. Mixtures of stones are also found. Most stones are radiopaque and detected by roentgenography.

When the stones block the flow of urine, hydronephrosis develops, and the constant irritation of the stone may be followed by a secondary infection, causing pyelonephritis, cystitis and so forth. Occasionally, stones in the kidney produce few symptoms; usually, however, there is a dull ache in the loin, and the patient passes increased amounts of urine containing blood and pus cells. A renal stone produces an increase in hydrostatic pressure and distends the renal pelvis and proximal ureter. Thus painful afferent sensations are initiated. Pain originating in the renal area radiates anteriorly and downward toward the bladder in the female and toward the testicle in the male. If the pain suddenly becomes acute, the loin exquisitely tender, and nausea and vomiting appear, the patient has an attack of *renal colic.*

When stones lodge in the ureter, acute shocking colicky pain is experienced, referred down the thigh and to the genitalia. There is usually a frequent desire to void, but very little urine is passed, and it usually contains blood because of the abrasive action of the stone as urine is passed. This group of

symptoms is called *ureteral colic.* The diagnosis is confirmed by intravenous urogram and/or retrograde pyelography.

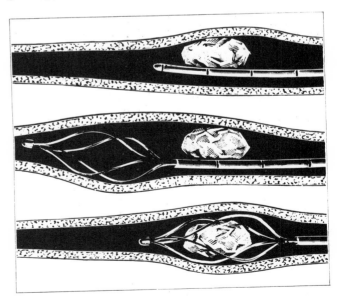

FIG. 25-11. (*Top*) A stone dislodger, inside a catheter sheath, is passed beyond or around the stone. (*Center*) Then the basket opening is controlled by the rod in the handle. (*Bottom*) Withdrawal by short to-and-fro movements engages the stone. (V. Mueller)

Most renal calculi will descend the urinary tract and are discovered in either the lower portion of the ureter or bladder. Urinary calculi must be removed to relieve recurring attacks of pain and to prevent the more serious secondary disease that their presence may lead to (hydronephrosis, secondary infection). The goal here is to preserve renal function.

If the stone is in the kidney, the operation performed may be a *nephrotomy* (simple incision into the kidney with removal of the stone), or nephrectomy, if the kidney is functionless due to infection or hydronephrosis. Stones in the kidney pelvis are removed by a *pyelotomy*, in the ureter by *ureterotomy*, and in the bladder by *cystotomy*. Sometimes an instrument is inserted through the urethra into the bladder, and the stone is crushed in the jaws of this instrument. Such an operation is called a *litholapaxy* (see Figs. 25-10, 25-11).

Medical, Surgical and Nursing Management. The basic principles underlying the management of the patient are to control the infection and relieve any obstruction that may be present. Infection and back pressure of obstructed urine can destroy the renal parenchyma.

Active treatment must be instituted for renal and ureteral colic. The immediate objective of treatment is to relieve the pain until its cause can be removed; morphine or meperidine hydrochloride will allay the pain. Hot baths or moist heat to the flank areas also are useful. Unless the patient is vomiting, fluids are encouraged, as this treatment tends to increase the hydrostatic pressure behind the stone and thus to assist it in its downward passage. Encouraging fluids also lowers the specific gravity of the urine. By keeping the urine dilute more solvent can be dissolved.

No time should be lost by the nurse in carrying out these treatments, because at times the pain suffered by these patients is so excruciating that shock and syncope result. A patient will be grateful for any relief. Cystoscopic examination and passage of a small ureteral catheter past the obstructive stone, whether in the ureter or the renal pelvis, immediately relieves back pressure upon the kidney and alleviates the intense agony. Whether this is done or not, the nursing care of patients with calculi require constant watchfulness for the spontaneous passage of a stone. All urine should be strained through gauze, as uric acid stones may crumble. Clots should be crushed and the sides of the urinal and bedpan inspected for clinging stones. When stones are recovered, the physician has them analyzed and then will prescribe a suitable diet to help to prevent further stone formation. Most stones consist of calcium oxalate or phosphate, and in such cases an acid ash diet may be given. Sometimes stones will cease growing simply by ensuring an adequate fluid intake and limiting certain articles in the diet that make up the main ingredient of the stone (e.g., calcium, phosphorus).

The lodgment of a stone in the ureter may at times cause complete suppression of urine, a condition termed *calculous anuria*. Unless this condition is relieved, renal failure develops, and death rapidly follows. If no urine is excreted within 36 hours, immediate operation is indicated. If the location of the stone is known, it may be searched for and removed; otherwise, the diseased kidney is incised and drained, and the stone is removed at a later operation when the patient is in better condition.

Patient Education. Inasmuch as urinary calculi may recur, it is necessary for the patient to understand this possibility and to follow a regimen of prophylaxis. This consists of maintaining a high fluid intake, avoiding infections, since toxins are eliminated by way of the kidney, and adhering to certain dietary restrictions. Food high in calcium should be avoided.

For patients who are inclined to develop phosphatic calculi, a limited amount of phosphorus should be ingested. To offset excess phosphorus, aluminum hydroxide gel often is ordered, since it combines with the excess phosphorus, causing it to be excreted through the intestinal tract rather than the urinary system.

Dehydration should be avoided because dehydration is a significant cause of renal stones. It is especially important to avoid occupations and sports (e.g., tennis) that produce excessive sweating that can lead to severe temporary dehydration. Patients should have their urine examined every 3 to 4 months and the urinary sediment evaluated for evidence of infection.

Renal Tumors and Cysts

Malignant tumors of the kidney may arise from embryonal defects of adrenal tissue in the kidney, hypernephroma, or from malignant degeneration of renal tissue. *The usual symptom that first calls attention to the tumor is painless hematuria.* Such a sign should be investigated immediately, for it may be the only early clue. Roentgen study usually confirms the diagnosis, and nephrectomy is performed if the tumor is operable. Radiation therapy is used in addition and as a palliative measure in inoperable tumors. However, renal tumors are usually radio resistant; chemotherapy and hormonal therapy are other treatment measures used. The patient who has had surgery for renal carcinoma should have a complete physical and roentgen examination of the chest yearly. These tumors may metastasize to the lungs or brain, and the patient's subsequent complaints should be evaluated with this in mind.

Cysts of the kidney may be multiple (polycystic) or single. Polycystic disease usually is congenital and involves both kidneys; therefore, it is only treated by surgery if infection occurs within the cysts. Solitary cysts often attain large size and are removed, and the defect in the kidney is repaired.

Congenital Anomalies

Congenital anomalies of the kidney are not uncommon. Occasionally, there is fusion of the two, forming what is called a horseshoe kidney. One kidney may be small and deformed and often is nonfunctioning. Abnormal vessels to the kidney may kink the ureter. Not infrequently there may be a double ureter or congenital stricture of the ureter. The treatment of these anomalies is necessary only if they cause symptoms, but it goes without saying that before renal surgery is attempted, it is important to know that the other kidney is present and functioning.

Kidney Trauma

Various types of crushing injuries of the loin may injure the kidney, producing tears in its structure. The kidneys receive half of the blood flow from the abdominal aorta; therefore, a fairly small renal laceration can produce massive bleeding. The appearance of blood in the urine following an injury to the loin is highly suggestive of an injury to the kidney; therefore, a urinalysis is always made.

The most common renal injury is simple contusion or small internal laceration of the kidney. In minor injuries to the kidney, healing may take place with conservative measures. The patient is kept on strict bedrest. Intravenous infusions may be necessary, because retroperitoneal bleeding may produce a reflex ileus. A sample of urine is saved from each voiding for laboratory analysis. The time voided and the volume should be recorded. Periodic hematocrits are also done. The vital signs are monitored to detect evidences of massive bleeding. When the kidney is injured sufficiently to cause hemorrhage of considerable amount, operation may be necessary. The damaged kidney usually has to be removed, although on occasions it is possible to repair it.

The Patient Having Kidney Surgery

Nursing Management—Preoperative and Postoperative. All operations on the kidney should be attempted only after a period of study and preparation. *Every effort is made to ensure that renal function is as good as possible.* This is the major preoperative objective. Fluids should be given in large amounts to promote increased excretion of waste products before the time of operation.

The preparation is described on pages 104 to 111. Usually, the incision is made in the loin, and the shaving should extend past the spine posteriorly and beyond the midline anteriorly, above the rib margin and well below the iliac crest. Apprehension should be allayed by gaining the confidence of the patient. Often the loss of a kidney may give the impression to him that he will be an invalid the rest of his life. This is not true in most instances, because normal function may be maintained by a single kidney.

The patient is placed on the operating table with a sand or air pillow under the loin of the unaffected side. The upper extremity corresponding to the side to be operated upon is extended to increase the size of the loin space. The lower extremity is flexed. The kidney is first exposed by an oblique incision, then delivered into the wound, and the appropriate operation is performed.

The general nursing care after operation is much the same as that after a laparotomy. Deep breathing, coughing and turning is especially essential for the patient having kidney surgery. These activities are very painful, because the incision is close to the diaphragm. The patient will voluntarily tend to splint his chest while breathing due to his pain. This in turn can lead to atelectasis and pneumonia. It is not wise to wait too long for pain control as the effect of the narcotic does not reach its peak for about 45 minutes after administration. Morphine sulfate and Demerol are usually given. If he is given the narcotic at proper intervals, the patient will be able to perform his coughing and deep breathing exercises more effectively. The patient may complain of muscular aches and pains resulting from his position on the operating table. Massage, moist heat and analgesic medications provide relief.

Adequate fluids should be given by vein, and by mouth when nausea ceases. An accurate intake and output chart should be kept. A normal diet may be given to these patients as soon as peristaltic activity is present. This is best indicated by passage of gas. Following such operations as nephrotomy, pyelotomy and ureterotomy, urine may drain from the wound for a time. This should not be mistaken by the nurse for hemorrhage. Often following these operations, drainage tubes have been placed directly in the kidney, the pelvis or the ureter; these will naturally divert the urine and keep the wound drier. The nurse should watch these tubes carefully after operation to see that there is no blockage, as from blood clot. Often following a nephrostomy, a surgeon will request periodic irrigation of the drainage tube. This is usually about 10 ml. of sterile saline, as the area to be irrigated is a small one. The nurse must be cautious in turning the patient on the operated side when a drainage tube is in place. A small pillow placed on either side of the tube makes a trough so that the tubing does not bend on itself. The character of the drainage and the number of milliliters eliminated should be tabulated every 12 to 24 hours. If the patient has more than one catheter, the output from each should be measured and recorded. Frequent changing of these dressings is necessary to prevent maceration of the skin and the offensive odor of urine that is uncomfortable and embarrassing to the patient and all concerned. The Montgomery strap dressing is conveniently used in this situation.

Occasionally, clamps are left in the incision following nephrectomy, because it may be impossible to ligate the renal vessels. On examination of the operative site the nurse may see the handles of these instruments extending from the dressings over the wound. In no circumstances should the clamps be dislodged. Obviously, such a patient is not permitted to lie on the operative side. Pillows placed strategically add to the comfort of this patient.

Following a nephropexy, the patient usually is placed in such a position that his chest is lower than his hips to facilitate the adherence of the kidney to its new position.

Drug therapy to combat infection may include penicillin and streptomycin. The nurse is expected to be able to recognize the toxic manifestations of these agents and to report such an occurrence.

When a patient who has had a kidney operation is ready for discharge, it is important that he know what his posthospital care should be. If he still has drainage tubes in place that require irrigation, as is true of a nephrostomy, he or some member of his family should be taught the care of this dressing and treatment. For postoperative nephrectomy, it is imperative that the patient refrain from lifting heavy objects for the first year.

Complications. *Hemorrhage.* Following nephrotomy and nephrectomy, the patient should be watched carefully for signs of hemorrhage. When inspecting the dressings, the nurse should remember that the ooze usually collects at the back and not on the anterior dressings. The constitutional signs of hemorrhage—an increasing pulse rate, restlessness and sweating—have been mentioned in Chapter 9. Because of the large vessels ligated, hemorrhages due to slipping of a ligature may be rapidly fatal. Therefore, the nurse should not hesitate to call the surgeon should the slightest suspicion of this complication arise.

Abdominal Distention. This complication occurs not infrequently after operations on the kidney and the ureter and is thought to be due to a reflex paralysis of intestinal peristalsis. In a weakened patient, the symptom may become very distressing, even causing embarrassment of the heart and respiration.

For relief of the abdominal distention, decompression by the use of a nasogastric tube gives rapid relief. The tube may be removed as soon as normal peristalsis and passage of gas are apparent.

Pain. Pain similar to renal colic is often a distressing symptom after operations on the kidney and the ureter. It is due commonly to the passage of clotted blood down the ureter. This symptom is usually of short duration but demands adequate doses of narcotics for its relief.

PROBLEMS AFFECTING THE BLADDER

The bladder is a muscular sac lined with mucous membrane, lying behind the symphysis pubis and covered above by peritoneum. It receives the urine from the ureters, and when it is sufficiently distended (the normal bladder capacity is about 500 ml.), sensations of discomfort are experienced. When the sphincters of the bladder are relaxed (voluntarily) urine is discharged through the urethra. This channel is short in the female, not more than 4 cm. (1½ in.) long, so that infection of the bladder by this route is not uncommon. In the male the urethra is much longer, passing through the prostate gland and the penis.

Bladder Injuries

Injury to the bladder may occur with a fracture of the symphysis pubis, and occasionally from a kick or blow in the lower abdomen when the bladder is full. The immediate result is extravasation of urine into the retropubic space or the peritoneum with pain, shock and an inability to void. What urine is obtained either by voiding or by catheter contains blood. If a rupture of the bladder is suspected, a cystogram will confirm the diagnosis. Early operative repair of the injured bladder is indicated. The patient has an indwelling catheter for approximately 10 days following surgery.

Cystitis

Cystitis is an inflammation of the urinary bladder that may be introduced from external sources or from the kidneys by way of the urine. A frequent cause of infection from an external source is unsterile catheterization. In hospital practice, cystitis occurs more frequently in women, probably due to the short urethra and to improper catheterization technique. The latter factor may be avoided by careful attention to the details of sterility and asepsis (see p. 552).

The cardinal symptoms of cystitis are 3 in number: (1) pain in the region of the bladder, which may be constant or occurs only during urination; (2) frequency of urination; and (3) changes (pus and often blood) in the composition of the urine.

Treatment. Pain and burning on urination may be alleviated somewhat by making the urine alkaline by the administration of sodium bicarbonate or sodium citrate 1.3 gm. (gr. 20) 3 or 4 times daily. Urinary antiseptics often are employed. These are usually sulfonamides (Gantrisin, specifically), streptomycin, tetracycline derivatives or chloramphenicol, depending on the organism. These measures, combined with a bland diet and a large amount of fluids, usually suffice to relieve the patient.

A urinary analgesic such as Pyridium helps to allay discomfort. Warm baths also are useful. If urgency is particularly troublesome, antispasmodics sometimes help.

When the cystitis is caused by a stone in the bladder or by some obstruction to the urethra, as a hypertrophied prostate or a stricture, an operation frequently is necessary to drain the bladder (cystostomy). This operation is discussed later.

The Female Patient With Urinary Infection

The female urethra is quite vulnerable to bacterial invasion, for in women, unless the personal hygiene of the patient is observed stringently, organisms migrating from the intestinal contents may gain ready entrance to the bladder and infect the urinary tract. If the infection remains confined to the bladder, it is termed "cystitis"; if the kidneys also are infected, the designations of "pyelitis" or "pyelonephritis" are applied, depending on whether the kidney pelves alone or both pelvis and parenchyma of these organs are involved.

Clinical evidences of urinary tract infection include urinary frequency, urgency and dysuria. Back pain also is to be expected if there is involvement of the ureters and the kidneys. Fever is a common and occasionally the sole clinical manifestation. Indeed, this is so often the case that the preliminary investigation of obscure fever invariably should include a search for pus in the urine, irrespective of the presence or the absence of symptoms indicative of urinary tract involvement.

Prevention and Nursing Care. This complication is almost entirely a problem of personal hygiene and nursing care. Although urinary infection in essence is quite simple, its requirements are very strict, namely, the complete removal of fecal material from the perineum following each defecation and during intervening periods the constant maintenance of thorough cleanliness of the perineum with respect to fecal contamination. It must be recognized that the techniques of perineal care customarily employed by healthy ambulatory girls and women may become totally inadequate during illness and bed confinement. Efficient lavage under these conditions is relatively difficult, even for patients who are not greatly incapacitated. Instructions must be issued by the nurse regarding the importance of thorough washing and the necessity for careful cleansing of the perianal region with soap and water after each defecation. Moreover, if there ever is reason to doubt the capacity of a patient to complete her own hygiene, the performance of this function must be undertaken personally by the nurse as one of the most important responsibilities associated with the care of the bed patient.

Urinary infections of the type described are ordinarily of brief duration, provided that there is no underlying renal disorder and no urinary obstruction, and assuming that the immune mechanisms are intact, and that repeated reinfection does not occur. Recovery is not invariably prompt and spontaneous, however, and the response of the infection to therapy may be very stubborn, particularly if there is an associated pyelonephritis.

Treatment. Therapy consists in the ample provision of fluids, i.e., 3 or more liters daily, unless this degree of hydration is contraindicated on other grounds, to assure a voluminous urine output. Specific chemotherapy with sulfonamides, streptomycin or another antibiotic agent, administered singly or in combination, is indicated.

Bladder Tumors

Tumors of the bladder occur commonly in older individuals. They arise as a cauliflowerlike growth in the bladder mucous membrane. Bleeding occurs when the tumor is traumatized by the contraction of the bladder in urination. A tumor is suspected when there is hematuria, frequency and dysuria, and the diagnosis is confirmed by direct examination of the bladder wall through the cystoscope.

Most tumors are small and are treated by electrocoagulation of the growth through a cystoscope. After irrigation of the bladder, it is distended with water or saline, and the coagulating needle is placed in the growth. Excellent results are reported by this method of treatment.

Bladder tumors may become quite large and obstruct the bladder neck or the ureteral orifices. The removal of the entire bladder is termed a *cystectomy*.

Neurogenic Bladder

The management of the neurogenic bladder is discussed on page 828.

THE PATIENT WITH URINARY DIVERSION

Common Methods of Urinary Diversion

The most common methods of urinary diversion are: (1) bringing the detached ureter through the abdominal wall and attaching it to an opening in the skin; this ureteral terminal ("bud") extends one ml. above the skin level and is surrounded by periureteral tissue in order to maintain maximal blood supply (Fig. 25-12); and (2) introducing the ureter into the sigmoid, which allows urine to flow through the colon

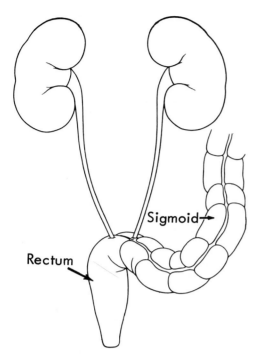

FIG. 25-12A. (*Left*) Ureterosigmoidostomy. This is performed for congenital malformations of the bladder (exstrophy of the bladder) and in some patients with carcinoma of the bladder and pelvic organs not involving the rectum. *Problems of the patient:* chronic and recurring infection of the urinary tract; reabsorption of urinary electrolytes; malignancy at the site of ureter implantation.

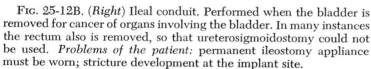

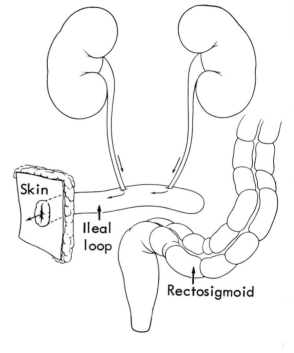

FIG. 25-12B. (*Right*) Ileal conduit. Performed when the bladder is removed for cancer of organs involving the bladder. In many instances the rectum also is removed, so that ureterosigmoidostomy could not be used. *Problems of the patient:* permanent ileostomy appliance must be worn; stricture development at the implant site.

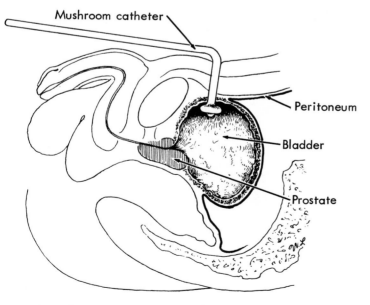

FIG. 25-12C. (*Left*) Cystostomy. Performed for obstruction of outlet of the bladder by prostatitis or prostatic carcinoma; following the removal of stones from the bladder; and in some cases of chronic cystitis. *Problems of the patient:* chronic infection of the bladder; stone formation.

FIG. 25-12. (*Continued on p. 573*) The major problems of the patient who has a urinary diversion operation. What are the underlying reasons for each of these problems? What measures may be taken by the physician to treat the patient? What are the functions of the nurse in caring for these patients? (Bloom, J., and Merrill, J. P.: Review of methods of urinary diversion, G.P. 23:91-97, 1961)

and out of the rectum (ureterosigmoidostomy) (Fig. 25-12). The advantages of the cutaneous ureterostomy over the sigmoid implant are several: the procedure is relatively simple from the surgeon's point of view, the danger of fecal contamination is eliminated, postoperative hydronephrosis is avoided, and there is an absence of an electrolyte imbalance from reabsorption of urine from the bowel. Still another advantage is the accessibility of the kidneys for irrigation and study. The disadvantages of cutaneous ureterostomy are the necessity of wearing leg urinals, the possibility of stenosis of the implanted ureter if catheters are not used continuously, the necessity of taking care of catheters if used, and the cumbersome apparatus and the ever-present possibility of leakage.

The ureters also may be transplanted to a section of terminal ileum, one end of which is brought to the abdominal wall as an ileostomy opening (Fig. 25-12). The loop of ileum is a simple conduit of urine from the ureters to the surface, and it is more convenient than a cutaneous ureterostomy, because an ileostomy bag may be used to collect the urinary excretion (pp. 484 and 574).

Nursing Care

The Patient With Cutaneous Ureterostomy. The deviations from routine care have to do with intelligent and satisfactory management of the mechanical and the physical problems involved and with strengthening the psychological adjustment of the patient, helping him to accept this permanent condition in as healthy a spirit as possible.

The cutaneous opening may be single, if only one ureter is involved, or double, if both are implanted. Various types of apparatus are available that are similar in principle to those used in the care and the management of an ileostomy. Skin care is essential, and the maintenance of a functioning aperture is vital. Because in many instances there is a danger of stenosis, indwelling catheters may be used. The patient must learn the sterile procedure involved in sterilizing and inserting a ureteral catheter. The important point is to position it properly: if the openings at the tip are inserted too far in the kidney pelvis, the catheter is beyond the source of urine and it will not drain. Likewise, if it is not inserted far enough, the openings of the catheter may be occluded by the wall of the ureter, and the catheter will not drain. A commercial apparatus is available in which a cap can be cemented to the skin surrounding the cutaneous "bud," and then the domelike covering is connected by rubber tubing to a rubber urinal worn on the leg. Specific instruc-

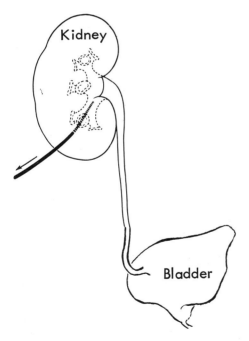

FIG. 25-12D. Nephrostomy. Indication for this is urinary obstruction in the lower urinary tract (prostate and prostatic obstructions, etc.) and in some cases of renal calculi in which the calculus is removed instead of performing a nephrectomy. *Problems of the patient:* chronic urinary infection; chronic pyelonephritis; renal deterioration; accidental dislodgement of the tube.

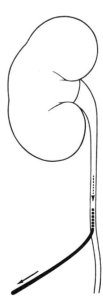

FIG. 25-12E. Ureterostomy. This is performed for stricture of the ureter and inflammatory obstruction. *Problems of the patient:* obstruction of ureter; ureteral stricture; periureteral abscess; leakage around appliance.

tions on the application and the care of apparatus are supplied.

The Patient With Ureterosigmoidostomy. Psychological preparation of the patient with bladder malignancy is important. The usual preoperative regimen is followed, and in addition the patient may be on a liquid diet for about 5 days preoperatively, so that the colon may be kept clean. Sulfathalidine or oral neomcyin sulfate may be given to lessen the number of intestinal organisms. The patient should be told that hereafter he will be voiding by rectum.

Postoperatively, a drainage tube may be in place in the rectum. Irrigations of this tube may be ordered at frequent intervals. Force never should be used because of the danger of introducing an infection into the newly implanted ureters.

Reassurance and encouragement should be a part of the care of the patient, for this is a new experience. When the rectal drain is removed, the patient begins to learn to control his rectal sphincter. At first, urination is frequent, and bedding may have to be changed. With patience, greater control is gained, and the patient will be able to ask for the bedpan "just in time." An understanding nurse can help this patient greatly.

The Patient With an Ileal Conduit (Ureterileostomy). Urinary resection in cases of cancer of the pelvis, or in other conditions in which the ureters become blocked, or in cases in which a total cystectomy must be performed often requires some form of urinary diversion. This can be accomplished in some cases by introduction of the ureter into the rectum or the sigmoid; or the urine is diverted by implanting the ureter into a loop of ileum, which is led out through the abdominal wall as an ileostomy (Fig. 25-12). This loop of ileum is known as an *ileal conduit.* It is a short piece of ileum that has been removed from the intestinal flow. The bowel continuity is obtained by anastomosis of the remaining ileum. Urine is collected in an ileostomy bag cemented to the abdominal wall. When the patient returns from the operating room, the ileostomy bag already has been applied. This is connected to a drainage tube and bottle. The nurse should measure and record the urinary volume hourly. The ileostomy appliance usually remains in place as long as it is watertight, and then it is changed. Eventually, a permanent rubber or plastic bag is used. The skin around the stoma may become irritated due to the secretion from the ileum or to urinary leakage. Therefore, it is important that the nurse inspect the application of the bag to be sure this irritation does not occur (p. 485).

The patient with constant urinary drainage utilizes the same principles of care in applying, wearing and maintaining an appliance as the ileostomy patient does (see p. 485 for specific nursing management measures). The patient may excrete a fairly large amount of mucus with his urine, owing to the urine irritating the mucous glands of the intestine. The patient should be reassured that this is a normal occurrence for one who has an ileal conduit.

The remaining care of the patient is essentially the same as for any intestinal resection (see pp. 496-497). As soon as bowel function resumes (as indicated by the passage of gas), the patient may have food and fluids by mouth, but until that time fluids and electrolytes are given intravenously.

The Patient With a Cystostomy. An operation whereby the bladder may be drained through an abdominal wound (suprapubic cystostomy) is indicated in the treatment of diseases causing obstruction of the urethra (prostatic hypertrophy, occasionally stricture) and for the removal of calculi and tumors from the bladder (Fig. 25-12).

In preparation for the operation the abdomen and the upper thighs should be shaved. This is the one abdominal operation in which it is not necessary to have the patient void immediately before operation. The patients often are aged and weakened by disease; hence, the operation frequently is performed under local or spinal anesthesia. The bladder is filled with fluid to carry the peritoneum upward, and the patient is placed in the Trendelenburg position. An opening is made into the bladder below the peritoneum, and the appropriate operation is performed within the bladder. Then a drainage tube is inserted and the bladder wall is closed round it.

The postoperative nursing care has much to do with the success of the operation. Especially in cases of prostatic hypertrophy, the patients are usually aged and rather poor operative risks. The vital signs are evaluated frequently until they are stabilized. Shock is not an uncommon postoperative complication. Fluids must be given by vein and by mouth until at least 2,500 to 3,000 ml. are taken daily. The diet should be soft at first and increased accordingly. Since older patients are prone to pulmonary complications, the nurse should turn the patient frequently from side to side and urge him to take deep breaths every hour. After 24 hours the head and the shoulders should be elevated. Skin care is an important adjunct to good nursing care in these patients. Frequent washing of the skin with soap and water and the application of petrolatum or zinc oxide ointment prevents excoriation.

The chief attention of the nurse, of course, should be directed toward keeping the patient and the bed dry. When a tube has been inserted into the bladder, it may be attached to a bottle at the side of the bed. With constant suction, the urine that collects in the bladder is removed and caught in a drainage bottle. This helps to prevent odors and keeps the patient dry, but it must be inspected frequently by the nurse.

Convalescence. A cystostomy may be temporary or permanent, depending on the original purpose of the operation. The patient often is sensitive about the "bottle and tube" that he carries with him. If he is with similar patients, the inconvenience and the awkwardness do not seem so great. However, if he is by himself or on a unit where he is the only one with such a device, diversional activity should be sought that will meet his particular interests. Odors are not a problem if the drainage tubing and the bottle are changed daily. They must be cleaned thoroughly with soap and water.

For the patient who is going home with a cystostomy, the use of a rubber or a plastic urinal is effective. This is an oval-shaped bladder. To one end of the bag a rubber or a plastic tubing is attached that can be connected to the drainage tube in the patient. The other end has a screw cap. The bag can be strapped to the inner aspect of the thigh or the calf in male patients or to the thigh in female patients. When it fills, it is quite easy to empty into the toilet by unscrewing the cap. The patient should be instructed regarding adequate cleaning of the bag with soap and water to prevent odors. At night he may use the drainage bottle at the side of the bed as the collecting unit; during this time the bag can be exposed to fresh air.

PROBLEMS AFFECTING THE URETHRA

Caruncle

A caruncle is a small, red, extremely vascular polypoid growth situated just within, and protruding from, the external urethral meatus of women, probably the result of long-continued infection or irritation of the mucosa at this point. On rare occasions it causes no subjective symptoms. As a rule it is acutely sensitive, causing a local burning pain exaggerated by exertion and frequency of urination, which is exquisitely painful. The caruncle should be removed by fulguration, clamp and cautery or excision.

Urethritis

Urethritis, or inflammation of the urethra, in the majority of patients is due to gonorrhea (see Chap. 37). Nongonorrheal urethritis may represent the extension of a chronic pyogenic prostatitis or follow direct injury to the urethra by instrumentation. (Never is it produced by strains, injuries or soiled toilet seats.) Nongonorrheal urethritis generally heals promptly, leaving no sequelae.

The symptoms of acute gonorrheal urethritis are frequency, burning urination, and, a discharge, which in the male is abundant and creamy but in the female, relatively scanty. In the discharge of acute cases the gonococcus easily is demonstrated; but in the very scanty discharge of more chronic infections this organism may be difficult to find, although it is always present.

The gonorrheal infection always involves the tissues around the urethra, often causing stricture, and the glands about the external genitalia, causing abscesses. It may spread to the bladder, causing cystitis; to the cervix of the uterus; to the fallopian tubes, causing the great majority of cases of pelvic abscess; and occasionally to the peritoneal cavity, giving rise to peritonitis. The gonococcus carried by the bloodstream causes one type of infectious arthritis, one form of acute bacterial endocarditis, and certain skin diseases.

Urethral Strictures

A urethral stricture is a narrowing of the lumen of the urethra owing to scar tissue formation and contraction. Strictures result from inflammation or trauma of the urethra. They produce symptoms of obstruction and retention of urine. One of the most common causes of inflammation is that produced by the gonococcus organism. It is important for the nurse to know if the disease is in its infectious stage, and if it is, to take the necessary precautions.

Treatment. The treatment may be palliative (gradual dilatation of the narrowed area with metal sounds) or operative (incision of the stricture—urethrotomy). If the stricture has become so small as to prevent the passage of a catheter, several small filiform bougies are used in search of the opening. When one bougie passes beyond the stricture into the bladder, it is fixed in place, and urine will drain from the bladder beside it. The stricture then can be dilated to larger size by the passage of a larger sound following behind the filiform as a guide. Sometimes a suprapubic cystostomy must be performed. The postoperative treatment of these patients is similar to that described for cystostomy, page 574.

PROBLEMS RELATED TO THE MALE REPRODUCTIVE SYSTEM

In the male, several organs serve both as parts of the urinary tract and of the reproductive system. Disease of these organs may produce functional abnormalities of either or both systems. For this reason diseases of the entire reproductive system in the male usually are treated by the urologist.

Anatomy and Physiology

The structures included in the male reproductive system are the testes, the vas deferens and the seminal vesicles, the penis, and certain accessory glands, such as the prostate gland and Cowper's gland. The testes are formed in embryonal life within the abdominal cavity near the kidney. During the last month of fetal life, they descend posterior to the peritoneum, to pierce the abdominal wall in the groin and to progress along the inguinal canal into the scrotum. In this descent, they are accompanied by blood vessels, lymphatics, nerves and ducts, which, along with supporting and investing tissue, make up the spermatic cord. This cord extends from the internal inguinal ring through the abdominal wall and the inguinal canal to the scrotum. As the testes descend into the scrotum, a tubular process of peritoneum accompanies them. This normally is obliterated, the only remaining portion being that which covers the testes, the *tunica vaginalis*. (When this peritoneal process does not obliterate but remains open into the abdominal cavity, a potential sac remains into which abdominal contents may enter to form an indirect inguinal hernia.)

The testes proper consist of numerous seminiferous tubules in which are formed the male reproductive elements, the spermatozoa. These are transmitted by a system of collecting tubules into the epididymis, which is a hoodlike structure lying on the testes and containing tortuous ducts that lead into the vas deferens. This firm tubular structure passes upward through the inguinal canal to enter the abdominal cavity behind the peritoneum and then extends downward toward the base of the bladder. An outpouching from this structure is the seminal vesicle, which acts as a reservoir for the secretion of the testes. The tract is continued as the ejaculatory duct, which then passes through the prostate gland to enter the urethra. The secretion of the testes is carried by this pathway to the end of the penis in the reproductive act.

The testes have a dual function. The primary function is reproduction—the formation of spermatozoa from the germinal cells of the seminiferous tubules. However, the testes are also important glands of internal secretion. This secretion is produced by the so-called interstitial cells and is called the male sex hormone, or testosterone, which induces and preserves the male sex qualities.

The prostate gland lies just below the neck of the bladder. It surrounds the urethra posteriorly and laterally and is traversed by the ejaculatory duct, the continuation of the vas deferens. This gland produces a secretion that is chemically and physiologically suitable to the needs of the spermatozoa in their passage from the genital glands.

The penis has a dual function of being the organ of copulation and of urination. Anatomically, it consists of a glans penis, a body and a root. The glans penis is the soft rounded portion at the end that retains its soft structure even when erect. The urethra opens at the extremity of the glans. The glans normally is covered or protected by an elongation of the skin of the penis—the foreskin—which may be reflected to expose the glans. The body of the penis is composed of erectile tissues that contain numerous blood vessels that may become distended during sexual excitement. Through it passes the urethra, which extends from the bladder through the prostate to the end of the penis.

Congenital Malformations. Many disturbances of normal growth may occur. The most common is a failure of the testes to descend into the scrotum. This condition is called *cryptorchism*. The testes may remain within the abdomen, may pass through the abdominal wall but be arrested in the inguinal canal, or may pass through the external abdominal ring but not descend into the scrotum. In almost all cases of undescended testicle, there is a potential if not a concomitant indirect inguinal hernia. In addition, the testicle not in the normal position may atrophy, and there is some evidence that such an organ may undergo malignant degeneration. In many boys the testicle may descend spontaneously shortly after puberty, and in other instances the descent may be brought about by hormonal therapy. In patients in whom the testicle does not descend normally, an operation often is performed to place it in the scrotum (p. 577).

Failure of the urethra to form normally in the penis is known as *hypospadias* when the urethral opening is on the lower wall of the penis; when it is a groove on its upper surface, the condition is called *epispadias*. These anatomic abnormalities may be repaired by various types of plastic operations. Unfortunately, all too often 2 or more attempts at repair are necessary, but frequently with good results.

Psychosocial Aspects of Care

The patient with a genitourinary problem deserves understanding and a dignified approach by the nurse in all her contacts with him. In many instances he is sensitive and embarrassed, and sometimes he even possesses a sense of guilt. His dignity, sensitivity and confidence can be maintained by the proper reponse and conduct of the nurse.

In caring for the male patient the successful nurse needs to know male psychology. She should be aware of the position her patient occupies in his family and community. Early in her contact with the elderly urologic patient, she should note all evidences of the aging process, such as hearing, chewing, habits and posture, especially in bed. By careful observation the nurse is able to determine his attitude toward life and toward his incapacity. Then from her assessment and evaluation she is able to know and to help him as an individual. At the same time she is equipped better to interpret the needs of the patient to the physician.

Conditions Affecting the Penis

Gonorrhea occurs as a result of an infection with the gonococcus, which penetrates the tissues of the urethra as a result of sexual exposure. The time elapsing from the moment of infection until the development of disease may be from 2 to 7 days, and sometimes longer. The infection produces a marked purulent, usually painful urethral discharge. At first the anterior portion of the urethra is invaded, but not infrequently the infection extends posteriorly to involve the prostate and to extend along the vas deferens to produce infection in the seminal vesicles and in the epididymis. The disease is diagnosed by the examination of a stained smear of the pus from the urethra. The gonococcus appears as a bean-shaped organism in pairs lying within the pus cells and staining in a characteristic manner (see p. 914).

Early treatment of the infection is most likely to prevent development of the complications of gonorrhea. It must not be forgotten that the transmission of the infection from the urethra to the eyes may produce a very marked ophthalmia. Penicillin prophylaxis and therapy have given excellent results.

Penile ulceration may be of several types, but because of the danger of chancre (syphilis), all lesions are considered to be syphilitic until proved otherwise. Diagnosis is made by a combination of history of the disease, a microscopic examination of a darkfield specimen removed from the lesions, and a blood serology examination. The treatment of penile ulceration varies greatly, depending on the cause of the ulceration. It is not started until the diagnosis is made.

Chancre is a firm ulceration that is the primary lesion of syphilis. It occurs as a result of sexual exposure. Local treatment usually is unnecessary other than a mild antiseptic and a protective dressing, the main portion of the treatment being confined to systemic measures that usually result in a rapid healing of the local lesion. Penicillin produces a rapid cure.

Chancroid is an ulceration produced by a mixed infection, usually associated with marked lymphadenopathy in the groin. Treatment often necessitates circumcision and cauterization of the ulceration.

Balanitis is an ulceration produced by a spirochete and a fusiform bacillus commonly found in the oral cavities. These organisms are largely anaerobic; therefore, the infection always occurs under the foreskin. Circumcision, cauterizing or oxidizing antiseptics frequently are used in the therapy.

Herpes of the glans penis begins as a small blister that produces secondary ulceration. This is not a venereal disease, and the ulcerations heal rapidly under protective dressing or with a mild antiseptic treatment.

Phimosis is a condition in which the foreskin is narrowed so that it cannot be retracted over the glans. It may be corrected by circumcision. The operation consists in the removal of the foreskin so that the glans penis is not covered. Many infants and adults are circumcised for hygienic or therapeutic reasons.

Carcinoma of the penis occurs in the skin of the penis and rarely, if ever, occurs in circumcised individuals. It represents about 3 per cent of all skin cancer. Local treatment or complete amputation of the penis may be necessary.

Conditions Affecting the Testes and Adjacent Structures

Undescended testis is a common congenital defect. The normal testis originates from embryonic tissue near the kidney, and as the fetus develops the testis moves downward into its normal position in the scrotum. If the testis does not descend, hormone therapy and/or surgery (*orchidopexy*) are employed to secure proper positioning.

In orchidopexy, an incision is made over the inguinal canal, and the testis is brought down and placed into the scrotum. To maintain proper position of the testis, traction may be applied to the thigh by means of a suture drawn from the lower end of the scrotum.

Epididymitis is due to an infection by pyogenic organisms or tubercle bacilli. It usually is secondary to prostatitis or infections in the seminal vesicles and the urethra. Any pathogens infecting the urinary tract may produce epididymitis. It may be a complication of gonorrhea. The infection passes upward through the urethra and the ejaculatory duct, and thence along the vas deferens to the epididymis.

The patient complains of pain and soreness in the inguinal canal along the course of the vas deferens and then develops pain and swelling in the scrotum and the groin. The epididymis becomes swollen and extremely painful; the temperature is elevated.

The patient should be placed on bed rest with the scrotum elevated to prevent tension on the spermatic cord. A scrotal support will accomplish this. Heat applications produce hyperemia and help to allay the infection. Antibiotics may be indicated.

Vasectomy. If the patient experiences recurrent acute epididymitis, a *vasectomy* (ligation and transection of the vas deferens) is done. This operation interrupts the pathway between the epididymis and prostate. The patient is sterile following the procedure, but not impotent. A vasectomy may be performed primarily as a sterilization procedure. The patient should receive a full explanation of the procedure and understand the consequences.

Orchitis is an inflammation of the testes that may occur as a result of some systemic infection. In addition, torsion of the spermatic cord or severe trauma may be factors in the production of orchitis. The symptoms are characteristic. The testicle becomes swollen, tense and painful, and the condition often is accompanied by high temperature, nausea and other systemic symptoms. The marked swelling inside the dense capsule of the testes may be sufficient to shut off the blood supply to the organ, so that gangrene of the testes is not infrequent. The sudden cessation of pain is a symptom of this complication.

Rest, elevation and the application of hot and cold compresses are the usual local measures. The general systemic infection causing the local lesion should be cared for. If suppuration occurs, incision and drainage often are necessary.

Tumors of the testicle usually occur in the adult during the years of greatest sexual activity. They are almost always malignant and most frequently arise as the result of congenital abnormalities in the testis itself. They are the most common form of neoplasm in men of the 20- to 35-year age group. The tumors tend to metastasize early to distant areas by direct extension and by way of the bloodstream and the lymphatics.

The symptoms appear very gradually with a gradual swelling of the testicle, followed by backache, pain in the abdomen, loss of weight, and general weakness. The metastatic growth may be more marked than the local testicular one. The enlargement of the testicle without pain is a significant diagnostic finding.

Removal of the testicle (orchiectomy), followed by supervoltage irradiation and retroperitoneal lymph node dissection, is the accepted method of therapy.

Hydrocele is a collection of fluid in the tunica vaginalis. It may be acute or chronic. The acute type occurs in association with acute infectious diseases of the epididymis or as a result of local trauma or of a systemic infectious disease, such as mumps. This type of hydrocele usually disappears spontaneously with improvement in the causative disease, and no local treatment is necessary. Chronic hydrocele is that which occurs as a result of a low-grade infection of the testes or the epididymis. It may occur also without any evident infection of these structures. The tunica vaginalis becomes widely distended with fluid; this lesion is differentiated from a hernia by the fact that it transmits light when transilluminated.

Treatment of the chronic type of hydrocele is sought because of the inconvenience of the large scrotal mass. Palliative therapy may consist of simple aspiration of the fluid; this usually results in a reaccumulation of the fluid, so that frequent aspirations are necessary.

In the surgical treatment of hydrocele, an incision is made through the wall of the scrotum down to the distended tunica vaginalis. The sac is opened and excised or everted around the testicle. In the postoperative care of these patients, a suspensory bandage usually is worn for a period of time. Such a support is made commercially and is obtainable in the pharmacy. However, gauze, muslin or adhesive suspensories can be improvised.

Variocele is a dilatation, elongation and tortuosity of the veins of the spermatic cord. This occurs most frequently in the veins on the left side in young adults. Very few if any subjective symptoms may be produced by the enlargement of the spermatic vein, and as a rule no treatment is required. When pain, tenderness and discomfort in the inguinal region are symptoms, therapy may be instituted. This usually consists in excision of the enlarged veins. In the postoperative care of these patients, a suspensory bandage is worn for a time.

Conditions of the Prostate

Benign Prostatic Hypertrophy. In many patients past 50 years of age, the prostate gland enlarges, extending upward into the bladder and producing obstruction to the outflow of urine by encroaching on the vesical orifice. This condition is known as enlargement of the prostate, or prostatic hypertrophy. Since this produces an obstruction to the flow of urine, a gradual dilatation of the ureters (hydro-ureter) and kidneys (hydronephrosis) results. The hypertrophied lobe extends upward into the bladder and forms a pouch that retains urine. This pouch is not emptied when voiding takes place, and the remaining urine (called residual urine) decomposes and may produce calculi or a cystitis. Considerable difficulty and frequency in urination develop gradually, and finally the patient is unable to void at all.

Carcinoma of the Prostate. Cancer of the prostate occurs in patients in the over-50 age group. With the exception of skin cancer, it is the most common malignant neoplasm of men in this country.

The symptoms may or may not be marked. If the neoplasm is large enough to encroach on the bladder neck or to cause obstruction of urine, then the patient has the same signs as those noted in benign prostatic hypertrophy. A needle biopsy or an excision of a segment of the prostate may be done to determine if a malignancy is present.

Every male over 50 should have a rectal examination as part of his annual checkup. Earlier detection is the clue to a higher cure rate. However, many pros-

Fig. 25-13A. Transurethral prostatectomy. A loop of wire connected with a cutting current is rotated in the cystoscope to remove shavings of prostate at the bladder orifice.

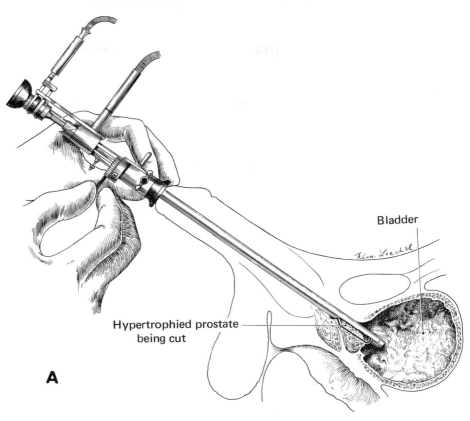

Bladder

Hypertrophied prostate being cut

A

tatic carcinomas are extremely malignant with few local symptoms and yet are widely disseminated. Metastases occur in bone, brain and lungs. On rectal examination, the prostate usually is found to be "stony hard" and fixed. Symptoms due to metastases are backache, loss of weight, loss of appetite and anemia.

Treatment for Benign Hypertrophy and Cancer of the Prostate. If a patient is admitted as an emergency because he is unable to void, the physician immediately tries to catheterize him. The ordinary rubber catheter frequently will be too soft and pliable to pass through the urethra into the bladder. A thin wire, called a *stylet*, then can be introduced into the catheter which will prevent the catheter from collapsing when resistance is met. The urologist often employs a catheter coated with wax whose end is upturned to form a slight angle (called a coudé-woven catheter).

In obstinate cases metal catheters must be employed. These have a curve more marked than the ordinary, called the *prostatic curve*. Sometimes, a suprapubic cystostomy is necessary to give adequate drainage (Fig. 25-12C). Treatment depends on the extent of disease. If the cancer has not invaded the capsule, then total radical prostatectomy by perineal or retropubic method is the procedure of choice. If

metastases are present, or the process has invaded beyond the capsule and the patient is having symptoms of urinary obstruction, then transurethral resection to allow an adequate channel for the passage of urine is indicated.

Preoperative Nursing Management. Estimation of kidney function, the administration of fluids in large quantities, and constant drainage of the bladder by triple lumen indwelling catheter are important parts of this regimen. During this time the nurse is able to help her older patient adjust to his environment. By conversation and observation she will note his idiosyncrasies, physical incapacities and mental attitude. The nurse should attempt to make his adjustment to surgery and its implications as smooth as possible. Any complications, such as cardiac and pulmonary, must be investigated before the patient has surgery. If the urinary obstruction has been nearly complete for a considerable period, a marked distention of the bladder occurs. If urine is relieved too suddenly, the patient may go into shock because of hemorrhage, or a renal shutdown may occur, producing uremia. For these reasons it may be desirable to remove urine gradually over a period of several days. The simplest method is to connect a urethral catheter or drainage tube with a Y-tube suspended on a bedside rack. Urine

Bladder

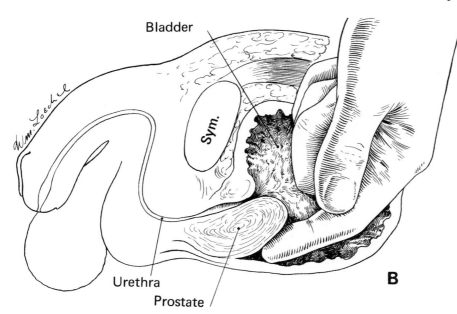

Sym.

Urethra

Prostate

B

FIG. 25-13B. Suprapubic prostatectomy. Diagrammatic drawing shows how the prostate is shelled out of its bed with the finger.

flows over the suspended Y-tube into the collecting bottle. At intervals the tubing is lowered until *bladder decompression* is accomplished.

In addition to one of the temporary measures (suprapubic cystostomy or indwelling catheter) to make the patient comfortable prior to major surgery, he is encouraged to take fluids and to eat a high-caloric diet. Eggnogs can be given between meals. Attention must be given to his own personal preferences and habits if he is to accept surgery favorably.

Prostatectomy. When the tests of the kidney show that the function has returned more nearly to the normal level, the patient is considered to be ready for operation. Four different approaches are possible in removing the hypertrophied fibroadenomatous portion of the prostate gland (see Table 25-1). The gland may be removed through an abdominal wound, a *supra-*

pubic prostatectomy. An opening is made into the bladder, and the gland is removed from above (Fig. 25-13). Such an approach can be used for a gland of any size, and few complications occur, although blood loss may be greater than with other methods. Another disadvantage is that an abdominal incision is required, with the concomitant hazards of any major surgical procedure.

In *perineal prostatectomy,* the gland is removed through an incision in the perineum (Fig. 25-13).. This approach is practicable when other approaches are blocked. It is good when open biopsy is needed. Postoperatively, the wound is contaminated easily because of the position of the incision. Incontinence, impotence or rectal injury are more likely as sequelae.

Instruments have been devised with an ocular and operating system that can be introduced through the

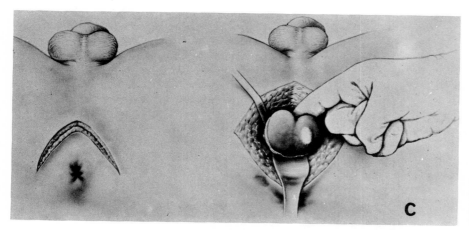

C

FIG. 25-13C. Perineal prostatectomy. Diagrammatic drawing shows the incision and how the prostate gland is removed in a perineal prostatectomy.

TABLE 25-1. Comparison of surgical approaches for prostatectomy

The operation of choice depends on (1) the size of the gland, (2) the location of the gland, (3) the age of patient, (4) the condition of patient, and (5) the presence of associated diseases

	Advantages	Disadvantages	Nursing Implications
Transurethral	Safer for surgical risk patient Shorter period of hospitalization and convalescence Useful for smaller gland Lower mortality rate	Requires highly skilled operator Not indicated for greatly enlarged prostate Recurrent obstruction may develop Delayed bleeding may occur	Watch for evidence of hemorrhage (drainage in bottle) Observe for symptoms of urethral stricture (dysuria, straining, small urinary stream)
Suprapubic	Technically simple Offers wider area of exploration Permits exploration for cancerous lymph nodes Allows more complete removal of obstructing gland Permits treatment of associated lesions in bladder	Requires surgical approach through the bladder Control of hemorrhage difficult Urinary leakage around suprapubic tube Convalescence more prolonged and uncomfortable	Watch for indications of shock Observe for hemorrhage Give meticulous aseptic attention to area around suprapubic tube
Perineal	Offers direct anatomic approach Permits gravity drainage Particularly efficacious for radical cancer therapy Allows hemostasis under direct vision Low mortality rate Less incidence of shock	Higher postoperative incidence of impotency and urinary incontinency Problem of damage to rectum Restricted operative field	Use drainage pads and bath towels to absorb excess urinary drainage Secure foam rubber ring for patient comfort
Retropubic	Most versatile procedure Permits easier control of hemorrhage Shorter period of convalescence	Cannot treat associated pathology in bladder Increased incidence of osteitis pubis	Watch for evidences of hemorrhage

urethra to the prostate. Under direct vision small pieces of obstructing gland tissue can be removed with an electric wire. This is called *transurethral resection of the prostate* (Fig. 25-13). The real advantage of this method is that there is no incision. It may be used for glands up to moderate size, and it is ideal for most poor-risk patients with small glands. This approach usually means a shorter hospital stay; however, strictures are more frequent, and repeat operations are more likely.

Another technique is to make a low abdominal incision and approach the prostate gland between the pubic arch and the bladder (without entering the bladder). This is called *retropubic prostatectomy*. This is suitable for large glands high in the pelvis. Blood loss is controlled more easily; however, inflammation of the pubic bone (osteitis pubis) is more likely.

Postoperative Nursing Management. As soon as the patient returns from the operating room, the nurse should check his pulse and his blood pressure, because the *immediate dangers following prostatectomy are shock and hemorrhage*. Bleeding may occur from the bed of the prostate, so that before completion of the operation many urologists pack the cavity or produce pressure on the walls by distending a small rubber bag attached to a tube which leads out through the urethra. In the suprapubic approach the packing or the bag is removed later through the abdominal wound. In spite of these precautions, the nurse must watch the patient carefully for signs of hemorrhage.

The drainage tube is connected to a piece of sterile plastic tubing placed in a closed drainage bottle near the patient's bed. At frequent intervals the nurse should inspect the urethral catheter for signs of obstruction. Any indications of kinking or compression of the drainage tubing must be avoided. A loop in the tubing may cause fluid to collect, thereby obstructing the flow. If the patient complains of pain, the nurse should check the drainage tubing and correct any obstruction before administering an analgesic.

An intake of fluids up to 3,000 ml. daily is encouraged. Obviously, an intake and output record is necessary. How rapidly a patient returns to a normal diet depends on the individual patient. Most patients are allowed bathroom privileges on their second postoperative day.

Following perineal prostatectomy, the urologist changes the dressing on the first day postoperatively; after that it may become the nurse's responsibility. Careful aseptic technique must be practiced, because the possibilities of infection are great. Dressings can be held in place by a double-tailed T-binder bandage. The tails can cross over the incision to give double thickness, and then each tail is drawn up on either side of the scrotum to the waistline and fastened. Rectal temperatures should not be taken, and a rectal tube should be used only on specific order by the physician. Any signs of oozing, infection, tenderness or pain should be reported.

Rehabilitation. As the days pass and drainage tubes are removed, the patient often shows signs of discouragement and depression because he is not able to gain control of his bladder immediately. There may be urinary frequency after the catheter is removed.

The following exercise is helpful for regaining urinary control. Tense the perineal muscles by pressing the buttocks together; hold this position; relax. This exercise, done 10 to 20 times each hour, can be performed while the patient is sitting or standing. It is important for him to know that regaining urinary control is a gradual process, and that even though he may be discharged from the hospital with "dribbling," it gradually should diminish. The patient's wife or some other responsible member of the family should be told of his condition. It is well for the family to realize that the patient should be encouraged to do as much for himself as possible. He needs mental stimulus to prevent boredom, despondency and physical lassitude. On the other hand, he must refrain from strenuous exercise, and he should avoid alcohol for at least a month. If any bleeding is detected, he should be advised to call his physician immediately.

When a cystostomy has been performed, the nursing care discussed on page 574 should be given carefully.

Inoperable Cancer of the Prostate. The principles underlying the treatment of inoperable cancer of the prostate are: (1) to maintain patency of the urethral passage; (2) to cause tumor regression; and (3) to control the pain.

To maintain patency of the urethral passage, repeated transurethral prostatectomies may have to be carried out until tumor growth is so rapid that surgical intervention becomes too frequent. When this is the case, catheter drainage is instituted by way of the suprapubic or transurethral route. The bladder should be irrigated daily or more frequently with a suitable anesthetic agent or preferably a wide spectrum antibiotic. The urine should be monitored for indications of cystitis.

Recent work does not confirm the supposed value of the time-honored use of orchiectomy, estrogens or both, to reduce tumor size. However this regimen is widely used because it provides pain relief. Initially, Stilbesterol is given in high doses that are gradually reduced over a period of weeks; the doses range from 30 mg. to 1 mg. per day. Ethinyl estradiol, 0.1 mg. 1 to 3 times a day, may be used. Chemotherapy has been reported effective: cyclophosphamide and vinblastine sulfate have been useful in some patients. Adrenal cortical hormone (prednisone) has also been used in doses of 20 to 100 mg. a day. Adrenalectomy and hypophysectomy have met with varying degrees of success, but these procedures have proved more useful in breast carcinoma. Radiation therapy has not been useful in producing tumor regression, but may control pain. Pain may be also controlled by the use of estrogens, narcotics and if necessary, severing spinal cord pain fibers by neurosurgery. Other symptoms arising from metastases are treated palliatively.

BIBLIOGRAPHY

Books

Bennington, J. L., and Kradjian, R. M.: Renal Carcinoma. Philadelphia, W. B. Saunders, 1967.

Brest, A. N., and Moyer, J.: Renal Failure. Philadelphia, J. B. Lippincott, 1967.

Campbell, M. F. (ed.): Urology. vols. 1, 2, 3. Philadelphia, W. B. Saunders, 1963.

Guyton, A. C.: Textbook of Physiology. pp. 470-542. Philadelphia, W. B. Saunders, 1966.

Hampers, C. L., and Schupak, E.: Long-Term Hemodialysis. New York, Grune and Stratton, 1967.

Hamm & Weinberg: Urology in General Practice. Philadelphia, J. B. Lippincott, 1962.

Harrison, T. R. (ed.): Principles of Internal Medicine. pp. 853-898. New York, McGraw-Hill, 1966.

Lalli, A. F.: Essentials of Urography. Springfield, Ill., Charles C Thomas, 1967.

Merrill, J. P.: The Treatment of Renal Failure. New York, Grune and Stratton, 1965.

Mitchell, J. P.: Urology for Nurses. Baltimore, Williams & Wilkins, 1965.

Rhoads, J., et al.: Surgery. Principles and Practice. Philadelphia, J. B. Lippincott, 1970.

Sussman, M. L., et al.: Urologic Roentgenography. Baltimore, Williams & Wilkins, 1967.

Symposium on Patient Care in Kidney and Urinary Tract Disease. Nurs. Cl. N. Amer., 4:No. 3 393-482, Sept., 1969.

Thornbury, J. R., and Culp, D. A.: The Urinary Tract. Chicago, Yearbook Medical Publishers, 1967.

Welch, C. E. (ed.): Progress in clinical renal homotransplantation. In Advances in Surgery. vol. 2, pp. 419-498. Chicago, Yearbook Medical Publishers, 1966.

Winter, C., and Roehm, M. M.: Sawyer's Nursing Care of Patients With Urologic Diseases. St. Louis, C. V. Mosby, 1968.

Kidney Problems

Becker, E. L.: The nephrotic syndrome in adults. Hosp. Med., 3:64-67, July, 1967.

Berlyne, G. M., *et al.:* The dietary treatment of acute renal failure. Quart. J. Med., 36:59-83, Jan., 1967.

Berman, L. B.: Selected topics in management of renal disease. GP, 35:127-137, June, 1967.

Cameron, J. S.: Renal disease I, II. Brit. Med. J., 2:811-813, 873-874, 1966.

Downing, S. R.: Nursing support in early renal failure. Amer. J. Nurs., 69:1212-1216, June, 1969.

Eisendrath, R. M.: The role of grief and fear in the death of kidney transplant patients. Amer. J. Psychiat., 126:381-387, Sept., 1969.

Gibbs, G. E.: Perineal care of the incapacitated patient. Amer. J. Nurs., 69:124-125, Jan. 1969.

Kark, R. M.: Renal biopsy and prognosis. Ann. Rev. Med., 18:269-298, 1967.

Kass, E. H.: How and why to treat urinary infections. Hosp. Med., 4:73-85, May, 1968.

Kazmin, M. H., *et al.:* Renal scan; the test of choice in renal trauma. J. Urol., 97:189-195, Feb. 1967.

Kolb, F. O. (ed.): Treatment of kidney stones. Mod. Treatment, 4:464-552, May, 1967.

Lee, D. A., *et al.:* Late complications of percutaneous renal biopsy. J. Urol., 97:793-797, May, 1967.

Levinsky, N. G.: The interpretation of proteinuria and the urinary sediment. Disease-A-Month, 3-30, March, 1967.

Mertz, J. H. O., *et al.:* Percutaneous renal biopsy utilizing cine-fluoroscopic monitoring. J. Urol., 95:618-621, May, 1966.

Monroe, J. M., and Komorita, N. I.: Problems with nephrosis in adolescence. Amer. J. Nurs., 67:336-340, Feb., 1967.

O'Flynn, J. D.: Advances in Urology. Practitioner, 197:503-510, Oct., 1966.

Rieser, C.: Diagnostic evaluation of suspected genitourinary tract injury. JAMA, 199:714-719, March, 1967.

Sanford, J. P.: Treatment and prevention of opportunistic infections of the urinary tract. Mod. Treatment, 3:1162-1170, Sept., 1966.

Techniques of renal biopsy. Lancet, 1:1368-1369, 24 June, 1967.

Tomskey, G. C., *et al.:* Injuries of the kidney. GP, 31:78-88, June, 1965.

Winter, C. C.: Renal calculi: Diagnosis and management. Hosp. Med., 2:31-36, Oct. 1966.

Yelderman, J. J., and Weaver, R. G.: The behavior and treatment of urethral strictures. J. Urol., 97:1040-1044, June, 1967.

Dialysis

————: Hemodialysis at home. Amer. J. Nurs., 66:1775-1778, Aug., 1966.

Albers, J.: Evaluation of blood volume in patients on hemodialysis. Amer. J. Nurs., 68:1677-1679, Aug., 1968.

Bluemle, L.: The artificial kidney. Med. Clin. N. Amer., 50:1351-1369, Sept., 1966.

Brand, L., and Komorita, N. I.: Adapting to long term hemodialysis. Amer. J. Nurs., 66:1778-1781, Aug., 1966.

Cohen, S. L., and Percival, A.: Prolonged peritoneal dialysis in patients awaiting renal transplantation. Brit. Med. J., 1:409-413, Feb. 17, 1968.

Fellows, B. J.: The role of the nurse in a chronic dialysis unit. Nurs. Clin. N. Amer., 1:577-586, Dec., 1966.

Johnson, W. J., *et al.:* Long-term intermittent hemodialysis for chronic renal failure. Mayo Clinic Proceedings, 41:73-94, Feb., 1966.

Kanter, A., *et al.:* Peritoneal dialysis: indications and technique in the surgical patient. Surg. Clin. N. Amer., 48:47-55, Feb., 1968.

O'Neill, M.: Peritoneal dialysis. Nurs. Clin. N. Amer. 1:309-323, June, 1966.

Redman, B. K., and Daly, S. M.: Patient teaching for home hemodialysis. *In* Bergerson: Current Concepts in Clinical Nursing. St. Louis, C. V. Mosby, 1969.

Versaci, A. A.: Hemodialysis: indications and techniques in surgical patients. Surg. Clin. N. Amer., 48:57-61, Feb., 1968.

Waterhouse, K., *et al.:* Intermittent hemodialysis for chronic renal failure. J. Urol., 97:426-431, March, 1967.

Watkins, F. L.: The patient who has peritoneal dialysis. Amer. J. Nurs., 66:1572-1577, July, 1966.

Kidney Transplantation

Bois, M. S., *et al.:* Nursing care of patients having kidney transplants. Amer. J. Nurs., 68:1238-1239; 1242-1247, June, 1968.

Borrowed time. (Editorial) New Eng. J. Med. 276:1206-1207, 25 May, 1967.

Hardy, J. D., *et al.:* Kidney transplantation in man. Ann. Surg., 165:933-946, June, 1967.

Martin, A. J.: Renal transplantation: Surgical technique and complications. Amer. J. Nurs., 68:1240-1241, June, 1968.

Merrill, J. P.: Present status of kidney transplantation. Med. Times, 95:403-415, April, 1967.

Shebelski, D. I.: Nursing patients who have renal homotransplants. Amer. J. Nurs., 66:2425-2428, Nov., 1966.

Bladder and Prostate

Abrams, H. J., and Neier, C. R.: Ureteral substitution with ileum. Amer. Surg., 33:437-442, June, 1967.

Cohen, S. M., and Persky, L.: A 10-year experience with uretero-ileostomy. Arch. Surg., 95:278-283, Aug., 1967.

Flint, L. D., and Hsiao, J-H: Radical prostatectomy for carcinoma: A review and perspective. Surg. Clin. N. Amer., 47:695-706, June, 1967.

Kasselman, M. J.: Nursing care of the patient with benign prostatic hypertrophy. Amer. J. Nurs., 66:1026-1030, May, 1966.

Katona, E. A.: A patient-centered, living-oriented approach to the patient with an artificial anus or bladder. Nurs. Clin. N. Amer., 2:623-634, Dec., 1967.

Patton, J. F., and Ross, G.: The painful testicle. Hosp. Med., 3:24-40, June, 1967.

PATIENT EDUCATION

Public Health Service
U.S. Department of Health, Education and Welfare
Washington, D.C. 20201
 Cancer of the Bladder. (HIS-145)
 Cancer of the Prostate. (HIS-127)
 Kidney Disease. (HIS-123)
 The Artificial Kidney. (Pub. Health Service Pub. No. 1409)

National Kidney Foundation
  315 Park Avenue South
  New York, New York 10010
    Five Warning Signs of Kidney Disease
    High Blood Pressure and the Kidney
    Some Facts to Remember
    Some Facts About Kidney Disease
    The Artificial Kidney Machine
    Your Kidneys
    Your Kidneys—Master Chemists of the Body

Johnson and Johnson, Inc.
  New Brunswick, New Jersey
    Hartman, M.: Home Care and the Incontinent Patient. 1966. (Booklet)

Nursing Division
  Memorial Hospital for Cancer and Allied Diseases
  444 E. 68th Street
  New York, New York 10016
    Home Care for the Patient After Urological Surgery. 1966. (Booklet on patient management of ureteral catheters, ureterostomy cups and ileal bladder bags.)

CHAPTER **26**

Nursing the Patient with a Gynecologic Condition

- *The Nurse and the Female Patient*
- *Gynecologic Examination*
- *Menstruation*
- *The Woman During Menopause*
- *Infertility*
- *Fertility Control*
- *The Patient Who has an Abortion*
- *Conditions of External Genitalia and Vagina*
- *Relation of Pelvic Muscles*
- *Conditions of the Uterus*
- *Conditions of the Ovaries and the Pelvic Cavity*

THE NURSE AND THE FEMALE PATIENT

Aspects of Feminine Hygiene

The nurse is in a key position to teach and to advise girls and women regarding the principles of good health and personal hygiene, specifically in the area of feminine hygiene, which is related to the care of those parts of the female body concerned with reproduction. The reproductive system, like any other part of the anatomy, will function well if the body has adequate nutrition, exercise, rest and elimination. The teaching of the nurse should extend into the areas of social diseases and prenatal and postnatal care as well.

It is important to recognize that concepts of feminine hygiene vary greatly with different cultures. What may be considered appropriate care for a European woman may be very different from that of an American or Japanese woman. An emphasis on cleanliness and neatness may be considered unnecessary by certain groups; climate and local customs may affect habits practiced. Even members of one family may have different opinions about personal tidiness.

Nurses need to understand the variations in attitudes and practices of hygiene and their relation toward sexual function. Because many methods of feminine hygiene are empirical, it is necessary to apply a common-sense approach. For example, whether a shower or tub bath is best is a matter of individual practice and preference; however, greater cleanliness can be assured by using a washcloth and sitting in a tub with the legs slightly apart to allow for free circulation of water. There is less enthusiasm for daily douching, but an occasional douche with a mild additive such as white vinegar (1 or 2 tablespoonfuls to 1 liter of water) may control odors and contribute to a feeling of cleanliness in some women. Too frequent douching may deprive the tissues of their natural protective secretions.

Deodorants and antiperspirants may be used providing they have been adequately tested for toxicity. New products should be used carefully. From general nursing courses, the student should recall the importance of good bowel hygiene and that, in wiping, the female begins at the urethral meatus and ends with the rectum. Otherwise, bacteria may be carried over the introitus and urethral meatus, which may predispose to vaginal and urinary tract infections.

585

Sex Education

An awareness of the differences between boys and girls begins early with most children; often it is heralded with the arrival of a new baby in the family. The wise parent answers correctly and simply the questions raised by the growing child.

The nurse is often an advisor to patients, parents, and friends; she may participate in sex education programs in school, church, or other groups. Filmstrips, movies and informative literature are available (see Patient Education, p. 614), and by being familiar with them, the nurse is able to be selective in meeting the needs of a particular group.

The Patient with a Gynecologic Problem

Complications of gynecologic disturbances can be prevented if proper medical care and supervision are available. The nurse is in a unique position to acquaint the lay person with the normal physiologic processes of menstruation and menopause. Many difficulties encountered by the young girl or the middle-aged woman usually can be corrected quite easily; if allowed to go untreated, they may cause irreparable damage. Danger signals that every woman should report to her physician are spotting, irregular or excessive bleeding, or any bleeding after menopause. Persistent painful menstruation, leukorrhea and urinary disturbances also ought to be investigated. Many of these early signs can be corrected simply and permanently. An annual pelvic examination is especially important for the woman who is past 30 years of age. The broad public health implications are a necessary part of gynecologic nursing.

Psychosocial Considerations. The gynecologic patient often calls for more understanding than other patients, because in addition to physical conditions there are many emotional factors governing the situation. She may resent any reference to her genitourinary system, feeling that she is suspected of questionable social or sexual habits. A real fear of venereal disease or of cancer may exist. All or any of these thoughts may manifest themselves in her conversation with the nurse, who by an understanding attitude can do much to dispel such anxieties.

Mixed emotional upsets can result from other fears. The suggestion of surgery as a means of treatment may raise a fear of disturbance of the reproductive process. Perhaps an explanation of the anatomy and the proposed treatment will clarify the situation. Any intention of sterilization must be explained carefully to the patient and her husband by the physician. Perhaps religious belief is more important to a patient than physical treatment. The decision rests with the patient, and, when it is made, it must be respected and supported.

Psychic factors may present themselves at the menopausal period. The loss of the reproductive capacity may cause disappointment if the woman has had no children. For a woman with a grown family, it may mean that she feels there is no further need for her. Present methods of mass production have left the individual with much less to do than formerly, and leisure time may hang heavily on her hands. However, the nurse continues to practice the principles of good nursing care and extends her energies to helping her patient orient herself to any change that may be necessary to make at this period.

An admonition to the gynecologic nurse is this: never talk about your patient or her disease. Gynecologic conditions often are of such a personal and a private nature that no patient would wish her nurse to tell other nurses, friends, or even her own family the details of her operation or treatment.

Special Nursing Considerations. Because many gynecologic diseases may be caused by highly infective organisms, especially the gonococcus, it is absolutely imperative that all instruments and equipment (catheters, douche nozzles, bedpans, rectal tubes and so forth) used in the treatment be sterilized both before and after their use. The nurse may protect herself by the use of rubber gloves, which should be cleansed and resterilized after treating each patient. Disposable sterile gloves are a satisfactory alternative. If gloves are not available, or the procedure does not require their use, it is wise to scrub the hands thoroughly. When possible, dressings, perineal pads and so forth should be handled with gloves or forceps, and the forceps should be sterilized after use.

GYNECOLOGIC EXAMINATION

Preparation of the Patient

The patient who is to have a gynecologic examination often has many fears and worries. Not only does she dislike the thought of being exposed and examined, but being placed in an embarrassing position can make the experience an unpleasant one. In addition, the concern and worry about what may be found by the physician serves to influence her reaction to the examination. She needs reassurance, understanding and tactful regard for her emotional as well as her physical problems.

Preparation includes voiding and evacuation of the bowels. Sufficient clothing should be removed to allow adequate exposure of the genitalia. All bands about the waist must be loosened and the girdle should be removed to permit examination of the abdomen. In preparation for the examination and in placing the patient on the examining table, the nurse should take special precautions to avoid exposing the patient. The nurse should be in attendance during the examination.

Positioning the Patient

The examination of the patient for a gynecologic condition is best made with the patient on the examining table. Three positions are employed commonly for these examinations. The most common is the dorsal position, with the knees and the hips flexed and the heels resting in foot rests. A sheet is draped diagonally over the patient, the lower corner being caught in the hands and gathered up so as to expose the vulva. A small towel then may be used to cover the exposed parts until the physician is ready to make the examination.

In Sims's position the patient lies on one side, usually the left, with her left arm behind her back. The right (uppermost) thigh and the knee are flexed as fully as possible, and the left leg is partly flexed. A sheet then is draped over the lower extremities and the hips in such a way as to expose the genitalia.

In the knee-chest position the patient kneels on the table so that the feet extend over the end. The knees should be separated and the thighs at right angles to the table. The head is turned to one side, and the arms grasp the sides of the table; the chest and the side of the face rest on a soft pillow.

If for any reason an examining table is not available, or the patient cannot be moved conveniently, these positions may be assumed in bed. Many physicians prefer to make the examination in the dorsal position with the patient across the bed, the hips extending slightly over the edge and the feet on the examiner's knees or on 2 chairs placed beside the bed. The cross-bed position must be used if instruments are to be used in making the examination. A sheet drape is used to cover the patient in the same way as for the table examinations.

Pelvic Examination

This includes first an inspection of the external genitalia for signs of inflammation, swelling, bleeding, discharge or local skin and epithelial changes. A speculum is inserted (Fig. 26-1) to enable the gynecologist to examine visually the vagina and cervix; a very small speculum may be used on a young virgin, or its use may be omitted altogether. The appearance of vaginal tissue and the nature of the cervix may be observed. The Papanicolaou smear and modified Schiller iodine tests described below can be done at this time. Then the gynecologist makes a bimanual examination, inserting 1 or 2 gloved fingers of the left hand in the vagina and palpating the abdomen with the right hand. In this way, the uterus and the adnexa are further examined. Lastly, a rectal examination is

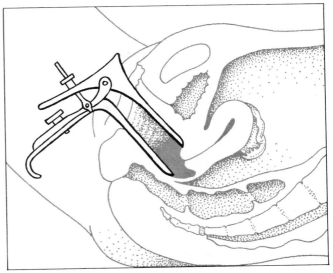

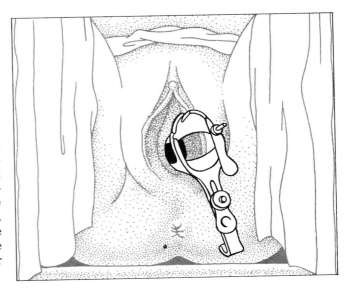

Fig. 26-1. The speculum in position. (*Top*) lateral view; (*bottom*) anterior view. (Smith Kline & French Laboratories)

made, often detecting abnormalities in the contour, motility and placement of adjacent structures and tissues.

During the examination, the nurse supports the patient, focuses the light, and assists the physician. At the conclusion of the examination, excess lubricating jelly or discharge should be wiped from the perineum before assisting the patient from the table. Both legs are removed from the stirrups simultaneously and the lower third of the table is brought to horizontal position. The elderly patient should be encouraged to sit upright for a minute or two and later should be

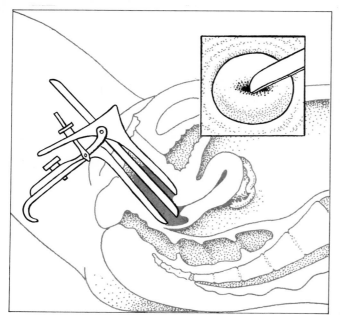

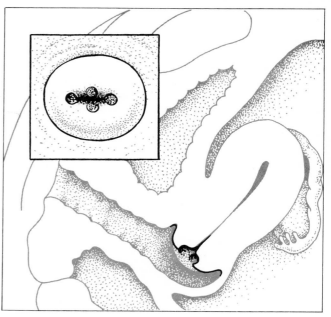

FIG. 26-3. Four biopsy sites. (Smith Kline & French Laboratories)

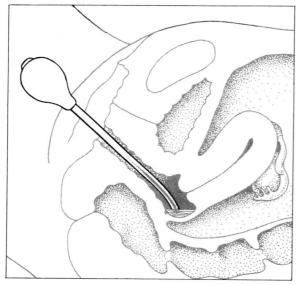

FIG. 26-2. (*Top*) Cell collection by scraping. (*Bottom*) Cell collection by aspiration (speculum not used). (Smith Kline & French Laboratories)

assisted to the dressing room. The woman may wish to rest before dressing. During this time, the nurse is available for answering questions or explaining further what the physician has told her; he may wish to see her before she leaves.

Cytologic Test for Cancer (Papanicolaou). This test is done for the purpose of diagnosing cervical cancer. It comprises the aspirating or the swabbing of vaginal secretions from the posterior fornix and making a smear on a glass slide (Fig. 26-2). The secretion usu-

ally is "fixed" immediately by immersing the slide in equal parts of 95 per cent alcohol and ether. The patient should be instructed not to take a douche before this examination, as such a treatment will wash away cellular deposits.

The pathologist examines and interprets the cytologic smear. The classification for cytologic findings as suggested by Papanicolaou is as follows:

Class 1. Absence of atypical or abnormal cells.

Class 2. Atypical cytology but no evidence of malignancy.

Class 3. Cytology suggestive of, but not conclusive for, malignancy.

Class 4. Cytology strongly suggestive of malignancy.

Class 5. Cytology conclusive for malignancy.

The finding of an abnormal smear (with the exception of Class 5) does not necessarily mean that the patient has cancer but points out that additional procedures, such as punch biopsies or a dilatation and curettage, are indicated. The patient will be grateful for this explanation.

Modified Schiller Iodine Test. A long cotton applicator is used to paint the cervix with 7 per cent tincture of iodine. A mahogany brown color covering the entire surface indicates a reaction between the iodine and the glycogen of normal cells. This test is considered negative. If abnormal, immature cells are present, tissues are not stained brown and the test is positive.

Cervical Biopsy and Cauterization

The results of the Papanicolaou test may indicate that further study of cervical tissue is necessary. This is scheduled for a time when the cervix is least vascular, usually a week after the end of the menstrual flow. The nature of this procedure is explained to the patient so that she will know that it is done in lithotomy position, that no anesthesia is required because the cervix does not have pain receptors, that usually an instrument with teeth (biopsy forceps) nibbles tissue (Fig. 26-3) and that some bleeding may occur and packing may be inserted. The cervical tissue is preserved in 10 per cent formalin before being properly labeled and sent to the laboratory.

If cauterization is required to control bleeding or to remove additional tissue, the placement of a lubricated lead plate under the patient in contact with her skin should be explained. Grounding of electrical charges is a safety measure. She should also be told that there may be an odor (burnt tissue) but this is usual and it will be over quickly.

There may be some discomfort during this procedure but after a brief rest, the patient is able to leave. Her instructions for home care include the following: avoid much, if any, work for the next 24 hours, rest and avoid heavy lifting. Packing should remain in place for as long as the physician recommends (usually 12 to 24 hours). There may be some bleeding, but excessive bleeding should be reported. The physician gives specific advice as to when sexual

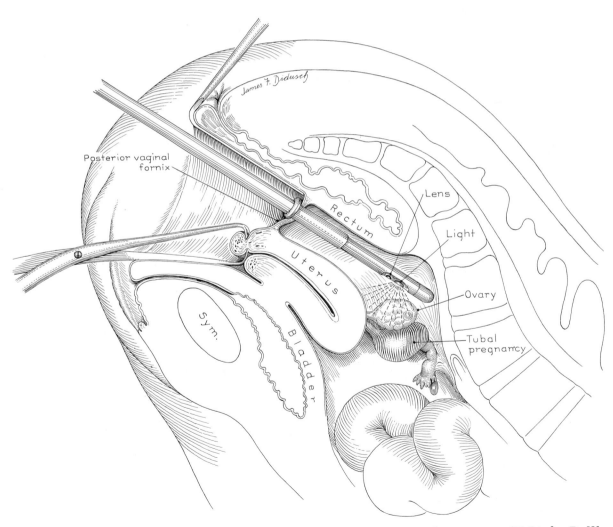

Fig. 26-4. Culdoscopy. Sagittal section showing culdoscope viewing pelvic viscera. (TeLinde, R. W.: Operative Gynecology, ed. 4, Phila., J. B. Lippincott, 1970)

relations may be resumed and when douching is permitted. Several days after a cauterization, there may be a discharge and odor because of tissue slough, but a daily bath should alleviate this.

Culdoscopy

In this diagnostic procedure, an incision is made in the posterior vaginal cul-de-sac to admit a tubular lighted instrument, the culdoscope; thus, this procedure is done in the operating room (Fig. 26-4). The patient is prepared as for a vaginal operation and anesthesia may be local, regional or general. With the patient in the knee-chest position, direct visualization of the uterus, tubes, broad ligaments, uterosacral ligaments, rectal wall, sigmoid and small intestine is possible. Following this examination, the scope is withdrawn and the patient is returned to her room. The incision heals easily without sutures.

Roentgen Studies

Hysterosalpingogram. A hysterosalpingogram is an x-ray study of the uterus and the fallopian tubes after the injection of a contrast media. This diagnostic procedure is done to study sterility problems, to evaluate tubal patency and to determine the presence of pathology in the uterine cavity.

The patient is placed in the lithotomy position, and the cervix is exposed with a bivalved speculum. A cannula is inserted into the cervix, and radiopaque dye is injected into the uterine cavity and the tubes. X-ray films are taken to show the path and the distribution of the contrast materials.

Pelvic Pneumoperitoneum (Nitrous Oxide Gynecogram.) This is a diagnostic procedure for the visualization of the female reproductive organs. Nitrous oxide gas is injected approximately 2 inches below the umbilicus into the pelvic cavity. This gas surrounds the organs of the pelvic cavity and thus outlines them on x-ray negatives. By changing the patient's position on the table the gas is displaced to all areas of the pelvic cavity. Originally intended as a diagnostic aid for the detection of Stein-Leventhal syndrome (polycystic ovaries), this test now is used to find other pelvic disorders.

The patient is informed that she will experience a feeling of fullness during the gas injection, which will be followed by a sensation of pressure under the diaphragm. She also may have spasmodic pains in the right shoulder due to severe irritation of the diaphragm from the gas displacement.

After the gynecogram the patient is placed in a Trendelenburg position for approximately 2 hours. This will help to relieve the shoulder spasm. A mild analgesic is usually all that is necessary to relieve any other discomfort.

MENSTRUATION

Physiology of Menstruation

If conception does not occur, the ovum dies, and the mucous membrane lining the uterus (the endometrium), which has become thickened and congested, becomes hemorrhagic. The upper layer of lining cells and the blood that appears in the uterine cavity are discharged through the cervix and the vagina. This flow of blood, mixed with mucus and cells, which occurs as a rule every 28 days during the sexual life of females, is called *menstruation*. The period of flow lasts usually 4 to 5 days, during which time from about 50 to 150 ml. of fluid is lost; most of this is blood but about one quarter is mucus, desquamated vaginal epithelium and fragments of endometrial cells. After the cessation of the menstrual flow the endometrium returns to an inactive state until stimulated again by ovulation. It is believed that ovulation usually occurs midway between menstrual periods.

The girl between the ages of 11 and 14 who is approaching the *menarche* or onset of menstruation should be instructed about this normal process. Psychologically, it is more healthy to refer to this event as "my period" rather than as "being sick" or "having the curse." With adequate nutrition, rest, exercise and good posture, there will be little discomfort. Some girls do experience breast tenderness and a feeling of fullness a day or two before the onset of menstruation. There may be a greater tendency to fatigue and some discomfort of the lower back, legs and pelvis on the first day; temperament and mood changes may be apparent. Slight deviations from the usual healthy pattern of daily living is permissible, but signs of excessive deviations may require investigation.

The perineal pad is the most widely used method of disposing of menstrual discharge; powder, cream, and spray deodorants for the pads are available. The use of tampons has increased recently, and there is no significant evidence of untoward effects from their use, providing there is no difficulty in inserting them. Should the "tail" string break and difficulty be encountered in removing the tampon, the woman's physician should be consulted. A third type of protection is the internal rubber cup, but this is used less frequently.

Psychosocial Considerations

As mentioned earlier, menstruation may be handled differently in different cultures. Some women believe that it is detrimental to change a pad (or tampon) too frequently; they believe that by allowing the discharge to accumulate, an increased flow is stimulated, which is considered desirable. For the nurse to insist that a pad be changed before the time the patient believes proper may cause conflict. These differences must be carefully reconciled so that proper understanding develops.

Other psychosocial aspects may need to be considered, such as vulnerability of the female to illness during menstruation. Many believe it is detrimental to swim, take a cold shower, receive a "permanent wave", get teeth filled, or eat certain foods during one's period. Such beliefs need to be understood and appraised. Many other examples of misunderstanding could be listed; however, the objective is to alert the nurse to these unexpressed, deep-rooted beliefs. Aspects of gynecological problems cannot always be expressed easily. The nurse needs to convey confidence and trust as well as to offer sound advice in order to set up a therapeutic environment.

Disturbances of Menstruation

There is a definite interrelation between the hormonal secretions of the ovary, the thyroid and the pituitary glands. A disturbance of this relationship by an increased or decreased function of one or more of these glands may influence the menstrual function. This is probably the most common cause of menstrual disturbances.

Dysmenorrhea (Primary). Dysmenorrhea, or painful menstruation, is a common condition found most often in unmarried women and women who have not borne children. The cause is not completely understood, and may involve emotional and psychologic factors. Pain may be due to uterine spasm caused by a narrowing of the cervical canal or perhaps as a result of endocrine gland dysfunction. The symptoms —acute cramp-like pains in the lower abdomen, often associated with chills, headache and perhaps vomiting—are most severe during the first day of the period. Women who have borne a child have a much lowered incidence of dysmenorrhea.

Treatment. This should be selective and varies with the individual and the severity of the problem. Many "old wives' tales" associated with the menses may have to be overcome before therapy can be effective. Proper preparation of young women before the menarche, so that this event is recognized as a perfectly normal part of development, helps to reduce or eliminate the problem of dysmenorrhea. Good posture plays an important role; exercises may be prescribed to improve posture and correct muscular imbalance. The emotional make-up of the woman may accentuate the discomfort. By understanding her problems in this area, psychotherapy alone or with pharmacotherapy may help.

A complete physical examination is done to rule out possible physical abnormalities, such as strictures of the cervix or vagina, imperforate hymen, and so forth. The patient is then treated on the basis of severity of symptoms (measured in terms of time lost from school or work). Fatigue and overexertion should be avoided. Often relief can be obtained by lying down and using heat on the lower abdomen. Salt restriction and a diuretic may control premenstrual edema. Hormonal therapy to suppress ovulation may be prescribed to break the cycle of dysmenorrhea. Mild analgesics will aid in controlling discomfort.

For the more severe problem, dysmenorrhea may be secondary to other pathology and surgery may be indicated. In surgical treatment, an effort is made to correct the conditions causing narrowing of the cervical canal and displacements of the uterus (p. 603). The cervical canal is dilated or stretched. Some physicians prescribe pelvic exercises, and others have treated the condition by cutting nerve fibers (presacral neurectomy).

A few patients may need psychiatric therapy. It is not uncommon to see dysmenorrhea disappear when an emotionally disturbed patient undergoes psychotherapy.

Amenorrhea. *Primary amenorrhea* (absence of menstrual flow) is the term used to signify the situation of a young girl who has not yet begun to menstruate at 16 or 17 years. This delayed menarche should be reported to and evaluated by the physician. The understanding nurse will provide an opportunity for such a patient to express her concerns and anxiety about this problem. She may feel that she is not like her peers and that she may not be able to fulfill her role as a woman. Amenorrhea may be caused by variations in anatomic development; it is treated according to its etiology.

Secondary amenorrhea occurs normally during pregnancy and lactation. However, extreme anxiety, acute or chronic disease, anemia or disease of the ductless glands and certain ovarian tumors (particularly arrhenoblastomas) may cause amenorrhea.

The treatment is directed toward the correction of the cause. Often there is a pituitary or thyroid dysfunction in the background that may be helped by appropriate measures. When a woman who is not pregnant misses periods, she should consult her gynecologist.

Menorrhagia. Menorrhagia is excessive bleeding at the time of the regular menstrual flow. In early life it may be due to endocrine disturbances, but menorrhagia with increase in duration of the menstrual periods in later life usually is due to inflammatory disturbances or tumors of the uterus. Emotional disturbance may affect bleeding also.

A woman with menorrhagia is encouraged to see her gynecologist and relate the nature of such excessive bleeding. Although difficult to measure, an estimate might be given in terms of numbers of pads or tampons used in excess of the regular flow.

Metrorrhagia. Metrorrhagia is the appearance of blood from the uterus between the regular menstrual periods or after the menopause. It is always the symptom of some disease, often cancer or benign tumors of the uterus; therefore, it merits early diagnosis and treatment. Metrorrhagia is probably the most significant form of menstrual dysfunction; the amount of blood loss is not important, but the fact that it occurred warrants further investigation.

THE WOMAN DURING THE MENOPAUSE

The menopausal period of a woman's life, usually occurring between the ages of 42 and 52, marks the end of her active reproductive life. Menopause is a physiologic and not a pathologic phenomenon. Menstruation then ceases, and as a result of the complete cessation of activity on the part of the ovaries, the reproductive organs and the mammary glands atrophy. No more ova develop and no ovarian hormones are produced. A similar situation prevails earlier if the ovaries are removed or destroyed by irradiation, giving rise to the artificial menopause. From the medical point of view this period is of concern because of certain more general manifestations—some temporary, some permanent—that may appear.

Usually, the menopause starts gradually and is recognized by the change in menstruation. The monthly flow becomes smaller in amount, then irregular and finally ceases. Often, the time between periods gets longer—there may be a lapse of several months between them. Any prolonged menstrual flow or bleeding between periods should be reported to the physician promptly.

Before and during these changes in the monthly periods, certain symptoms may appear, e.g., hot or warm flushes, dizziness, weakness, nervousness, insomnia. Many women have very mild symptoms; some have none at all; with a few, the discomfort is very severe. The symptoms are caused by the diminution of the female sex hormone that the ovaries produce. The same symptoms occur when the ovaries are removed surgically because of disease (surgical menopause). After a period of months, or even a year or two, the body adjusts itself, and the symptoms disappear. While this adjustment is taking place, hot flushes, etc., can appear.

The menopause is not a complete change of life. The normal sex urges remain, and women retain their usual reaction to sex long after the menopause. There is nothing abnormal about the change of life and nothing unusual about the continuation of happy marital relations afterward. Many women enjoy better health after the menopause than they have had for years. This is especially true with persons who have always suffered pain during their menstrual periods.

Management and Education of the Patient

The majority of patients will respond to a program of education, reassurance, modification of their living habits, and an improved regimen of health. In some patients mild sedatives and tranquilizers are necessary to control nervousness and to counteract depression. Mental depression is not at all unusual at this time. Sometimes, it becomes so deep that even an everyday problem seems too much to cope with.

Interest has increased in the possible amelioration of certain disease conditions associated with the menopause by administration of exogenous estrogen therapy. The existence of a direct causal relationship between certain disorders and diminished estrogen secretion has not been established. However, beneficial effects in the prevention of atherosclerosis and osteoporosis have been claimed to accompany estrogen therapy. With such therapy, re-epithelialization of the reproductive tract is produced; itching and burning of atrophic vaginitis is relieved and atrophic changes in the urethra are reversed.

Restraint in the use of estrogen therapy for all menopausal women must be exercised, because of the concern that protracted estrogen treatment will induce neoplastic changes in estrogen-sensitive aging tissues. Therefore, during hormone therapy, the emphasis is placed on close periodic evaluation by the gynecologist. An individualized approach provides the most effective and safe way to guide a woman through another stage of life.

The physician and the nurse should take the time to explain to the patient that the cessation of the menses is a normal physiologic function that is not necessarily accompanied by extreme nervous symptoms and various illnesses. Measures should be taken to promote her general health. Since many patients are in the menopausal age group, the following factors should be stressed in patient teaching:

1. The climacteric period is normal and self-limiting.

2. Overfatigue and environmental problems exaggerate the symptoms.

3. A nutritious diet and avoidance of overweight will improve the physical condition.

4. Interest and participation in outside activities help to absorb anxiety and to lessen tension.

5. The menopause does not mean a termination of the sex life.

6. An annual physical examination is essential to the maintenance of continuing good health.

The current expected lifespan after menopause for the average woman is 30 to 35 years. This is an optimistic thought, since it encompasses as much as the child-bearing phase of her life.

Other effects of aging include a tendency to gain weight, particularly around hips, thighs and abdomen. Paying increased attention to good grooming tends to give the woman a lift when it is most needed. The individual woman's evaluation of herself and her worth now and in the future certainly affects her emotional reaction to this change in her life.

INFERTILITY

Infertility is the inability to conceive; it may be remedied. However, should the condition persist, it is referred to as *sterility*. In the United States, one out of every 8 to 10 couples are childless because of infertility; it is a major medical and social problem. Both husband and wife are urged to seek medical attention for complete examinations and evaluation, since almost as many men as women may cause a sterile marriage. It is usually recommended that the male be evaluated first, because tests for the female are more expensive and time-consuming. Such tests may require the services of a urologist, gynecologist, endocrinologist and internist.

In the female, the organs of reproduction and the glands influencing them are evaluated. Among the causative factors may be displacement and tumors of the uterus, genital infantilism and inflammation. To allow fertilization of an ovum, it is necessary that the vagina, cervix and uterus to be patent and have mucosal secretions receptive to the sperm. Semen is alkaline, as is cervical secretion; normal vaginal secretion is acid. Treatment is directed toward correcting the deficiencies encountered in the individual patient. The following tests assist the gynecologist in delimiting the problem.

Rubin Test. This procedure is to determine the patency of the fallopian tubes by introducing carbon dioxide through a sterile cannula into the uterus, the tubes and then into the peritoneal cavity. By listening with a stethoscope on the abdomen, the physician may hear the gas swishing into the abdomen. The patient may feel referred pain under the scapula or shoulder on the side of the patent tube, indicating that gas is under the diaphragm (irritating the phrenic nerve). If the pressure gauge reaches 200 mm. of mercury, an occlusion may be suspected.

Salpinogram; Hysterosalpingogram. A radiopaque substance is often used to determine the site of tubal obstruction; an x-ray picture then shows the outline of the tubal lumen. Such insufflation may be therapeutic in itself, by stretching a tube to permit passage of a fertilized ovum.

In preparation for a salpingogram, the intestinal tract is prepared by a laxative and an enema so that gas shadows do not distort the roentgenograms. An analgesic is prescribed for comfort, since some patients experience nausea, vomiting, cramps and faintness. Following the test, it may be advisable for the patient to apply a perineal pad for several hours, because the radiopaque medium may stain clothing. To relieve "gas pains" after the examination, the knee-chest position or lying on the abdomen with the head lower than the feet will allow the gas to rise to the lower abdomen.

Huhner Test. Within an hour or two after intercourse, the physician aspirates cervical secretions with a long cannula. The woman had been instructed not to void, bathe or douche between coitus and the examination; a perineal pad is worn until she is placed in lithotomy position in the examining room. Aspirated material is placed on a slide and examined under the microscope for presence and viability of sperm cells. If sperm cells are being killed, proper douche solutions or antibiotics are prescribed to produce the proper vaginal flora at the time of ovulation so that it is more receptive to the spermatozoa.

Treatment

The treatment of sterility is a difficult matter, because it may be caused by a combination of several factors. Efforts are made to build up the general health of the patient, supplying lacking glandular hormones as indicated. Operative treatments include removal of obstructions and plastic operations to restore tubal patency. Unfortunately, these are not too successful; in addition there is a high incidence of tubal pregnancy following such operations.

The psychic and social factors of infertility must not be overlooked. Among some religious groups and nationalities, it is important to have blood descendants; adopting children is not acceptable in these families. In other family groups, the man's virility or woman's femininity are suspected when a couple fails to have children. Many pregnancies have occurred after an infertile couple has adopted a child, moved to another location, or the husband had a change of jobs.

FERTILITY CONTROL

No attempt will be made to examine the pros and cons of population control. Much investigation and public attention recently has been directed toward "population explosion" and the student is referred to the library for additional references covering legal, moral and social implications.

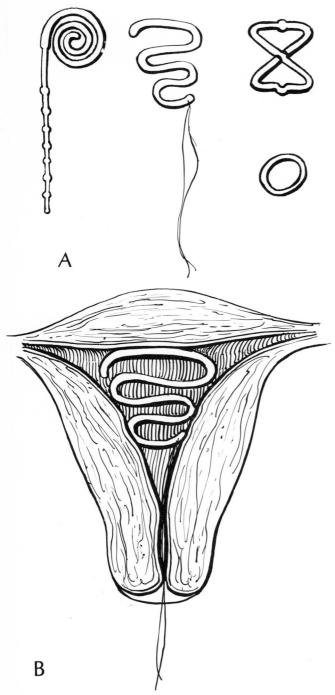

A

B

Fig. 26-5. (A) Intrauterine devices (IUDs) include, from left to right, Margulies spiral, Lippes loop and Birnberg bow (all of plastic), and the Hall stainless steel spring ring. (Consumers Union of U.S., Inc.) (B) Drawing showing IUD in place in the uterus.

Various forms of fertility control are available to individuals; it is their right to select the method most appropriate and acceptable to them. Of 100 women of proved fertility, 80 become pregnant in a year when no attempt is made to interfere with the control of conception.

With advanced scientific knowledge and greater dissemination of contraception information, the traditional methods (withdrawal, household spermicides, and douches) of contraception have given way to proved methods of prevention. *Condoms, diaphragms,* vaginal *jellies,* and *foams* are all safe and fairly reliable. At present, considerable attention is being given to intrauterine contraception and oral ovulating-inhibiting steroid—the "Pill."

Rhythm Method

The rhythm method of contraception, to be sure, has discrepancies because it is based on a woman's being able to determine her time of ovulation. The fertile phase (which requires sexual continence) is estimated to occur about 14 days before menstruation. It is assumed that spermatozoa can fertilize for 48 hours after intercourse and that the ovum can be fertilized for about 24 hours after it leaves the ovary. Studies reveal that of 100 women practicing the rhythm method, 15 will conceive during a year. This is a considerable reduction when compared with statistics of women taking no precautions.

Intrauterine Devices (IUD)*

Intrauterine devices (IUD)* in principle are not new; however, the modern pioneer was a German physician, Ernst Graefenberg, who around 1920 inserted silkworm gut and later silver or gold wire coils into the uterine cavities. In the United States, 4 main types of intrauterine devices are currently in use; these are made of materials nonreactive with body tissues. Three IUD's, shaped respectively like a spiral, a loop, and a bow (Fig. 26-5) are of molded plastic. One is a spring ring of stainless steel.

The device is positioned in a narrow straight stylet that is introduced by the physician through the cervical os. The plunger forces the IUD into the uterine cavity. Most devices have nylon thread tails that are useful in removing the IUD, as well as in determining whether it is still in the uterus. Of the 4 devices, the double S-shaped Lippes loop appears to be superior to the other 3. Pregnancy rates of users vary from 5 to 7.5 per 100 years (i.e., of 100 women of proven fertility, 5 to 7.5 will become pregnant in a year).

The advantages of this method is that it reduces

* Sometimes referred to as *IUCD*—intrauterine contraceptive device.

the factor of patient error, which makes it suitable for large-scale use in lower socioeconomic groups. The disadvantages are that such a device may be expelled unnoticed, and there is the possibility of infection and rupture of the uterus. Expulsion of an IUD, if it occurs at all, takes place during the first, second, or third menstrual period after insertion. If the device is retained beyond this time, it is likely to remain in position indefinitely. IUD's probably can remain in the uterus for several years without being changed; however, many American physicians prefer to replace the IUD every year or two and request annual check-ups.

Oral Fertility Control—The "Pill"

Oral synthetic steroid preparations of estrogen and progesterone tend to block the central nervous system stimulation of the ovary by preventing the release of the follicle-stimulating hormone (FSH) from the anterior pituitary. In the absence of FSH, a follicle does not ripen and ovulation does not take place; this is the basis of operation of oral contraceptives. A single pill is taken on the fifth day of menstruation and each day thereafter for 20 days; this is repeated on the fifth day of each ensuing menstrual period. There are 2 kinds of therapy: "combined" and "sequential"—the difference lies in the dosage of progestogens. In the combined therapy, estrogen and progestogen are present in every pill. Progestogen interferes with cervical mucus production and prevents uterine endometrium from fully developing to receive the fertilized ovum, resulting in a lighter than normal menstrual flow. In the sequential therapy, only estrogen is contained in the first 15 pills and the combined hormones comprise the next 5 or 6 pills. Thus, there is a closer approximation of the normal menstrual cycle. According to 100 women-years of exposure, the pregnancy rate with the combined steroid program was 0.1, whereas it reached 5.0 with the sequential method.

Oral contraceptives can have adverse effects on some women; therefore, they should be administered responsibly. Each woman should have a complete physical examination before the drug is prescribed and a check-up every 6 months after using the "pill." Side-effects continue to be studied. The metabolism of certain sugars and starches appear to be altered in some women, but how and why this occurs is not yet known. There also appears to be a cause-and-effect relationship between oral contraceptives and the development of thromboembolism, but in view of its low frequency of occurrence, there does not appear to be a general contraindication to the use of such contraceptives at this time. Meanwhile, research and experimentation continue in order to develop a single monthly pill or injection that would be safe as well as effective.

Patient Education

Much has been written about family planning and the availability and use of contraceptive devices. The nurse is in a strong position to help patients understand the physician's advice. Religious groups have made clear their teachings and dogma regarding birth control, and these need to be respected and understood as each couple makes its decision. Research is changing the methods used in fertility control, and more acceptable and longer lasting types are sought. The nurse should be familiar with the information as it comes out. A valuable source of information is the American College of Obstetricians and Gynecologists, 79 West Monroe Street, Chicago, Illinois.

THE PATIENT WHO HAS AN ABORTION

Interruption of pregnancy or expulsion of the contents of the pregnant uterus before the fetus is viable is called *abortion*. Viability is usually considered to be any time after the sixth month of gestation; however, legal periods of viability vary in different states in the U.S. *Miscarriage* is the lay term for this condition, whereas "abortion" is suggestive of something illegal. It is important for the nurse to be cognizant of the lay person's interpretation of abortion, since professionally it does not carry an illegal connotation.

The aborted fetus weighs less than 1,000 gm.; if more than this weight, the baby is usually viable and the term *premature labor* is used instead of abortion to describe the situation. It is estimated that one out of every 5 or 10 conceptions results in abortion. Most of these occur because of an abnormality in the fetus and abortion is nature's method of rejection. Other causes may be due to systemic diseases, hormonal imbalance or anatomic abnormalities.

Spontaneous Abortion

Spontaneous abortion occurs naturally with no known cause. There are various kinds of spontaneous abortion, depending upon the nature of the process (threatened, inevitable, incomplete, and complete). Uterine bleeding and pain (uterine contractions) are suggestive of an abortion in a woman of child-bearing age. In such a *threatened abortion*, the cervix does not dilate; with bed rest and conservative treatment, it can be prevented. If it cannot be prevented, an *inevitable abortion* is imminent. If some of the tissue but not all is passed, the abortion is referred to as *incomplete*; however, if the fetus and all related tissue is expressed, the abortion is *complete*.

Habitual Abortion

Habitual abortion is successive (3) repeated abortions of unknown cause. Ultraconservative measures are employed in an attempt to save the pregnancy, such as complete bed rest, administration of stilbestrol and progesterone to prevent sloughing of the endometrium, thyroid extract therapy, and psychotherapy. In the condition known as "incompetent cervical os," the cervix dilates painlessly in the second trimester of pregnancy and spontaneous abortion may occur. A surgical procedure called the Shirodkar operation is designed to prevent the cervix from dilating prematurely. A purse-string suture of nylon or fascia is placed in the submucous layer. It is most important that this patient and nurses attending her, including those in public health agencies and industry, know when such a suture is in place. As soon as labor occurs, the physician should be notified immediately so that the suture can be cut and labor allowed to proceed; otherwise, the uterus may possibly rupture. Usually delivery is by caesarean section.

Therapeutic Abortion

Under certain circumstances, the physician may consider terminating a pregnancy; such a termination is called a *therapeutic abortion,* and is performed by skilled medical personnel in a hospital. Legislation regarding indications for therapeutic abortion vary among states and countries. Besides consulting with the patient and her husband, the physician usually consults with at least one other physician.

The policy adopted by the American College of Obstetricians and Gynecologists in 1968 gives as medical indications for a therapeutic abortion:

1. When continuation of the pregnancy may threaten the life of the woman or seriously impair her health. In determining whether or not there is such risk to health, account may be taken of the patient's total environment, actual or reasonably foreseeable.

2. When pregnancy has resulted from rape or incest: in this case the same medical criteria should be employed in the evaluation of the patient.

3. When continuation of the pregnancy is likely to result in the birth of a child with grave physical deformities or mental retardation.

In coming to such a difficult decision, the religious beliefs of the parents must be respected.

Criminal Abortion

The illegal termination of a pregnancy by the patient or others is a criminal abortion. Accurate figures are not available regarding the extent of such practices, however, estimates place the total at a million a year in the United States. Over 10,000 deaths result annually from infection or overdosage of drugs connected with criminal abortion. The nurse is obligated to refer any woman who does not want her child to agencies prepared to help. Such agencies offer shelter, anonymity, services of social workers and possible placement of the child with an adopting agency.* If at all possible, the mother-to-be should be encouraged to continue through her pregnancy since there is no safe way to induce an abortion and cope with possible complications outside of hospital facilities. When unskilled attempts to end a pregnancy are made, the methods usually include the taking of large amounts of drugs (effects are toxic and never really evacuate the uterus) or the performance of a curettage, with an associated high risk of rupturing the uterus, hemorrhage or infection.

Medical and Nursing Management

Signs of a threatening abortion are vaginal discharge or bleeding and abdominal cramps. The woman is encouraged to see a physician who will probably recommend bed rest, light diet and no straining on defecation. All tissue passed vaginally is to be saved for examination by the physician. Sedation or tranquillizers may be prescribed and if infection is suspected, antibiotics may be given. In the hospital, all personnel caring for the patient will be alerted to save the contents of the bedpan for possible placental tissue or fetus. If there is much bleeding, the patient may require transfusions. The nursing staff may be asked to count and record the number of perineal pads used per 24 hours to estimate blood loss. For an incomplete abortion, ergot may be given and the patient will probably have a dilatation and evacuation (D and E). Such an *evacuation of retained secretions* (ERS) requires the same nursing care as a dilatation and curettage (see p. 604).

Inasmuch as this patient experiences a severe emotional reaction, the component of "caring" for her is an important aspect of nursing. The cause of the abortion colors the problem and the patient's reaction. If the response of the woman who desperately wants the baby is quite different from that of a woman who does not want to be pregnant but may be frightened of the possible consequences of the abortion, providing opportunities for the patient to talk and vent her emotions will allow the nurse to help her.

Ectopic Pregnancy

Ectopic pregnancy is a pregnancy in which the fertilized ovum does not reach the cavity of the uterus but becomes caught and embedded in the fallopian tube or, occasionally, in the ovary or the abdomen. As the fertilized ovum increases in size, the tube becomes more and more distended until finally, from 4 to 6

---

* Information can be obtained from such agencies as: Salvation Army, 546 Avenue of the Americas, New York, New York 10011; Florence Crittenton League, 307 East 12th Street, New York, New York 10003.

weeks after conception has occurred, rupture takes place and the ovum is discharged into the abdominal cavity. The symptoms may start with attacks of colicky pain on the affected side due to distention of the fallopian tube. When tubal rupture occurs, the patient experiences agonizing pain, faintness, shock and air hunger. It is recognized at once that the patient is desperately ill; all the signs of hemorrhage—rapid, thready pulse, subnormal temperature, restlessness, pallor, sweating—are in evidence. By vaginal examination the surgeon is able to feel a large mass of clotted blood that has collected in the pelvis behind the uterus.

The treatment of ectopic pregnancy always is surgical—removal of the tube (salpingectomy), and the ovary if necessary, on the affected side. However, many patients are in such a shocked condition that immediate operation cannot be performed. Measures then should be instituted to combat the shock and hemorrhage (see Chap. 9). When the operation is performed early, practically all such patients recover with remarkable rapidity, but without operation the mortality is 60 to 70 per cent.

After operation the treatment is the same as that for any laparotomy, plus transfusions to combat the acute anemia.

CONDITIONS OF EXTERNAL GENITALIA AND VAGINA

Vulvitis and Abscess of Bartholin's Glands

Vulvitis, an inflammation of the vulva, may occur as a result of uncleanliness, irritating discharges, or infection. Besides the gonococcus, other organisms invade the gland and cause inflammation. The most frequent of these are *Escherichia coli*, staphylococcus, streptococcus, and *Trichomonas vaginalis*.

The symptoms of the disease may be very slight, but in the typical case the patient complains of a constant burning pain that is worse during urination and defecation. The genitalia become red and edematous, and there is a profuse purulent exudate in which the offending organism may be found by examination of a smear.

The infection usually involves Bartholin's glands, the glands in the floor of the urethra and those in the cervix of the uterus. Not infrequently, the infection of Bartholin's glands leads to the formation of an abscess (vulvovaginal) that is characterized by more acute throbbing pain and swelling between the labia.

In the treatment of such a condition, broad spectrum antibiotics or combination therapy, such as tetracycline or penicillin and streptomycin, are most effective. Hot packs and sitz baths may provide comfort; analgesics add to the relief from pain. Not infrequently, the in-

flammatory reaction may subside, but there usually is a recurrence later if the gland is not excised. The duct of the gland often may be occluded after subsidence of the inflammation. As the gland continues to secrete, a Bartholin's cyst is formed. These cysts usually are removed surgically.

Once the acute stage of the infection has passed, the disease tends to become chronic. Bartholinectomy is recommended if cancer is feared or there are large, painful recurrences with obstruction at the introitus. Postoperatively, the application of ice packs intermittently for 24 hours reduces the likelihood of edema and provides comfort. Thereafter, warm sitz baths or a perineal heat lamp are effective.

Fistulas of the Vagina

A fistula is an abnormal, winding opening between 2 internal hollow organs or between an internal hollow organ and the exterior of the body. The name of the fistula indicates the 2 areas that are connected abnormally: a *ureterovaginal* fistula is an opening between the ureter and vagina; a *vesicovaginal* fistula, between the bladder and the vagina; and a *rectovaginal* fistula, between the rectum and the vagina. Fistulae may occur congenitally, but in the adult, the breakdown often occurs because of tissue damage resulting from an invasive carcinoma.

The immediate problem becomes one of infection and resulting excoriation. For example, the patient who has a vesicovaginal fistula has a continuous trickling of urine into the vagina. With a rectovaginal fistula, there is fecal incontinence, and flatus is discharged through the vagina. When such a discharge combines with a leukorrhea, a malodorous condition develops that is difficult to control. The woman quite naturally tends to withdraw from social contacts. Deodorant sprays and vaginal pads are temporary measures until surgery is performed. Unfortunately, because of the poor condition of the tissues, surgical repair may not be possible.

Treatment and Nursing Management. If surgery is contemplated for the repair of a vaginal fistula, the tissues of the patient are treated so that they are in the most optimal condition possible. This is brought about by proper nutrition with an increase in vitamin and protein content of meals, local cleanliness by means of douching and enemata, rest, and intestinal chemotherapy. When inflammation and edema have subsided, surgical repair may be attempted. Of the different kinds of fistulae, the rectovaginal are the most difficult for the patient to handle and many times surgical correction is not possible.

Postoperatively, following repair of a rectovaginal fistula, bowel activity is limited by keeping the patient on clear liquids for several days before progressing to low-residue and then full diet. More rest is required for this person than most postoperative patients because of a higher incidence of debilitation and the delicate as well as sensitive nature of the tissues. Warm perineal irrigations and controlled heat lamp treatments are effective in stimulating the healing process.

For the patient who has had a repair of a vesico-vaginal fistula, a Foley catheter is usually inserted. Drainage is observed carefully and its proper functioning must be maintained. If the catheter becomes clogged, urine may collect in the bladder to cause pressure that may damage the repaired tissue. Bladder irrigations and vaginal irrigations are done gently with minimal pressure.

Effective measures to assist the woman whose fistula cannot be repaired must be planned on an individual basis. Cleanliness, frequent sitz baths, and deodorizing douches are required, as well as the use of perineal pads and rubber pants. Particular attention to skin care is necessary to prevent excoriation. Bland creams or a light dusting of cornstarch may be soothing. Morale boosters and attention to the social and psychological needs of this patient are essential components of effective care.

Vaginal Infection

Leukorrhea and Simple Vaginitis. *Leukorrhea* is a whitish vaginal discharge, which in slight amount is considered normal at the time of ovulation, just prior to the menarche or onset of menstruation. The vagina is protected from infection by its acid secretion (pH 3.5 to 4.5) and the presence of Doderlein's bacilli. If the resistance of the patient is lowered and organisms, such as *Escherichia coli*, staphylococci and streptococci, invade the vagina, a more profuse and yellowish mucoid discharge is present and a simple *vaginitis* or inflammation of the lining of the vaginal wall develops. Often vaginitis is accompanied by an urethritis, because of the proximity of the urethra. The discharge may cause itching, redness, burning and edema, which may be aggravated by voiding and defecation.

Treatment may be directed toward enhancing the natural flora of the vagina. This can be accomplished by a weak acid douche (1 tablespoon of white vinegar to 1 quart of warm water). In addition, beta-lactose, a sugar, can be administered as a vaginal suppository. Upon insertion into the vagina, the suppository dissolves with body heat; the sugar stimulates the growth of Doderlein's bacilli. An additional objective is to initiate chemotherapy. Local intravaginal applications may be dispensed from a tube with an applicator. This is inserted into the vagina and medication is expressed in the desired amount. Chemotherapeutic cream may be applied locally after douching or sitz

baths as prescribed. Cleanliness after voiding and defecation are stressed.

Trichomonas vaginalis is a protozoan that infects the vagina and produces a profuse frothy white irritating leukorrhea. The organism thrives in an alkaline media and is detectable under microscopic examination as a pear-shaped mobile flagellate. Persistence is required in the treatment of this condition because of its resistance. Remissions under treatment may occur, the organism being harbored in the urinary tract or other parts of the lower urogenital tract not as accessible to local treatment. The male partner may have the organisms in his urogenital tract and he may cause reinfection of his mate.

The most effective treatment appears to be metronidazole (Flagyl) given as a tablet orally 3 times a day for 10 days. For stubborn infections, oral therapy is combined with a vaginal insert of the same medication. Local treatment varies with physician preference. Some prefer a thorough cleansing of the vaginal tract with a soap solution containing hexachlorophene, using cotton balls on a long Kelly clamp, to be followed by local use of suppositories, jellies or powders containing antibiotics or sulfonamides. If the bladder is involved, instillation of silver protein (Argyrol) may be used.

Monilial vaginitis is a fungal infection caused by *Candida albicans*. It is seen commonly in patients with poorly controlled diabetes mellitus, which supports the fact that this fungus thrives in an environment rich in carbohydrate. Monilia is also found in patients who have been on antibiotic or steroid therapy for a while, probably reducing the number of natural protective organisms usually present in the vaginal tract.

The vaginal discharge is irritating and watery, containing white cheesy particles. It causes itching and sometimes severe yeast vaginitis. White material is noted adhering to the vaginal walls. Treatment is directed toward controlling the diabetes, if present. Locally, gentian violet (5 per cent) swabbing of the vagina may be done 3 times a week or more often. A perineal pad should be worn to prevent staining of clothing. In addition, other useful antibiotics are nystatin (Mycostatin) and tetracycline. Antiseptic medications such as Hexetidine (Sterisil) and Propion Gel, which contains calcium and sodium propionate, are also useful.

Atrophic (Senile) Vaginitis. A common postmenopausal occurrence is atrophy of the vaginal mucosa, which then becomes more prone to infection. An annoying vaginal discharge causes itching and burning. Treatment is similar to that of simple vaginitis. In addition, estrogenic hormones taken orally or

TABLE 26-1. The patient with a vaginal infection

Condition	Cause	Signs and Symptoms	Objectives of Treatment
Trichomonas vaginalis	*Trichomonas vaginalis* (protozoan)	Inflammation of vaginal epithelium, producing burning and itching Greenish-yellow or yellowish-white vaginal discharge	To remove exudate, relieve inflammation, restore acidity and reestablish normal bacterial flora: vinegar or pHisoHex douches; insert Floraquin tablets To destroy infective protozoa: insert chlortetracycline capsules q. 2 n. x 7
Monilial infection	*Candida albicans* (fungus)	Inflammation of vaginal epithelium producing itching, reddish irritation White cheeselike discharge clinging to epithelium	To eradicate the fungus: Local applications of gentian violet; Mycostatin vaginal suppositories To relieve other causative factors: Stop antibiotic therapy; determine if diabetes or other systemic disease is present
Infection of Bartholin's gland	*Escherichia coli* *Trichomonas vaginalis* Staphlyococcus Streptococcus Gonococcus	Erythema around Bartholin's gland Swelling and edema Development of Bartholin's abscess	To drain the abscess: Antibiotic therapy; surgical drainage; excision of gland in patients with chronic bartholinitis
Cervicitis— acute and chronic	Gonorrhea Streptococcus Many pathogenic bacteria	Profuse purulent vaginal discharge Backache Urinary frequency and urgency	To determine the cause: Cytologic examination of cervical smear To eradicate the gonococcus, if present: Penicillin, 600,000 units daily, or chloromycetin therapy if indicated To eradicate other causes: cervical cauterization
Postmenopausal vaginitis (atrophic vaginitis)	Lack of estrin effects	Loss of redness, tissue folds, and epithelial covering of the vagina Itching and burning	To provide estrogen therapy for vaginal epithelialization: Topical estrogen therapy; improve nutrition

applied locally as an ointment are effective in restoring epithelium.

Patient Education and Nursing Management. *Vaginal Irrigations.* Douches are common therapeutic measures in the treatment of patients with gynecologic diseases. They are used both before and after operation and are of 2 types: vulvar and vaginal.

Vaginal irrigations are used therapeutically to cleanse or disinfect the vagina and adjacent parts both before and after operation. They may be used also to soothe inflamed tissues and to stimulate relaxed tissues. Occasionally, hot or cold douches are indicated in the treatment of oozing from the parts.

The patient is prepared for a vaginal douche in the same manner as for a vulvar douche. Commonly used solutions include sterile water, normal saline, and antiseptic solutions.

Douches should be given at a temperature of 43.3° C.

(110° F.) or as ordered. To give the douche, the patient is placed in the dorsal position on the bedpan and covered to prevent chilling. The tube leading from the douche bag is clamped, and the end of the tube with the douche nozzle is inserted into the reservoir, which then is hung on the standard. The reservoir should be not more than 2 feet above the level of the patient's hips. The nurse then puts on the sterile gloves, and, separating the labia with the thumb and the forefinger of the left hand, cleans the vaginal orifice and inserts the douche nozzle gently into the vagina for a distance of 2 inches, the tip being directed toward the hollow of the sacrum. The clamp then is removed from the tube, and the solution is allowed to flow. Pressure should be avoided to prevent douche fluid refluxing through the uterus and the tubes. The solution can be allowed to flow intermittently until at least 1 liter of solution has been used. The treatment should not be done hastily if therapeutic benefits are to be achieved; it should take from 20 to 30 minutes. At this time the nozzle may be removed, and the patient should be asked to strain as if trying to move the bowels. This act tends to expel the fluid remaining in the vagina. The bedpan then is removed, and the parts are dried with cotton. The patient should be instructed to remain flat on her back for at least an hour after a hot douche. After the douche has been completed, the apparatus should be cleansed and sterilized again, including the bedpan. When done at home, the patient usually lies in the bathtub and follows the same principles just described.

Vulvar irrigations are indicated chiefly after operations on the perineum. They should be given after each urination or bowel movement in an effort to keep the incision free from infection. The patient should be brought to the side of the bed and placed on the bedpan in the dorsal position, with the knees apart and the labia separated. The bed should be protected by placing a rubber or plastic sheet under the pan. Warmed sterile water then is poured gently over the vulva from a sterile pitcher. The area is dried with sterile gauze or cotton, and a sterile dressing or pad is applied and held in place with a T-binder.

Vaginal antiseptic jellies have been available for local application since the advent of chemotherapy, sulfa and penicillin jellies. By means of an applicator, the patient is able to administer such medication. Creams or jellies can be used before and after operation, and in many instances they are substituted for the therapeutic and cleansing douche. It may be necessary for the patient to wear a perineal pad during the course of the application.

Conditions of the Vulva

Pruritus (Itching of the Vulva). In young women this problem usually accompanies chronic infections of the genital tract such as trichomoniasis, yeast infection or gonorrhea, or it may be caused by strong chemical douches. Symptoms are itching, which causes scratching and a thickening of tissues. The patient often appears nervous. Management of these patients requires a conscientious search for the cause. Glycosuria and urinary incontinence need to be controlled and cleanliness must be scrupulous. Soothing lotions and ointments offer temporary relief.

Condylomata. Condylomata are warty papillary excrescences that appear on the external genitalia. They are the result of irritation and infection. There are 2 usual types: those of the pointed type are associated with gonorrhea; the flat condylomata usually are considered syphilitic in origin. The condylomata of themselves cause few symptoms, but nearly always there is an associated leukorrheal discharge that causes maceration and irritation.

Kraurosis and Leukoplakia. Kraurosis is a disease of the vulva in which the skin over these structures becomes thin, dry, white and easily fissured. As the disease advances, the structure of the vulva may be shrunken and leathery in appearance. The chief symptom is marked itching. Often it leads to the development of cancer of the vulva.

Ovarian extract, antihistaminics and vitamin A have been used with some success in the treatment of these patients, but often in advanced cases vulvectomy is recommended.

Leukoplakia is a somewhat similar condition characterized by grayish-white patchy thickening of the vulvar skin with itching and burning. It is treated as is kraurosis.

The Patient with Cancer of the Vulva. Cancer of the vulva represents about 5 per cent of all malignancies of the female reproductive organs; it usually occurs in elderly women. Although it begins on the skin surface and is easily noticed as a small ulcer that becomes infected and causes pain, women so affected seem reluctant to seek medical attention. Procrastination causes more extensive involvement, jeopardizing cure. Early treatment may be curative; uncorrected, the cancer may spread to the inguinal lymph nodes.

Medical and Nursing Management. Carcinoma of the vulva is best treated by surgery *(vulvectomy)* including excision of the superficial and deep inguinal lymph nodes. In addition to the nursing care described on p. 101, wide preparation of the skin includes perineal, pubic and inguinal regions. This patient must be allowed time to talk and ask questions. Fear of mutilation and loss of function is lessened when a woman of child-bearing age learns that the possibility of having sexual relations is good, as is the possibility of her becoming pregnant following a simple vulvectomy. Of course, the nurse must know what the physician has told the patient in this regard. Radical vulvectomy is more extensive and may require a second trip to the operating room for skin grafting.

Upon returning from the operating room, perineal dressings are more likely to remain in place and be comfortable for the patient if a T-binder is used. Groin wounds may be exposed or covered with simple dressings. Because of serous drainage, dressings need to be changed frequently for the first 3 days. Care must be taken to prevent dislodgement of Penrose or other drains. Since stitches may be taut because of the surgeon's attempt to approximate tissues, comfortable positioning is required. Perhaps a low Fowler's position, or occasionally a pillow placed under the knees, will relieve tension on the incision. Turning is important and comfort may be achieved with a pillow placed strategically between the legs and against the lumbar region. Moving from one position to another requires time and patience on the part of both patient and nurse. Ambulation may be attempted on the second or third day.

Major nursing objectives are to prevent wound and bladder infection. The wound is cleansed daily with soap solution containing hexachlorophene, dilute hydrogen peroxide, or warm saline. After a *gentle* cleansing, a warm water spray is pleasant, nontraumatizing and enhances circulation. The wound should be exposed to the air at frequent intervals. While stitches are in, some physicians prefer dry heat from a heating lamp and later, perineal packs or soaks.

A low residue diet helps to prevent straining on defecation and wound contamination. Of particular concern is urethral and catheter care, inasmuch as an indwelling catheter is usually in place. The incidence of infection is high, which emphasizes the need for the best in nursing intervention. Many nursing researchers frown on the use of sitz baths for vulvectomy patients because of the likelihood of reinfecting the wound.

Analgesics are given as required for comfort. Because the healing process is slow and the nature of the surgery disquieting to a female, this patient is apt to be discouraged. The nurse must be aware of the patient's uneasiness about being "caught" unduly exposed when visitors arrive or someone enters the room. She will tend to be sensitive and apologetic about odors; cleanliness, deodorant sprays, immediate removal of soiled dressings, and adequate ventilation contribute to a more pleasant environment.

Posthospital care requires the transference of complete instructions to the visiting nurse or family member who will care for this patient at home. Gradual resumption of physical and social activities is to be encouraged.

RELAXATION OF PELVIC MUSCLES

Cystocele

Cystocele is a downward displacement of the bladder toward the vaginal orifice (Fig. 26-6). It is caused occasionally by tissue weakness, but most often it is a result of injuries received during childbirth. The condition appears as a bulging downward of the anterior vaginal wall that causes a sense of pelvic

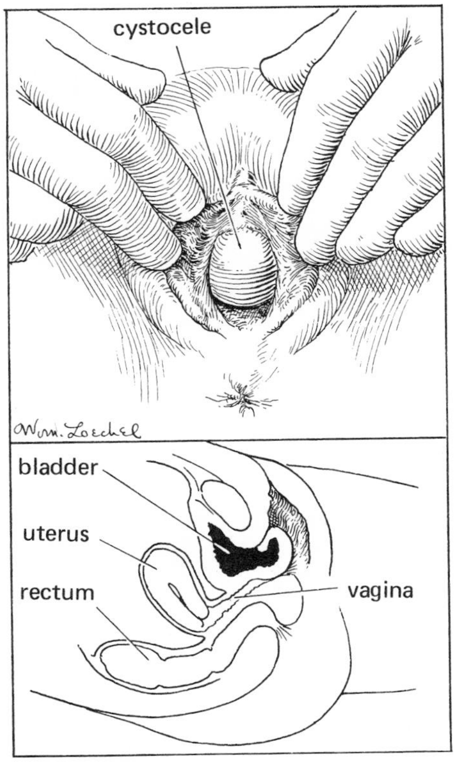

Fig. 26-6. Cystocele. Relaxation of the anterior vaginal wall permits downward bulge of bladder on straining.

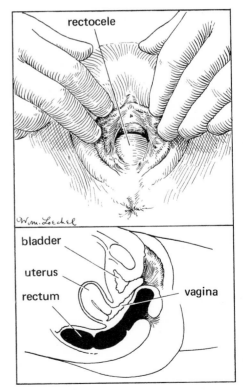

Fig. 26-7. Rectocele. Relaxation of the posterior vaginal wall permits bulging of the rectum with the vagina on straining.

pressure, easy fatigue and often such urinary symptoms as incontinence, frequency and urgency of urination.

The treatment of the condition is surgical, the operation for the repair of the anterior vaginal wall being termed *anterior colporrhaphy*. Perineal exercises sometimes are prescribed and help to strengthen the weakened muscles. These are more effective in the early stages of a cystocele.

Rectocele and Lacerations of Perineum

Injuries to the muscles and the tissues of the pelvic floor frequently occur at the time of childbirth. Due to tears in muscles below the vagina, the rectum may pouch upward, pushing the posterior wall of the vagina in front of it. This condition is termed a *rectocele* (Fig. 26-7). The lacerations may extend at times so as to sever completely the fibers of the anal sphincter (complete tear). The symptoms of this condition are similar to those given for cystocele, substituting for the urinary symptoms those of constipation and incontinence of gas and liquid feces in patients with complete tears.

The operation for the repair of these patients is called a *perineorrhaphy* or a *posterior colporrhaphy*. Anterior and posterior colporrhaphies often are classed together under the term *plastic operations*.

Nursing Management Before and After Perineal Surgery. The chief problem is to encourage women with these problems to see a gynecologist. There is a tendency to procrastinate, to feel embarrassed, to expect that in time it will take care of itself, or to even believe that this is a natural consequence of childbearing that has to be accepted. They need to know that the condition can become more restricting; it cannot cure itself, but can lead to complications such as infections, cervical ulceration, cystitis, hemorrhoids and other problems.

When the patient is admitted to the hospital, it may be part of the plan for optimal operative preparation to allow a day or two for relaxation in bed. Low Fowler's position lessens congestion and edema. Usually this patient has been very busy caring for children or she is older and probably has other physical problems. In either event, the rest may be welcome. For a posterior colporrhaphy, it is important to have the intestinal tract empty; therefore, a cathartic and enemas are in order.

Postoperatively, the objectives of care are to prevent pressure on the suture line and prevent infection. This will require perineal care and may preclude the use of dressings. Voiding is to be encouraged. The patient always is urged to void within a few hours after operation, and every 4 to 8 hours thereafter. The bladder should not be allowed to accumulate more

than 150 ml. of urine for the first few days, especially after operations for cystocele and complete tear. If the patient does not void within the above period, or if she feels uncomfortable or has pain in the region of the bladder before 6 hours, catheterization should be performed. Some physicians prefer to have an indwelling catheter in place for 2 to 4 days. There are various other methods of bladder care.

After each urination or bowel movement, the perineum should be irrigated with warm sterile saline (see vulvar douche, p. 600) and the area blotted dry with sterile cotton.

There are several methods used in caring for the sutures. In one method, the stitches are left alone until healing occurs, i.e., for 5 to 10 days, and daily vaginal douches of sterile saline are given thereafter during the period of convalescence. In another method—the wet method—small douches of sterile saline are given twice daily, beginning on the day after operation and continuing throughout convalescence. Of course, the method to be used depends on the preference of the surgeon.

A heat lamp may be used to help dry the area and enhance the healing process. Commercially available sprays containing a combination of antiseptic and anesthetic solutions are soothing and effective. An ice pack applied locally may relieve discomfort. A plastic bag filled with ice chips is effective; allow the weight of it to rest on the bed and not on the patient.

The routine postoperative care is much like that after an abdominal operation. The patient is placed in bed with the head and the knees elevated slightly. Liquid diet (many surgeons omit milk) is given on the first day and then a full diet as soon as desired.

Patients after operations for a complete perineal laceration (through the rectal sphincter) require special care and attention. The bladder should be emptied by catheterization if the patient is having discomfort. She should be kept flat in bed with the head raised on a pillow. Most surgeons prefer that the patient have no bowel movements for 5 to 7 days. A rectal tube should not be introduced during this period, and enemas never are used. Liquid diet without milk is given, and, in order to reduce peristalsis and inhibit bowel function tincture of opium (paregoric) (15 minims) may be administered. On the sixth or the seventh day give 1 ounce of mineral oil, followed at the first inclination for a bowel movement by a small oil enema (3 or 4 ounces) that should be retained for a few minutes.

Throughout the convalescence of all patients who have had plastic surgery, liquid petrolatum or other stool-softening agent is given each night after a soft diet is begun. Instructions are given regarding douching and when to return to see the gynecologist.

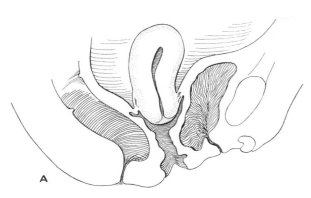

(A) First-degree prolapse of the uterus and the vagina. Note uterus dipping into vaginal vault.

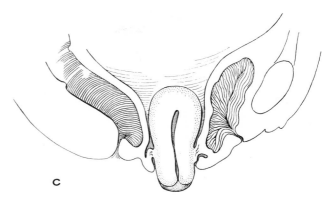

(C) Third-degree prolapse. Uterus protrudes outside of body.

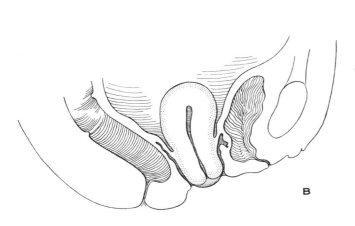

(B) Second-degree prolapse. Extension of cervix beyond vaginal os.

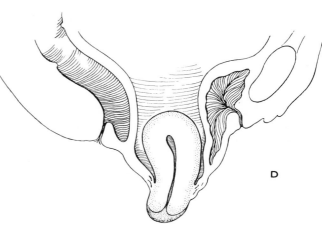

(D) Procidentia.

Fig. 26-8. Prolapse of the uterus and the vagina. (Gray, L. A.: Postgrad. Med. *30*:208-209)

Displacements of the Uterus

The uterus lies normally with the cervix at right angles to the long axis of the vagina and with the body inclined slightly forward. However, it is freely movable, owing to the requirements of pregnancy. The strain of this physiologic function, the formation of adhesions or a weakening of its natural supports may produce changes in the normal position that usually causes no trouble to the patient, but may give rise to many troublesome symptoms.

Backward Displacements. The backward displacements (retroversion and retroflexion) may give rise to such symptoms as backache, a sense of pelvic pressure, easy fatigue, and leukorrheal discharge. More retrograde displacements are asymptomatic rather than symptomatic.

The treatment of backward displacements is surgical only if the condition is incapacitating. The uterus is brought forward into its normal position by way of an abdominal incision and maintained there by shortening its ligaments. Some patients with retroversion may be treated by the use of pessaries. These are S-shaped instruments of hard rubber or crystal-clear Plexiglas that keep the uterus forward by exerting pressure on ligaments attached to the posterior wall of the cervix. They are of great value as a test of the patient's symptoms and often effect a cure. Pessaries must be removed and cleaned by the gynecologist at frequent intervals.

Prolapse and Procidentia. Due to the weakening of the supports of the uterus, most often brought about by childbirth, the uterus may work its way down the vaginal canal (prolapse; Fig. 26-8) and even appear outside the vaginal orifice (procidentia; Fig. 26-8).

In its descent the uterus pulls with it the vaginal walls and even the bladder and the rectum. The symptoms caused are similar to those mentioned for backward displacements, plus urinary symptoms (incontinence and retention) from displacement of the bladder. These are aggravated when the woman coughs, lifts a heavy object or stands for a long while. Normal activities are troublesome tasks; even walking up the steps may aggravate the problem. Nurses can encourage friends and relatives with such difficulties to seek medical attention, because time is not likely to correct these conditions. Public health and industrial nurses are in particularly opportune situations to encourage women to have displacements repaired.

The best treatment is operative: the uterus is sutured back into place. Postmenopausal patients may have the uterus removed (hysterectomy). Many patients may be treated by pessaries when, because of age or disease, operation is not feasible.

Patients with prolapse or procidentia should be kept flat in bed for 2 or 3 days with a vaginal pack or a pessary in place. This treatment serves to take the tension off the strained ligaments and allows the surgeon to proceed with greater ease.

CONDITIONS OF THE UTERUS

Lacerations of the Cervix

Lacerations of the cervix may occur as a result of childbirth. When healing takes place, a considerable portion of the mucous membrane, which normally lies in the cervical canal, is everted. It practically always becomes infected and causes an annoying leukorrhea. Most surgeons believe that cervical lacerations predispose to cancer of the cervix, and for this reason these lacerations should be repaired, particularly in the fifth decade, when cancer is most likely to occur.

Dilatation and Curettage

A dilatation and curettage (D and C) is the widening of the cervical canal with a dilator and the scraping of the uterine endometrium with a curette. It is done to secure endometrial or endocervical tissue for cytologic examination, to control abnormal uterine bleeding and as a therapeutic measure for incomplete abortion.

Since this procedure is done under anesthesia and requires surgical asepsis, it is done in the operating room. Explanations as well as psychological and physical preparations are done by the nurse. The patient has a right to know what will be done (usually explained by her gynecologist) and what to expect in the way of postoperative discomfort, drainage or incapacity. Many physicians do not require perineal shaving, but voiding and evacuation by small enema of the intestinal tract is usually desired.

In the operating room with the patient in the lithotomy position, the cervix is dilated with an instrument and scrapings of the endometrium are obtained by means of a curette. Tissue for biopsy also may be obtained by cutting with an electric needle or by using a punch biopsy forceps. A cone of tissue may be obtained with a cautery or scalpel. Packing is placed in the cervical and vaginal canal; a sterile perineal pad is placed over the perineum.

Postoperatively, a sanitary belt is positioned to hold the pad in place. When the pad requires changing, a sterile pad is used during the time packing is in place (usually 24 hours). Excessive bleeding in any event needs to be reported. After operation the patient usually prefers to rest the remainder of the day. She may get up to go to the bathroom. Her diet is what she desires.

Discomfort in the form of pelvic and low back pain is usually relieved by mild analgesics.

Endocervicitis

Endocervicitis is an inflammation of the mucosa and the glands of the cervix. It is a fairly common problem in which organisms can gain access to the cervical glands after abortion, intrauterine manipulation or delivery. It is an infection which, if untreated, may extend into the uterus, tubes, and pelvic cavity. In the majority of cases the inflammation is caused by the ordinary pyogenic organisms, but gonorrheal infection of the glands can occur. Inflammation can cause erosion of the cervical tissue, causing spotting or bleeding. The chief symptom is a thick purulent leukorrheal discharge, at times associated with sacral backache, low abdominal pain and disturbances in menstruation.

Palliative treatment consists of douches and the application of antiseptics to the cervix, but often a cure is effected only after destroying the cervical glands with a cautery or excising the diseased tissue. Anesthesia may or may not be required, since cauterization is a painless procedure. Following cauterization, the patient should rest more than usual for the next few days. The nature of vaginal discharge should be explained to the patient so that she can expect a grayish-green, malodorous discharge for up to three weeks, because of sloughing cervical tissue. A follow-up visit is recommended by the gynecologist in 2 to 3 weeks, when the cervix is checked for possible stenosis, which may require dilatation. Usually, 6 to 8 weeks are required for healing. Sexual relations are resumed upon recommendation of the physician.

For more severe chronic cervicitis, conization may be done, which may require over-night hospitalization. Anesthesia is optional. In the operating room, the tip of an electric instrument is inserted into the external os of the cervix and rotated to cut and coagulate a cone of tissue. After-care may require packing, but otherwise it is similar to that following electric cauterization. The patient should note any excess bleeding and report it to her physician.

The Patient Having a Hysterectomy

Psychological Considerations

The psychosocial problems faced by women undergoing gynecologic surgery are those discussed in the beginning of this chapter, on page 586. Moreover, when hormonal balances are upset, as often occurs in disturbances of the reproductive system, the patient may exhibit depression and heightened emotional sensitivity to people and situations. Each patient must be understood in the light of such factors, and approached and evaluated individually. This understanding must be shared by her family as well as the paramedical personnel. The nurse who exhibits interest, concern and willingness to listen to the patient's fears will add immeasureably to the patient's progress through her surgical experience, however temporary or prolonged that may be.

Preparation of the Patient

This differs little from the details described for the preparation of a patient for a laparotomy. The lower half of the abdomen and the pubic and the perineal regions should be carefully shaved and cleansed with soap and water. The bowels and the bladder should be empty before the patient is sent to the operating room. This is most important.

Abdominal Hysterectomy

The midline incision is usually made under general anesthesia. In a *subtotal hysterectomy,* the fundus of the uterus is removed but the cervical stump remains. A *total hysterectomy* involves the removal of the entire uterus, including cervix; the tubes and ovaries remain. In a *panhysterectomy,* the entire uterus, tubes and ovaries are removed.

Postoperatively, the principles of general postoperative care for abdominal surgery apply (p. 129). In addition, because of the proximity of the surgical intervention to the bladder, problems of voiding may be expected; edema or nerve trauma may cause temporary atony and an indwelling catheter may be used.

If no catheter is in place, catheterization may be necessary if the patient has not voided after 8 hours. If the catheter is in place, it is usually removed on the third or fourth day. Bladder infection may result from the pooling of residual urine; therefore, the patient is catheterized after each voiding.

To combat the discomfort of abdominal distention, a nasogastric tube may be inserted in the operating room, especially if the surgeon realizes that excessive handling of viscera took place, or if a large tumor was present, its excision could cause edema because of the sudden release of pressure. Postoperatively, fluids and food may be restricted for a day or two. If there is abdominal flatus, a rectal tube may be prescribed as well as heat to the abdomen. When peristalsis begins, the patient is served additional fluids and soft diet. Ambulation facilitates the return to normal.

Vascular disorders, such as phlebitis, thrombosis or edema, must be guarded against. Frequent changes of position and avoidance of high Fowler's position and pressure under the knee will minimize stasis and pooling of blood. The nurse must be particularly alert if the patient has varicose veins in her legs. Special leg exercises to promote circulation and the application of elastic bandages help.

In patients in whom there is anemia due to the loss of blood caused by a tumor, convalescence may be hastened by a high-protein diet supplemented by iron salts. If the tumor has been so large as to produce marked relaxation of the abdominal walls, often it is wise to advise the patient to wear an abdominal support or a girdle for a time after the operation. The surgeon usually orders the application of an abdominal binder after surgery for such patient, to be worn until the support is obtained.

In anticipation of posthospital care, the nurse provides opportunities for the patient to ask questions. The patient should be aware of the nature of her surgery and the immediate and long-range limitations, if any, imposed by it. For example, a subtotal hysterectomy does not stop menstruation, whereas a total hysterectomy produces a surgical menopause. In the latter situation, the gynecologist directs the patient in hormonal replacement. The patient needs to know when sexual relations and her usual physical activities can be resumed. Annual or more frequent physical examinations, including gynecologic evaluation, are imperative for maintaining peace of mind and detecting early evidence of pathology.

Vaginal Hysterectomy

In older individuals and especially in individuals in whom prolapse has occurred, the uterus may be removed through the vagina. The abdomen is not entered in the vaginal hysterectomy, but the entire

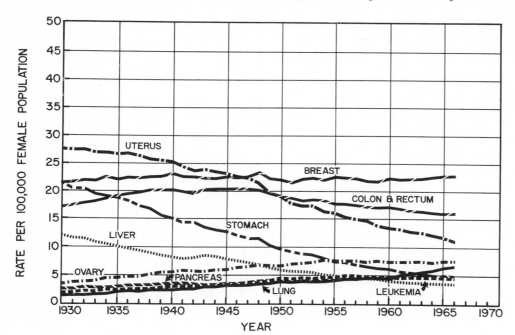

Fig. 26-9. Female cancer death rates by site.

procedure is carried out through the vagina. In these patients either the uterus alone may be removed, or the uterus including the fallopian tubes and the ovaries may be taken away. Postoperative care of such patients is similar to that of those patients who have had plastic surgical procedures performed (see p. 602).

Tumors of the Uterus

Incidence and Patient Education

In this country, malignant tumors of the female reproductive system (excluding the breast) rank as the second cause of death, accounting for approximately 23,000 deaths in 1968. However, the death rate for uterine cancer has been showing a steady decline, which has been attributed to the education of women to seek annual check-ups, including the Papanicolaou test (see p. 588). When it is realized that 13 million women have heard of this test but have not yet had it performed, while another 7 million have never heard of it nor have had it performed, much remains to be done.

Why a woman who knows about the Papanicolaou test does not have it performed is a question to be explored by all those concerned with public health. Are women who feel and look healthy afraid to "look for trouble"? Is getting to the clinic or physician inconvenient, because of hours, transportation, or babysitting difficulties? Not only is the continued dissemination of information necessary, but it may be necessary for health personnel to "go more than half-way" in order to ensure the broadest possible application of

this test. Perhaps a routine Papanicolaou test could be a required part of pre-employment examinations, applications for marriage license, admissions to a hospital, and applications for insurance. Perhaps the professional nurse could be trained to do the test, to make it more available. Perhaps someday a "do-it-yourself" kit will be available, so that a woman could follow simple instructions to get her own specimen and send it properly preserved to the laboratory. Whatever measures are followed to increase the number of women having this simple, painless test will save lives that otherwise would be claimed by cancer.*

Cancer of the Cervix

Cancer of the cervix is the most common cancer of the reproductive system in women. It may occur at any age, but it is most common between the ages of 30 to 50. This disease is almost always curable in its preinvasive state. Early cancer of the cervix is usually asymptomatic. Therefore, to discover the disease early, every woman over 35 years of age should have a thorough gynecologic examination yearly.

Statistics seem to indicate that sexual activity has some relationship to the incidence of cancer of the cervix, its being found most often in women who have married young and have had children. Studies made on its incidence among prostitutes also tend toward this conclusion. Chronic infections and erosions of the

* A sound and color film, *Time and Two Women*, is an effective teaching tool for use in women's groups. Available from the local American Cancer Society.

cervix seem to play a significant part in its development. It may become a large cauliflowerlike growth or a deep, ulcerating crater before giving many symptoms of its presence.

The classification in Table 26-2 has been widely accepted. In studying this table one has the sobering realization that the prognosis of the patient with Stage 4 cancer of the cervix is poor, and that the patient's problems are many.

Symptoms. The 2 chief symptoms of early carcinoma of the cervix are leukorrhea and irregular vaginal bleeding or spotting. For a long time the leukorrhea may be the only abnormal symptom. The discharge increases gradually in amount, becomes watery and, finally, dark and foul-smelling because of necrosis and infection of the tumor mass. The bleeding occurs at irregular intervals, between the periods (metrorrhagia) or after the menopause. It may be very slight, just enough to spot the undergarments, and it is noted usually after some form of trauma (intercourse, douching or defecation). As the disease continues, the bleeding may become constant and increase in amount.

As the cancer advances, the tissues outside the cervix may be invaded, including the lymph glands anterior to the sacrum. In one-third of patients with invasive cervical cancer, the disease involves the fundus. The nerves in this region become involved, producing excruciating pain in the back and the legs that is relieved only by large doses of narcotics. The final picture is one of extreme emaciation and anemia, often with irregular fever due to secondary infection and abscesses in the ulcerating mass.

Medical and Surgical Mangement. In situ cancer of the cervix is confined to the mucosal layer of the cervix. If the patient is of child-bearing age, the surgeon may perform an extensive conization procedure in which the substance of the cervix surrounding the entire length of the cervical canal is dissected free of its epithelial coverings and removed, like the core of an apple, together with the involved mucosa. Following this procedure, however, the patient has to have periodic cytologic smears and close follow-up supervision. In the majority of patients a simple hysterectomy is preferred for cancer in situ.

Radical surgery is advocated by some authorities, especially when a patient is unable to withstand the effects of radiation or has a radiation-resistant cancer. The type of surgery may vary from a radical hysterectomy with bilateral dissection of nodes to a total exenteration of the pelvic organs. The latter operation is performed occasionally when distant metastasis has not occurred, and the disease is confined to the pelvis. The pelvic lymph nodes, the uterus, the vagina, the bladder, and the rectum are removed, and the

TABLE 26-2. International classification of carcinoma of the uterine cervix

Stage 0. Carcinoma in situ. The carcinoma is limited to the epithelial layer with no evidence of invasion.

Stage 1. The carcinoma is confined strictly to the cervix.

Stage 2. Parametrial cancer. The carcinoma infiltrates the parametrium on one or both sides, but does not invade the pelvic wall.

Stage 2. Vaginal cancer. The carcinoma infiltrates the vagina, but does not involve the lower third.

Stage 2. Corpus cancer. The endocervical carcinoma has spread to the corpus.

Stage 3. Parametrial cancer. The carcinomatous infiltration of the parametrium invades the pelvic wall on either one or both sides. On rectal examination, no cancer-free space is found between the tumor and the pelvic wall.

Stage 3. Vaginal cancer. The carcinoma involves the lower third of the vagina.

Stage 3. Isolated pelvic metastases. Isolated carcinomatous metastases are palpable on the pelvic wall (irrespective of the extent of the primary cervical growth).

Stage 4. Bladder extension. The carcinoma involves the bladder; determined by cystoscopic examination or by the presence of a vesicovaginal fistula.

Stage 4. Rectal extension. The carcinoma involves the rectum.

Stage 4. Distant spread. The carcinoma spreads outside the true pelvis (below the vaginal inlet, above the pelvic brim and now includes distant metastases to other organs).

urinary stream is diverted into an isolated ileal loop or to the skin surface of the abdomen. The patient and her husband are advised before the operation about the permanent colostomy stoma and the diversion of the urinary stream.

Radiation Therapy. Patients with more extensive cancer usually are treated with radiation therapy. Radium, radioactive cobalt (^{60}Co) or iridium (^{192}Ir) is introduced into the endocervical canal for a period of time as prescribed by the radiotherapist. This treatment may be supplemented by external radiation therapy with supervoltage machines directed over the pelvis in an effort to eliminate the spread of cancer by way of the lymphatic system. A protective shield is placed over the intracavitary area receiving radium. The therapy is individualized according to the patient's stage of disease and her response and tolerance for radiation.

The preparation of the patient should begin as soon as she is told that radiation therapy is recommended. Usually, several days of testing is done, perhaps on an

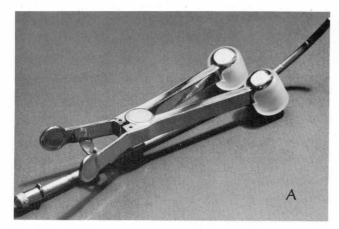

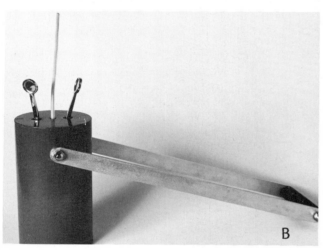

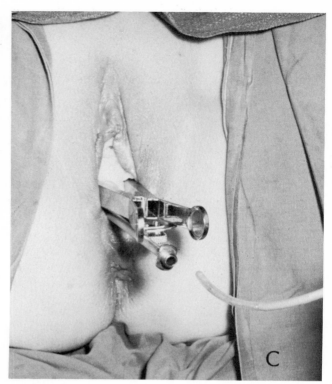

FIG. 26-10 (A) Close-up showing relationship of tandem and ovoids with tandem in place. (B) Lead pot containing the radium carrier for the ovoids and tandem. (C) Applicator in position ready to be loaded. (Hilkemeyer, N.: Nursing care in radium therapy. Nurs. Clin. N. Amer., March, 1967)

outpatient basis, and might include cervical and endometrial biopsies, blood studies, electrocardiogram, chest x-ray and cystoscopy. Making herself available for questions, the nurse can explain the nature of the tests and what is expected of the patient. The patient is usually admitted to the hospital the day before radiation therapy begins. The intestinal tract is cleansed with enemata and the vaginal tract by douche, such as 1 oz. Betadine per 1,000 ml. water. Anesthesia is usually general, and the required medications and surgical preparations are done.

Several applicators are manufactured for radiation treatment of carcinoma of the cervix and the uterus. The Ernst applicator is commonly used for cervical carcinoma (Fig. 26-10). It consists of a central portion (tandem) that is inserted into the uterus. The tandem contains 1 to 3 radium tubes. Surrounding the cervix in the vaginal vault are radium-loaded capsules called *ovoids*. The ovoids and the intrauterine tandem are fixed together in one applicator. Different sections of the tandem and the ovoids are loaded with tubes of radium in the radiotherapy department and

transported to the operating room in a long-handled lead cart.

An indwelling catheter is inserted to keep the bladder empty. Under anesthesia the cervix is dilated in the same manner as in a dilatation and curettage. The applicator is inserted, the tandem being placed in the uterus and the ovoids in the vaginal vault (Fig. 26-10). Then vaginal packing is inserted to maintain the position of the applicator. The objective of treatment at this time is to keep the tandem and the ovoids at certain anatomic points so that the radiation remains at a fixed dosage and is not to be changed during the period of treatment.

Another method of radium application is the *afterloading technique*. In this procedure, the radium is not inserted in the operating room, which reduces the exposure of many individuals to the radium. In surgery, the tandems and ovoids as well as packing are inserted (Fig. 26-10); the patient emerges from anesthesia in the recovery room and then is taken to the x-ray department for anterior-posterior and lateral x-rays before being returned to her room. At

FIG. 26-11. Sagittal section through the uterus showing an Ernst applicator in treatment position. Gauze packing usually is placed on the anterior and the posterior sides of the applicator to hold it firmly in position. This may produce a sensation of pressure in the bladder and the rectum. (Radium Chemical Co., Inc., New York, N. Y.)

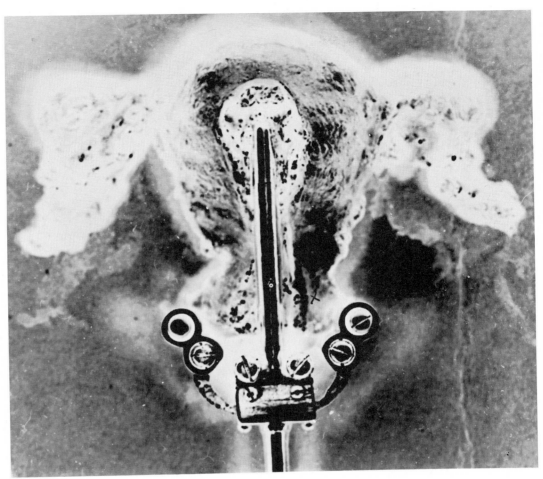

this time, she is placed in the lithotomy position. The radium curator brings the radium carrier (Fig. 26-10) and the surgeon removes the radium from the lead pot and inserts them in the already-positioned apparatus.

Nursing the Patient Receiving Radium Treatment. *While the radium is in place, all nursing measures are geared to keeping the radium applicator in the uterine canal and to preventing a change in the position of the applicator during the course of treatment.* Usually, the patient is on a low-residue diet to prevent the bowels from moving and possibly dislodging the radium. The nurse should inspect the catheter frequently to make sure that it is draining properly. *The chief hazard of improper drainage is that the bladder may become distended and be in the path of radiation.*

The patient is observed for evidence of temperature elevation, nausea or vomiting. These symptoms should be reported to the physician, as often they are indicative of radiation sickness. Although antiemetic drugs may be given to the patient at this time, the radiotherapist usually modifies the dosage schedule, as these symptoms may indicate that the patient is reaching her point of tissue tolerance. These patients often have poor appetites and need to be encouraged to eat and to drink.

Usually the patient is permitted to lie on either side or on her back with the head of the bed elevated about 30°. Back care is much appreciated by the patient, but adequate care is given with a minimum of time spent at the bedside. The nurse must remember to protect herself from excessive radiation. While appearing unhurried, she should care for the patient's needs in as efficient manner as possible. Hence, visits to the patient should not be aimless, and these nurse-patient contacts should provide opportunity for the patient to talk, relieving her anxiety and fear.

Radium Removal. At the end of the prescribed period, the nurse should notify the surgeon that it is time for the removal of the radium. Sterile gloves, long forceps and a waste basin should be provided for his use.

A linen bag is kept in the patient's unit, and any soiled linen is stored there until the radium has been removed and accounted for. Radium is the most expensive metal in common use today. The tiny amount used in the application often is valued at thousands of dollars, so that extreme care is necessary in handling the tubes after their removal from a patient. The number of tubes applied should be noted on the operating sheet, and the nurse should be sure that the same number is removed. After removal from the filters, the tubes should be placed in small lead or brass bottles supplied for the purpose and taken immediately to the hospital repository. Burns may be obtained by an over-dosage; that is, by not removing the radium at the end of the prescribed time or by too frequent handling of radium tubes. For this reason they should be removed promptly from the patient at the end of the prescribed period and handled not directly, but with long forceps, preferably behind a lead shield. After the patient has had the radium removed, usually she is given a cleansing enema, and then she may be out of bed. (See p. 201, Radiation Therapy).

Postirradiation Care. Unfortunately, before x-rays can reach the tissue that requires treatment, they must pass through healthy tissue. The skin is especially vulnerable to x-rays, and caution must be practiced to avoid burns. The skin is kept dry; the use of soap on irradiated areas is avoided. For a dry, desquamating reaction to radiation, a light dusting of a soothing powder that does not contain heavy metals, such as cornstarch, relieves itching and discomfort. When areas of erythema occur, a bland ointment such as aloe vera ointment, white petrolatum, or vitamin A and D ointment may relieve the irritation. No ointment should be used unless ordered by the physician. With supervoltage x-ray units, large tumorcidal doses can be given with less skin reaction.

Following large doses of x-rays, the patient may show anorexia, nausea and vomiting. Some studies have shown that nausea often occurs when it has been suggested that it might occur. Because of this, the likelihood of nausea should not be mentioned. Diarrhea and tenesmus are symptoms of radiation injury to the intestine. These symptoms should be reported to the physician, who will decide whether treatment should continue.

During treatment the nurse should encourage her patient to drink citrus-fruit juices. For meals, small, frequent servings may be more appetizing than large servings. Pyridoxine orally is helpful in minimizing discomfort.

In preparing the patient for discharge, the nurse will afford her an opportunity to ask questions. The patient should know how much activity is permissible at home, whether she can use a douche or vaginal cream, when she can resume sexual relations, and when she should return for follow-up visits. She should also know what reactions are worthy of her calling to the attention of her physician. Of course, the nurse must be aware of the extent of information the physician has already given the patient, and should refer her back to the physician if necessary.

Nursing the Patient with Advanced Cancer of the Cervix. Unfortunately, not every patient will be seen by a physician and treated early. Only palliative treatment is suitable when the disease is advanced. The patient's major problems will arise from pain, vaginal bleeding and a foul-smelling discharge, intestinal obstruction, and urinary or fecal fistulae.

Mild analgesics, such as salicylates, provide symptomatic relief at first, but later in the course of the disease, opiates are necessary. Radiation therapy may help to control the pain. If not, a chordotomy may be effective.

Bleeding may be controlled by external or internal radiation, the insertion of local packing into the uterus, or by a bilateral hypogastric artery ligation. The malodorous discharge that is so distressing to the patient may be relieved by cleansing douches. Antibiotic therapy allays secondary infection. The soiled perineal pads should be changed frequently, wrapped in paper, and removed from the room immediately.

When an intestinal obstruction occurs, a colostomy may be necessary. Surgery or radiation therapy may cause the formation of urinary or fecal fistulae. If operative repair is not feasible, a diversion of the urinary or the fecal stream may be done (see page 571).

The nurse must be able to cope with the despair and the despondency manifested by these patients. It is important that the nurse help the patient to feel that her case is not "hopeless," and that she is not being neglected. Keeping the environment cheerful, promoting the intake of a nutritious diet, and encouraging the family to give extra little attentions will help to brighten the patient's day and to raise her morale.

Cancer of the Fundus

Cancer of the fundus of the uterus is seen only about one third or one fourth as often as cancer of the cervix. About 50 per cent of all patients with postmenopausal bleeding have cancer of the fundus. Its progress is slow, metastasis occurs later, and the symptom of irregular vaginal bleeding often appears early enough in the disease to allow cure by the removal of the uterus. In late cases, radium and roentgen rays are the usual therapeutic measures.

The major emphasis for the nurse is to encourage all women, particularly those over 40, to have annual check-ups including a gynecologic examination. More detailed nursing care following surgery or radiation therapy is found on p. 128 and p. 195.

Pelvic Exenteration*

Radical Pelvic Surgery. Pelvic exenteration or evisceration may be performed in both men and women when other forms of therapy prove to be ineffective in checking the spread of cancer. These patients are selected carefully on the basis of their likelihood to survive the surgery as well as to adjust to and accept the imposed limitations.

Anterior pelvic exenteration is the removal of the bladder and lower part of the ureters. In addition, in women the vagina, the adnexa, the pelvic lymph nodes and the pelvic peritoneum are removed. The ureters are implanted in the colon or the small intestines.

Posterior pelvic exenteration is the removal of the colon and the rectum. In addition, in women the uterus, the vagina and the adnexa are removed. The pelvic lymph nodes may or may not be excised.

Total pelvic exenteration is the removal of the rectum, the distal sigmoid colon, the urinary bladder, the distal portion of the ureters and the internal iliac artery and vein. In addition, in the female all pelvic reproductive organs, lymph nodes, and the entire pelvic floor, including the pelvic peritoneum, levator muscles, and perineum are removed. Both urinary and fecal diversion are necessary in this procedure; hence, the patient will have a colostomy, and a substitute bladder will be made from a segment of ileum.

Nursing Considerations. Although the following discussion considers pelvic exenteration from the perspective of the female patient, similar considerations apply to male patients who have undergone like procedures. This patient has probably faced surgery before and is aware of most of the physical preparation required before going to the operating room. However, the most important preparation is psychological. The needs of this patient are courage, the ability to realize what is about to happen, and the fortitude to be able to accept it. Consent to have the operation may have been given without question, since it may be clearly evident that this is a life-saving procedure.

However, the full impact of adjustment may come several days postoperatively. Expressions of the patient may offer clues to her feelings that will give direction to subsequent care. Usually, the patient's reaction takes 1 of 3 courses: (1) she may adjust very well without any abnormal complications; (2) she may become depressed, listless, and wish to die (this reaction may be altered with antidepressant medications; meanwhile, the nurse continues to emphasize the *positive* features of the patient's future); (3) there

---

* An excellent 18-page publication is: *Hemipelvectomy with Total Pelvic Exenteration: The Challenge and the Response.* A Nursing Clinical Conference presented by the Nursing Department of the Clinical Center, National Institutes of Health, Clinical Center, Bethesda, Maryland 20014.

may be an insidious reaction in which the patient exalts her disfigurement, assuming an almost martyr-like pose. By being preoccupied with herself and centering her attention on her disability, she may show pettiness, be selfish in her demands, and withdraw interest from her family. The nurse's hope here is to try to turn the patient's thoughts from herself to others and to direct the patient to see her body in its proper perspective, focusing more attention on the intact parts.

This patient requires intensive care postoperatively. Because satisfactory body function depends on adequate fluid balance, particular attention needs to be given to an accurate intake and output record. Proper functioning of the gastrointestinal tract may not return for several days. The nurse is referred to colostomy and ileostomy care on pages 484 to 493. Likewise, in the care of a patient with radical surgery, the likelihood of complications is greater; therefore, the nurse must be aware of the signs and the symptoms of postoperative complications as well as the ways and means of avoiding such problems.

Teaching and rehabilitation are a continuous part of the care of the patient with a pelvic exenteration. This should be gradual, moving from the simple to the more complex. The family should be included as the convalescence of the patient continues. Cognizance of the patient's own reaction and day-by-day progress is observed carefully; encouragement and understanding go a long way in helping her to achieve as many goals as possible.

Myomata or Fibroid Tumors

Myomatous or fibroid tumors of the uterus are benign tumors arising from the muscle tissue of the uterus. They are very common, occurring in at least 40 per cent of all women. They develop slowly between the ages of 25 and 40, and often they attain large size after this period. There are instances where such a tumor causes no symptoms. The most common symptom is menorrhagia. Other symptoms are due to pressure on surrounding organs—pain, backache, constipation and urinary symptoms—and the tumors often cause metrorrhagia and even sterility.

Treatment and Nursing Care. The treatment of uterine fibroids depends to a large extent on their size and location. The patient with minor symptoms is watched closely. If she is desirous of having children, treatment is as conservative as possible. As a rule, large tumors producing pressure symptoms should be removed. Usually, the uterus is removed (hysterectomy), the ovaries being preserved, if possible. If the tumor is small, it may be removed (myomectomy), the wound in the uterus being closed. This is the procedure of choice in young women. If the tumor is producing excessive bleeding, the uterus and the tumor are removed (hysteromyomectomy).

Principles of nursing management of the patient having a hysterectomy are on pages 605-606.

CONDITIONS OF THE OVARIES AND THE PELVIC CAVITY

Ovarian Cysts and Tumors

The ovary is a frequent site for the development of cysts. These may be simply pathologic enlargements of normal ovarian constituents, cysts of the graafian follicle or corpus luteum, or they may arise from abnormal growth of ovarian epithelium. These are considered benign tumors with a possibility of becoming malignant.

Dermoid cysts are tumors that are believed to arise from parts of the ovum that disappear normally as ripening (maturation) takes place. As their origin is unsettled, all that can be said is that they are tumors made up of undifferentiated embryonal cells. They are slow-growing and at operation are found to contain a thick yellow sebaceous material arising from a skin lining. Hair, teeth, bone, brain, eyes and many other tissues often are found in a rudimentary state within these cysts.

Treatment and Nursing Management. The treatment of ovarian cysts is surgical removal. However, if malignant degeneration has taken place, with invasion of the abdomen and emaciation (general carcinomatosis), operation is of little benefit. The patient may be given roentgen therapy and testosterone. The abdomen may be tapped to relieve distention from ascites.

The postoperative nursing care after cystectomy is similar to that for abdominal surgery, except for one particular. The marked decrease in intra-abdominal pressure incidental to the removal of a large cyst often leads to considerable abdominal distention. This complication may be prevented to some extent by the application of a pad and an abdominal binder.

Endometriosis

Endometriosis is a benign lesion in which cells resembling those lining the uterus are found growing aberrantly in the pelvic cavity outside of the uterus. Endometriosis affecting the uterine lining is referred to as *adenomyosis*. (This is discussed on p. 611—the condition is somewhat different.) In order of frequency, pelvic endometriosis attacks the ovary, uterosacral ligaments, the cul-de-sac, uretervesical peritoneum, cervix, umbilicus, laparotomy scars, hernial sacs and appendix. The misplaced endometrium responds to ovarian hormonal stimulation, and, indeed, depends on this for survival. When the uterus goes through the process of menstruation, this ectopic tissue bleeds—mostly into areas having no outlet—which then causes pain and adhesions. At surgery, these lesions are typically small, puckered, brown or blue-black, indicating concealed bleeding. If the endometrial tissue is within an ovarian cyst, there is no outlet for the bleeding and the formation is referred to as a *chocolate cyst*. Symptoms vary and may be misleading, since extensive endometriosis may cause few symptoms whereas an isolated lesion may produce considerable symptomatology. The following patient experienced some typical symptoms:

> Mrs. Esther Salinas, age 29, complained of acquired dysmenorrhea and an acquired progressive dyspareunia (painful sexual relations). She recalled painful defecation, some premenstrual staining and frequency of urination with occasional hematuria. So far all attempts for Mrs. Salinas to become pregnant have failed (infertility).

Several theories have been advanced regarding the origin of these lesions: (1) reflux menstruation, which is the backflow of menses, causes endometrial tissue to be transported to extopic sites through the fallopian tubes; (2) during surgery, endometrial tissue inadvertently may be transferred by way of instruments; (3) such tissue may possibly be spread by lymphatic or venous channels; and (4) tissue that covers the pelvic peritoneum and ovaries is a remnant of embryonic tissue. A combination of such factors may be responsible.

Pelvic endometriosis, rarely encountered in Negroes, occurs in about 25 to 30 per cent of women. It is thought to be the cause in 30 to 40 per cent of all cases of infertility. Upon bimanual examination, fixed tender nodules may be detected and the uterus may be restricted in motility, indicating adhesion formation.

Medical and Nursing Management. This depends upon the severity of the symptoms and the age group of the patient. Medical management is initiated with hormonal therapy that blocks ovulation. This relieves dysmenorrhea and postpones surgical intervention. When the function of child-bearing is to be considered, as with Mrs. Salinas, conservative therapy is preferred, preserving as much of the reproductive tract as possible. Procedures of choice are resection of cysts and lysis (cutting) of adhesions. The likelihood of recurrence of endometriosis is high; however, the desire for and possibility of pregnancy takes priority. In women aged 35 to 45 years, ovarian tissue is saved when possible; after age 45, more radical procedures are undertaken. Total hysterectomy (p. 605) usually alleviates most of the symptoms.

The nurse's role in patient education is to dispel false fears, such as a causative relation between the use of tampons and endometriosis—this is not true. In order to combat the upward trend of endometriosis, women need to be encouraged to have regular physical examinations. Unusual menstrual bleeding patterns need to be reported and investigated.

Adenomyosis. In this condition, endometriosis involves the uterine wall; the incidence is highest in women from 40 to 50 years of age. Symptoms are hypermenorrhea (excessive and prolonged bleeding), acquired dysmenorrhea, polymenorrhea (abnormally frequent bleeding) and premenstrual staining. On physical examination, the uterus is felt to be enlarged, firm and tender. Treatment depends upon severity of bleeding and pain; hysterectomy offers greater relief than more conservative forms of therapy.

Pelvic Inflammatory Disease

Pelvic inflammatory disease (P.I.D.) is an inflammatory condition of the pelvic cavity that may involve the fallopian tubes (salpingitis), ovaries (oophoritis), pelvic peritoneum, or pelvic vascular system. This disease may be acute or chronic and may be caused by the staphylococcus, streptococcus, or venereal organisms. These pathogenic organisms usually are introduced from the outside, pass through the cervical canal and the uterus and into the pelvis by way of lymphatic channels, uterine veins or fallopian tubes. When pelvic infection is caused by the tubercle bacilli, it is usually conveyed by way of the bloodstream from the lungs.

Medical and Nursing Management. In order to give effective care, the nurse must know the cause, signs and symptoms of pelvic infections, as well as methods of spread. The main objective of care is to control the spread of infection within the patient, to the nurse and to others. Symptoms may include abdominal pain, nausea and vomiting, elevation of temperature, malaise, malodorous purulent vaginal discharge and leukocytosis. The patient assumes the semi-Fowler position (dependent drainage). Catheterization and the use of tampons are avoided. In addition, the patient is supported nutritionally and with selective antibiotic therapy. Spread of infection to others can be controlled in many ways: employment of safeguards in handling perineal pads, such as using an instrument or gloves, and depositing the soiled pad in a paper bag for proper disposal; careful handwashing procedures, using hexachlorophene soaps; adequately disinfecting utensils, bedpans, toilet seats, and linen as indicated by the procedure for the control of the specific organism. The patient must be informed and take part in plans to prevent contamination of others as well as reinfection of herself.

For comfort, heat can be applied to the abdomen externally and hot douches may be ordered to improve circulation. Proper recording of vital signs, patient's physical and mental response to treatment, and nature and amount of vaginal discharge are necessary to guide the physician in future therapy.

If untreated, pelvic inflammatory disease can lead to chronic pelvic discomfort. Scar tissue may close the fallopian tubes, resulting in sterility. Ectopic pregnancy could occur if a fertilized egg is unable to pass the stricture. Adhesions are a common development that eventually may require removal of the uterus, tubes and ovaries.

The "caring" for the patient with pelvic inflammatory disease is just as important as the "curing." This infection may be very distressing, both physically and mentally. Such a patient may feel well one day and develop vague symptoms and discomfort the next; she suffers from constipation and menstrual difficulties. These patients are frequently unjustly labeled "neurotic." The nurse must also keep in mind the social aspects of venereal diseases, which may cause pelvic inflammatory disease (see p. 918).

BIBLIOGRAPHY

Books

Ball, T. L.: Gynecological Surgery and Urology. ed. 2. St. Louis, C. V. Mosby, 1963.

Brewer, J. I., Molbo, D. M., and Gerbie, A. B.: Gynecologic Nursing. St. Louis, C. V. Mosby, 1966.

Calderone, M. S.: Manual of Contraceptive Practice. Baltimore, Williams & Wilkins, 1964.

Editors of Consumer Reports: The Consumers Union Report on Family Planning. Mt. Vernon, New York, Consumers Union of U.S., Inc., 1966.

Fitzpatrick, G. M.: Gynecologic Nursing. New York, Macmillan, 1965.

Hawkins, J.: Shaw's Textbook of Operative Gynecology. ed. 3. Baltimore, Williams & Wilkins, 1968.

Kleegman, S. J., and Kaufman, S. A.: Infertility in Women. Philadelphia, F. A. Davis, 1966.

Miller, N. F., and Avery, H.: Gynecology and Gynecologic Nursing. Philadelphia, W. B. Saunders, 1965.

Miller, R. A.: Feminine Forever. New York, M. Evans, 1966.

Planned Parenthood Federation of America, Inc.: Memos for Nurses—The Nurse and Family Planning. New York, Planned Parenthood—World Population, 1965.

TeLinde, R. W.: Operative Gynecology. ed. 3. Philadelphia, J. B. Lippincott, 1962.

General Articles

Dillon, H. B.: The woman patient. Nurs. Clin. N. Amer., 3:195-203, June, 1968.

Durbin, M. S., Jr.: Geriatric gynecology. Nurs. Clin. N. Amer., 3:253-261, June, 1968.

Franklin, R. R., and McIlhaney, J. S., Jr.: Anomalies of the female genital tract. Nurs. Clin. N. Amer., 3:205-215, June, 1968.

Gold, J. J.: Symposium on treatment of menstrual disorders. Mod. Treatment, 2:117-212, Jan., 1965.

McCulley, L. B.: Health counseling of women. Nurs. Clin. N. Amer., 3:263-273, June, 1968.

Newt, M.: Feminine hygiene. Amer. J. Nurs., 64:100-102, Dec., 1964.

Menopause

Blanchet, J.: Estrogen and the menopause. Canad. Nurse, *63:* 38-39, Feb., 1967.

McEwen, D. C.: Estrogen replacement therapy at menopause. Canad. Nurse, *63:*34-37, Feb., 1967.

Infertility

Cohen, M. R.: A simplified plan for the infertile couple. Postgrad. Med., *36:*337-342, 1964.

Fertility Control

Arnold, E.: Individualizing nursing care in family planning. Nurs. Outlook, *15:*26-27, Dec., 1967.

Bennett, E. A.: Abortion. Nurs. Clin. N. Amer., *3:*243-251, June, 1968.

Buxton, C. L.: One doctor's opinion of abortion laws. Amer. J. Nurs., *68:*1026-1027, May, 1968.

Eichner, E.: Progestins. Amer. J. Nurs., *65:*78-81, Sept., 1965.

Fischman, S. H.: Choosing an appropriate contraceptive. Nurs. Outlook, *15:*28-31, Dec., 1967.

Fonesca, J. D., and Buxton, C. L.: Induced abortion. Amer. J. Nurs., *68:*1022-1028, May, 1968.

Hall, R. E.: A comparative evaluation of intrauterine contraceptive devices. Amer. J. Obstet. Gynec., *94:*65-77, Jan., 1966.

Manisoff, M. T.: Counseling for family planning. Amer. J. Nurs., *66:*2671-2675, Dec., 1966.

Milton, I. C.: Contraceptive practices past and present. Canad. Nurse, *63:*29-31, Oct., 1967.

Mitchell, H. D.: How do I talk?—family planning. Amer. J. Pub. Health, *56:*738-741, May, 1966.

Willson, J. R., and Ledger, W. J.: Complications associated with the use of intrauterine contraceptive devices in women of middle and upper socio-economic class. Amer. J. Obstet. Gynec., *100:*649-661, 1968.

Vaginal and Vulvar Problems

Anderson, N. J.: Vulvectomy: Nursing care. Amer. J. Nurs., *60:*668, May, 1960.

Graham, J., and Carpenter, R.: Cancer of the vulva. Geriatrics, *23:*176-178, May, 1968.

Hesseltine, H. C.: Vaginal "infections." Hosp. Med., *4:*68-73, April, 1968.

Hofmeister, F. J., and Reik, R. P.: Vulvectomy. Amer. J. Nurs., *60:*666-667, May, 1960.

McGowan, L.: New ideas about patient care before and after vaginal surgery. Amer. J. Nurs., *64:*73-75, Feb., 1964.

McKeown, M., and Hesseltine, H. C.: Vulval carcinoma. Postgrad. Med., *41:*204-208, Feb., 1967.

Sweeney, W. J., III: Perineal shaves and bladder catheterizations; necessary and benign, or unnecessary and potentially injurious? Amer. J. Obstet. Gynec. *21:*291-295, 1963.

Cervix and Uterus

Alford, D. M.: Nursing care of the patient with endometriosis. Nurs. Clin. N. Amer., *3:*217-227, June, 1968.

Alpenfels, E. J.: Cancer in situ of the cervix—cultural clues to reactions. Amer. J. Nurs., *64:*83-86, April, 1964.

Chalfant, R. L.: Diagnosis and treatment of cancer of the uterus. Nurs. Forum, *4:*67-75, No. 3, 1965.

Gusberg, S. B.: Cancer in situ of the cervix—treatment as preventive medicine. Amer. J. Nurs., *64:*76-79, April, 1964.

Hilkemeyer, R.: Nursing care in radium therapy (uterine cancer). Nurs. Clin. N. Amer., *2:*83-95, March, 1967.

Lewis, G. C., Jr.: Cancer in situ of the cervix—screening and diagnosis. Amer. J. Nurs., *64:*72-75, April, 1964.

Mayo, P., and Wilkey, N. L.: Prevention of cancer of the breast and cervix. Nurs. Clin. N. Amer., *3:*229-241, June, 1968.

Robbins, L. C., and Walker, E.: Cancer in situ of the cervix—problems of control. Amer. J. Nurs., *64:*80-83, April, 1964.

Suit, H. D., *et al.*: Modification of Fletcher ovoid system for afterloading, using standard sized radium tubes. Radiology, *81:*126-131, July, 1963.

PATIENT EDUCATION

Sex Education

Booklets available from:

American Medical Association
535 N. Dearborn Street
Chicago, Illinois 60610

Public Affairs Pamphlets
381 Park Ave., South
New York, New York 10016

Personal Products Corp.
Milltown, New Jersey 08850

Tampax Inc.
161 E. 42nd Street
New York, New York 10017

Kimberly-Clark Corp.
Neenah, Wisconsin 54956

Family Planning

Public Affairs Pamphlets (address above).
Duvall, E.: Building Your Marriage. (No. 113)
Mace, D. R.: What is Marriage Counseling? (No. 250)
Mace, D. R.: What Makes a Marriage Happy? (No. 290)
Ogg, E.: A New Chapter in Family Planning. (No. 1360)

Planned Parenthood—World Population
(Planned Parenthood Federation of America)
515 Madison Avenue
New York, New York 10022
The Churches Speak Up on Birth Control. 1967.
Questions and Answers about Intrauterine Devices. 1967.
The Ethics of Family Planning. 1966

Association for Voluntary Sterilization, Inc.
14 West 40th Street
New York, New York 10018

Abortion

Association for the Study of Abortion, Inc.
120 West 57th Street
New York, New York 10019

CHAPTER **27**

Patients with Problems of the Breast

- *The Female Breast*
- *Diagnosis of Breast Lesions*
- *Conditions Affecting the Nipple*
- *The Patient with an Inflammation of the Breast*
- *Fibrocytic Disease*
- *Tumors of the Breast*
- *Reconstructive and Plastic Surgery*
- *Diseases of the Male Breast*

THE FEMALE BREAST
Development and Physiology of the Breast

Up to the time of puberty it is impossible to find microscopically any difference in the breasts of the 2 sexes. At puberty, some slight swelling appears in the male breast. At the same time, a pronounced increase in size occurs in the female organ. This begins about the tenth year and increases rapidly up to the fourteenth and the sixteenth years. The development of the mammary gland is a result of hormone action that begins with puberty in the female. At this time, the nipple takes on its natural protruding form. In the male, contrary to some statements, breast tissue always exists and may grow.

The breast is a glandular organ with many lobules; its secretion passes through collecting ducts to the nipple. In some women, there is a cyclic engorgement of the breasts, associated with tingling and tenderness; this is due to a hormonal disturbance. The symptoms begin usually in the latter part of the menstrual cycle and disappear when menstruation occurs. About 8 weeks after a woman conceives, her breasts enlarge greatly, the nipples become more prominent and sensitive, and the breast is prepared to nourish the infant. When pregnancy is over and lactation has ceased, the breast shrinks, loses its excessive fat and often becomes flabby and flattened.

Psychosocial Implications

In Western cultures, the breast is considered a significant component of feminine beauty. Shapeliness is a quality much desired and is emphasized in a woman's choice of clothing. Particularly in the United States, the social value placed upon looking young has led to consumer demands for foundation garments that further contribute to a trim, fit look. Thus, any actual or suspected disease of or injury to her breast is interpreted by a woman within the context of the social significance placed upon that organ. Not only do social values play a significant role in the rehabilitation of a patient who has undergone radical breast surgery, but the fear of disfigurement may prevent a woman from seeking immediate medical attention after she has detected suspicious signs or changes in her breast.

A major objective of the health professions is to spread sound advice regarding the prevention of illness and the detection of disease in its early stages. Every woman should be alerted to the early signs of breast pathology, and each should have sufficient information about what to do about suspicious changes. The nurse has great responsibility in the area of prevention and early detection of breast diseases, and in handling the concomitant psychosocial concerns of the patient. The nurse's contacts in industry, diagnostic

615

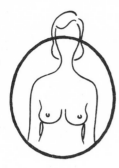

(1) Sit or stand in front of your mirror, with your arms relaxed at your sides, and examine your breasts carefully for any changes in size and shape. Look for any puckering or dimpling of the skin, and for any discharge or change in the nipples.

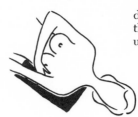

(5) Now bring your left arm down to your side, and still using the flat part of your fingers, feel under your armpit.

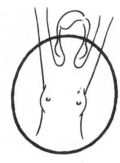

(2) Raise both your arms over your head, and look for exactly the same things. .See if there's been any change since you last examined your breasts.

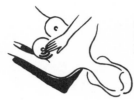

(6) Use the same gentle pressure to feel the upper, outer quarter of your breast from the nipple line to where your arm is resting.

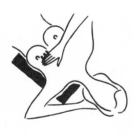

(3) Lie down on your bed, put a pillow or a bath towel under your left shoulder, and your left hand under your head. (From this Step through Step 8, you should feel for a lump or thickening.) With the fingers of your right hand held together flat, press gently but firmly with small circular motions to feel the inner, upper quarter of your left breast, starting at your breastbone and going outward toward the nipple line. Also feel the area around the nipple.

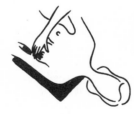

(7) And finally, feel the lower outer section of your breast, going from the outer part to the nipple.

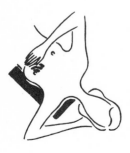

(4) With the same gentle pressure, feel the lower inner part of your breast. Incidentally, in this area you will feel a ridge of firm tissue or flesh. Don't be alarmed. This is perfectly normal.

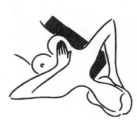

(8) Repeat the entire procedure, as described, on the right breast.

FIG. 27-1. Self-examination of the breast. (American Cancer Society, Inc., N.Y., N.Y.)

clinics, public health and community agencies offer opportunities to teach and disseminate information.

Incidence of Disease

Although the majority of the disorders of the female breast are benign in character, the breast is one of the two female organs that are most frequently primary sites of cancer. The breast normally changes during menstruation, pregnancy, lactation, and menopause, and these variations need to be differentiated from pathologic changes. Although the breast is fairly accessible to examination, the detection and accurate diagnosis of breast disease can be difficult.

About one-fourth of all women have irregular areas in their breasts at some time. Just before menstruation, irregularities produced by hyperplasia and involution occur; these feel granular or finely nodular and usually occur in the upper outer quadrants. Some women have persistently irregular breast tissue that feels shot-like or plaque-like between periods. Such masses are not considered true in the sense that they usually are bilateral and do not increase in size or consolidate. On the other hand, true masses do not fluctuate in size and are usually unilateral. Ninety-five per cent of all true masses are cysts, fibroadenomas and carcinomas.

The benign lesions, represented in the order of frequency and the common ages at which they occur, are: fibrocystic disease (20 to 25 years), fibroadenoma (20 to 39 years), and intraductal papilloma (35 to 45 years). By way of contrast, cancer of the breast is manifested chiefly in the menopausal and postmenopausal years; approximately 75 per cent occur in patients over the age of 40; less than 2 per cent occur before the age of 30.

In 1968, approximately 65,000 new cases of malignant breast tumors were discovered, according to the American Cancer Society, and approximately 28,000 women died from the disease. The survival rate for all breast cancer patients, whether treated or untreated, is roughly 50 per cent; the sooner women seek treatment and the lesion is recognized, the greater the possibility of survival.

DIAGNOSIS OF BREAST LESIONS

Self-Examination

Because 95 per cent of breast cancers are detected by women themselves, top priority must be given to teaching all women how and when to examine their breasts. The nurse is in a unique position to offer this advice and to arrange for showings of the film *Breast Self-Examination*, available from local chapters of the American Cancer Society. The method of self-examination of breasts, which should be performed monthly,

TABLE 27-1. X-ray appearance of breast masses*

	Benign	Malignant
Shape	Round, oval	Variable, ragged, spicular, tentacled
Border	Regular, smooth, well-circumscribed	Irregular, poorly circumscribed
Size	Same as palpable mass	Smaller than palpable mass
Density	Homogeneous	Nonhomogeneous, hard
Surrounding Tissue	Displaced, not invaded	Infiltrated, nipple retracted
Calcifications	Few, isolated or widely scattered, coarse	Numerous, uncountable, confined to area of lesion
Secondary Signs	None	Frequently present

* Egan, R. L.: Mammography. Amer. J. Nurs., *66*:108-111, Jan., 1966.

is shown in Figure 27-1. In addition, breast examination by palpation should be included in the annual complete physical examination of all women. A breast examination should be done twice a year in women who have a family history of breast cancer.

Mammography

Mammography is a roentgenography of the breast without the injection of a contrast medium. It is a safe, simple, nontraumatic, gross diagnostic procedure. It complements but does not substitute for physical examination. With mammography, breast cancer can be demonstrated before signs and symptoms are present; however, it requires skilled roentgenologists to interpret the findings. Egan* offers the following indications for mammography: (1) signs and symptoms of breast disease, (2) previous breast biopsy, (3) familial history of breast cancer, (4) survey of remaining breast after mastectomy, (5) lumpy or large pendulous breasts, difficult to examine, (6) cancerophobia, and (7) adenocarcinoma, site undetermined. Usually 3 views are taken. For the craniocaudal view, the patient is seated while an x-ray is taken from above looking downward. The other 2 views are mediolateral and axillary (Fig. 27-2).

Thermography

Abnormal circulatory signs may be detected by infrared photography. The patient is placed in a room under basal conditions (i.e., the room has been cooled to 21°C. or 70°F.) for 20 to 30 minutes. By means of a sophisticated heat-sensing apparatus, it is possible to

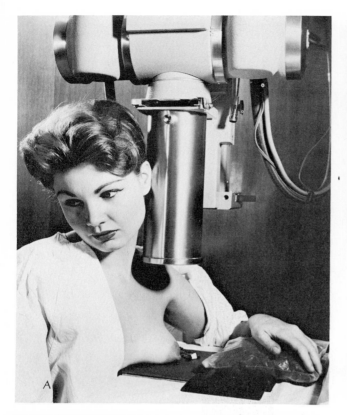

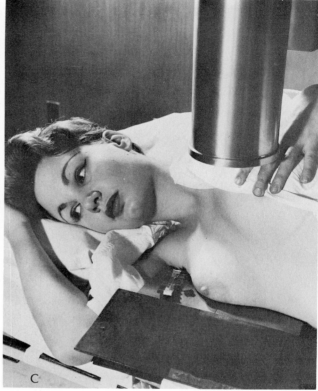

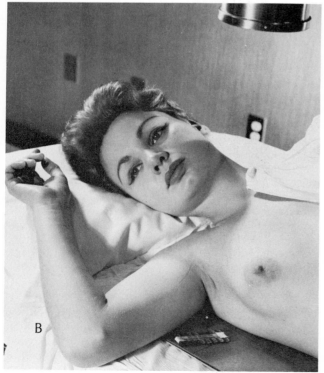

Fig. 27-2. Mammography: A diagnostic adjunct. (A) The craniocaudal view. The patient sits comfortably at the end of a roentgenographic table; the breast is positioned on the film holder and the radiographic tube brought into position as shown. (B) The axillary view. The central beam is centered below the apex of the axilla and parallel to the retromammary space. This position allows maximum visualization of the axilla by reducing the number of skin folds. (C) The mediolateral view. The patient lies on her side; the breast is supported on a wooden block and the film holder. The film markers are placed toward the axilla. The only variable is the distance needed to visualize the entire breast. (Egan, R. L.: Experience with mammography in a tumor institution. Radiology, 75:894-900, 1960)

detect minute amounts of heat generated in and around areas of increased blood supply. This method requires a well-trained radiologist to interpret abnormal patterns. A diagnosis is made only within the context of a thorough history and complete physical examination. With improved devices and techniques, thermography may prove a valuable diagnostic adjunct.

Xerography

In xerography, a selenium-coated plate is subjected to an electrical charge, the x-ray exposure is made, and the plate is then developed by a special process under careful monitoring. The result is a xerogram in which all tissues of the breast, including skin, are portrayed in a bas-relief effect. Although disadvantages exist with regard to the painstaking processing, xerography appears to hold promise in detecting early cancer. However, it has not yet been established as a routine diagnostic procedure.

Biopsy

Aspiration. This procedure can be done in the outpatient department or physician's office. Following the injection of a local anesthetic, a No. 18 needle is directed into the site to be sampled. Upon suction of a syringe, tissue is drawn into the needle. This material is spread on a glass slide, fixed and stained before being sent to the laboratory.

Incisional. Incisional biopsies are usually done in the operating room under general anesthesia, and may comprise the entire lesion. Tissue is sent to the laboratory where it is frozen rapidly; very thin slices containing a good cross-section of tissue are stained with a dye to facilitate microscopic observation.

CONDITIONS AFFECTING THE NIPPLE

Fissure of the Nipple

Fissure of the nipple is a longitudinal ulcer that tends to develop in any woman who is nursing a baby. The ulcer is irritated constantly by the act of suckling and causes the mother considerable pain, often associated with bleeding of the nipple. Prophylactic treatment, cleanliness and washing and drying of the nipple after each nursing usually prevent the occurrence of this condition. In the prenatal period, the woman can wash, dry and lubricate the nipples in preparation for nursing, thereby helping to prevent fissure development. If a fissure develops, it should be washed at frequent intervals with sterile saline solution, and nursing should continue only with the use of an artificial nipple. If healing does not occur promptly, or if the case is severe and painful, nursing should be stopped and a breast pump substituted for it. Persistent ulceration suggests carcinoma or a primary luetic lesion.

Bleeding or Bloody Discharge From the Nipple

At times, a bloody discharge may be noted on the clothes, which upon investigation is found to be coming from the nipple. Often, there may be one area at the edge of the areola where pressure produces the discharge. Although a bloody nipple discharge may occasionally be caused by malignancy, it is most commonly due to a wart-like papilloma growing in one of the larger collecting ducts just at the edge of the areola. This bleeds on trauma and the blood collects in the duct until it is pressed out at the nipple. The duct can be identified in the nipple and traced down, so that the duct and the papilloma can be excised through a small periareolar incision.

Paget's Disease

This disease of the nipple is seen most frequently in women over 40; usually, it is unilateral. Most often it begins as a mild eczematoid condition of the nipple that may spread over the areola and even part of the breast; later, it may become ulcerated or eroded. In the more advanced stages, there may be retraction of the nipple. This is a true carcinoma of the ducts of the breast that converge at the nipple.

When any lesion of the nipple has not healed after a few weeks of treatment by simple cleansing and protective measures, a suspicion of Paget's disease should be confirmed by biopsy examination. This disease demands early and total removal of the mammary gland.

THE PATIENT WITH AN INFLAMMATION OF THE BREAST

Acute Mastitis

This disease may occur at the beginning or the end of lactation. Mastitis may result from the transfer of microorganisms to the breast by the hands of the patient or those of the personnel caring for her. The baby with an oral, eye or skin infection may be a source of infection. Mastitis is also caused by blood-borne organisms. An infection of the ducts results, causing stagnation of milk in one or more lobules. The breast becomes tough and doughy, and the patient complains of dull pain in the region affected. A nipple that is discharging pus, serum or blood demands investigation.

Treatment consists of taking the baby off the breast temporarily. Heat and cold are used to treat the inflammatory process. A saline cathartic is usually administered and the patient may be given a broad-spectrum antibiotic.

Progesterone has been found to reduce breast congestion, which in turn relieves the pain. The patient should wear a firm breast support and follow good habits of personal hygiene.

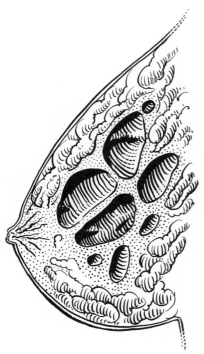

Fig. 27-3. Chronic fibrocystic disease of the breast.

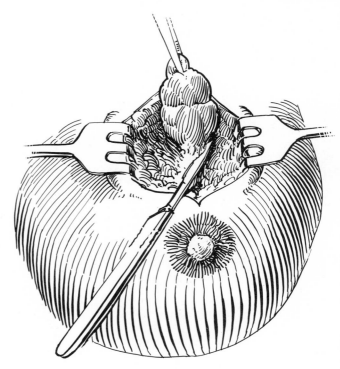

Fig. 27-4. Excision of a fibroadenoma of the breast.

Mammary Abscess

Breast abscess usually develops as a sequela of an acute mastitis, although it may occur independent of lactation. The area affected becomes very tender and dusky red, and pus may be expressed from the nipple. Chemotherapy and antibiotic therapy are being used with success; however, incision and drainage may be performed when fluctuation indicates the presence of pus. Dressings soaked in hot solution increase the drainage and hasten resolution. The use of the suction cup has proved to be valuable in the treatment of such abscesses.

Chronic Cystic Mastitis

In this condition of the breast, many small cysts are produced owing to an overgrowth of fibrous tissue about the ducts. The disease occurs most commonly between the ages of 30 and 50 and is characterized by an uncomfortable feeling in the breast, the presence of small nodules that feel like tiny lead shot, and, occasionally, by shooting pains.

Any mass in the breast should raise a suspicion of malignancy, and for that reason surgical advice should be obtained. If the disease occurs before the age of 38, when it is important to preserve the function of the breast, the lesion may be kept under close observa-

tion for a time. In older women, and in younger women when doubt exists as to the diagnosis, it is safer to remove the mass for pathologic examination.

FIBROCYSTIC DISEASE

Retention Cysts

There is a continuous secretion from the epithelium of the mammary ducts that is so small in amount that it escapes unnoticed at the nipple under normal conditions. With advancing age and the cyclic changes that occur in the breast with each menstrual period, a mammary duct may become obstructed by fibrosis, with the result that the secretion of the duct behind the obstruction collects and dilates the duct to form a retention cyst. These are most prone to appear near the menopause and in women whose breasts have not functioned in lactation and nursing.

These cysts appear as firm, smooth, round masses in the breast and often are tender on palpation or pressure. The cyst itself rarely has any malignant potential, although breasts containing cysts may be more prone to develop cancer than are normal breasts. Most cysts can be treated by simple aspiration of the fluid under local anesthesia. No surgery is required.

Fig. 27-5. Signs of cancer of the breast. (1) Bleeding from the nipple arising from a papilloma in the duct. This may be a benign lesion at first, but it is definitely considered to be a premalignant lesion. (2) Deformity or asymmetry of the breast. (3) Skin attachment at the site of a malignant mass. (4) Retraction of the nipple when cancer appears at the center of the breast. (5) Elevation of the breast involved due to contraction and shortening of the fibrous tissue trabeculations brought about by the malignant tumor. (American Cancer Society, New York)

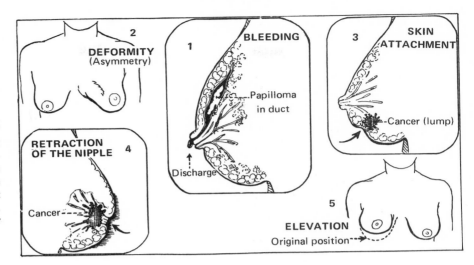

TUMORS OF THE BREAST

Every tumor of the breast should be viewed with suspicion and should be removed unless there is a contraindication.

Fibroadenomata

These are firm, round, movable, benign tumors of the breast, usually appearing in the breasts of girls in their late teens and early twenties. They cause no pain and are not tender. They can be removed through a small incision and have no malignant potential (Fig. 27-4).

Carcinoma

The breast is one of the two most frequent sites of development of carcinoma in the female (see p. 183 for incidence). It is so common that one author states that most tumors of the breast in women over 40 years of age are carcinomatous. Of tumors diagnosed as benign before operation, 10 per cent are found after removal to be cancerous.

The causes of breast carcinoma are not known. It occurs more frequently in women having a family history of breast cancer, in the higher economic levels, and in those having a late menopause. It is not believed that injuries lead to malignancy.

Course of Disease. The tumor is located most frequently in the upper outer quadrant of the breast. As it grows, it becomes attached to the chest wall or the overlying skin. If no treatment is given, the tumor invades the surrounding tissues and extends to the lymph glands of the adjacent axilla. When the tumor arises in the medial half of the breast, its extension may involve the lymph nodes within the chest along the internal mammary artery. Metastases may occur in the lungs, bone, brain or liver. In untreated cases death usually results in 2 or 3 years.

The situation of the patient with an inoperable cancer of the breast is a most distressing one. It is distressing also to the surgeon, who realizes that there was a time when the tumor may have been curable, but that the patient, perhaps through ignorance, neglect or fear, appeared for treatment when it was too late. The situation of the inoperable patient also is distressing because the tumor spreads to such areas as the brain, the lungs, the liver and bone and causes symptoms that are hard to relieve.

Symptoms. The symptoms of the disease, unfortunately, are insidious. A nontender lump, which may be movable, appears in the breast, usually the upper outer quadrant. Pain usually is absent, except in the very late stages. Eventually, a dimpling or "orange peel" skin may be observed. On examination in the mirror, the patient may note asymmetry and an elevation of the affected breast. Nipple retraction may be evident. Later, the breast becomes more or less fixated on the chest wall and nodules appear in the axilla. Finally, ulceration occurs and cachexia becomes prominent.

Medical and Nursing Management. *Physical and Psychosocial Preparation.* The treatment of carcinoma of the breast is removal or destruction of the whole tumor. It is evident that complete removal of the tumor can be accomplished most surely when the cancer still is confined to the breast. This is borne out by clinical experience, which shows a rate of cure better than 70 per cent if the tumor is confined to the breast. When it has spread to the nodes of the axilla, the cure rate falls to 40 per cent.

Surgical removal of the breast and the muscles of the chest wall beneath it, as well as of the lymphatic

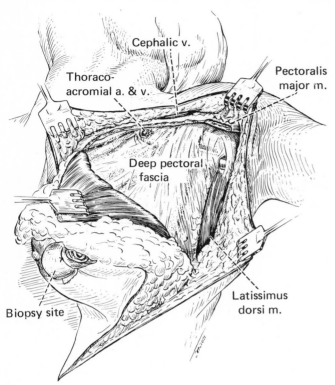

FIG. 27-6A. Radical mastectomy. Area of dissection in intermediate stage. The pectoralis major muscle has been reflexed and the deep pectoral fascia exposed. (Garside, E., and Mella, L.; Radical mastectomy, S. Clin. North Amer. *41*:183)

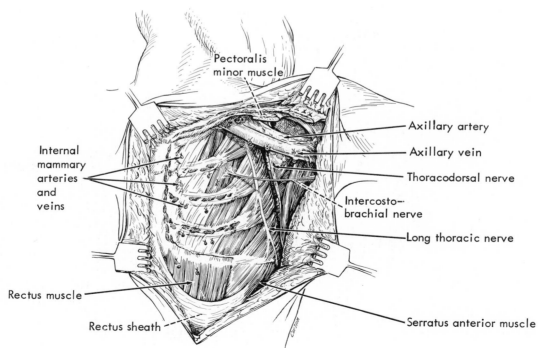

FIG. 27-6B. Radical mastectomy. Dissection completed. (To the student: [1] Why is the drainage so profuse following a radical mastectomy? [2] Why is the dissection subcutaneously so extensive?) (Garside and Mella, p. 184)

pathways if the cancer has spread to the axilla, is looked upon as the best method of treatment in operable cases.

Emotional preparation of the patient begins at the time she is told that hospitalization and biopsy with possible other surgery may be required. Actually all women, when being informed regarding detection of breast disorders, should be prepared to follow through on suspicious findings. As indicated earlier in this chapter, the identification of femininity is strongly related to the breast (p. 615). Upon admission to a hospital for a questionable tumor of the breast, most women have a real fear of cancer. Unfortunately, many times this fear has made them delay seeking treatment until the tumor has metastasized. Fear also stems from the emotional trauma of knowing that the breast may be removed.

The nurse can help greatly in the psychologic preparation of the patient for breast surgery. She can point out that loss of the breast as against loss of life is a small price to pay in a physical sense. It must be recognized that a mastectomy is a significant threat to her femininity. Because of this, the nurse must be available to listen to and support the patient. She may be able to allay the patient's fear of disfigurement by describing artificial appliances that can be used. Such concealment alone, however, may not be enough to erase deep-seated concerns. These must be recognized and accepted by the patient before she can adjust positively to her altered image.

The only delay before operation should be that necessary to check the physical and the nutritional needs of the patient. If radical surgery is anticipated, in which there may be fluid and blood loss, blood replacement must be available. The patient is told by the surgeon that there is a possibility of radical surgery if it is indicated. The support of the husband is sought if it is determined that he can genuinely help through his understanding. No patient should go to the operating room anticipating a half-inch incision for a tumor excision and return having had a radical mastectomy. Because the emotional factor is a significant one, encouragement and reassurance must be given all along the way.

A hypnotic is administered and the usual physical preoperative preparation is carried out. Skin preparation should be extensive enough to meet the maximal possible surgery. If it is known that radical surgery, including a skin graft, is to be done, the donor skin area (usually the anterior aspect of the thigh) must be shaved and cleaned.

Surgery. About 50,000 mastectomies are performed each year in the United States. After receiving general anesthesia, the patient is placed in the supine position

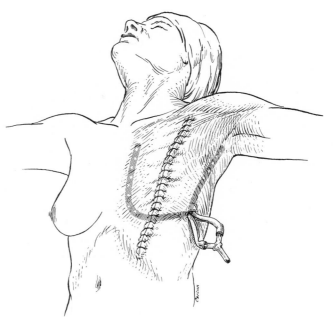

Fig. 27-7. Radical mastectomy. Wound closure with suction tube in place. (Garside and Mella, Radical mastectomy. S. Clin. N. Amer., *41*:186)

on the operating table, the arm of the affected side being positioned upward to expose the axilla. Following a biopsy, the entire field is redraped and a new set of instruments are used so that the possibility of transferring cancer cells from the biopsy site to the other areas of the wound is avoided. A *simple mastectomy* is the removal of a breast without lymph node dissection. A *radical mastectomy* comprises removal of the breast and the underlying muscles down to the chest wall after removal of the nodules and the lymphatics of the axilla (Fig. 27-6). Such a radical operation is necessary to remove the tumor and the area of lymphatic spread. Bleeding points are ligated and the skin is closed as well as possible over the chest wall. Skin grafting is done if the skin flaps are not of sufficient size to close the wound. Pressure dressings usually are applied. A drainage tube usually is placed in the axilla; Hemovac drainage may be preferred by some surgeons. A blood transfusion often is given during the operation to compensate for blood loss.

Postoperative Management. The anesthetic of choice usually is general for a radical mastectomy. Postoperative care is given with special attention to pulse and blood pressure, as they are valuable indices in detecting shock and hemorrhage. Dressings must be inspected for bleeding, especially under the axilla and the area on which the patient is lying.

After the patient has recovered from the anesthesia, sedatives are given for the relief of pain, and the patient is encouraged to turn and take deep breaths to avert pulmonary complications. The dressing usually is fairly snug; however, it should not be so tight that lung expansion is restricted. Some surgeons prefer to include the arm (flexed at the elbow) in the dressing to give added pressure. In other instances, gauze fluffs or foam rubber sponge may be added to the dressing within the binder to provide pressure.

In many patients a drainage catheter is inserted through a stab wound into the axilla; then this catheter is attached to a suction machine and drained into a trap bottle. By this means serum and blood collected are aspirated rapidly, and the skin flap is held tightly against the chest wall. Thus, serum collections and hematomas are avoided. Some surgeons eliminate pressure dressings early in the postoperative period and use Hemovac suction instead. However, dressings over incision and donor graft areas usually are not changed for several days.

Positioning of the patient depends on the dressing; semi-Fowler usually is desirable. The arm, if free, should be elevated with each joint positioned higher than the more proximal joint. Thus, gravity helps to remove the fluid by the lymphatic and the venous pathways. Whether the arm is flexed or extended depends on the orders of the physician. Such elevation helps to prevent lymphedema, which may be a postoperative occurrence due to interference with the circulatory and the lymphatic systems. Whether or not there will be satisfactory postmastectomy lymph drainage depends upon the existence of adequate collateral lymphatic avenues not destroyed during surgery.

The patient usually is allowed out of bed on the second or the third day after operation; the arm on the affected side may be held in a sling for a time to prevent tension on the wound. Assistance is given only when it is needed; the nurse supports the patient from the unoperated side. A normal diet may be given unless nausea is a symptom. If a drainage tube has been inserted, it is removed usually on the second or the third day. The patient may be advised to have radiotherapy after operation to try to destroy cancer cells that may have escaped removal at operation. Anorexia, nausea and vomiting are not infrequent symptoms after irradiation; to abstain from eating and drinking 3 hours before and after these treatments often helps.

Physical and Mental Rehabilitation. The full impact of the meaning of a mastectomy may not be felt by the patient until several days after surgery. Meanwhile, a gesture that offers real support to this patient is the nurse's making it understood that she has time to talk or listen to the patient whenever the patient expresses the need for this. Frequent questions are these: Is it normal to drain so much? Will the swelling of my arm go down? How will my husband react to my deformity? Will I be able to wear a regular bathing suit? Will people be aware that I am a cripple? Will I be able to swim, play tennis or golf, drive a car? After studying this chapter, the nurse should be able to answer these questions intelligently. Her attitude should not be impersonal; this patient needs someone with whom she can share her troubling thoughts. Psychological reaction, however, is expressed differently by different women. This must be understood inasmuch as a patient may appear to be adjusting unusually well and yet deep within be extremely troubled.

The preparation of the husband should not be overlooked. An example of this need is illustrated by the husband who thought that he was being kind by not looking at his wife, whereas she interpreted his reaction as one of rejection and repulsion. If time had been taken to tell the husband how he might help his wife in making her adjustment, such an experience would have been avoided.

After 24 hours, the arm on the affected side should begin active exercise. This can be increased each day with the patient doing more herself by brushing her teeth, washing her face, and combing her hair with the hand on the affected side. Failure to encourage such exercises as "climbing the wall with the fingers" may prolong the disuse of the arm and promote the development of a contracture. Exercise should not be accompanied by pain; if the patient has plastic reconstruction or the incision was closed with considerable tension, such exercises are limited greatly and done very gradually.

Many hospitals promote classes for the postmastectomy patient; this encourages women who would otherwise remain passive and inactive in their own rooms. At the bedside, pulley-type ropes from the over-bed or curtain frame can be used for one kind of exercise. Turning a jump rope that is attached to the door knob can be arranged easily (see muscle training exercises, Fig. 27-8). In all exercises, it is important to emphasize bilateral activity. Likewise, the value of proper posture must be emphasized; to hunch over and favor the affected side as one combs her hair may defeat the purpose of the exercises.

Patient Education for Effective Posthospital Progress. *Care of the Incision Site and Prosthesis.* The surgeon outlines to the patient her plan of care to be followed at home. If the nurse is present, she can later reinforce and clarify the directions for the patient. The nature of the incision, how it looks and feels now and how it will gradually change are explained. The patient needs to know that the newly healed area may have lessened sensation because nerves have been severed; however, it should be bathed gently and blotted dry to avoid injury. Signs of irritation and possible infection should be described, so that if they occur, the patient will know to inform her physician. When talking about the incision, the nurse should refer to it by that term and not as a "scar," since scarring connotes defect, deformity and ugliness in the minds of most persons.

Gentle massage of the healed incision with cocoa butter helps to increase the elasticity of the skin and encourages circulation. When a prosthesis is prescribed, its effect on the incision site needs to be observed. To offset irritation, a layer of lamb's wool is effective when pressure is exerted. The kind of prosthesis suitable for the patient is suggested on an individual basis by the physician. Skilled fitters from reliable companies are available and they usually have many helpful suggestions, literature and an optimistic, understanding approach that is most encouraging to postmastectomy patients.

In preparation for an individualized prosthesis, a temporary make-shift padded brassiere can be designed and stitched by the nurse with the patient's participation. Loose cotton covered with gauze can be stitched loosely into the patient's own brassiere;

A. *Wall hand-climbing.* Stand facing the wall, with the toes as close to the wall as possible — feet apart. With elbows somewhat bent, place the palms on the wall at shoulder level. By flexing the fingers, work hands up the wall until arms are fully extended. Work hands down to starting point.

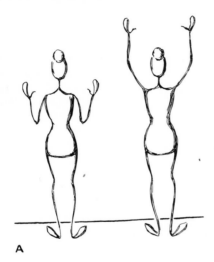

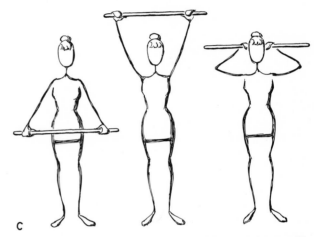

C. *Rod or Broom.* Grasp rod with both hands, held about 2 feet apart. With arms straight, raise rod over the head. Bend elbows, lowering rod behind the head. Reverse maneuver, raising rod above head, then to starting position.

B. *Rope turning.* Stand facing the door. Take free end of light rope in hand of the operated side. Place other hand on hip. With arm extended and held away from the body —nearly parallel with the floor—turn rope, making as wide swings as possible. Slow at first—speed up later.

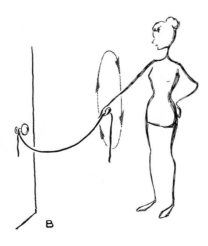

D. *Pulley.* Toss rope over shower curtain rod or doorway curtain rod. Stand as nearly under rope as possible. Grasp an end in each hand. Extend arms straight and away from body. Pull left arm up by tugging down with right arm, then right arm up and left down—like a seesaw.

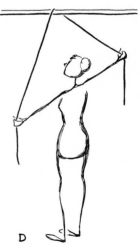

FIG. 27-8. The purpose of the exercise program is to secure a complete range of motion of the affected shoulder joint. (Adapted from Radler: A Handbook for Your Recovery. New York, The Society of Memorial Center)

snaps can be used in making a pocket to fit the "falsie." Ingenuity and resourcefulness can fashion effective padding from sanitary pads, nylon stockings, and shredded foam rubber.

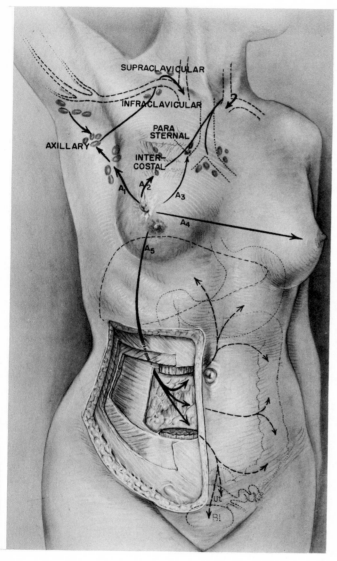

FIG. 27-9. Lymphatic drainage of the mammary gland. Metastases from cancer of the mammary gland may follow several lymphatic pathways: A_1. Upper outer quadrant to axillary, infraclavicular, supraclavicular nodes, etc. A_2. Upper inner quadrant to intercostal and parasternal nodes. A_3. Upper inner quadrant directly to parasternal nodes. A_4. Directly across midline to opposite breast. A_5. Lower quadrants, particularly inner aspect, through pectoralis major, external oblique and linea alba to subperitoneal lymphatic plexus, followed by abdominal and pelvic spread. (MacBryde: Signs and Symptoms, Phila., J. B. Lippincott, 1964)

There are many types of breast prostheses available: sponge rubber, air-filled and fluid-filled. A properly fitted brassiere is essential to a well-fitted prosthesis. Breasts readily follow the law of gravity and change their contour and position with every body motion. Therefore, the most satisfactory prostheses are those filled with a slow flowing, thick fluid. Often, when a patient knows that such appliances are available, her fear of disfigurement is eliminated. No prosthesis should be worn until the physician has authorized it.

Exercise and Lymphedema. The exercises done in the hospital and illustrated in Fig. 27-8 can be related to household activities. Putting dishes on a shelf, dusting, window washing, typing and piano playing are maneuvers that promote and maintain muscle tone.*

Although 9 out of 10 postmastectomy patients escape massive lymphedema, this complication would occur even less frequently if nurses impressed their patients with the importance of elevating and massaging the affected arm for 3 or 4 months postoperatively. Movement increases circulation and thus helps to prevent edema.

As part of treatment for lymphedema, the physician may order a diuretic. An elastic sleeve going from the wrist to the shoulder, similar to an elastic stocking, may be ordered to give extra support to the tissues. Other valuable suggestions that the nurse can offer to her patient about lymphedema treatment at home are: Elevate the arm frequently; do exercises and massage ordered by the physician; swing the arm while walking; wear loose or nonconstricting clothing; keep mastectomy site, underarm and arm scrupulously clean; wear gloves when gardening.

Follow-Up Visits are very important to evaluate incision healing, mental outlook, general physical condition, and to look for evidences of recurrence. If there is a need for public health nurse consultation, the availability of such a service should be pointed out to the patient.

Palliative Treatment and Concern. Occasionally, when a breast tumor is inoperable so far as cure is concerned, the surgeon may remove the breast to free the patient from a foul, ulcerating lesion. There are other methods of treatment, however, that are used in addition to surgery or by themselves. Radiotherapy may be used before and after operation. Radium needles may be introduced into the tumor mass in inoperable cases. There is evidence to support the belief that ovarian hormones influence the growth of breast carcinoma. In some instances, surgical or x-ray castration may be performed, especially in menstruat-

* *After Mastectomy* is a film by the American Cancer Society available from local chapters that is helpful for the postmastectomy patient.

ing women. Male sex hormone (testosterone) has been found helpful, especially in the treatment of metastasis (Fig. 27-9). In some patients removal of the adrenal glands or the pituitary gland has produced regression of the recurrent growth. There is no reason to believe that any of these measures will produce a cure of breast carcinoma, but they may have a palliative effect for a time.

The patient who is admitted to the hospital with an inoperable carcinoma of the breast calls for the utmost in sympathy and understanding: her physical and mental comfort is the primary goal. Details of care follow the regimen used in terminal carcinoma of any part of the body (see p. 193).

RECONSTRUCTIVE AND PLASTIC SURGERY OF THE BREAST

Hypertrophy of the Breast

The breasts are such an important part of the female figure that abnormalities often lead to requests for their surgical correction. The abnormalities most often encountered are breasts that are too large or too small. Those that are too large are said to be hypertrophied; when the condition occurs in early life, it is called virginal breast hypertrophy. The condition is usually bilateral, but may occur on only one side. The hypertrophied breasts that occur in later life are always bilateral.

Symptoms of Breast Hypertrophy. These patients complain of tender breasts, diffuse pains and fatigue. The tenderness and pain is particularly marked at the time of the menstrual periods. The weight of the breasts causes a dragging sensation on the shoulders, and efforts to support these tremendous breasts with brassieres are hopeless. Most patients with virginal hypertrophy also have deep grooves dug into the shoulder tissue by brassiere straps.

Not only are physical symptoms present, but psychological difficulties develop, especially in girls and younger women. They become too embarrassed to wear bathing suits, sweaters or evening gowns. This restricts their social life and they become introverts, avoid social contacts and even marriage. Because they think that they are unattractive, married women develop a sense of insecurity, fearing loss of their husband's affection and, possibly, divorce. These are very real difficulties that cause mental repercussions which may be very serious.

Mammoplasty. The operation performed to reduce the size of the breasts is termed a reduction mammoplasty. In this operation, the surgeon makes one incision beneath the breast and a similarly curved incision in the skin of the anterior breast. The nipple is transplanted to a new location after cutting away the redundant tissue. The remaining skin edges are approximated with sutures and the nipple is sutured to its new location. Drains are placed in the incision and remain for only a day or two. Simple gauze dressings are used without pressure.

Postoperative care following mammoplasty is simple. These patients sit up in bed the day after operation and may be out of bed on a normal diet thereafter. The results of these plastic operations are good as far as relief of symptoms is concerned. There is no recurrence of the hypertrophy and the operation is not a serious one. The newly transplanted nipple will turn black and be covered by a dry scab. This is to be expected, but the scab will come away after a week or 2 as the nipple regains a blood supply in its new location. It must be accepted that the breast cannot function after such an operation.

Operations to Enlarge or Uplift the Female Breast

These operations are fairly frequently requested of plastic surgeons. Although padded brassieres and other devices are available, these do not always give the desired result. The operations are performed through an incision along the undermargin of the breast. The breast is elevated and a pocket is formed between it and the chest wall into which are inserted various types of plastic and synthetic materials intended to enlarge and uplift the breast. These operations are not serious, but they are not always without complications in that the inserted substance may have to be removed.

DISEASES OF THE MALE BREAST

The male breast is subject to the same diseases as the female breast. Very occasionally they develop cancer; not infrequently, there may be hypertrophy of one or both breasts. Hypertrophy in the male is called *gynecomastia* and is frequently the cause of embarrassment in gymnasiums and swimming pools. The enlarged mammary glands are often removed through a small periareolar incision.

BIBLIOGRAPHY

Books

American Cancer Society: A Cancer Source Book for Nurses. New York, American Cancer Society, 1966.
————: Cancer of the Breast, A Report on Research. New York, American Cancer Society, 1968.
Lewison, E. F.: The Total Care of Your Mastectomy Patient. Rev. 1967. (Brochure available to the nursing profession when requested on official stationery.) Identical Form, Inc., 17 West 60th Street, New York, New York 10023.
Moore, F. D., et al.: Carcinoma of the Breast. Boston, Little, Brown & Co., 1968.

Southwick, H. W., Slaughter, D. P., and Humphrey, L. J.: Surgery of the Breast. Year Book Medical Pub., 1968.

Spratt, J. S., and Donegan, W. L.: Cancer of the Breast. Vol. V of Major Problems in Clinical Surgery. Philadelphia, W. B. Saunders, 1967.

Articles

Baker, T. J.: Cosmetic surgery for small breasts. Amer. J. Nurs., *61*:77-78, 1961.

Berens, J. J., and Polson, D. A.: Axillary dissection without mastectomy. Surg. Gynec. Obstet., *124*:123-126, Jan., 1967.

Current Concepts in Cancer: Carcinoma of the breast Stage I—Surgical Spectrum. J.A.M.A., *199*:732-746, 1967.

Egan, R. L.: Mammography. Amer. J. Nurs., *66*:108-111, Jan., 1966.

Gershon-Cohen, J.: Mammography, thermography, and xerography. CA, *17*:108-112, May-June, 1967.

Graham, J. B.: Palliative aspects of gynecological cancer. *In* Hickey, R. C.: Palliative Care of the Cancer Patient. Boston, Little Brown, 1967.

Gribbons, C. A., and Aliapoulios, M. A.: Early carcinoma of the breast. Amer. J. Nurs. *69*:1945-1950, Sept., 1969.

Hartley, I. O., and Brandt, E. M.: Control and prevention of lymphedema following radical mastectomy. Nurs. Res., *16*:333-336, Fall, 1967.

Hickey, R. C.: Palliation of breast cancer. *In* Hickey, R. C.: Palliative Care of the Cancer Patient. pp. 155-185. Boston, Little Brown, 1967.

Is breast cancer really two separate diseases? Med. World News, *8*:30-31. April 21, 1967.

Leis, H. P.: Prophylactic removal of the second breast. Hosp. Med., *4*:45-55, Jan., 1968.

Lewison, E. F.: The nurse's role in early detection of cancer of the breast. Nurs. Forum, *4*:82-86, No. 3, 1965.

Mayo, P. and Wilkey, N. L.: Prevention of cancer of the breast and cervix. Nurs. Clin. N. Amer., *3*:229-241, June, 1968.

Nosanchuk, J. S.: Silicone granuloma in breast. Arch. Surg., *97*:583-585, Oct., 1968.

Quint, J. C.: Mastectomy: Signpost in Time. J. Nurs. Ed., *2*:3-34, Sept., 1963.

Shimkin, M. B.: End results in cancer of breast. Cancer, *20*: 1039-1043, July, 1967.

Wolf, E. S.: Nursing care of patients with breast cancer. Nurs. Clin. N. Amer., *2*:587-598, Dec., 1967.

Zimmer, T. S.: Pitfalls and limitations of breast examinations. Hosp. Med., *4*:13-18, Aug., 1968.

PATIENT EDUCATION

Pamphlets and Information

American Cancer Society
(Local Chapter)
The Nurse and Breast Self-Examination.
Cancer of the Breast.
After Mastectomy.
Help Yourself to Recovery.

U. S. Government Printing Office
Superintendent of Documents
Washington, D.C.
Cancer of the Breast. (PHS Publication No. 576.)

Identical Form, Inc.
17 West 60th Street
New York, New York 10023
Radler, H. B.: A Handbook for Your Recovery. A 16-page booklet describing and illustrating exercises and activities for the patient who has had a radical mastectomy.
The above booklet has an insert on Fashion Suggestions from the Leading Pattern Companies.
An additional supplement is a pamphlet, Man to Man, which physicians find helpful for the husband of the woman who is recovering from a mastectomy.

Reach to Recovery
666 Fifth Avenue
New York, New York 10019
Lasser, T.: Reach to Recovery. (Booklet for postmastectomy patient.)

S. H. Camp & Co.
Jackson, Michigan 49204

Films

1. Breast Self-Examination. (16 mm. sound, color, 15½ min.)
2. Breast Cancer. The Problem of Early Diagnosis, (16 mm. sound, color, 34 min.)
3. After Mastectomy. (16 mm. sound, color, 20 min.)
Available from State Health Department or the State Division of the American Cancer Society.

CHAPTER **28**

Patients with Dermatologic Problems

- *The Skin*
- *Nursing Responsibilities in Dermatology*
- *Secretory Disorders*
- *Seborrheic Dermatoses*
- *Infections and Infestations of the Skin*
- *Noninfectious Inflammatory Dermatoses*
- *Systemic Diseases with Dermatologic Manifestations*
- *Ulcers and Tumors of the Skin*
- *Disorders Involving Hair*
- *Dermatologic Surgery and Plastic Reconstructive Surgery*

THE SKIN

The skin is an indispensable structure for human life. Because it forms a barrier between the internal organs and the external environment, the skin participates in many vital functions of the body. Its outer surface consists of stratified layers of dead, *keratinized* cells that form an effective protective covering against the penetration of noxious substances from the outside environment. The protective function is further enhanced by the oily and slightly acid secretions of the *sebaceous glands*, which discourage the growth and multiplication of many harmful bacteria.

Underlying this tough outer layer (the *epidermis*) are the *dermis* and *subcutaneous* tissues that, far from being homogeneous, are composed of a multitude of tissues, i.e., glandular, vascular, nervous, muscular and fatty, which are supported and maintained in proper relation to one another by means of *fibrous* and *elastic connective tissue*. Obviously the skin, rather than being a single organ, consists of groups of organs, each responsive to its own particular stimuli and each vulnerable to any harmful influences that would threaten it elsewhere in the body.

Many skin lesions originate as a result of some injurious contact in the external environment, such as an infective organism, a toxic chemical or physical trauma. Other lesions result not so much from the activity of the external agent itself, but rather to the sensitivity or response of the particular individual to that particular agent, which may be perfectly harmless to other, nonsensitive individuals. A damaging reaction of this sort may take the form of a local inflammatory lesion, an ulcer or an abscess, and accounts for a substantial proportion of all such lesions.

The nurse, whose professional activities necessitate intimate and frequent contact with patients affected by skin diseases, soon discovers the importance of *emotional stress* as a factor influencing the course of the disease. The emotions apparently exert their influence through the autonomic nervous system, which controls the caliber of the skin vessels. Recognizing that dilatation of an arteriole must lower the resistance to blood flow through that vessel, it follows that the blood pressure in the distal capillaries must increase, indeed, as much as tenfold. It is not difficult to imagine that such great pressures can produce a plasma leakage and/or hemorrhage through the capillary wall, causing lesions that damage or destroy the overlying skin.

Pruritus ("the itch") is clearly instrumental in prolonging and aggravating existing skin lesions and, perhaps, producing them as well by compelling the patient to scratch. Itching is "detected" by the free

```
┌─────────────────────────────────────────────────────┐
│ Definition of terms commonly used in dermatology     │
│                                                       │
│ Annular—ring-shaped                                   │
│ Arcuate—in the form of an arc                         │
│ Circinate—circular                                    │
│ Confluent—lesions run together or join               │
│ Discoid—disc-shaped                                   │
│ Discrete—lesions remain separate                     │
│ Eczematoid or eczematous—inflammation with a ten-    │
│    dency to thicken, scale, vesiculate, crust or weep │
│ Erythema—red                                          │
│ Generalized—widespread eruption                       │
│ Grouped—lesions clustered together                   │
│ Guttate—drop-like                                     │
│ Gyrate—twisted spiral                                 │
│ Iris—circle within a circle                           │
│ Keratosis—circumscribed horny thickening             │
│ Keratotic—horny thickening                            │
│ Linear—in lines                                       │
│ Moniliform—beaded                                     │
│ Multiform—more than one kind of skin lesion          │
│ Polymorphous—more than one kind of skin lesion       │
│ Serpiginous—snake-like, creeping                      │
│ Telangiectasia—relatively permanent dilatation of super-│
│    ficial vessels                                     │
│ Universal—entire skin affected                        │
│ Zosteriform—linear arrangement along a nerve         │
└─────────────────────────────────────────────────────┘
```

From Lewis, G. M., and Wheeler, C. E.: Practical Dermatology. P. 85. Philadelphia, W. B. Saunders, 1967.

nerve endings in the upper portions of the skin, but the mechanisms causing the nerve endings to respond are not known in most instances. However, the importance of emotions in the symptom complex of pruritus is abundantly clear.

There is very little constancy or uniformity in dermatologic practice as regards the details of therapeutic procedures. Therefore, instead of describing particular treatments at length and in great detail, only basic principles of therapy are stressed; principles that can be accepted, on the whole, as valid and that are obviously important in the planning and execution of treatment and nursing care of patients with dermatologic conditions.

NURSING RESPONSIBILITIES IN DERMATOLOGY

Psychological Aspects

The nurse should accustom herself as quickly as possible to the less attractive aspects of dermatologic disease and overcome as completely as possible her personal (and natural) sense of repugnance when in close proximity to dermatologic patients. Conscious effort in that direction will make such contact progressively easier. She must never betray a reluctance to touch her patient, which would only add to his anxiety, frustration and humiliation, but must cultivate an attitude that promotes a sense of security and tends to restore optimism.

Patients with skin disease frequently are embarrassed and self-conscious as a result of unattractive or disfiguring lesions or because of the necessary display of conspicuous dressings. Also, they may be depressed and frustrated by the protracted course of the disease and being constantly scrutinized by people who might be repelled by and fearful of the disease. These psychological aspects of dermatologic practice require expert management on the part of the attending nurses, who must exhibit an understanding and unending patience and offer tireless encouragement to their patients.

Persistent pruritus, with resultant sleeplessness, may be a potent contributing factor to an anxiety state, which in turn inevitably reinforces discomfort and fatigue.

Clinical Observations

Many systemic conditions may be accompanied by dermatologic manifestations. In fact, any patient hospitalized with a medical or surgical condition may suddenly develop itching and a rash. The nurse must be able to describe the dermatosis (abnormal condition of the skin) clearly and in detail. The following questions are pertinent: What is the color of the lesion? Is there redness, heat, pain or swelling? Is the eruption macular, papular, scaling or oozing? How large an area is involved? When did the patient first notice the eruption? How does he describe his sensations? Are there itching, burning, tingling or crawling sensations, or is there a loss of sensation? Was the appearance of the eruption related to the intake of food? What drugs is the patient receiving that might possibly have caused this reaction?

Primary lesions that do not produce a break in the skin include the following:

Macule—a spot on the skin that is not raised or depressed

Papule—a solid elevation of the skin

Vesicle—a small elevation of the skin that is filled with clear fluid

Pustule—an elevation in the skin that contains pus

Wheal—an area of transitory edema in the skin

Secondary lesions that break the skin include scales, crusts, excoriations, fissures and ulcers.

PLATE 1

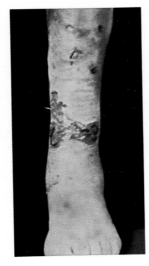
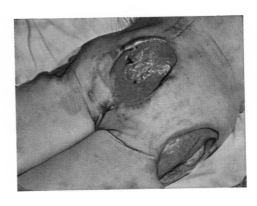

Ischemic necrosis of the skin. (Left) A "stasis ulcer," occurring as a complication of venous pooling and tissue edema in a leg with varicose veins (see p. 336). (Right) Multiple, extremely extensive decubitus ulcers that have developed in vulnerable pressure areas as a result of prolonged ischemia and as a direct consequence of failure to sustain peripheral blood flow in a debilitated, paralyzed patient (see p. 168). (Herbert Mescon, M.D., Boston)

PLATE 2

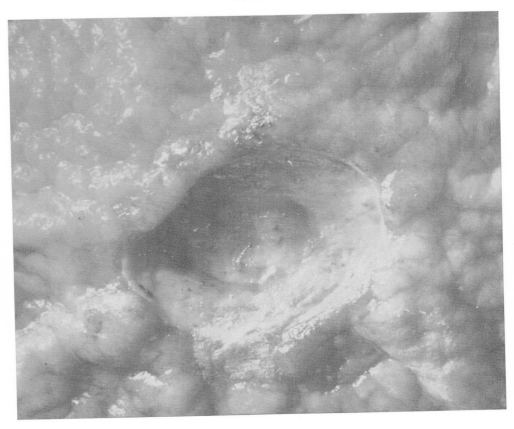

A well-defined gastric ulcer (see p. 460). (From L. Kraeer Ferguson, M.D.)

PLATE 3

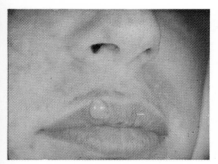

Herpetic vesicle of the lip.
(See p. 433.)

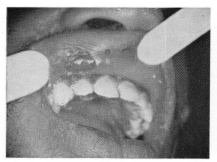

Chancre of the lip.
(See p. 919.)

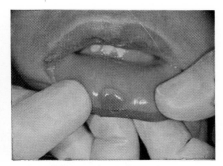

A syphilitic patch on the oral mucosa.
(See p. 919.)

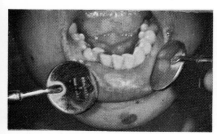

Oral and dermal manifestations of
acute syphilis.
(See p. 919.)

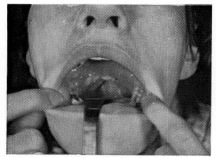

Vincent's angina.
(See p. 433.)

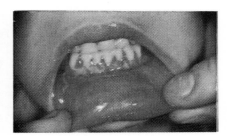

Tuberculous lesions of mucosa
and gums.
(See p. 639.)

(Burket, L. W.: Oral Medicine, ed. 3, Philadelphia, Lippincott)

PLATE 4

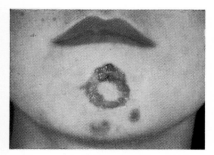

Impetigo contagiosa.
(See p. 637.)

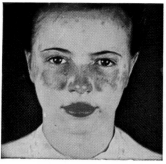

Lupus erythematosus.
(See p. 643.)

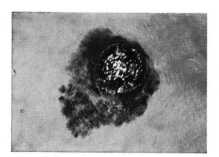

Malignant melanotic sarcoma.
(See p. 644.)

(Herbert Mescon, M.D., Boston)

PLATE 1

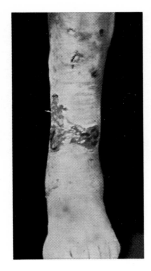
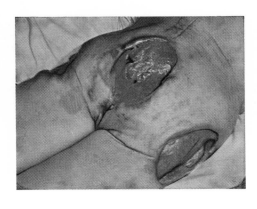

Ischemic necrosis of the skin. (Left) A "stasis ulcer," occurring as a complication of venous pooling and tissue edema in a leg with varicose veins (see p. 336). (Right) Multiple, extremely extensive decubitus ulcers that have developed in vulnerable pressure areas as a result of prolonged ischemia and as a direct consequence of failure to sustain peripheral blood flow in a debilitated, paralyzed patient (see p. 168). (Herbert Mescon, M.D., Boston)

PLATE 2

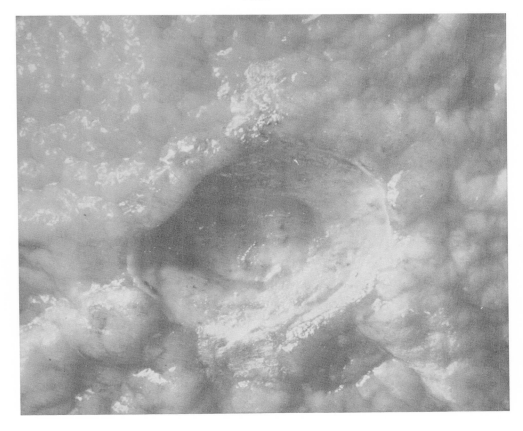

A well-defined gastric ulcer (see p. 460). (From L. Kraeer Ferguson, M.D.)

PLATE 3

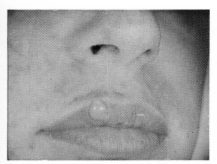

Herpetic vesicle of the lip.
(See p. 433.)

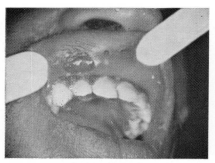

Chancre of the lip.
(See p. 919.)

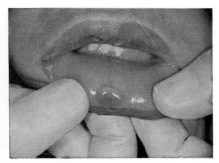

A syphilitic patch on the oral mucosa.
(See p. 919.)

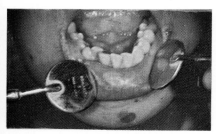

Oral and dermal manifestations of
acute syphilis.
(See p. 919.)

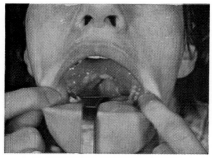

Vincent's angina.
(See p. 433.)

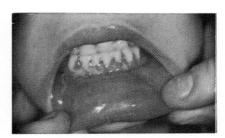

Tuberculous lesions of mucosa
and gums.
(See p. 639.)

(Burket, L. W.: Oral Medicine, ed. 3, Philadelphia, Lippincott)

PLATE 4

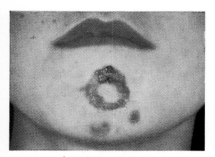

Impetigo contagiosa.
(See p. 637.)

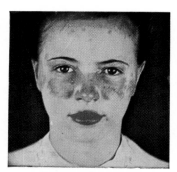

Lupus erythematosus.
(See p. 643.)

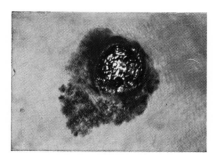

Malignant melanotic sarcoma.
(See p. 644.)

(Herbert Mescon, M.D., Boston)

PLATE 5

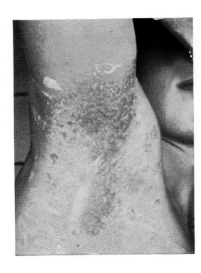

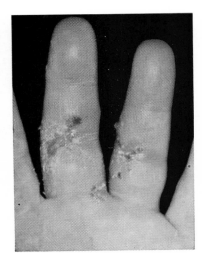

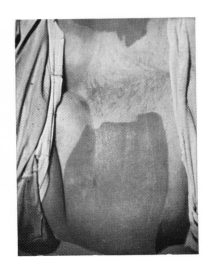

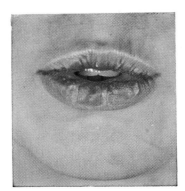

Contact dermatitis exhibited by four sensitized individuals, and occurring as a manifestation of skin allergy in response to a specific antigen, i.e. a cream deodorant (upper left); a soap (upper middle); an adhesive plaster (upper right); and a lipstick (lower left). (See p. 678.) (Herbert Mescon, M.D., Boston)

PLATE 6

Secondary stage of early syphilis—maculopapular rash. (See p. 919.) (Kampmeier, R. H.: Essentials of Syphilology, Philadelphia, Lippincott)

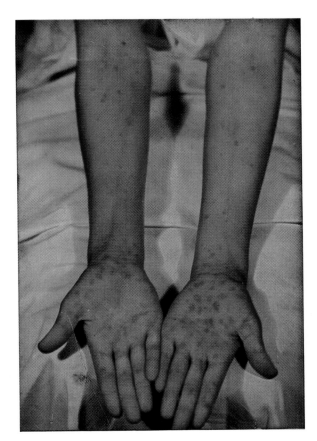

PLATE 7

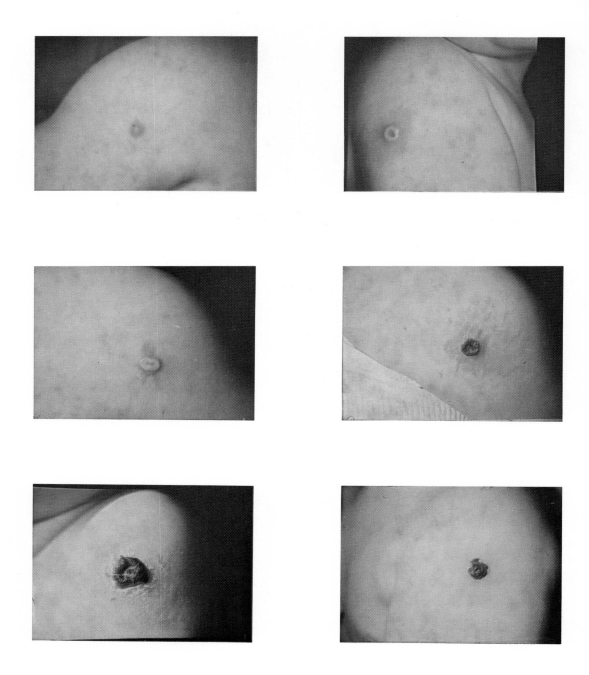

Evolution of vaccinia. (See p. 901.) (Top, left) Day 3. (Top, right) Day 6. (Center, left) Day 9. (Center, right) Day 15. (Bottom, left) Day 20. (Bottom, right) Day 30.

Care of the Skin

Remember that even perfectly normal skin is vulnerable to damage by the blandest of soaps unless the soap is completely removed by rinsing before the skin is dry. If soap remains in an area of skin that tends to be moist, the damage is greater and occurs more promptly. Residual soap is an important predisposing factor and, perhaps, the principal cause of common lesions such as "diaper rash." It may be pointed out, in this connection, that any substance in prolonged contact with moist skin can excite an inflammatory reaction that will result in damage and desquamation of the skin in the area of contact. There is one, and only one, outstanding exception to this rule, namely, water.

Principles of Dermatologic Therapy

There is very little constancy or standardization in dermatologic therapy, and there is much variation among clinics in the nursing techniques prescribed. In the following paragraphs it is proposed to offer no precise description of any particular type of treatment but, rather, to include certain general principles regarded as important in the nursing care of patients with skin diseases.

In hospitals where patients are bathed as a matter of routine on admission, specific exceptions must be made for patients presenting skin lesions. Some skin disorders are markedly aggravated by soap and water, and, for this reason, the procedure is postponed until ordered by the physician. Alternate modes of cleansing may be indicated, and the technique depends on the character of the disease.

Denuded skin, whether the area of desquamation is large or small, is excessively prone to damage by chemical means and, also, as a result of trauma. The friction of a towel, if applied with vigor, is sufficient to excite a brisk inflammatory response that causes any existing lesion to flare up and increase in extent. Thus, the essence of skin care and protection in bathing a patient with abnormal skin is to ensure the complete removal of the soap when rinsing, then to dry the area gently with a soft cloth and light touch.

The use of pledgets saturated in olive oil aids in loosening crusts, removing exudates or freeing an adherent dry dressing. The latter also may be saturated with sterile physiologic salt solution or dilute (3 per cent) hydrogen peroxide, which softens it and permits it to be pulled away gently.

Potentially infectious skin lesions should be regarded strictly as such, and proper precautions should be observed until the diagnosis is established. Rubber or disposable polyethylene gloves are worn by the nurse and the physician. (Oil causes rubber to deteriorate rapidly; therefore, if oil is used on the patient, the gloves must be cleansed promptly.) Dressings removed from infected skin should be enclosed securely in paper wraps and burned as soon as possible.

Application of Wet Dressings

Wet dressings are employed for many types of lesions. Owing to water evaporation, wet dressings have a cooling effect and relieve inflammation, burning and itching. They are especially helpful for oozing, crusting types of skin conditions. Characteristic solutions, occasionally indicated, include physiologic saline, aluminum acetate (usually 0.5 per cent), boric acid, magnesium sulfate (approximately 3 per cent) and potassium permanganate (perhaps 1:4,000). These should be prepared in sterile water. For some patients it may be desirable to keep the dressing warm; for others, cool. Some dressings must be covered to prevent evaporation, whereas most are allowed to remain open. The *open dressing* requires frequent changing, because evaporation is, of course, rapid.

The *closed dressing* is changed less frequently, and there is always a danger that it will cause not only softening but actual maceration of the underlying skin. Moisture is maintained satisfactorily by the use of fluffs, gauze roll or abdominal gauze. Absorbent cotton should not be applied directly adjacent to the skin; however, because it retains moisture quite efficiently, it is a useful component of a wet dressing if employed in thin sheaths between layers of gauze. Areas of normal skin that may be exposed to moisture for any extended period should first be coated with petroleum jelly, a silicone oil or zinc oxide paste.

Preparation of Wet Dressings. A dressing may be rinsed in the appropriate solution before application (this is the preferable procedure if warmth is desired), or the solution may be added—for example, with an Asepto syringe—after it is in place. Care must be taken lest the dressings become excessively soaked and the solution runs over into normal areas. Sterile towels hold the dressings in place; they may be protected further by plastic film secured with bandage, if necessary. So arranged, the temperature of the dressing can be maintained for several hours. The use of external heating appliances is not only unnecessary but undesirable, because the danger of burning the skin is very real.

A stocking may be converted into a convenient wet dressing for the leg, and a glove similarly prepared for the hand. Face lesions should be dressed with gauze fashioned into a mask and applied in several thicknesses. If wet dressings are required to cover extensive areas of the body, flannel pajamas soaked in

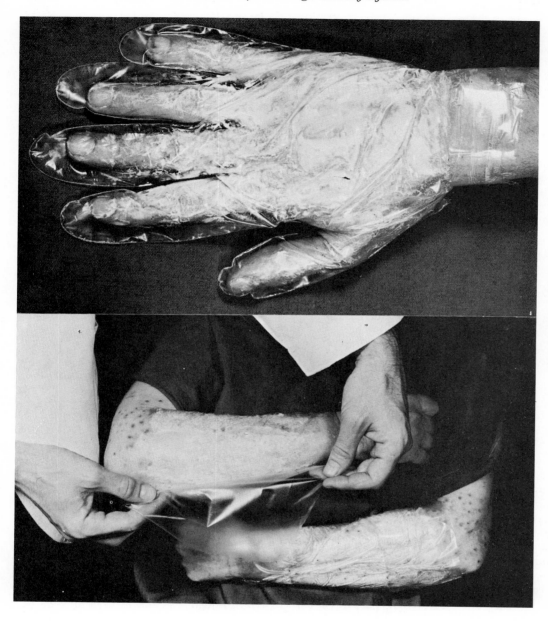

Fig. 28-1. (*Top*) The use of a thin plastic occlusive dressing over the hand assures better contact of medication with the skin lesion and is convenient and less cumbersome for the patient. (*Bottom*) After the affected areas have been cleansed and a layer of prescribed ointment or cream applied, the arm is covered with the occlusion dressing, fastened with adhesive or cellophane tape and wrapped with a lightweight cotton dressing to hold the plastic dressing in place. (Eli Lilly, Indianapolis, Indiana)

the solution serve as a useful form of dressing. The full bath may be used as a total wet dressing if it is desirable to treat the whole skin surface, care being observed to avoid chilling.

Remoistening of the dressing may be accomplished by removing the protective cloaks and pouring solution over the gauze, or the gauze may be removed completely, immersed again in the solution and then reapplied. If the remoistening is done without removal of the gauze, applications of sterile water are alternated with those of solution, particularly if the solution contains a metallic salt, which becomes continuously more concentrated through evaporation. If an exudate is present, the dressing should, of course, be changed completely at frequent intervals.

Therapeutic Baths

Baths are useful as a means of applying medications to large areas of the skin, removing crusts and scales and relieving itching that accompanies acute dermatoses. Usually the temperature of the water is 35 to 38° C. (95 to 100° F.). Caution the patient against slipping in the tub, especially after emollient preparations have been used. See Table 28-1.

THE PATIENT WITH A DERMATOSIS
Objectives and Principles of Nursing Management

I. To control itching and relieve pain
   A. Examine area of involvement
     1. Attempt to discover the cause of discomfort
     2. Record observations in detail, using descriptive terminology
   B. Encourage rest and immobility to reduce stimuli of pain and itching, and to raise the threshold of discomfort
   C. Eliminate foods and beverages that produce flushing, e.g., condiments, coffee and alcohol
   D. Employ measures that produce vasoconstriction
     1. Maintain cool environment
     2. Reduce excess bedding or personal clothing
     3. Provide tepid, cooling baths
     4. Apply cool wet dressings
   E. Apply anesthetic lotions or ointments
   F. Supply analgesic and antipruritic medications as indicated
   G. Administer tranquilizing agents or sedative drugs, as necessary, to control intense pruritus or other discomfort
   H. Instruct patient to refrain from self-medication with salves or lotions that are commercially advertised
   I. Assist the anxious patient to improve his insight, identify his problems and find their solution

II. To treat an inflammatory lesion
   A. Apply continuous or intermittent wet dressings to reduce intensity of inflammation
   B. Remove crusts and scales before applying topical medications

   C. Use topical applications containing corticosteroid drugs, as indicated
     1. Rub topical medicaments well into skin to enhance penetration
     2. Observe lesion periodically for changes in response to therapy

III. To control oozing and prevent crust formation
   A. Provide tub baths and wet dressings to loosen exudates and scales
   B. Remove medications with mineral oil before reapplying
   C. Use mildly astringent solutions to precipitate proteins and decrease oozing
   D. Supply a high protein diet if oozing is voluminous and serum loss substantial
   E. Administer antibiotics by topical application or by mouth, as indicated

IV. To avoid damage to skin
   A. Protect healthy skin from maceration when applying wet dressings
   B. Remove moisture from skin by blotting gently and avoiding friction
   C. Guard carefully against risk of thermal trauma from excessively hot wet dressings

V. To ensure efficacy of topical applications
   A. Use occlusive dressings, as needed, to retain medication in constant contact with affected skin
   B. Elicit the patient's cooperation in performing his own dermatologic treatments
   C. Instruct patient clearly and in detail to ensure that treatments are carried out as prescribed

Dermatologic Medications and Dressings

Medications in the form of powders, lotions, creams and ointments are used to treat skin lesions. In general, lotions and emulsions are used for the more acute dermatoses when large areas of skin are involved. Lotions exert a cooling action through water evaporation; they also have a protective effect and are applied easily with a soft paintbrush. Powders are dusted on the skin with a shaker or with cotton sponges. Although their medical action is brief, powders absorb moisture and reduce friction between the skin and the bedding. Pastes are mixtures of powders and ointments and are used in inflammatory conditions. Ointments retard water loss and are preferred in the more chronic or localized skin conditions. Pastes and ointments are applied with a wooden tongue depressor. The patient should be taught to apply them gently but thoroughly.

Many of these topical applications are greasy and require a covering with dressings to prevent soilage of clothing. If it is to be satisfactory, a dressing must be comfortable as well as protective. Plastic film is advantageous because it is thin and adapts itself readily to anatomic structures of all shapes and sizes. (See Fig. 28-1.) Stretchable cotton dressings (Surgitube, Tubegauze) likewise are excellent covering materials.

Corticosteroids are being widely used in the treatment of many dermatologic conditions. Topical steroids frequently are used to suppress inflammation, thus relieving pain and itching. Instruct the patient to use only small quantities of steroid cream and to rub it in thoroughly. If the area covered by the steroid cream is wrapped with an occlusive dressing,

TABLE 28-1. Dermatologic baths

Type of Bath*	Uses
1. Zinc (0.028%) and copper sulfate (0.08%)	1. Oxidizing, disinfecting and deodorizing. Useful particularly in exudative, vesicular and bullous dermatoses.
2. Tar	2. Antipruritic, mildly keratolytic. Coal tar and oil of cade emulsions are most frequently used. They are valuable in the chronic dermatoses.
3. Colloid	3. Soothing bland baths are used to calm and relieve irritated, inflamed or pruritic skin conditions. They are usually prepared from cornstarch, oatmeal or colloidal oatmeal. Colloidal oatmeal requires no boiling to extract the colloid.
4. Emollient	4. These baths include emollient oils to soften and lubricate dry, scaly or lichenified skin.

* Modified from Franks, A. G.: Dermatologic uses of baths. Amer. Pract., *9*(No. 12):998-2000, 1958.

the humidity under the dressing rises and increases the penetration of the steroid. Plastic film occlusion thus increases the efficacy and reduces the expense of topical steroid treatment. Corticosteroids are also used in intralesional therapy and are given systemically.

Disposable polyethylene gloves make acceptable coverings for patients who require finger and hand dressings. When large body areas require covering, disposable diapers are useful. The plastic side is placed next to the skin and the diaper is held in place by being pinned to the underclothing.* These plastic covers are useful as occlusive dressings to keep local creams, ointments or soaks moist and effective for prolonged periods.

The patient with a dermatologic problem has to take an active part in his treatment. He must be able to apply and remove his medications and dressings. Therefore, he must be indoctrinated fully regarding treatment techniques and the observations he is expected to report to his physician. In short, he participates in his own therapy as an assistant to the physician and the nurse.

PRURITUS

Pruritus (itching) is a very common complaint. Although it is a symptom of many skin diseases such as eczema or urticaria, it may also occur in the absence of any visible skin lesions. Thus, it may be the first

* Witten, V. H., and Sulzberger, M. B.: Newer dermatologic methods for using corticosteroids more efficaciously. Med. Clin. N. Am. *45*:857-868, 1961.

indication of serious internal diseases such as diabetes mellitus, leukemia or cancer. Itching may also accompany pregnancy and renal, hepatic and thyroid diseases. Dry skin, particularly that of elderly patients, often itches intensely. Pruritus may be caused by certain medications taken internally, the external application of certain drugs, soaps and chemicals, prickly heat (miliaria), and contact with woolen garments. Among the secondary effects of pruritus that are caused by scratching are excoriations, erythema, wheals, infections of the skin and changes in pigmentation.

Treatment

The cause of the pruritus, if known, should be removed. In some instances, patients are relieved by changing from a meat to a vegetable diet; in others, by substituting silk or cotton for woolen or nylon underwear. Soothing baths may contain sodium bicarbonate, starch, bland oils, bran or menthol. At first the water is tepid and then cooled, and the skin is dried without rubbing. Phenol (about 2 per cent) and menthol (0.25 to 0.5 per cent) lotions are cooling and can be applied externally. Some patients, particularly those with dry skin, are relieved by frequent applications of bland lubricating creams or ointments to the involved areas. Corticosteroids in cream form have proved to be effective in some patients with itching. Excessive warmth should be avoided, bed covers being reduced to the minimal number consistent with comfort and safety, and the room kept cool. The patient should be urged to avoid scratching; if he cannot desist, or excoriates himself while asleep, he may need to wear mitts and receive heavy sedation.

Pruritus of *the anal and the genital regions* may be caused by local irritants, such as scabies and lice; local lesions, such as hemorrhoids; nicotinic-acid deficiency (pellagra); infection with certain fungi and yeasts and pinworm infestation. It occurs also in postmenopausal women and in conditions such as diabetes mellitus, the anemias, hyperthyroidism and pregnancy. The treatment is removal of the local cause, use of the soothing applications mentioned above, sitz baths and local heat.

SECRETORY DISORDERS

Sweat and sebum inhibit the growth of bacteria, and serve to defend the skin against bacterial invasion. Disturbances of sweat secretion produce increased or decreased moistness of the skin, and are best judged by the condition over the chest or the axillae, since sweating of the hands and the feet is controlled by other factors. Thus cold, wet hands often indicate emotional tension. As a rule, moist skin is warm, and dry skin is apt to be cool. However, sweating and vasomotor dilatation are not always associated. The nurse has ample opportunities to observe cold sweats, the warm, dry skin of a dehydrated patient, and the very hot, dry skin peculiar to some febrile states.

Hyperhidrosis

Normally, temporary hyperhidrosis (excessive sweating) is associated with subcutaneous hyperemia. It may be due to exercise, exposure to heat and exposure to certain light rays. However, a cold sweat often accompanies fright, shock or very severe pain such as that of angina pectoris. Temporary hyperhidrosis is a response to the action of certain drugs, such as pilocarpine, ammonium acetate and various coal-tar products (the so-called *antipyretics*).

Persisting hyperhidrosis, increased still more by hot weather and physical exertion, is natural to some persons. It affects the general body surface, but always is marked in those regions where sweating normally is most active.

In certain diseases of the central nervous system, excessive sweating occurs over limited areas, as over half the face or on one side of the body. Profuse general sweating, most marked over the head, the face and the neck, is one of the sequelae of epidemic encephalitis.

Hyperhidrosis of the palms and soles often is an indication of emotional stress. It may also be part of the symptom complex of a vasomotor disturbance such as Raynaud's phenomenon.

Treatment. The underlying disease should be diagnosed and treated. Temporary relief may be obtained by cooling baths, shake powders or the judicious application of mild astringents.

SEBORRHEIC DERMATOSES

Seborrhea

The result of functional hyperactivity of the sebaceous glands, *seborrhea* is a condition normal to some persons. Clinically, there are patches of sallow, greasy-appearing skin with or without scaling and slight erythema, predominantly on the forehead, nose, and scalp. The thin, grayish scales often present in the scalp are commonly designated as "dandruff." Seborrhea is seen most frequently in dark-complexioned persons who tend to have a coarse pore pattern. The mild forms of the disease are asymptomatic. When scaling is present, it is often accompanied by pruritus that may lead to scratching and result in secondary complications such as infections and excoriations.

Seborrhea may be controlled by the use of medicated shampoos once or twice weekly and by the application of topical preparations containing sulfur and salicylic acid. Corticosteroid creams applied several times daily usually bring about rapid improvement of the lesions. It should be emphasized, however, that treatment is not curative but rather serves to bring the disease under control. Thereafter, less frequent applications of medications keep the condition in check.

Acne Vulgaris

Acne vulgaris is a common chronic disorder of the sebaceous (oil) glands, characterized by the presence of blackheads (comedones), whiteheads, pustules, nodules and cysts. It occurs predominantly on the face, chest, back and upper arms. It usually appears between the ages of 12 and 30 but becomes more marked at puberty and during adolescence, perhaps because at that age certain endocrine glands of the body are at their peaks of activity, which influences the secretions of the sebaceous glands. Acne may become worse during periods of emotional stress, during the premenstrual phase and, perhaps, when the diet contains an excess of fats.

The earliest and commonest lesions of acne are comedones (blackheads), which represent accumulations of increased amounts of sebum (the natural oil of the skin) in the follicular openings. Since the sebum can escape to the surface, there is no accompanying inflammation. Whiteheads, on the other hand, are comedones in which the follicular opening is so tiny that it prevents the escape of the oily contents to the surface. Such lesions may act as foreign bodies in the skin, resulting in inflammatory changes that may present as papules, pustules, or cysts which may cause scarring on healing.

Treatment. The objectives of treatment are (1) to prevent follicular obstruction, (2) to reduce inflammation and combat secondary infection, and (3) to eliminate factors that may predispose to acne. Thorough cleansing of the involved areas with soap and water twice daily is recommended. Mild drying and peeling agents such as weak salicylic acid and resorcin may be beneficial. Skin surface bacteria that may play a role in secondary infection can be reduced by the local application of 70 per cent alcohol. Ultraviolet light or natural sunlight is of benefit, probably because of the mild peeling of the skin that follows exposure.

The tetracyclines have proven useful. Long-term therapy may be necessary because of the chronic nature of this condition. It is thought that tetracycline has not only a bactericidal effect, but may reduce the fatty acids in the sebaceous glands. Estrogen therapy has been found to suppress sebum formation and reduce skin oiliness in women. Oral contraceptive compounds may be given on a prescribed cyclic regimen. Corticosteroids have an anti-inflammatory effect and may be helpful in the treatment of some patients. More recently, small amounts of corticosteroids have been injected into or just below the chronic papular lesions. This therapy has resulted in the flattening of the lesions within a few days. Thus, *intralesional injection* of acne cysts is a valuable tool in dermatologic therapy for some patients.

In some instances, reduction of dietary fats results in improvement. If the patient has observed that certain foods make his disease worse, then these may be restricted. It is of great importance that problems of the young patient be taken seriously by those caring for him. He needs understanding, reassurance and support. He should be cautioned not to squeeze the lesions, because secondary infection with scarring might ensue. Lesions may be opened and blackheads removed with a comedo extractor, but this procedure should be done by the physician rather than the patient or anyone else.

INFECTIONS AND INFESTATIONS OF THE SKIN

Bacterial Infections

Furuncles

The staphylococcus is a common inhabitant of the skin surface and the circulating air. Frequently it causes surface infections by invading a hair follicle or the duct of a gland. The infection may be a very slight one, characterized by a small, red, raised, painful "pimple" that may subside very rapidly with the drainage of a tiny drop of pus. Frequently, however, the infection may progress and involve the skin and the subcutaneous fatty tissue in a tense, raised, reddened mound termed a *furuncle,* known familiarly as a boil. The area of redness and induration represents an effort of the body to keep the infection localized. The bacteria produce necrosis of the invaded tissues, and, in a few days, the characteristic pointing appears. When this occurs, the boil is popularly said to have "come to a head."

Treatment and Nursing Care. If treated conservatively, the body may control the infection by eventual evacuation of the central necrotic core and the pus contained in this necrotic center. Hot moist applications will hasten this process. These may be applied in the form of hot compresses or poultices. In the conservative treatment of staphylococcic infections it is important not to rupture or destroy the protective wall of induration that has localized the infection. Therefore, the boil or pimple should never be squeezed, and it is well, when possible, to apply a splint to immobilize the part and thus protect the wall from being destroyed by movement. This procedure relieves the pain, as movement of the part produces tension on the infected area.

Local applications of neomycin or bacitracin ointment may help to limit the surface spread of the infection. If spreading still occurs or if the area of involvement poses a risk of complications (see below), systemic antibiotic therapy is indicated, employing Methicillin, Oxacillin or another of the agents that are effective against the staphylococcus, the selection of drug being governed in most cases by the results of sensitivity studies.

Sometimes a furuncle is so intensely painful that it is wise not to wait for localization and spontaneous evacuation of the necrotic material. In such cases a crucial incision may be made through the area of infection to permit relief of tension and more direct evacuation of the pus and slough. The patient should be instructed to cover a draining or moist lesion with a dressing. Soiled dressings should be wrapped in paper and burned.

Special precautions must be taken with boils on the face, for the skin area drains directly into the cranial venous sinuses. Sinus thrombosis, with fatal pyemia, has been known to develop after manipulation of a boil in this location. Bed rest is advised for patients having boils on nose, lip, groin, perineum or about the anal region, and a course of systemic antibiotic therapy is indicated to control the spread of the infection.

Carbuncles

These are staphylococcic infections similar to boils, except that the infection spreads widely in the subcutaneous fatty tissues, producing numerous sites of pointing and, therefore, a much more extensive area of acute inflammation. Carbuncles appear most commonly in areas in which the skin is thick and the subcutaneous tissues are more fibrous; therefore, they are seen most frequently on the back of the neck and less frequently on the back and other parts of the body. They are more apt to occur in older and debilitated people, and they are especially frequent in diabetics. So frequent is this latter association that every patient past middle age with a carbuncle should be suspected of diabetes until it is disproved. In carbuncles, the extensive inflammation frequently is not associated with a complete walling-off of the infection, so that absorption with production of high fever, leukocytosis and even extension of the infection to the bloodstream may occur.

Treatment and Nursing Emphasis. In many cases a carbuncle may subside rapidly following the administration of the antibiotic to which the infecting organism is sensitive. The antibiotic must be continued until the infective process is controlled. If the process already has gone on to form pus, incision and drainage may be necessary.

In caring for patients with carbuncles, the nurse

must consider not only the surgical lesion but also the general care of a frequently toxic patient. Furthermore, since many of these patients are diabetic, the question of diet, the administration of insulin and intravenous glucose and the complications of diabetes, such as keto-acidosis, must be borne in mind.

Carbuncle of the Upper Lip

This is an unusually serious disease because of the danger of thrombosis and embolism of the veins of the face and the nose. Some of these vessels drain into the cavernous sinus, a large venous channel in the skull, and an extension of the process in that direction is attended with grave consequences. Neither the nurse nor any one else should ever attempt to squeeze or manipulate the lesion, because of the danger of breaking the protective wall and thus producing an extension of the process. Rapid death may result from an intracranial extension causing septicemia or meningitis. Therefore, this apparently minor condition must be regarded as a very serious disease with a potentially high mortality.

Impetigo Contagiosa

Impetigo is a superficial infection of the skin caused by streptococci, staphylococci, or both. The lesions begin as discrete, thin-walled vesicles that soon rupture and become covered with a loosely adherent, honey-yellow crust. These crusts are easily removed and reveal smooth, red, moist surfaces on which new crusts soon develop. The face and the hands are the areas most frequently involved. As its name implies, it is contagious and may spread to other parts of the patient's skin or to other members of the family by fingers or towels soiled with the exudate of the lesions.

Although impetigo contagiosa is seen at all ages, it is particularly common among undernourished children living in poor hygienic conditions. It is acquired by children in schools and by adults in barber shops, beauty shops, or swimming pools. Often it appears secondary to pediculosis capitis, scabies, cold sores, insect bites, poison ivy or eczema.

Treatment and Nursing Care. Strict cleanliness is imperative to prevent the spread of the disease and, also, to protect children against further outbreaks. To hasten the curative process, the crusts first may be sponged with hydrogen peroxide, softened with olive oil and then removed by forceps. Topical ointments (bacitracin, neomycin, or polymyxin) are then applied. In severe cases, systemic antibiotic therapy may be indicated in addition to local therapy. Care must be taken lest the disease be spread from one skin area to another or from one person to another. Each patient should be instructed to keep his own towels and boil them before laundering. Children with this condi-

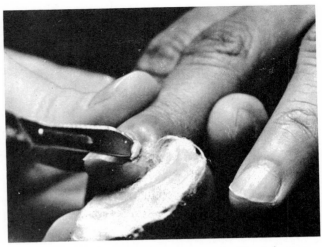

Fig. 28-2. Paronychia or runaround. The infection lies between the soft tissues and the side of the nail. Drainage by inserting the tip of a scalpel along the edge of the nail is customary surgery.

tion are excluded from school. Printed directions for hygienic care are distributed to these patients in skin clinics.

Infections of the Hand

Minor Injuries. Trivial accidents in daily living often result in cuts, pricks and abrasions of the skin, particularly of the hands and fingers. Although these wounds are potentially infected, they rarely become seats of infection if ordinary precautions are taken. Mechanical cleansing with soap and tap water and protection with a Band-aid or other form of dressing are usually all that is required to permit healing without infection. Antiseptics may be used if desired, but their role in preventing infection is much less important than is ordinary washing with soap and water.

Infections of the fingers and the hand are of extreme importance to the nurse, not only because she must know how to take care of these lesions, but also because frequent accidents in nursing may lead to the development of such infections in the nurse herself. Therefore, it is important that she know the cause and, especially, the prophylactic treatment of these infections, because they may lead to serious disability if not to fatal consequences.

Since almost all of hand and finger inflammations are due to infection, it is important to identify the organism and to determine its sensitivity to antibiotics. In the treatment of these infections, the appropriate antibiotic properly administered permits rapid subsidence of the inflammatory process; it may abort the infection in some cases, and in other well-established infections it hastens resolution of the infection.

Paronychia (runaround) is a common pyogenic infection involving the folds of tissue at the base of the fingernail. It results most often from an infection of a hangnail and is seen frequently after manicuring. The infection extends between the soft tissues and the nail on the dorsum of the fingertip and forms a tense, painful, throbbing area of inflammation at the side of the nail. If the infection is allowed to go untreated, it may progress underneath the eponychium (cuticle) and then invade the space underneath the base of the nail. This gives this infection its common name.

Cleanliness of the hands and careful care of the nails are the best prophylaxis against paronychia. If the infection does occur, it is treated by hot soaks and by lifting up the soft tissues from the edge of the nail with the tip of a scalpel (Fig. 28-2). Once the pus is evacuated, the inflammation usually subsides with the use of hot moist applications. The discharge is cultured and appropriate antibiotics may be given. If the infection is due to monilia, amphotericin B lotion is applied locally.

Infections of the pulp of the fingertip usually are the result of a puncture wound, the stick of a pin or a needle, when bacteria are carried into the layers of the skin or into the fatty tissues underlying it. When the infection lies between the layers of the skin, the abscess formed is spoken of as an *epidermal abscess.* This lesion is diagnosed easily, because it forms a small, tender, blisterlike mound at the site of the pinprick. Puncture and removal of the overlying skin may be performed without anesthesia, exposing the true skin below. In workmen and in others in whom the surface skin is thick, the infection may not progress to the surface so readily and, instead, may perforate through the true skin and invade the subcutaneous fatty tissues. This process is known as a *collar-button abscess,* one abscess cavity lying between layers of the skin connected by a narrow tract and a second abscess lying below the skin. In the treatment of such abscesses it is important to drain both the superficial and the deep collection by incision.

Felon (Distal Closed Space Infection). The most common and serious type of infection of the fingertip is that due to the streptococcus in the pulp of the finger. There usually is a history of needleprick or pinprick or some other form of puncture, followed several days later by throbbing pain, which may be of such intensity as to prevent sleep. The swelling and the edema produced by the infection may be sufficient to impair or shut off completely the arterial supply to the soft tissue, so that rapid necrosis and even invasion of the bone may occur. The resulting disability often is great because of the extreme importance of the fingertips in the use of the hand and the fingers.

Treatment. Early incision and drainage prevent the progress of the necrosis; therefore, wide incision often is practiced for what may appear to be a relatively small area of infection. It is surprising to note that radical incision is the conservative therapy in dealing with infections of the pulp of the finger.

After incision, the wound is held open by rubber dam or gauze drainage and immobilized by an appropriate splint. Warm moist dressings are used until the area of slough has separated entirely, after which time healing may be permitted to take place.

Prophylaxis. In the prophylaxis of fingertip infections, the nurse who has pricked her finger with a needle or a pin should report it to the head nurse at once. Occasionally, a slight enlargement of the incision or cauterization of the needle puncture with phenol may abort a serious infection. If throbbing pain becomes a prominent symptom, no time should be wasted before consulting a surgeon. The appropriate antibiotic must be administered.

Infections of Tendon Sheaths—Tenosynovitis (Whitlow). Infections of the tendon sheaths on the palmar surface of the hand occur most frequently from puncture wounds. Most often they are caused by the streptococcus. They are serious, because they may lead to a rapid destruction of the tendon itself and, therefore, to a marked finger and hand disability. An infection may involve the sheaths of the tendons in the fingers and the thumb; it may invade the fascial spaces of the hand, or it may advance along the tendon sheaths of the thumb and the fifth finger and invade the bursal space through which the tendons pass at the wrist. It produces a tense swelling of the involved finger with extreme pain when motion is attempted.

Treatment. Early incision and drainage are necessary to prevent necrosis of the tendon. Petrolatum gauze usually is laid in the wound to provide drainage.

The specific antibiotic is administered. In the early phases of the infection, the antibiotic may prevent necrosis and the necessity for incision. After incision, it is used to prevent extension of the infection and to hasten healing.

Postoperative Nursing Care. In the postoperative care of these patients, the nurse usually finds the part bandaged and on a splint, and for a time hot moist applications are applied through the dressings directly or through tubes fastened in them. The nurse must be extremely careful to observe sterile technique in moistening the dressings because of the danger of producing a mixed infection, which usually is associated with the extension of the inflammatory process. Elevation of the part must be enforced to reduce the inflammatory edema and to give comfort to the patient. This usually is accomplished by means of pillows, which should always be protected with a plastic cover.

Fig. 28-3. Fungal infection of the fingernails. (Ralph E. McDonnell, M.D., New Haven)

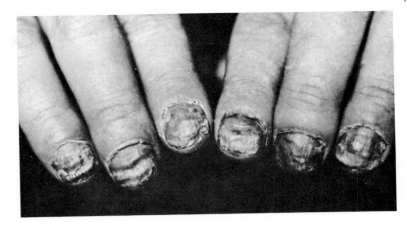

After the acute inflammatory process has been controlled, the infected hand often may be treated in a warm saline bath 2 or 3 times daily. The basin and the solution should be sterilized and the solution placed in the basin at a temperature as warm as the patient can stand comfortably. This temperature is maintained as well as possible by adding more solution at intervals. The bath usually is continued for at least 30 minutes. Its purpose is to apply heat to aid in the discharge of the necrotic materials from the wound. After removal from the bath the hand is placed in a sterile towel, and dry heat may be continued by the use of an electric light in a bed cradle. The nurse must be careful to avoid scalding or burning.

Skin Tuberculosis

Fortunately, skin tuberculosis is rare in the United States. Its most frequent manifestation is called lupus vulgaris, in which there are reddish-brown, nodular, infiltrated patches, occurring predominantly on the face. As a rule, these lesions are asymptomatic. Under pressure with a glass slide, small translucent nodules of apple-jelly color may be seen within these patches; this peculiarly is of great diagnostic significance. If untreated, the lesions usually progress slowly and produce severe scarring and mutilation.

Less frequently encountered forms of skin tuberculosis include tuberculous ulcers found chiefly in and around the mouth, the anus, and the genitalia. These are almost always associated with tuberculosis of the internal organs of the body. The ulcers are shallow, indolent and often covered with a purulent, soggy crust.

A wart-like tuberculous lesion may develop on the fingers or hands, more rarely elsewhere, in persons who handle infected animals or who come in close bodily contact with tuberculous patients. There is little tendency for the infection to spread to other parts of the body, and it usually heals within several months with scar formation.

Scrofuloderma is the term applied to all tuberculous skin lesions that are direct extensions of deeper tuberculous processes. It develops over scrofulous cervical lymph nodes and surrounding the orifices of sinuses from tuberculous bones and joints. These lesions are oval-shaped or linear-shaped ulcerations with undermined edges; the ulcerations are covered with reddish granulations that often are crusted, are more or less edematous and produce considerable exudate. Upon healing, they leave hypertrophic scars and cicatricial bands.

Treatment. Antituberculous chemotherapy, described in detail in Chapter 16, is applicable and used to good effect in patients with tuberculosis of the skin. General supportive care is important, with special heed to the nutritional and hygienic needs of the patient.

Fungal Infections

The fungi, tiny representatives of the plant kingdom, are responsible for a variety of common skin infections. In most cases they affect only the skin and its appendages (i.e., hair and nails), but in others, involvement of the internal organs is found. In the latter instance fungal disease may be so serious as to constitute a threat to life. Superficial infections, on the other hand, rarely cause temporary disability and respond readily to treatment. The diagnosis is made by direct microscopic examination of the infected skin and by growing the offending organism in culture.

Tinea Pedis (Athlete's Foot)

This relatively common superficial fungal infection may manifest itself as an acute, inflammatory, vesicular process, or as a chronic scaling, dusky erythematous rash involving the soles of the feet and the interdigital web spaces. The toenails may or may not be affected; if involved, they are apt to be discolored, brittle, and heaped-up. As a rule there is moderate to severe itching. Lymphangitis and cellulitis may be seen occasionally when bacterial superinfection occurs.

Treatment. The infected areas should be kept clean and dry. During the acute (vesicular) phase, potassium permanganate or saline soaks twice daily help to relieve pruritus and promote healing. As the acute stage subsides, fungistatic creams and ointments such as undecylenic acid preparations may be applied to the involved skin. Since moisture encourages the growth of fungi, the feet should be kept as dry as possible by frequent applications of absorbent powder and, if necessary, a change of socks during the day. In selected cases, an antifungal antibiotic, griseofulvin, is given orally.

Tinea Capitis (Ringworm of the Scalp)

Fungal disease of the scalp is the main cause of hair loss in children. Clinically, there are one or several round patches of redness and scaling. Small pustules or papules may be seen at the edges of such patches. As the hairs in the affected areas are invaded by the fungi, they become brittle and often break off at or near the surface of the scalp, resulting in areas of baldness. Most cases of tinea capitis heal without scarring, hence the hair loss is only temporary. Sometimes a boggy swelling somewhat resembling a furuncle occurs in an area of involvement; this lesion is known as a *kerion*. Tinea capitis is contagious.

Treatment. Griseofulvin, an antifungal antibiotic given orally, is indicated in all cases of tinea capitis. In addition, topical antifungal preparations are often used to reduce dissemination of the organisms. The nurse, being aware of the contagious nature of the disease, may assist the patient or his family in setting up a hygienic regimen for home use. Brushes and combs used by the patient should not be used by other members of the family. The hair should be kept short and shampooed frequently, and a stockinette cap may be worn at night. The physician often wants to examine

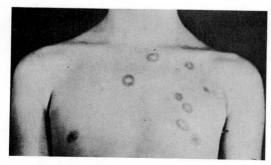

FIG. 28-4. Tinea circinata. This boy contracted the lesions by carrying a kitten under his shirt. (Paterson, D., and McCreary, J. F.: Pediatrics, p. 439, Philadelphia, Lippincott)

other members of the family for tinea capitis, because familial infections are relatively common.

Tinea Corporis (Ringworm of the Body)

Superficial fungal infection of the nonhairy skin usually presents as sharply outlined, round to oval, scaly, erythematous patches, occurring singly or severally. As a rule, there is an elevated border consisting of small papules or vesicles, whereas the central part of the patch may show a tendency to clear. Coalescence of individual rings may result in large patches with bizarre scalloped borders.

Tinea Barbae (Ringworm of the Beard)

This uncommon fungal infection is always associated with inflammation that causes tenderness, swelling and considerable pain. The lesions vary from pustules or nodules to boggy areas of inflammation similar to those seen in kerion. Bacterial superinfection is common. Treatment is essentially the same as that for tinea capitis. Bacterial superinfection is treated with the appropriate antibiotics.

Parasitic Infestations

Pediculosis

Three varieties of lice (pediculi) infest man, and their very itchy bites are the cause of many skin troubles.

The head louse (*Pediculus capitis*) parasitizes the hairy scalp, attaching its eggs (nits) to the hair shafts. The eggs are visible to the naked eye as greyish, glistening oval bodies that are not easily removed from the hair. The bite of the insect causes intense itching, and the resultant scratching often leads to complications such as impetigo, furuncles and enlarged cervical lymph nodes. The disease is more common in children, particularly in girls, and poor hygiene is an important contributing factor.

Treatment and Nursing Care. The application of benzyl benzoate emulsion to the scalp and the hair is effective. The next day the hair is shampooed. The treatment may have to be repeated if the infestation is severe. Kwell and topocide may also be used in a similar fashion.

The body louse (*Pediculus corporis*) lives chiefly in the seams of undergarments, to which it clings as it pierces the skin with its proboscis. Its bites cause characteristic minute hemorrhagic points and, on sensitive skins, evanescent wheals. Among the secondary lesions produced are hyperemia, parallel linear scratches, a slight degree of eczema and, in persistent cases, a general pigmentation that sometimes is as dark as that of Addison's disease. The areas of skin chiefly involved are those that come in closest contact with the undergarments—i.e., neck, trunk and thighs. Sterilization of

FIG. 28-5. Psoriasis of the leg and the knee. (Sauer, G. C.: Manual of Skin Diseases, p. 84, Philadelphia, Lippincott)

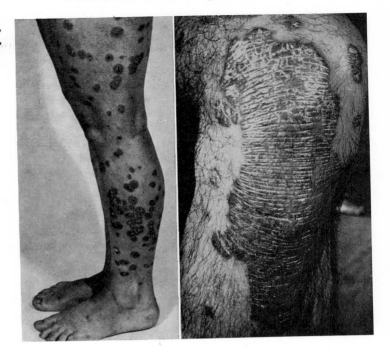

infested clothing by boiling or pressing with a hot iron destroys the parasite and its eggs. An alternate method is treatment of the garments with 10 per cent DDT powder.

The pubic louse *(Phthirus pubis)*, is most often found in the pubic area, although involvement of the eyelashes, eyebrows, and rarely, axillary hair, has been noted. Its bites result in scratching that may cause excoriations, secondary infection and eczematization. Treatment is the same as that described for head lice.

Scabies

Scabies is an infestation of the skin by the itch mite *(Acarus scabiei)*. It is a disease of overcrowding and poor hygienic conditions. The characteristic lesion is the burrow, produced by the female mite as it penetrates into the upper layers of the skin. The burrows are short, wavy, brownish or blackish, thread-like lesions most commonly observed between the fingers, on the flexor surfaces of the wrists, the palms, and around the nipples. This disease is invariably accompanied by itching, characteristically more pronounced at night after the patient retires since the increased warmth of the skin has a stimulating effect on the parasites. Secondary lesions, which are quite common, include vesicles, papules, pustules, excoriations and crusts. Bacterial superinfection or eczematization may complicate the picture.

Treatment. Benzyl benzoate is applied topically and allowed to remain on the skin for 24 hours. Following this application the patient bathes and changes his clothing and bedding.

Bedbugs

The bites of the bedbug *(Cimex lectularius)* produce purpuric spots, often occurring in irregular clusters of 3, 4 or more. The hemorrhagic spots may be associated with papular or wheal-like lesions, and on close inspection a tiny red point is often found, marking the original site of the bite. The legs, particularly the ankles, are the regions most often bitten, and the patient experiences variable degrees of itching and burning. Phenol and menthol-containing lotions have a soothing effect. Elimination of the insect may be accomplished by impregnating the bed with powder containing DDT and pyrethrins and spraying the walls and the floor with a similar solution.

NONINFECTIOUS INFLAMMATORY DERMATOSES

Psoriasis

Psoriasis is an eruption of circular patches of all sizes, sharply defined against the normal skin and covered with abundant dry, silvery scales (Fig. 28-5). Scrape off these scales and one exposes the dark red base of the lesion covered with a thin white membrane which, if scratched, bleeds. These patches are not moist and may or may not itch. They enlarge slowly, until, after many months, by coalescing they form extensive, irregularly-shaped patches.

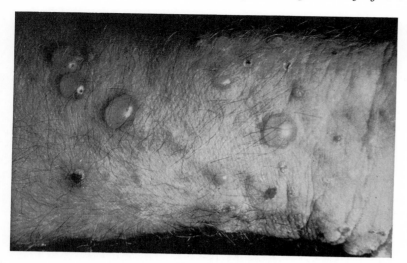

Fig. 28-6. Pemphigus vulgaris bullae on the wrist. (Sauer, G. C.: Manual of Skin Diseases, p. 84, Philadelphia, Lippincott)

Psoriasis appears most often on the extensor surfaces of the arms and the legs (especially about the knees and the elbows), on the scalp and the ears and over the sacrum. The face, the back of the hands, the palms and the soles are seldom affected; the tongue and the mucous membranes, never. Psoriasis per se causes no subjective symptoms, nor does it affect the general health. There is a hereditary predisposition to this disease. Approximately 3 per cent of the population in the U.S. have psoriasis.

The condition, however, not infrequently is accompanied by rheumatoid arthritis. It has a marked tendency to improve and then recur, even throughout life; yet many cases stop spontaneously. The etiology is unknown although it is thought to be related to a hereditary biochemical defect that causes an overproduction of keratin.

Therapeutic Management. The treatment of psoriasis is individualized, because what is helpful to one patient may not have any value to another. The objective of management is to reduce the scaling and redness. Sometimes this can be accomplished by exposure to sunlight during the summer months. However, with more widespread psoriasis, tar ointments or tar baths combined with carefully graded doses of ultraviolet radiation may be beneficial. (The application of tar to the skin increases its sensitivity to ultraviolet rays.) The patient is taught to remove the excess scales by scrubbing with a soft brush while he is bathing.

Intralesional injections of triamcinolone acetonide into patches of psoriasis have provided remissions for 6 to 12 months. The application of topical steroids under occlusive plastic film dressings (p. 632) may give relief to those patients with particularly troublesome symptoms. Anthralin (a psoriacide) has shown to be a useful therapeutic agent for resistant psoriasis.

The hands should be washed after handling this medication, because it can produce a chemical conjunctivitis. The use of Valisone cream has also reportedly been successful.

Exfoliative Dermatitis

Generalized exfoliative dermatitis is characterized by a universal, obstinate, very itchy scaling of the skin, frequently accompanied by the loss of hair and nails. It may develop as a primary condition. It may arise secondary to other chronic skin diseases, such as eczema and psoriasis, particularly if these are treated with irritating ointments over a long period of time. Exfoliative dermatitis may appear as a part of the lymphoma group of diseases and may actually precede the appearance of lymphoma. It also appears as a severe reaction to a wide number of drugs, including penicillin.

This condition starts acutely as either a patchy or generalized erythematous eruption accompanied by fever, malaise and, occasionally, gastrointestinal symptoms (possibly due to similar lesions involving the gastrointestinal epithelium). The skin color changes from pink to dark red, then after a week the characteristic exfoliation begins, usually in the form of thin flakes which leave the underlying skin smooth and red, new scales forming as the older ones exfoliate. Relapses are the rule. Death, perhaps the result of secondary infection, occasionally occurs.

Treatment and Nursing Care. The treatment of this condition is most unsatisfactory; it includes bed rest and soothing applications in the form of baths, wet compresses and calamine or corticosteroid cream to the skin. Antihistamines and sedatives give symptomatic relief for this distressing condition. Systemic administration of corticosteroids lessen the severity of exacerbations and give the patient considerable relief.

The patient is likely to become extremely irritable because of the severe itching. In response, however, his nurse should be calm, good-natured, reassuring and sympathetic. She must carefully avoid exhibiting any trace of revulsion excited by his appearance, for he will be quick to detect unfavorable reactions on her part.

Pemphigus

Pemphigus is a serious disease of the skin characterized by the appearance of variously sized blisters (bullae) on apparently normal skin and mucous membranes. The bullae enlarge, rupture, and leave eroded areas that eventually become crusted. Bacterial superinfection is common. Prior to the availability of corticosteroids, the disease was always fatal.

Since patients with pemphigus are invariably hospitalized at one time or another during exacerbations of the disease, the nurse is exposed to such patients in her hospital work and soon discovers that pemphigus is perhaps the most debilitating skin disease of all. The constant misery of the patient and the foul smell of the lesions makes good nursing a real challenge to any individual assigned to the care of such patients. The nurse should accept this challenge wholeheartedly, no matter how repulsive the patient might seem to her at first. Her task will be easier if she fully realizes that proper nursing care is of utmost importance to bring about clinical improvement.

Treatment and Nursing Management. In pemphigus the use of steroid hormones is fully justified. Internally administered corticosteroids are given initially in high dosages until the disease is under control, as evidenced by the disappearance of the bullous lesions. The patient is usually hospitalized during this period. Essential to his therapeutic management are daily evaluation of body weight, measurements of blood pressure, testing of urine for glucose, and recording of the fluid balance. (High-dosage corticosteroid therapy has its own serious toxic effects.) The nursing supervision has been likened to that required for a patient with an extensive burn; particular attention is given to assessing the patient for signs of local and systemic infection, maintaining protein and electrolyte balance and keeping the nutrition and hematologic status at physiologic levels. As the disease becomes controlled, the corticosteroid dosage is gradually decreased and the patient is kept on low maintenance dosages or the therapy is discontinued after a prolonged period. The patient is given a high protein, high caloric diet. Keep the skin protected against secondary infections. There is a significant loss, through the skin, of tissue fluids and, therefore, of sodium chloride. This salt loss is responsible for many of the constitutional symptoms associated with the disease and must be combated with administration of adequate saline, parenterally or otherwise.

Systemic antibiotics may be given when cutaneous infection is present. Plasma and whole-blood transfusion may be used to maintain the blood volume, as well as the hemoglobin and plasma protein concentrations.

Wet dressings or mild antiseptic lotions are protective and soothing. Patients with large areas of blistering have a characteristic odor that is lessened when secondary infection is controlled. Meticulous oral hygiene is important, since lesions in the mouth are common in pemphigus and add greatly to the patient's misery. The patient is usually depressed. The nurse should strive to give him the small but important "extras" that serve to lift the morale.

SYSTEMIC DISEASES WITH DERMATOLOGIC MANIFESTATIONS

Lupus Erythematosus

There are 2 apparently related conditions for which the term *lupus erythematosus* is used. *Discoid lupus erythematosus* denotes a chronic eruption of the skin which, although often disfiguring, does not pose a threat to life. On the other hand, *systemic lupus erythematosus* with or without skin manifestations is a serious disease affecting many organs of the body and often terminating fatally. The etiology of this condition is not understood; its clinical and pathologic features, its course, its response to corticosteroid therapy and some of the laboratory findings associated with it suggest that it may be a disease based on autoimmunity.

Systemic lupus erythematosus (S.L.E.) attacks persons predominantly of the younger age group and chiefly those of the female sex. Outstanding clinical characteristics include long-continued, low-grade fever; arthritis, akin to rheumatoid arthritis (page 870); a skin rash with butterfly distribution involving the face; telangiectasis of the vessels in the nail beds; anemia; leukopenia; thrombocytopenia, similar to that in idiopathic thrombocytopenic purpura (page 323); and evidences of nephritis, notably proteinuria, pyuria and signs of renal insufficiency. A sterile endocarditis often develops, and cardiac failure is not infrequent. The disease is characterized by remissions and exacerbations. One factor that may produce the latter is exposure to sunlight. A fatal termination because of renal failure is to be anticipated eventually, but a specific prognosis is impossible, so variable is the course of the disease. It is possible to control the disease indefinitely and fairly satisfactorily by the administration of steroid hormones. Salicylates and the antimalarial drug chloroquine likewise are useful for symptomatic relief and retardation of the progression of lupus, but eradication of the process has yet to be achieved.

Of some diagnostic value is the observation of phagocytosis of leukocytes by other leukocytes in preparations that contain these cells in high concentration. This phenomenon is the basis of the so-called "L.E. test."

Lupus erythematosus occurs without signs of systemic involvement, manifested only by a butterfly rash on the face, which is probably related in its pathogenesis to the disseminated form. Discoid lupus erythematosus occurs without overt signs of systemic involvement. The face, the external ears, the scalp, and the neck are commonly affected. At times the rash occurs on both upper cheeks and over the bridge of the nose, giving it a "butterfly" pattern. The individual lesions are erythematous patches with sharply outlined borders and prominent follicular plugging. After persisting for a variable length of time, the lesions characteristically heal with atrophy, scarring and pigmentary changes. Scalp lesions usually result in permanent hair loss in the affected sites.

Periarteritis Nodosa

This condition, possibly another example of autoimmunity, attacks persons of all ages and both sexes. It is a disease of the smaller arteries, usually of many organs. The walls of the vessels are involved by spotty inflammation, with resulting changes in circulation and tissue damage. Approximately 25 per cent of patients with periarteritis nodosa have skin manifestations, usually in the form of painful nodules that may ulcerate. The clinical manifestations commonly encountered are quite similar to those enumerated in the foregoing description of systemic lupus erythematosus. The patient is prone to exhibit signs of prolonged fever, hypertension, nephritis, peripheral neuritis, palpable nodules along the arterial trunks and eosinophilia. Infrequently, aneurysms appear. These are the result of focal weakening of the arterial wall, and are most likely to develop in the abdomen. Periarteritis is apt to run a course of several years' duration, death finally occurring as a result of either renal decompensation or hypertension.

It has been noted that some patients had experienced allergic phenomena in response to sulfonamide therapy at some time prior to the development of the disease, which lends further emphasis to the importance of avoiding the use of such agents, unless based on specific indications.

Treatment. Systemic corticosteroids have been used successfully to achieve control of the disease, but this is not always possible.

ULCERS AND TUMORS OF THE SKIN
Ulcerations

The superficial loss of surface tissue due to death of the cells is called an *ulceration*. A simple ulcer, such as is found in a small superficial second-degree burn, tends to heal by granulation if kept clean and protected from injury. If exposed to the air, the serum that escapes from it will dry and form a scab, under which the epithelial cells will grow and cover the surface completely. Certain diseases cause characteristic ulcers—thus, one can distinguish between tuberculous ulcers and syphilitic ulcers.

Ulcers of the skin arise usually either from infection or from an interference with the blood supply. Infectious ulcers are not uncommon. They develop usually from an infection with anaerobic streptococci or from a combination of infections in which hemolytic anaerobic streptococci live in symbosis with staphylococci. Ulcers of this type tend to progress peripherally and are seen often on the lower extremty or on the abdomen or the chest after operation. They are characterized by an overhanging edge, and culture from them usually shows the type of organism causing the infection. These ulcers tend to resist ordinary forms of treatment, but the application of zinc peroxide, which liberates oxygen over a long period of time, converts the anaerobic portions of the wound into an aerobic area. Penicillin locally or intramuscularly also is highly effective. Healing occurs rapidly owing to the inability of the anaerobic streptococci to live in an unfavorable environment.

Ulcers due to a deficient arterial circulation are seen in patients with peripheral vascular disease, arteriosclerosis, Raynaud's disease and frostbite. In these patients, the treatment of the ulceration must be carried out in conjunction with the treatment of the arterial disease. The danger is from secondary infection. Frequently, amputation of the part is the only effective therapy. (See varicose ulcers, p. 336.)

Tumors
Cysts

Epidermal cysts are common, slowly growing, firm, elevated tumors found most frequently on the back. They probably arise from an invagination of the epidermis into the dermal tissues.

Sebaceous cysts, which are less frequent, occur predominantly on the scalp. Their clinical appearance is identical to that of epidermal cysts. Both are commonly referred to as *wens*. As a rule these lesions are asymptomatic but occasionally they may become secondarily infected. Malignant degeneration is rare. The treatment consists of surgical excision under local anesthesia.

Benign Tumors

Verrucae (warts) are common benign skin tumors caused by a virus. All age groups may be affected, but the condition is more frequent in children. As a rule, warts are asymptomatic except when they occur on weight-bearing areas such as the soles of the feet. They may be treated with salicylic acid plasters, electrodesiccation, or the application of cantharidin.

Angiomas (birthmarks) are benign vascular tumors involving the skin and the subcutaneous tissues. They may occur as flat, violet-red patches (port-wine angiomas) or as raised, bright red nodular lesions (strawberry angiomas). The latter have a tendency to involute spontaneously. Port-wine angiomas, on the other hand, usually persist indefinitely and are not easily treated. Most patients use masking cosmetics (Covermark) to camouflage the defect.

Pigmented nevi (moles) are common skin tumors of various sizes and shades ranging from yellowish to brown to black. They may be flat macular lesions or elevated papules or nodules that occasionally contain hair. The great majority of pigmented nevi are harmless lesions. However, in rare cases, malignant changes supervene and a melanoma develops at the site of the nevus. Therefore, some authorities recommend that nevi located at sites of repeated trauma should be removed as a preventive measure against possible malignant changes.

Keloids are benign overgrowths of fibrous tissue at the site of a scar or trauma. They appear to be more prevalent among the colored races. Keloids are asymptomatic but may cause disfigurement and cosmetic concern. Occasionally they involute spontaneously. They may be treated with irradiation or intralesional injection of corticosteroids.

Dermatofibroma is a common benign connective tissue tumor that occurs predominantly on the extremities. It is a firm dome-shaped papule or nodule that may be skin-colored or of a pinkish-brown hue. Excisional biopsy is the recommended method of treatment.

Multiple neurofibromata occur in von Recklinghausen's disease. Any area of the body may be involved, and the number and size of the lesions is extremely variable. Small freckle-like spots and larger, lightly pigmented patches are common additional findings.

Cancer of the Skin

Cancer of the skin has a greater incidence than cancer of any other organ. It comprises 22 per cent of all cancers in men and 12 per cent of all cancers in women. Although 5,000 people die of this disease yearly, there is still a 95 per cent cure rate. The high curability is due to early diagnosis (the skin is accessible to direct visualization), the slow progression of most skin cancers and the effective methods of treatment available.

Skin cancer is diagnosed by biopsy and histologic evaluation. The 2 most common types of skin cancer are *basal cell epithelioma* and *squamous cell carcinoma*. The earliest lesion of basal cell epithelioma is a small waxy nodule that slowly enlarges and undergoes central ulceration. These cancers are slow-growing and are called rodent ulcers. They are characterized by invasion and erosion of contiguous tissues but they rarely metastasize. The lesions appear most frequently on the face, especially the temples. There are 6 clinical types of basal cell epitheliomas; other lesions of this disease may appear as shiny, flat, gray or yellowish plaques.

Squamous cell carcinoma is less frequently seen but of greater concern because it is a truly invasive carcinoma. The lesions may be primary or develop from a precancerous condition such as actinic keratosis or leukoplakia. It appears as a shallow ulcer around which is a border that is wider, more infiltrated and more inflammatory than is the border of basal cell carcinoma. Secondary infection can occur. A careful evaluation of regional nodes must be made for evidences of metastases. Exposed areas, especially of the upper extremities and of the face, lower lip, ears, nose, and forehead, are common sites.

Metastatic Skin Tumors. The skin is an important although not common site of metastatic cancer. All types of cancer may metastasize to the skin, but car-

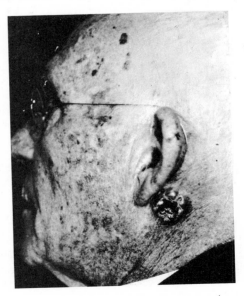

Fig. 28-7. Basal cell carcinoma (rodent ulcer) originating from one of the numerous senile keratoses observed over the head and the neck. (Ralph E. McDonnell, M.D., New Haven)

cinoma of the breast is the most frequent source. Next to carcinoma of the breast, cancers of the stomach, the uterus, and the lungs give rise to the majority of metastatic skin tumors. The clinical appearance of metastatic skin lesions is not distinctive except perhaps, in some cases of breast cancer where diffuse brawny hardening of the skin of the involved breast is seen ("cancer en cuirasse"). In most instances, metastatic lesions occur as single or multiple cutaneous or subcutaneous papules or nodules of varying size that may be skin-colored or show different shades of red.

Malignant Melanoma. Malignant melanoma may arise either in a pre-existing pigmented lesion or it may develop on previously normal skin. The clinical appearance is usually that of a gradually enlarging pigmented nodule surrounded by redness. The nodule tends to bleed on even slight trauma and eventually it ulcerates. Numerous secondary nodules sometimes cluster around the primary tumor, crowding together in patches. Metastases to distant sites are common. In some patients, the first evidence that a mole has become malignant is metastatic enlargement of the regional lymph nodes or the appearance of distant metastases. In most instances, however, there are clinical signs of malignant transformation such as bleeding, crusting, increase in size, or change in color of a given lesion.

The treatment of melanoma is to excise with a wide margin all pigmented moles which, being subject to friction, pressure or other forms of irritation, have shown evidence of growth, color changes, ulceration or bleeding. Dissection of the regional lymph nodes commonly is combined with radical local removal of the melanoma.

Treatment and Nursing Management. Each person with cancer of the skin has to be evaluated and treated individually. The treatment depends on the size of the lesion, and its cell type, location and depth, and whether or not it is invasive and metastatic nodes are present. The most common modalities of treatment are surgical excision, irradiation or curettage followed by electrodesiccation. Malignant melanoma, being radioresistant is treated surgically.

The nursing care consists of the application of sterile dressings to the lesion and careful observation for any signs of hemorrhage. Hemorrhage often occurs after operation, but it may result simply from the erosion of a large vessel without any reference to operation.

The nurse can explain the nature of radiotherapy to the patient receiving this treatment for the first time. Being alone in a small room with a huge machine is less frightening when the patient has some understanding of it. Reassure the individual who fears that this treatment will cause sterilization that it will not. Explain to him that he may experience some reddening and perhaps blistering of the treated skin. Lanolin or any soothing lubricant will keep the skin soft after radiation therapy is completed. The patient should know that he always will have delicate skin; therefore, he must protect it from excess exposure to the sun, cold and so forth. The importance of follow-up care must be stressed, because there is always the possibility of recurrence or of a new primary lesion.

Prevention and Patient Education. The cause of most skin cancer is thought to be overexposure to sunlight. Outdoor workers such as sailors and farmers who have been chronically exposed to solar rays have a higher incidence; there is also a greater number of cases in geographic areas having intense sunlight. Chronicity as well as intensity of exposure definitely contribute to the development of skin cancer. Light complexioned persons are also more susceptible. Other influences that can promote the development of skin cancer are radiation exposure, industrial chemicals and exposure to tar and tar products.

The following factors are important in the education of patients in prevention:

1. Avoid unnecessary exposure to the sun, especially during times when ultraviolet radiation light is most intense (10 a.m. to 2 p.m.).
2. Wear appropriate protective clothing (e.g., broad-rimmed hat, long-sleeved garments).
3. Use shading devices (e.g., umbrella over a tractor).
4. Apply a protective sunscreen cream or lotion if an activity requires long periods of exposure.
5. Have moles treated that are accessible to repeated friction and irritation (palms of hands and soles of feet).
6. Watch for indications of potential malignancy in moles (e.g., increase in size, ulceration, bleeding or serous exudation).

DISORDERS INVOLVING THE HAIR

Alopecia

Alopecia (loss of hair) may involve any hairy area of the skin, but it is most commonly seen on the scalp. Temporary alopecia sometimes occurs after febrile illnesses (notably typhoid fever), severe emotional trauma, or after childbirth. A peculiar type of patchy hair loss, characterized by thinning of the hair in many small ill-defined areas, is associated with secondary syphilis ("moth-eaten alopecia"). The common type of hair loss seen in the male, in which there is thinning of hair on the vertex of the scalp and a receding hairline on both sides of the forehead, is largely under hormonal control and cannot be satisfactorily treated despite thousands of claims to the contrary. Severe dandruff and other local scalp conditions may also cause thinning of the hair.

Alopecia areata is a common disorder of unknown

TABLE 28-2. Common cosmetic plastic operations

Operation	Purpose	Surgery	Postoperative Expectations	Hospital Discharge
Rhinoplasty (Nose)	To improve the shape of the nose in relation to the rest of the face	1 to 1½ hours. Excess bone or cartilage is removed; nose is reshaped	Nasal splint; soft intranasal packing; foam rubber dressings	1-5 days
Mentoplasty (Chin)	To improve the profile, such as is necessary with a receding chin	Incision approach is within the mouth. Silicone or plastic implant is positioned	Healing complete in a week	1-2 days
Rhytidoplasty (Face lift)	To remove wrinkles caused by loose skin and to tighten fatty tissues	Incision line is anterior to ear; facial skin is undermined and drawn taut	Improvement lasts from 5 to 10 years	1 week
Glabellar rhytidoplasty	To remove 2 vertical furrows between eyebrows	Dermabrasion and excision; skin graft may be required		3-5 days
Otoplasty (Ear)	To correct deformed, flattened or protruding ears	1 to 1½ hours. Silicone or plastic implant may be used	Ear bandaged for a week; protection during sleep required for 3 weeks	1-2 days
Blepharoplasty (Eyelid)	To remove wrinkles and bulges caused by aging or inheritance	1 to 1½ hours. Two incisions; one on upper lid and one on lower lid	Swelling and discoloration subsides in about 10 days	1-2 days

cause characterized by sharply circumscribed areas of complete hair loss. The scalp, the eyebrows, and the beard are the usual sites of involvement. The disease occurs most commonly in children and young adults. The patchy hair loss may be relatively sudden, i.e., occurring within a few days, but usually it develops within several weeks. The skin in the involved areas appears normal, and there are no symptoms except for occasional mild pruritus. As a rule, the patches first spread peripherally and then remain stationary for many weeks to months. In extensive cases the patches may coalesce and result in almost total loss of hair. In most instances, however, regrowth of hair occurs within 6 to 12 months. At first the hair is apt to be finer and of a lighter shade, but eventually it resumes its normal texture and color.

Treatment. Except in cases associated with an underlying treatable disease, the management of baldness is largely unsatisfactory. Local scalp conditions such as dandruff should be brought under control. In some cases of alopecia areata, intralesional injections of corticosteroid hormones have resulted in relatively rapid regrowth of hair.

DERMATOLOGIC SURGERY AND PLASTIC RECONSTRUCTIVE SURGERY

Reconstructive surgery is performed to repair extravisceral defects and malformations, both congenital and acquired, and to restore function as well as to prevent further loss of function. Occasionally, plastic surgery is done primarily for aesthetic and cosmetic improvement; it is applicable to many parts of the body and to numerous structures such as bone, cartilage, fat, fascia, mucous membrane, muscle, nerve and cutaneous structures. For bone it includes bone inlays and transplants for deformities and nonunion; muscle can be transferred; nerves can be reconstructed and spliced; and cartilage can be replaced. Lastly, but as important as any, is the reconstruction of the cutaneous tissues around the neck and the face; this is usually referred to as *cosmetic surgery.*

Living tissue may be transferred from one part of the body to another or it may be obtained from one person for use in another. A *graft* is a piece of tissue separated completely from its normal and original position and transferred by one or more stages to correct a distant defect. Transfers or transplants from the same person are termed *autografts;* from a different person *homografts.* The former type is much better, being safer and more likely to be successful. Some transplant tissues may have been stored in "banks," for example, cornea of the eye, bone, fascia and collagen. At times tissue may be used from other animal sources, such as calf bone.

Beginning in the 1950's, kidney, lung, liver and heart transplants have been performed with varying degrees of success. With all transplants, the recipient reacts to the new tissue as to a foreign invader; the graft acts as an antigen causing the host to produce antibodies. The autoimmune reaction of the body is not fully understood, but attempts are made to avert such a reaction by immunosuppressive drugs.

Inert substances have long been used in plastic surgery. Such materials must not irritate the tissues of the

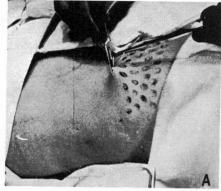
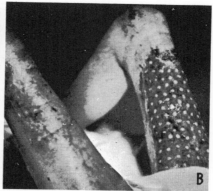
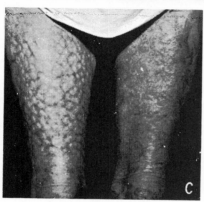

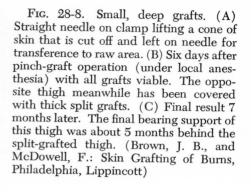

FIG. 28-8. Small, deep grafts. (A) Straight needle on clamp lifting a cone of skin that is cut off and left on needle for transference to raw area. (B) Six days after pinch-graft operation (under local anesthesia) with all grafts viable. The opposite thigh meanwhile has been covered with thick split grafts. (C) Final result 7 months later. The final bearing support of this thigh was about 5 months behind the split-grafted thigh. (Brown, J. B., and McDowell, F.: Skin Grafting of Burns, Philadelphia, Lippincott)

recipient, nor must they alter in shape or consistency. On the other hand, the substance ought to match the quality of the part being replaced and provide proper function and cosmetic appeal. In the fascinating history of plastic surgery, a variety of substances have been used, such as metal, ivory, boiled inert bone, rubber and wax. More recently, silicone and inert plastic materials such as Teflon and Dacron have been used with amazing results.

The field of reconstructive and plastic surgery has been expanded to such an extent that often the problem requires the team work of several specialists, such as an orthopedist, a neurosurgeon and a plastic surgeon to replace an extremity that had been accidently severed. Maxillofacial reconstruction requires the work of an oral surgeon, a reconstructive surgeon and an ear, nose and throat specialist. In addition to the nurse, the services of a sociologist, a psychologist and a psychiatrist are often required.

Availability of Facilities

The patient who is in need of plastic or reconstructive surgery may not know that such help is available. In this situation, therefore, the nurse may be in a position to disseminate information. Parents who have a congenitally deformed child often delay in seeking assistance either because of guilt feelings, conviction

that they must bear their own burden, false beliefs that perhaps the child will outgrow his handicap, or ignorance about what can be done. Scars or port-wine stains are not uncommon; their presence may affect adversely an otherwise healthy personality and result in a maladjusted person whose future happiness is jeopardized.

Children and individuals up to the age of 21 with congenital defects are eligible for financial support to meet the costs of plastic or reconstructive surgery. Plans for medical care of crippled children are available in each state; these, in turn, are partially supported by the Children's Bureau of the United States.

Preparation of the Patient

As in any other form of treatment, it is necessary to evaluate the patient as a whole and the patient's problem in its entirety. What is his problem? Is his defect a threat to his position or security among his daily contacts? Does the defect affect his personality? Are personality changes out of proportion to the size or the nature of his physical problem?

The emotional reaction of the patient to his disfigurement or abnormality is most significant, and must be understood if the repair process is to be progressive. The status of an adolescent girl may be threatened if she does not "look like" most of the other

Fig. 28-9. The Brown-Electro Dermatome is operated electrically to obtain the desired thickness graft in widths from 1¾″ to 3″. Blades are disposable; the apparatus is easily operated. (Zimmer Manufacturing Co., Warsaw, Ind.)

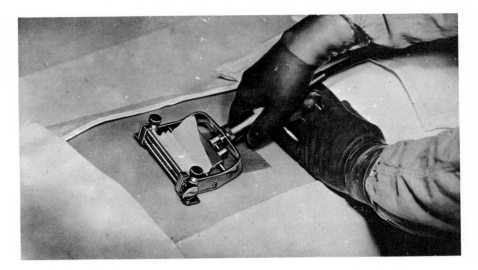

girls. The young man's scars may lead him to feel "inferior" to the other members of his class. The personality is affected, which in turn may affect the level of performance and adjustment to the meaningful experiences of life. Feeling withdrawn and threatened, this person may lash out against his family, friends and society. Some individuals have long blamed a history of disappointments, limited achievement and unhappiness on a deformity or disfigurement, and believe surgical repair will rechannel the future into a more wonderful course. The personality of the patient and his expectations must be clearly understood and guided, sometimes with professional assistance, so that the best possible results are obtained with the patient, nurse and surgeon all following the same plan of therapy.

The patient should be told that immediate postoperative appearances of a wound are temporary and that it may take days for changes to take place before the site takes on its eventual appearance. Redness, distortion, swelling and unattractive suture lines are characteristics that change with time. The family needs to be informed of the postoperative appearance, the condition and the recovery plans of the patient. Their genuine encouragement and support can mean a great deal to the apprehensive patient.

Physically, the patient is assessed for nutritional status. Increased vitamin and protein intake may be recommended to facilitate tissue healing. Hemoglobin and clotting time are noted, because their levels can affect the healing process. It is important that the tissues concerned be free of infection, and that other conditions, such as syphilis, tuberculosis, and diabetes mellitus, be under control. The general condition of the patient with regard to nutrition, age and morale should be at optimal levels.

Donor and recipient sites are prepared as for any

surgical incision. The patient needs to know those aspects of postoperative care that are significant in helping him to have a smooth recovery. The fact that wound appearances may be unattractive, red, distorted and puffy at first does not mean that the incision will not change. The fact that the size of the bandages (such as used with pressure dressings) may be voluminous does not mean that the surgery was correspondingly worse. Whether mirrors in the room should be removed would depend upon the circumstances. Of course, the family is to be aware of the postoperative appearance of the patient so that their surprised or disturbed expressions will not be conveyed to the patient on the first postoperative visit.

Skin Grafting

Since this type of reconstructive or plastic surgery most often is found necessary to correct unsightly and embarrassing deformity around the face, the mouth and neck, attention is given especially to the maxillofacial technique and nursing care.

So that the operation may be a success, the area to be covered with grafts must be free of infection and sloughs, because grafts "take" or grow only on a clean "granulating" surface. Therefore, a period of preparation of the wound usually is necessary before the operation can be undertaken. Warm saline or penicillin dressings often are used, and penicillin usually is given systemically. The donor area most often is the anterior thigh, but, because the nurse cannot tell where it is to be, she should ask for specific instructions. The preparation of the donor area consists of a shave and thorough cleansing by a germicidal soap and water.

Several types of grafts are in common usage. To cover small surfaces, the *Reverdin* or *pinch graft* often is used. Bits of skin are picked up on the point of a needle or with forceps and cut off with the scissors;

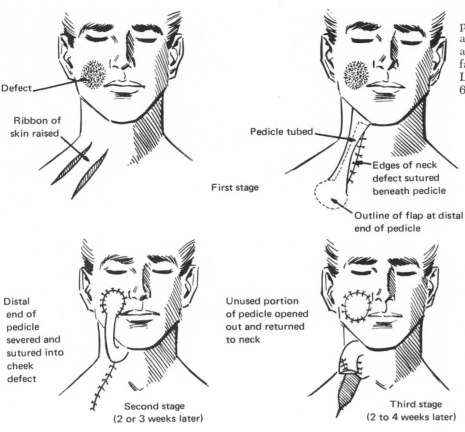

Defect

Ribbon of skin raised

First stage

Pedicle tubed

Edges of neck defect sutured beneath pedicle

Outline of flap at distal end of pedicle

Distal end of pedicle severed and sutured into cheek defect

Second stage (2 or 3 weeks later)

Unused portion of pedicle opened out and returned to neck

Third stage (2 to 4 weeks later)

these "islands" are applied to the area to be grafted (Fig. 28-8). This operation may be performed easily under local anesthesia.

Nature of Flaps and Grafts. In all reconstructive work, tissue to fill the defect must be obtained from either a distant site or nearby. This is accomplished by using a flap or graft. A *flap* is a piece of tissue used to cover or fill a defect. It has been lifted from its bed but still has a partial attachment by a pedicle, from which it receives its blood supply until healed in its new location.

The *Ollier-Thiersch graft* is used to cover larger surfaces. Strips of superficial skin are shaved off with a razor and applied to the granulating wound. This type of graft is relatively difficult to handle, because of its tendency to contract and wrinkle. On the other hand, it is the type most likely to grow in areas where the blood supply is poor, e.g., over bony prominences, and its donor site is re-epithelialized rapidly.

Split-thickness grafts are grafts of approximately one half the thickness of the skin, removed by a knife or a dermatome (Fig. 28-9). These grafts are handled more easily and, as in the case of the Ollier-Thiersch graft, skin at the donor site regenerates quickly.

Wolfe-Krause grafts differ from the previous types in that they consist of the full thickness of the skin. These are taken when the matching of skin color and texture is important. Obviously, more problems are to be expected with this type of graft, because of the difficulty of establishing a blood supply.

In the treatment of contractures from scars of old burns or injuries, especially those of neck and chin, it is necessary often to excise a large amount of contracted (scar) tissue. The area thus denuded most often is covered with a *pedicle* or *Gillies tube flap.* This flap is so cut that a tube or pedicle may be left attached through which the graft may obtain its blood supply. The flap is applied to the surface to be covered with the pedicle still attached. After the flap is well united to its new location, blood vessels grow into it and the pedicle can be removed (Fig. 28-10).

Other areas of the body may require plastic work of greater surface magnitude, in patients with extensive burns, mutilated limbs and crippling scar contractures. Here will arise the problem of donor areas for Reverdin, Ollier-Thiersch or sliding grafts. The Thiersch type may be made with a sharp razor blade or by the Padgett dermatome for the larger sheets of skin split of a definite thickness. When a cavity such as the orbit, the mouth or the nostril is to be relined,

FIG. 28-11. Commonly employed sites for donor areas of skin grafts. (From Converse, J. M., and Brauer, R. A.: Reconstructive Plastic Surgery, Philadelphia, 1964, W. B. Saunders Co.)

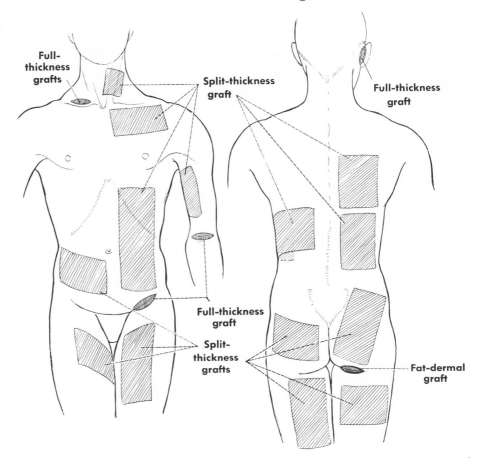

the graft may be sutured round a previously fashioned mold of dental rubber or plastic material.

In some circumstances, instead of free grafts or pedicle flaps, "sliding" flaps of skin and subcutaneous tissue from the surrounding area can be used. One application of the sliding flap method is the Z-plasty, very useful for relieving comparatively narrow scar contractures about the neck or about joints such as the axilla, the elbow, the knee or the wrist. The application of the Z-plasty to a scar contracture is shown in Figure 28-12.

Fascial transplants have numerous uses. They are obtained generally from the fascia lata of the thigh and are adaptable for use as suture material, for repair of hernia defects and for replacement of tendon loss. Cartilage transplantation may be immediate and direct, taken from the costal cartilages and transferred to the nose. Bone grafts demand meticulous aseptic technique and rigid fixation in their new site. They may be taken from the crest of the tibia, the upper border of the iliac bone or a rib.

All donor areas should receive the same careful treatment given any other surgical wound. If pos-

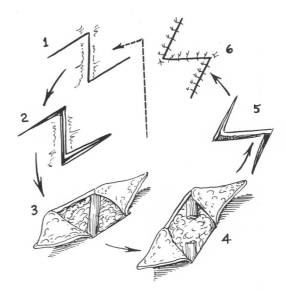

FIG. 28-12. Application of the Z-plasty to a scar contracture.

sible to close safely by suture, such is done. For the raw, wide area left from the Thiersch method, paraffin mesh, Albolene or petrolatum gauze permits a painless dressing within 8 to 10 days. The area from which the free graft is to be taken, usually the anterior surface of the thigh or the abdomen, is designated by the surgeon for preparation. The hair should be shaved from it, but generally no antiseptics are used until the patient is taken to the operating room.

After the application of the grafts, a dressing that will effect rapid epithelialization is appled. A perforated plastic or fine-mesh gauze appears to be ideal, particularly if it is impregnated with a thin layer of a dry type of ointment such as paraffin; this acts as a scaffold on which new tissue grows. Frequently, more adequate pressure is maintained by incorporating in the dressings sponge rubber, moist sea sponge or cotton waste. No redressing is necessary for 3 to 5 days, at which time only the gauze is removed, the paraffin mesh being left in place. Care must be exercised in removing the dressings so as not to disturb the grafts.

Nursing Management of the Patient With Maxillofacial Problems

The face is a part of the body that every person desires to keep at its best; many individuals try to improve on nature by various and sundry methods. When the face becomes disfigured, an emotional reaction occurs. Consequently, the victim of an automobile accident, whose face is injured, presents a problem that demands the utmost in understanding by the nurse. The patient's reaction to his problem, to his family and to the medical and the nursing personnel are all indices of his inner feelings that are most significant if appropriate measures are to be taken to help him.

Preoperative Attention. The patient may have a good meal the evening before, and a light breakfast or fluid up to 4 hours before the operation. For the comfort of the patient, operation is done best in the morning.

The mouth should be made as clean as possible to lessen the danger both of lung complications after general anesthesia and of infection in the wound. Preoperative medication is ordered with specific regard to relaxing the patient and reducing mouth secretions. If the patient is a man, the skin of the face should be shaved closely and, of course, well cleansed with soap and water. If the operative field extends up toward the scalp, this should also be shaved as far as is necessary.

Postoperative Management. Immediate postoperative care is concentrated on maintaining an adequate airway. Care must be taken to prevent disturbance or soilage of dressings. Observe for impairment of circulation and edema.

Occasionally, after an operation within the mouth, the nurse may be alarmed by undue bleeding from the gums. All ordinary hemorrhage of this nature can be controlled by inserting a gauze pad in the mouth against the bleeding part of the jaw and bringing pressure of the opposing teeth to bear against it. If the patient is conscious, he can be made to bite on the pad. This pressure of the jaw often can be applied even when no teeth are present. In case of difficulty, the nurse should make pressure with the pad until the doctor arrives. The gauze pad can be changed as it becomes soaked with blood or saliva. After plastic operations on the face, frequently no dressings are used. If the incisions have been closed accurately with sutures, no dressings are necessary unless it is desired to control oozing of blood by pressure. Particularly near the mouth, dressings tend to become soaked with saliva and food, which may lead to infection of an otherwise clean wound. Slight oozing of blood from the incisions generally occurs for a short time after operation. If this blood is allowed to clot on the wound, infection may occur under the clot and spoil the cosmetic result. For the first hour or so after operation the nurse should wipe the blood that oozes from the incision with an alcohol sponge so that it will not clot on the surface.

In plastic operations the flaps sometimes become blue and congested, due to partial obstruction of the venous circulation. The surgeon sometimes scarifies the surface of the flap, making numerous small openings to relieve the blood congestion and avoid gangrene of the flap. The blood flow from these small incisions then can be kept up by the continuous application for several hours of hot fomentations of 1 per cent sodium citrate. These must be applied in an aseptic manner in order not to infect the flap. Probably the most convenient way is for the nurse to drop some of the warm sodium citrate solution on the dressings from time to time with a syringe.

Pain is more likely to follow operations involving the jaw bones than the soft tissues alone. For postoperative pain, either a hot-water bag or an ice bag may give relief. Whichever works best in the individual patient is employed. Analgesics ranging from aspirin to morphine may be required.

Maxillofacial patients need not be denied fluids for any length of time after operation, as may be the case after abdominal operations. The patient may have cracked ice or water as soon as postanesthetic vomiting is over, and liquid diet may be started as soon as the patient has a desire for food. Very often soft diet is started the day after operation.

When there is a wound of the mouth, the mouth should be cleansed after each feeding. It is not sufficient always for the patient to use a mouthwash.

Frequent swabbing of the gums and the teeth with cotton on applicators soaked in hydrogen peroxide will accomplish a great deal in keeping the mouth clean. The mouth, and especially the wounded or diseased part, should be irrigated 3 or 4 times a day with some antiseptic fluid. The syringe should require only one hand to operate it, leaving the other hand free to retract the cheek or hold a light. A very convenient syringe is the one used for irrigating eyes. This consists of a fairly large rubber bulb and a small glass nozzle of the medicine dropper type. An all-rubber ear syringe or a power spray also may be used. When very frequent irrigation is required, a reservoir (bag or douche can) may be suspended over the head of the bed, not more than 2 feet above the patient's head, and the fluid carried to the mouth through a plastic nozzle. Sometimes the patient himself can use this.

Gauze packing frequently is placed in mouth wounds. This should not be allowed to remain longer than 48 hours without change. If no packing is used in the mouth, no treatment other than frequent irrigation is required.

Suppurating superficial wounds can be cleansed with hydrogen peroxide. Granulating surfaces are treated by application of penicillin solution and covered with petrolatum gauze.

Nutrition. The diet for maxillofacial patients is very important. Many of them, particularly those with fractures of the jaws, have to have the upper and the lower teeth fastened together for weeks and, therefore, can take only liquid food. Others are able to take soft food, but are unable to masticate. These patients are not to be classed with the ordinary postoperative patient on liquid diet, to whom the liquid is given in small amounts because he is in no condition to assimilate more, and to whom a soft and, finally, a full diet is given after a short time.

In patients obliged to remain for a long time on liquid diet because of an injury to the jaw, sufficient quantity and quality should be given to maintain them in a state of good nutrition. Under this regimen a loss of weight will be noted at first, but, if properly carried out, it is possible to obtain a gain in weight. Much can be accomplished with the liberal use of stewed fruits and fruit juices, soft cereals, malted milk, cocoa, coffee, tea and so forth. A proper vitamin content must not be overlooked. The soft diet for patients able to manage it also demands careful preparation. The usual routine soft diet in hospitals is not always suitable for patients unable to masticate. All meat, vegetables and cooked fruits should be divided finely or mashed. The patient must be fed often in order to obtain the equivalent of a full diet.

Psychological Support. The nurse is in a unique position to help these patients to accept their many experiences more easily. Rehabilitation is often a combination of both physical and mental aspects. Such rehabilitation depends not only on eradication of a physical scar but also on the correction of psychic trauma that is so markedly influenced by the patient's social and emotional background. An understanding of these factors helps greatly in promoting the progress of this patient to the ends desired.

Many times, the ultimate objective requires a number of operations separated by long intervals of time. Patience is a real factor. Recreational, occupational and spiritual therapies need to be explored fully with the interests of the individual patient kept intact.

Often, the kinds of dressings that have to be worn, the unusual positions that have to be maintained and the temporary incapacities that must be experienced can be very upsetting to the most stable person. The nurse must be able to offer hope and encouragement and to combine this with a wholesome sense of humor. Tact and patience, and attention to small details will make the nurse an invaluable colleague as the patient regains his self-assurance and more normal usefulness and appearance.

Surgical Planing (Dermabrasion)

Dermal abrasion, or surgical planing of the skin, is done in selected patients with facial disfigurements from scars resulting from acne, trauma, tattoo, nevi, freckles and chickenpox or smallpox. The procedure involves the removal of the epidermis and some superficial dermis while preserving enough of the dermis to allow re-epithelialization of the dermabraded areas. Results are best in the face, because it is rich in intra-dermal epithelial elements. Planing is performed either manually with coarse abrasive paper, or mechanically with an abrader or a rapidly rotating wire brush.

Patient Instruction and Preparation. The primary reason for undergoing dermabrasion is to improve appearance. The surgeon explains to the patient what he can expect from dermabrasion. The patient should also be informed about the nature of the postoperative dressing, what discomfort he may experience, and how long it will take before his tissues look normal. The extent of the surface to be planed will determine whether the procedure takes place in the surgeon's office, the clinic or the hospital; most often a general anesthetic is used and the patient is hospitalized.

The skin is thoroughly cleansed with pHisoHex for several days before surgery. Shaving is not necessary in the female; however, the male shaves the morning of surgery.

In addition to general anesthesia, the use of a topical spray anesthetic (such as Frigiderm) for stabilizing and stiffening the skin may be desirable. The depth of planing can be readily gauged and the anesthetized

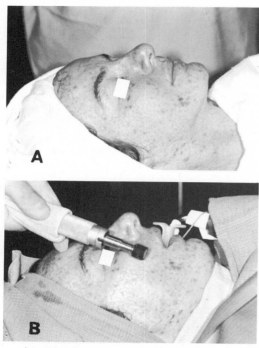

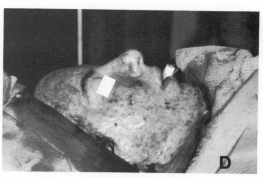

(D) The appearance of the skin after bleeding is controlled by pressure. Upper lip, eyelids and nostril rims have not yet been abraded.

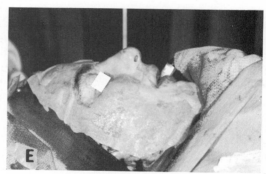

(A, B) The patient with acne before the dermabrasion procedure.

(E) A layer of petrolatum dressing is applied.

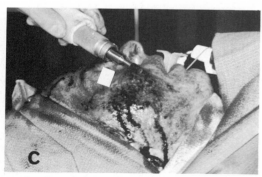

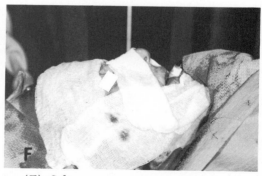

(C) Iverson Dermabrader being used to abrade superficial epithelium.

(F) Saline compresses are applied over the petrolatum dressing. This is done to absorb oozing and clotting which are subject to infection.

FIG. 28-13. Dermabrasion procedures. The saline compresses are discontinued after 12 to 24 hours and the petrolatum dressing is allowed to air dry in place. It is removed in 3 to 5 days. The skin will remain red for 6 to 8 weeks.

area is momentarily bloodless. The superficial layers of skin are removed by an abrasive machine (Dermabrader) or sandpapering. During and after planing, copious saline irrigations remove debris and allow for inspection.

Postoperative and Convalescent Care. Usually, petrolatum gauze or perforated plastic-faced (Telfa) bandages are applied. Pressure dressings are often used. Edema occurs during the first postoperative day, which may even cause the eyes to close. The patient should be informed that this will subside within a day. After about 48 hours, the dressings are removed and the sensation is one of a recent sunburn. When the crust forms, lanolin, cocoa butter or hypoallergic cream relieves the sensation of tightness. When no dressings are used, oozing may be noticed. In some clinics, the drying process is facilitated by using a hair dryer turned to warm and the air allowed to flow gently over the area. Within 14 days the crusts have separated, and although the skin is still red, most of the scars are gone. The patient is advised to avoid direct sunlight for 3 to 4 months. Repeat treatments are usually advocated. The patient's chief complaint is that the procedure is more annoying than discomforting. The effects produced are well worth the inconvenience.

BIBLIOGRAPHY

Books

Allen, A. C.: The Skin. New York, Grune and Stratton, 1967.

Behrman, I. T., and Labow, T. A.: The Practitioner's Illustrated Dermatology. New York, Grune and Stratton, 1965.

Converse, H. M. (ed.): Reconstructive Plastic Surgery. Philadelphia, W. B. Saunders, 1966.

Fisher, A. A.: Contact Dermatitis. Philadelphia, Lea & Febiger, 1967.

Lewis, G. M., and Wheeler, C. E.: Practical Dermatology, Philadelphia, W. B. Saunders, 1967.

Montgomery, H. (ed.): Dermatopathology. vols. 1 and 2. New York, Harper and Row—Hoeber Medical Division, 1967.

Sauer, G. C.: Manual of Skin Diseases. Philadelphia, J. B. Lippincott, 1966.

Stewart, W. D., Danto, J. L., and Maddin, S.: Synopsis of Dermatology, St. Louis, C. V. Mosby, 1966.

Wood-Smith, D., and Porowski, P. (eds.): Nursing Care of the Plastic Surgery Patient. St. Louis, C. V. Mosby, 1967.

Dermatology

Baird, K. A.: A new and effective treatment for psoriasis. Dermat. Internat., 4:155-158, July-Sept., 1965.

Bolton, P. S.: Anti-inflammatory corticosteroids in cutaneous medicine. App. Therap., 9:247-250, March, 1967.

Christianson, H. B., and Applewhite, M. L.: Cutaneous diseases of the aged. Geriatrics, 22:153-164, Nov., 1967.

Farber, E. M., et al.: Psoriasis; a questionnaire survey of 2,144 patients. Arch. Derm., 98:248-259, Sept., 1968.

Freeman, R. G., and Knox, J. M.: Skin cancer and the sun. CA, 17:231-238, Sept.-Oct., 1967.

Hackney, V. C., and Norins, A. L.: How we treat seborrheic dermatitis. Postgrad. Med., 43:242-243, Feb., 1968.

Higdon, R. S., and Elgart, M. L.: How we treat dermatitis herpetiformis. Postgrad. Med., 42:A120-A123, Dec., 1967.

James, A. P. R. (ed.): Common dermatologic disorders. Clin. Symposia, 19:39-65, April-June, 1967.

Knox, J. M., and Freeman, R. G.: Detection and diagnosis of skin cancer. CA 15:216-225, 1965.

————: et al.: Treatment of skin cancer. South. Med. J., 60:241-246, March, 1967.

Lea, W. A., Jr., and Falconer, H. S.: Cutaneous diseases. Postgrad. Med., 39:488-493, 1966.

Lehman, J. A., Jr., et al.: Clinical study of 49 patients with malignant melanoma. Cancer, 19:611-619, 1960.

Leonard, R. R.: Prevention of superficial cutaneous infections. Arch. Dermat., 95:520-523, May, 1967.

Lyell, A.: Management of warts. Brit. Med. J., 2:1339-1402; 1576-1579, 1966.

Martyn, D.: Radiation therapy for skin cancer. Canad. Nurse, 63:48-50, Feb., 1967.

McCallum, J. L., et al.: Seminar on nevi and melanomata. App. Therap., 7:375-385, 1965.

Mundth, E. D., et al.: Malignant melanoma: A clinical study of 427 cases. Ann. Surg., 162:15-28, 1965.

Recent advances in dermatology. Med. Clin. N. Amer., 49, May, 1965.

Rook, A.: Advances in treatment of diseases of the skin. Practitioner, 197:442-446, Oct., 1966.

The skin and internal disease. Postgrad. Med., 41, May, 1967.

Snyderman, R. K., et al.: Complete replacement of port-wine stains. N.Y. State J. Med., 66:1905-1910, 1966.

Trice, E. R.: A rational approach to the management of acne vulgaris. Virginia Med. Monthly, 94:338-341, June, 1967.

Wexler, L.: Gamma benzene hexachloride in treatment of pediculosis and scabies. Amer. J. Nurs., 69:565-566, March, 1969.

Whelan, C. S.: Electrocoagulation in the treatment of skin cancers about the head and face. Surgery, 62:1017-1020, Dec., 1967.

Reconstructive Surgery

Castillo, P.: The younger look—rhytidectomy. AORN J., 8:41-45, Nov., 1968.

Conway, H.: Skin grafts: The techniques. Amer. J. Nurs., 64:94-97, Nov., 1964.

Edwards, B. F.: Endoprostheses in plastic surgery. Amer. J. Nurs., 64:123-125, May, 1964.

Nayer, D.: Skin grafts: The patient. Amer. J. Nurs., 64:98-101, Nov., 1964.

Ohlwiler, D. A.: The use of silicone implants in plastic surgery. Nurs. Clin. N. Amer., 2:495-501, Sept., 1967.

Pickrell, K. L.: Reconstructive plastic surgery of the face. Clin. Symposia, 19:71-99, July-Aug.-Sept., 1967.

Spira., M., Gerow, E. J., and Hardy, S. B.: Cervicofacial rhytidectomy. Plastic Recon. Surg., 40, Dec., 1967.

Zarem, H. A.: Silastic implants in plastic surgery. Surg. Clin. N. Amer., 48:129-142, Feb., 1968.

PATIENT EDUCATION

U.S. Government Printing Office
Superintendent of Documents
Washington, D.C. 20402
    U.S. Dept. H.E.W.: Cancer of the Skin. 1968. (Nat. Institutes of Health Pub. No. 28)

American Cancer Society
(Local Chapter)
    Cancer of the Skin. 1967.
    Sense in the Sun. 1967.

Ayerst Laboratories
New York, New York 10017
    Getting Around the Problem of Ringworm Fungi. 1966.

American Academy of Facial Plastic and Reconstructive Surgery, Inc.
322 California Company Bldg.
1111 Tulane Avenue
New Orleans, Louisiana 70112
    Plastic Surgery.

CHAPTER 29

Nursing the Patient with Burns

- *The Problem of Burns*
- *Pathophysiology of Burns*
- *Evaluations of a Patient's Burn Injury*
- *Local Care of a Burn*
- *Medical and Nursing Management of the Burn Patient*

THE PROBLEM OF BURNS

Approximately 8,000 persons die of burns each year in the United States. In addition, hundreds of thousands experience pain, disability and disfigurement as a result of burns. Some authorities estimate that, practicing reasonable caution and well-known safety measures, 75 per cent of all burns could be prevented.* By taking advantage of opportunities to teach and to promote legislation for safety practices, the nurse can play an active part in preventing fires and burns.

Four major objectives relating to human burns are:

1. Prevention;
2. Institution of life-saving measures in the severely burned person;
3. Prevention of disability and disfigurement through early specialized, individual treatment;
4. Rehabilitation of the individual through reconstructive surgery and rehabilitative programs.

* The National Institute of Health has established a six member registry for the purpose of compiling statistics with regard to cause of burns, place of origin, extent of burned area of the body, complications, and so forth. Significant research data will be forthcoming from this compilation. Members are Universities of Texas, Michigan, Cincinnati, Med. College of Va., Brooke Army Medical Center and Cook County Hospital.

Prevention

Four-fifths of all burn accidents in the United States occur in the home and are caused primarily by ignorance, carelessness or the impulses of children. The nurse in the public health field is in a unique position to assist families in correcting unsafe practices in the home. The National Fire Protection Association points out that there is no mystery about most home fires:

A carelessly discarded cigarette is left to smoulder in an overstuffed chair, a portable oil heater is refilled while burning, hot liquids are overturned, electric circuits are overloaded. Uncleared rubbish becomes a breeding place for fire. Fire deaths occur when simple rules of safety are violated—smoking in bed, leaving children alone, neglecting to teach youngsters that matches and lighters are not playthings.

Where do home fires start? Studies give these percentages:

Living room	27%	Basement	10%
Kitchen	27%	Closets	14%
Bedroom	12%	Attics	5%
	Concealed spaces	5%	

Legislation has been passed to require the observance of some fire safety measures. Fire hazard inspections and regulations in hospitals, nursing homes, hotels, and buildings where large numbers of people congregate are required by law. Products that are flammable must carry a label indicating the precautions necessary for safe handling. The observance of the following safety measures would help to prevent the occurrence of fires and burns in the home:

1. Never empty an ash tray until you know the contents are cold.
2. Use a flashlight, never an open flame, to illuminate dark spaces.
3. Adequate electric wiring is a must. Circuits that were safe 25 years ago may be dangerously overloaded with today's appliances. A jungle of wires leading to one outlet is a fire hazard.
4. Keep burners and broilers of the kitchen stove clean. Accumulated grease may catch fire.
5. Never hang a curtain where it may blow over an open flame.
6. Do not smoke in bed or when sleepy.
7. Use fuses of correct size—15 amperes for most circuits.
8. Cluttered stairways, closets and storage spaces are fire hazards.
9. Never use gasoline or similar fluids indoors.
10. Chimneys and flues should be cleaned and repaired regularly.
11. Don't store paints or other burnable materials near the furnace.
12. Flimsy, fast-burning fabrics are dangerous for children's clothing.
13. Teach children the basic facts of fire safety as soon as possible. Never leave young children alone.
14. Oily rags, mops and other burnable odds and ends may ignite spontaneously or help spread a fire.
15. Gasoline and other burnable fluids should be stored in safe containers, not breakable bottles.
16. Be aware of the dangers involved in mishandling plastic and paper products, especially clothing made of these materials.

Long before the first smoke is detected, each family should have a plan of what to do in case of a fire. Escape routes should be devised and equipment, such as extinguishers, ropes and ladders, maintained and periodically checked. Family fire drills should be carried out, and plans made regarding where members of the family should meet.

Intelligent action during a fire requires knowledge about what happens when a building is on fire. Bare wood will ignite at 800° F. in 30 seconds. A blaze can produce temperatures of 800 to 1,000° F. very quickly, by building up super-heated gases that rise and spread. Thus, fires do not spread inch by inch; they build up heat, then leapfrog. Smoke and gases produced by fire, which contain carbon monoxide and many other toxic gases, are major causes of death, frequently taking the lives of people on upper levels that are not even touched by the flames:

The following are good measures to observe in the event of a fire:

1. Get everybody out of the house, if possible.
2. Call the fire department.
3. Battling a roaring fire with an extinguisher is not only dangerous but futile.
4. If smoke is smelled, *never* fling open a door to investigate. Remember those deadly gases. If the door is very warm to the hand, leave it closed. Otherwise, brace a hip against the door and open slightly; if a hot draft is felt, slam it shut.
5. Normally, windows are the best escape routes. If the window leads to a garage or porch roof, wait there for help. If it is necessary to leave, back over the edge, hold on the edge, hang down and drop with knees bent. If you are trapped in a room, open a window for air to breathe, but keep the door shut to prevent draft. Hang a sheet out to alert rescuers.
6. Do not walk upright in a burning building, but crawl on the floor to avoid inhaling toxic gases. Take short breaths and cover the face with a damp cloth to filter out the smoke.

Emergency First Aid

Once a burn has been sustained, the application of cold is the best first aid measure. Soaking the burned area in ice water or applying cold towels gives immediate and striking relief from pain, and restricts local tissue edema and damage. The burn should also be covered as quickly as possible, to minimize bacterial contamination and decrease pain by preventing air from coming into contact with the injured surface. Sterile dressings are best, but any clean, dry cloth can be used as an emergency dressing. Ointments and salves should not be used.

Chemical burns, which result from contact with a corrosive material, should be irrigated immediately. Most chemical laboratories have a high-pressure shower for such emergencies; if at home, a quick shower or a soaking in a running bath will work well. If a chemical gets in or near the eyes, they should be flushed with cool clean water. Following this, 2 or 3 drops of a mild oil (mineral or olive) should be instilled, and a physician promptly consulted. When clothes catch on fire, quench the flames by having the victim fall to the floor or ground and roll him in a rug or blanket. Standing still would force him to breathe flames and smoke, and running would fan the flames. After the flames are extinguished, soak the hot clothing with cold water and notify the physician, who in turn will alert the proper hospital personnel. Thus, life-saving measures can be initiated immediately by a trained team with no time lost.

As a burn victim awaits transportation to the hospital, he should remain lying down; no attempt should be made to remove clothing. Exposed burned surfaces can be covered with the cleanest material available to prevent exposure to air and contamination; covering the person with a blanket will prevent loss of body heat. For pain, ice or cold water bottles can be placed strategically around him. If the hospital cannot be reached within an hour, the physician will probably initiate fluid therapy intravenously. Otherwise, an effective first-aid measure would be to give the conscious patient fluids to drink, if he can tolerate them. To a quart of water, add one teaspoon (3 gm.) of salt and a half teaspoon (1.5 gm.) of soda bicarbonate. (Salt provides sodium and soda bicarbonate helps to combat acidosis.)

As a rule, the physician will give some form of pain relief, such as codeine or morphine, before transportation to the hospital. It is essential that such medication be clearly recorded and the record sent along to the hospital with the patient. Neglect of this precaution may lead to death from overdosage of narcotics, if the hospital physician, unaware of a previous narcotic administration, orders additional doses to be given.

PATHOPHYSIOLOGY OF BURNS

Burns are wounds produced by various kinds of thermal, electrical, radioactive or chemical agents. These agents kill cells by changing the protein substance of the cell. Because they attack the organism from its environment, the tissues in direct contact with that environment (e.g., the skin and mucosa of the respiratory tract and the upper alimentary tract) are the first to be damaged.

The pathophysiology of a burn may be divided into 4 stages. These stages overlap one another, but in general they are: (1) the stage of neurogenic shock, (2) the stage of fluid-loss shock, (3) the stage of infection and slough of burned tissue, and (4) the stage of repair.

Stage of Neurogenic Shock

This is the first stage of a burn episode, and it may be lethal. It includes the fright, terror and hysterical reaction of the individual, and especially the pain produced by the irritation of thousands of nerve endings in the skin. The factors of this stage are enough to produce a precipitous fall in blood pressure to shock

levels, from which the patient may never recover. This is especially true of the young and the old.

Stage of Fluid-loss Shock

Although the local effects of a burn are the most immediately evident, the systemic effects pose a greater threat to life. These may be more easily understood if they are traced in the order of their occurrence. The first effect of a burn is to produce a dilatation of the capillaries and small vessels in the area, thus increasing capillary permeability. Plasma seeps out into the surrounding tissues to produce blisters and edema. The type, the duration and the intensity of the burn affects the amount and duration of the fluid loss. Fluid loss reduces the blood volume, so that the blood becomes thicker, i.e., the volume of the cellular elements of the blood increases in relation to the volume of fluid (plasma) of the blood. This change makes the circulation less efficient. The loss of fluid volume is reflected in the fall of the blood pressure, causing shock. The relative increase in cell volume is reflected in the increasing hematocrit, which is a fairly accurate and reliable measure of the systemic effect of the burn. The hematocrit reading is used as a guide to estimate the fluid requirements of the patient; the aim is to provide enough fluids to bring the hematocrit back to normal. The amount of urinary output also indicates the amount of fluid loss from the blood. When the blood is concentrated by fluid loss and the hematocrit elevated, the urinary output is reduced. Fluid administration during this period is adjusted so that a urinary flow of at least 25 to 40 ml. per hour is obtained.

Stage of Burn Slough and Infection

The third stage of a burn is the period when the tissue killed by the burn (eschar) separates from the underlying viable tissue by a process of liquefaction called slough formation. This leaves a large open wound that is usually infected. The infecting organisms vary; in the upper part of the body, they are more apt to be those found in the nose and throat. The lower part of the body often has colon bacilli as the infecting organisms. The infection does not occur suddenly; it probably begins soon after the burn occurs and then gradually grows in the sloughing tissue (a good culture medium). The infection reveals itself by gradually increasing fever and local tenderness, tachycardia, and often by lymphangitis. Because infection is almost always a factor in burn treatment, antibiotics are usually added to the intravenous solutions from the first. Cultures are made and sensitivity tests carried out, and the appropriate antibiotic selected.

Stage of Repair

This stage of a burn may be divided into (1) repair of the burned area and (2) systemic repair. The repair of a large wound left by a burn cannot begin until the area is free of sloughing tissue. In some cases the death of skin tissue may not have included deeper epithelial elements, so that some degree of epithelialization may occur from these remains of skin cells. When the entire thickness of the skin has been destroyed by the burn, repair must begin at the edges of the wound. This takes a long time in large burns, and permits an overgrowth of granulation (scar) tissue to occur. To avoid this excessive overgrowth of granulation, the burn wound is covered with skin grafts, which also allows earlier healing. Sometimes the burn wound may be covered with cadaver skin preserved in banks; this provides an excellent temporary covering that may last a month or more but eventually sloughs away, and must be replaced by grafts of the patient's own skin.

Systemic repair includes such measures as blood transfusions to overcome the anemia that always develops in the later stages of large burns, and a high caloric, high protein diet to aid in replacing the nutritional elements lost from the draining wound and from the decreased food intake during the early phases of burn treatment.

EVALUATION OF PATIENT'S BURN INJURY (BURN APPRAISAL)

Initial evaluation of a burned victim is necessary to select the best method of treatment, to develop a guide for fluid management, and to determine the resources (personnel and equipment) available for patient care. A burn is evaluated by determining the cause of the burn, the condition of the patient, the extent of surface area involved, and the depth of the burn.

The Cause of the Burns

The cause of the burns may be:

1. *Thermal*—moist, as from steam or boiling water; dry, as from a flame, a hot-water bottle, hot metals, hot grease.

2. *Chemical*—strong acids, such as sulfuric or nitric; strong alkalies, such as caustic soda (lye). Other strong chemicals include phosphorus, mustard gas, etc.

3. *Electrical*—the effects vary widely, depending on the type, voltage and amperage of the current. Burns usually are noted both where the current enters and where it leaves the body. In addition to these local effects, systemic changes that produce respiratory, circulatory and central nervous system disturbances may be noted.

4. *Irradiation*—may be caused by ultraviolet rays, x-rays and radium. Sunburn and burns from ultraviolet lamps usually are superficial and produce short-lived effects. Burns from x-rays and radium are slow to appear, and the most marked effects, such as ulceration, may not occur for years.

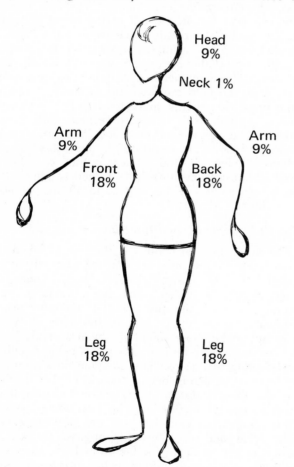

Fig. 29-1. "Rule of Nine" chart for calculating per cent of body burns in the adult. (Actual values have been modified for practical purposes.)

The Person with a Burn

The general condition and state of health of a burn victim, his approximate age, and when he was burned are important factors that may modify his treatment. The elderly and very young are more susceptible to shock than the young adult. The case of a debilitated 60-year-old man who fell asleep with a lighted cigarette that ignited the sofa would present a different problem than that of a 38-year-old man whose clothing caught fire while he burned leaves. Diabetes, emphysema or other diseases add complicating factors that must be considered in planning care. The nurse has a

TABLE 29-1. Evaluation of depth of a burn.

Degree	Nature of Burn	Skin Involvement	Symptoms	Appearance	Course
First	Sunburn Low-intensity flash	Epidermis	Tingling Hyperesthesia Painful Soothed by cooling	Reddened; blanches with pressure Minimal or no edema	Complete recovery within a week Peeling
Second	Scalds Flash flame	Dermis	Painful Hyperesthesia Sensitive to cold air	Blistered, mottled red base, broken epidermis, weeping surface Edema	Recovery in 2 to 3 weeks Some scarring and depigmentation Infection may convert to third degree
Third	Fire Prolonged exposure to hot liquids	Subcutaneous tissue	Painless Symptoms of shock Hematuria and hemolysis of blood likely	Dry; pale white or charred Broken skin with fat exposed Edema	Eschar sloughs Grafting necessary Scarring and loss of contour and function

responsibility to learn as much as possible about the patient, including his preburn weight and state of health, from his relatives and friends.

Where the accident happened, such as a particular industrial plant, and what first aid measures were employed also are significant to the physician.

Extent of Surface Area Burned

An estimation of the total body surface area (TBSA) involved as a result of a burn is simplified by dividing the body into multiples of 9. The initial evaluation should be revised on the 2nd and 3rd postburn days, since the demarcation usually is not visible until then (Fig. 29-1).

Depth of Burn

This is often difficult to determine. Classification of burns by degrees is helpful for description and identification (see Table 29-1). *First-degree* burns are not serious unless large areas of the body are involved. They produce redness of the burned area. *Second-degree* burns are those associated with blister formation (vesicles). The superficial layers of skin have been destroyed, but the deeper layers have escaped injury. Patients with large areas of second-degree burns require hospitalization. Skin healing can take place from the deeper skin cells that have remained viable. *Third-degree* burns imply a destruction of the full thickness of the skin and often of the underlying fat, muscles, and even bone. Rapid transportation to the hospital is important.

In determining depth of a burn, it is important that the following be known: (1) the causative agent, such as flame, scalding milk, etc., (2) the duration of exposure, and (3) the thickness of the skin. Hematuria and high plasma hemoglobin suggest deep burns. Burns are classified as major if 2nd-degree burns involve over 30 per cent of the body and if 3rd-degree burns involve over 10 per cent.

Survival Prediction

The best survival expectancy with burns is obtained in the young adult group, ages 15 to 45 years of age. However, in this group, burns of over 40 per cent of the body are likely to be fatal. A burn of over 20 per cent of the body endangers life. The following chart* gives a clear picture of the effect of age and per cent of the body burned on survival rate:

Age	Per Cent of Body Burned	Survival	Mortality
5 and under	30%	30%	70%
15 to 45 years	50%	45%	55%
	65% & over	0%	100%
65 years and over	20%	0%	100%

Prognosis depends on the depth and extent of the burn as well as the condition and age of the patient. Problems encountered are shock, infection, circulatory and renal difficulties. Although much progress has been made in recent years, the medical and nursing professions continue to seek better methods of treatment and management.

* From Baxter; Burns. *In*: Conn: Current Therapy. p. 748 Philadelphia, W. B. Saunders, 1967.

TABLE 29-2. A method of classifying burns.

Degree	Minor	Classification Moderate	Major (Critical)	
Second	Less than 15%	15 to 30%	Over 30%	Burns complicated with fractures, respiratory tract injury, major soft tissue injury.
Third	Less than 2%	Less than 10% (excluding face, feet, hands)	Over 10% or deep burns of face, feet or hands	

LOCAL CARE OF THE BURN

Conscientious management of the burned area itself is of vital importance. The major cause of death in patients with extensive burns who have survived the first few days is infection occurring within the burn site. A few of the bacteria ever-present in our environment contaminate the wound; these bacteria (staphylococci, *Proteus*, *Pseudomonas*, *E. coli* and *Klebsiella* enterobacteria) find optimal conditions for growth within the burn. The burn eschar is a nonviable crust with no blood supply where polymorphonuclear leukocytes and antibodies cannot reach. Phenomenal numbers of bacteria—over one billion per gram of tissue—may appear and subsequently spread to the bloodstream, or they release their toxins, which reach distant sites. Through the years, various approaches have been devised to combat these problems. Several approaches are presented here, although all have their advantages and their disadvantages. The most promising and increasingly popular method at present is the application of silver nitrate solution.

"Open Air" or Exposure Method

This method became popular when large numbers of people had to be taken care of in disasters and dressings could not be applied to burns. It is most frequently used to treat burns of the face, neck, perineum and extensive areas of the trunk. By exposing a burn to the drying effect of air, the exudate dries to form a hard crust in about 3 days; this protects the wound. In a 2nd-degree burn, regeneration of skin beneath the crust takes 2 to 3 weeks, at which time the crust falls off. In a 3rd-degree burn. epithelization occurs beneath the eschar and takes 4 to 5 weeks; the crust loosens and cracks in 2 to 3 weeks. Because such cracks are an invitation to bacteria, some surgeons prefer to remove the crusts and apply skin grafts.

The success of this method depends upon keeping the immediate environment free of organisms: everything that comes in contact with the patient must be sterile. He lies on sterile linens and those who come in direct contact with him wear masks, sterile gowns and gloves. Visitors are instructed to wear gowns and masks and to not touch the bed nor hand the patient anything. A cradle may be placed over the patient to prevent sheets from touching him, to minimize the effects of air currents to which a burn patient is unusually sensitive, and to provide him with some form of covering. (Some persons are sensitive to being unduly exposed.) The use of a sterile "burn pack" facilitates the care of this patient and may contain sheets, pillowcases, wash cloth, bath blanket, loin cloth, halter, and perhaps, a gown and mask for the attendant.

The room should be kept scrupulously clean; windows should have screens to keep out flies and other insects. Damp dusting and mopping is preferable to dry dusting and sweeping. Regulation of the room temperature and humidity are necessary for the patient's comfort and for optimal crust development. The patient feels temperature changes more acutely and is most comfortable when the room is kept at 24.4° C. (76° F.). By monitoring the patient's temperature, the room temperature can be adjusted to his needs. A temperature that is too warm may cause him to lose fluids through perspiration and in addition, promote bacterial growth. If the temperature is too cool, a blanket may be spread over the cradle or small light bulbs may be placed in the tent. With these lights, the patient may want to wear sunglasses or an eye shade. The preferred humidity range of the room is between 40 and 50 per cent. A room that is more dry will cause burn crusts to crack and cause pain, whereas a room too moist will encourage softening and premature separation of crusts. Portable electric humidifiers or dehumidifiers are effective in controlling humidity.

A light sprinkling of sterile cornstarch on the lower sheet helps prevent a burn area from sticking to the sheet. When linens are changed, care must be taken not to pull adherent parts; by wetting such an area with sterile saline, the sheet may be freed gently. Turning is encouraged to prevent pneumonia and contractures and to promote circulation. The patient may prefer to do this without assistance; if help is required, the sterile gloved hands of the nurse should handle nonburn areas, preferably.

The advantages of the exposure method are: (1) there are no painful dressing changes; (2) less equipment is used; (3) infection can be detected early; and

FIG. 29-2. (A) Technique of application of an occlusive dressing. After initial cleansing and removal of all debris and detached epithelium, the surface should be covered with fine-mesh gauze. In this instance, lightly impregnated petrolatum roller gauze was used. Individual strips were applied in a circular fashion. When a continuous circular bandage is used, it does not conform evenly to the part and may become constrictive if excessive edema occurs. It is important that this first layer be applied smoothly and without wrinkles. (B) Large abdominal pads have been placed beneath the leg. The petrolatum-impregnated gauze has been fixed in place with a single layer of dry 4- by 8-inch gauze pads, and a large layer of fluffed gauze is being placed over the extremity. (C) A final layer of large abdominal pads is placed over the bulky layer of fluffed gauze. Although the foot was not involved, the dressing extends down over the foot. When the terminal portion of the extremity is not incorporated in the bandage, there is a tendency for excessive edema formation. (D) The occlusive dressing has been completed by an outer layer of conforming bandage. This bandage has been applied in such a way that there is even, resilient compression over all areas. A bulky dressing of this type immobilizes the extremity, and a splint is unnecessary. Adhesive tape has been used to anchor the dressing in place. By labeling the dressing, information is always readily available as to the time of burn, time of application of the dressing, and the type of immediate covering of the wound. (Artz, C. P., and Moncrief, V. A.: The Treatment of Burns. Philadelphia, Saunders, 1969, p. 153)

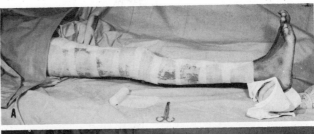
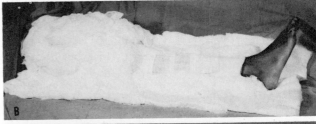
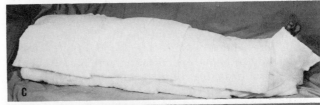
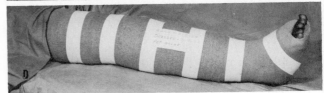

(4) large numbers of patients can be treated, making this particularly suitable for disaster situations.

Disadvantages of this method are: (1) it is not suitable for burns of the hands and feet because proper alignment and elevation are difficult to maintain; (2) it is unsuitable when the patient must be transported any distance, as from a battlefront to a base hospital; and (3) it is less effective when other injuries exist that require the patient to be turned frequently. Bandaging would be preferable in these instances.

Occlusive (Pressure) Dressings

These dressings are used primarily for burns of the feet and hands. Petrolatum gauze is applied lightly to the cleansed burn area. Precautions are taken to prevent two body surfaces from touching, such as fingers or toes, ear and scalp, under the breasts, or at flexion or genital folds. Functional body alignment positions are maintained; thus, the fingers and thumb curve over fluffed gauze or a bandage roll, the foot is positioned to avoid pronation and drop foot, and support is placed under the knees. On top of the petrolatum gauze is placed sterile absorptive fluffed or washed gauze in such a way that lumping is mini-

mized. Some physicians fix the loose gauze in place with elastic bandage or stockinette; others apply abdominal pads before applying the conforming bandage. Evenly distributed pressure is desired with no constriction to hinder circulation. Circulation may be checked every 3 or 4 hours by noting pulse, color, warmth and signs of paresthesia (Fig. 29-2).

Dressings are changed every 4 to 8 days (sooner in some clinics). This may be done in the patient's unit or in the operating room with the patient anesthetized. If exudate stain is noted, indicating moisture, the wet dressings are replaced to encourage drying and to prevent the growth of microorganisms. Signs of infection are increased pulse, elevated temperature and, possibly, odor.

Burns of the extremities are elevated to prevent edema; this may be accomplished by using pillows or, in the case of a hand, by improvising a bucket-handle suspension device.

Treatment With 0.5 Per Cent Silver Nitrate Solution

At the Hartford Burn Unit, Washington University School of Medicine in St. Louis, Dr. Moyer and his staff have proposed a method of treating severe burns by the use of dressings saturated with 0.5 per cent silver nitrate. (Concentrations above 1 per cent produce tissue necrosis, whereas those below 0.5 per cent are ineffective antiseptically.) They believe that the bacteriostatic action of the silver nitrate solution on burn wounds is so effective that cross infection does not occur; therefore, isolation technique is not necessary. Caps, masks and gowns are not worn, and relatives are permitted to visit freely and even feed the patient. However, cleanliness and hand washing are stressed. Clean (not sterile) strips of gauze are cut from large rolls and used as dressings. These practices are a departure from the usual practice, but they have been carried out in order to develop an effective bacteriostatic agent that may be used in case of war or in disasters where large numbers of burns must be treated, and they have proved to be successful.

The Treatment of the Primary Shock. A burn of more than 20 per cent of the body surface produces a period of primary shock due to the pain of the burn and the physiologic changes associated with it (loss of fluid leading to hemoconcentration and loss of heat by vaporization from the burned surface). During the period of shock, large amounts of fluids (as much as 10 to 20 liters, preferably of Ringer's solution with sodium lactate) are given through an indwelling plastic cannula in the vein. The amount and speed of injection is gauged by the urinary output from an indwelling catheter and the rate of flow should be fast enough to maintain a urinary flow of at least 30 to 50 ml. per hour. This means that the nurse must collect, measure and record the flow from the indwelling catheter every hour. Additional gauges of the fluid requirements include hematocrit and hemoglobin determinations. Blood samples for these examinations and for the determination of electrolytes are withdrawn at frequent intervals. If the hematocrit and hemoglobin determinations decrease or if the urinary output is more than 50 ml. of urine per hour, the speed of flow of the intravenous solution may be decreased.

Often as much as 2 million units of aqueous penicillin are added to the first liter of Ringer's solution. Immunization against tetanus is carried out, using tetanus toxoid if the patient has been immunized before, or human antitetanus serum if he has not previously received toxoid.

If nausea or vomiting occurs, a nasogastric tube is introduced into the stomach and attached to a suction apparatus. After the period of shock is over and the patient can take fluids by mouth, a solution of 4 gm. of sodium chloride and 1.5 gm. of sodium bicarbonate in 1 liter of iced water (Moyer's cocktail) is provided as a drink for 24 to 36 hours. No water, tea or coffee is given during this time. At the end of this period,

water is substituted for the saline solution and a general diet is given.

Local Treatment of Extensive Burns. While the primary shock is being treated, the local treatment of the burn is also started. The patient is placed on a bed sheet, and after cutting away the remnants of clothing, all loose epidermis is removed from the burned surface. This means cutting away all blisters and wiping off shreds of skin that overlie deeper burns.

Every 2 days the patient is placed in a sterile bath of warmed Locke's solution* and all greases and ointments are carefully removed from the burn area; this may require up to an hour. The patient enjoys the comfortable and relaxing bath and is able to exercise joints without experiencing pain. The burns are then covered with gauze dressings thoroughly soaked with 0.5 per cent silver nitrate solution. These dressings are kept wet with the silver nitrate solution, using bulb syringes. The best dressings are composed of 6 to 8 layers of 4-ply gauze applied dripping wet and held in place with bandages of bias-cut wide stockinette. The gauze of the dressing should not contain cotton between the layers because this interferes with the efficient action of the silver nitrate solution. Catheters may be incorporated into the thick dressings to permit saturation every 2 to 4 hours. The dressings are changed daily. The patient is covered with 1 or 2 dry sheets and a dry cotton blanket. These dry layers prevent or reduce the heat loss produced by vaporization from the wet dressings and from the burned surface. When the coverings become moist, they are changed. The patient is turned frequently to provide pressure and wetness to all areas. For the severely burned patient, the Stryker frame or circular bed may be used.

Moyer has shown from his studies that the high mortality of extensive burns does not result from toxins produced by the burn, as was believed for a long time, but rather from inanition and overwhelming infection of the burn surface and the loss of heat from the burn surface by vaporization. He found that covering the burn with continuous wet dressings of 0.5 per cent silver nitrate solution effectively controls the infection. The dry sheet and blanket coverings

---

* Modified Locke's solution for the sterile bath for the burned patient is a combination of various salts. It is best prepared from 2 stock solutions that are mixed at the time the bath is prepared.

Solution A—gm./L.		*Solution B—gm./L.*	
NaCl	175.5	$NaHCO_3$	73.3
KCl	9.0	$NaH_2PO_4 \cdot H_2O$	3.8
$CaCl_2 \cdot 2\ H_2O$	11.1		
$MgCl_2 \cdot 6\ H_2O$	9.13		

Add 1 volume of Solution A, followed by 1 volume of B, to 23 volumes of water.

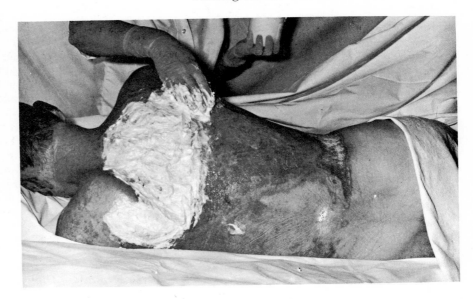

Fig. 29-3. Photograph of back of patient with deep second-degree burn being treated with Sulfamylon. The Sulfamylon cream is put on in a thick layer with the gloved hand. (Artz, C. P., and Mancrief, V. A.: The Treatment of Burns. Philadelphia, Saunders, p. 163)

prevent heat loss that would occur from vaporization.

The use of 0.5 per cent silver nitrate solution dressings is not without danger, because electrolytes, especially sodium and potassium, are withdrawn from the body fluids and pass into the dressings impregnated with silver nitrate solution. The withdrawal of sodium may occur very rapidly, especially in cases of extensive burns and in children, producing an acute electrolyte imbalance. For this reason, in the early phases of the burn treatment, blood must be drawn at frequent intervals—every 2 to 4 hours—for determinations of sodium, chloride, potassium, and calcium. These electrolytes must be replaced either by the ingestion of the saline and sodium bicarbonate iced drink mentioned previously or by the intravenous administration of the Ringer's solution with sodium lactate. After the patient can take a normal diet, salt is added to the diet. The depression of calcium is treated by the addition of calcium lactate or gluconate to the diet, and potassium depression, by the administration of potassium gluconate elixir. Deficits in these constituents of the blood electrolytes naturally are more marked in more extensive burns comprising 50 to 80 per cent of the body surface.

The silver nitrate solution has the disadvantage of turning black in the sunlight. This means that everything wet with the solution becomes indelibly stained black, including clothes, hands, floors and other objects. The nurse attending a patient being treated with silver nitrate solution must wear rubber gloves, not to prevent the spread of infection, but to protect her hands from the silver nitrate stains.

In order to facilitate the removal of the burned tissue and the eschar, the patients are immersed in warmed sterile baths of Locke's solution for 2 to 6 hours 1 to 3 times a week. Often, it is possible to remove the eschar without causing pain or bleeding after such an immersion. After removal of the eschar and before granulation tissue develops, thin split-thickness skin grafts are applied to the open burn wounds. The silver nitrate solution dressings are continued even after the skin grafts are applied to the burn, and are also applied to the area from which the grafts had been taken. These applications do not appear to hinder the growth of the grafts or the healing of the donor areas. During this treatment, no oily or ointment dressings are used, because they prevent the silver nitrate solution from reaching the wound surface and so permit the development of infection.

Other important measures employed during the treatment of burns include the administration of iron and penicillin for at least 2 months after the burn wound has healed. This prevents infection in the tender, newly formed skin, which may occur with slight trauma. As described, the silver nitrate treatment has markedly reduced the mortality from extensive burns, but it requires meticulous attention to details of therapy. In this effort the nurse plays a most important role.

Topical Chemotherapy

Mafenide Hydrochloride (Sulfamylon Hydrochloride) and Mafenide Acetate (Sulfamylon Acetate). Physicians have been searching for a chemotherapeutic agent that will penetrate the eschar to kill infecting organisms, inasmuch as thrombosis and damage of the vascular channels prevent systemic antibodies from reaching the burn wound, the area of need and primary source of sepsis. Mafenide hydrochloride and mafenide acetate are used in some clinics. In ointment form, these agents diffuse rapidly through the burned skin and are relatively nontoxic. However, they are strong carbonic anhydrase inhibitors and may adversely affect the blood pH level. With mafenide hydrochloride, the patient has a tendency to absorb the chloride ions, which can initiate severe metabolic acidosis; mafenide acetate lessens this danger. The cream is applied in a thick layer and a fine mesh gauze is applied in strips directly to the burn and changed daily or washed off in a whirlpool bath. A disadvantage to this form of treatment is the burning pain experienced by the patient for a few minutes following its application.

Gentamycin Sulfate Ointment (Garamycin). This ointment is impregnated in fine mesh gauze and applied directly to the burn wound. Dressings are changed daily, after the patient has soaked in a tub. Garamycin appears to inhibit all organisms except *Pseudomonas aeruginosa.*

MEDICAL AND NURSING MANAGEMENT OF THE BURN PATIENT

Room Prepared to Receive the Burn Patient

In preparing the bed, the mattress is completely covered with a plastic sheet; this is covered with a sterile bottom sheet. Three sterile draw sheets (top, middle and bottom) are placed to permit changing by the nurse with minimal discomfort to the patient. Caps, masks and sterile gowns and gloves are available for those attending the patient. Equipment most likely to be required should be in the room, including: intravenous therapy equipment, with polyethylene catheters and fluids; blood withdrawal syringes, needles, and tubes; catheterization tray and drainage equipment; tracheostomy set; suction and oxygen therapy equipment; packaged sterile sheets; overbed cradle; side rails. The particular procedure to be followed in wound care determines additional needs.

In some clinics, patients with severe burns of the trunk are placed in circular beds and rotated from prone to supine position every 3 hours. The Stryker frame also may be used if it meets the individual patient's needs.

Immediate Patient Care

Upon admission to his bed in the hospital, the patient has his clothes carefully removed and he is placed on or between sterile sheets. Concern for this patient, who is usually frightened and may be in emotional shock, needs to be demonstrated by those in attendance. Encouragement is offered and explanations are given when necessary; should the patient express the desire to see a spiritual advisor, one should

be notified. Attending personnel wear masks, caps and gowns; sterile gloves are worn when handling the burn area. The physician evaluates the general condition and burns of the patient, determines the priorities and directs the individualized plan of treatment, which is divided into systemic management and local care of the burned area.[*] A well-organized professional team does many things simultaneously during the first hour of intensive care. These activities are directed toward life-saving and comfort measures. One physician may perform a tracheostomy while another initiates fluid therapy and a third cares for the burned area. The nurse assists the physicians, attends to the patient's needs and cares for his family. The patient's vital signs are taken at frequent intervals; temperatures over 38.3° C. (101° F.) or below 36.1° C. (97° F.) are reported.

Respiratory Difficulties

Of prime concern is an assessment of the patient's respiratory status. Whether the patient has inhaled smoke, steam, gases or fire should be determined early; such may be suspected if the victim appears hoarse, has a dry cough, labored respiration, singed nasal hair, red sore throat, blood tinged or blackened sputum and moist rales. Since such a condition may lead to pulmonary edema and respiratory difficulties, a tracheostomy may be performed. The nursing care of a tracheotomized patient is described on p. 222; however, remember that the individual with a possible respiratory burn has a more sensitive tract than other patients.[†] Suction should not be on when the tracheal catheter is moved; lower pressure is used to avoid causing tissue damage and edema. Meticulous aseptic technique is required in this infection-prone patient. Deep breathing is also encouraged to inflate collapsed alveoli.

Pathology at various levels of the respiratory tree may result from inhaling noxious fumes given off when painted wood burns; these include sulfuric acid, carbon monoxide and hydrocyanic acid. It may be necessary to follow intensive bronchopulmonary cleaning through the tracheostomy tube with IPPB (intermittent positive pressure breathing) and continuous nebulization of warm water-saturated air. Cyanosis is a sign that may be overlooked, but must be watched for. Oxygen therapy may prevent irreparable brain damage.

---

[*] A photograph may be taken of the burn areas at this time and periodically throughout the treatment. In this way, progress of healing may be determined quickly. Such evidence is invaluable in insurance claims and courts of law.

[†] Because of this, some clinics prefer high humidity and oxygen therapy for burn patients with respiratory damage rather than tracheostomy.

Fluid Derangement (Plasma-to-interstitial fluid shift)

Next to handling respiratory difficulties, the most urgent need is to replace lost fluid and to prevent irreversible shock. In extensive burns, a systemic derangement of fluid balance occurs. This begins with the loss of fluid into the tissues surrounding the burn area to produce vesicles, and loss of fluid from the surface of the burn. This produces a decrease in the circulating fluid of the entire body. Extravasation of fluid into the tissue begins within an hour and reaches its peak in 4 to 6 hours; fluid loss continues into the tissues up to 48 hours postburn. (There is no known way to stop the outpouring of fluids, but replacement of fluids is possible.) The result is a relative increase in the ratio between blood cells to the blood fluid—in other words, an increase in the *hematocrit,* causing a less efficient circulation and a fall in the blood pressure. Shock is likely to occur and the patient is seriously ill.

The physician calculates the projected fluid requirements for the first 24 hours through his evaluation of the patient's burn injury, p. 660). Three types of fluid may be considered: (1) colloids: whole blood, plasma, and plasma expanders; (2) electrolytes: physiologic sodium chloride, Ringer's solution, Hartmann's solution; (3) nonelectrolyte fluids: distilled water with 5 per cent glucose.

Formulas have been evolved for estimating fluid loss based on the estimated per cent of body surface area burned and the weight of the patient.* These are modified by physicians and individualized to meet the requirements of each patient. During the first 24 hours, one half of the planned fluids are given in the first 8 hours, followed by a quarter in each of the remaining 8-hour periods. One half of the fluids given in the first 24 hours are given during the 2nd day. Usually the colloids and electrolytes are reduced, whereas metabolic needs are met by increasing the nonelectrolyte fluids.

In the critically burned patient, some physicians withhold all oral fluids for 2 or 3 days, and insert a Levine tube to reduce the possibility of paralytic ileus and gastric retention.

Venipuncture equipment needs to be available to draw blood for typing, cross-matching, hemoglobin and hematocrit. Fluids prescribed for intravenous therapy are ordered; the nurse assists the physician and patient during the procedures. Conscientious recording of all fluid administered as well as all fluid output aids the physician in determining the needs of the patient.

* See "Postburn Electrolyte Therapy," p. 672.

TABLE 29-3. Water and electrolyte changes in the first 48 hours of major burns
Fluid accumulation phase (shock phase)
Plasma ——→ Interstitial fluid (edema at burn site)

Observation	Explanation
1. Generalized dehydration	Plasma leaks through damaged capillaries
2. Reduction of blood volume	Brought about by plasma loss, fall of blood pressure
3. Decreased urinary output	Secondary to: Fluid loss Decreased renal blood flow Increased secretion of ADH (antidiuretic hormone) Sodium and water retention caused by increased adreno-cortical activity Hemolysis of red blood cells, causing hemoglobinuria
4. Potassium excess	Massive cellular trauma causes release of K^+ into extracellular fluid (ordinarily, most K^+ is intracellular)
5. Sodium deficit	Large amount of Na^+ is lost in trapped edema fluid and exudate (ordinarily most Na^+ is extracellular)
6. Metabolic acidosis (base bicarbonate deficit)	Loss of bicarbonate ions accompanies sodium loss
7. Hemoconcentration (elevated hematocrit)	Liquid blood component lost

Adapted from Metheny, N. M., and Snively, W. D.: Nurses' Handbook of Fluid Balance. p. 161. Philadelphia, J. B. Lippincott, 1967.

Pain

Intravenous morphine, 8 to 10 mg. in adults, is usually prescribed. Subcutaneous or intramuscular routes are less effective because of impaired circulation. For individuals with burns of the head and neck, barbiturates are preferred to morphine, which can depress respiration.

Pain is more severe in 2nd degree burns than in 3rd degree burns, because the nerve endings are destroyed in the latter. Exposed nerve endings are sensitive to cool moving air; therefore, a sterile covering can help reduce pain. Fright, hysteria and severe pain can later cause neurogenic pain. Intravenous morphine or other narcotics are prescribed as needed, but large doses are avoided because of the danger of respiratory depression and the possibility of masking other symptoms.

Shock (Burn)

Restlessness and disorientation may suggest the onset of shock. Vital signs are taken hourly. Blood pressure may vary; this determination may be a problem in the patient who has extensive burns of the extremities. To compensate for decreased blood volume, the heart beats faster (tachycardia). Because of generalized cellular dehydration, the patient may exhibit extreme thirst. Other signs may be oliguria and drowsiness. When the physician is made aware of these symptoms, he can adjust fluid therapy to correct the problem. Fluids by mouth are given only as prescribed; usually this is the salt-soda bicarbonate drink described on p. 659 or a similar oral electrolyte preparation. The nurse must know the maximal amount of fluid the patient is allowed to have, which is usually 200 cc. per hour. Sipping of fluids helps prevent gastric distention that may cause vomiting—an undesirable development, since more fluid is lost.

Renal Function

Initial catheterization is done (using a indwelling catheter) and a specimen is sent to the laboratory. The retention bag is filled with 5 ml. sterile saline and the indwelling catheter is allowed to drain into a calibrated receptacle. Drainage is measured and recorded every hour; the presence of hematuria must be reported to the physician. Should the urine output fall below 30 ml./hour (suggesting marked fluid loss) or exceed 100 ml./hour (which may cause pulmonary edema), the physician should be informed, since he may have to adjust fluid intake.

Other Nursing Care and Observation

Attendance by the nurse is needed constantly. It is important to recognize that the patient may be sensitive about his appearance and may be deeply concerned about disfigurement. Attendants need to remember that any indication of revulsion or shock on their part is noticed by the patient.

Any and all changes must be reported promptly—such as restlessness, level of consciousness, change in vital signs. Signs of water intoxication also must be watched for: tremor, twitching, nausea, diarrhea, salivation, disorientation. The complete recording of fluids, patient appearance and reaction, signs and symptoms, therapy and treatment will give a progressive accounting of the patient's condition which will be invaluable to the physician.

Infection Prevention

The primary source of bacterial infection appears to be the environment. (See p. 659.) Antibiotics are usually given prophylactically. Penicillin, streptomycin and erythromycin are preferred. Sensitivity to antibiotics should be determined prior to administration.

Ordinarily, mask, cap and gown are worn while caring for the patient with extensive burns to prevent infection. Aseptic technique is replaced by clean technique when silver nitrate dressings are used (see p. 663). Aseptic technique is practiced in caring directly for burn wounds. The patient may be required to wear a mask to protect his wounds from organisms present in his own respiratory tract.

Wound cleaning and débridement are performed by the physician and he determines the extensiveness of such a procedure. Warm soap solution or a detergent such as pHisoHex may be used for cleansing; at which time, débridement may also be done.

Because burns are considered as contaminated wounds, adequate tetanus prophylaxis is given. If the patient has been immunized or has had no booster dose in the preceding 4 years, he will receive 3,000 units of antitoxin and a booster dose of toxoid (0.5 ml.). If he has never had immunizing toxoid, he should receive hyperimmune human antitetanus serum. The amount he receives should depend on the extent of the burn and the environment of the injury. If he has rolled on the earth or has been lying on the earth, the danger of tetanus is increased, hence larger doses of antiserum are used.

Postburn Patient from 2 to 5 Days

Pathophysiology

Following the shock period, the patient moves into the fluid remobilization phase (48 to 72 hours). At this time, the response of the patient is shifting from a position of defense and emergency response to a position of repair of damages and mobilization for recovery. During this period, fluid is reabsorbed from the area of edema and moves into the bloodstream, increasing the blood volume. An extra strain is placed on the heart; urinary output is greatly increased and fluid back-up into the lungs may cause pulmonary edema. The physician should be made aware of these changes, because it is imperative that fluid intake be restricted, particularly intravenously.

The nurse's observation and assessment of these changes are important. She must be especially alert for respiratory distress, moist rales, coughing of frothy liquid and cyanosis, since they may herald a fatal pulmonary edema.

Fluid, Electrolyte and Blood Needs

The loss of fluids through burned skin area may reach 3 to 5 liters. The determination of water replacement can be measured by maintenance of a normal serum sodium; a reading higher than 132 to 136 mEq./L. (normal) would suggest the need for water. More frequently, serum hyponatremia (sodium below

132 mEq./L.) occurs between the third and the tenth day with rapid fluid mobilization from the burned area.

Other indications helpful in determining water replacement are urinary output and weight loss, which should not exceed 1 Kg. per day. If the patient is not able to stand on a scale at the bedside, a bed scale might be used.

On the 2nd or 3rd postburn day, blood transfusions are begun to combat anemia. Observing the patient for possible transfusion reaction is a nursing responsibility (p. 94).

Nutrition Management and Gastrointestinal Disturbances

Gastric dilatation and paralytic ileus occur frequently, and are indicated by vomiting and distention; therefore a Levine tube is passed early in the treatment. The nursing responsibility in this instance is to administer oral fluids *slowly*. The patient's tolerance is noted, and if vomiting, distention or diarrhea do not occur, fluids may be slowly increased. In the immediate emergency treatment, electrolyte solutions are given, but as the body needs change, the nature of fluids is changed. Fruit juices that contain potassium are given after the serum potassium levels decrease. High-protein drinks are offered, and provide an excellent means of supplementing the diet. A diet containing more solid food is usually begun toward the end of the first week, when the patient's tolerance for food improves. The catabolic response of the body is great, with daily caloric expenditures of 5,000 to 6,000 calories a day. This means that, to meet nutritional demands, the patient must build up his nutritional intake to a similar number of calories; he needs approximately 3 gm. of protein per Kg. of body weight, 20 per cent of the needed calories in the form of fats and the remainder in carbohydrates.

Provimalt is a good protein supplement, causing fewer side effects or vomiting, diarrhea and abdominal cramps. However, ordinary foods such as meat, potatoes, eggs, etc. are best. Oral fat emulsion (e.g., Lipomul) is available; vitamins (ascorbic acid, thiamine, riboflavin and nicotinamide) supplements are also necessary. Physician preference and patient tolerance determine the choices. As the patient progresses, every effort must be made to stimulate his appetite and provide for his needs. Imagination and ingenuity will be required to stimulate his sluggish appetite.

The incidence of gastrointestinal tract ulcer (Curling's ulcer) is in proportion to the extent of the burn area. This condition may first be manifested by hemorrhage, detected in blood tinged contents from nasogastric suction or in the stool. A sudden drop in hemoglobin concentration may be diagnostic even before the hemorrhage is evident. Gastric surgery may be indicated. This is a rare complication.

TABLE 29-4. Water and electrolyte changes beginning 48 hours after major burns
Fluid remobilization phase (state of diuresis)
Interstitial fluid ⟶ plasma

Observation	Explanation
1. Hemodilution (decreased hematocrit)	Blood cell concentration is diluted as fluid enters the vascular compartment; loss of red blood cells destroyed at burn site
2. Increased urinary output	Fluid shift into intravascular compartment increases renal blood flow and causes increased urine formation
3. Sodium deficit	With diuresis, sodium is lost with water
4. Potassium deficit (occurs occasionally in this phase)	Beginning on the 4th or 5th postburn day, K^+ shifts from extracellular fluid into cells
5. Metabolic acidosis	

Adapted from Metheny, N. M., and Snively, W. D.: Nurses' Handbook of Fluid Balance. p. 162. Philadelphia, J. B. Lippincott, 1967.

Urinary Output

After diuresis is established, the amount of urine is measured and recorded every 8 hours and daily specimens are sent to the laboratory.

Proper Positioning and Mobilization

The prevention of pneumonia, the control of edema, and the prevention of pressure sores and contractures are guiding principles. Deep breathing, turning and proper repositioning are essential nursing practices modified to meet individual needs. Early ambulation may be encouraged according to the capability of the patient. Both passive and active range-of-motion exercises are initiated in this period and continued after grafting.

Bathing

Wound care in many clinics includes immersion of the patient in an electrolyte, soapy, or germicidal bath. This may be a tub bath, regular or walk-in type, or a whirlpool bath. The agitation in the latter aids in cleansing and gently massaging of the tissues. Temperature of the bath is maintained at 37.8° C. (100° F.).

Psychosocial Response

As the burn victim progresses through the second phase, he is aware of daily improvement and begins

THE PATIENT WITH BURNS
Objectives and Principles of Medical and Nursing Management

I. To prevent and treat burn shock

  A. Provide for blood, fluid, electrolyte and colloid replacement immediately

    1. Weigh the patient on admission (if possible) and daily thereafter

    2. Insert an indwelling catheter

      a. Measure hourly urinary output

      b. Describe the appearance and the color of the urine

    3. Encourage the patient to drink sodium chloride and sodium bicarbonate mixture if ordered

    4. Prepare the patient for cannulization of vein for continuous I.V. therapy

    5. Have accessible and labeled the daily ordered I.V. fluids

    6. Maintain a detailed intake record of oral and I.V. fluids

    7. Know and be alert for the symptoms of dehydration and overdehydration

    8. Increase and decrease the rate of intravenous fluid flow according to the symptoms of fluid shift and the clinical response of the patient

    9. Notify the physician immediately if symptoms of overhydration or dehydration occur

    10. Give I.V. analgesics with caution if patient is in shock

  B. Maintain careful nursing observation during transfusion therapy

II. To evaluate the patient's response to the injury

  A. Watch the patient's systemic reaction and his response to therapy

    1. Keep sphygmomanometer cuff on accessible artery

    2. Record vital signs hourly

    3. Ensure that blood samples are obtained by the laboratory personnel at specified times

      a. Watch for rising hematocrit or hemoglobin

      b. Report changes in serum protein, blood urea nitrogen and serum electrolyte levels

    4. Obtain 24-hour urine specimens for 17-ketosteroid and 17-hydroxysteroid tests if requested

  B. Keep the patient physically comfortable and emotionally supported

    1. Elevate the burned extremities

    2. Control the patient's pain

    3. Maintain the patient in physiologic positions

    4. Allay the patient's fear and anxiety

III. To prevent complications

  A. Guard against infection

    1. Keep burned areas covered with sterile dressings if indicated

      a. Mask, gown and glove personnel during dressing changes

      b. Employ rigid aseptic technique during dressing changes

    2. Keep the environment free of pathogens

      a. Use isolation precautions

      b. See that room is damp-dusted periodically

      c. Restrict visitors

    3. Obtain wound cultures as ordered

    4. Maintain optimal personal hygiene for the patient

      a. Give frequent oral hygiene

      b. Wash unburned areas with hexachlorophene soap or detergent and water

      c. Give meticulous attention to the patient's eyes, ears, nares and nails

      d. Shave pubic and axillary areas if near burned area

      e. Cleanse area around meatus and catheter at intervals

    5. Keep the patient's nutritional status at optimal level

    6. Give antibiotics as ordered

  B. Observe for symptoms of sinus tachycardia

    1. Watch the patient's pulse rate and volume carefully

    2. Give digitalis as ordered

  C. Watch for symptoms of respiratory embarrassment

    1. Evaluate the respiratory rate, chest movements and respiratory symptoms

    2. Determine whether or not the nasal hair is singed, the pharynx is red, the voice is hoarse, the patient is coughing, or respiratory stridor is present

    3. Prepare for tracheostomy if needed

    4. Keep the room air humidified if respiratory problems become apparent

    5. Encourage the patient to cough frequently

    6. Have oxygen equipment accessible

  D. Prevent contractures and deformities; maintain good body alignment

  E. Observe for untoward elevations of body temperature

IV. To promote wound healing

  A. Maintain the patient in the best condition possible for future surgical procedures

    1. Assist with local wound care

      a. Provide sterile equipment for cleansing and débridement of wound

THE PATIENT WITH BURNS (*Continued*)

IV. To promote wound healing (*Continued*)
    b. Provide dressing for occlusive therapy or sterile sheets, etc., for exposure method of treatment
  2. Prepare the patient for grafting procedures when indicated
  3. Maintain the nutrition of the patient
    a. Encourage the intake of a high protein diet
    b. Give supplementary protein feedings
    c. Record the amount of diet eaten

V. To promote the rehabilitation of the patient
  A. Maintain the patient in a correct position
    1. Use a foot board
    2. Splint affected hands and utilize hand rolls
    3. Provide posterior splints for affected legs
    4. Keep burned extremities elevated and immobilized in a position of function
    5. Utilize bed cradles

B. Employ passive and full range-of-motion exercises at the earliest possible time as indicated by the surgeon
  1. Use tilt table to provide for early weight-bearing activity
  2. Apply elastic bandages to the legs of the ambulatory patient with burns of the lower extremities

C. Assist the patient to adjust to his physical limitations
  1. Provide self-help devices for eating and other activities
  2. Encourage the patient to participate in his own care
  3. Assist the patient to develop realistic future goals
  4. Refer the patient to the proper agencies for follow-up care

---

to exhibit basic concerns: Will I be disfigured? How long will I have to be in the hospital? What about my job and family? Will I ever be independent again? How can I pay for my care? Was this the result of my carelessness? As he expresses his concerns, the nurse should take time to listen and to encourage him.

The nurse should prepare the patient's family for their first visit not only by advising them about aseptic techniques, but also in preparing them for the appearance of the patient. Edema can cause distortions, bandaging can appear voluminous, and certain treatments, such as silver nitrate, are most unattractive. Visitors must conceal their own shocked expressions from the patient.

Recovery, Convalescence and Rehabilitation

Nutritional Aspects

Weight loss is the most obvious change in the patient recovering from a severe burn. Reserve fat deposits were tapped during the shock phase, fluids were lost and caloric intake was limited. Because of his low resistance to infection and disease, the nurse is challenged to improve the patient's nutritional state even though he has a poor appetite and is still weak. Semisolid and then solid foods are offered early in the 2nd week and increased rapidly as he tolerates and accepts more. Encouraging him, catering to his preferences, and offering protein and vitamin supplement snacks are part of the nurse's subtle attempts to increase gradually his intake from 3,000 to as many as 6,000 calories a day.

TABLE 29-5. Water and electrolyte changes after 5 days Convalescent phase

Observation	Explanation
1. Calcium deficit	Since calcium may be immobilized at the burn site in the slough and early granulation phase of burns, symptoms of calcium deficit may occur rarely.
2. Potassium deficit	Extracellular K^+ moves into the cells, leaving a deficit of K^+ in the extracellular fluid.
3. Negative nitrogen balance (present for several weeks following burns)	Secondary to: Stress reaction Immobilization Inadequate protein intake Protein losses in exudate Direct destruction of protein at burn site
4. Sodium deficit	

Adapted from Metheny, N. M., and Snively, W. D.: Nurses' Handbook of Fluid Balance. p. 162. Philadelphia, J. B. Lippincott, 1967.

Wound Care and Skin Grafting

As the crusts of 2nd degree burns give way to tender, new pink skin, the patient participates in the physical therapy program to recondition his muscles and stimulate circulation.

After a week or two, the burned tissue tends to separate from the remaining normal tissue. The burned area forms an *eschar*; this can be separated from the underlying viable tissue (débridement), leaving a granulating, painful, bleeding wound. Many of these wounds, which appear to be very deep, will be found to have some epithelium still remaining in them, and healing can take place from these islands of skin. In other areas where the skin is completely destroyed, nature must have some help to heal the tremendous wounds left by the burn. It is in these patients that skin grafts are most effective.

In the preparation of the burned area for skin grafts, warm saline baths are frequently used. The patient may be immersed in such a bath for an hour at a time, while the burned areas are washed gently to remove the debris that is usually attached to them. As soon as the burn wound becomes a red, granulating area without slough, skin grafts may be used. During the care of the patient in the bath, the nurse should wear a cap, a mask and sterile gloves in order not to infect the burned area.

The split-thickness type of skin graft is most often used to cover the area left after removal of the eschar. (See p. 649 for skin grafting management.) Nursing care is most important to adjust the part to its most comfortable position and to prevent the skin graft from being dislodged. Skin loss in areas such as the neck, the elbow, etc. produce scars that contract and cause marked deformities. It is in these areas especially that early skin grafting is most efficacious.

Large areas of burn often require a considerable time in the hospital to permit healing. This is a trying time for the patient, and diversional therapy is most helpful. Occupational therapy and other types of therapy that take the patient's mind away from his troubles are very helpful.

POSTBURN ELECTROLYTE THERAPY* †

First 24 Hours Postburn

The Evans Formula:

1. Colloids (blood, plasma, dextran): 1 ml. times per cent burn times Kg. body weight
2. Electrolytes (saline): 1 ml. times per cent burn times Kg. body weight
3. 5 per cent glucose in water, 2,000 ml.

Second and 3rd-degree burns totaling over 50 per cent are calculated on the basis of 50 per cent. In any event, 10,000 ml. of total fluids is the maximal amount to be given in a 24-hour period. One half of the calculated fluid is given in the first 8 hours postburn; the remainder is spread evenly over the next 16 hours.

---

* Artz, C. P., and Reiss, E.: The Treatment of Burns. Philadelphia, W. B. Saunders, 1957.

† Evans, E. I., *et al.*: Fluid and electrolyte requirements in severe burns. Ann. Surg., *135*:804, 1952.

The Brooke Army Hospital Formula:

Differs from the Evans formula only in that the colloid fraction is reduced from 1 ml. to 0.5 ml. and the electrolyte fraction increased from 1 ml. to 1.5 ml. Instead of saline, the electrolyte preferred is lactated Ringer's solution because of its lower chloride content.

The Second 24 Hours Postburn

Fluid requirement for combating shock after the first 24 hours is roughly one half of the amounts of colloids and electrolytes calculated for the preceding period. For metabolic needs, again add 2,000 ml. of 5 per cent glucose in water.

After 48 Hours

At this time fluid resorption begins, hence intravenous fluids are restricted. Oral fluid intake is encouraged. Serum sodium and potassium determinations are helpful at this stage. A sodium level of 132 to 136 mEq./L. indicates adequate hydration; levels higher than this indicate need for additional electrolyte-free water. Hypokalemia may occur at this time. Unless adequate oral intake of food and liquids is possible, give 80 to 100 mEq./day of potassium.

BIBLIOGRAPHY

Books

Artz, C. P., and Moncrief, J. A.: Burns. Philadelphia, W. B. Saunders, 1969.

Metheny, N. M., and Snively, W. D.: Nurses' Handbook of Fluid Balance. pp. 157-175. Philadelphia, J. B. Lippincott, 1967.

Moyer, C. A., and Butcher, H. R., Jr.: Burns, Shock, and Plasma Volume Regulation. St. Louis, C. V. Mosby, 1967.

Order, S. E., and Moncrief, J. A.: The Burn Wound. Springfield, Ill., Charles C Thomas, 1965.

Articles

Artz, C.: The burn patient. Nurs. Forum 4(No. 3): 87-92, 1965.

Artz, C. P., Fitts, C. T., and Hargest, T. S.: Use of a new nonadherent dressing. Amer. J. Surg., *114*:973, 1967.

Boswick, J. A.: Current concepts in the clinical management of the burn patient. Surg. Clin. N. Amer., 47:49-60, 1967.

———: Long-term management of the burn patient. Mod. Treatment 4:1282-1290, Nov., 1967.

Boswick, J. A., and Stone, N. A.: Methods and materials in managing the severely burned patient. Surg. Clin. N. Amer., 48: 177-190, 1968.

Brown, W. A.: Thermal burns. Canad. Nurse, *61*:365-367, May, 1965.

Burgess, R. E.: Fluids and electrolytes. Amer. J. Nurs., 65:90-95, Oct., 1965.

Collentine, G. E., Jr.: How to calculate fluids for burned patients. Amer. J. Nurs., *62*:77-79, March, 1962.

Conway, H., and Hugo, N. E.: Local care of the burn wound. Surg. Clin. N. Amer., 47:1049-1057, 1967.

Fay, N. C., and Demes, L. C.: Care of severely burned patients. *In*: Bergersen, N. S., *et al.*: Current Concepts in Clinical Nursing. St. Louis, C. V. Mosby, 1967.

Henley, N. L.: Sulfamylon for burns, Amer. J. Nurs., *69*:2122-2123, Oct., 1969.

Larson, D., and Gaston, R.: Current trends in the care of burned patients. Amer. J. Nurs., *67*:319-327, Feb., 1967.

Lindberg, R. D., *et al.*: The successful control of burn wound sepsis. J. Trauma, *5*:601-616, 1965.

Luschen, M.: Technique and temperament made the difference. Amer. J. Nurs., *64*:103-104, Oct., 1964.

McCrady, M., and Mitchell, C.: Nursing care: a patient with burns. Canad. Nurse, *61*:371-374, May, 1965.

Maxwell, P., Linas, M., McDonnough, P., and Kinder, J.: Routines on the burn ward (silver nitrate treatment of burns). Amer. J. Nurs., *66*:522-524, Mar., 1966.

Monafo, W. W.: The treatment of burns with compresses wet with 0.5% silver nitrate solution. Surg. Clin. N. Amer., *47*: 1029-1037, 1967.

Monafo, W. W., and Moyer, C. A.: Effectiveness of dilute aqueous silver nitrate in the treatment of major burns. Arch. Surg., *91*:200-210, 1965.

Moncrief, J. A.: The status of topical antibacterial therapy in the treatment of burns. Surg., *63*:862-867, 1968.

Moyer, C. A., *et al.*: Treatment of large human burns with 0.5% silver nitrate solution. Arch. Surg., *90*:812-867, 1965.

Noonan, J., and Noonan, L.: Two burned patients in flotation therapy. Amer. J. Nurs., *68*:316-319, Feb., 1968.

Ousterhout, D. K., and Faller, I.: Occult gastrointestinal hemorrhage in burned patients. Arch. Surg., *96*:420-422, 1968.

Price, W. R., and Wood, M.: Operating room care of burned patients treated wtih silver nitrate. Amer. J. Nurs., *68*:1705-1707, Aug., 1968.

Quinlan, E.: Dietary treatment in burns. Canad. Nurse, *61*:375, May, 1965.

Sherman, R. T.: Burn fluid management. Nurs. Forum, *4*(No. 3): 93-98, 1965.

Simeone, F. A.: Shock: its nature and treatment. Amer. J. Nurs., *66*:1287-1294, June, 1966.

Strathie, N., and Swanson, C.: Problems in one patient's care (silver nitrate treatment of burns). Amer. J. Nurs., *66*:524-527, Mar., 1966.

Waters, W. R.: The patient with severe burns. Canad. Nurse, *61*:367-371, May, 1965.

Wood, M., Kenny, H. A., and Price, W. R.: Silver nitrate treatment of burns. Amer. J. Nurs., *66*:518-527, March, 1966.

NATIONAL AGENCIES

National Fire Protection Association
  60 Batterymarch Street
  Boston, Massachusetts

National Safety Council
  425 N. Michigan Avenue
  Chicago, Illinois 60611

CHAPTER **30**

Nursing the Patient with an Allergic Disorder

- *The Allergic Reaction*
- *Respiratory Allergies*
- *Allergic Dermatoses*
- *Gastrointestinal Allergy*
- *Desensitization, Antihistaminics, and Hormones in Allergy*
- *Serum Disease*
- *Anaphylactic Shock*

THE ALLERGIC REACTION

The term *allergy,* in its broadest sense, refers to any activity occurring in human or animal tissue as the result of an interaction between an antigen and an antibody. An *antigen* is any substance which, in the course of repeated contacts with the body, stimulates the body to produce another substance, a globulin, called an *antibody,* capable of combining with it in a very specific manner (p. 899). This antibody may circulate freely in the blood or may be "fixed" in the tissues. Antigens likewise differ, and there are corresponding differences between various antigen-antibody reactions with respect to their location, the manner in which they operate and how their operations are manifested. These reactions, the basis of so-called allergic phenomena, involve the preliminary sensitization of a particular tissue or organ, and this, in turn, implies previous contact with the antigenic substance, or *allergen.*

The human body is menaced by a host of potential invaders—for the most part, microbial organisms—which are constantly threatening its surface defenses. Having penetrated those defenses, these agents compete with the body for its nutrients and, if allowed to flourish unimpeded, disrupt its enzyme systems and destroy its vital tissues. Against these agents, the body

is equipped with an elaborate blockade system. The first line of defense consists of the epithelial cells that coat the skin and compose the lining of the respiratory, the gastrointestinal and the genitourinary tracts. The structure of these surfaces and the effects of their penetration have been discussed in connection with specific infections.

One of the most effective of the body's defense mechanisms is its capacity to equip itself rapidly with weapons individually designed to meet each new invader, namely, specific protein antibodies. Antibodies react with foreign protein materials in a variety of ways: (1) by coating their surface, if they are particulate substances; (2) by neutralizing them, if they are toxic, or (3) by precipitating them out of solution, if they are dissolved. In any event, the antibodies make the foreign materials safe for handling by the phagocytic cells of the blood and the tissues.

Antibody-antigen reactions are not invariably protective and beneficial to the body. In certain instances, their only obvious effect is to cause tissue damage or, at least, considerable discomfort to the individual. Under certain circumstances an antibody is produced that reacts not only in response to the presence of some noxious agent but also against materials that are ordinarily harmless, although similar in chemical composition to the original antigen. Such a reaction apparently serves no useful purpose and should be regarded as an unfortunate by-product of what is otherwise an invaluable defense mechanism.

Moreover, certain individuals have an abnormal tendency to become sensitized to miscellaneous foreign proteins, particularly after repeated exposure to certain areas of the body surface, such as the respiratory mucosa or the gastrointestinal mucosa. This situation does, in fact, apply in a considerable number of cases: specifically, in about 7 per cent of the population. These individuals apparently are sensitized with unusual ease, producing antibodies against any number of substances that are prevalent in the environment but excite no response in most people. The resulting antigen-antibody reactions are responsible for a number of clinical disorders. Included among these is a dermatitis, in which inflammatory lesions develop on the body surface in areas that have been in direct contact with a specific substance to which the patient is "sensitive." Other disorders include those types of hay fever and asthma caused by airborne allergens such as pollens, mold spores, animal danders and house dust. The role of allergy is equally clear-cut in cases of urticaria and gastrointestinal disturbances associated with the ingestion of particular foods. Allergies such as these are apparently based on a hereditary susceptibility to sensitization; often several members of the patient's family exhibit allergies. The term *allergy* is similarly applicable in another group of conditions, including serum disease, dermatitis venenata (for example, poison ivy) and certain drug reactions. Likewise in this category are the local skin lesions that appear following the inoculation of killed bacteria, or bacterial products, for diagnostic purposes, exemplified by the tuberculin reaction.

Many diseases are classed tentatively as allergic disorders, despite the fact that no antigens have been identified in relation to their causation. These include some cases of vasomotor rhinitis and certain cases of asthma, eczema and urticaria. Whereas these conditions may have originated from antigen-antibody reactions, the principal cause, in each instance, appears to be an excessive reactivity on the part of the particular tissue or organ involved. These disorders, and those in which an immunologic mechanism is demonstrable, often are grouped together under the term *atopic disease*.

Special problems complicate the nursing care of the allergic patient. For example, persons with symptomatic allergy are inclined to be apprehensive to a degree that is nearly unique. Their state of mind is likely to be concealed in a manner that belies their anxiety, conveying instead an impression of impatience, lack of consideration, aggressiveness, even frank hostility—or they may display merely the attributes of "high strung"

individuals. The nurse must understand her allergic patient, offering her services and lending an interested, friendly ear, but remembering that, so far as her own emotional reactions are concerned, empathy remains the keynote! In the course of her many contacts with her patient, she may garner enough data and impressions to characterize him accurately from the psychological standpoint, to discern with clarity the environment in which he habitually dwells, and therefore to discover what factors are most important from the standpoint of "triggering" attacks. The nurse also must be prepared to meet the dangerous emergency that allergy creates on occasion in the form of anaphylactic shock or fulminating asthma, when swift and effective countermeasures may spell the difference between life and death.

RESPIRATORY ALLERGIES

Hay Fever

Hay fever (allergic coryza; pollinosis) is a rhinitis induced by airborne pollens and, therefore, characterized by a seasonal occurrence. The spring type, the so-called *rose cold*, apparently stimulated by the pollens of certain trees (oak, elm, poplar and others), occurs from late March to early June; the summer type is induced by the pollens of certain grasses (such as timothy or red top); and the fall type, which develops from the middle of August to the first frost, is stimulated particularly by pollens of the ragweed family. Each year the attacks begin and end approximately the same dates. Usually the rhinitis starts in the mucous membrane of the nose, which may become so edematous and swollen that the nostrils are closed completely. The nasal mucous membrane itches, burns and secretes a thin irritating discharge. Violent paroxysms of sneezing are the rule. The eyes, usually also involved, become red, burn and lacrimate.

Sensitivity Tests. The patient's hypersensitivity to the pollens that induce his attacks often, but not always, may be confirmed by proper skin, conjunctival or intradermal tests. Though spectacular, these reactions are not necessarily specific. The dosage of the pollen injected is important, and the majority of patients are hypersensitive not to one but to several pollens, and under testing conditions, they may not react to the specific pollens that induce their attacks. Ragweed seems to be the most potent of all.

Treatment. The best treatment of hay fever, if the nasal passages and the paranasal sinuses otherwise are normal and, especially, if the attacks began in childhood, is a seasonal change of climate. When and to where, however, depends on the experience of the individual case. Nasal sprays containing ephedrine help some persons. Sinusitis or other nasal lesions that may be present should be treated thoroughly during the free seasons. Various eyewashes relieve the conjunctivitis.

Prophylactic injections of extracts of the pollens that seem to be involved in each case (usually, mixed vaccines of nonspecific proteins are used), given once each week, beginning each successive year several months before and continuing during the attacks, relieve the coryza symptoms in a fair percentage of cases but do not cure the condition. Antihistamine therapy during the active phase is of symptomatic benefit in the majority of patients.

Vasomotor Rhinitis

Vasomotor rhinitis, one of the commonest of allergic manifestations, is a form of noninfectious rhinitis induced by certain foods (such as milk, eggs, fish or shellfish) and by certain medicines (such as quinine), when these are ingested. In some patients it is caused by the toxins of germs growing within the body, particularly in the paranasal sinuses. Symptoms of vasomotor rhinitis can be aggravated or produced by overuse of vasoconstrictor nose drops and sprays. This "yo-yo effect" is produced by shrinkage and rebound congestion of the membranes.

The symptoms of vasomotor rhinitis in many patients are quite similar to those of hay fever, but some persons have paroxysms of sneezing only, while others merely develop temporary nasal obstruction with or without discharge, due to sudden turgescence of the mucous membrane of the nose. However, the rhinitis that follows the ingestion of foods to which the person is hypersensitive is usually a minor part of a general reaction, other features of which are urticaria, asthma and gastrointestinal disturbances. Vasomotor rhinitis is difficult to distinguish from infectious coryza. However, the former has no prodromal period with malaise, and the discharge does not present the same changes as that of the common cold.

Bronchial Asthma

Asthma is a form of paroxysmal dyspnea, predominantly expiratory in type, which is characterized by wheezy breathing. A hereditary tendency seems to be present in two thirds of all cases. The hay fever attacks of about 50 per cent of all patients end as asthma.

The stimuli of essential asthma may be extrinsic or intrinsic. Of the extrinsic stimuli, pollens and dusts are the most common for adults, and foods (especially egg white, cereals or cow's milk) for children. The stimuli of intrinsic cases are abnormalities in the respiratory tract (such as adenoids, spurs or sinus infections), infected tracheobronchial lymph nodes and pulmonary infections. Adults previously free from asthma have developed it after repeated bronchial infection or long-continued exposure to mildly irritating dusts.

The asthmatic attack starts suddenly with cough and a sensation of tightness in the chest. Then slow, laborious, wheezy breathing begins. Expiration is always much more strenuous and prolonged than inspiration, which forces the patient to sit upright and use every accessory muscle of respiration. He becomes blue from hypoxia and breaks out into a profuse sweat; his pulse is weak; his extremities are cold; there may be fever, and, occasionally, pain, nausea, vomiting and diarrhea. The cough at first is tight and dry, but it soon becomes more violent and raises with difficulty a distinctive sputum of thin mucus in which swim small round gelatinous masses. These are the "pearls of Laënnec," which are molds of the smaller bronchi and contain Curschmann's spirals. The attack may last from one half to several hours. Finally it subsides, and the tired patient can breathe again without undue effort. Such attacks are rarely fatal. Occasionally "status asthmaticus" occurs in which therapeutic measures fail and the patient has repeated attacks or continuous asthma. This condition is life-threatening.

Related Reactions. Among allergic reactions related to asthma are eczema (present at some time during life in 75 per cent of asthma patients), urticaria and angioneurotic edema (present in 50 per cent of the patients). Emotional stress may bring on an attack in the susceptible person.

Patient Evaluation. A clear history of hypersensitivity to some known substance that may be inhaled or ingested, such as a pollen, a particular type of food, feather, animal hair, face powder, etc., or a history suggesting the probability of such a sensitivity, is very important in determining the type of asthma presented in any given patient. The close association of the attacks with simple hay fever or vasomotor rhinitis, together with the discovery, during the attack, of marked pallor and swelling of the nasal mucous membrane, aids in establishing the case as one of extrinsic allergic asthma. The finding of an abnormally high count of eosinophilic cells in the blood or the sputum tends to confirm this diagnostic impression. However, "all that wheezes is not asthma," and it is important to be able to rule out congestive cardiac failure or bronchial obstruction due to a foreign body or a tumor as the underlying cause or precipitating factor that may explain the attack. Hence the necessity for careful radiologic and, often, bronchoscopic examination in every case of doubtful origin.

Treatment and Nursing Care. It should be remembered that asthma is a syndrome in the production of which many widely different factors may enter. Not the least of these is emotional hyperexcitability and stress, and the importance of mental relaxation in the

THE PATIENT WITH ASTHMA

Objectives and Principles of Medical and Nursing Management

The Problem: During an acute asthmatic episode, the ventilatory processes are altered due to airway obstruction. The ensuing hypoxia can be life-threatening to the patient.

I. To treat the patient during the acute asthmatic episode

  A. Relieve the airway obstruction

    1. Give the medications as directed

      a. Isoproterenol administered by nebulizer to oropharynx

      b. Intravenous aminophylline (250 to 500 mg.) administered slowly

      c. Epinephrine (0.2 to 0.5 ml. of 1:1000 sol.) subcutaneously

    2. Evaluate patient's reaction to medication

    3. Observe for symptoms of congestive failure

    4. Prepare for bronchoscopic aspiration to eliminate bronchial obstruction if indicated

  B. Relieve the hypoxia

    1. Use intermittent positive pressure breathing (p. 252) to assist respirations

    2. Use oropharyngeal oxygen with caution

    3. Observe for symptoms of carbon dioxide narcosis

  C. Liquefy the bronchial and the respiratory secretions

    1. Add sodium iodide (0.5 gm.) to intravenous solutions as directed

    2. Humidify the room

    3. Replace fluid and electrolyte losses

    4. Encourage oral intake of fluids as soon as possible

  D. Alleviate the patient's anxiety and exhaustion

    1. Use mild sedatives cautiously

    2. Give corticosteroids if needed to combat effects of prolonged stress

    3. Promote the comfort of the patient

      a. Use supportive devices for orthopneic position

      b. Keep the environment cool and quiet

      c. Restrict visitors

      d. Have a positive and calm approach to the patient

      e. Ensure that patient sleeps undisturbed following attack

II. To individualize the patient's therapy to prevent future attacks

  A. Avoid precipitating factors that will trigger an asthmatic attack

  B. Remove the patient from allergic material

  C. Carry out a program of desensitization

  D. Conduct the program of maintenance therapy

    1. Bronchodilators

    2. Sedatives

    3. Corticosteroids

    4. I.P.P.B. treatments

  E. Control secondary infections

    1. Teach patient to call physician at first symptoms of respiratory infection

    2. Observe the color of respiratory secretions

    3. Treat "minor" respiratory infections vigorously

    4. Avoid persons with colds and infections

  F. Promote the rehabilitation of the patient

    1. Teach patient to call physician at first symptoms

    2. Teach patient to avoid irritants

    3. Keep environmental air humidified and filtered when possible

    4. Refer to state office of vocational rehabilitation when needed

    5. Institute balanced program of nutrition, rest and exercise

    6. Encourage the patient to express his anxieties

    7. Assist the patient to have insight into his situational problems

---

therapy of the acute attack cannot be overestimated. Often a mere change of environment, such as from home to hospital, is sufficient to halt a severe attack. The patient should be isolated from relatives and friends; he should be placed in a quiet room and surrounded with an atmosphere of calm and encouragement. Mild sedatives—for example, a barbiturate—may be indicated at times, but they should be administered cautiously if the patient is exhausted as a result of prolonged respiratory difficulty, because death may ensue from respiratory failure. If cyanosis is present oxygen with helium may be given with caution, particularly if the patient has obstructive lung disease

(see p. 249). Adrenalin chloride, injected either subcutaneously in 1:1,000 solution of sprayed intratracheally in a strength of 1:100, or Isuprel Hydrochloride administered in the form of a 1:200 to 1:100 solution by means of a nebulizer or by oxygen-aerosolization, usually bring prompt relief. The inhalation of steam, unmedicated or with benzoin tincture, also may be effective. The patient requires adequate hydration to liquefy his thick tenacious sputum.

The corticosteroids, e.g., prednisone in oral doses of 10 to 30 mg. per day, terminate dramatically the majority of asthmatic attacks, regardless of their severity. Moreover, the frequency and the severity of recurrent attacks are reduced in most instances by the continued administration of these drugs.

Respiratory efficiency may be improved and comfort increased during an acute asthmatic attack by elevating the head of the bed and supporting the pillows in position by strapping. The patient is likely to be most comfortable leaning forward, with arms supported on a pillow-upholstered over-bed table. Every opportunity for sleep and rest should be fostered after an acute asthmatic attack.

These patients are prone to perspire excessively, introducing the need for protection against chilling. Covers made of flannel are preferred, and frequent changes of gown should be carried out as needed.

Special dietary orders, for patients on elimination diets, and prescriptions concerning fluid intake are to be observed with care during the acute phases of the illness and precise instructions transmitted to the patient (and his family) with respect to food and fluids permitted after discharge from the hospital. Detailed and accurate instructions are also to be provided in connection with: (1) injections or aerosol inhalations to be administered at home; (2) permissible activities and contraindicated activities; (3) types of contact that are considered potentially provocative of asthmatic attacks and are, therefore, to be avoided; and (4) the scheduling of return visits for observations during and following convalescence. The social worker may assist in securing new employment if a change of occupation is desirable.

Complications of Asthma. The acute asthmatic attack per se is seldom serious, although occasionally it does prove to be fatal through respiratory exhaustion, which is particularly possible if sedatives are administered too freely.

Complications of asthma include emphysema, chronic and recurrent acute bronchitis, bronchiectasis, pulmonary hypertension and hypertrophy of the right side of the heart with right heart failure (pulmonary heart disease). Chronic hypoxia due to these complications leads to mental symptoms and personality changes.

Prevention. In every case of recurrent asthma, evidence should be sought that might implicate a foreign protein to which the patient is hypersensitive and that might precipitate his attacks. If attacks chiefly occur at night when the patient is in bed, he should be skin-tested with the material composing his mattress and pillows, and, if hypersensitivity to these becomes evident, substitutions should be carried out. If attacks appear to be associated with the presence of a particular species of animal, such as a horse or a cat, similar skin tests should be made with an antigen composed of hair or skin scrapings from the animal concerned. The physician should search for foci of bacterial infection, e.g., of chronically infected sinuses or teeth, because their eradication may be strikingly beneficial in certain patients. A seasonal incidence of attacks in a patient suggests an air-borne antigen as the chief etiologic agent. In such cases, therapy may be attempted with pollen vaccines. Air conditioning offers possibilities in the prevention of attacks, depending on the extent to which the patient can restrict his life to air-conditioned rooms during the asthma season. A complete change of climatic environment to a locality with different flora during that period is the most satisfactory solution when feasible.

Asthmatic children should be provided with the best available facilities for good mental and physical hygiene, including proper rest, nourishment and any social readjustments that may be indicated.

Psychotherapy. It is important to remember that asthmatic attacks, once started, may continue as an asthma habit: that in some patients suggestion alone can induce them. The asthma paroxysms of some adults begin after a period of mental stress and strain, and they cease after the reason for the anxiety has been removed. Children without intent may develop asthma by imitating the attacks of others, and persons who voluntarily practice asthmatic breathing may later suffer from spontaneous attacks whenever they catch cold.

ALLERGIC DERMATOSES

Contact Dermatitis

Contact dermatitis (dermatitis venenata) is an inflammatory, often eczematous condition caused by a skin reaction to contact with a variety of irritating or allergenic materials. Almost any substance can produce contact dermatitis. Poison ivy is probably the most common and best example; cosmetics, soaps, detergents and industrial chemicals are frequent offenders. The skin sensitivity may develop after brief or prolonged periods of exposure and a clinical picture may appear hours or weeks after the sensitized skin has been exposed. The symptoms are itching,

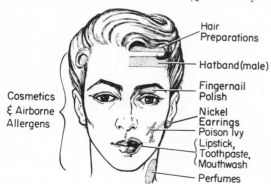

Fig. 30-1. Contact dermatitis of the face. (Sauer, G. C.: Manual of Skin Diseases, p. 42, Philadelphia, Lippincott)

burning, erythema, vesiculation and edema, followed by weeping, crusting and finally a drying up and peeling of the skin. In very severe responses, hemorrhagic bullae may develop. Repeated reactions may be accompanied by the development of thickening of the skin and pigmentary changes.

Secondary invasion by bacteria may develop in skin abraded from rubbing or scratching. Usually there are no systemic symptoms unless the eruption is widespread.

Diagnosis may sometimes be made easily by the location of the eruption and history of exposure. But in cases of obscure irritants or an unobservant patient, diagnosis may be extremely difficult and many trial-and-error procedures may be involved before the etiology is correctly determined. Patch tests on the skin with suspected offending agents may clarify the picture.

The most important aspect of treatment is to remove the patient from further contact with the irritant or allergen. Burow's solution soaks (aluminum acetate) soothe the blistered erythematous skin and may be followed by corticosteroid ointments or creams. Antimicrobials are given if secondary invasion is present.

Atopic dermatitis is chronic, pruritic, familial and allergic in nature, and principally involves the skin of the neck, the face and the antecubital creases. It waxes and wanes in activity. Family history is usually positive for allergies such as hay fever, asthma or eczema. It has a more prolonged course than simple contact dermatitis. Drying of the skin is an aggravating factor; wool and lanolin commonly irritate the skin of these patients. Allergy to foods has probably been overstressed but is, nonetheless, a factor. Emotional stress and nervousness aggravate the condition. The principles of treatment are the same as for dermatitis venenata.

Drug Reactions (Dermatitis Medicamentosa)

Dermatitis medicamentosa is the term applied to skin rashes induced by the internal administration of certain drugs. While, as a rule, certain drugs tend to induce eruptions of similar types, individuals react differently to each of them.

In general, it may be said that drug rashes appear suddenly, have a particularly vivid color, present characteristics that are more spectacular than the somewhat similar eruptions of infectious origin and, with the exception of the bromide and the iodide rashes, disappear rapidly after the drug is withdrawn. Some drug rashes are accompanied by constitutional symptoms. Upon discovery of a drug allergy, the patient should be warned that he reacts peculiarly to a particular drug and should be advised not to take it again. The nurse has a very important responsibility in relation to drug eruptions, for these lesions offer a

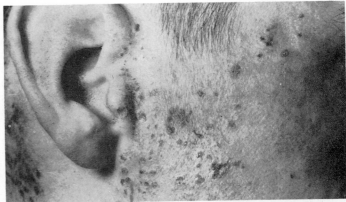

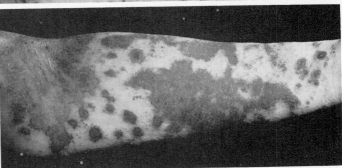

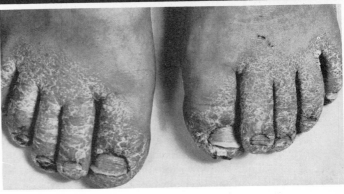

Fig. 30-2. Atopic eczema. (Sauer, G. C.: Manual of Skin Diseases, p. 50, Philadelphia, Lippincott)

warning of serious trouble pending, and she is in a position to detect the signal before anyone else. She must be on the alert for it and report its appearance at once, so that the physician will omit the offending drug without unnecessary delay.

Urticaria and Angioneurotic Edema

Urticaria (hives) is an allergic affection of the skin characterized by the sudden appearance of pinkish edematous elevations, variable in size and shape, which itch and smart. They may involve any part of the body, including the mucous membranes, especially those of the mouth, the larynx (occasionally with serious results) and the gastrointestinal tract. Each hive remains for a few minutes to several hours, then disappears. For hours or days, crops of these lesions may come, go and return in a most capricious manner. If this sequence continues indefinitely, the condition is called *chronic urticaria;* if the individual lesions themselves persist for several days, it is known as *urticaria perstans.*

The swellings of angioneurotic edema vary in size from a few millimeters in diameter to several centimeters. On occasion, one may be seen that covers the entire back. The skin over them may appear normal, but often it has a reddish hue. It does not pit on pressure as ordinary edema does. The regions most often involved are lips, eyelids, cheeks, hands, feet, genitalia and tongue; also, the mucous membranes of the larynx, the bronchi and the gastrointestinal canal, particularly in cases of the hereditary type. An eye may be completely closed; one lip may become so large that eating is impossible; one hand may become so huge that the fingers cannot be flexed. These swellings may appear suddenly in a few seconds or minutes, or slowly, in 1 or 2 hours. In the latter case, their appearance often is preceded by itching or burning sensations. Seldom does more than a single swelling appear at one time, although one may develop while another is disappearing. Only infrequently do they recur in the same region. The individual lesions usually last from 24 to 36 hours. On rare occasions they recur with a remarkable periodicity at intervals of 3 or 4 weeks.

The swellings of angioneurotic edema along the gastrointestinal canal may cause acute crises of pain with vomiting, which suggest acute appendicitis, acute cholecystitis, renal colic or intussusception; those in the throat, edema of the glottis; those in a primary bronchus, massive pulmonary collapse.

Treatment. Many patients are relieved by antihistamine drugs; others require injections of epinephrine. Corticosteroids usually give rapid resolution. Tracheotomy becomes necessary if laryngeal edema threatens to obstruct the glottis.

GASTROINTESTINAL ALLERGY

To a few persons, certain common foods are veritable poisons. There are those who cannot eat strawberries or shellfish without an attack of urticaria; or pork, or cheese, no matter how well disguised these foods may be, without vomiting promptly; or, if the food is retained, without diarrhea often accompanied by considerable pain (owing, it is surmised, to urticarial lesions along the gastrointestinal mucosa). Often asthma and urticaria result as well.

DESENSITIZATION, ANTIHISTAMINICS AND HORMONES IN ALLERGY

It is of the utmost importance that the nurse become familiar with certain general concepts regarding therapy in allergic diseases, since she is very apt to find herself an active participant in their treatment and will almost certainly be in the position of advisor to patients who are potential candidates for one or another of these procedures.

The commonest method of treatment employs the serial injection of one or more antigens which are selected in each particular case on the basis of *skin tests.* Skin testing entails the simultaneous intradermal inoculation (or superficial application), at separate sites, of several solutions containing individual antigens, comprising an assortment of those allergens deemed most likely to be implicated in the patient's disease. A positive reaction, evidenced by the appearance of an urticarial wheal or by localized erythema in the area of inoculation or contact, is regarded as evidence of sensitivity to the corresponding antigen. Skin tests lend important weight to other evidence obtained from the patient's history, indicating which of several antigens are most likely to provoke his symptoms and providing some clue to the intensity of his sensitization. (On the other hand, it should be recognized that the skin test is a test of skin reactivity, and any deduction that might be drawn from it relative to allergic phenomena in other tissues, such as the respiratory or gastrointestinal mucosa, is largely a matter of correlation and conjecture.)

A positive skin test may be regarded as an indication for a series of desensitizing (hyposensitizing) injections, a course involving the repeated inoculation of the suspected allergen in graded doses and at regularly spaced intervals. The value of such injections has been fairly well established in those cases of hay fever and asthma that are clearly due to sensitivity to one of the common pollens or molds or to house dust. Although referred to as a "desensitization" procedure, the effects are very probably attributable to the opposite process, i.e., immunization, for it appears to stimulate the production of a new antibody with the capacity of neutralizing the allergy-provoking properties of the responsible antigen.

One approach to the symptomatic treatment of allergic disorders has been the administration of certain chemical agents called "antihistaminic drugs." These, most of which are derivatives of aminoethanol and ethylenediamine, are capable of neutralizing histamine, a substance that is liberated in the course of tissue antigen-antibody reactions and has been considered to be responsible, in part at least, for the symptoms of allergic reactions. In actual practice, the effectiveness of these drugs is sharply limited to certain cases of hay fever, vasomotor rhinitis, urticaria and mild asthma; they are rarely effective in other conditions or in severe conditions of any sort.

Administration of the steroid hormones dramatically eliminates any allergic phenomena that happen to be in progress at the time. The reason for their effectiveness in allergic disorders appears to be related to their inhibiting effect on inflammatory reactions in general. In this sense, their beneficial effect in allergic patients must be classed as nonspecific, bearing no relation to any specific antigen-antibody reaction that may be responsible for the disorder. Certain circumstances justify the administration of these hormones.

SERUM DISEASE

Serum disease is an acute malady that not uncommonly follows the injection of a serum—usually an antiserum prepared from horse or rabbit blood. Also, it develops occasionally after a course of penicillin injections. Its characteristic features, which appear after an incubation period of 6 to 12 days, include urticaria, enlargement of the regional lymph nodes, mild fever and pain in the joints—symptoms that disappear entirely in a few days to 3 weeks. In severe cases the skin rash is purpuric in character, the temperature for a week or 10 days ranges irregularly from 39.4° C. (103° F.) to 40° C. (104° F.), the lymphadenitis is general, the spleen is enlarged, and the joints are as red and swollen as in acute rheumatic fever. Other features often present are headache, abdominal pain, vomiting, diarrhea, proteinuria and cylindruria. This is potentially a serious complication, not to be regarded as a mere annoyance. Not only does it share many of the clinical characteristics of rheumatic fever and periarteritis nodosa, but it is also known to produce pathologic lesions very similar to those found in the two conditions.

One of the rarer consequences of serum sickness, which can produce permanent disability is peripheral neuritis. The nerves most often involved are components of the brachial plexus. Their damage results in atrophy and weakness of muscles in the shoulder and the upper arm (Erb's palsy). It may affect the muscles of respiration, with potentially fatal results.

Treatment. Serum sickness, with all of its manifestations, including neuritis, if present, responds promptly to the administration of the steroid hormones. The speediest recovery can be anticipated after the parenteral administration of hydrocortisone in doses of 200 to 300 mg. or dexamethasone, 8 to 12 mg., given intravenously over periods of 12 to 24 hours. Mild cases, exhibiting merely urticaria and arthralgia, may respond satisfactorily to one of the antihistaminic drugs, supplemented by aspirin and codeine.

Prevention. Avoidance of allergic phenomena following the administration of horse serum is possible to a large extent if each prospective recipient is questioned closely regarding the possibility of sensitivity to horse dander, and if a skin test is carried out with horse serum. If either yields positive results, it still may be feasible to employ the antiserum if the patient first can be desensitized by a series of small injections.

When contemplating the inoculation of a virus or rickettsial vaccine, it must be borne in mind that the materials incorporate egg yolk and, therefore, are a source of grave danger to individuals who are sensitive to eggs.

ANAPHYLACTIC SHOCK

Anaphylactic shock, one of the so-called *serum accidents*, is the immediate shock-like and sometimes fatal reaction that follows the administration of an animal serum to an individual who, because of a previous injection, has become sensitized to that foreign protein.

The onset of serum shock may be immediate, almost before the needle is withdrawn. There are local edema, itching, sneezing and prickling feelings in the throat. Soon there appear edema of the face, hands and even of the whole body, cyanosis, a choking cough and violent asthma. The pupils dilate, the pulse is weak; there may be fever and in some cases, convulsions. Death may follow in 10 minutes to several hours, or the illness may follow the course of a serious case of serum disease.

No serum ever should be administered without a previous sensitivity test. This applies especially to those patients who have ever had asthma or hay fever, or who recently had received an injection of horse serum. If he is found to be sensitive, the patient should be desensitized by a series of frequently repeated subcutaneous injections, in ascending doses, of the serum to be used, and the use of the serum should be preceded by a 50-mg. to 100-mg. dose of an antihistaminic drug. Epinephrine, in doses of from 0.5 to 1 ml. (1:1,000), is a specific remedy for this type of accident.

BIBLIOGRAPHY

General Articles

Feinberg, A. A.: Allergies and air conditioning. Amer. J. Nurs., *66*:1333-1336, June, 1966.

Gottlieb, P. M.: Broadening horizons of allergy. JAMA, *194*:890-892, 1965.

Green, M. A.: The family physician's role in allergy. GP, 38:96-101, 1968.

Henderson, L. L.: A special article: anaphylaxis. Ann. Allergy, 23:525-528, 1965.

Horesh, A. J.: Allergy and infection—a new concept. Ann. Allergy, 23:621-635, 1965.

Milton, C. F.: Seasonal allergies. Postgrad. Med., 44:76-80, 1968.

Pruzansky, J. J., *et al.*: Immunologic changes during hyposensitization therapy. JAMA, 203:805-806, 1968.

Dermatologic and Gastrointestinal Allergies

Rothenborg, H. W., *et al.*: Allergy to perfumes from toilet soaps and detergents in patients with dermatitis. Arch. Derm., 97:417-421, 1968.

Sheffer, A. L.: Hypersensitivity and the gastrointestinal tract. Med. Clin. N. Amer., 50:393-416, 1966.

Respiratory Allergy

Brown, E. B.: Hyposensitization therapy in respiratory allergy. Mod. Treatment, 3:845-865, July, 1966.

Carryer, H. M.: Corticosteroid drugs in the management of asthma. JAMA, 194:1122-1124, 1965.

Freedman, S. O. (ed.): Symposium on treatment of respiratory allergy. Mod. Treatment, 3:813-932, July, 1966.

Frouchtman, R.: Psychosocial aspects of bronchial asthma. Dis. Chest, 53:227-228, Feb., 1968.

Itkin, I.: The pro's and con's of exercise for the person with asthma. Amer. J. Nurs., 66:1584-1587, July, 1966.

Larsen, W. G.: Hyposensitization for allergic rhinitis. Arch. Derm., 96:586-587, Nov., 1967.

Miller, A.: A statistical review of double-blind studies on ragweed hay fever injection threapy. Ann. Allergy, 26:339-347, July, 1968.

PATIENT EDUCATION

Public Health Service
U.S. Department of Health, Education, and Welfare
Washington, D.C. 20201
    Allergy. (HIS-32)
    Asthma. (HIS-19)
    Hay Fever. (HIS-17)

VOLUNTARY AGENCIES

Asthmatic Children's Foundation
Denver U.S. National Center
Denver, Colorado 80202

International Allergy Association
133 East 58th Street
New York, New York 10022

National Foundation for Asthmatic Children
5601 Trails End
Tucson, Arizona 85702

CHAPTER 31

Nursing in Endocrine and Metabolic Disorders

- *Physiology of Endocrine Glands*
- *The Thyroid Gland*
- *The Parathyroid Glands*
- *The Pancreas*
- *The Adrenal Gland*
- *The Pituitary Gland*
- *The Patient with Gout*

PHYSIOLOGY OF ENDOCRINE GLANDS

No organism as complex as the human body could possibly function with any degree of efficiency without precision equipment for the integration and the control of its innumerable metabolic activities. Designed specifically for this purpose is the endocrine system, comprising a series of ingenious regulating devices which are fully automatic and operate in accordance with the most advanced principles of cybernetics. Its functioning components are the endocrine glands. These units can function individually, in series or in parallel, their activities being integrated closely. Communication with each other and with the tissues under their control is established by means of chemical signals, or *hormones*, which they produce, store and release as required, and which are distributed throughout the body by means of a mechanical conveyor, the circulating blood.

These glands, with two exceptions, have no means of communicating with other tissues excepting by way of the bloodstream, depending exclusively on chemical signals for their own regulation. In most instances the agent stimulating or inhibiting their activity is the hormone produced by the corresponding target gland, an arrangement calculated to ensure stability of operation.

The two exceptions are the adrenal medulla and the posterior pituitary gland. These glands are connected with the autonomic nervous system, secreting their hormones in response to electrical stimuli originating in higher centers in the brain and reaching them by way of the nerve fibers that link them to that system. Stimulation of the posterior pituitary causes the prompt secretion of *vasopressin*. Stimulation of the adrenal medulla results in the immediate release of *epinephrine* (Adrenalin) and *l-norepinephrine* (l-norepinephrine) also is liberated at the terminal ends of all sympathetic nerve fibers in response to electrical stimulation.

These hormones, in contrast with all others, have widespread effects that are achieved almost instantaneously and involve many organs. Their net objective is to fortify the body against disaster and to compensate for bodily injury. The effect of epinephrine is to increase the efficiency of the circulatory and respiratory systems; to mobilize quick-energy from glucose storage depots into the circulating blood; to improve the acuity of vision; and to reinforce the clotting mechanism, in anticipation of massive bleeding. It even goes so far as to set into motion a series of reactions that would have the effect, a few hours later, of lessening the severity of the body's responses to any tissue damage that might be incurred in the interim! Norepinephrine in the circulating blood produces constriction of all arterioles throughout the body, except those within the heart muscle. As a result of this action, the systolic and diastolic arterial pressures are elevated, and blood flow through the myocardium is increased.

Vasopressin helps the body to survive severe hemorrhage and to correct the resulting deficiency in blood volume. Through its antidiuretic action, this hormone prevents further loss of body water through excretion in the urine. By causing smooth muscle everywhere to contract, it forces the evacuation of all hollow viscera, and has an effect on the uterus. It also reduces the capacity of the vascular bed and tends to maintain the arterial pressure in the heart and the brain at functional levels until the blood volume can be restored.

The remainder of the endocrine system includes the following secretory tissues: the anterior portion of the pituitary gland, the thyroid, the parathyroids, the adrenal cortex, the pancreas, the ovarian follicles and the interstitial cells of the testes. Their secretions, as a group, are concerned with tissue growth and metabolism, the storage and the utilization of fuel substances, the processes of reproduction and other phases of the bodily economy. One gland, the anterior pituitary, integrates the activities of the entire system. This gland, either through its own secretions, or through other glands that are among its targets, exerts a potent influence on every phase of metabolic activity throughout the body. The action of each individual hormone from the anterior pituitary, however, and from all other glands in this group as well, is highly selective and strictly limited, in marked contrast with the effects of adrenalin and vasopressin.

Secretions of the anterior pituitary gland number at least eight protein or peptide hormones. *Somatotropin* (growth hormone) regulates cell division, hence organ and body growth. It also elevates the concentration of glucose in the blood by decreasing the rate at which glucose is consumed by the tissue cell and by preventing its deposition in the liver, effects that may be described as "diabetogenic." *Luteotropin* (luteotropic hormone, LTH) prepares the breasts for lactation during pregnancy and stimulates milk production after the fetus is delivered.

The remaining hormones have as their targets individual endocrine glands, whose hormones inhibit, in each case, the production of that particular stimulant by the anterior pituitary. *Corticotropin* (adrenocorticotropic hormones, ACTH), for example, stimulates the adrenal cortex to produce hydrocortisone, aldosterone and other steroid hormones, while the rate of ACTH production, in turn, is regulated by the concentration of those hormones in the circulating blood. *Thyrotropin* (thyrotropic or thyroid-stimulating hormone, TSH), by stimulating the enzymatic breakdown of stored thyroglobulin, forces the liberation of thyroxine from the thyroid gland. The resulting level of thyroxine in the blood determines the amount of thyrotropic hormone that is produced by the anterior pituitary at any given time.

There are two *gonadotropic* hormones from the anterior pituitary. One of these, the *follicle-stimulating hormone* (FSH), is responsible for the development of graafian follicles in the ovary and for the proliferation of spermatozoa by the testis. The other, called *luteinizing hormone* (LH, or interstitial-cell-stimulating hormone, ICSH), causes the follicle to atrophy and to undergo metamorphosis into another structure known as the corpus luteum. In the adolescent and adult male, LH stimulates the interstitial cells of the testis to increase production of *testosterone*, the male sex hormone. *Melanocyte-stimulating hormone* (MSH) stimulates the synthesis of melanin; an abnormal increase in this hormone, as occurs in patients with Addison's disease (see page 706), is responsible for the brown pigmentation of the skin associated with spontaneous adrenal insufficiency or operative adrenalectomy. Finally, a *fat-mobilizing hormone* has been isolated from the anterior pituitaries of certain animals, the effect of which is to provoke a rise in the circulating free fatty acids; this may play a role in the regulation of lipid metabolism in man.

Thyroxine and *triiodothyronine*, the hormones of the thyroid gland, speed oxidative reactions that energize all cellular activities. The parathyroids and their product, *parathormone,* regulate the metabolism of calcium and phosphorus and direct the migration of these ions between the bones and the blood. Pancreatic *insulin* enables the glucose that is contained in the circulating blood to penetrate the membranes and enter the cytoplasm of tissue cells, thus providing these cells with ready access to this vitally needed fuel. Another pancreatic hormone, *glucagon,* speeds the liberation of glucose from its storage form, namely, glycogen, thereby increasing its concentration in the blood. The *hormones of the adrenal cortex* perform a variety of functions, including the conversion of proteins into glucose (gluconeogenesis), the control of lymphocyte production, the development of secondary sex characteristics and the prevention of sodium loss in the urine, causing the cells of the renal tubules to extract this ion from the glomerular filtrate and return it to the blood.

The testes and the ovaries are likewise an integral part of the endocrine system. Their secretory functions, controlled by the pituitary through its gonadotropic hormones, are responsible for the formation of the secondary sex characteristics, the functional and anatomic changes that are involved in the process of menstruation and the changes that occur during pregnancy.

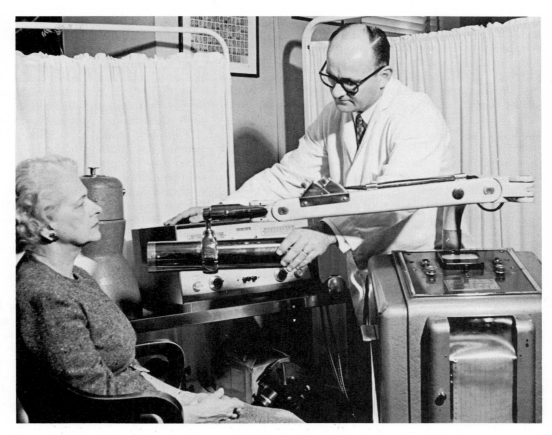

Fig. 31-1. Performance of 24-hour iodine uptake test. The physician has centered the scintillation probe and is measuring the energy transmitted from the gamma emissions by means of a pulse-height analyzer. (Photo by Caroline Bailey)

THE THYROID GLAND

Thyroid Physiology

The thyroid gland sits astride the trachea just below the larynx, its two lobes clasping the trachea on either side and the intermediate portion, or "isthmus," overlying that structure anteriorly. The lobes of the normal gland usually can be felt as they elevate during the act of swallowing. If the thyroid is enlarged significantly it produces a visible swelling in the neck, or *goiter.*

This gland affects the rate at which all tissues metabolize. It regulates the speed of their chemical reactions, the volume of oxygen they consume and the amount of heat they produce. Thus, the thyroid gland is an "energizer," so to speak, stimulating the tissue cells to whatever level of activity is required to maintain the total body temperature at a preset level. In the absence of the thyroid gland, metabolism continues, but at an exceedingly retarded pace (see p. 687).

The thyroid achieves its stimulating effect through the production and distribution of two hormones, one of which is called L-*thyroxine* and the other, *triiodothyronine.* Both compounds contain iodine that is protein-bound. According to present evidence, the function of thyroxine is to maintain the body's metabolism in a steady state, and at a level suitable for an individual who is situated in a stable, normal environment. Whenever there is a sudden need for a substantial increase in heat production, some of the thyroxine is converted into a more active agent, namely, triiodothyronine, which is approximately 5 times as potent as thyroxine.

The manufacture of thyroid hormone requires small amounts of iodine intake by the body, lack of which leads to thyroid deficiency (hypothyroidism), a hypometabolic state and goiter (thyroid gland enlargement). The thyroid stores its hormone and releases it as needed. If too much, or too rapid a release occurs, a state of hyperthyroidism or thyrotoxicosis develops. The same picture can be produced by ingestion of excessive amounts of thyroid substance (thyrotoxicosis factitis).

Tests of Thyroid Function

In the majority of thyroid disorders, the most prominent signs and symptoms are those that reflect an excessive or inadequate production of thyroid hormone. These signs provide a useful basis for evaluating the activity of the gland.

Protein-bound Iodine. A very reliable and definitive index of thyroid function is the concentration of protein-bound iodine (PBI) in the blood. Normal values range from 3.5 μg. to 7.5 μg. (0.0035 to 0.0075 mg.) per 100 ml. of plasma. Values above 7.5 μg. indicate thyroid overactivity; conversely, concentrations below 3.5 μg. are considered evidence of hypothyroidism.

Ingestion of drugs or the administration of dyes containing iodine (as for gallbladder studies) impairs the usefulness of the PBI study. Other drugs, such as mercurial diuretics or estrogens, also cause inaccurate results of the test. Pregnancy impairs the test.

Radioiodine (^{131}I). The rate of ^{131}I uptake by the thyroid gland, the plasma clearance of ^{131}I and the urinary excretion of this isotope furnish reliable criteria of thyroid activity. Moreover, the distribution of radioactivity in the thyroid and elsewhere in the body after the administration of radioiodine affords a means of distinguishing malignant from benign thyroid nodules and a method for the detection of metastatic thyroid cancer.

The T-3 test using radioactive iodine, is a newer and safer test and is done in vitro (within the test tube). No radioactive material is given to the patient. Normal levels are 28 to 35 per cent; higher values indicate overactivity of the gland, and lower levels indicate hypothyroidism. Pregnancy impairs the test.

^{131}I *Uptake.* The usual procedure is to administer orally to the fasting patient a solution of sodium iodide^{131} (or a capsule prepared with an internal coating of ^{131}I) in a dose of 5 to 50 microcuries. After a standard time interval, e.g., 24 and 48 hours, the ^{131}I that has been assimiliated by the thyroid gland is measured on the basis of the radioactive counts per minute that are detected at a point above the isthmus of the thyroid gland. Hyperthyroid individuals accumulate a high proportion of the ^{131}I, in some cases approximately 90 per cent, whereas hypothyroid individuals exhibit a very low uptake (Fig. 31-1).

Thyroidal Iodide Clearance. The ^{131}I clearance test measures the quantity of circulating blood that is cleared completely of iodide per unit time. After the intravenous injection of radioiodine, the radioactivity over the thyroid gland is measured continuously for 30 to 60 minutes, and the total amount of ^{131}I accumulated by the gland per minute is computed. In addition, the plasma ^{131}I content is measured in samples of blood collected 45 and 70 minutes after injection; these values are averaged. Thyroid ^{131}I, divided by the mean plasma ^{131}I, equals thyroid clearance (ml. of plasma cleared of iodide per minute). The mean clearance value for normal (euthyroid) individuals is 25 ml. per minute; for hyperthyroid patients, 250 ml. per minute; and hypothyroid patients, 1.6 ml. per minute.

^{131}I *Excretion.* Another test of thyroid activity using radioiodine involves measuring the urinary output of this isotope during the 24- to 48-hour period after its ingestion. A subject whose thyroid activity is normal (i.e., euthyroid individual) excretes 40 to 80 per cent of the ingested iodine in 24 hours. Hyperthyroid individuals almost invariably excrete less than 40 per cent, and patients with hypothyroidism excrete more than 80 per cent of the tracer dose.

Thyroid "Scan". In addition to quantitative measurement of iodine uptake by the thyroid gland, the latter may be subjected to external scanning by means of a handheld scintillation counter or by a mechanical scanning device for evidence of irregularity in the deposition of radioactive iodine. The scintillation crystal is electromechanically linked to a recording device that automatically maps the activity in the scanned area, producing a so-called "scintogram," "scanogram" or "gammagram." Discovery of decreased ^{131}I uptake in a localized area of the thyroid is construed as evidence of a malignancy. Scanning of the entire body to obtain the total body profile may be carried out in a search for a functioning thyroid metastasis.

Role of the Nurse in ^{131}I Thyroid Tests. Although the nurse may not be involved directly in the performance of these tests, their validity may depend on her participation. Except for nursing vigilance throughout the 24-hour observation period, the iodine excretion test would prove worthless in a high proportion of cases. Valid results require the salvaging and pooling of every urine specimen voided during that interval. Experience has demonstrated that one specimen at least is unintentionally discarded and lost in 25 per cent of tests despite clear-cut directions given in advance by the physician and despite the desire of the patient to cooperate.

Another source of error that may increase the iodine uptake, clearance and excretion tests is prior exposure of the patient to iodine. Such exposure, whether acquired in the form of a prescribed medication containing an iodide salt or as the result of the injection of an iodine-containing contrast medium in a bronchogram, venogram, pyelogram or gallbladder study, or an application of iodine to the skin, reduces the uptake of ^{131}I and invalidates these tests. Other sources of iodine may be antiseptics, cough syrups and nail strengtheners. Thus, as soon as the physician is informed that a radioiodine excretion test or uptake test is in prospect, he should systematically eliminate any chance of such contact in the interim.

Basal Metabolic Rate. A semiquantitative estimation of thyroid activity is possible from the basal metabolism rate, or B.M.R. The term "basal metabolism" refers to the oxygen consumption of an individual who is at rest, whose body temperature is normal and who has fasted for at least 14 hours in order to escape the stimulating effect of recently ingested food. From the volume of oxygen that is absorbed in a standard period of time under these conditions, it is possible to compute the rate at which heat is produced by the body. An average adult male produces heat at a rate of approximately 1,500 calories, and an average adult female, 1,300 calories, per 24 hours. Expressed in terms of heat production per square meter of surface per hour, the average metabolic rate for a normal individual under basal conditions is approximately 40 calories, depending on sex and age.

The B.M.R. should be determined in the morning, while the patient is reclining quietly. Ambulatory patients should rest in bed quietly for an hour immediately before the test is performed. The entire procedure, which involves breathing through a rubber tube for several minutes with nostrils clamped shut, should be described fully to the patient in advance, because apprehension and emotional excitement, through stimulation of the sympathetic nervous system, increase the oxygen consumption (that is, metabolism) and the result is a high figure for the B.M.R. not at all indicative of thyroid overactivity.

B.M.R. Values

Normal	−10% to +10%
Hypothyroidism	−15% to −40%
Hyperfunctioning adenoma	+20% to +30%
Hyperthyroidism	+35% to +60%

This test is less popular than previously; when it is used, the results are evaluated in relation to other thyroid function tests.

Hypothyroidism and Myxedema

If the thyroid gland is removed surgically, is destroyed by disease or becomes inactive for any reason, the metabolism of the patient declines proportionately as the production of thyroid hormone is reduced. Complete extirpation of this organ is followed by a steady drop in the B.M.R., which in approximately 3 months' time stabilizes at a level of about −40 percent.

The Hypothyroid Patient.

Mrs. Robinson at 29 no longer made "different" sandwiches each day for the children's school lunches —now it was always peanut butter and jelly. Nor did she have a daily "catch" with her 12-year-old son, a baseball enthusiast. She became *lethargic* and *forgetful* and frequently *dozed* during the day. Her *skin* and *hair* became noticeably *dull* and *dry*. The children were aware that she was *hypersensitive to cold*. She blamed her *lack of pep* on *frequent headaches*. All of these symptoms of hypometabolism improved remarkably after the diagnosis was established and she was started on thyroid replacement therapy.

With severer grades of this disorder the temperature and the pulse rate become subnormal and the patient begins to gain weight. The skin becomes thickened, because a mucilaginous substance (the origin of the term *myxedema*) accumulates in the subcutaneous tissues. Menorrhagia is apt to develop; the hair thins and falls out; the expression of the face becomes stolid, stupid and masklike. At first the patient may be irritable, but as the condition progresses she becomes completely complacent, the emotional responses subdued and the mental process dulled. The advanced myxedematous state is one of utter bovine placidity, much less distressing to its possessor than to his associates. It is not without its complications, however, because there is an associated tendency to the rapid development of arteriosclerosis, with all the undesirable features of that disease; also anemia and poor reaction to anesthetic agents.

Medical and Nursing Management. One of the most brilliant of all medical discoveries has been the discovery that thyroid deficiency can be remedied by giving animal thyroid tissue extracts by mouth. This replacement therapy now is provided in the form of desiccated thyroid extract or synthetic crystalline L-thyroxine by mouth. Preparations of thyroid extract, standardized and of uniform potency, are available in tablet form. It is administered in one daily oral dose of 15 to 300 mg. (¼ to 5 grains), the usual initial dose for adults being 60 mg. (1 grain). L-thyroxine (Synthroid) is distributed in tablet form, a 0.15-mg. tablet being equivalent in potency to 60 mg. (1 grain) of the extract. The dosage range for this product is 0.025 mg. to 0.5 mg. daily.

The dosage for either material is scheduled on the basis of the patient's metabolic response, as ascertained by repeated measurements of the B.M.R. or of the ^{131}I uptake. If replacement therapy is adequate, the symptoms of myxedema disappear and normal metabolic activity is resumed.

Skillful nursing judgment and action are required in caring for patients with myxedema because of the possibility of several complications:

1. Severe untreated hypothyroidism is attended by an *increased susceptibility to all hypnotic and sedative drugs*. These agents, even in small doses, may induce profound somnolence lasting far longer than anticipated. Moreover, they are prone to cause respiratory depression, which could easily prove fatal. With this in mind, the dosage of any such drug should be most conservative, e.g., no more than a half or one third the dosage ordinarily employed in patients of similar age and weight who are not myxedematous. Drugs in this category should not be used at all unless the indications are very specific and, if they are given,

the nurse must be unusually watchful for signs of impending narcosis or respiratory failure.

2. *Myocardial ischemia* or *infarction* may occur in response to therapy in patients with myxedema. Any patient who has been myxedematous for a long period of time is almost certain to have coronary sclerosis of some degree. As long as metabolism is subnormal and the tissues, including the myocardium, require relatively little oxygen, a reduction in blood supply is tolerated very well. However, when thyroid hormone is given the situation changes: the oxygen requirements are greater, but its delivery cannot be speeded up unless, or until, the arteriosclerosis improves, which will occur very slowly, if at all. The signal that the oxygen needs of the myocardium are outstripping its blood supply is angina pectoris.

The nurse must be alert for that signal, especially during the early phase of treatment, and if detected, it must be heeded at once if a fatal myocardial infarction is to be averted. Obviously, the administration of thyroid hormone must be discontinued immediately, and later, when it can be resumed safely, substitution therapy should be applied with caution, at a lower level of dosage and under the close observation of the physician and the nurse. Elderly arteriosclerotic patients may also become confused and agitated if their metabolic rate is raised too quickly in myxedema.

Marked clinical improvement follows the administration of desiccated thyroid, L-thyroxine or L-triiodothyronine. Signs of myxedema disappear promptly; maturation and linear growth of the skeleton proceed rapidly, but mental retardation persists.

The term 'cretinism' applies to patients born with thyroid deficiency of mothers likewise deficient. In these patients, prenatal development has not proceeded normally, and the results are irreparable. The reader is referred to a pediatric textbook for further discussion.

The Patient with Hyperthyroidism

Spontaneous hyperthyroidism constitutes a well-defined disease entity, variously designated as *Graves' disease, Basedow's disease* and *exophthalmic goiter.* This disease occurs more commonly in women than in men. Its etiology is unknown, but it is believed to represent a dysfunction of the pituitary gland, whereby this gland produces an excess of thyrotropic (thyroid-stimulating) hormone. The disorder may appear after an emotional shock, nervous strain or an infection—particularly one involving the upper respiratory tract—but the exact significance of these relationships is not understood.

Symptoms. Patients with well-developed hyperthyroidism exhibit a characteristic group of symptoms and signs. Their presenting symptom is often nervousness. They are emotionally hyperexcitable, their state of mind is apt to be irritable and apprehensive; they cannot sit quietly; they suffer from palpitation; and their pulse is abnormally rapid at rest as well as on exertion. They tolerate heat poorly and perspire unusually freely; the skin is flushed continuously, with a characteristic salmon color, and is likely to be warm, soft and moist. A fine tremor of the hands may be observed. Many patients exhibit bulging eyes (exophthalmos), lending a startled expression to the countenance. (This is the only sign exhibited by these individuals that cannot be ascribed to thyroid overactivity *per se* or to the pituitary thyrotropic hormone; its mechanism remains obscure.)

The thyroid gland invariably is enlarged to some extent. It is soft and may pulsate; a thrill often can be felt over the thyroid arteries—a sign of greatly increased blood flow through the organ. Other important symptoms include an increased appetite (unless gastrointestinal symptoms develop), progressive loss of weight, abnormal muscular fatigability and weakness, amenorrhea and changes in bowel habit, either to constipation or diarrhea. The pulse rate of these patients ranges constantly between 90 and 160; the systolic, but characteristically not diastolic, blood pressure is elevated; atrial fibrillation may appear and cardiac decompensation is common, especially in elderly patients. In the more advanced cases, the diagnosis is established readily on the basis of the symptoms and the tests described previously: an elevated B.M.R., which declines over a period of several days on iodine therapy; an increase in protein-bound iodine in the blood; and an increased ^{131}I uptake by the thyroid (45 per cent to 90 per cent).

The course of the disease may be mild, characterized by remissions and exacerbations and terminating with spontaneous recovery in the course of a few months or years. On the other hand, it may progress relentlessly, the untreated patient becoming emaciated, intensely nervous, delirious—even disoriented—and the heart eventually "racing itself to death."

Medical and Nursing Management. As yet, no treatment for hyperthyroidism has been discovered that combats its basic cause. However, reduction of thyroid hyperactivity provides effective symptomatic relief and removes the principal source of its most important complications.

Three forms of treatment are available for the control of excessive thyroid activity: (1) pharmacologic, employing antithyroid drugs that interfere with the synthesis of thyroid hormones; (2) radiation, involving the administration of the radioisotope ^{131}I for destructive effects on the thyroid gland; and (3) surgical, accomplishing the removal of most of the thyroid gland.

Pharmacologic Treatment. Certain drugs effectively block the utilization of iodine by the thyroid gland and therefore prevent the synthesis of thyroid hormone, to the great benefit of the patient with hyperthyroidism. Propylthiouracil or methylthiouracil (Methiacil) may be prescribed orally in 100 mg. doses or methimazole (Tapazole) in 10 to 15 mg. doses, until the patient is *euthyroid* (i.e., neither hyper- nor hypothyroid). Therapy is controlled on the basis of clinical criteria, including changes in pulse rate, pulse pressure, body weight, size of the goiter and basal metabolic rate. Toxic complications of propylthiouracil are relatively uncommon; nevertheless, periodic examinations cannot be neglected in view of the possibility that drug sensitization, followed by fever, rash, urticaria or even granulopenia, may develop in its recipients. With any sign of infection, especially pharyngitis, the patient is advised to have a blood examination. Pharmacologic therapy for thyrotoxicosis may have to continue for several years.

Radioactive Iodine. Practically all of the iodine that enters and is retained in the body becomes concentrated within the thyroid gland. This applies to the radioactive isotopes of iodine as well, providing the basis for a very effective device for the selective inhibition of thyroid activity, namely, the administration of radioiodine (^{131}I). The objective of this treatment is the irradiation of the gland, which is accomplished by this technique without jeopardizing other radiosensitive tissues. Radioactive iodine has been used successfully in most varieties of thyrotoxicosis and is especially preferred for the treatment of patients over 25.

Surgical Intervention. The surgical removal of about five sixths of the thyroid tissue (subtotal thyroidectomy) practically assures a prolonged remission in most cases of exophthalmic goiter. Before surgery the patient is given propylthiouracil until signs of hyperthyroidism have disappeared. Iodine also is prescribed, either before or after a full remission has been achieved with propylthiouracil. The effect of iodine is to reduce the size and the vascularity of the goiter. It may be given in the form of potassium iodide or hydriodic acid. Patients receiving this medication must be watched for evidence of iodine toxicity (iodism), the appearance of which is the signal for immediate withdrawal of the drug. Symptoms of iodism include swelling of the buccal mucosa, excessive salivation, coryza and skin eruptions.

Thyroidectomy usually is scheduled within a few days after the patient's basal metabolic rate has been reduced to normal.

Thyroiditis

Subacute or *granulomatous thyroiditis*, an inflammatory disorder of the thyroid gland, presents as a painful swelling in the anterior neck that lasts 1 or 2 months, then disappears without residual effects. Women in their 50's are affected predominantly. The thyroid enlarges symmetrically and painfully. The overlying skin is often reddened and warm. Swallowing may be difficult and uncomfortable. Irritability, nervousness, insomnia and weight loss—manifestations of hyperthyroidism—are common, and many patients experience chills and fever as well. X-ray irradiation of the thyroid and steroid therapy have been applied with reported benefit.

Chronic thyroiditis, predominantly a disease of women in their 50's and 60's, has been classified as "Hashimoto's struma" or "Riedel's struma," depending on the histologic appearance of the inflamed gland. In contrast with acute thyroiditis, the chronic varieties are unaccompanied by pain, pressure symptoms or fever, and thyroid activity is apt to be normal or low, rather than increased. Steroid therapy likewise has been recommended for these patients.

There is evidence to suggest that thyroiditis, acute and chronic alike, may represent disorders of "auto-immunity" analogous to acquired hemolytic jaundice (see p. 511), as evidenced by the presence of antithyroid antibody in the serum of these patients.

Thyroid Tumors

Tumors of the thyroid gland are classified on the basis of their benign or malignant character, the presence or the absence of thyrotoxicosis associated with them and the diffuse or irregular quality of the glandular enlargement. If the enlargement is sufficient to cause a visible swelling in the neck, the tumor is referred to as a "goiter."

All grades of goiter are encountered, from those that are barely visible to those producing an unsightly disfigurement. Some are symmetrical and diffuse, others nodular. Some are accompanied by hyperthyroidism, in which case they are described as "toxic"; others are associated with a euthyroid state and are called "non-toxic" goiters.

Endemic (Iodine-Deficient) Goiter. The most common type of goiter, encountered chiefly in geographic regions where the natural supply of iodine is deficient (e.g., the Great Lakes area of the United States), is the so-called *simple* or *colloid goiter.* It represents a compensatory hypertrophy on the part of the entire gland, presumably due to stimulation by the pituitary gland. Thus, the pituitary gland produces a hormone controlling thyroid growth, and this production is excessive if there is subnormal thyroid activity, as when insufficient iodine is available for production of the thyroid hormone. Such goiters usually cause no symptoms except for the swelling in the neck, which, however, may result in tracheal compression when excessive. Many goiters of this type recede after treatment with thyroid extract, which tends to depress the pituitary's thyroid-stimulating activity. The operative removal of very large goiters occasionally is desirable.

Prevention. This is accomplished by providing children in iodine-poor districts with iodine compounds. If the mean iodine intake is less than 40 μg. per day, the thyroid hypertrophies. The World Health Organization recommends that salt be iodized to a concentration of one part in 100,000, which is adequate for the prevention of endemic goiter. In the U.S., salt is iodized to one part in 10,000.

Nodular Goiter. Certain thyroid glands are nodular because of the presence of one or several areas of *hyperplasia* (overgrowth) that appear to develop under conditions similar to those responsible for the colloid goiter. No symptoms may arise as a result of this condition, but, not uncommonly, these nodules slowly increase in size, some descending into the thorax and there causing local pressure symptoms. Some nodules become malignant and some become associated with a hyperthyroid state. Thus, many nodular thyroids eventually require surgical attention.

Thyroid Cancer. Benign thyroid tumors, or "adenomas," become cancerous in a significant percentage of patients. Thus, between 8 and 20 per cent of individuals with single thyroid nodules are discovered to harbor a carcinoma when the gland is removed and examined microscopically. The most vicious form of thyroid cancer is the rapidly growing, widely metastasizing adenocarcinoma, which occurs predominantly in middle-aged and elderly individuals. This cancer may respond briefly to one course of x-ray irradiation, but is otherwise refractory to treatment, and few patients survive longer than 2 years after its initial appearance. The second group comprises the "papillary cancers" (papillary adenocarcinomas), encountered with about equal frequency in all age groups. Its growth is slow, and its spread usually confined to the lymph nodes that drain the thyroid area. The chance of cure is excellent after surgical removal of the thyroid gland and involved nodes.

The rarest and most peculiar type of thyroid cancer is familiarly known as "benign metastasizing goiter" or "metastasizing adenoma." Each metastatic nodule, like the parent gland itself, takes up iodine with great avidity, a property that renders it vulnerable to detection and localization after the administration of ^{131}I and simple scanning with a Geiger tube. By the same token, the administration of radioactive iodine in large doses offers a practical and effective means of irradiating the tumor therapeutically, a procedure of great palliative value, especially when carried out in conjunction with thyroidectomy.

The Patient Undergoing Thyroidectomy

Preoperative Nursing Management. Patients suffering with exophthalmic goiter cannot be operated upon without requisite preoperative preparation. These extremely nervous individuals must have a period of rest in bed in the most quiet atmosphere possible. They must be protected from disturbing sights and should be placed so that they will not come in contact with very ill patients. For psychological reasons, it may be well to place this patient beside one who has made a satisfactory recovery from operation.

The nurse should see that this patient has an abundance of fresh air and an ample amount of carbohydrate and protein foods. Usually he is embarrassed about his unusually large appetite and may hesitate to ask for another helping. The nurse should recognize this dietary need, caused by increased metabolic activity and the rapid depletion of glycogen reserves. A daily caloric intake of 4,000 to 5,000 calories is not only desirable but essential. Supplementary vitamins, particularly thiamine and ascorbic acid, are necessary. Tea or coffee is not given without the permission of the physician because they are stimulants.

The nurse should gain the complete confidence of her patient and attempt to keep him free from worry and anxiety. Some forms of occupational therapy are quieting and are given at the direction of the surgeon.

The patient with hyperthyroidism often comes from a home made tense and unhappy by his restlessness, nervousness and loss of efficiency. It is necessary to protect the patient from a continuance of such unpleasantness and unhappiness. If there is any evidence of nervous upsets by visits of family or friends, it may be advisable to limit the visiting privileges during the preoperative period.

Sedatives (bromides and phenobarbital) are administered frequently, and because many older patients with hyperthyroidism have associated cardiac disease, digitalis may also be given.

Surgical Intervention. The immediate preparation of thyroid patients for surgery includes a good night's rest the preceding night, adequate shaving of the neck and upper chest (see p. 107), nothing by mouth after midnight and a preanesthetic hypodermic about 20 or 30 minutes before surgery. The operation is performed with the patient in the dorsal position, with a sandbag or air pillow under the shoulders and the head low (neck hyperextended) to make the neck more prominent. The patient's hair should be enclosed in a cap. Through a transverse incision in the lower part of the neck the thyroid is exposed and excised, leaving only a small amount of glandular tissue on the posterior capsule of the gland on each side. This small amount of thyroid tissue is all that is necessary for normal function, and an inadequate removal of the gland predisposes to a recurrence of hyperthyroidism. The wound usually is closed with clips and often is drained for a day or two.

Postoperative Nursing Management. The patient should be moved carefully, care being taken to support the head so that no tension is placed on the sutures. The most comfortable position is the semi-Fowler with the head elevated and supported by pillows. The utmost quiet is observed, and morphine is given hypodermically to relieve the painful effects of the operation. Occasionally the patient is placed in an oxygen tent for the first few hours to facilitate breathing. The nurse should anticipate apprehension in the patient and inform him that by being in the tent his breathing will be easier, and he will be less tired. Fluid may be given by vein, but water may be given by mouth as soon as nausea ceases. The nurse should inspect and reinforce the dressings when necessary, remembering that when the patient is in the dorsal position, evidences of bleeding should be looked for at the sides and the back of the neck as well as anteriorly. In addition to checking the pulse and the blood pressure, it is also important to be on the alert for complaints from the patient of a sensation of pressure or fullness at the incision site. These may indicate hemorrhage and should be reported. In many hospitals, ice bags are routinely applied over the dressing to help in bleeding control. Usually, there is a little difficulty in swallowing, and in this condition cold fluids and ice may be taken better than other fluids. Often patients prefer a soft diet to a liquid diet. Occasionally, difficulty in respiration occurs, with the development of cyanosis and noisy breathing, owing to an edema of the glottis or to an injury to the recurrent laryngeal nerve. Since this complication demands the insertion of a tracheostomy tube, the surgeon should be summoned at once.

Little talking should be permitted, but when the patient does speak, the nurse should note any voice changes, which might indicate injury to the recurrent laryngeal nerves that lie just behind the thyroid next to the trachea.

When the nurse is not in constant attendance, an overbed table is a great comfort to the patient. On it may be placed materials that are needed frequently, such as paper wipes, water pitcher and glass, small emesis basin, etc. These are kept within easy reach so that the patient is not required to turn the head in search of them. It is also convenient to use this table when inhalations are given for the relief of excessive mucous secretions.

The patient usually is permitted out of bed on the first postoperative day and has a choice of diet. A well-balanced high-caloric diet is prescribed to regain any weight loss. Sutures or skin clips usually are removed on the second day. By the fifth day, the average patient is ready for discharge from the hospital.

Complications. Hemorrhage, edema of the glottis and injury to the recurrent laryngeal nerve are complications that have been reviewed previously. Occasionally, in thyroid operations the parathyroid glandules may be injured or removed. This produces a disturbance of the calcium metabolism of the body. As the blood calcium falls, there appears a hyper-irritability of the nerves, with spasms of the hand and the feet and muscular twitchings; this group of symptoms is termed *tetany*, and its appearance should be called to the attention of the surgeon at once. Tetany of this type usually is relieved by the administration of parathyroid extract or calcium in some form.

Posthospital Care. The patient should not be permitted to resume his former activities or responsibilities in full until thyrotoxicosis has been eliminated. The necessity for rest, relaxation and nutrition is explained to both the patient and his family at the time of discharge. Specific instructions are issued regarding follow-up visits to the physician or the clinic, which are inevitably necessary and invariably important.

Responsibilities and factors relating to the home environment that engender emotional tension often have been implicated as precipitating causes of thyrotoxicosis. The patient's hospitalization affords an opportunity for a fair evaluation of these factors and perhaps alterations in the environmental situation. This is the most favorable time for establishing a close rapport with the patient and for supplying him with whatever psychological support and assistance in emotional readjustments that he may require.

THE PARATHYROID GLANDS

The parathyroid glands are 4, 6 or 8 small, bean-sized structures embedded in the posterior of the thyroid gland. These bodies furnish *parathormone*, which influences the concentrations of calcium and phosphorus in the blood and the migration of these elements between the blood and the bones. Its basic function is to promote the urinary excretion of phosphorus by preventing reabsorption of the phosphate ion by the kidney tubules.

Pathophysiology

If parathormone is inadequate, as in hypoparathyroidism, too much phosphate re-enters the blood from the renal tubules; the blood phosphate level becomes abnormally high. A reciprocal relationship exists between phosphate and calcium levels in the blood. Accordingly, in hypoparathyroidism, the blood calcium declines to an abnormally low level, to the extent that the patient may experience muscular hyperirritability and uncontrollable spasms, i.e., hypocalcemic tetany. If parathormone is excessive, too little phosphorus is retrieved from the glomerular filtrate and an excessive amount escapes in the urine. The concentration of phosphorus in the blood, therefore, declines, causing some of the calcium phosphate contained in the bones to dissolve in the blood. This additional phosphorus also is removed with dispatch by the kidneys; however, the calcium is not cleared with the same rapidity, and an elevated blood calcium results.

In summary, the net effect of parathormone is to depress the concentration of phosphorus and to increase the concentration of calcium in the blood.

Hyperparathyroidism

Hyperparathyroidism, due to an overgrowth of the parathyroid glands, is characterized by bony decalcification, the development of calcium phosphate stones in both kidneys and a depression of the neuromuscular apparatus. Parathyroid hyperactivity with similar manifestations also occurs in patients with chronic nephritis and so-called "renal rickets," presumably as a result of phosphorus retention. These patients experience symptoms of apathy, fatigue, muscular weakness, nausea, vomiting, constipation and cardiac arrhythmias, all attributable to an increased concentration of calcium in the blood.

The formation of stones in both kidneys, related to the increased urinary excretion of calcium and phosphorus, is one of the important complications of hyperparathyroidism. The renal damage that results from the precipitation of calcium phosphate in the renal pelves and parenchyma (nephrocalcinosis) often is responsible for pyelonephritis and uremia and explains many of its most prominent clinical manifestations.

The skeletal changes, however, are the characteristic hallmark of hyperparathyroidism, whether this occurs as a primary disorder or as a secondary complication of calcium and phosphorus retention in patients with chronic renal disease. There are two aspects of this bony involvement to be considered: (1) demineralization of the bones, resulting in skeletal pain and tenderness, pain on weight-bearing, pathologic fractures, deformities, shortening of body structure and the formation of bony cysts; (2) the development of bone tumors, composed of benign giant cells and representing an overgrowth of osteoclasts. This variety of neoplasm is encountered occasionally on dental examination as a tumor of the jaw, in which location it is referred to as an "epulis."

The diagnosis is established by the clinical picture, by persistently elevated serum calcium, and by skeletal changes detected by x-ray pictures. Only occasionally can a parathyroid tumor be palpated.

Treatment. The treatment of hyperparathyroidism is the surgical removal of enough parathyroid tissue to restore the calcium-phosphorus metabolism to normal. The nursing management is essentially the same as that for a thyroidectomy patient (p. 690). The patient must be closely watched to detect signs and symptoms of tetany, which is usually an early postoperative occurrence.

Hypoparathyroidism

This condition follows the operative removal of too much parathyroid tissue; also, it is encountered in association with idiopathic atrophy. Its symptoms and signs are due to a deficiency of parathormone, which results in an accumulation of phosphorus in the blood and a decrease in the concentration of blood calcium.

Tetany. The chief symptom of hypoparathyroid disease is tetany, by which is meant a general muscular hypertonia with tremor and spasmodic or incoordinated contractions following any effort to make a voluntary movement. In typical cases, there is tonic flexion of the arms at the elbows, of the wrist and of the fingers at the metacarpophalangeal joints. The muscular irritability is so great that a muscle goes into spasm following pressure on its vessel or a tap on its nerve. Spasm of the larynx and even convulsions may occur.

Tetany is caused by the low blood calcium and resembles, so far as the nervous system signs are concerned, the phenomenon that occurs in alkalosis caused by hyperventilation or that results from severe acute chloride loss from persistent vomiting.

Treatment. The treatment of hypoparathyroidism consists in elevating to normal the blood calcium level by the oral or parenteral administration of calcium salts; by injections of parathyroid extract; and by supplying ample quantities of vitamin D (or of dihydrotachysterol, a substance related chemically to vitamin D).

Patients with acute hypocalcemic tetany should promptly receive calcium lactate intravenously (e.g., 10 to 30 ml. of 10% calcium lactate in normal saline, injected as often as necessary to control symptoms). Simultaneously, 50 to 150 units of parathormone solution (0.5 to 1.5 ml.) may be given subcutaneously, intramuscularly or intravenously, and vitamin D (50,000 to 100,000 units daily) should be given by mouth. Dihydrotachysterol (AT 10, or Hytakerol), 0.5 to 1.0 ml. daily by mouth, provides a satisfactory substitute for vitamin D in maintenance therapy. The dosages of calcium, parathormone and vitamin D (or

AT 10) are controlled on the basis of serum and urinary calcium levels. The Sulkowitch test for urinary calcium (p. 546), which the patient can perform very easily, provides a reliable guide for maintenance therapy.

THE PANCREAS

The pancreas manufactures and secretes into the bloodstream two hormones, *insulin* and *glucagon*. Insulin is required for the utilization of glucose by the tissue cells as the principal source of energy for their metabolic activities. It apparently affects the transport of glucose through the cell membrane. Glucagon serves to prevent excessive drops in blood glucose concentration (hypoglycemia). Secreted in response to the development of hypoglycemia, this hormone stimulates the rapid conversion of liver glycogen to glucose (glycogenolysis), the effect of which is to elevate promptly the blood sugar.

The Patient with Diabetes Mellitus

Diabetes mellitus is a disease complex featured most prominently by hyperglycemia—an abnormally high level of blood sugar—owing to a relative insufficiency of insulin or to excessive inactivation of this hormone by chemical inhibitors or "binders" in the circulation. There are two distinct types of diabetes: juvenile diabetes and maturity onset diabetes. These forms differ not only in age of onset, but in their clinical courses and complications, and thus in their clinical management. People with juvenile diabetes usually lack insulin and require exogenous insulin therapy; those having maturity onset diabetes have insulin circulating in the blood and respond more satisfactorily to oral hypoglycemic drugs, such as tolbutamide and phenformin. Both types of diabetes produce deleterious effects on every tissue and organ system, notably, on the nervous and the vascular systems. Hyperglycemia in the absence of diabetes mellitus, having entirely different implications, occurs temporarily in people suffering from head injuries, starvation, and other conditions. Corticosteroid therapy may unmask a latent or subclinical diabetes.

Pathophysiology

Insulin promotes the storage of blood glucose as glycogen in the liver and tissue utilization of this sugar, possibly by enhancing the transport of glucose across the cell wall. In the absence of sufficient or effective insulin, partial compensation is achieved by increasing the blood sugar in order to enhance glucose transfer into the cell. Glucose in the blood comes from ingested carbohydrates or from the conversion of amino acids and fatty acids to glucose by the liver. The latter activity is called *gluconeogenesis* and is

TABLE 31-1. The nurse as a case finder

Individuals in whom diabetes mellitus should be suspected:

1. Relatives of known diabetics

2. Obese individuals

3. Mothers delivered of large babies or those who have had an abnormal obstetrical history

4. Persons with early onset of arteriosclerosis
   (a) Premenopausal women with myocardial infarction
   (b) Men having myocardial infarctions before the age of 40

5. Persons with frequent or chronic infections (gallbladder disease, pyelonephritis, pancreatitis, etc.)

6. Patients exhibiting temporary loss of glucose tolerance during stress (myocardial infarction, infection, trauma, surgery)

7. Patients developing glucose intolerance during drug therapy (thiazides, glucocorticoids, ovulatory suppressants)

8. Persons with retinopathy, nephropathy or other vascular manifestations

under the control of the adrenocortical hormones. Therefore protein and fat are mobilized rather than stored or deposited in cells; the circulation of large quantities of fats may exert an influence upon blood vessels. Ketone bodies are acid substances formed by the incomplete metabolism of fats. In diabetes, excessive amounts of ketone bodies appear in the circulation, causing acidosis. Attempts by the body to compensate for the acidosis result in hyperventilation and the loss of sodium, potassium, chloride and water. Thus, the net metabolic result is loss of fat stores, liver glycogen, cellular protein, electrolytes and water. If the intake of these substances is insufficient, acidosis and electrolyte imbalance develop. If the concentration of glucose in the blood is sufficiently high, the kidney does not reabsorb all of the filtered glucose and it appears in the urine (*glycosuria*).

Incidence

The importance of diabetes mellitus is obvious from its prevalence alone. There are now almost 4 million diabetics in the United States—that is, one out of every 50 persons in this country is diabetic. Almost half of these persons are unaware of their affliction. At the present rate of increase, it has been predicted that the number of people who will develop diabetes may exceed 10 per cent. Diabetes ranks seventh as a cause of death in the United States.

The prediction and prevention of diabetes are based on the theory that diabetes is a recessive Mendelian trait. At least one third of all patients describe the occurrence of the disease among their relatives. In fact, if both parents of an individual are diabetic, there is a 100 per cent probability that he will develop the disease. Therefore, *blood relatives of known diabetics should maintain lifelong vigilance for this condition.* Obese persons are especially susceptible to diabetes; 85 per cent of diabetics are overweight or have been overweight prior to the onset of their disease. Persons over 45 appear to be more vulnerable. Diabetes may be suspected in mothers who have delivered large babies. These high risk persons (Table 31-1) should be examined regularly for evidences of diabetes. The nurse has an important role as a case finder and in encouraging people to seek medical evaluation.

Symptoms and Course

The juvenile type of diabetes (which may occur in adults as well as children) usually has a fairly abrupt onset with weight loss, weakness, polyuria, polydipsia and at first polyphagia, although the hearty appetite may soon depart as the metabolic situation becomes unbalanced. These patients may have measurable circulating insulin early in the course of the disease, but it soon disappears. They are prone to develop ketosis and often the diagnosis is first made when they are brought to the hospital in acidosis or coma. Their diabetes is unstable even with good care and they require insulin injections for control.

The maturity onset type of diabetes usually occurs after the age of 40; 75 per cent of the patients are overweight when the condition is first discovered. Onset is insidious and symptoms may be mild. Excessive fatigue, tendency to drowse after a meal, irritability, nocturia, itching of the skin (especially about the vulva in the female), skin wounds that heal poorly, blurring of vision, loss of weight and cramps in the muscles are all warning symptoms of diabetes. In about 10 per cent of the patients, the discovery is made as the result of a routine urinalysis. In mild cases there may be no symptoms, and only a metabolic stress such as surgery or a febrile illness will call forth enough hyperglycemia to result in glycosuria. Often blood sugar tests are normal with hyperglycemia being seen only postprandially (following a meal) or as a result of a glucose tolerance test. These patients have serum insulin, but it comes forth poorly and may be somewhat abnormal.

The intensity of diabetes mellitus, as measured by blood sugar levels, tends to wax and wane, and depends on the patient's general state of health, stresses of life, dietary control, weight control, activity and other factors, many of which are not well understood. Therefore, treatment in type and amount is variable throughout the course of the disease, necessitating lifelong care if good results are to be obtained. Poorly controlled or neglected diabetes is attended ultimately with the frequent and premature development of atherosclerosis, affecting the heart, kidneys, brain and peripheral vessels. Neuropathy may develop and resistance to infections is decreased—a picture of early aging. On the other hand, meticulous control of the diabetes retards the development of these chronic complications, although it does not completely prevent them.

Diagnosis

The presence of sugar in the urine does not invariably signify diabetes mellitus. The patient may simply have a low renal threshold for sugar or have some other nondiabetic melituria. The finding of glycosuria is a signal to take further diagnostic measures. The fasting blood sugar is elevated in many cases of diabetes, but not in the milder ones. A far better test is the blood glucose taken one to two hours after a full meal or after the administration of 100 gm. of glucose. The best diagnostic test of all is the standard three-hour glucose tolerance test. This is performed by having the patient on a high-carbohydrate diet for three days preceding the test and an overnight fast the night preceding the test. On the morning of the test, a fasting blood sugar is drawn, 100 gm. of glucose is given and specimens of blood for glucose determination are taken at half-hour, one-hour, two-hour and three-hour intervals after the glucose ingestion.

Urine Testing for Glycosuria

Sugar (glucose) is present in small traces in normal urine, but not enough to be detected by ordinary tests. In certain conditions, notably untreated diabetes mellitus, much larger amounts are present.

Each nurse and each diabetic patient should be able to examine the urine for sugar. The Clinitest method, currently in wide use, involves the addition of a tablet to 5 drops of urine and 10 drops of water, measured and delivered by a medicine dropper into a test tube. The tube is placed in a rack and left undisturbed until the solution has ceased to boil. After an interval of at least 15 seconds, the color of the material is compared with a color chart, which indicates the sugar concentration.

A simple, convenient and highly specific color test for glycosuria has become available* which employs a paper strip that has been impregnated with 3 reagents: the enzymes, glucose oxidase and peroxidase, and an indicator dye, orthotolidin. The strip is merely moistened with urine, and subsequently indicates the presence of glucose.

---

* Tes-Tape; Uristix; Clinistix.

Medical and Nursing Management

The objectives of treatment are (1) to correct the biochemical and metabolic abnormalities; (2) to attain and maintain optimal body weight; and (3) to prevent the progression of the disease and avoid or postpone the complications usually associated with diabetes. Depending upon the individual patient, these objectives are accomplished by careful dietary treatment alone, or by diet and injections of insulin, or by diet and the use of oral hypoglycemic agents. With a program of *continuing* education, the health team endeavors to help the patient develop insight into his condition and live a productive and normal life. If the diabetes is under good control, the patient will have no symptoms and reactions and have a normal fasting or postprandial blood sugar and little or no glycosuria.

Diet

The dietary regimen is an important aspect of treatment. The objective of dietary management is to meet the basic nutritional requirements of the individual patient with proper proportions of protein, carbohydrates and fat in a well-balanced diet that will promote optimal body weight. The major dietary restriction is on concentrated sources of carbohydrates. The diabetic patient must consume the same number of prescribed calories daily and eat his meals at regular times. The menu is varied, with the emphasis placed on what the patient is allowed rather than on what is forbidden. Obesity is corrected as rapidly as the patient's condition permits. Some patients, particularly those who are overweight, achieve normoglycemic levels with dietary treatment alone.

In planning the diet, the first problem is ascertaining the patient's basic caloric requirement, which varies according to age, body weight and degree of activity. Generally, the normal adult leading a sedentary existence requires a diet that furnishes 30 Cal. per Kg. of body weight per day; an adult at light work, 35 to 40; and the heavy laborer, 40 to 50 (or more).

The distribution in the diet between carbohydrate, fat and protein should not deviate greatly from the usual normal well-balanced diet. However, deviation is required in the carbohydrate intake, which almost always is restricted. The usual protein allowance for the adult patient is 1.0 to 1.2 Gm. per Kg. of body weight, or 70 to 100 Gm. daily. During the process of regulation, it is important that the patient eat all, and nothing except, the diet specified for him. Food that is refused should be identified and its quantity evaluated, so that appropriate corrections can be applied in calculating the amount of protein, fat and carbohydrate actually ingested. Vomiting, or the refusal of any significant portion of the diet, should be reported to the physician. The American Diabetes Association has developed a booklet, "Meal Planning with Exchange Lists" that describes various meal plans. The foods are arranged in groups of "exchanges," and the patient is able to modify his prescribed diet by exchanging one item with another item on the same list. The foods in each exchange list have approximately the same sugar content; this facilitates the individual's meal planning and makes his diet more acceptable.

As soon as it is practicable, the diabetic patient is offered a systematic course of instruction in dietetics. Participants in this educational program, which is of paramount importance in diabetic care, are the physician, the dietitian, and the nurse, who must be sufficiently well versed in the subject to discuss its problems intelligently with the patient and to furnish his family with whatever instructions they may require relating to his diet. Responsibility for the care of the diabetic is not ended until the patient's ability to plan and follow his prescribed diet is assured.

Exercise

Exercise is very important in the treatment of the patient with diabetes mellitus because it promotes metabolism and the utilization of carbohydrates. Thus, insulin requirements of the body are diminished. There should be reasonable uniformity in the amount of exercise done from day to day.

Insulin Therapy

Many obese patients with mild, uncomplicated diabetes may control their disease solely by means of a low-caloric diet, without insulin. Many patients who are not obese, whose diabetes is mild and who have experienced the onset of diabetes during their adult years, can control it satisfactorily by diet plus one of the oral hypoglycemic drugs, such as Orinase (tolbutamide). However, all diabetic children, all diabetic adults who have lost an excessive amount of weight, all diabetics with acute complications and all individuals with severe diabetes require regular hypodermic injections of insulin.

The major physiologic action of insulin is the lowering of the blood sugar by facilitating the uptake and utilization of glucose by the tissues. It also affects fat and protein metabolism as well as electrolytes.

Seven insulin preparations are available for therapeutic administration. Insulin preparations are prescribed in units and are available in various concentrations (U 40 and U 80 concentrations are the most frequently used). Which preparation the physician selects depends on the onset of action desired, time of

TABLE 31-2. Insulin preparations

Action	Type of Insulin	Time of onset (hr.)	Peak (hr.)	Duration (hr.)	Time when hypoglycemia most apt to occur
Rapid	Crystalline Zinc (regular)	Within hour or less	2-4	5-7	Before lunch
	Semi-lente	1	6-10	12-16	Before lunch
Intermediate	Globin	2-4	6-12	18-24	Late afternoon
	NPH	2-4	8-12	24-28	Late afternoon
	Lente	2-4	8-12	24-28	Late afternoon
Slow	Protamine Zinc	3-6	14-20	36+	During night and early morning
	Ultralente	8	16-24	36+	During night and early morning

peak effect required and the duration of action. It is important that both the patient and the nurse know when insulin is having its effect. Knowing when hypoglycemia is most apt to occur will assist the nurse in assessing the patient's symptoms and behavior. (See Table 31-2.)

Teaching the Patient Self-injection of Insulin. As soon as the need for insulin therapy has been established, patient education should begin. From the very beginning the patient is instructed in the technique of self-injection. It is natural for a person to be reluctant to inject himself with a needle; the nurse should anticipate this reluctance. An optimistic approach will offer the patient encouragement.

Give the patient the prepared syringe containing the prescribed dose of insulin and instruct him to hold it like a pencil. The nurse can prepare the skin with alcohol. Show the patient how to hold the skin taut on the anterior surface of the thigh. If the patient is very thin, a skin fold is formed by picking up sub-

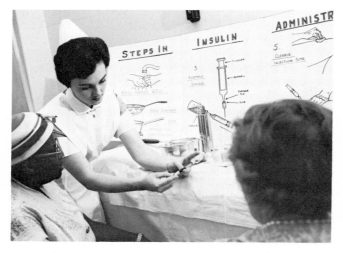

Fig. 31-2. The nurse is using charts and demonstration to teach self-administration of insulin to patients. This will be followed by a return demonstration. (The Bryn Mawr Hospital School of Nursing)

cutaneous tissue between two fingers. The skin fold is released after the needle is inserted (Fig. 31-3B). If necessary, steady the patient's hand and assist him to insert the needle with a quick thrust up to the hub at a right angle to the skin surface (see Fig. 31-3A). The patient then exerts slight traction on the plunger to be sure that the needle is not in a blood vessel and then pushes the plunger with a downward motion. The insulin is injected into deep subcutaneous tissue. After the patient has mastered the injection technique, he can be taught care and sterilization of the syringe, how to withdraw the insulin from the vial, and so forth. A member of the patient's family should also be instructed in this important phase of diabetic management.

Injection sites should be systemically rotated to prevent scar tissue from developing, which would interfere with subsequent absorption of insulin (see Fig. 31-4). Have the patient keep a record of each injection site and emphasize avoiding the use of the same site for two weeks. There is now available a preset attachment for insulin syringes that limits the dosage to a predetermined amount. Thus a patient with a visual handicap is able to load his own syringe. If the patient continues to be fearful about injecting himself, an automatic injector can be used.

Regulation of Dosage. The dosage of insulin is adjusted according to the presence (or absence) and the degree of glycosuria, and its time of appearance in relation to insulin injections and meals. The regulation of insulin dosage is aided further by determinations of the blood sugar level, which should be measured periodically during the period of hospitalization. The results of these tests should be charted each time for evaluation. In preparation for this task, hospitalized diabetics should have ample opportunity to observe and rehearse the method of urinalysis that they will use after discharge. Indeed, it is good practice to conduct these tests, occasionally at least, at the patient's bedside from the very beginning.

In the absence of complications, treatment may be

started with 10 to 20 units of NPH insulin, given subcutaneously just before breakfast; this dosage may be increased at 2- to 7-day intervals, if necessary, by additions of 5 to 10 units until glycosuria is absent throughout the day and the night and the fasting blood sugar level is normal. If the diabetes is obviously severe, larger doses are employed from the outset and are increased as rapidly as necessary. Patients receiving NPH insulin who exhibit glycosuria during the daytime only may receive supplementary injections

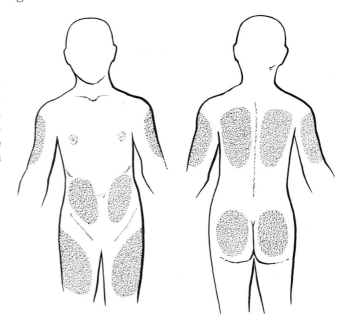

Fig. 31-4. Sites for insulin injection.

of regular or crystalline zinc insulin. The latter is given in an initial dosage of 4 to 8 units, 2 to 8 units more being administered each day until glycosuria is controlled completely. The dosage of NPH insulin meanwhile is lowered, if necessary, in order to reduce the risk of delayed hypoglycemic reactions, which can be very dangerous, especially if they occur at night while the patient is asleep.

This regimen usually provides adequate control of the diabetes, especially if the carbohydrate intake is distributed appropriately. These patients should receive bedtime nourishment consisting of 10 to 20 gm. of carbohydrate, together with whatever fat and protein may be required to make this nourishment palatable. The remainder of the carbohydrate quota is divided as follows: one fifth for breakfast, two fifths for lunch and two fifths for supper. Those patients receiving combinations of NPH and crystalline (or regular) insulin before breakfast may be allotted one third of their carbohydrate quota at breakfast time, one third at lunch and one third at supper time, but a portion of the noon allotment (e.g., one serving of fruit) is prescribed as a midmorning snack, and an equal or larger portion of the evening meal is deferred until bedtime. Patients receiving NPH or globin insulin should have a midafternoon snack.

Complications of Insulin Treatment. *Hypoglycemic Reactions.* These are likely to occur when for any reason the blood sugar falls below 60 mg. per 100 ml. of blood. They result usually from the omission of a meal or the vomiting of a meal after taking insulin.

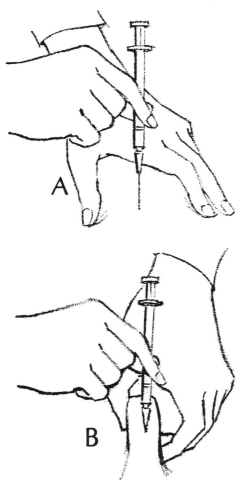

Fig. 31-3A. The insulin syringe is held perpendicular to the stretched skin before the needle is thrust into the subcutaneous tissue. (B) A skin fold is formed for the injection when a patient has only a thin layer of subcutaneous fat. This technique ensures that the needle tip is inserted into the subcutaneous tissue and outside the muscle. (From Coates, F. C., and Fabrykant, M.: An insulin injection technique for preventing skin reactions. Amer J. Nurs., February, 1965)

If unconscious or acting strangely I may be having a reaction to insulin or to an oral medicine taken for diabetes.

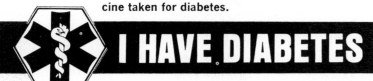

I HAVE DIABETES

If I can swallow give me sugar, candy, fruit juice or a sweetened drink. If this does not bring recovery or I can not swallow call a physician or send me to a hospital quickly for administration of glucose or glucagon.

Distributed by
AMERICAN DIABETES ASSOCIATION, INC. • 18 East 48th St. • New York, N.Y. 10017

NAME		PHONE	
ADDRESS			
	(Street)	(City)	(State)
PHYSICIAN		PHONE	
ADDRESS			
	(Street)	(City)	(State)

INSULIN	DOSAGE	TIME	ORAL MEDICATION	DOSAGE	TIME
Regular			Orinase		
PZI			Diabinese		
Globin			Dymelor		
NPH			Tolinase		
Lente			DBI		
Semilente			DBI-TD		
Ultralente					
	DATE			© 1966	

Fig. 31-5. A sample identification card carried by diabetics on insulin to ensure the correct diagnosis and treatment if found in hypoglycemic shock.

Some attacks follow undue exertion. The majority of attacks occur in the morning and in the early evening.

These reactions begin 5 to 20 minutes following an injection of regular insulin, but not for several hours after NPH insulin is given. *The symptoms and the signs should be familiar to every nurse, and the warning symptoms should be described carefully to every diabetic patient receiving insulin.* If the blood sugar falls to a level between 70 and 50 mg. per 100 ml., general muscular weakness develops, together with mental confusion, restlessness, profuse sweating, vertigo, pallor or flushing of the face, trembling and, occasionally, hunger pangs in the epigastrium. If the level drops rapidly to below 50 or 40 mg. per 100 ml., the patient may become comatose. Some patients experience hypoglycemia so rapidly that the symptoms progress almost without warning to those of epileptiform convulsions. Hypoglycemic reactions exhibited by patients receiving NPH insulin may not follow this typical pattern; instead of pallor and sweating, the skin may be flushed, hot and dry, the patient disoriented and psychotic, or merely drowsy.

For immediate treatment, when the warning symptoms appear, the patient should take a drink containing sugar or eat a piece of candy. All patients on insulin should carry a chocolate bar, a few lumps of sugar or several crackers in their pockets. Such carbohydrate ingestion checks the reaction within a few minutes. If the patient is unconscious, *glucose* may be injected intravenously. A subcutaneous injection of *epinephrine* (0.3 to 0.5 ml. of a 1:1,000 solution) or *glucagon hydrochloride* (0.5 to 1.0 mg.) may be administered with the object of raising the blood sugar sufficiently to restore the patient to consciousness long enough to accept a sweetened drink, the effect of which will become manifest after perhaps 10 minutes and will terminate the attack.

In order to be assured of a correct diagnosis and prompt treatment if discovered in a hypoglycemic state, every diabetic receiving insulin always should carry on his person an identification card similar to the type shown in Figure 31-5.

Local Allergic Reactions. These consist of erythematous wheals, which usually disappear in the course of a few days. They may follow injections of insulin during the beginning stages of therapy. If such reactions continue to occur, crystalline insulin should be tried, because many of these allergic manifestations represent a sensitivity on the part of the patient to beef or pig protein present in the regular, but absent in the crystalline, product.

Insulin Lumps. These may appear at spots where injections are repeated at too frequent intervals. In these areas, absorption is diminished, and there is an increased susceptibility to local infection.

Localized Fat-tissue and Muscle-tissue Atrophy. This develops on rare occasions at the sites of injection and requires several months for restoration. Trials with other insulin preparations—for example, those prepared from other animals or the crystalline product—are indicated. Injection of insulin into these sites is to be avoided.

Local Abscess of Fat Necrosis. Occasionally, fat tissue necrosis and abscesses may develop at a site of repeated insulin injection. These lesions are characterized by swelling, fluctuation, redness and pain, depending upon whether infection is present or not. Incision and drainage are usually necessary.

Oral Hypoglycemic Agents

Effective control of diabetes mellitus by orally administered medication has become possible for some diabetic patients with the development of orally effective hypoglycemic agents. These drugs are of two types:

1. Sulfonylureas, which appear to act by stimulating the pancreas to produce or release insulin. These are tolbutamide (Orinase), chlorpropamide (Diabinese), acetohexamide (Dymelor) and tolazamide (Tolinase).

2. Biguanide compounds exemplified by phenformin (DBI and its long-acting form, DBI-TD), whose mode of action is not known. Table 31-3 shows the tablet size and dose range of these compounds. The major difference among the sulfonylurea drugs is their duration of action, the Orinase being the shortest in action (6 to 12 hours) chlorpropamide, the longest (24 to 60 hours), and the others in between. DBI lasts 4 to 6 hours, and DBI-TD, 8 to 12 hours. DBI-TD given at 12-hour intervals has pretty much replaced the short-acting DBI.

The oral agents are not useful for every diabetic. (See p. 695 for patients requiring insulin injections.) Overweight diabetics should receive neither oral agents nor insulin (except in emergencies), but should reduce their body weight by proper diet. Oral hypoglycemic agents function best in those diabetics with the maturity type onset who are over 40 years of age and who require less than 40 units of insulin daily.

TABLE 31-3. Oral hypoglycemic agents

Agent	Tablet Size	Usual Daily Dose
Sulfonylurea Group		
1. Tolbutamide (Orinase)	0.5 gm.	0.5-2 gm.
2. Chlorpropamide (Diabinese)	100 mg.; 250 mg.	100-500 mg.
3. Acetohexamide (Dymelor)	250 mg.; 500 mg.	250 mg.-1.5 gm.
4. Tolazamide (Tolinase)	100 mg.; 250 mg.	100 mg.-1.0 gm.
Biguanide Group		
1. Phenformin (DBI)	25 mg.	50-200 mg.
2. Phenformin, long-acting (DBI-TD)	50 mg. (capsule)	50-200 mg.

These agents have no place in the treatment of diabetes during acute complications or at the time of surgery and they cannot prevent the development of ketosis in such situations.

All the sulfonylurea agents can produce hypoglycemia, but this is more likely to occur with chlorpropamide than with the other agents and more likely to occur in the elderly than in the young. Phenformin does not cause hypoglycemia, but tends to provoke gastrointestinal upsets. "Secondary failures" of up to 30 per cent have been reported with these agents after one year's use, but only 7 to 10 per cent of these are truly drug failures. The rest are really dietary failures and the unhappiest consequence of oral therapy for diabetics is the unconscious or conscious dietary relaxation on the part of the patient. The disciplinary effect of the daily injection is gone.

Complications of Diabetes

Acidosis and Coma

One of the most important functions of the nurse engaged in diabetic management is to be on the lookout for symptoms suggesting the onset of coma, the most severe complication of diabetes mellitus, yet one that is entirely preventable and, if treated promptly and energetically, in most patients, curable. Patients with severe cases of diabetes are constantly faced with this threat. Its onset may be precipitated by many factors, including infections of all types, exposure and dietary indiscretions. The early symptoms include thirst, anorexia, nausea, vomiting, abdominal pain, headache, listlessness, drowsiness, weakness, vertigo, ringing in the ears, visual disturbances, excitement or delirium. Coma is ushered in with symptoms of air hunger (Kussmaul breathing), characterized by

COMPARATIVE STUDY OF DIABETIC KETOACIDOSIS AND HYPOGLYCEMIA

The Patient with Diabetic Ketoacidosis

Definition

A lack of insulin resulting in a derangement of carbohydrate, fat and protein metabolism with dehydration and electrolyte imbalance.

Symptoms and Signs

Restlessness
Dry skin
Flushed face
Thirst
Vomiting
Abdominal pain
Appears hot, dry, flushed

Drowsiness
Rapid pulse
Deep respirations
Lowered pulse pressure
Coma

Objectives and Principles of Management

I. To restore carbohydrate utilization and correct electrolyte imbalance

  A. Secure blood and urine samples immediately
    1. Insert indwelling catheter (if so ordered by physician)
    2. Obtain specimen at prescribed times
    3. Report blood glucose, CO_2, pH, electrolyte, acetone, BUN and hematocrit levels

  B. Administer rapid acting insulin: ⅓ of initial dose I.V. and ⅔ subcutaneously; all insulin thereafter, subcutaneously
    1. Report blood glucose levels to the physician
    2. Give doses of insulin as ordered

  C. Replace fluids and electrolytes
    1. Give isotonic saline/sodium lactate solution I.V. to replace sodium loss
    2. Give supplementary potassium if ordered
    3. Measure and record intake and output
    4. Offer potassium-rich and sweetened fluids (orange juice) as soon as tolerated

  D. Treat for circulatory collapse if present
    1. Record vital signs every ½ hour
    2. Elevate the lower extremities
    3. Administer vasopressors as ordered

  E. Prepare for gastric lavage if ordered

  F. Obtain electrocardiograms as ordered

Objectives and Principles of Management

II. To prevent the recurrence of diabetic ketoacidosis
  A. Avoid infection
  B. Make insulin and dietary adjustments during the periods of illness

The Patient with Hypoglycemia

Definition

Low blood sugar, usually resulting from excessive insulin caused either by excessive insulin intake or by absorption from a tumor of an islet of Langerhans.

Symptoms and Signs

Headache
Nervousness
Hunger
Faintness
Sweating
Tremor
Appears cool, moist, pale

Tachycardia or
  bradycardia
Slurred speech
Irrational behavior
Convulsion
Coma

Objectives and Principles of Management

I. To restore normal cerebral function as quickly as possible

  A. Secure blood and urine samples

  B. Prepare intravenous injection of 50 per cent glucose

  C. Prepare glucagon for subsequent use if necessary

  D. Obtain intravenous equipment for glucose infusion

  E. Remain with patient until he regains consciousness

  F. Have oral carbohydrates available

  G. Watch patient closely for evidences of recurrent hypoglycemia

Objectives and Principles of Management

II. To prevent the recurrence of a hypoglycemic reaction
  A. Reduce insulin dose
  B. Test the urine 4 times daily for sugar and ketone
  C. Adjust the patient's diet according to the patient's clinical response

COMPARATIVE STUDY OF DIABETIC KETOACIDOSIS
AND HYPOGLYCEMIA (*Continued*)

The Patient with Diabetic Ketoacidosis (*Continued*)	The Patient with Hypoglycemia (*Continued*)
Objectives and Principles of Management (*Continued*)	Objectives and Principles of Management (*Continued*)

The Patient with
Diabetic Ketoacidosis (*Continued*)

Objectives and Principles of Management (*Continued*)

C. Teach the patient to:
  1. Accept responsibility for following his plan of care
  2. Keep in balance his regimen of diet, insulin, and exercise
  3. Keep his urine sugar free
  4. Eat prescribed diet regularly
  5. Increase his food during periods of exercise
  6. Inform his physician when infection, vomiting, or diarrhea are present

The Patient with
Hypoglycemia (*Continued*)

Objectives and Principles of Management (*Continued*)

D. Plan exercises according to the patient's individual needs

E. Teach the patient to:
  1. Understand and develop an awareness of the actions of insulin
  2. Keep in balance his regimen of diet, insulin, and exercise
  3. Eat when the symptoms of hypoglycemia *first* occur
  4. Carry candy or lump sugar in his pocket
  5. Have available vials of injectable glucagon hydrochloride

*To facilitate recognition and treatment, instruct the patient
to carry an identification card on his person at all times* (Fig. 31-5).

very deep, yet not labored, respiratory movements—a symptom of profound acidosis. The breath has a sweetish odor. The patient is drowsy and soon becomes comatose. Examination of the blood at this time reveals a high sugar concentration (and often an elevated N.P.N.), a low CO_2-combining power and increased acidity. The urine output may be diminished, and urinalysis shows marked glycosuria and the presence of ketone bodies. The situation at this stage is serious, but if therapy is initiated at once and pursued vigorously, improvement in most patients is evident within a few hours, and recovery is complete within 1 to 3 days.

The patient with incipient coma should be put to bed, kept warm and immediately given 25 to 50 units of insulin subcutaneously. Thereafter insulin is injected at intervals of one-half to 2 hours in doses of 15 to 50 units, depending on the degree of glycosuria and ketonuria. Larger doses are safe only if the blood sugar level can be determined before each injection. If the patient is unable to void, catheterization is advisable because of the necessity for repeated collections and tests of the urine at this stage of treatment. Parenteral fluids are supplied in liberal amounts and consist of electrolyte repair solutions containing sodium, chloride and potassium ions and dextrose, because death in diabetic coma usually is attributable to dehydration and electrolyte imbalance. Norepinephrine is kept available in anticipation of the advent of vascular collapse.

Complete Diabetic Coma. This necessitates exactly the same procedure, except that all fluids have to be given parenterally, and the insulin should be given at more frequent intervals (perhaps every hour). Ideally, each dose should depend on a blood sugar and blood ketone determination. Once the glycosuria begins to decrease, glucose should be added to the parenteral fluids so that hypoglycemia does not supervene. Decreasing ketonemia signals an increase in insulin sensitivity and requires a decrease in insulin dosage.

Another immediate need of the patient in diabetic coma is for sodium, which may be injected intravenously in the form of sodium chloride. For the treatment of acidotic patients with renal failure, the physiologically correct proportions of sodium and chloride ions (approximately 3 to 2) are provided in the intravenous solution.

Another dangerous possible occurrence is a deficiency in the concentration of potassium in the blood, giving rise to paralytic complications. This occurs because of the rapid migration of potassium ions from the body fluids into the cells. In order to maintain its concentration in the blood, Butler's mixture or another source of potassium is included among the parenteral fluids administered. By about the sixth hour of therapy, the electrocardiogram and serum potassium levels will indicate potassium need.

Electrolyte solutions are injected continuously until dehydration and acidosis are controlled, the urine output has improved and the patient is no longer comatose. Procrastination in fluid replacement may be responsible for the complication of hemoglobinuric nephrosis, with the patient perhaps recovering from his stupor, electrolyte imbalance, hyperglycemia and dehydration, only to relapse and finally succumb in terminal uremia.

Nursing Problems. Constant nursing care is an extremely important aspect of treatment in cases of diabetic coma, which is to be regarded in all respects as an emergency situation and treated as such. The patient is protected from excessive cooling by the application of extra blankets, and with the addition of an external heat source if the situation warrants.

The nurse is responsible for seeing that all necessary equipment has been assembled and all preparations made for emergency treatment, such as gastric lavage, catheterization, collection of venous blood, enemas, intravenous or subcutaneous infusions, blood transfusions, insulin injections, and parenteral stimulants. Frequent recordings are made of the blood pressure and the pulse rate, and the total amounts of parenteral fluid and insulin received and the time of their administration are noted. The nursing notes should provide a concise description of the current situation, including the patient's clinical status and details regarding any change for better or for worse.

Treatment, unless hopelessly delayed, should be successful in the vast majority of cases, consciousness being restored and all metabolic disturbances corrected within 24 to 48 hours. The problem then becomes one of diabetic regulation, the various aspects of which have been considered. The precipitating cause of the coma and the manner of its onset must be investigated to prevent a recurrence.

Infections

Infections are more difficult to treat in the diabetic, both because susceptibility to them may be increased and because the diabetes itself becomes temporarily more severe in the course of infections. Every means must be utilized to prevent infections, and their early diagnosis is imperative. Chest roentgenograms should be taken in the course of the diabetic study to rule out tuberculosis; they should be part of the routine examination of all diabetics, among whom the incidence of tuberculosis is significantly higher than it is among the general population. Its prognosis, however, if both the infection and the carbohydrate metabolism are well controlled, is probably no less favorable than in the absence of diabetes. Once a local infection is present, it is difficult to control. Moreover, the usual insulin treatments may be ineffective in an acute spreading infection. In these cases, it may be necessary to determine blood sugar every 12 hours to have an accurate picture of the diabetic state and to guide treatment.

Chronic Complications

The chronic complications of diabetes mellitus are primarily vascular in nature and affect the arteries throughout the body, particularly the eyes (diabetic retinopathy), the kidneys (diabetic nephropathy), the heart (coronary atherosclerosis) and the extremities (peripheral atherosclerosis and peripheral arterial insufficiency). The peripheral and the autonomic nervous systems may be involved either directly or by changes in their vascular supply, causing diabetic neuropathy. The vascular changes of the aging process seem to be accelerated in the diabetic. Myocardial infarction and arteriosclerotic gangrene occur far more frequently and they occur earlier in the diabetic than in the general populace. Good control of the diabetes may retard their development, but such complications cannot be prevented with certainty.

Education of the Diabetic Patient

Diabetes mellitus is a chronic disease requiring skillful, exacting and continuous care. Controls can never be relaxed; therefore, since professional supervision is only occasional, the responsibility for carrying out treatment must rest with the patient himself to a large extent. As long as the course of the disease is uneventful, the patient functions as his own physician, nurse and laboratory technician. In preparation for this role, the patient must be well educated, not only in the problems of diabetes, but also in matters pertaining to nutrition, preventive medicine, general health and hygiene. This educational program is extended whenever possible to include at least one responsible member of the patient's family.

Patient's Conception of the Disease

The patient must have a clear conception of the general character of diabetes. He must realize that his body metabolism is, and always will be, embarrassed by a deficiency in a chemical required for normal food utilization, but that this defect can be met satisfactorily by means of certain dietary adjustments, supplemented, if necessary, by the administration of certain drugs. He should understand that, provided he follows faithfully the regimen prescribed for him, his prospects for a long, happy and effective life are excellent. Optimism along these lines, tempered with caution, is highly beneficial to build morale and to provide a motive for self-discipline. On the other hand, avoid the implication that the patient is "one of the afflicted": an individual set apart, unable to identify with the normal group.

A completely favorable prognosis, would imply that no irreversible damage to the vascular system had occurred before treatment was begun and that future damage can be prevented by perfect regulation of the diabetes. Unfortunately, however, this may not be the case; diabetic patients are unusually subject to the development of arteriosclerotic vascular disease, which in many instances is well-established before medical attention is sought. Obviously, irreparable disabilities already present should not be emphasized unnecessarily. On the other hand, the patient must be familiar with the preventable complications of diabetes in order to understand his own responsibilities in connection with their early recognition and their prevention.

Social service departments are usually instrumental in providing the equipment needed for insulin injections and urinalyses, if they cannot be secured otherwise because of economic reasons. The public health nurse often serves an important role in the education of the diabetic patient, instructing him in hygienic precautions, the interpretation of urine tests and the self-administration of insulin. Group instruction has proved to be an effective method of education, and diabetic clinics organized on this basis by physicians, hospitals and public health departments have contributed much to the comfort, welfare and security of these patients. A summary of the major elements of treatment that the diabetic patient must know about appears on page 704.

Prognosis

No conclusive evidence exists of a cure of diabetes mellitus. Prolonged amelioration of the disorder has been observed; this, however, does not result from therapy but is related to metabolic changes in the individual (e.g., associated with the correction of obesity or the healing of an infection). However, although the underlying metabolic disorder may persist indefinitely, it can be compensated for satisfactorily by means of a proper diet and insulin regimen. These measures, together with those designed to improve the general condition of the patient, restore to the diabetic a metabolic state that is essentially normal. If treatment is begun early, before arteriosclerotic changes have appeared, and is directed skillfully and followed faithfully, there is every reason to anticipate a reasonable life expectancy.

Hyperinsulinism

This disorder develops as a result of the overproduction of insulin by the pancreatic islets. Its symptoms resemble those that follow excessive doses of insulin and are attributable to the same mechanism—an abnormal reduction in the concentration of blood sugar. Clinically, it is characterized by episodes during which the patient experiences unusual hunger, nervousness, sweating, headache and faintness; in severe cases, convulsive seizures and episodes of unconsciousness may occur. The findings at operation or postmortem examination may indicate hyperplasia (overgrowth) of the islets of Langerhans, or a benign or malignant tumor involving the islets and capable of producing large amounts of insulin. Occasionally, tumors of nonpancreatic origin produce an insulin-like material that can cause hypoglycemia. This condition occasionally is responsible for epileptiform seizures, convulsions coinciding with decreases in the blood sugar concentration to levels which are inadequate to sustain normal brain function (i.e., below 30 mg. %).

As in patients with hypoglycemia due to insulin therapy, all of the symptoms that accompany the spontaneous variety are relieved by the oral or parenteral administration of glucose. Surgical extirpation of the hyperplastic or neoplastic tissue from the pancreas offers the only successful method of treatment. About 15 per cent of people with spontaneous (functional) hypoglycemia eventually develop diabetes mellitus.

Hypoglycemic shock due to injections of insulin has been discussed as a complication of diabetic management. Its purposeful induction in nondiabetic patients has been employed with some success in treating certain mental diseases, notably schizophrenia, although its therapeutic value in these patients has not been satisfactorily explained.

Special Nursing Emphasis

Any infection in a diabetic is a source of potential danger, because organisms thrive and spread more rapidly when blood sugar content is above normal. Whether the patient with diabetes has had surgery or is to have surgery, the principles of care remain the same. Essentially, trauma to tissues must be minimized and the metabolic balance must be maintained. Otherwise, the patient risks the hazards of spreading infection with necrosis and experiences the metabolic imbalances of diabetic coma or insulin shock. When a wound is present, aseptic technique must be followed in an attempt to prevent infection from spreading.

The nurse is responsible for serving an attractive diet. She should note and report what has not been eaten, so that a proper substitute may be made to maintain metabolic balance. She is also responsible for the collection of urine and blood specimens and their proper disposition to the laboratory. These two functions are as important as the giving of medications.

The diabetic surgical patient may face any one or all 3 of the following disturbances which interfere with a properly balanced metabolism: (1) vomiting—this should be inspected for food loss and reported so

PATIENT EDUCATION
The Patient with Diabetes Mellitus

The diabetic must accept a major role in the management of his disease. His education must be amplified, reinforced and updated continuously, since diabetes is a lifelong disease.

Objective: To maintain the best possible control of diabetes.

I. To become familiar with diabetes and how it affects the body
   A. Visit the physician on a regular basis
   B. Study and review available literature from reputable sources (physician, A.M.A.)
   C. Secure booklets and pamphlets from the American Diabetes Association
   D. Attend available classes

II. To maintain health at an optimal level
   A. Maintain a daily routine that is fairly consistent
   B. Get adequate rest and sleep
   C. Exercise regularly and consistently
      1. Avoid "spurts" of arduous exercise before meals
      2. Exercise 1½ hours after meals
      3. Keep some form of carbohydrate (sugar, candy, orange juice) available during exercise periods
   D. Seek employment with regular hours

III. To follow the prescribed dietary regimen
   A. Consume a constant daily diet three times a day
   B. Become thoroughly familiar with the "Meal Planning Booklet"
   C. Learn how to follow a calculated diet
   D. Know the caloric value of foods frequently eaten
   E. Use household measures or a gram scale until serving sizes can be judged accurately
   F. Avoid concentrated carbohydrates
   G. Keep weight at optimal level
      1. Weigh weekly
      2. Keep a weight record
   H. Eat extra calories when unusual physical activity is anticipated, (if taking insulin)
   I. Eat a bedtime snack, when taking insulin if permissible

IV. To be aware of the degree of diabetic control
   A. Test urine for both *sugar* and *acetone* at each testing
   B. Test urine upon arising, before lunch, in late afternoon and at bedtime while control is being attained or during periods of illness
   C. Test urine at least once daily during periods of good control
   D. Test only freshly voided urine
   E. Keep a daily record of urine sugar tests (date, hour, color reaction)
   F. Take the record of urine tests to physician at appointed times
   G. Know that acetone in the urine indicates need for *more insulin*
   H. Avoid handling reagent tablets
   I. Protect test tapes from light, moisture and heat

V. To become familiar with all aspects of insulin usage
   A. Know when the prescribed insulin is having its peak action
   B. Adjust insulin dosage according to urine sugar tests as prescribed
   C. Rotate the sites of insulin injections in a systematic manner
   D. Keep the sterile syringe and needle in the same place
   E. Keep an extra insulin syringe available
   F. Know the conditions that produce insulin reactions
      1. Omission of a meal
      2. Unaccustomed or strenuous exercise
      3. Too much insulin
   G. Know the symptoms of an insulin reaction
      1. Any unfamiliar or peculiar sensation
      2. Hunger, perspiration, palpitation, tachycardia, weakness, tremor, pallor
   H. Know how to combat an impending insulin reaction
      1. Eat carbohydrates (sugar, orange juice, candy) when symptoms first occur
      2. Test urine
      3. Carry extra carbohydrate at all times (sugar lumps, candy)
      4. Eat extra carbohydrate before strenuous exercise and during periods of prolonged exercise
      5. Eat a snack at bedtime
   I. Carry diabetic identification card

PATIENT EDUCATION (*Continued*)

VI. To take prescribed oral hypoglycemic medication

    A. Adhere faithfully to the prescribed diet

    B. Test the urine daily

    C. Take the medication exactly as directed

VII. To appreciate the importance of proper foot care

    A. Inspect the feet carefully and routinely for calluses, corns, blisters and abrasions

    B. Bathe the feet in warm (never hot) water daily

    C. Massage the feet with a lanolin preparation, except between the toes

    D. Prevent moisture between the toes
       1. Insert lamb's wool between overlapping toes
       2. Use powder in the web spaces

    E. Wear the correct shoe and sock sizes

    F. Trim the toenails straight across

    G. Go to a podiatrist on a regular basis if corns, calluses and ingrown toenails are present

    H. Avoid injuries to the feet

    I. If an injury occurs to the feet
       1. Wash the area with soap and water
       2. Cover with a dry sterile dressing *without* adhesive

       3. Call the physician

    J. Do foot exercises regularly

VIII. To maintain diabetic control during periods of illness

    A. Call physician when any unusual symptoms become evident

    B. Make dietary adjustments during illness according to physician's directions

    C. Continue taking insulin

    D. Test urine for sugar and acetone more frequently

    E. Know the conditions that bring about diabetic acidosis
       1. Nausea and vomiting
       2. Failure to increase insulin when urine sugar is increasing
       3. Failure to take insulin
       4. Dietary excesses

    F. Know how to combat impending diabetic acidosis
       1. Examine urine for sugar and acetone, and report results to physician
       2. Take additional insulin as advised by physician
       3. Go to bed and keep warm
       4. Alert someone to be in attendance
       5. Drink a glass of liquid hourly if possible

---

that essential food value may be replaced intravenously; (2) starvation—prior to surgery, a patient is placed on nothing by mouth. Infusions of glucose and injections of insulin are used to maintain balance; (3) febrile reactions—these are sufficient to upset carbohydrate metabolism, and appropriate steps must be taken to maintain metabolic balance by increasing insulin. In addition to the above, an adequate protein reserve must be established prior to operation and the salt and water balance must be maintained.

Diabetes with the threat of coma or insulin shock requires close attention and observation on the part of the nurse. She should have insulin and intravenous glucose solution on hand for immediate use in any possible emergency. Moreover, nondiabetic complications, such as coronary artery thrombosis, tend to occur in the older diabetic patient.

The Diabetic Patient Undergoing Surgery

Surgery is not used to treat diabetes; however, diabetics may require surgery for other conditions, some of them complications of diabetes. A patient with diabetes is usually considered a poor operative risk. This is due, in part, to the fact that the majority of

such patients are elderly and already in a state of general decline, or are prematurely "old" because of early arteriosclerosis. Resistance to infection is low, healing is usually delayed, and serious diabetic complications, such as coma, often follow minor infections and even minor operative procedures. With the advent of insulin and the facilities for chemical analysis of the blood, the prognosis for the diabetic has improved materially. The metabolic problems that previously complicated nearly every surgical operation now can be handled by proper pre- and postoperative treatment.

Insulin and the administration of glucose, either by mouth (orange juice) or intravenously, are the usual preoperative measures. Fluids should be supplied in abundance. For minor surgery, the only change in the diabetic patient's routine may be the intravenous administration of 1 liter of 5 per cent glucose in water in place of a meal prior to surgery. For major surgery it is preferable to place the patient on a "4 equal feeding regular insulin program" the day before surgery; this program is continued postoperatively until he is stabilized and able to resume his ordinary regimen. This program divides the 24-hour day into equal intervals of 6 hours each (such as 7 A.M., 1 P.M., 7 P.M. and

1 A.M.). Testing of the urine for sugar and acetone and the administration of regular insulin and ¼ of the 24-hour total caloric allowance orally or intravenously are carried out at these hours. This program allows more precise control of the diabetes, and the surgical procedure may be performed whenever desired or required. The feeding prior to surgery should be parenteral glucose. After the patient is stabilized postoperatively and afebrile, he may resume the former 3-meal program and his former insulin program. This 4-equal-feeding-program is also useful in acute nonsurgical situations, such as pneumonia, myocardial infarction, labor and delivery.

Whenever possible, local anesthesia is generally preferred for diabetics; however, in major procedures, any of the usual general anesthetics are acceptable when administered by a skilled anesthesiologist using modern techniques.

Postoperatively, food and fluids are given as soon as possible, with sufficient insulin to prevent acidosis. Because postoperative vomiting may often occur, it is the practice in some clinics to pass a nasogastric tube before or immediately after operation. Fluids and liquid foods may be given slowly by this method almost immediately after operation. The operations most commonly performed on diabetics are amputations for gangrene. The utmost care must be employed in dressing the wounds of diabetics to prevent infection.

Gangrene of the toes and the foot is the most frequent surgical complication of the diabetic, resulting from the early development of arteriosclerosis. See page 330 for measures in the care of the feet. It results from the early development of arteriosclerosis. The cold and painful extremities that are the premonitory signs of gangrene are often carelessly treated by heat, and burns, which occur too often, may mark the onset of gangrene. The treatment of early gangrene has been described elsewhere (p. 344).

THE ADRENAL GLAND

Each adrenal gland represents in fact two different glands having different anatomic characteristics and different functions in the endocrine system. In some animals, these structures are actually separate in location; in man, however, they are fused together and incorporated in one organ, forming the cortex and medullary portion of each adrenal gland.

The medulla of the adrenal gland is the sole source of epinephrine and produces about ½ of the total supply of 1-norepinephrine in the body, both hormones being secreted in response to nerve impulses transmitted by way of the sympathetic nervous system. The cortex of the adrenal, on the other hand, receives its controlling stimuli by way of the bloodstream, delivered in the form of a hormone from the anterior pituitary gland (i.e., the adrenocorticotropic hormone, or ACTH).

The Adrenal Cortex

Among the hormones produced by the adrenal cortex are hydrocortisone, the chief glucocorticoid, 10 to 20 mg. daily; aldosterone, the chief mineralocorticoid, 0.2 to 0.4 mg. daily; and corticosterone and 11-oxy-17-ketosteroids, which are delivered in very small quantities.

Hydrocortisone is concerned with organic metabolism. It enhances the metabolic breakdown of body proteins and fat to form glucose, thereby providing a source of quick energy at times of stress and duress. It tends to retard reticuloendothelial growth and activity, thus limiting the vigor of immune responses and restricting the intensity of inflammatory reactions.

Aldosterone regulates salt and water metabolism, one of the mechanisms by which the concentrations of sodium and potassium are adjusted individually and maintained at physiologic levels. Corticosterone has both glucocorticoid and mineralocorticoid properties; 11-oxy-17-ketosteroids serve many functions in relation to organic metabolism and to the development of secondary sex characteristics. Both androgenic and estrogenic compounds are produced by the adrenal cortex.

Addison's Disease

Addison's disease, caused by a deficiency of cortical hormones, results when the adrenal cortex is destroyed, often the result of tuberculous infection of the gland. This hormonal deficiency gives rise to a characteristic clinical picture. The chief signs and symptoms include muscular weakness, anorexia, gastrointestinal symptoms, fatigue, emaciation, generalized dark pigmentation of the skin, low blood pressure, low blood sugar, low B.M.R., low blood sodium and high blood potassium. Most of the symptoms arise from the disturbance of sodium and potassium metabolism, with depletion of the sodium and water through the urine and severe chronic dehydration.

Diagnostic Evaluation. The diagnosis of Addison's disease depends on the proper identification of the signs of adrenocortical insufficiency. These include a decrease in the concentrations of blood sugar and sodium (hypoglycemia and hyponatremia), an increased concentration of blood potassium (hyperkalemia) and lymphoid hyperplasia. Particular importance is attached to the decreased concentration of sodium in the blood.

A valuable contribution to the diagnosis of Addison's disease is the artificial stimulation of the adrenals by an injection of potent pituitary adrenocorticotropic hormone. Unless the adrenal cortex is destroyed or is incapable, for any reason, of responding to this stimulus, a fall in the circulating eosinophils and an increase in uric acid excretion may be expected to occur in about 4 hours; in Addison's disease, the response is diminished or absent. ACTH injection fails to cause the normal rise in plasma cortisol and urinary 17-ketosteroids.

Treatment and Nursing Management. Treatment of Addison's disease consists of an attempt to restore the normal electrolyte balance, first with a high-sodium, low-potassium diet and fluids, and second by the administration of hydrocortisone (17-hydroxycorticosterone). Patients in addisonian crisis should receive this hormone in injectable form (e.g., Solu-Cortef; Hydrocortone Phosphate) by the intravenous route in 50 to 100 mg. doses, as required. Effective replacement therapy may be supplied on a long-term basis by the daily ingestion of hydrocortisone in 30- to 40-mg. doses.

Nursing Precautions. During hospitalization a close watch is kept for changes in the vital signs. Any symptoms such as cyanosis, nausea, vomiting or sudden fall in blood pressure suggest a sudden exacerbation of the disease (addisonian crisis). Even slight overexertion, exposure to cold, acute infections, a decrease in the salt intake or diarrhea from overenthusiastic purgation may lead to circulatory collapse: the systolic pressure falls to 40 or 50 mm. of mercury, the pulse is weak, the skin is cold and clammy, and the patient is in danger of death. In this situation the blood volume must be increased as soon as possible by means of blood transfusions, intravenous injection of sodium chloride solution and the administration of cortical extract or hydrocortisone. External heat is applied, and circulatory stimulants are injected. Patients frequently recover from these crises of adrenal insufficiency, but may die unexpectedly when apparently quite well.

The nurse has a particular responsibility in the accurate calculation and recording of the salt intake and the urine output. Emphasis is placed on getting adequate rest and warmth and the avoidance of overexertion, catharsis and exposure to cold. A high salt intake, adequate diet, cortical hormone and care of underlying tuberculosis, if present, are of paramount importance. With proper therapy the prognosis is favorable for extended periods of time.

Cushing's Syndrome

Cushing's syndrome is the antithesis of Addison's disease, its clinical characteristics reflecting excessive, rather than deficient, adrenocortical activity. The basic lesion responsible for Cushing's syndrome may be a tumor arising in the cortex of one of the adrenal glands or a basophilic adenoma of the pituitary gland (see p. 799) involving an overgrowth of pituitary cells producing the adrenocorticotropic hormone (ACTH). The syndrome may also result from excessive administration of cortisone or ACTH, or hyperplasia of the adrenal cortex.

The outstanding features of this syndrome include an increase in blood sodium and blood sugar and a decreased concentration of potassium, a reduction in the number of blood eosinophils and a disappearance of lymphoid tissue.

Levels of 17-hydroxycorticoids and 17-kerosteroids in the urine may be elevated. Plasma cortisol is elevated. Plasma ACTH is elevated in those cases caused by pituitary tumor.

When overproduction of the adrenal cortical hormone occurs in childhood, precocious puberty occurs, and in females of all ages, masculinization, or "virilism," is produced. Virilism is characterized by the appearance of masculine and the recession of feminine physical and mental traits. There is an excessive growth of hair on the face (hirsutism), the breasts atrophy, and menses cease, the clitoris enlarges, and the patient's voice and habits approach the masculine. If these changes occur in utero, a true hermaphrodite may result. If the change begins in early childhood, pseudohermaphrodism results. Arrhenoblastoma of the ovary (a very rare tumor) stimulates the above symptom complex.

The clinical picture of Cushing's syndrome in the adult shows a characteristic "central type obesity," with a fatty "buffalo hump" in the neck and supraclavicular areas, heavy trunk and relatively thin extremities. The skin is thinned and fragile; ecchymoses and striae develop. The face is rounded, plethoric, oily and hirsute. The patient complains of weakness and lassitude. Menses become irregular and scanty and libido is lost. Muscles are wasted because of excessive protein catabolism. Osteoporosis occurs, resulting in the characteristic kyphosis, backache and sometimes compression fractures of the vertebrae. Hypertension commonly develops and congestive heart failure may occur. Changes occur in mood and mental activity and these patients may occasionally develop a psychosis. They have an increased susceptibility to infections. If a pituitary tumor is the cause, visual disturbances may exist.

Treatment is directed toward removal of the cause if possible, such as removal of an adrenal or pituitary tumor. If hyperplasia of the adrenals is responsible, adrenalectomy is performed and replacement therapy given as needed.

Primary Aldosteronism

The principal action of aldosterone is to conserve body sodium. Under the influence of this hormone, the kidneys excrete less sodium and more potassium and hydrogen ions.

Excessive production of aldosterone, which occurs in some patients with functioning tumors of the adrenal gland, causes a distinctive pattern of biochemical changes and a corresponding set of clinical signs and symptoms that are diagnostic of this condition. Such patients exhibit a profound decline in the blood levels of potassium (hypokalemia) and hydrogen ions (alkalosis), as demonstrated by an increase in its pH and carbon-dioxide-combining power. The blood sodium is elevated (hypernatremia). Hypertension is present.

Hypokalemia is responsible for the periodic development of marked muscle weakness in patients with aldosteronism, as well as an inability on the part of their kidneys to acidify or concentrate the urine. Accordingly, the urine volume is excessive; these patients complain of polyuria. Their blood sodium, by contrast, becomes abnormally concentrated, which explains their excessive thirst (polydipsia) and may account for arterial hypertension. Tetany and paresthesias are to be expected in such patients, as complications of alkalosis. Cure usually follows surgical removal of the adrenal tumor.

Therapeutic Applications of Corticotropin (ACTH) and the Corticosteroids

Of the many notable achievements of medical science during the past few years, among the most outstanding have been the chemical identification, synthesis and large-scale production of agents that share the endocrine properties of the adrenal steroid hormones. As a group, these compounds are referred to as the "corticosteroids." They include *cortisone* (17-hydroxy-11-dehydrocorticosterone), *hydrocortisone* (17-desoxycorticosterone), *prednisone* (Δ1-cortisone), *prednisolone* (Δ1-hydrocortisone), *triamcinolone* (9α-fluoro-16α-hydroxyprednisolone) and *dexamethasone* (9α-fluoro-16α-methyl prednisolone). The availability of pituitary extracts with potent corticotrophic activity (ACTH) and the advent of these synthetic corticosteroid drugs represent a therapeutic milestone. These drugs, possessing the endocrine activity of the adrenal cortex, and ACTH, which activates the adrenal cortex, offer remarkable benefits in many diseases. Their value, as therapeutic agents, is poorly understood but appears to rest on their ability to suppress inflammation. Inflammatory processes, and processes of repair, although basically protective, may sometimes be damaging.

In the presence of these drugs, inflammatory reactions are reduced in severity or completely prevented, whether they are excited in response to chemical irritants, antigenic foreign proteins or microorganisms. This action on the part of the adrenocortical hormone provides the rationale for its use in such inflammatory disorders as rheumatic fever, rheumatoid arthritis, lupus erythematosus disseminata, periarteritis nodosa, severe allergic reactions involving the skin, the respiratory tract and the gastrointestinal tract of inflammatory lesions within the eye. Depression of antibody production is one of the reasons for its effectiveness in acquired hemolytic jaundice and in idiopathic thrombocytopenic purpura, caused by red cell and platelet antibodies respectively. Moreover, in purpura of all types, as in all varieties of inflammation, the presence of this hormone appears to improve the stamina and to maintain the integrity of the smaller blood vessels, thus preventing their leakage or rupture.

The inhibiting effect of the hormone on reparative processes stems from its ability to prevent the congregation of reticulum cells, as well as local accumulations of lymphocytes and fibroblasts. Not only does it impede production, but it aso favors disintegration of reticulum and fibrous tissue in areas of inflammation, thereby forestalling their disabling activities in vulnerable regions, such as the joints and the eyes. The "lympholytic" action of the hormone is used to advantage in treating the lymphoid tumors, including lymphatic leukemia, lymphosarcoma and the lymphomas.

Other disorders that are reportedly benefited by the administration of adrenocortical hormone include chronic ulcerative colitis and idiopathic steatorrhea, the granulomatous lung lesions of sarcoid and beryllium poisoning and poisoning by animal venoms. These drugs are also useful in the treatment of some types of malignant tumors. The adrenal hormone also is said to facilitate drug withdrawal in cases of addiction and to speed recovery from delirium tremens.

The biologic products and synthetic drugs that currently are available for corticosteroid therapy are listed below, together with details concerning their administration.

ACTH (corticotropin, Acthar), in contrast with the adrenal hormones, is available not as a pure synthetic compound but as a complex mixture of proteins extracted from animal pituitary glands. Given intramuscularly once or twice daily, its anti-inflammatory effect is approximately equal, milligram for milligram, to that of hydrocortisone. The most efficient but least convenient method of giving ACTH is in the form of a constant intravenous infusion.

Cortisone usually is given by mouth in the form of tablets containing cortisone acetate. A microcrystalline suspension of this material in physiologic saline is available for intramuscular injection. For the topical application of cortisone to the eye, one may utilize a microcrystalline suspension of the acetate, or an ophthalmic ointment consisting of a petrolatum base and containing cortisone acetate.

Hydrocortisone likewise is available in tablet form as the acetate ester (Cortef). This product is twice as potent as cortisone, and its dosage is correspondingly smaller. For purposes of intravenous or intramuscular administration hydrocortisone phosphate (Hydrocortone, Cortiphate) or succinate (Solu-Cortef) may be selected. A microcrystalline suspension of hydrocortisone acetate in saline is available for intra-articular injection in cases of noninfectious inflammatory diseases of the joints. A collyrium for the local treatment of inflammatory lesions in the anterior segment of the eye may be prepared by diluting this suspension with 4 parts of physiologic saline solution, or with a 1:5,000 solution of aqueous Zephiran Chloride.

Prednisone (Meticorten, Deltra, Deltasone) and *prednisolone* (Meticortelone, Meprolone, Cordex) are entirely comparable as regards potency, therapeutic efficacy and side-effects. Their anti-inflammatory and antiallergic actions are approximately 5 times as powerful, but their salt-retaining effect is less pronounced than that of cortisone. These compounds are absorbed readily and are rapidly effective after oral ingestion. Aqueous suspensions of prednisolone acetate are available for injection into joint cavities and bursae, and prednisolone sodium hemisuccinate is distributed as a sterile, pyrogen-free soluble powder, ready for solution and intravenous injection.

Triamcinolone (Aristocort, Kenacort), a fluorinated derivative of prednisolone, exhibits 50 per cent more anti-inflammatory, antiallergic and antirheumatic activity than prednisone or prednisolone. It is approximately 4 times as effective therapeutically as hydrocortisone and 6 times as effective as cortisone. On the other hand, triamcinolone has little or no tendency to cause sodium retention, edema or potassium excretion.

Dexamethasone (Decadron, Deronil) is the most potent anti-inflammatory agent in the pharmacopeia. Another fluorinated derivative of prednisolone, this drug is 4 to 5 times as effective as triamcinolone (30 to 40 times as potent as hydrocortisone), and its dosage is computed accordingly.

Nursing Activities Related to Steroid Therapy. Many potential hazards attend the use of these powerful endocrine agents, each complication being based on one or more of the physiologic properties of the adrenocortical hormone that have been described.

Prolonged administration of the corticoids results in complete suppression of ACTH formation by the pituitary. An abrupt cessation of steroid therapy, therefore, is dangerous from the standpoint of precipitating adrenocortical failure, i.e., the equivalent of an addisonian crisis.

The suppressive effect of this therapy on inflammatory lesions strips the patient of some very important defenses against bacterial invasion. Moreover, it tends to obscure the presence of an infection. Latent tuberculosis may be reactivated and spread extensively, or a virulent bacterial pneumonia may develop with complications of bacteremia, yet remain entirely unrecognized and unsuspected until death. All candidates for this endocrine therapy should be questioned with care, and have their lungs examined by x-ray before treatment is started, in order to exclude pulmonary tuberculosis. After treatment has begun, each patient should be scrutinized daily by the nurse and the physician in search of any evidence that might suggest the onset of some infectious complicaton.

Interference with inflammation implies interference with tissue repair, introducing an important problem in the care of any patient who has sustained a traumatic wound or who may require surgical treatment. It also favors the reactivation of peptic ulcer as well as the penetration of a peptic ulcer into or through the visceral wall, without warning. With this in mind, patients with a present or past history suggestive of peptic ulcer should receive steroids only if the therapeutic indications are compelling, and provided that appropriate studies have been completed to exclude the presence of a lesion.

The effect of the adrenal cortex on water and electrolyte metabolism constitutes a potential danger in patients with diminished cardiac reserve because of the risk of promoting edema through excessive sodium and water retention. All patients receiving ACTH, cortisone or hydrocortisone should be restricted in their sodium intake. Moreover, such patients should be weighed and examined for edema each day in order to detect any signs of water retention. Because it is responsible for the wastage of potassium in the urine, the patient's diet should be supplemented with potassium in the form of 2 to 3 gm. of potassium chloride each day. The nurse should determine whether this supplement has been received and ingested; moreover, she should be on the alert for signs of potassium deficiency, notably generalized muscular weakness.

Certain complications may be of less serious import, and yet may be the principal source of anxiety for the patient and require explanations by the nurse. In the course of steroid therapy the skin tends to become more darkly pigmented. Moreover, the skin becomes thinned, sometimes to the point of uncovering pigmented striations in the region of the thighs, the buttocks and the abdomen. Acne may erupt on the face and the trunk. Female patients may be very disturbed by the discovery of an appreciable growth of facial hair and may be further concerned by the appearance of her face, if the typical "moon facies" has become pronounced.

A complication that occurs not uncommonly, and may present unusual difficulties from the nurse's standpoint, is the development of a psychological disturbance following the onset of steroid therapy. No uniform pattern is evident in these manifestations, except that they often appear to represent an exaggeration of some pre-existing personality aberration.

Psychiatric complications of steroid treatment, like its other complications, are reversible in time, but the length of time required for complete return to the pretreatment status may extend to 2 or 3 months, and, meanwhile, the patient may be in serious jeopardy as a potential suicide. Every patient on steroid or ACTH therapy should be regarded by the nurse as a potential psychiatric casualty until his response to therapy has become stabilized and he can be evaluated psychologically. If there appears to be no essential change from his earlier status, he may be given a good prognosis as regards his psychological integrity.

A potential hazard associated with steroid therapy is the chance that treatment may be discontinued abruptly as a result of inadvertent omission of the appropriate orders. This error may be made when a patient on maintenance therapy is first admitted to the hospital. It also can occur when a patient is transferred from one hospital service to another or, in the case of postoperative patients, when a new set of orders is written. Thus, in preparation for surgery, a patient receiving oral steroid therapy will have all oral medications omitted as a matter of hospital routine. Parenteral steroids, for example, in the form of intramuscular hydrocortisone, can be substituted for the oral hormone. Forty-eight hours later all parenteral therapy is discontinued, including parenteral fluids, nutrients, stimulants, sedatives and hydrocortisone. It is not difficult to imagine that the hydrocortisone may be dealt with in the same manner as are the other injected drugs and materials, without thought of continuing its administration in another form. When this happens, the patient's postoperative course becomes very stormy indeed: blood pressure drops to levels that are alarmingly low; he becomes febrile, complains of fever, weakness and abdominal pain, and may experience vomiting, diarrhea or both. The longer the patient has been maintained on steroids and the higher the maintenance dose, the more severe are the withdrawal symptoms, and before the situation is recognized, he may die in an addisonian crisis. The nurse is in a position to minimize the risk of such tragedies and should be alert to the possibility of its occurrence in any case whose preoperative or operative orders have included steroid therapy.

The Adrenal Medulla

The medullary portion of the adrenal gland is the source of two powerful stimulants, *epinephrine* and *norepinephrine,* which are secreted instantly in the event of an emergency, real or threatened, placing the individual in a state of readiness for "fight or flight."

These two hormones function jointly to speed the delivery of fuel to organs whose activities are of immediate importance, and facilitate the removal of wastes, including excess heat, from those organs. Norepinephrine causes all arterioles, except those in the heart muscle, to constrict, thereby raising the systolic and diastolic pressures. The effect of epinephrine is to increase the pulse rate and cardiac output. It also counteracts the vasoconstricting action of norepinephrine in crucial areas, such as the brain, the muscles of the trunk and the extremities and the skin, causing all vessels in those organs to dilate. The net effect of both hormones, therefore, is to increase both the flow rate and the volume of blood flowing through the brain, the muscles, the myocardium and the skin.

Epinephrine causes the liver to unload some of its carbohydrate stores, with the result that the level of blood sugar is increased. It induces sweating, which, together with hyperemia of the skin, permits more rapid cooling of the blood. It also dilates the ocular pupils, assuring maximal acuity of vision. Finally, among its other effects, epinephrine stimulates the anterior pituitary gland to produce adrenocorticotropic hormone (ACTH) and thereby forces the release of hydrocortisone and aldosterone from the adrenal cortex. The latter is the basis of the so-called "alarm reaction," which reduces the severity of tissue responses, in general, to injury.

Pheochromocytoma

Functioning tumors of the adrenal medulla, or *pheochromocytoma,* cause arterial hypertension and other cardiovascular disturbances. The nature and severity depend on the relative proportions of epinephrine and norepinephrine in its secretions.

The hypertension may be paroxysmal or chronic. If it is of chronic, sustained type, it may be difficult to distinguish from the so-called "essential hypertension." In addition to hypertension, the symptoms are essentially the same as those encountered after the administration of epinephrine in large doses, namely, tachycardia, excessive perspiration, tremor, nervousness and hyperglycemia.

The clinical picture of pheochromocytoma usually is characterized by acute, unpredictable attacks, lasting several hours or only a few seconds, during which the patient feels excessively anxious, tremulous and weak and suffers from headache, vertigo, blurring of vision, tinnitus and air hunger. Other symptoms include polyuria, nausea, vomiting, diarrhea and abdominal pain.

Diagnosis and Treatment. The diagnosis of pheochromocytoma is suspected if signs of sympathetic overactivity occur in association with marked elevations of blood pressure. Diagnostic proof may require surgical exploration, but a presumptive diagnosis is often possible before operation with the aid of tests that depend on the reaction of the blood pressure to *provocative* drugs and to *adrenergic blocking* drugs. Provocative agents are those that stimulate a sharp rise, and adrenergic blocking drugs a definite fall, in arterial pressure in patients with this disease. The provocative drugs include histamine, tetraethylammonium chloride (or bromide) and methacholine (Mecholyl). The testing agent of choice among the adrenergic blocking agents is phentolamine (Regitine), which neutralizes the action of epinephrine. Injections of this material in patients with epinephrine-secreting tumors cause a precipitous fall in the arterial blood pressure. Determinations of the catecholamines in urine and blood offer the most direct and conclusive test for overactivity of the adrenal medulla. VMA (vanillylmandelic acid) determination in particular is preferable (normal urinary values: 2 to 6 mg./24 hrs.)

Patients with pheochromocytoma may be cured by excision of the tumor. In anticipation of surgery, attempts are made to localize the tumor by the injection of air into the retroperitoneal tissues. By this injection the retroperitoneal structures may be outlined on an x-ray film. The pheochromocytoma presents as an enlargement of the shadow of the adrenal on the side of the tumor.

Adrenalectomy

For Adrenal Tumors

All of the endocrine disturbances associated with a functioning tumor of the adrenal cortex or medulla can be relieved completely, and the patient improved dramatically, by surgical removal of the involved gland. Adrenalectomy is performed through an incision in the loin or the abdomen. In general, the postoperative care resembles that given for any abdominal operation. Some patients with adrenal cortical tumors may require the temporary administration of a steroid hormone, such as hydrocortisone, after operation. More serious problems may attend and follow adrenalectomy for pheochromocytoma, manipulation of this tumor at operation often producing extreme fluctuations in arterial pressure that must be counteracted by appropriate drugs. After ligation of the vessels leading from the tumor, an abrupt fall in blood pressure is apt to occur, which may require the administration of large amounts of epinephrine intravenously. Nursing care in the postoperative state often involves frequent estimation of blood pressure and the regulation of vasopressor intravenous drugs for 24 to 48 hours.

For Malignancy of Breasts or Prostate (see also pp. 578 and 621)

Certain malignancies, notably those of the breast and the prostate, are affected by the hormones produced by endocrine glands. Thus the ovary is known to have an effect on carcinoma of the breast, and the testes on carcinoma of the prostate. In some cases, even after ablation of endocrine stimulation, the hormones are still present, and they have been found to arise from adrenal glands. For this reason bilateral adrenalectomy is often performed in an effort to control or benefit recurrent carcinoma of the breast or the prostate. The adrenals are approached either transabdominally or through the bed of the 12th rib from behind. Postoperatively, adrenal cortical hormone must be administered in appropriate dosage to overcome the sudden deprivation of those hormones by the operation. The dosage of adrenal cortical hormone may be reduced gradually as the body adjusts itself to its new plane of hormone production.

For Hypertension

Since the adrenal is an important organ in the production of epinephrine, which constricts blood vessels and increases blood pressure, the adrenals have been removed in an effort to treat hypertension and sometimes in conjunction with the division of splanchnic and sympathetic nerve trunks. The postoperative care of these patients, in addition to the regulation of blood pressure by administration of vasopressor drugs intravenously, requires that adrenal cortical hormone be given as substitution therapy until the body adjusts itself to a new plane of blood pressure and hormonal balance.

THE PITUITARY GLAND

The pituitary gland is a small organ, approximately the size of a cherry, situated immediately below the midbrain and just posterior to the plane of the orbits. It is composed of three parts, the most anterior having a glandular structure, and the posterior being composed largely of nervous tissue. The central area is best described as a thin sheet of epithelial tissue, the structure and the vascularity of which do not indicate either a secretory or a nervous function. The posterior lobe is the source of two hormones: (1) *oxytocin,* the injection of which causes contraction of the smooth muscles and elevates blood pressure, and (2) *vasopressin,* which causes marked reduction in urine volume. The activity of the anterior lobe is more diverse, furnishing hormones that stimulate growth, the secretion of milk and the activity of the thyroid and the adrenal glands. The development of the ova and the sperm and the production of the ovarian and testicular hormones also are regulated by the anterior portion of the pituitary gland.

Diabetes Insipidus

Diabetes insipidus is a disorder of water metabolism caused by deficiency of vasopressin, the antidiuretic hormone (ADH). Its predominant symptom is an enormous daily output of 6, 8 or even 40 liters of very dilute urine, in appearance like water, with a specific gravity of 1.001 to 1.005. The urine contains no abnormal substances, such as sugar and albumin. Some cases of this disease are secondary to lesions of the brain (tumor, fracture of the skull, gumma, etc.) all in the region of the pituitary gland, on which, if possible, the treatment should be centered. Other cases are called *primary*, since no demonstrable lesion can be found and may be caused by circulatory changes in the kidneys, secondary to a deficiency of a posterior lobe hormone or to a lesion in the midbrain.

The primary symptoms may begin at birth. Polyuria in adults may have an insidious onset, but sometimes it occurs suddenly and may be related to a fright or an injury. The general health and duration of life are little affected by this disease.

Symptoms. In general, polyuria, not excessive thirst (polydipsia), is the primary symptom in diabetes insipidus. The disease cannot be controlled by limiting the intake of fluids. Attempts to do this causes the patient to suffer extremely from an insatiable craving for fluid. Great embarrassment, inconvenience and interference with daily activities are occasioned by the urgent need to allay thirst and pass urine.

Treatment. The administration of vasopressin is the only remedy to control the polyuria. This drug may be given by subcutaneous injection, by spray or by

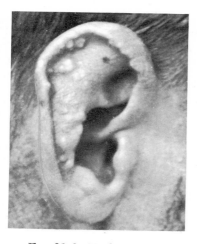

Fig. 31-6. Tophi of gout.

pledgets of cotton inserted into the nasopharynx. The amount of urine voided daily, as the result of this treatment, is reduced from 10 to 12 or more liters to perhaps 3 or less, thus assuring these unhappy patients of more restful days and nights.

Panhypopituitarism (Simmonds' Disease)

The destruction of the pituitary gland by surgical excision, a tumor or a vascular lesion removes every stimulus that is normally received by the thyroid and the adrenal glands. The resulting endocrinopathy, called Simmonds' disease, is characterized by extreme weight loss, emaciation, atrophy of all organs, hair loss, impotence, amenorrhea, hypometabolism, hypoglycemia, eventual coma and death.

Hypophysectomy for Metastatic Carcinoma

In an effort to alter the hormonal milieu of the body to create a hormonal environment hostile to the continued growth of a neoplasm, removal of the pituitary gland may be performed. This type of treatment affects only endocrine-dependent tumors, especially carcinoma of the breast, and it is used as a palliative measure in patients with metastatic disease.

The rationale of hypophysectomy for carcinoma of the breast is not completely clear, but it is known that certain pituitary hormones influence the growth of the normal breast and the function of the ovaries and the adrenal glands. Hypophysectomy removes the hormonal influences of these glands. About half of the patients experience regression of the tumor and its metastasis for 6 months or longer after operation.

Pituitary Tumors

Tumors of the pituitary gland are of three principal types: those representing an overgrowth of (1) eosinophilic cells, (2) basophilic cells or (3) chromophobic cells (i.e., cells with no affinity for either eosinophilic or basophilic stains).

Eosinophilic tumors, if they develop early enough in life, produce gigantism. The individual thus affected may be over 7 feet tall and large in all proportions, yet so feeble that he can hardly stand. If the disorder begins during adult life, the excessive skeletal growth occurs only in certain portions of the body, notably in the feet, the hands, the superciliary ridges, the molar eminences, the nose and the chin, giving rise to the clinical picture called *acromegaly*. Enlargement, moreover, is not confined to the skeleton, but involves every tissue and organ of the body. Many of these patients suffer from severe headaches and become partially blind because of pressure of the tumor on the optic nerves. Decalcification of the skeleton, muscular weakness and endocrine disturbances, similar to those occurring in patients with hyperthyroidism, also are associated with tumors of this type.

Basophilic tumors give rise to the so-called *Cushing syndrome* (see p. 707), with features largely attributable to hyperadrenalism, including masculinization and amenorrhea in females, girdle obesity, hypertension, osteoporosis and polycythemia. Since this type of tumor rarely enlarges to the extent characteristic of eosinophilic adenomas, local pressure symptoms such as headaches and blindness are uncommon.

Chromophobic tumors produce no hormones but destroy the rest of the pituitary gland, causing hypopituitarism. Patients with this disease are inclined to be obese and somnolent, exhibiting fine, scanty hair, dry soft skin, pasty complexion and small bones. They also experience headaches, loss of libido and visual defects progressing to blindness. Other symptoms include polyuria, polyphagia, a lowering of the basal metabolic rate and a subnormal body temperature.

THE PATIENT WITH GOUT

Gout is a metabolic disturbance in which little masses of sodium urate crystals, called *tophi*, become deposited in the vicinity of joints (particularly the great toe), in the ears (Fig. 31-6) and on the knuckles. Most gouty patients are men beyond middle age.

In so-called "primary gout" the basic problem appears to be a genetic defect in purine metabolism, or possibly a genetic defect in amino acid metabolism, which results in the constant overproduction of uric acid, chronic hyperuricemia (elevated blood uric acid) and progressive accumulation of uric acid in the tissues. In patients with "secondary gout," representing about 5 per cent of all cases, the source of hyperuricemia is excessive breakdown of cellular nucleoprotein, which may be split to purine ribosides and then oxidized to uric acid. Such is the situation in many patients with acute and chronic granulocytic leukemia, polycythemia vera, myeloma and other hematologic malignancies. In both types of gout, the patient progressively loses the capacity to excrete uric acid; he therefore is in a constant state of uric acid imbalance. Uric acid continues to accumulate in greater and greater excess in the body. Its concentration in the blood is almost always high, and, because of its low solubility, it tends to precipitate and form deposits at various sites where blood flow is least active, including the cartilaginous tissues.

Symptoms

An attack of acute gout usually begins in the early morning, with agonizing pain in the first joint of the big toe and later in the other joints of the foot. These joints become swollen, red, hot and exquisitely sensitive; the patient feels as if the foot were in a vise.

The superficial veins of the foot are swollen. The patient has a fever. Later in the morning the pain abates or even disappears, so that the patient can walk about, although the joints may still appear acutely inflamed. The following night the pain returns, and this pattern is repeated for 5 to 8 days, the severity of the pain gradually diminishing each time. These attacks usually recur, often with intervals of several months. Almost any joint may be involved, but the great toe rarely escapes.

Following repeated acute attacks, some of which may be very mild, the gout may become chronic, leaving certain joints (particularly those of the hands) permanently disabled, much deformed and painful. Among other symptoms are gastrointestinal disturbances with pain, vomiting, diarrhea and constipation; skin diseases, especially eczema; and all the symptoms of chronic nephritis and arteriosclerosis. The deposits of uric acid sometimes form knobs on the knuckles that may ulcerate through the skin (chalk stones).

An infallible sign of gout is the presence in the skin of tophi (Fig. 31-6), from which one may aspirate the typical crystals of sodium urate. Roentgenograms of the joints likewise may give a positive diagnosis. In the absence of tophi, the presence of gout is indicated when the uric acid in the blood rises to 5 mg. per 100 ml. or over, provided that the urea and the creatinine levels of the plasma are not simultaneously increased. If they are, renal decompensation may be suspected, and the occurrence of gout under these circumstances is a complication of uric acid retention caused by failure of the diseased kidney to excrete this material.

Therapeutic and Nursing Management

An acute attack of gouty arthritis can be terminated, in a high proportion of patients, by the administration of colchicine, 0.5 to 1.0 mg. of the crystalline product being given at 2-hour intervals for a total dose of 6 to 10 mg. The first dose may be administered by intravenous injection. Anorexia, nausea, vomiting and diarrhea are common in recipients of colchicine.

The corticosteroid drugs (e.g., prednisone or dexamethasone) speedily reduce the inflammation and eliminate the pain of acute gouty arthritis, and their administration on a short-term basis for this purpose is beneficial and fully justified. Likewise effective in the relief of acute gout is phenylbutazone (Butazolidin). This drug, ingested in doses of 100 mg. 4 times a day, reduces the fever and eliminates the inflammatory joint changes within a period of 48 hours. However, serious complications, including bone marrow depression and reactivation of peptic ulcer, have occurred in patients receiving phenylbutazone for extended periods of time. Its use, therefore, is limited to a small minority of patients who have proved to be both refractory to colchicine (or unusually susceptible to its toxic effects) and poor candidates for corticosteroid therapy (e.g., because of severe arterial hypertension or diabetes).

During the acute phase of gouty arthritis, the patient's symptoms confine him to complete bed rest. Bed covers should be raised out of contact with the extremely sensitive joints by means of a bed cradle, and the joints themselves should be positioned in semi-flexion, thereby reducing the intra-articular pressure to a minimum and affording the greatest comfort possible to the patient.

Hot or cold applications may alleviate pain to a significant extent, and deserve a cautious trial. Fluids are to be encouraged, in the attempt to avoid the precipitation of urate crystals in the urinary tract. Urinalysis data should be charted promptly.

Following subsidence of the acute attack and as soon as the patient shows a readiness to receive instruction, he should be informed regarding the long-term management of his disease.

Long-term Management of Gout

Patients with gout should acquire regularity in all habits of living, including habits of eating, exercise and rest. Intake of preformed purine bases should be limited. Foods containing more than 100 mg. of purine bases per 100 gm. of tissue include meat extracts, glandular meats, roe, shellfish, sardines and brains. Other foods to be especially avoided, or ingested in relatively limited amounts, include kidney, liver, sweetbreads, squab, meats in general, fowl, beans, mushrooms, peas and spinach. A low-purine diet would contain eggs, fat-free milk, cottage cheese, cereals, fruit and vegetables other than those mentioned.

An increase in blood uric acid and the precipitation of acute gouty arthritis in susceptible individuals have been demonstrated following the ingestion of fatty foods and ethyl alcohol, the implications of which are obvious.

Drugs of value in the management of chronic gout tend to prevent the accumulation of uric acid in the body and therefore diminish the likelihood of acute recurrences; these are the so-called "uricosuric agents" that promote the excretion of uric acid in the urine. Such a drug is p-dipropylsulfamyl benzoic acid (Benemid), effective in daily doses of 0.5 to 1.5 gm. by mouth, apparently with no more significant side-reaction than an occasional mild gastrointestinal upset and a tendency to constipation. This drug is not to be given in conjunction with aspirin or any other salicylate, because each tends to offset the action of the other. Another useful uricosuric drug is sulfinpyrazone (Anturane), which is given orally in daily doses of 200

to 800 mg. Anturane and the salicylates are also mutually antagonistic and must not be administered together.

Following the initiation of uricosuric drug therapy, the urinary concentration of urates may rise to such heights that crystals may precipitate out of solution, causing urolithiasis and renal colic. To avoid this complication, the patient should receive fluids in ample quantities and sufficient alkalies to render the urine alkaline during the early phase of treatment.

A new approach to the treatment of hyperuricemia and an important advance in the therapeutic management of gout has been the development of a chemical compound that blocks the production of uric acid by the body. This agent, allopurinol, inhibits the enzyme (xanthine oxidase) responsible for converting hypoxanthine into xanthine, and xanthine, in turn, into uric acid. The administration of allopurinol generally produces a prompt fall in both serum and urinary uric acid. It has proved most useful in patients with gouty nephropathy, in patients who tend to form uric acid stones, and in patients with severe gouty arthritis. Many persons with chronic gout have been relieved of their joint pain and have experienced increased joint mobility. Tophaceous deposits cease to form and draining urate sinuses tend to heal on this regimen. The average dose is 200 to 300 mg. per day for patients with mild gout, and 400 to 600 mg. for those with moderately severe tophaceous gout, the total daily requirement being divided into 2 or 3 portions and ingested after meals. The fluid intake should be adjusted to assure a 24-hour urinary output of at least 2 liters. Maintenance doses of colchicine should be prescribed prophylactically with the institution of allopurinal therapy to avoid a temporary exacerbation of acute gout.

BIBLIOGRAPHY

Books

Grollman, A.: Clinical Endocrinology and its Physiologic Basis. Philadelphia, J. B. Lippincott, 1964.

Guyton, A. C.: Textbook of Medical Physiology. ed. 3, pp. 1069-1083. Philadelphia, W. B. Saunders, 1966.

Harrison, T. R., et al.: Principles of Internal Medicine. pp. 489-512. New York, McGraw-Hill, 1966.

Joslin, E. P., et al.: The Treatment of Diabetes Mellitus. ed. 10. Philadelphia, Lea & Febiger, 1959.

Lilly Research Laboratories: Diabetes Mellitus. Indianapolis, Eli Lilly and Co., 1967.

Moyer, C. A., et al.: Surgery. Principles and Practices. ed. 3. pp. 856-884. Philadelphia, J. B. Lippincott, 1965.

Rosenthal, H., and Rosenthal, J.: Diabetic Care in Pictures. ed. 4. Philadelphia, J. B. Lippincott, 1968.

Warren, S., et al.: The Pathology of Diabetes Mellitus. Philadelphia, Lea & Febiger, 1966.

Adrenal Conditions

Frohman, L. P.: The adrenocorticosteroids. Amer. J. Nurs., *64*: 120-123, Nov., 1964.

Greenblatt, R. B., and Malts, J. C., Jr.: Addison's disease. Amer. J. Nurs., *60*:1249-1252, Sept., 1960.

Lanes, P.: Primary aldosteronism. Amer. J. Nurs., *61*:46-47, Aug., 1961.

Lustscher, J. A.: Aldosteronism. Disease-A-Month, May, 1964.

Nelson, D. H. (ed.): Treatment of adrenal disorders. Modern Treatment, 3:1328-1334, Nov., 1966.

Reich, B. H., and Hwalt, L. P.: Nursing care of the patient with Addison's disease. Amer. J. Nurs., *60*:1252-1255, Sept., 1960.

Shea, K., *et al.*: What and how to teach a patient with adrenal insufficiency. Amer. J. Nurs., *65*:80, Dec., 1965.

Taylor, F. H.: Diagnostic problems in adrenal cortical malfunctions. Disease-A-Month, March, 1965.

Diabetes Mellitus

Bregman, D.: Current concepts in management of the surgical diabetic patient. Med. Times, *94*:441-447, April, 1966.

Coates, F. C., and Fabrykant, M.: An insulin technique for preventing skin reactions. Amer. J. Nurs., *65*:127-128, Feb., 1965.

DeLawter, D. E., and Moss, J. M.: Aids in diabetic management. G. P., *33*:78-86, May, 1966.

Donaldson, J. B.: Current concepts in the treatment of diabetes mellitus. Med. Clin. N. Amer., *49*:1349-1360, 1965.

Dowling, H. (ed.): Newer concepts in diabetes mellitus, including management. Disease-a-Month, Sept., 1965.

Frawley, T. F. (ed.): Treatment of diabetes mellitus. Mod. Treatment, 2:693-696, July, 1965.

Hodges, R. E.: Present knowledge of nutrition in relation to diabetes mellitus. Nutrition Rev., *24*:257-260, Sept., 1966.

Krysan, G. S.: How do we teach four million diabetics? Amer. J. Nurs., *65*:105-107, Nov., 1965.

Levine, R.: Diabetes mellitus. Clinical Symposia, *15*:103-132, Oct.-Nov.-Dec., 1963.

Martin, M.: Diabetes mellitus: current concepts. Amer. J. Nurs., *66*:511-514, March, 1966.

Root, H. F.: Preoperative medical care of the diabetic patient. Postgrad. Med., *40*:439-444, 1966.

Sharkey, T. P.: Recent research developments in diabetes mellitus. J. Amer. Dietetic Assoc., *48*:288-293, April, 1966.

Shuman, C. R. (ed.): Treatment of complications of diabetes. Mod. Treatment, 4:13-109, Jan., 1967.

Smith, A. G., and Casingal, E. L.: Management of diabetic patients with foot lesions. Surg. Gynec. Obstet., *128*:85-87, Jan., 1969.

Watkins, J. D., and Moss, F. T.: Confusion in the management of diabetes. Amer. J. Nurs., *69*:521-524, Mar., 1969.

White, P. (ed.): Symposium on diabetes. Med. Clin. N. Amer., *49*:855-1161, 1965.

World Health Organization: Diabetes mellitus. Technical Report Series No. 310, pp. 1-44, 1965.

Thyroid Conditions

Garde, Sister Mariana: Cancer of the thyroid. Amer. J. Nurs., *65*:98-102, Nov., 1965.

Nordyke, R. A.: The overactive and the underactive thyroid. Amer. J. Nurs., *63*:66-71, May, 1963.

Rawson, R. W.: The thyroid gland. Clinical Symposia, *17*:35-63, Apr.-May-June, 1965.

Roe, C. F.: New equipment for metabolic studies. Nurs. Clin. N. Amer., *1*:624, Dec., 1966.

PATIENT EDUCATION

American Diabetes Association, Inc.
18 East 48th Street
New York, New York 10017

ADA Forecast (Bimonthly magazine)
ADA Forecast Reprint Series. (Reprints of articles selected for their long-term value to people with diabetes and their families.)
Meal Planning with Exchange Lists.
A Cookbook for Diabetics.
Facts About Diabetes.
Identification Card. (Bears the official Emergency Identification Symbol of the American Medical Association.)
The Nurse and the Diabetic.

Public Health Service
Audiovisual Facility
Atlanta, Georgia 30333

Just One in a Crowd. (Six-part filmstrip series presenting basic information for diabetes patient education. Each 15-minute session is complete. The series comes in a set, with instructor's manual, in slide or filmstrip format with the audio portion available on both tape and record. Color, 35 mm frames, for use in standard slide projectors. On loan, free of charge.

The Upjohn Co.
7171 Portage Road
Kalamazoo, Michigan 49002
You and Diabetes. 1964.

U.S. Government Printing Office
Supt. of Documents
Washington, D.C. 20402
Foot Care for the Diabetic Patient. 1965. PHS Publication No. 1153.

Weller, C., and Boylan, B. R.: How to Live with Hypoglycemia. Garden City, Doubleday, 1968.

CHAPTER **32**

Patients with Problems of the Eye

- *The Nurse and Eye Health Education*
- *Anatomy and Pathophysiology*
- *Examinations and Diagnostic Procedures*
- *Eyeglasses and Contact Lenses*
- *Psychological and Physical Needs of the Eye Patient*
- *The Patient with Trauma to the Eye*
- *The Patient Having Eye Surgery*
- *Corneal Transplantation (Keratoplasty)*
- *The Patient with a Detached Retina*
- *The Patient with a Cataract*
- *The Patient with Glaucoma*
- *Enucleation*
- *The Nurse and the Newly Blind*

THE NURSE AND EYE HEALTH EDUCATION

The eye is such an important organ that its care and protection are a major consideration. Care begins at birth and is continued throughout life. The nurse, as an important member of the health team, is looked on as a teacher and a practitioner of sound health habits. One of the most vital fields in health education is the care of the eyes and the prevention of eye diseases.

Since many problems and health habits begin in childhood, sound principles of safe care need to be stressed at this time. Complaints such as these need to be investigated: headaches, dizziness, tiredness after close eye work, "can't see well," letters "jump" or "run together," eyes that feel scratchy or itch. The appearance of inflamed or watery eyes, red rimmed, encrusted or puffy lids, recurring styes, crossed eyes and unequal pupils may be significant. Unusual behavior also should be noted—such as holding a book too close, frowning, blinking, skipping words, squinting, rubbing the eyes, stumbling, and failing in school work. A combination of these signs may be of short duration and often expected with an upper respiratory infection; however, persistence of these complaints indicates the need for an eye examination.

Faulty diet may account for the onset of many eye difficulties. For instance, deficiencies of vitamins A and B may cause changes in the retina, the conjunctiva and the cornea. Sensible eating habits can correct some problems; however, prolonged lack of vitamins A and B may produce irreversible eye damage.

Just as the eyes often reflect a systemic problem, an eye weakness may affect the total well-being of a person. The concept of total health care must be recognized by the nurse. An individual may complain of a minor visual disturbance and pass it off as something that may clear by itself. Such procrastination may have serious consequences.

The recognition of the importance of eye care has extended to industry and industrial art schools. Protective devices are a necessity in procedures in which there is danger of injury from foreign bodies. Safety glasses should be worn when the task at hand requires it. Eyes should be protected from bright sun, sun lamps, ultraviolet rays and even hair sprays. In the home, ammonia and alkali products, such as lye, present a particularly dangerous hazard for both children and adults. These agents can produce severe eye burns.

Eyes need to rest after being used for close work for a period of time. Occasionally glancing out the window or around the room allows relaxation. Adequate sleep each night prevents the tired feeling of the eyes when one stays up too late.

The importance of adequate and well-placed light in preventing eyestrain is essentially no longer a medical problem but one of general, industrial and social concern.

Recommended Room Lighting

All parts of a room absorb and reflect light; consequently, the room itself (walls and accessories) is a secondary source of light. The more light there is, the greater the reflection. The darker the surface, the greater the absorption. Interiors are more pleasant when dark colors are used to compensate other colors to produce recommended reflectances.

Recommended Reflectances

Ceiling	60-90%
Walls	35-60%
Floor	15-35%

Two lighting arrangements are suggested for a room: general and local. *General* or "fill-in" lighting is a low, though not even, amount of light throughout an area. It is light for moving about, for most housekeeping, and for softening pools of local light. Such lighting is achieved by ceiling fixtures, lighted wall-brackets or valances, or groupings of open-top, white lined portable lamps. Combinations of fixture types are desirable.

Local or functional lighting is used for visual tasks. This is provided in living areas by portable lamps close to the user, and in utility areas, by fixtures. Local sources should also contribute to general lighting.

Recommended Foot-candles (minimal)	Visual Task
10-20	Card playing
20-30	Casual reading; good type on white paper. Easy sewing, such as basting with contrast thread.
30-50	Household activities in kitchen and laundry.
40-70	Prolonged reading. Study. Hand sewing on medium-colored fabric. Machine stitching. Shaving. Benchwork.
100-200	Fine sewing. Hobbies with small details.

The National Society for the Prevention of Blindness and other medical groups have been responsible for the dissemination of invaluable information on eye care. It is important for the nurse to become familiar with them so that she may offer sound advice when a patient asks her such questions as: Will watching television damage my eyes? Are tinted glasses helpful for night driving? What kind of sun glasses are safe to wear?

Eye-Care Specialists

Public misunderstanding of the specific function of eye specialists is widespread. The nurse can clarify their roles and direct individuals intelligently for proper care. The importance of adequate eye examination cannot be emphasized too strongly. Too often we find patients using a pair of glasses that belonged to a relative or was purchased at the local variety store.

The care of the eye is undertaken by 4 groups of specialists:

1. The *oculist*, the *ophthalmologist* or the *ophthalmic physician* is a medical doctor who is skilled in the treatment of all conditions and diseases of the eye. Because of training and experience, he is able to make a more thorough and complete examination of the eye for refractive errors and other changes.

2. The *optician*, not a physician, whose concern it is to grind, mount and dispense lenses.

3. The *optometrist*, who is licensed to examine for refractive errors in the eye by mechanical means and to provide appropriate corrective lenses. He is not a physician, and he does not use drugs in the examination of the eyes.

4. *Ocularist* is a technician who makes artificial eyes and other prostheses used in ophthalmology.

ANATOMY AND PATHOPHYSIOLOGY

Anatomy

The eyeball is a spherical organ situated in a bony cavity called the *orbit*. It is rotated easily in all the necessary directions by 6 muscles attached to its outer surface; these are similar to the reins on a team of horses. The muscles are located not only on each side of the eye, but also on the top and the bottom of the eye. Each of these 4 muscles leads back to the apex of the orbit and turns the eye in or out, up or down; these are the *rectus* muscles. The 2 other muscles of

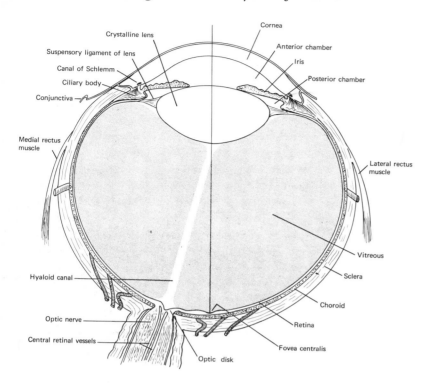

Fig. 32-1. Transverse section of right eye (× 3½). (Chaffee, E. E., and Greisheimer, E. M.: Basic Physiology and Anatomy, Philadelphia, J. B. Lippincott)

the eye run from the globe toward the medial wall of the orbit; these are the *oblique* muscles.

For the purpose of study, the eyeball may be divided into 3 coats or tunics. The dense white fibrous outer coat is called the *sclera*. Anteriorly, the sclera becomes continuous with the *cornea*, the translucent structure that bulges forward slightly from the general contour of the eye. Posteriorly, the sclera has an opening through which the optic nerve passes into the eyeball. The nerve spreads out over the posterior two thirds of the inner surface of globe in a thin layer called the *retina*. In it are situated the tiny nerve endings, which, when properly stimulated, transmit visual impulses to the brain that are interpreted as sight.

Between the sclera and the retina is the pigmented middle coat known as the *uveal tract*. This tract is composed of 3 parts. The posterior part, the *choroid*, contains most of the blood vessels that nourish the eye. The anterior part is a pigmented muscular organ, the *iris*, which gives the characteristic color to the eye (blue, brown and so forth). The circular opening at its center, the *pupil*, is made smaller of larger according to the intensity of the light, by two sets of muscle fibers. Contraction of the circular fibers constrict the pupil; the radial fibers enlarge it. Between the iris and the choroid is the third portion of the uveal tract, a muscular body known as the *ciliary body*. It is composed of radial processes arising from a triangular-shaped muscle (ciliary muscle). Between these pro-

cesses and to them are attached delicate ligaments that pass centrally and become inserted in the capsule of the crystalline lens.

The *lens* is a semisolid body enclosed in a transparent elastic capsule. It is capable of being modified to varying degrees of convexity by the contraction and the relaxation of the ciliary muscle, thus changing the focus of the eye as it looks from one object to another.

The cavity within the eye is divided by the lens into 2 parts. The posterior part contains a jellylike translucent substance called the *vitreous humor*, which is the chief factor in maintaining the form of the eyeball. The anterior part contains a clear, watery fluid, the *aqueous humor*, which is secreted by the ciliary processes. It bathes the anterior surface of the lens, escapes at the pupil and enters the space between the iris and the cornea known as the *anterior chamber*. Finally it is drained from the eye through lymph channels (the canal of Schlemm) located at the junction of the iris and the sclera.

Appendages. The eyelids are the protective coverings of the eye. Lining the lids and entirely covering the anterior part of the eye is a highly sensitive membrane, the *conjunctiva*, the surface of which is kept moist by a constant flow of lacrimal fluid (tears). This fluid is excreted from the lacrimal gland, which is located in the upper and outer part of the orbit. It flows downward and inward across the eye and drains

FIG. 32-2. Diagrams on the left illustrate rays of light converging in the normal (A), myopic (B), and hypermetropic (C) eye. X indicates the point of convergence of the light rays. On the right, the correcting lenses permit the rays of light to converge on the retina. (Adapted from Kimber, D. C., Gray, C. E., Stackpole, C. E., and Leavell, L. C.: Anatomy and Physiology, New York, Macmillan)

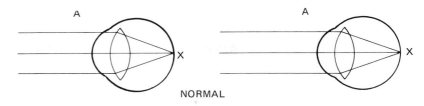

NORMAL

Rays brought to focus (X) on retina   No correction necessary

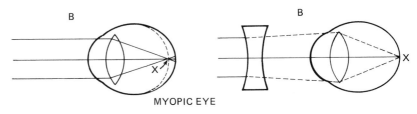

MYOPIC EYE

Rays focus (X) in front of retina   Concave lens corrects myopic error

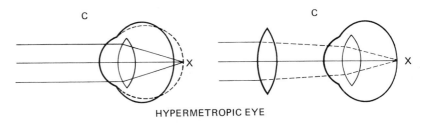

HYPERMETROPIC EYE

Rays focus (X) behind retina   Convex lens corrects hypermetropic error

into tiny channels (lacrimal punctae). By these channels it is conducted to the lacrimal sac and duct, which pass downward, backward and outward and open into the nasal cavity beneath the inferior turbinate bone.

Pathophysiology and Refractive Errors

Vision is made possible by the passage of rays of light from an object through the cornea, the aqueous humor, the lens and the vitreous humor to the retina. In the normal eye, rays coming from an object at a distance of 6 meters or more are brought to a focus on the retina by the lens while perfectly at rest. If, under the same conditions, the rays of light are brought to a focus in front of the retina, the condition is spoken of as *myopia*, or nearsightedness, and if the rays are focused behind the retina, the condition is called *hyperopia* (farsightedness) (Fig. 32-2). In such conditions glass lenses are prescribed. These, in association with the lenses of the eye, will correct the fault and restore a normal focus at the retina.

Rays from objects situated at shorter distances (less than 6 meters) require a "stronger" lens to focus them on the retina. This is brought about by a contraction of the ciliary muscle that relaxes the lens capsule and causes the lens to become more convex. This function is called *accommodation,* and by its means objects at different distances from the eye may be seen distinctly. With increasing age, the elasticity of the lens decreases, and accommodation for near vision is not complete. For example, it is common to see older people reading a paper held at arm's length; this condition is called *presbyopia.* "Reading glasses" may be prescribed for these patients to enable them to focus rays from near objects on the retina.

Astigmatism results from uneven curvature of the cornea—instead of curving equally in all directions, the cornea is shaped somewhat like the bowl of a spoon. Two foci thus occur instead of one and, as a consequence, the patient is unable to focus horizontal and vertical rays on the retina at the same time. These defects may be corrected with lenses called cylinder lenses. A patient may be myopic or hyperopic and also

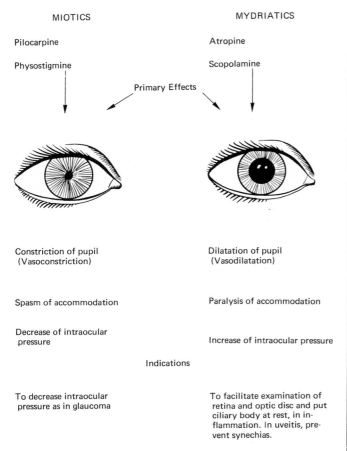

MIOTICS	MYDRIATICS
Pilocarpine	Atropine
Physostigmine	Scopolamine

Primary Effects

Constriction of pupil (Vasoconstriction)	Dilatation of pupil (Vasodilatation)
Spasm of accommodation	Paralysis of accommodation
Decrease of intraocular pressure	Increase of intraocular pressure

Indications

To decrease intraocular pressure as in glaucoma	To facilitate examination of retina and optic disc and put ciliary body at rest, in inflammation. In uveitis, prevent synechias.

FIG. 32-3. Effects and indications of miotics and mydriatics.

ABBREVIATIONS AND TERMS USED IN OPHTHALMOLOGY

O.D. or R.E. (ocular dexter)—right eye
O.S. or L.E. (ocular sinister)—left eye
O. U. or O_2 (ocular unitas)—both eyes together
D. (diopter)—unit of measurement of strength or refractive power of lenses. (A 1-diopter lens brings parallel light rays to a focus at 1 meter from the lens.)
E.O.M.—extra ocular muscles
H (hyperopia, hypermetropia)—farsightedness
HT (hypertropia)—upward deviation of one eye
ST (esotropia)—inward deviation of one eye
XT (exotropia)—outward deviation of one eye
+ —plus or convex
− —minus or concave
Diplopia—seeing one object as two ("double vision")
Ectropion—turning out (eversion) of eyelid
Entropion—turning in of eyelid
Ptosis—drooping of upper lid
Epiphoria—excessive production of tears
Hemianopsia—blindness of one-half the field of vision
Photophobia—abnormal sensitivity to light
Presbyopia—lessening of power of accommodation owing to aging process

---

have astigmatism. In such a situation, a compound sphero-cylinder lens is ordered from the optician.

EXAMINATIONS AND DIAGNOSTIC PROCEDURES

External Examination

The eye can be examined with relative ease both as to its function and its structure. A functional examination includes the ability to move in the orbit and the reaction of the pupil to light and accommodation. The function of the eye may be tested in several ways. The patient may be asked to identify illuminated letter or objects of varying sizes on what is known as the Snellen chart.

The examiner observes the viewer rather than the chart, because the patient may attempt to squint to improve (abnormally) his vision. A narrowed aperture or squeezed lids gives "pin-hole" or camera-like vision. A patient with an amblyopic eye would move his head slightly to see with his better or unoccluded eye; this does not give a true picture of the patient's vision and is to be discouraged.

Usually each eye is tested alone. Letters or objects are of the size that can be seen by the normal eye at a distance of 20 feet from the chart. Rows of letters of larger sizes are designated as 30, 40 and so on. These really are letters of a size that should be seen by the normal eye at distances of 30 feet, 40 feet and so on. When an eye can identify letters of size 20 at 20 feet, the eye is said to have 20/20 vision. The mathematical principle behind the size of letters is that the normal eye can resolve 5 minutes of arc. Therefore the big "E" subtends 5 minutes of arc at 200 feet. This vision is called 20/200. The big "E" should be seen by the normal eye at 200 feet. If the person can identify only the letters of the number 40 line, he is said to have 20/40 vision. (The figure 6/6 is the same as 20/20 in the metric system. Instead of using 20 feet, this method uses 6 meters, which equals 20 feet.)

The *visual fields* are spot tested by a perimeter, an

instrument that tests the peripheral or side vision with the eye fixed at a central point. Tests for *color vision* are made by having the patient identify various colors or wool yarn or figures or letters that can be seen only if the patient can identify colors in a color plate.

Refraction. The normal eye, by reason of its lens apparatus and the cornea, is able to refract parallel rays of light so that they focus on the retina. Due to abnormalities in the eye structure or in the lens structure, defective vision may occur because objects are not focused correctly on the retina.

The drug atropine paralyzes the nerve endings that function in accommodation, and for this reason "drops" of this drug or homatropine, a short-acting derivative, are placed in the eye before an examination for "glasses." The ophthalmologist thus can ascertain the function of the eye with the lens completely at rest (see p. 725).

By various examinations and tests with trial lenses, the ophthalmologist can determine the strength and the type of lens that will overcome the refractive error. In the case of presbyopia, two different types of lenses may be used—bifocals—one for far distance and one for near vision and reading. Trifocal lenses are also available; these add a third segment that gives sharp focus in the 27-inch to 50-inch range. Most lenses are prescribed for use in "glasses," but in some cases the lens may be applied directly to the surface of the eye (contact lens).

Internal Examination

Examination of the structural part of the eye may be made in several ways. Tension within the eyeball is measured by a tonometer. In certain diseases, especially glaucoma, the tension in the eyeball is increased markedly. (Normal tension is approximately 11 to 22 mm. Hg.) The surface of the eyeball and the conjunctiva may be more closely inspected by the magnifying loupe. This also is used in the search for foreign bodies. The slit-lamp is an instrument that projects a beam of light into the anterior segment of the eye for detection of disease.

With the *ophthalmoscope,* a small beam of light is reflected through the pupil and, through a small opening in the mirror, the examiner may view the interior of the eye. The instrument is fitted with a series of lenses that permit examination of structural changes. Thus, in certain diseases of the brain, the optic nerve may be pushed forward into the eyeball. This is spoken of as *choking of the disk* and, by means of the lenses in the ophthalmoscope, the amount of choking may be estimated and described in diopters (e.g., "choked disk of 3 diopters"). In addition, the blood vessels of the interior of the eye may be visualized.

Since this is the only area in the body in which blood vessels can be observed by direct vision, it is an important source of information, not only in diseases of the eye but also in many systemic conditions, such as hypertension and diabetes.

A *binocular ophthalmoscope* allows the examiner to use both his eyes and thus has in-depth perception of the interior of the eye under examination. Better detail can be seen.

By means of a contact glass and a magnifying device, the angle of the anterior chamber may be seen (*gonioscopy*). Such visualization is desirable in congestion, inflammation, tumors, cysts, trauma, glaucoma and congenital anomalies. It is particularly helpful in diagnosis, management and surgery of glaucoma.

EYEGLASSES AND CONTACT LENSES

The stigma of wearing glasses has been removed in the past decade with the advent of attractive designs. The shape, the color, and the decorative features of eye glasses are selected by the wearer to enhance his physical features as well as personality. Thus there are glasses for study and business wear and other styles for more formal occasions. They are adapted to the needs of all age groups. Plastic lenses are more durable for young school-age children. Children, and perhaps one-eyed people, should always wear shatterproof lenses, either case-hardened glass or plastic lenses. However, a case could easily be made for the argument that *all* people should wear shatterproof lenses.

Contact Lenses

The corneal lens is made of light-weight, paper-thin plastic about 10 mm. or less in diameter. Scleral lenses are larger and are used for special medical conditions and some sports. When properly fitted, contact lenses "float" on the fluid layer of the eyeball and are held loosely in place by the capillary attraction of the tears and the upper lid. The lens moves with the eye and is centered over the cornea.

The popularity of contact lenses continues to increase with the development of better techniques for measuring the eye and better supervision and instruction in the use of the lenses. They are particularly effective in certain occupations, and are desirable for cosmetic reasons in many others. However, there are many individuals for whom contact lenses should not be recommended; all potential candidates should be thoroughly screened by an ophthalmologist.

Medical conditions in which corneal lenses are recommended include absence of lens (aphakia), absence of iris (aniridia), congenital absence of pigment, myopia and hyperopia, some types of astigmatism, cone-shaped deformity of the cornea (keratoconus), and turned-in eyelashes. Contraindications include allergic and inflammatory conditions (such as chronic blepharoconjunctivitis, corneal infection, iritis, uveitis), epiphora (abnormal overflow of tears), presbyopia, severe exophthalmus, pterygium or local neoplasm.

Contact lenses have many advantages over framed lenses: they do not steam up when the wearer goes from the cold outside to a warm room; they are automatically cleaned with each blink of the eyelid; they can be worn safely during sports; they eliminate the need for less attractive lenses; peripheral vision is increased; and the incidence of breakage is extremely low.

Some disadvantages and dangers in wearing contact lenses include the following: contact lenses are more expensive than framed lenses; the adjustment period in learning to use them properly is longer; contact lenses can be lost easily, such as down the sink drain or in a swimming pool; in the event of a chemical splash to the eye, the chemical agent may seep beneath the lens to cause extensive damage before the contact lens can be removed. The wearer of contact lenses should carry a card indicating that he wears contact lenses. This may help in an encounter with the police, if his license happens to be marked "must wear glasses." Should he be involved in an accident or become unconscious and unable to remove the lenses, prolonged wearing may be injurious to the cornea. Emergency room attendants should have available a suction device to remove such a lens when the patient cannot do it.

Briefly, recommendations for the wearers of contact lenses are:

1. Wash hands thoroughly before touching the lenses, whether applying them or removing them
2. Cleanse lenses only with the recommended sterile solution (noncaustic)
3. Dry the lenses when they are removed and to be stored
4. Keep the storage kit clean
5. Do not wear lenses beyond the prescribed time (maximal average is 10 to 16 hours)
6. Do not wear lenses when sleeping or suffering from an eye infecton.

The improper use of contact lenses can cause corneal abrasions and ulcerations, which result from poorly fitted lenses, improper technique in applying or removing the lenses, and insufficient tear circulation under the lenses. Although the advantages outweigh the disadvantages, precautions and safeguards must be understood by the nurse, the wearer and his employer. The contact lense must be regarded as a medical prosthesis, not a cosmetic device. The care and precaution given to any medical prosthesis must be used with contact lenses.

PSYCHOLOGICAL AND PHYSICAL NEEDS OF THE EYE PATIENT

It is well to remember that a patient with an eye problem may have other problems as well. Often other physical conditions are primary and affect the eye as a consequence. The appearance of the eye can alert the patient and the physician to difficulties in some disturbances of other parts of the body even before other symptoms present themselves. The mental anxiety frequently experienced by the ophthalmic patient requires as much consideration as does his physical condition.

One's dependence on sight is emphasized when one faces a temporary or possible permanent loss of this vital sense. Worry, fear and depression are common evidences of a patient's concern. Tension, resentment, anger and rejection may develop. By encouraging the patient to express his feelings, the nurse may discover the basic problems caused by his physical condition. When these basic problems are known, assistance in solving them can be secured.

When permissible, the nurse should use such means as the radio and occupational therapy to keep the patient's mind occupied. She should not be oversolicitous, but she should show interest, empathy and understanding. Because of differences of personality, her approaches in overcoming the mental anxiety of individual patients should vary. When permanent blindness is apparent, re-education may be done by similarly afflicted persons or by specially-trained people.

The daily care of ophthalmic patients should be the same as for other patients. The patient should be assisted as much as possible; at the same time, he should be encouraged to help himself so that he will become self-sufficient and not consider himself a burden. A patient who cannot see should be fed, but if he is accustomed to feeding himself, he should be supervised. Proper elimination should be promoted by proper diet, cathartics or enemas, as ordered. Ambulatory patients should have a daily rest period in the afternoon.

Ophthalmic patients should not read, smoke or shave unless given permission by the physician. They must be cautioned against rubbing their eyes or wiping them with a soiled handkerchief. All patients receiving atropine should wear dark glasses.

Reduction of Light

Because light causes pain in many conditions of the eye, and because the eyes should be rested as much as possible before and after undergoing operation, it is well to treat the ophthalmic patient in a darkened room. Dimmed artificial lights may be used by the nurse for her own needs.

Eyedrops

Solution of various drugs are employed in the treatment of nearly every kind of eye disease. The administration of these drops often is the responsibility of the nurse, and often she has to instruct others in the technique.

Before instilling drops the nurse must be sure that she has the prescribed drug and identifies the affected eye. Some drugs (for example, atropine and eserine) act in exactly opposite ways. Therefore, if one of these drugs is indicated in the treatment of a certain eye disease, the other is contraindicated. It may seem needless to emphasize this warning, but experience has taught how easy it is in a dimly lighted room to pick up the wrong bottle from a tray containing similar vials.

The nurse then should inspect the solution for color changes or sedimentation. These signs are evidences of decomposition, and, if present, the solution should be discarded and a fresh one ordered and sterilized for use. The importance of using fresh medicines can be stressed with patients who often use drugs that have been in the medicine cabinet at home for months or years. However, this problem is diminishing with the advent of small sterile disposable containers.

An eyedropper usually is employed for the instillation of drops. This instrument is composed of a glass or plastic pipette fitted with a small rubber or plastic bulb. The glass part is washed and sterilized easily, but the rubber undergoes gradual deterioration, and for this reason only a small amount of solution should be drawn into the pipette. The dropper never should be inverted or filled too full, as there is risk of contaminating the solution by contact with fine particles of rubber found in the bulb. An excess of solution remaining after instilling the drops should be discarded because of the possibility of contamination if it is returned to the bottle. Eyedrops may be packaged in single-dose plastic containers, thus eliminating the need for a dropper and a stock bottle of medication. This is the most desirable procedure.

Instillation. The lids and the lashes are cleansed before instilling the medication. Then the head of the patient should be tilted backward (Fig. 32-4) and inclined slightly to the side, so that the solution will run away from the tear duct. This latter precaution is especially necessary when poisonous solutions, such as atropine, are employed, because absorption of the excess drug by way of the nose and the pharynx may lead to toxic symptoms. In most cases it is well to press the inner angle of the eye after instilling the drops to prevent the excess of the solution from entering the nose. The lower lid is depressed with the fingers of the left hand, the patient is told to look upward, and the solution is dropped on the everted lower lid. Care must be taken that the pipette does

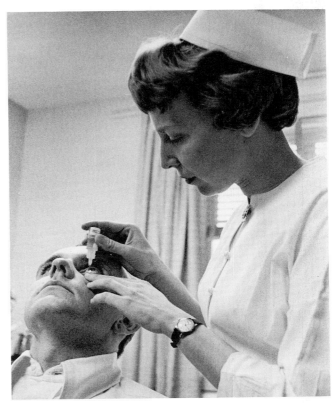

Fig. 32-4. Instilling drug into the eye. Note that the nurse, in using the dropper, rests her right hand against the patient's forehead and with her left hand depresses the lower lid. The eyedropper is held directly above the sulcus, between the lower lid and the eyeball. (Clinical Center, National Institutes of Health)

not touch any part of the eye or the lids to guard against contamination of the dropper and injury to the eye. After placing the drops (1 or 2 at most) in the eye, the lid is released and any excess of fluid is sponged gently from the lids and the cheeks with sterile cotton. After the medicaton is instilled, the nurse can tell her patient to close his eyes gently; this patient often has a tendency to "squeeze" his eyes closed, thereby expelling the medication.

After using the dropper, if contamination has been avoided, it may be replaced in the bottle, but in no circumstances should it be used for other solutions until it has been cleansed thoroughly.

Ointments

Ointments of various kinds are used frequently in the treatment of inflammatory diseases of the lids, the conjunctiva and the cornea. Those ordered most commonly are sulfonamides, bacitracin, neomycin, chlor-

TABLE 32-1. Medications used frequently in eye conditions

Medication	Action
LOCAL ANESTHETICS	
Tetracaine hydrochloride (Pontocaine), 0.5%	Commonly used topical anesthetic Anesthesia produced in 1 to 2 minutes
Proparacaine hydrochloride (Ophthaine), 0.5%	More rapid in action Less discomfort during instillation
Benoxinate hydrochloride (Dorsacaine), 0.4%	Fewer allergic reactions than tetracaine
Cocaine hydrochloride, 0.5, 2 and 10%	Produces a more profound corneal anesthesia than tetracaine To be used sparingly
Procaine hydrochloride, 1 and 2%	Commonly used for injection in eye surgery Lasts about 45 minutes
Lidocaine hydrochloride (Xylocaine), 2%	Some favor this over procaine because its action is more rapid and it lasts longer
ANTIMICROBIAL AND CHEMOTHERAPEUTIC AGENTS	
Neomycin sulfate (Mycifradin)	Topical application for external infections
Neomycin sulfate with polymyxin and bacitracin (Neosporin)	Broad-spectrum, ointment or solution Only disadvantage is its allergenic nature
Chloramphenicol (Chloromycetin), 10 to 15% sol.; topically used in ¼% and ½%	Good penetrating power Very effective May sensitize a patient for future sytemic use
Penicillin	Primarily used in newborns in ointment form Occasionally used for intraocular infection Primarily reserved for systemic use
Sodium methicillin (Staphcillin)	Used for penicillinase-producing organisms
Bacitracin, 500 units/gm. ointment	Good as a penicillin substitute for local eye uses against gram-positive organisms
Erythromycin	Effective as a penicillin substitute against resistant staphylococcal organisms

Sulfonamides:
  Sulfisoxazole (Gantrisin), 4% sol. or ointment
  Sulfacetamide sodium (Sulamyd Sod.)
	Used in treatment of conjunctivitis

DYES (For corneal staining to detect superficial abrasions)	
Fluorescein sodium	NOTE: Because *Pseudomonas aeruginosa,* highly pathogenic for corneal tissues, grows well in fluorescein solutions, the sterile single-dose containers or sterile Kimura fluorescein papers are recommended.
Merbromin (Mercurochrome), 2%	Less effective as a dye than fluorescein but less likely to become contaminated.
Rose Bengal, 2%	Selective dye to stain conjunctiva
CARBONIC ANHYDRASE INHIBITOR (Carbonic anhydrase is an enzyme present in body tissues. In the ciliary body, it is directly involved in the production of aqueous humor.)	
Acetazolamide (Diamox)	A sulfonamide used as a diuretic and also effective in decreasing production of aqueous humor by ciliary body in glaucoma. Because of side effects (gastric distress, shortness of breath, acidosis, tingling of extremities, dermatitis, ureteral stones), it is prescribed cautiously for selected patients.

TABLE 32-1. Medications used frequently in eye conditions (*continued*)

Medication	Action
SYMPATHOMIMETIC DRUGS (Used primarily for mydriasis and occasionally as vasoconstrictors)	
Phenylephrine hydrochloride (Neo-Synephrine), 2.5 to 10%	Action lasts 3 hours
Hydroxyamphetamine hydrobromide ophthalmic solution (Paredrine), 1%	Action lasts 3 hours
Epinephrine hydrochloride (Adrenalin), 1:1000; (Glaucon), 2%	Lowers intraocular pressure in open-angle glaucoma (inhibits aqueous production)
Epinephryl borate (Eppy), 1%	

Medication	Action
PARASYMPATHOMIMETIC DRUGS (Used as miotics for controlling intraocular pressure in glaucoma)	
Group I—Act directly on myoneural junction:	
Pilocarpine hydrochloride, 0.5, 1, 2, 3, 4, and 6%	Drug of choice in glaucoma Action lasts 6 to 8 hours
Carbachol (Doryl), 1.5 to 3%	Used if pilocarpine is ineffective
Group II—Cholinesterase inhibitors:	
Physostigmine salicylate (Eserine), 0.25 and 0.5%	Action lasts 6 to 8 hours Because it is allergenic, unstable, and short in its action, it is gradually being replaced by Phospholine.
Echothiophate iodide (Phospholine Iodide), 0.06, 0.125, 0.25%	Water soluble Causes less local irritation Action lasts 24 hours
Isofluorophate (diisopropyl fluorophosphate) (DFP) (Floropryl), 0.0025% ophthalmic ointment; 0.1%—ophthalmic solution	Oil soluble miotic May produce side-effects; watch for vomiting, diarrhea, tenesmus

Medication	Action
PARASYMPATHOLYTIC MEDICATIONS (Used as mydriatics to facilitate ophthalmoscopic examination and for mydriasis and cyclopegia in refraction and in treatment of uveitis)	
Mydriatics:	
Epinephrine (Epitrate), 1 to 2%	Action lasts 12 hours
Eucatropine hydrochloride (Euphthalmine), 5.0%	Short-lived action Can dilate pupil without affecting accommodation
Cycloplegics:	
Homatropine hydrobromide, 2 and 5%	A popular drug for cycloplegic refraction Action lasts 24 to 36 hours Allergic reactions rare
Scopolamine hydrobromide (hyoscine), 0.2% to 0.5%	Used in children's refraction Used in treating uveitis Because of low allergic reaction, it is preferred to atropine May cause dizziness and disorientation in older persons
Atropine sulfate, 0.5, 1, and 2%	Most powerful of this group Action lasts 10 to 14 days, during which eyes must be protected from bright light Used in treating uveitis Used in refraction of children Contraindicated in primary glaucoma 5% of persons are sensitive to it (Symptoms: difficulty in swallowing, dizziness, flushed skin with circumoral pallor, rapid full pulse, delirium)
Cyclopentolate hydrochloride, (Cyclogyl), 0.5 and 1%	Action is less than 24 hours Very popular drug for cycloplegic refraction
Tropicamide (Mydriacyl), 0.5 to 1%	Newer, shorter acting—lasts 6 hours

TABLE 32-1. Medications used frequently in eye conditions (*continued*)

Medication	Action
ADRENAL CORTICOSTEROIDS (Effective in treating inflammatory conditions of the eye: uveitis, episcleritis, chemical burns. Decreases vascularization and scarring following burns, trauma and severe inflammation.)	
Cortisone acetate, 0.5 to 2.5%—suspension; 1.5%—ointment	Least expensive
Hydrocortisone, 0.5 to 2.5%—suspension; 1.5%—ointment	Greater potency than cortisone, so it can be used in lower concentrations
Prednisone, prednisolone, dexamethasone and betametkasone	These are thought to be more potent than hydrocortisone
Fludrocortisone acetate (Florinef, Alflorone, F-Cortef), 0.1%	NOTE: These are highly dangerous when used in the presence of herpes simplex keratitis. Definitely, the patient should be under the care of an ophthalmologist with these medications. All steroids are now known to produce glaucoma in certain predisposed patients. Use of steroids locally or systemically must be carefully supervised.

amphenicol, Terramycin, steroids, and combinations. These are applied best by pulling down gently the lower lid and expressing a small amount of the ointment from the tube to the conjunctiva of the lower lid. Care is taken not to touch the eye or the eyelid with the tube. The lid then may be massaged gently in such a way as to distribute the drug over the eyeball.

Ocular Irrigations

Ocular irrigations are indicated in various inflammations of the conjunctiva, in the preparation of the eye for operation and in the removal of inflammatory secretions. Also, they are used for their antiseptic effect. The fluid to be employed depends on the condition present. Irrigation should be warmed before using.

The irrigating apparatus is simple, consisting of a commercially prepared plastic irrigating bottle containing sterile ophthalmic solution (Blinx, Dacriose), and a small curved basin and cotton for catching the fluid and the secretions.

The patient should be flat on his back or sitting with the head tilted backward and inclined slightly toward the side to be treated. The basin may be held by the patient, if sitting, or so placed that when he is lying down it will catch the fluid as it runs from the eye. The nurse stands in front of the patient.

After carefully cleansing the lids of dust, secretions and crusts, she holds them open with the thumb and the fingers of one hand, and with the other hand she flushes the eye gently, directing the stream away from the nose. The fluid should never be directed toward the nose, because of the danger of spilling over into the other eye. The procedure should be continued until the eye is entirely free of secretions. It must be remembered that very little force should be used, be-

cause of the danger of injury. For the same reason and to prevent contamination, no part of the irrigator should touch the eye, the lids or the lashes. When the irrigation has been completed, the eye and the cheek should be dried gently with cotton. Each patient should have his own solution in a plastic dispenser with cap.

Continuous Irrigation of the Eye. Continuous irrigation is indicated in chemical burns, resistant corneal ulcers, enophthalmitis, uveitis, socket infections after enucleation, or conditions in which constant medication or débridement are indicated. An effective method of continuous eye irrigation has been devised by Houser and Stokes.* After infiltrating the tissues of the lower lid with local anesthesia, a 16-gauge cannula is then passed through the inferior cul-de-sac and threaded with a sterile miniature polyethylene T-tube. By removing the cannula and attaching an adapter to the T-tube, an irrigating container is connected to provide the desired irrigating solution. This method provides greater patient comfort while assuring maximal therapy. Drug administration is atraumatic as indicated by fewer incidences of blepharospasm. Such an irrigation provides continuous gentle débridement. Since the lids can be closed comfortably, there is less chance of infection.

Drugs are usually mixed in a solution of physiologic saline and the irrigation rate is 1 or 2 drops per minute. The irrigation can usually be drained by way of the punctum lacrimalis; however, if the medication irritates the alimentary tract, it may be necessary to occlude the punctum. Drainage may be directed to the side of the face, where an absorbent folded hand towel can be placed on a plastic square. The irriga-

---

* Dr. Ben P. Houser, Jr., Wills Eye Hospital, Phila. and Dr. Hunter R. Stokes, U.S. Army Hospital, Camp Zama, Japan.

tion may be stopped while the patient has his meals, goes to the bathroom and so forth. Nursing problems are lessened and the patient is more comfortable.

Hot Compresses

Heat relieves pain and increases the circulation, thereby promoting absorption and reducing tension in the eye. It is especially valuable for the deep-seated inflammations of the eyeball, iritis, acute glaucoma and so forth, as well as for such superficial inflammations as keratitis and conjunctivitis. Heat is best applied in the form of compresses composed of 7 or 8 thicknesses of gauze or cotton, just large enough to cover the eye.

The patient is moved to the side of the bed, and a towel is used to cover the chest. The skin of the lids and the adjacent cheek may be anointed with cold cream or petrolatum. The compresses then are moistened in a basin of water or any other prescribed solution that has been heated by an electric hot plate placed on a table beside the bed. The fluid, which should be kept at a temperature between 115° and 120° F., should be expressed from the pad and, after being tested for temperature on the back of the hand, the compress is placed gently over the closed lids. The pads should be changed every 30 to 60 seconds for 10 or 15 minutes, and the application should be repeated every 2 or 3 hours. At the completion of the period of application, the lids should be dried gently with cotton. New pads should be used for each application and, if the eyes have a purulent secretion, the compresses should be applied to one eye at a time, the solution and the basin being changed between applications in order not to carry infection from one eye to the other.

Cold Compresses

Cold causes a capillary constriction that tends to reduce the amount of secretion and relieve pain during the early stages of acute inflammatory conditions of the conjunctiva. It is indicated also in the treatment of injuries or after operations on the eye, as it tends to reduce swelling and to retard bacterial growth. Cold compresses are useful in relieving itching due to allergic conjunctivitis.

The patient is prepared in the same manner as for the application of hot compresses. The pads are moistened in boric-acid solution and placed in rows on a block of ice suspended by a gauze sling over a basin. They are applied to the closed lids and are changed every 15 to 30 seconds, for a period of 5 to 15 minutes each hour. Cold compresses are never used in the treatment of deep-seated inflammations of the eye (iritis, keratitis), because cold, by constricting the capillaries, interferes with the nutrition of the cornea.

THE PATIENT WITH TRAUMA TO THE EYE

The prevention of eye injuries is a phase of child and adult education that cannot be emphasized too strongly. Children need to be reminded frequently of the dangers of sticks, arrows and darts, BB guns, "sparklers," sling shots, rubber bands, and even harmless looking toys. Precautions that should be taken when using power tools need to be explained to the teenager. Protection is necessary from very bright lights, sun shining on the snow, fumes of chemicals, sprays, and flying chips of wood. The use of goggles give protection against most foreign bodies, but specially designed safety goggles or glasses with impact resistance lenses are preferable if there is danger of flying metal or wood objects that may break the glass. Elderly persons or those unsure of their footing need safeguards where there is a possibility of injury.

General measures to follow in caring for patients with eye injuries are: (1) irrigate the eye with saline solution; (2) instill 1 drop of fluorescein solution—the yellowish-green dye used to detect abrasions and ulcers; (3) irrigate the eye again; (4) evaluate and treat injury; and (5) employ follow-up care.

Foreign Bodies

Foreign bodies (dust, cinders and so forth) frequently cause considerable discomfort by irritating the sensitive conjunctiva. If the body has been in the eye only a short time, it may be removed by a nurse. The lower lid should be everted, the patient instructed to look up and the lower half of the conjunctival sac examined.

If the body is not found, the upper eye should be examined by everting the upper lid. The nurse stands in front of the patient and instructs him to look down at his feet. She then takes the lashes between thumb and fingers of one hand and with the other places a matchstick, an applicator or a toothpick across the upper part of the lid. The lashes are pulled downward and forward away from the eye as the applicator is pressed downward gently. The foreign body may be removed by touching it gently with a small applicator tipped with cotton and moistened in saline solution.

If removal by this method is unsuccessful, or if the offending particle has been in the eye for a considerable time, the nurse should not attempt to remove it. It may have become embedded in the cornea and there is considerable danger of serious injury if removal is attempted by unskilled hands. The ophthalmologist usually requires local anesthesia, a hand lens, fluorescein, an eye spud, normal saline for irrigating the eye and, as a prophylaxis against infection, an antibiotic solution to instill after removal of the offending

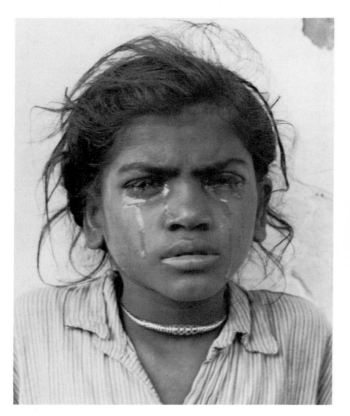

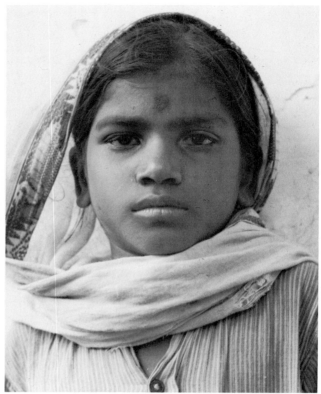

FIG. 32-5A. Tears of trachoma (India). When the eye is infected by the virus of trachoma, the delicate membranes called "conjunctiva" are the site of small granulations that give them a characteristic, roughened appearance. Indeed, the term *trachoma* comes from a Greek word meaning *roughness*. (World Health Organization)

FIG. 32-5B. Ten days later. Treatment with Aureomycin ointment has given back their sparkle to the young patient's eyes. Other commmon eye inflammations of tropical regions make it easier for trachoma to take root. A large number of countries have launched antitrachoma campaigns with help from WHO. (World Health Organization)

particle. If the particle is known to be a metal, the doctor may use a magnet to remove it.

Acid and Alkali Burns

Careless use of hair sprays and other spray-on products is increasing the incidence of chemical burns. Whenever acid or alkali get on the lids or in the eye, an emergency exists in which there is frequently no time to wait for the physician. In such a condition, *the lids, the conjunctiva and the cornea must be flushed copiously!* The easiest and quickest way for this to be done may be the best, i.e., simply immerse the patient's head in a bucket or a basin of water. More satisfactory is to flush the eye using a syringe, if available, taking care not to contaminate the other eye if it has not already been contaminated. Continuous flushing for at least 15 minutes is desirable. Plain tap water is adequate under such circumstances.

Actinic Trauma

Excessive sunlight or a welder's arc can cause ultraviolet ray damage to the cornea. This injury may also be known as "welder's flash" or snow blindness. In the home, it may occur from use of a sun lamp. Treatment consists of patching both eyes and instilling anesthetic drops.

Contusions and Hematoma ("Black Eye")

Hemorrhage into the orbit from trauma is a frequent occurrence. The bleeding that takes place into the loose tissues of the orbit spreads rapidly and produces a discoloration of lids and surrounding skin. In itself the injury is not too serious, but frequently it is frightening to patients because of discoloration and marked swelling in such a prominent site. The bleeding usually stops spontaneously, but it may be reduced in amount and the swelling made less by the application of cold compresses. Absorption of the blood may be hastened after the first 24 hours by the use of hot compresses applied 15 minutes at a time at intervals throughout the day. Drugs are now available to help hasten absorption of hematomas.

Corneal Abrasions

Lacerations of the cornea can be detected after being stained with sodium fluorescein. Usually a local anesthetic and antibacterial drops are administered and an eye patch is applied for 24 to 36 hours. The patient is instructed to keep the eyes at rest for comfort and to facilitate the healing process. A few physicians recommend no eye dressing. The danger to be guarded against with an abrasion is the development of a corneal ulcer.

Lacerations

Lacerations of the eyelids are not serious unless they are accompanied by an injury to the eyeball. Injuries to the lids are treated in the same way as any other wound but, because of his special training, the ophthalmologist usually is requested to care for them. Lacerations of the eyeball are more serious because of the danger of the production of visual defects, and more extensive injuries may even endanger the entire eye. These are referred invariably to the ophthalmologist for appropriate care. Such injuries may entail transplantation of conjunctival flaps to prevent leakage of ocular fluids, excision of prolapsed iris and, in severe injuries, even removal of the eye.

CONDITIONS OF THE EYELIDS

Blepharitis

By maintaining cleanliness and preventing excessive dryness, this common disorder of the lids can be controlled. It is frequently associated with dandruff; therefore, attempts are made to keep the scalp clean. Daily cleaning of the eyelids by rubbing gently with a clean wet washcloth helps to remove scales. Usually, an anti-infective ointment is prescribed, such as nitrofurazone (Furacin) or sulfisoxazole (Gantrisin), to be applied to the lid margin at bedtime.

Sty (External Hordeolum)

A *sty* is an infection of the Zeis's or Moll's glands that empty at the free edge of the eyelid. The area becomes swollen, red, tender and painful. An eyelash will be found in the center of the yellow point that appears. Hot compresses, applied in the early stage, hasten the pointing of the abscess. Removal of the central lash often is followed by drainage of pus, but incision sometimes is necessary. Antibiotic therapy hastens control of the infection.

Chalazia

A *chalazion* is a cyst of the meibomian glands. It occurs as a small lump, hard and painless, in the lid. Occasionally, such a cyst may become infected. When this occurs, hot compresses are used; an incision and a drainage may be necessary. Massage may help resorption of an uninfected cyst; however, the usual treatment is to make a small incision and express the cyst.

Trachoma

This chronic, highly communicable disease of the eyelids (Fig. 32-5) is one of the most common diseases of man and affects about 15 per cent of the world's population. It is bilateral and is caused by a virus of the psittacosis-lymphogranuloma venereum group. Trachoma is common in China, India, Japan and countries around the Mediterranean; individuals may suffer with trachoma for months and years when untreated. In the United States, it is rare except among American Indians and Mexicans.

After an acute inflammatory process, follicles appear on the conjunctiva. Due to scar formation, the eyelid turns in, which causes the lashes to scratch the cornea, thereby irritating and infecting it. This inflammation often leads to ulceration and blindness.

Trachoma is spread by direct contact; therefore, personal cleanliness is a key factor in prevention. By isolating known cases, encouraging solitary sleeping and initiating antibiotic therapy early, the disease may be controlled. The World Health Organization is making great strides in eliminating this curable disease. It has almost been eliminated in Japan and the Philippines.

THE PATIENT WITH AN INFLAMMATION OF THE EYE

Conjunctivitis

Conjunctivitis may result from bacterial infection, allergy, trauma, and viral, rickettsial or chemical injury. However, no matter what the cause, the symptoms are similar: redness, pain, swelling and lacrimation. The amount and the nature of discharge depend on the offending organisms; for instance, the pneumococcus and the gonococcus cause an abundant purulent discharge. Frequent saline irrigations are required to remove the discharge. Warm compresses are recommended, to be applied for 15 minutes 3 or 4 times a day. Ointments such as sulfacetamide (Sulamyd) or sulfisoxazole (Gantrisin) may be instilled, which clear the infection in 1 to 3 days. Untreated, the infection usually subsides in a week to 10 days. Precautions must be taken to prevent dissemination of infection to the other eye as well as to other persons. Hands should be kept clean when treating the eye; individual clean washcloths and towels should be used.

TABLE 32-2. Differential diagnosis of inflamed eye

	Acute Conjunctivitis	Acute Iritis	Acute Glaucoma	Corneal Ulcer or Trauma
Incidence	Very common	Common	Not common	Common
Vision	Normal	Some blurring	Marked blurring	Blurred (usually)
Pain	None	Moderate	Severe	May have pain
Intraocular pressure	Normal	Normal or low	Elevated	Normal
Cornea	Clear	Clear	Steamy	May have abrasion, foreign body or ulcer
Ocular discharge	Moderate to copious	None	None	Watery and perhaps purulent
Pupillary response to light	Normal	Weak	Weak	Normal
Pupil size	Normal	Small	Dilated	Normal or small
Conjunctival vessels dilated	Yes	Mostly circumcorneal	Yes	Yes
Prognosis	Self-limited; 3 to 5 days	Poor	Without Proper Treatment Poor	Poor

Uveitis

Uveitis is a general term for inflammatory conditions of the uveal tract (iris, ciliary body, choroid). It may affect one or all parts; causative agents are multiple. *Anterior uveitis* refers to *iritis* and *iridocyclitis,* whereas *posterior uveitis* refers to *choroiditis* and *chorioretinitis; panuveitis* involves the entire uveal tract. The most frequent form of uveitis (iritis) is usually unilateral and is characterized by pain, photophobia, blurring of vision, redness (circumcorneal flush) and a constricted pupil.

Some authorities prefer to classify the various forms of uveitis into granulomatous and nongranulomatous. In some aspects, the two forms are similar, but in others, there occurs a significant difference (see Table 32-3).

It is important for the nurse to recognize the significance of uveitis because of the complications and

TABLE 32-3. Comparison between granulomatous and nongranulomatous uveitis

	Granulomatous	Nongranulomatous
Location	Any portion of uveal tract but predilection for posterior part	Anterior portion; iris, ciliary body
Onset	Insidious	Acute
Pain	None or minimal	Marked
Circumcorneal flush	Slight	Present
Course	Chronic	Acute
Prognosis	Fair to poor	Good

sequelae should it go untreated. Anterior uveitis may produce adhesions that impede aqueous outflow at the anterior chamber angle, causing *glaucoma.* In posterior uveitis, adhesions develop that hinder the flow of aqueous from the posterior to the anterior chamber. This in turn interferes with lens metabolism and sometimes causes *cataract.* Even *retinal detachment* may occur as a result of traction exerted on the retina by vitreous strands.

Treatment and Management of Uveitis. Because the ophthalmologist can differentiate among the various forms of uveitis in his diagnosis, treatment is directed to each specific type of involvement. Atropine is used to reduce the likelihood of adhesion formation. Local steroids such as methylprednisolone (Medrol) are effective for anti-inflammatory and antiallergic action. Occasionally, systemic steroids are used. Medications for comfort and relief of pain are also prescribed.

Nongranulomatous uveitis subsides with treatment in a few weeks. Granulomatous uveitis may last months and even years in spite of treatment.

Sympathetic Ophthalmia

Fortunately, this is a rare condition, but it may be suspected when there is a history of a penetrating eye injury in one eye (exciting eye) and the patient complains of photophobia, blurring vision and injection in the other eye (sympathizing eye). Sympathetic ophthalmia is a severe granulomatous bilateral uveitis that may occur from 2 to several years after an eye injury.

Medical management is directed in 1 of 2 directions: corticosteroids are administered both locally and systemically, as well as atropine locally. This treatment has proved effective. The other, more radical procedure is to suggest preventive enucleation of the severely injured eye before sympathetic ophthalmia develops. This decision is a difficult one; often, a patient can think more clearly and reach a satisfactory decision if he has the time and opportunity to express his thoughts and rationalizations. In such a case the nurse needs to understand the nature of the problem, the patient's ability and condition, and the desired goals of the ophthalmologist. Untreated, the disease progresses to cause bilateral blindness.

Pterygium

Pterygium is a triangular fold of membrane that extends onto the cornea from the white of the eye; it always occurs nasally. It is thought to be caused by chronic irritation, as from dust or wind. Surgical interference prevents its growth and protects against loss of vision. In some eye clinics, surgery is followed by beta radiation therapy, which helps prevent recurrence of pterygium. Patients often erroneously refer to pterygium as a cataract.

THE PATIENT HAVING EYE SURGERY

Preoperative Nursing Management

(Review Psychological and Physical Needs of the Eye Patient, p. 722.)

The preparation of the patient for an ophthalmic operation must be carried out with the most scrupulous care. The lower bowel is evacuated in the morning of the day of operation, and only liquid diet is given after that. The hair of female patients should be so arranged that it will remain in place for several days and bandages may be applied over it. Usually, long hair is plaited into 2 braids that may be pinned up over the head. Before preparing the eyes for operation, the head of the patient should be covered with a stockinet cap. The male patient should have his face shaved. The eyebrow above the eye to be operated upon is shaved only in special cases ordered by the surgeon. The eyelashes of the eye to undergo operation are cut with blunt scissors covered with petrolatum in order to catch the lashes. Both eyelids, the nose, the forehead and the cheeks are scrubbed thoroughly with pHisoHex and then are rinsed with saline solution; sterile cotton sponges and forceps are used. After this procedure both eyes are irrigated with 2 per cent saline solution, followed by drops of an antiseptic or antibiotic solution into the eye to be operated on. This procedure varies in different clinics. A small cross mark then is made with a colored solution on the forehead over the eye to be operated on. Both closed eyes then are covered with eye patches wet with boric acid solution, and the eyes and the forehead are protected with sterile gauze dressings bound in place with a 2-inch bandage. In the preparation of patients for operations on the eye, no adhesive should be used on the skin.

Before the patient is taken to the operating room, precautions as to the removal of artificial eyes, dentures and so forth must be taken. These are the same as those described for any other surgical operation. If the patient is to have local anesthesia, he should be instructed to hold his head still and to look up or down as directed by the ophthalmologist. He should be cautioned not to "squeeze" the eye during or after operation.

Postoperative Nursing Considerations

After operation the patient is returned to bed to lie in the supine position with a small pillow under the head. Pillows on each side of the head are used to keep the head quiet. Where possible, the patient should have a call bell at hand and should be instructed to ring when necessary rather than to move or strain in an attempt to be self-sufficient. Inasmuch as the patient often has both eyes covered, it is well for any person who enters his unit to announce himself. The application of bed sides to the bed of a patient with bandaged eyes frequently gives him a sense of security.

The ophthalmologist should be notified immediately if the patient is restless, if he coughs, turns, develops a rhinitis, has excessive pains or disturbs the dressing.

The mouth should be swabbed twice daily, but the teeth should not be brushed until permission is given by the ophthalmologist. Female patients should not have their hair combed until they are allowed out of bed. When the patient complains of abdominal discomfort due to gas, a hot-water bottle to the abdomen and the insertion of a rectal tube often give relief. Catheterization may be necessary when there is difficulty in voiding. Morphine should never be given to ophthalmic patients unless it is certain that vomiting will not injure the eye.

Diversional or recreational therapy is important, but should be of such a nature that the eyes are not fatigued in any way. Even the environment of this patient is an important consideration. The walls and the ceiling should be painted in soft pastel shades. Light should be regulated so that it is not bright and does not produce a glare.

Before the patient leaves the hospital, he must be informed thoroughly by the physician regarding medications, eye aids (glasses), the type of work he can do and his follow-up visits.

STRABISMUS (SQUINT)

Strabismus or *squint* is a condition in which one eye deviates from the object at which the person is looking (lay term "crosseyed"). The deviating eye may turn in *(esotropia)* or out *(exotropia)*. It may result from paralysis of the nerves supplying the extraocular muscles, due to injury or disease. Double vision or diplopia results. In children, a strabismus due to ocular defects often develops. It is characterized by single vision, usually because the image seen by the divergent eye is suppressed involuntarily.

The strabismus in children often may be corrected by the wearing of properly fitted glasses. Orthopedic training for muscle disturbances such as strabismus is successful in some instances without operation. It consists of a series of muscle exercises carried out by means of various instruments, cards and test objects. Patients with a marked degree of squint usually undergo operation after having had some training; after the eyes are straightened, the exercises are employed again. Early detection and immediate medical consultation are to be encouraged if the defect is to be corrected satisfactorily.

CORNEAL TRANSPLANTATION (KERATOPLASTY)

A keratoplasty may be done to repair a corneal opacity (scar) or for keratoconus. The circular segment of cornea removed from the patient must be exactly matched and replaced by a similar segment of cornea from a donor eye. For best results, the graft should be removed within 5 or 6 hours following the death of the donor (to prevent softening of the cornea) and transplanted within 2 days.* Recently, a method of freezing corneal tissue at a controlled rate to −190° F. has made older corneal tissue as suitable as fresh tissue. Older preserved grafts (frozen, dehydrated, or in glycerine) may be used for lamellar rather than penetrating transplants.

The graft may be total penetrating (including all layers of the cornea), partial penetrating, or lamellar (involving only the outer layers of the cornea).

Medical and Nursing Management

Preoperative and Intraoperative Care. Since this is elective surgery, the patient is probably aware of the nature of the operation and the postoperative limita-

* The national eye bank (Eye-Bank for Sight Restoration, Inc., 210 E. 64th St., New York, N. Y. 10021) was founded in 1945. Eyes have been donated from persons all over the country and distributed to qualified ophthalmologists throughout the United States.

tions; he is no doubt optimistic about the likelihood of improved vision. The nurse, nevertheless, must allow time for the expression of concerns or questions that the patient may still have. Psychological and cultural concerns regarding his disability may have to be explored before he is in optimal condition for surgery. Freedom from respiratory or eye infections promotes postoperative healing.

Usually a transplant is done under general anesthesia. A trephining instrument, having an end similar to that of a cookie cutter but the size of the cornea, is placed over the opacity and the cornea is removed. A set of instruments identical in size is used to remove the donor cornea. Usually 8 sutures fix the transplant in place. About 80 per cent of patients with keratoconus receive improved vision with this procedure; for scarring, the improvement is from 30 to 70 per cent, according to Vaughan.

Postoperative Care. Objectives of postoperative patient care are (1) to avoid intraocular pressure as well as pressure upon the operated eye; (2) to provide rest for the eye so that healing progresses smoothly; and (3) to employ measures that will prevent infection of the eye.

To avoid increasing the pressure in the eye, the nurse must be cognizant of those activities that can elevate pressure (see p. 738). Loss of aqueous humor through the suture line by increased pressure could cause dislocation of the newly transplanted cornea, prolapse of the iris, adhesions of the iris to the cornea, or malformation of the anterior chamber. As the patient is transferred from the operating table to his bed or stretcher, adequate personnel are required in order to move him horizontally in one smooth shift, giving adequate support to his head.

Both eyes are covered to provide rest, which enhances healing. If one eye is uncovered, its movement would affect the operated eye, because they move in unison. Healing is slow because the cornea is avascular, which also makes the possibility of infection greater. Dressing changes may be done daily by the physician, who will instill a miotic and an antibiotic. Bilateral dressings usually are in place up to a week. Unabsorbable sutures (silk) are removed in about 21 to 25 days; absorbable (surgical gut) sutures do not have to be removed. Meticulous sterile technique is followed in dressing changes to protect the susceptible corneal epithelium from infection.

A patient with a penetrating type of corneal transplant requires bed rest much longer than one with the nonpenetrating type. His restrictions mean that he must be fed and bathed, and depends upon the nurse for mouth care and being placed on the bed pan. His head may be elevated slightly toward the unoperated side. Passive range-of-motion and regular deep breathing exercises are encouraged to prevent circulatory and respiratory complications.

The individual with a nonpenetrating corneal transplant may be allowed out of bed with assistance to sit in a chair for short lengths of time; his eyes are bandaged.

Medications, fluid, and a diet that will prevent urinary retention, straining with defecation or constipation are given. Usually codeine and aspirin can alleviate complaints of pain. If such discomforts remain unrelieved, the physician should be informed, because they may indicate that the transplant has shifted, hemorrhage has occurred, or the dressing is too tight.

As healing progresses, activity increases. When the unoperated eye is uncovered, more liberties are allowed. Those activities that produce strain are still forbidden. The patient's vision will still be poor when the dressing is removed, but it will improve gradually as the inflammation and edema diminish. At night, he should wear a protective shield. Instructions for home care include precautions to be taken as well as information about signs that indicate complications. Periodic visits to the ophthalmologist will ensure that the progress is going in the right direction.

CORNEAL ULCERS

Inflammation of the cornea is called *keratitis* and, if this process is associated with a loss of substance, a corneal ulcer results. The inflammatory reaction often spreads deeper to the iris (iritis), with the result that pus is formed and collects as a white or yellow deposit behind the cornea (hypopyon). If the ulceration perforates, the iris may prolapse through the cornea, or other serious complications may follow.

Because of the importance of the cornea to vision, any ulceration must be considered as a most serious condition. Scarring or perforation due to corneal ulceration is a major cause of blindness; 10 per cent of all blindness is caused by corneal ulcers. The healing of any but very superficial ulcers is attended with some degree of opacity of the cornea and, therefore, with some diminution of vision.

Symptoms

The symptoms of corneal ulceration are pain, marked photophobia and increased lacrimation. The eye usually appears somewhat injected or "bloodshot."

Treatment

Prevention is much simpler and easier than cure. Therefore, the nurse must realize that prompt removal of foreign bodies and early treatment of infec-tions may prevent the occurrence of a corneal ulcer.

Dark glasses are provided to relieve the photophobia. Mydriatics are given at frequent intervals. Tetracaine (Pontocaine) may be used to relieve pain. Fluorescein generally is used to outline the ulcers before the application of the healing solutions. Antibiotic solutions and chemotherapeutic agents are prescribed for the specific type of infection, inasmuch as the microorganism may be bacterial, viral, or fungal. Warm compresses help greatly to relieve the pain of this condition.

THE PATIENT WITH A DETACHED RETINA

A retinal detachment is a separation of the retina from the choroid. The retina, one may recall, is that layer that perceives light and transmits impulses from its nerve cells to the optic nerve. Normally, the choroid and retina are not joined, but are in close apposition. Tears or holes in the retina may result from trauma or from degeneration, as may occur in myopia. It may happen suddenly or develop slowly. Recent studies have shown that approximately 6 per cent of the population have small holes or tears in the retina. Aging weakens these spots. A tear in the retina allows vitreous humor and transudate from the choroidal vessels to seep behind the retina and separate it from the choroid. Diagnosis is not too difficult for the ophthalmologist; surgery is the only effective treatment if done fairly early.

The usual symptoms include flashes of light and blurred or "sooty" vision sudden in onset; the patient may have the sensation of particles moving in his line of vision. Definite areas of vision may be blank and in a few days the patient may have the sensation of a veil coming up or down in front of the eye, finally resulting in loss of vision.

The suddenness of the incapacity creates confusion and apprehension in most patients, as well as a fear of blindness. Usually, it means that the man must abandon his business or the woman her activity, with little or no time to make plans. The patient is treated with bed rest and has both eyes bandaged, in the hope that the retina will fall back into place as much as possible before surgery.

The area of detachment should be in the dependent position. For example, a patient with a superior temporal detachment (the most commonly affected) in the right eye should be supine with the head turned to the right. For a left inferior nasal detachment of the retina, he should sit up with the head turned to the right. Sedation and the tranquilizing drugs keep the patient comfortable and quiet.

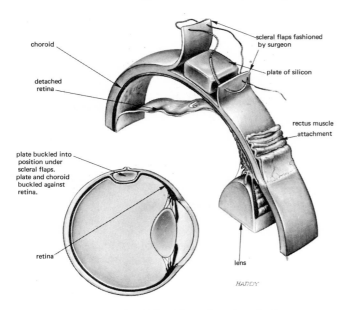

FIG. 32-6. Scleral buckling for detached retina. (Ethicon, Inc.)

Surgical Intervention

The objective in surgical treatment is to create a scar that seals the retina in place as it heals. Such treatment may be accomplished in one of several ways: electrodiathermy, cryosurgery, photocoagulation, or scleral buckling.

1. In *electrodiathermy,* an electrode needle is passed through the sclera, allowing the subretinal collection of fluid to escape. Because an exudate forms from the choroid, the torn retina adheres to the choroid, which in turn adheres to the sclera.

2. A supercooled probe (*cryosurgery* or *retinal cryopexy*) is applied to the sclera, causing minimal damage; the choroid and retina adhere as a result of the scarring. The advantage of this method over the use of diathermy is the reduced damage to the sclera.

3. By directing a strong beam of light from a carbon arc source through the dilated pupil, a small burn causing a choroid retinal inflammatory exudate can be formed. The *laser beam* (light amplification by stimulated emission of radiation) can be used in *photocoagulation.* This method of treatment is used for limited retinal detachments and also may be used postoperatively to reattach small areas.

In *scleral buckling,* the idea is to shorten the sclera to enhance contact between the choroid and retina. After the subretinal fluid is withdrawn, the detachment is treated by one of the methods described above. Then the treated area is indented to "buckle" inward toward the vitreous (Fig. 32-6).

Postoperative Management and Prognosis

The patient has both eyes bandaged and is kept in bed for several days. This routine varies with the surgical procedure; patients with scleral buckling operations are permitted out of bed much sooner than those having diathermy. Precautions are taken to prevent bumping the head. After a gradual resumption of function, the patient may resume his usual activities in 3 to 5 weeks.

The psychological nursing care of this patient is of major importance. Diversion that is relaxing is desirable, such as conversation, listening to music, having someone read a favorite book and so forth.* These individuals become depressed easily; therefore, every attempt should be made to prevent this reaction. The nurse should be sure that the patient understands all instructions for posthospital care and follow-up visits.

The prognosis for untreated retinal detachment is increasing detachment and eventual blindness. About 75 per cent of patients can be cured with electrocoagulation. Some patients may require a second operation, which may be performed about 10 to 14 days after the first one. Twenty-five per cent of all detachments are or will become bilateral.

THE PATIENT WITH A CATARACT

A *cataract* is an opacity of the crystalline lens or its capsule. Occasionally it occurs at birth (congenital cataract), it may occur in younger individuals as a result of trauma or disease, but most commonly it occurs in adults past middle age (senile cataract).

Pathophysiology

The normal lens is a clear, transparent, button-like structure lying back of the iris; it possesses strong refractive powers. Physical and chemical changes may produce a loss of transparency of the lens. Swelling fibers, for example, cause a distortion of the image. Chemical change in lens protein may cause coagulation, thereby producing a cloudy appearance. Metabolic changes that result in a reduction of vitamins C and B_2 in the lens also contribute to the formation of opacities. Although cataracts can be produced in the laboratory in many ways, the real cause of senile cataracts is still unknown.

Symptoms

Because the rays of light entering the eye must pass through the pupil and the lens to reach the retina, any opacity in the lens behind the pupil will produce alterations in vision. Objects may seem distorted; in

---

* Recordings of books may be obtained from the public library or local association for the blind.

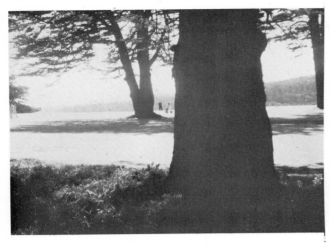 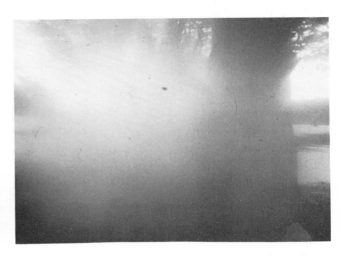

FIG. 32-7. The photograph on the left is a view seen by a person with normal vision. The photograph on the right is reproduced as if seen by a person with a moderately advanced senile cataract (note that the opacity is more dense in the center). (Vaughan, Cook and Asbury: General Ophthalmology. ed. 5. Lange Medical Publications, 1968)

bright light, the patient may be annoyed with glare. With cataract, halos may appear around light. The patient experiences no pain, and visual loss is gradual (Fig. 32-7). In time, the degenerative processes cause more opacification of the lens, and opacity becomes complete. Ordinarily, the lens is not visible; however, when a cataract develops, the pupil, which is normally black, becomes gray and later milky-white. The cataract can be cured only by operation.

Patient Preparation for Surgery

In patients with uncomplicated senile cataracts, about 95 per cent will regain satisfactory vision with surgery. Surgery for cataract is done at the convenience of the patient; usually he requests it when the sight in his better eye causes problems for him. Because this particular surgery can be performed safely on elderly patients, even those in their nineties, the nurse is in a position to dispel family beliefs that the patient may be "too old" for the procedure. Improvement of a visual defect may make a person more independent and happier.

The patient is oriented to his room, personnel and other patients in such a way that his personal needs are considered. For example, the nurse could place his bedside table on the side of his eye that has better vision. The patient can then see his belongings with a minimum of head movement.

Prior to coming to the operating room, the patient receives medications such as secobarbital and meperidine, which make him drowsy. Local anesthesia is administered in the operating room.

Surgical Intervention

Two general types of lens extraction may be performed: extracapsular and intracapsular. *Extracapsular extraction* is more often performed for congenital and traumatic cataracts than for senile cataracts. An incision is made through the sclera barely outside of the cornea, the lens capsule is excised and the lens is expressed by pressure on the eye from below with a metal spoon. It is more conservative and simple to perform than the intracapsular extraction; however, in about 30 per cent of patients, a secondary membrane forms that requires *discission* (a needling or dividing of the membrane).

The *intracapsular extraction* consists of removing the lens and the capsule which encases it. This is the procedure of choice for senile cataracts.

Operative Procedure. To hold the eyelids apart, a speculum (self-retaining retractor) is placed inside the lids. Guide line and traction sutures are placed before the conjunctival incision is made at the 12 o'clock position; this incision is then extended to 3 and 9 o'clock positions. The lens capsule is grasped and delivered and final suturing is done. If necessary, the surgeon reforms the anterior chamber with an injection of saline. Usually an iridectomy is performed at the time of cataract extraction.

When difficulty is expected in freeing the capsule of its zonules, a fibrinolytic and proteolytic enzyme, α-chymotrypsin, is injected into the anterior chamber under the iris. The lytic action is completed in 2 or 3 minutes and allows the lens to be extracted more easily.

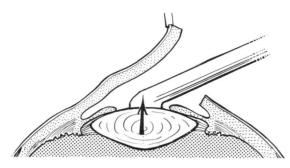

The direction of the initial pull is straight upward toward the ceiling.

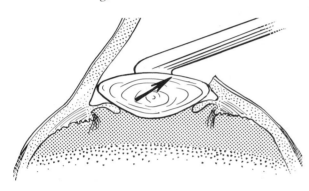

The direction of pull is changed as indicated only when the lens feels free and ready to detach.

FIG. 32-8. Cryosurgery for cataract extraction. (Croll, M., and Croll, L. J.: A new cryoslide technique for cataract removal. Amer. J. Ophthal., *62*:83-88, 1966)

Cryosurgery. Cryosurgery is a recently devised approach to the extraction of cataracts. Many instruments and techniques have developed since Kelman first introduced the cryostylet in the United States in 1962. All cryosurgical instruments operate on the principle that a cold metal adheres to a moist object. A thick pencil-like instrument with a metal probe tip (straight or curved) is activated so that the temperature of the tip ranges from −30° C. to −40° C. The conjunctival flap is prepared and dissected as for a regular intracapsular extraction, after which the cryosurgical instrument is placed directly on the lens capsule (Fig. 32-8). An ice ball forms in seconds, causing the capsule to adhere to the probe. A gentle upward and then sideward force frees and delivers the lens. The corneal flap is sutured back in place.

Cryoextraction is indicated for hypermature cataracts, which have a high incidence of capsular rupture, and in patients in whom a capsular rupture may exacerbate a glaucoma or uveitis.

Nursing implications both pre- and postoperatively are the same as for the conventional intracapsular extraction. In the operating room, the nurse must know about the care and handling of the special instrument. Some are operated thermo-electrically while others are self-contained disposable units.

Postoperative Nursing Management

The eye is kept bandaged for 5 to 10 days and an eye shield is worn over the dressing to protect the eye from injury. Both eyes may be covered, but usually only the operated eye is covered.

The patient is permitted a low firm pillow immediately after operation and may have the head of the bed raised 30° to 45°. Any strain felt by the patient may be relieved somewhat by placing pillows under the knees for short intervals and a small pillow under the small of the back. Liquid diet is supplemented with custards, junkets, gelatin and so forth. Iced water, fruit juices, milk and other gas-producing foods are avoided. Soft diet or diet of choice usually is resumed on the second day.

Pain usually is slight after cataract extraction but, should it become severe, the surgeon should be notified at once, since it may be the symptom of a serious complication such as hemorrhage.

The patient is allowed out of bed in 24 to 48 hours, depending on his condition and his physician's orders. However, he is advised to move cautiously and slowly and to avoid straining for at least 3 weeks. For example, he ought not to stoop, pick up objects from the floor, or lift anything. Slip-in slippers will avoid the necessity to bend to tie laces. Even if the patient has vision in one eye, he should not walk through corridors alone; this will prevent his being bumped because of an inability to see objects or persons on the operated side.

The surgeon usually dresses the eye 24 hours after operation and once daily thereafter until the seventh or the eighth day. When the sutures are removed, the eye is anesthetized with 1 per cent pontocaine; sterile eye speculum, forceps and scissors are required. The patient is discharged when his eyes have become accustomed to ordinary daylight (about the tenth day).

About 3 weeks postoperatively, the aphakic (without lens) patient receives a temporary pair of thick convex glasses. Adjustment to these is gradual. The sides curve inward, the bottom curves upward and the top curves down. Only through the center of the glass will the patient have clear vision. He must learn to turn his head to bring an object into central vision. The patient needs practice in judging distances, such as when climbing stairs or pouring liquids. Objects appear one third larger than they really are. Contact lenses reduce this size discrepancy and allow adjustment to binocular vision more readily.

THE PATIENT WITH CATARACT SURGERY
Objectives and Principles of Nursing Management

I. To prepare the patient for cataract surgery
   A. Orient the patient to his new environment
      1. Walk with the patient around the unit
      2. Explain the plan of care
      3. Provide side rails on bed if patient is elderly
   B. Begin rehabilitation measures as soon after admission as possible
      1. Teach patient to breathe deeply, move extremities and do quadriceps muscle setting without moving his head
      2. Instruct the patient how to close his eyes slowly without squeezing the lids
   C. Reduce the conjunctival bacterial count
      1. Obtain a conjunctival culture
      2. Use local broad-spectrum antibiotics as ordered
      3. Use aseptic technique when doing eye treatments and procedures
   D. Prepare the affected eye for surgery
      1. Instill local mydriatic if ordered
      2. Determine whether the pupil is dilated after the instillation of a mydriatic is completed

II. To give optimal nursing care postoperatively
   A. Reorient the patient to his surroundings
   B. Prevent increased intraocular pressure and stress on the suture line
      1. Instruct the patient not to cough, sneeze, or move too rapidly
      2. Position the patient on his back and unoperated side
      3. Elevate the head of the bed 30° to 45° for comfort
      4. Keep the eye shield on the operated eye to protect it from injury

   C. Promote the comfort of the patient
      1. Position him to relieve back pain
      2. Give mild analgesics to control pain
      3. Maintain a quiet and relaxed environment
      4. Inform the patient when you enter the room
   D. Observe and treat for complications
      1. Nausea and vomiting
         a. Support the patient's head when he is vomiting
         b. Use antiemetic drugs and cold compresses to throat
      2. Hemorrhage
         a. Notify physician immediately if patient complains of sudden pain in eye
         b. Observe for and try to allay restlessness

III. To promote the rehabilitation of the patient
   A. Encourage the patient to become independent
      1. Teach him to increase his activities gradually
      2. Walk with him when he first becomes ambulatory
   B. Instruct the patient and his family about the use of eyedrops
   C. Refer the patient to proper agencies if home assistance is needed
   D. Assist the patient to participate in a program of diversional activities during the convalescent period
   E. Inform the patient that:
      1. Dark glasses may be used after the eye dressing is removed
      2. Temporary corrective lenses may be prescribed during the convalescent period
      3. Permanent lenses will be prescribed 6 to 8 weeks after surgery

However, not all individuals can adjust to contact lenses. In about 8 weeks, permanent lenses are ordered. By this time, the patient should be making a satisfactory psychological, physical and visual adjustment.[*]

Some eye surgeons substitute a plastic lens for the real lens when it is removed. The introduction of the plastic lens into the eye dispenses with the need to wear eyeglasses or contact lenses postoperatively. However, this technique is complicated and not accepted by all ophthalmologists. Much more study is needed before this procedure can be used generally.

[*] Read Cockerill, E. E.: Reflections on my nursing care. Amer. J. Nurs., 65:83-85, May, 1965. This is an excellent paper written by a person who experienced cataract surgery. The psychological aspects are described particularly well.

THE PATIENT WITH GLAUCOMA

Glaucoma means sea green, which is the color of the light reflex from the pupil after vision has been destroyed. Glaucoma was known to Socrates four centuries before Christ. The disease is not hopeless, but the degree to which treatment for it can be successful depends on how early it is detected and how cooperative the patient is.[*]

The second most common cause of blindness in the United States is glaucoma; it is estimated that 1 million Americans have undiagnosed glaucoma. The health professions have a responsibility to encourage eye check-ups in conjunction with an annual physical

[*] Headland, M. F.: I'm winning my fight against glaucoma. Today's Health, 34:44.

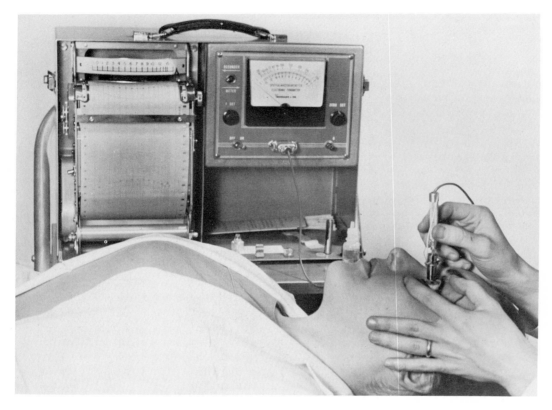

Fig. 32-9. A patient is about to have the tonometer footplate placed on her cornea, centrally and vertically. In addition to the indicator on the right side of the electronic tonometer showing the intraocular pressure, the left side of the machine (tonographer) can graphically produce a 4 minute permanent record showing pressure changes. (Thomas Czerner, M.D., Chicago Wesley Memorial Hospital and V. Mueller)

examination, because *early detection could substantially reduce the incidence of blindness from glaucoma.*

Glaucoma is a disease characterized by increased tension or pressure within the eye. This disease ordinarily occurs in individuals past 40 and may be classified as primary or secondary:

1. *Primary:*
   a. Chronic simple glaucoma (wide-angle)
   b. Congestive glaucoma (narrow-angle)
      (1) Acute
      (2) Chronic

2. *Secondary:*

   Many types secondary to such conditions as trauma, aphakia, iritis, tumor, hemorrhage, etc.

The cause of primary glaucoma is unknown, although it often is associated with emotional disturbances, endocrine imbalance, allergy or vasomotor disturbance. Evidence is accumulating that chronic simple glaucoma, the most common form, is inherited. A recently devised steroid test can show whether an individual has a predisposition to develop this type of glaucoma.

Pathophysiology and Diagnostic Assessment

Intraocular pressure increases when the patient exerts energy as in running, climbing the stairs, bending over to pick up an object, sneezing, or turning the head suddenly. It occurs when one is emotionally upset (e.g., apprehension about the nature and prognosis of surgery may cause an increase in pressure). Also likely to affect pressure are such common-place maneuvers as rubbing the eyes, brushing the hair, squinting or closing the eyes tightly because of a bright light or flying dust and dirt. Apparently, both physical and emotional factors are involved in increasing pressure within the eye. This knowledge is significant to the nurse as she assesses the needs of the patient who has an eye problem, whether it occurs preoperatively or postoperatively.

The total volume and pressure of intraocular fluid is regulated by the balance between formation and reabsorption of aqueous humor. Ordinarily, the pressure-regulating mechanism maintains an almost constant balance throughout life. The exact operation of this mechanism is not known; however, pathologic changes at the irido-corneal angle usually increases intraocular pressure.

Measurement of Intraocular Pressure. Increased intraocular pressure or hardening of the eyeball may be noted with the fingers, but more accurately it is measured by means of a *tonometer*. This is a simple and painless test in which the patient tilts his head back and looks to the ceiling. The cornea of the eye is anesthetized with a drop of 0.5 per cent ophthaine. The sterile footplate of the tonometer is placed on the cornea; a small pressure is applied to the central plunger, causing the central cornea to be displaced inward. Pressure within the eye exerts a force that moves an indicator (Fig. 32-9). A normal reading is 12 to 22 mm. Hg.

Electronic tonometry can be done, but it involves expensive equipment. Tonography units are available in which a graphic presentation of intraocular pressure is documented for a 4-minute test period (Fig. 32-9). This is a valuable index that assists the physician in determining movement of the aqueous humor.

Acute (Narrow-Angle) Glaucoma

When pressure increases rapidly, severe pain occurs in and around the eye. Artificial lights appear to have a rainbow around them. Vision becomes cloudy or blurred. Nausea and vomiting as well as pupil dilatation may be noted. This is an emergency situation, which, if left untreated, may lead to blindness.

Pharmacotherapy. By the use of miotic drugs the pupil is contracted and the iris is drawn away from the cornea, thus allowing the aqueous humor to drain through the lymph spaces into the canal of Schlemm. Pilocarpine, eserine or DFP (diisopropylfluorophosphate) are the drugs employed. Dosage and frequency of drops are regulated to meet the individual requirements.

Another kind of medication (carbonic anhydrase inhibitor) restricts the action of the enzyme that is necessary to produce aqueous humor. Diamox and Neptazine are examples of such an agent. These may aid in getting some patients in better condition for surgery and may control tension in other patients to such an extent that surgery is not necessary.

Osmoglin or ordinary U.S.P. glycerine reduce intraocular pressure through the mechanism of osmotic balance exchange. Glycerine has a high osmotic pressure; it withdraws fluid from the eye through the membrane and lowers pressure.

Surgical Intervention. In acute narrow-angle glaucoma, an incision is made through the cornea so that a portion of the iris may be drawn out and excised (*iridectomy*). This may be peripheral or total (keyhole) iridectomy. By doing this, the iris is prevented from bulging forward to crowd the chamber angle and permits drainage of aqueous humor from the anterior

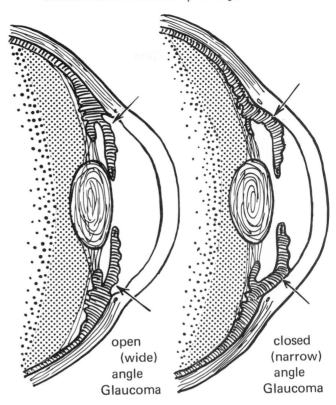

open (wide) angle Glaucoma

closed (narrow) angle Glaucoma

FIG. 32-10. The arrows point to the angle between the root of the iris and the cornea through which the aqueous humor drains back into the circulation. The two kinds of glaucoma require different kinds of treatment. Open angle glaucoma responds well to miotics whereas narrow angle glaucoma requires surgery. (Gordon, D. M.: Diseases of the Eye, Clinical Symposia. Summit, N.J., Ciba Pharm. Co., Dec. 1962)

chamber, thereby reducing intraocular tension. Other operations on the iris (*iridencleisis*) are modifications having the same objective, that is, to permit fluid to escape.

Chronic (Wide-Angle) Glaucoma

This is the most common form of glaucoma. Symptoms are insidious and develop slowly. The patient may have mild discomfort, such as a tired feeling in the eye. Impairment of peripheral vision occurs long before any effects are noted on central vision. The patient may become aware of his peripheral visual impairment by bumping into things at his side that he did not see; driving a car may be a hazard to others because he may not be able to see pedestrians or approaching vehicles laterally. The patient may also note halos around lights.

Pharmaco- and Surgical Therapy. Chronic (wide-angle) glaucoma often is treated by combining miotics with carbonic anhydrous inhibitors. Remissions may occur, but, if there is no improvement, surgery may be done. In the preoperative treatment of these patients, irrigations of both eyes are often prescribed, and weaker solutions of pilocarpine are instilled in the unaffected eye.

The surgeon makes a small opening with a circular knife at the junction of the cornea and the sclera. This operation, called *corneoscleral trephining,* leaves a permanent opening through which aqueous humor may drain. Usually it is covered by a flap of conjunctiva.

After operation, the patient is kept flat and relatively quiet for 24 hours in order to prevent prolapse of the iris through the incision. A liquid diet is permitted. Narcotics or sedatives may be given if necessary. After the first dressing is changed, the patient is allowed more freedom. Usually, he is discharged on the fifth day. He is expected to visit the ophthalmologist regularly, since glaucoma is a condition that must be followed periodically.

Patient Education

Although glaucoma cannot be cured, it can be controlled to a great extent. Whether the patient has had surgery or not, he needs to know what he can do safely and at what point limitations must be set.

Activities that may increase intraocular pressure and should be avoided are:

1. Worry, fear, anger and excitement
2. Tight clothing, such as a tight belt, collar or girdle
3. Heavy lifting
4. Upper respiratory infections
5. Using a mydriatic, such as atropine (accidental use of such a drug may cause blindness)
6. Excessive fluid intake

Recommended activities are:

1. Moderate use of the eyes, as when reading
2. Exercise in moderation to promote general circulation
3. Maintenance of regular bowel habits (straining raises eye pressure)
4. Promotion of oral cleanliness
5. Use of eye medications or washes only with the consent of the ophthalmologist
6. Carrying a card or "dog tag" indicating that the individual has glaucoma

ENUCLEATION

Removal of the eyeball is called *enucleation.* It is necessitated by such trauma that the contents of the globe escape, by infections and by other injuries which threaten the development of sympathetic ophthalmia (see p. 730). During the removal of the eye, muscles are cut as close to the globe as possible. These muscles are approximated with sutures to a plastic prosthesis, thereby providing the means for coordinated motion of the prothesis with the patient's real eye. A plastic, gold or teflon ball is placed in the area of the removed eyeball to form a stump on which the ocularist fixes the prosthesis. This prosthesis is colored to match the patient's eye. In successful cases, it is difficult to distinguish the prosthesis from the normal eye.

In certain cases, the sclera can be retained and the rest of the contents of the eye "scooped" out; this procedure is known as *evisceration.* The main advantage of evisceration is that it provides better motion to the artificial eye.

Exenteration is usually performed in advanced malignancy or severe war injuries. In this procedure, the eyelids, the eyeball and all contents of orbit are removed down to the bone. This operation is *very* disfiguring, and although the ocularist may attempt to build a prosthesis, it very often appears rather poor and unlifelike. These patients usually wear a black patch.

THE NURSE AND THE NEWLY BLIND

There are about 1,000,000 blind persons in America, and each year nearly 40,000 more go blind. Of these newly blind cases, approximately half could have been prevented with our present knowledge.

When an individual has marked visual impairment or is newly blind, he needs a great deal of help in making a healthy adjustment. For the most part, this help is entrusted to those skilled in such rehabilitation. However, a nurse can follow certain practices as she cares for such a person.

A blind person always should be treated with the dignity accorded a normal human being. Avoid expressions of pity. Keep the patient from becoming discouraged by seeing to it that he has someone with whom he can talk or some other form of diversion such as a radio. Help him to overcome his feeling of awkwardness as he performs simple activities.

If he is allowed out of bed, the blind person should survey his room by walking around and touching the furniture. Thereafter, the nurse should be sure that the furniture remains in the same position. Never leave a door half-open; it should be either open or shut. When walking with a blind person, allow him to follow you by lightly touching your elbow; do not push him ahead of you. When he walks alone, he should learn to use a lightweight, white walking stick to warn him of obstacles.

Personal appearance is a significant part of the patient's care. He should be allowed to dress by himself; a woman even can learn to fix her hair and use cosmetics. Table etiquette, writing and so forth all are activities that can be acquired with practice. The nurse should be familiar with the programs offered by such groups as The Seeing Eye, Inc., Morristown, N. J., where blind persons learn to work with a dog guide.

BIBLIOGRAPHY

Books

Adler, F. H.: Textbook of Ophthalmology. ed. 7. Philadelphia, W. B. Saunders, 1962.

Guyton, A. C.: Textbook of Medical Physiology. Chaps. 49-51. Philadelphia, W. B. Saunders, 1966.

Hughes, W. F.: The Yearbook of Ophthalmology. Chicago, Year Book Medical Publishers, 1967-68.

U. S. Dept. of H.E.W.: Research Profile: Summary of Progress in Eye Disorders. Washington, D.C., P.H.S., 1966.

Vaughan, D., Cook, R., and Asbury, T.: General Ophthalmology. ed. 5. Los Altos, Cal., Lange Medical Publishers, 1968.

General Articles

Abrahamson, I. A., Jr.: Chalazion. G.P., 38:83-87, July, 1968.

Ballen, P. H.: Ophthalmic surgery: The nurse's role. A.O.R.N. J., 6:35-44, Aug., 1967.

Gordon, D. M.: Diseases of the eye. Clinical Symposia, Oct.-Nov.-Dec., 1962.

Haddad, H. M.: Drugs for ophthalmic use. Amer. J. Nurs., 68:324-327, Feb., 1968.

Snyder, J.: Newer concepts in ophthalmic surgery. Nurs. Clin. N. Amer., 3:539-541, Sept., 1968.

Contact Lenses

Bixler, D. P.: Bacterial decontamination and cleaning of contact lenses. Amer. J. Ophthal., 62:324-329, Aug., 1966.

Brueggen, S. L.: Contact lenses. Amer. J. Nurs., 65:92-94, Sept., 1965.

Dixon, J. M.: Ocular changes due to contact lenses. Amer. J. Ophthal., 58:424-443, Sept., 1964.

Dixon, J. M., and Lawaczeck, E.: Some disadvantages of contact lenses. Eye, Ear, Nose, Throat Monthly, 43:62-63, Sept., 1964.

Gould, H. L., and Inglima, R.: Corneal contact lens solution. Eye, Ear, Nose, Throat Monthly, 43:39-49, April, 1964.

Magoon, R. C., and Sexton, R.: Wet or dry contact lens storage. Arch. Ophthal., 77:197-199, Feb., 1967.

Obear, M. F., and Winter, F. C.: Bacteriologic culture of wet and dry contact lenses storage cases. Amer. J. Ophthal., 57:441-443, May, 1964.

Riegelman, S.: Bacterial testing of contact lens solutions. Amer. J. Ophthal., 64, Letter to Editor, Sept., 1967.

Shumate, R. E. L.: What the industrial nurse should know about contact lenses. Amer. Ass. Ind. Nurses, J., 9:21-22, Dec., 1961.

Cornea

Bosanko, L.: Patients with corneal transplants. *In* Bergersen, B. S., *et al.*: Current Concepts in Clinical Nursing. pp. 3-15. St. Louis, C. V. Mosby, 1967.

Epstein, D. L., and Paton, D.: Keratitis from misuse of corneal anesthetics. New Eng. J. Med., 279:396-399, 1968.

Stoeker, F. W., and Bell, R.: Corneal transplantation and nursing care of the patient with corneal transplant. Amer. J. Nurs., 62:65-70, 1960.

Cataract

Callahan, A.: Direct zonulolysis with stripper for cataract extraction. Amer. J. Ophthal., 63:316-319, Feb., 1967.

Cockerill, E. E.: Reflections on my nursing care. Amer. J. Nurs., 65:83-85, May, 1965.

Croll, M., and Croll, L. J.: A new cryoslide technique for cataract removal. Amer. J. Ophthal., 62:83-88, July, 1966.

Johnson, R., and Kara, G. B.: Cryophake, a disposable cryoextractor for cataract surgery. Eye, Ear, Nose, Throat Monthly, 45:48-50, June, 1966.

Nordstrom, W.: Adjusting to cataract glasses. Amer. J. Nurs., 66:1578-1579, July, 1966.

Glaucoma

Starin, I.: Need for routine glaucoma screening by hospitals and physicians. Pub. Health Rep., 81:12-16, Jan., 1966.

Retina

Shea, M., and Dickson, D.: Thermoelectric retinal cryosurgery. Canad. J. Ophthal., 1:138-146, April, 1966.

National Agencies

American Foundation for the Blind
15 W. 16th Street
New York, New York 10011

American Printing House for the Blind, Inc.
1839 Frankfort Avenue
Louisville, Kentucky 40206

Guide Dogs for the Blind, Inc.
San Rafael, California 94902

Howe Press of Perkins School for the Blind
Watertown, Massachusetts 02172

Library of Congress
The Division for the Blind and Physically Handicapped
Washington, D.C. 20542
(Available through state libraries)

Office of Vocational Rehabilitation
U. S. Dept. Health, Education, and Welfare
Washington, D.C. 20402

Readers Digest Assoc., Inc.
Pleasantville, New York 10570

National Society for the Prevention of Blindness
16 East 40th Street
New York, New York 10016

Recording for the Blind, Inc.
121 East 58th Street
New York, New York 10022

The Seeing Eye, Inc.
Morristown, New Jersey 07960

CHAPTER **33**

Patients with Problems of the Ear and the Mastoid

- *The Person with a Hearing Difficulty*
- *Hearing Tests*
- *General Hygiene of the Ear*
- *Patients with Problems of the External Ear*
- *Patients with Problems of the Middle Ear*
- *Patients with Problems of the Inner Ear*
- *Classification of Hearing Loss*
- *Rehabilitation*

The ear is a very complex sense organ for hearing and equilibrium. The early detection and the accurate diagnosis of ear disease are important both in children and in adults. Among those who take an important part in the diagnosis of patients with auditory disorders are pediatricians, otolaryngologists, psychiatrists, neurologists, psychologists, speech pathologists, educators and audiologists. Before a child can speak, he must first be able to hear, then interpret what he hears, and, lastly, be able to express himself in speech. Occurrences during birth, disorders due to birth injury, bacterial and virus infections in childhood, toxic drug effects, damage to the ear by noise, and changes in the ear as the result of aging are only a few of the problems confronting the otologist in diagnosis, treatment and rehabilitation.

THE PERSON WITH A HEARING DIFFICULTY

Impairment of hearing may cause changes in a person's personality and attitude, in his ability to communicate, in his awareness of his surroundings, and even his ability to protect himself. In a classroom, a student with impaired hearing may show disinterest, inattention, and failing grades. A woman at home may think the "world is dead" because she no longer can hear the clock chime, the refrigerator hum, the birds sing, or the traffic pass. A pedestrian may attempt to cross the street, having failed to hear the approaching car. The person with hearing loss may miss parts of conversations and allow suspicions to arise that people may be talking about him. Many individuals are not even aware that their hearing is gradually becoming impaired.

Not infrequently, a person with a hearing loss refuses to seek medical attention, because he interprets hearing loss as a sign of advancing age. Many people refuse to wear a hearing aid for this reason; others are sensitive when they do wear an aid.

The nurse must be aware of these attitudes and behavior. In her contacts with all individuals, she should offer assistance and advice when she suspects hearing loss. The hearing difficulty may be due to impacted cerumen (wax), which is readily treated; however, proper evaluation is best done by an otologist. The *otologist* is a physician who specializes in the diagnosis and treatment of problems of the ear. An *otolaryngologist* is a physician who specializes in problems relating to the ear, nose and throat. An *audiologist* is a person who specializes in nonmedical evaluation and rehabilitation of hearing disorders; his preparation usually includes an M.A. or Ph.D. degree.

Fig. 33-1. An audiogram presents a graphic outline of the individual's hearing as measured by tones of different pitches ranging from 125 through 8000 cycles per second (cps or Hz). Thresholds for these different tones as heard by air and bone conduction are plotted on this graph. The information is important for determining the type of hearing loss. Also, by testing through the critical speech range (approximately 300 to 3000 cps), one can predict how much difficulty there may be in hearing and understanding speech. (From Nilo, E. R.: Hearing Impairment. *In* Saunders, W. H., *et al.*: Nursing Care in Eye, Ear, Nose, and Throat Disorders. ed. 2. St. Louis, C. V. Mosby, 1968)

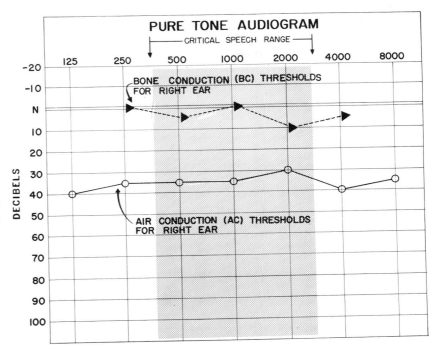

HEARING TESTS

Hearing tests not only help to determine the particular type of hearing defect present but also establish the potential of the patient's hearing.

Tuning Fork

This inexpensive instrument can differentiate between *conductive deafness* (caused by a disorder in the auditory canal, the eardrum or the ossicles) and *sensorineural (perceptive) deafness* (due to a disorder of the organ of Corti or the auditory nerve).

In the *Weber test*, the fork is placed on the forehead in order to compare hearing in the two ears. For example, in normal hearing or in deafness that is equal on both sides, the patient indicates that he hears the vibrations in the middle of his head. Variations suggest hearing inequality. In conductive hearing loss, bone-conducted sounds shift to the poorer ear. In sensorineural hearing loss, sounds are heard louder in the better ear.

The next step is the *Rinne test*. In this test, after striking the tuning fork, the doctor first places the handle against the mastoid process, behind the external auditory opening. Then he holds the tines beside the ear and asks the patient to tell where he heard the sound better or longer. A "Rinne positive" result means that the tone was heard longer by air conduction—this indicates perceptive loss. A "Rinne negative" result occurs when the tone is heard longer by bone conduction—this indicates conductive loss.

"Rinne equal" means that the tone is heard the same by air and bone conduction.

These two tests do not give quantitative information, which is obtained by audiologic study (audiogram).

Audiogram

In deafness, the audiometer is the single most important diagnostic instrument. Audiometric testing is of two kinds: (1) pure-tone audiometry, in which the sound stimulus consists of a pure or musical tone (the louder the tone before the patient perceives it, the greater the hearing loss; the unit of measure of loudness of sound is the *decibel*); (2) speech audiometry, in which the spoken word is used to determine the ability to understand and discriminate sounds.

For accuracy, audiometric tests should be done in a soundproof room. The patient wears earphones and is instructed to signal when he hears the tone and again when he no longer hears it. When the tone is applied directly over the external auditory opening, air conduction is measured. When the stimulus is applied to the mastoid bone, thereby bypassing the conductive mechanism, nerve conduction is tested.

The normal human ear perceives sounds ranging from about 20 cycles per second (cps or Hz) to 20,000 cycles per second; however, only the frequencies from 500 to 2,000 are important in understanding everyday speech. Clinically, this range is referred to as *speech range*. The critical level of loudness is around 30 decibels. In treating patients surgically to improve

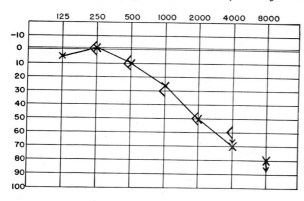

(A) Audiogram typical of presbycusis (hearing loss due to age). Air and bone conduction are equally affected, and loss is mainly in higher tones. No improvement can be expected from surgery.

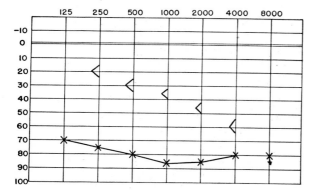

(B) Severe mixed hearing loss. Although a great differential exists between air conduction and bone conduction, considerable high-tone deafness is inescapable, regardless of the results of surgery.

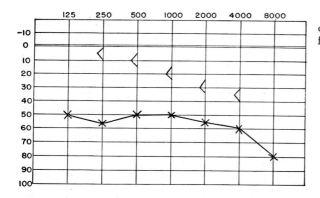

(C) Moderately severe mixed hearing loss. Hearing may be considerably improved by surgery, but perception of the higher frequencies may be inadequate.

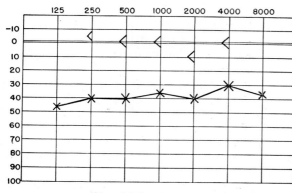

(D) This audiogram illustrates a pure conduction loss because of uncomplicated otosclerosis. In such a case, surgery should give excellent results.

Fig. 33-2. Conventional audiograms. (From Ciba, Clinical Symposia, Vol. 14, No. 2)

hearing loss, the aim is to improve the hearing level to 30 decibels or better within the speech frequencies (Figs. 33-1 and 33-2).

GENERAL HYGIENE OF THE EAR

Cleansing of the external auditory canal by the introduction of matches, hair pins and other implements is dangerous, since trauma to the skin may result in accidental infection of the skin or damage to the eardrum. Wax deposits may be softened by the instillation of a few drops of warmed glycerine daily, followed by irrigation at body temperature, using a bulb syringe or a special ear syringe. The inner ear is easily stimulated with water temperatures either below or above body temperature, creating annoying vertigo. After irrigation, the canal is dried carefully with a sterile applicator and cotton. The removal of impacted cerumen or earwax may require the skilled attention of the physician (see p. 746).

Vigorous blowing of the nose or douching of the nose may be dangerous during acute infection, such as the common cold. Middle ear infection by way of the eustachian tube is not uncommon. Patients with a history of ear infection, and particularly those with perforations of the drum, should avoid contamination of the ear with water at bathing, swimming or diving. The patient is instructed to plug the ear with cotton or lamb's wool saturated with petrolatum and to wear a rubber cap at the time of ocean bathing or swimming.

Noise

One of the waste products of the 20th century is noise (unwanted sound). In recent years, the sheer volume of noise that surrounds us daily has grown from being simple annoyance into a potentially dangerous source of physical damage. Acoustical authorities claim that noise cuts down on work efficiency, and conversely, the elimination of noise increases efficiency. In one factory located near a boiler plant, workers made 60 mistakes in assembling 80 temperature regulators. Moved to a quiet room, they made only 7 mistakes. Quietness is more conducive to peace of mind; in the hospital, patients are happier and less upset when noise is reduced by carpeting, soundproofed ceilings and quiet elevator doors.

Scientists measure sound *intensity* (pressure exerted by sound) in decibels. For example, the shuffling of papers in quiet surroundings represents about 15 decibels; a low conversation, 40 decibels; and a jet plane 100 feet away about 140 decibels. Sound above 80 decibels begins to grate harshly upon the human ear (Fig. 33-3).

Over the past 30 years the loudest sounds to which men have been exposed have grown from 120 decibels (the roar of a small 2-engine prop plane) to 150

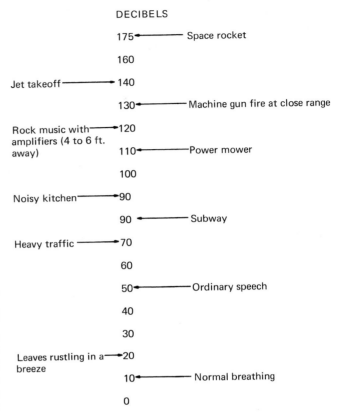

DECIBELS

175 ◄—— Space rocket
160
Jet takeoff ——► 140
130 ◄—— Machine gun fire at close range
Rock music with ——120
amplifiers (4 to 6 ft. away)
110 ◄—— Power mower
100
Noisy kitchen ——►90
90 ◄—— Subway
Heavy traffic ——►70
60
50 ◄—— Ordinary speech
40
30
Leaves rustling in a ——►20
breeze
10 ◄—— Normal breathing
0
Threshold of Hearing
DECIBELS (dB)

FIG. 33-3. Intensity range of human hearing.

decibels (the blast of a giant 4-engine jet). Experiments have shown that 160 decibels are lethal for small fur-bearing animals. Research at many universities shows that exposure to noise of 90 decibels or more can cause the skin to flush, the stomach muscles to constrict and tempers to be short.

Frequency refers to the number of sound waves emanating from a source per second—cycles per second (cps or Hz). *Pitch* refers to frequency, so that a tone with 100 cps or Hz is considered low pitch, whereas 10,000 cps or Hz is of high pitch. Generally, a young adult can distinguish frequencies from 16 cps to 20,000 cps.

One of the obvious effects of our noisy world is the amount of deafness it produces. In the early 1900's, hearing loss was described as "boilermakers ears" because deafness then was found more often among boilermakers and railroad men. Today, compensation claims for deafness acquired on the job amount to over 2 million dollars a year.

The individual's reaction to noise varies greatly. At least 3 factors are involved: (1) the intensity of sound, (2) the time the subject is confined in a noisy environment and (3) individual tolerance of noise. No one would want to live in a world completely without sound. However, the noise level inside a home should not exceed 35 or 40 decibels. This can be achieved by proper construction and the use of absorptive materials such as heavy carpets and draperies. For sound sleep, some people have learned to use ear protectors. These are now widely used in industry to provide protection when noise exceeds 80 decibels, and in the Armed Forces when the critical point of continuous noise experienced is 85 decibels or higher.

PATIENTS WITH PROBLEMS OF THE EXTERNAL EAR

The auricle or external ear varies in size, shape and position on the head, and it aids in the collection of sound waves and their passage into the external auditory canal. The external auditory canal is a skin-lined tube that ends at a disklike structure, also lined with skin, the eardrum. The skin of the canal contains highly specialized glands that secrete a brown wax-like substance, *cerumen* (earwax). This material serves as a protection for the skin. There are also hair follicles and sweat glands.

Infections (External Otitis)

Bacterial or fungal infections may result from an abrasion of the ear canal or from swimming in contaminated water; they appear more commonly during the summer. Such infections are painful, therefore treatment is directed toward relieving this symptom. Even touching or moving the auricle increases pain. (In a middle ear infection, movement of the auricle does not increase pain.) Aspirin, codeine and applications of heat provide comfort. If the tissues are edematous, it may be necessary to insert gently a wick of cotton through the canal to the eardrum so that liquid medications may be introduced. Later, these medications may be given by dropper at room temperature. Such medications usually are combinations of antibiotics and agents to soothe the inflamed membranes. Systemic antibiotic therapy may be required. The patient is cautioned to avoid swimming or allowing water to enter the ear when shampooing or showering.

Furuncle of the External Canal

In this condition, there is an infection of the skin and the subcutaneous tissue of the external canal. Usually great pain, marked tinnitus, deafness and ear noise in the affected ear occur. There may be fever, severe headache and enlargement of the local lymph nodes. This disorder may be mistaken for mastoid infection. The early administration of antibiotics is usually followed by definite improvement, but surgical drainage may be necessary by incision of the furuncle. After incision, wet dressings are applied and are important to facilitate drainage and relieve pain.

Cerumen in the Ear Canal

Earwax normally accumulates in the ear, with the amount and color varying with the individual. Ordinarily, it does not have to be removed, but it may occasionally became impacted and interfere with hearing. An irrigation of the external auditory canal may loosen the cerumen; the fluid must be at room temperature and the flow directed toward the top of the canal so that the wax is more likely to be dislodged. Most physicians prefer to do this with a large syringe for irrigation, although some prefer to use a cerumen spoon, which is directed through an aural speculum. (See p. 747 for irrigation of the external auditory canal.) It may be necessary to precede an irrigation with a softening agent such as carbamide (urea) peroxide in glyceryl (Debrox), to be instilled twice a day for 3 or 4 days.

Foreign Bodies in the External Canal

Small objects are inserted into the ear, usually by young children and mentally retarded persons. Such objects may be nonirritating and remain for years without symptoms. An insect in the ear may be disturbing, but can be easily managed by instilling oil drops that smother the insect and allow it to be floated or flushed out.

Vegetable foreign bodies have a tendency to swell, so irrigation is contraindicated. Attempts at removal may be dangerous in unskilled hands, because the body may be pushed completely into the bony portion of the canal, lacerating the skin of the canal and perforating the drum. Serious infections of the middle ear and the mastoid, with ensuing deafness, may result. Instrumental removal should be done under general anesthesia in the very young; when skillfully performed, there are no sequelae.

Deformities

Deformities of the ear and the external canal occur as congenital malformations and may be manifested as abnormal size or protrusion of the ear, atresia or closure of the external canal. Acquired deformities, such as cauliflower ear in the boxer and loss of a part or all of the ear, result from accident or injury. These disorders can be aided or cured with appropriate plastic surgery.

Earlobe Piercing

Women and particularly young girls desire pierced earlobes so that they can wear earrings without fear of losing them. Goldman and Kitzmiller recommend the following as the best technique for cosmetic purposes. It is suggested that a physician perform this procedure rather than risking the dangers of performing it yourself: Use a large (18-gauge) straight needle, with a sterilized and flexible gold wire inserted into the bevel and inside of the needle. With a little local anesthesia, the needle is inserted through the back of the earlobe, then withdrawn, leaving the wire in the ear. The wire is tied loosely in place—serving as a type of primitive earring—and is removed 10 days to 2 weeks later. During this time, the area is cleansed daily with soap and water, followed by a mild antiseptic ointment, and the wire is moved from time to time to ensure patency of the opening in the patient's earlobe.

Some difficulties have been experienced with all types of ear–piercing procedures, among them, premature closure of the puncture, hemorrhage into the earlobe, secondary infection, and keloid formation. With this particular procedure, the only difficulty reported has been tangling of the hair in the loose ends of the wire.

Irrigation of the External Auditory Canal

Various types of equipment may be used to irrigate the ear, but the most acceptable is an irrigating container and tubing with an irrigating tip. Usually up to 500 ml. of solution is used. The purposes for irrigation may be varied: to clean the ear when discharge is present, to remove a nonvegetable foreign body from the external canal and to apply heat in order to localize infection or to relieve pain. The solutions for irrigating the ear should be at a temperature of about 105° to 110° F.* Solutions that are too hot or too cold or are used with too much force may cause pain or dizziness. The patient may sit or lie with his head tilted toward the side of the affected ear. He may support the curved basin under his ear to receive the returning solution. To be effective the fluids must reach the eardrum, and to this end the nurse is advised to pull the auricle upward and backward in order to straighten the external auditory canal. (In children this canal may be straightened by pulling the auricle down and back.) Extreme gentleness should be used, and care must be taken that the fluid has free exit so that it is not driven into the middle ear. After the irrigation, the external opening should be plugged lightly with sterile cotton, which is changed

* 40.6° to 43.3° C.

when necessary. After the procedure, the patient is instructed to lie on the affected ear so that gravity facilitates drainage. Note: If injury to the tympanic membrane is suspected, irrigation should not be performed.

PATIENTS WITH PROBLEMS OF THE MIDDLE EAR

Function of the Middle Ear

The middle ear, with its ossicles and ligaments and their connection to the eardrum, is vitally concerned in the function of hearing. The middle ear connects with the posterior portion of the nose by means of the eustachian tube; thus equal air pressure is maintained on both sides of the eardrum. The tube, normally closed, opens by action of the muscles of the palate on yawning or swallowing. The tube serves as a drainage channel for normal and abnormal secretions of the middle ear and equalizes pressures in the middle ear to that of the atmosphere. When the membrane of this tube is inflamed, it offers an easy passage for infection into the middle ear.

Sound waves transmitted by the drum to the ossicles of the middle ear are transferred to the *cochlea,* the organ of hearing, lodged in the labyrinth or inner ear. An important ossicle is the stapes, which rocks on its posterior portion, not unlike a piston, and sets up vibrations in fluids contained in the labyrinth. These pressure waves, passed through the cochlea, produce sound stimuli by setting into vibration hair cells in the organ of Corti, which in turn are passed along the auditory nerve to the cerebral cortex in the brain, where sound is analyzed and interpreted.

Serous Otitis Media

Exudates in the middle ear may be retained after acute inflammation that has been treated with antibiotics. Symptoms such as ear pain and fever may subside, and, although the exudates in the middle ear have been rendered sterile, because of tubal inflammation they are not evacuated. Deafness and a sense of fullness in the ear caused by the exudates persists. Simple myringotomy, or incision of the drum, evacuates the contents of the middle ear, and healing takes place in a few days, with complete resolution and relief of symptoms. This condition, known as secretory otitis media, is commonly seen today in patients treated with wide-spectrum antibiotics. When unrecognized, it can be a common cause of persistent deafness in children and in adults.

Aero-otitis media is a form of serous otitis media in which fluid and/or air is trapped in the middle ear due to sudden descent in an airplane. The condition usually lasts a short time, but it may continue for days. Many individuals avoid flying when they have an upper respiratory infection for this reason. Preventive measures to be taken by flight passengers are to chew gum, suck on hard candy, yawn or swallow several times during descent of the plane. Those flying should be taught to inflate the ears by the so-called Valsalva method. In this technique the nostrils are held tightly, and the ears are inflated by vigorous blowing; thus pressure in the middle ear is equalized to relieve annoying symptoms.

In some clinics, the aeration of the middle ear is accomplished by inserting a small plastic button or hollow tube in the eardrum. This affords relief even when the eustachian tube is blocked.

Acute Otitis Media (Abscess in the Ear)

The essential cause of acute otitis media is the entrance of pathogenic bacteria into the normally sterile middle ear when the resistance is lowered or the virulence of the organism is great enough to produce inflammation. Bacteria commonly found, in the order of importance, are: the hemolytic streptococcus, the pneumococcus, the staphylococcus and the influenza bacillus. The mode of entry of the bacteria in most patients is spread by way of the auditory canal or the eustachian tube during the indiscriminate use of nose drops or nasal douching, forcible blowing of the nose or sneezing; in rare cases, infection may enter after fracture of the skull. The symptoms may vary with the severity of the infection and may be either very mild and transient or very severe and fraught with serious complications. Pain in and about the ear is the first symptom. It may be intense and is relieved after spontaneous perforation of the drum or after myringotomy. Fever varies and in severe cases may range between 104° and 105° F.* Deafness, ear noises, headache, loss of appetite, nausea and vomiting are other symptoms.

The end-results of otitis media depend on the virulence of the bacteria, the efficiency of the therapy and the resistance of the patient. With early and appropriate wide-spectrum antibiotic therapy, otitis media may clear with healing, and no serious sequelae result. The condition may become subacute, with long-persistent purulent discharge from the ear. Healing may take place with permanent deafness. Perforation as the result of rupture of the eardrum may persist and develop into a chronic form of otitis media. Secondary complications, with involvement of the mastoid, and other serious intracranial complications such as meningitis or brain abscess, may result.

The nurse should be alert to the fact that symptoms

* 40.0° to 40.6° C.

may be masked by the antibiotic therapy, and that during the course of treatment of an acute middle ear infection, symptoms such as headache, slow pulse, vomiting and vertigo are all significant and should be recorded carefully for evaluation by the otologist. The appropriate antibiotic, often determined by culture and sensitivity tests, is important to the prognosis for eventual cure.

Myringotomy. In mild cases treated early, myringotomy may not be necessary. However, if pain persists, this procedure is important for promoting surgical drainage and it offers a ready means of identification of the type of organism present to test its sensitivity to chemotherapeutic agents.

An incision is made in the posterior inferior aspect of the tympanic membrane. Even though a sweeping incision is made to relieve pressure and pus from a middle ear infection, the incision heals rapidly and hearing is not impaired. This procedure is now performed much less frequently than it was before the advent of antibiotic therapy.

Chronic Otitis Media and Mastoiditis

Chronic otitis media results from repeated attacks of otitis media causing persistent perforation of the drum, and it is due to particular virulence of the infecting organism or to bacterial resistance to antibiotic therapy. The chronically infected ear is characterized by persistent or recurrent purulent discharge, with or without pain, and varying degrees of deafness. Most chronic otitis media begins in childhood and may persist to adult life.

The condition is divided into 2 forms, both of which have entirely different significance: (1) simple chronic otitis media, which is caused by central perforation of the drum with the presence of a mucuslike discharge, this being the so-called nondangerous type of otitis media, and (2) chronic otitis media, with marginal perforation of the drum membrane and the presence of *cholesteatoma* (the formation of a soft, white ball of dead skin). Cholesteatoma is caused by an ingrowth of skin from the perforation in the drum, and fills the area in the mastoid and the middle ear. By its encroachment, the cholesteatoma may involve vital structures, such as the facial nerve, the labyrinth and the adjoining areas of the brain.

The symptoms of chronic otitis media may be minimal, with mild deafness and the presence of a persistent or intermittent foul-smelling discharge of variable quantity. The diagnosis is corroborated by the physical finding, but, in addition, roentgenograms of the mastoids usually show pathologic changes. In the nondangerous type of chronic otitis media, treatment often is successful, bringing about cessation of the foul discharge and, in some patients, improvement of hearing.

Local treatment can be effective, but antibiotics, while often tried, are largely disappointing because most of the organisms present in this chronic malady are resistant, and it is difficult to get the drug into prolonged contact with infected areas in sufficient concentration. In chronic otitis media of the dangerous type, with cholesteatoma, surgery may be indicated, based on clinical and x-ray findings. There is usually no pain unless complications ensue. Serious complications as a result of chronic disease may be protracted or sudden in onset. Symptoms such as sudden facial paralysis, unusually profound deafness or dizziness, onset of headache with dizziness and stiff neck may intimate beginning meningitis or brain abscess. Surgical intervention may be elective but in the event of serious complications may represent a serious emergency.

Simple Mastoidectomy. Mastoid cells, a honeycomb of bone that adjoins the middle ear, must be removed when positive signs exist of disease in the mastoid process. In acute cases marked swelling, redness and tenderness behind the ear over the mastoid occur. The operation is performed when there are recurrent or persistent tenderness, fever, headache, and discharge from the ear.

Preparation of the Patient. The patient is prepared as for any operation. The field is made ready by clipping the hair, then shaving the scalp for 1½ inches about the ear—for the incision behind the ear (the postauricular approach). In patients in whom the approach to the mastoid is by the endaural route, in which the incision is made from the canal of the ear outward, the hair is shaved above the ear. In the operation, the infection is removed completely from the mastoid process, with drainage from the middle ear, thus preventing spread of the infection to surrounding structures. The middle ear can be saved from further damage and the possible resulting permanent hearing loss.

Nursing Care. Sedatives usually are indicated after the operation and during the first postoperative days to control pain and restlessness. Fluids are given freely when the anesthetic reaction clears. The mastoid is packed with gauze for drainage, and the packing is usually removed at the end of 3 to 4 days. Dressings are done with sterile precautions every day or every other day, as indicated by the surgeon. Granulation tissue fills in the defect during the healing process.

A complication after mastoidectomy is facial paralysis, and the nurse may be the first to note this serious indication of facial nerve inflammation or injury. The patient shows immobility of the side affected, so that the eye cannot be closed and the mouth droops. He is unable to drink without water dripping from the mouth, and he is unable to whistle. On speaking or grimacing, the facial paralysis is more pronounced, due to the immobility of the paralyzed side. When there is evidence of facial paralysis, cortisone derivatives are useful in restoring the nerve to function. The continued use of antibiotic agents is important for combating the infection and aiding healing.

Radical Mastoid Operation. The purpose of this operation is the removal of all disease from the mastoid and the middle ear; through surgery, the external canal, the middle ear and the mastoid are merged into one cavity. The operative preparation and the postoperative care are essentially the same as for the simple mastoid operation. The surgery is carried out by either the postauricular or the endaural technique, and in some instances the mastoid wound is lined by skin, muscle or fascial grafts. Segments of skin are removed from either the arm or the leg, preceded by the appropriate skin disinfection.

The nurse should be on the alert for unusual symptoms that may intimate complications. Vertigo may be present for several days because of inner ear disturbance. Persistent headache, unusual rise in temperature accompanied by chills, stiff neck, nausea and vomiting should alert the attending nurse to the possibility of serious sequelae. If the stapes has been removed or dislodged, hearing is lost. If the stapes or cochlea have sustained no damage, the patient regains hearing with the assistance of a hearing aid.

Perforations of the Eardrum

Etiology and Pathology. The most frequent cause of permanent perforation of the tympanic membrane is infection. Perforations of the drum membrane that fail to heal are often the end-result of acute or chronic suppurative otitis media.

Before the advent of antibiotics, clinicians were often confronted with acute otologic complications of eruptive diseases in children. In patients with acute fulminating streptococcal infection, spontaneous rupture of the drum followed by necrosis could result in a perforation so large that only the thicker rim portion of the drum remained. In chronic otitis media, infection of the middle ear and the mastoid perpetuates the purulent otorrhea and prevents healing of the perforation.

Second to infections of the middle ear, trauma may be a cause of permanent perforation of the drum. Blast effect of high explosives or intense compression caused by a severe blow on the ear can rupture the drum. Burning of the drum by a welder's spark is no rarity. Less frequent causes are perforation of the drum by foreign objects, water, burns of the face that include the external ear and the drum membrane, and postmyringotomy defects.

Medical Management. Most accidental perforations of the drum membrane heal spontaneously. Some persist because of the growth of scar tissue over the edges of the perforation, thus preventing extension of the epithelial areas across the margins and final healing. Central perforations of the drum lend themselves to medical treatment for eventual closure, except in patients who have only a rim of the drum membrane remaining. In some patients, persistent care consisting of cauterization of the perforation with trichloroacetic acid at frequent intervals and the use of a prosthesis will result in a completely healed drum membrane by scar.

Surgical Management. See Tympanoplasty, Type I (Myringoplasty), page 751.

Tympanoplasty

Tympanoplasty denotes a number of reconstructive operations on middle ear structures that have become diseased or are congenitally deformed (see Table 33-1). The procedure entails the construction or the preservation of the conductive mechanism to maintain or improve hearing. The impetus that led to this work has been due largely to advances in surgical techniques with the illuminated binocular microscope. This surgery has been helped by the protection of the antibiotics to ensure a sterile procedure in uninfected patients and the use of these drugs to eradicate chronic otitis media and mastoiditis.

Physiologic Principles Underlying Sound Conduction. The conductive function of the eardrum and the ossicles transforms sound waves from airborne vibrations to mechanical stimulation of the endolymphatic fluids. At present, the prevailing physiologic concept holds that the ratio of the large tympanic membrane to the smaller oval window, combined with the lever action of the ossicles, transforms stimuli from the air to the inner ear fluids with great increase in force. It is calculated that the lever ratio for the tympanic membrane to the oval window is 22. Obviously, defects in the tympanic membrane or interruption of the ossicular chain will disturb that mass relationship to the oval window and will cause a loss of the sound-pressure ratio, resulting in hearing loss.

The functional physiology of the round and oval windows plays an important role as well. The oval window is bordered by the annular ligament and the unimpeded motility of the stapes foot-plate receives impulses transmitted by the incus and the malleus from the drum membrane. The round window, opening on the opposite side of the cochlear duct, permits motion of the endolymphatic fluids with sound-wave stimulation. With the normally intact drum mem-

TABLE 33-1. Tympanoplastic procedures

Type	Damage to Middle Ear	Methods of Repair
I	Perforated tympanic membrane with normal ossicular chain	Closure of perforation; same as myringoplasty
II	Perforation of tympanic membrane with erosion of malleus	Closure with graft against incus or remains of malleus
III	Destruction of tympanic membrane and ossicular chain *but with* intact and mobile stapes	Graft contacts normal stapes; also gives sound protection for round window
IV	Similar to type III, but head, neck, and crura of stapes missing; foot-plate mobile	Mobile foot-plate left exposed; air pocket between round window and graft provides sound protection for round window.
V	Similar to type IV plus *fixed* foot-plate	Fenestra in horizontal semicircular canal; graft seals off middle ear to give sound protection for round window.

(From DeWeese, D. D., and Saunders, W. H.: Textbook of Otolaryngology. ed. 3, St. Louis, C. V. Mosby, 1968.

brane, sound waves stimulate the oval window first, and a lag occurs before the terminal effect of the stimulus reaches the round window. This phase lag, normally present with an intact drum, is changed by a perforation of the drum that is large enough to allow sound waves to impinge on both the round and oval windows simultaneously. This effect cancels the lag and prevents the maximal effect of labyrinth fluid motility and its subsequent effect in stimulating the hair cells in the organ of Corti.

Pathophysiology. Pathologic sequelae vary after otitis media, with minimal or large defects remaining in the tympanic membrane. In protracted or virulent infections, necrotic involvement of the ossicles may occur. Involvement of motility may result with fibrosis or necrosis of all or part of the ossicular chain. The malleus commonly is involved, the handle lost by osteonecrosis as the perforation in the drum enlarges. The lenticular process of the incus often is involved, because of its tenuous blood supply. Osteonecrosis may involve the entire ossicular chain, so that the stapedial foot-plate is the only portion remaining. The oval and round windows may be impeded functionally by granuloma, polyps, fibrous or bony plaques. Otosclerosis may exist along with the pathologic sequelae of otitis media. Obstruction of the tympanic orifice of the eustachian tube by pathologic tissue deposits or fibrotic stenosis may result in dysfunction of this structure.

Tympanoplasty, Type I (Myringoplasty). Myringoplasty is a plastic surgical procedure designed to close perforations of the tympanic membrane. The operation has a dual purpose: to create a closed middle ear cavity by graft over the perforation, and to improve hearing.

Indications and Contraindications. The most important advantage of the closed tympanic membrane is the avoidance of the risk of contamination of the middle ear during bathing, swimming or diving. The reactivation of a chronic otitis media and/or mastoiditis thus may be prevented. Dramatic improvement in hearing may result from closure of a perforation if there is no involvement of the ossicles. The probability of improved hearing after closure of the drum membrane can be prognosticated to some degree by an audiometric study with evaluation of the air–bone conduction levels. Preoperative testing, with and without a patch prosthesis over the perforation, usually provides a fairly accurate estimate of the degree of hearing levels. Temporary patching of the defect with glazed paper, latex, or a cotton collodium disk should be a routine maneuver during the preliminary examination of the patient. When the patching of a perforation of the drum is not followed by audiometric improvement, one must consider involvement of the ossicular chain. During the surgical repair of a perforation, a careful inspection of the middle ear contents, with particular attention to the continuity of the ossicles, is important.

Medical or surgical closure of perforations of the drum in the presence of an active infection usually is contraindicated. In chronic disease of the middle ear with malfunction of the eustachian tube, and therefore inadequate drainage from the middle ear (the only avenue for egress of discharges), surgery is contraindicated. Involvement of the nasopharynx because of chronic infectious discharge from sinusitis or allergy, plus a history of acute exacerbations of otitis media, is an obvious contraindication.

Surgical Approach. Tympanoplasty Type I was previously done by taking skin from the postauricular area and placing it over the denuded remaining part of the tympanic membrane. Otologists, however, now prefer to use epithelium from the ear canal because it contains fewer glands and is thinner. This may be a free graft or a pedicle-type graft (see p. 650).

Some surgeons use vein grafts from the hand or forearm to repair a perforated member. Such a graft is placed either on the outside or inside of the eardrum. Saline-soaked Gelfoam is used to hold the graft against the drum. Within weeks the graft becomes well-attached to the edges of the perforation and hearing is improved. Another tissue popular for grafting is fascia obtained from the temporal muscle.

Postoperative Management and Instructions. An antibiotic is administered routinely for at least 5 days after surgery. The patient remains in the hospital for 3 or 4 days at the most, and the dressing is left undisturbed except for the external bandage, which may be changed if it becomes soiled from bleeding. The gauze strip is removed from the canal on the 7th day; the Gelfoam is left undisturbed. No suction or probing is carried out at this time.

On the 12th day, capillary suction can be used carefully to remove the Gelfoam or crusted debris. Gentle inflation may be carried out to test the efficiency of the closure of the perforation by the graft. Eardrops never are used, and the only topical treatment is a dusting powder of Neosporin or Chloromycetin-Boric.

The patient is seen at 5-day intervals and is instructed to avoid contaminating the ear by shampooing or showering. Antibiotics are given for 1 week, but may be continued if there is evidence of complicating respiratory infection. An antihistaminic with an ephedrine derivative is used routinely for 1 month postoperatively. In those patients with known seasonal or perennial rhinologic allergy, an antihistaminic is continued.

Tympanoplasty (Types II to V). These operations are described in Table 33-1; they are procedures with modifications designed to correct additional problems in the middle ear.

Preoperative Care. The bacterial flora in all patients shoud be studied by culture and sensitivity tests. In those whose treatment is accompanied by the parenteral administration of an appropriate antibiotic, the postoperative morbidity is less. Infection due to resistant organisms may be treated postoperatively with the use of a catheter placed in the wound, by which one can instill the topical antibiotics. This often facilitates healing. Topical and systemic antibiotic treatment should precede surgery on the patient whose ear is continuously or frequently discharging.

Operative Procedure. Part of the tympanoplastic procedure includes the restoration in the continuity of the sound mechanism, when it is involved. Ossicular interruption is most frequent in otitis media, but problems of reconstruction occur with malformations of the middle ear and ossicular dislocations due to head injuries.

Polyethylene tubing, stainless steel wire, bone and cartilage have been used as replacements, either to utilize the remaining parts of the ossicles or to create a columella (little column) effect for the transmission of impulses from the tympanic graft to the oval window.

A 2-stage procedure may be necessary—the first for the surgical eradication of all pathology and to achieve a healed, dry middle ear, and the second for the reconstructive process. The ear should remain dry for 2 or 3 months before the second stage for the exploration of the window niches and the restoration of a conductive mechanism. Remaining parts of the ossicular chain may be repositioned to establish impulse transmission to the oval window.

Postoperative Care. Outer dressings may be reinforced if soiled with blood or drainage, but the inner dressing is undisturbed. The patient is hospitalized for 3 or 4 days. The nurse assists him when he first gets out of bed, because a typical reaction is dizziness and nystagmus. The physician may prescribe medications to combat vertigo and nausea. The patient is cautioned to avoid nose blowing and wetting the dressings during bathing. Eventually he will be permitted to resume showering and swimming.

Clinical Results. Patients with a lengthy history of disease may achieve hearing gains as great as those with less protracted infections. In patients whose otitis media has been healed and the ear dry for a lengthy period, hearing improvement may be marked after tympanoplasty. Younger patients achieve better results than older patients. The simpler the surgery, the better the chance for hearing gain; this, of course, relates directly to the functional integrity of the ossicular chain and the efficiency of the newly-created tympanic covering.

Continued research is being done to improve tympanoplasty procedures. In some instances, clinical failures have been due to infection, poor technique and tissue rejection of graft or prosthesis.

Otosclerosis

Otosclerosis is the term applied to a form of progressive deafness caused by the formation of new spongy bone in the labyrinth, fixing the stapes and preventing sound transmission by the vibrating ossicles to the inner ear fluids. The cause of this condition is unknown, but it occurs most commonly in women, beginning after puberty, and it has a hereditary basis. The condition begins with insidious loss of hearing, with ringing or buzzing ear noise, and both ears usually are involved about equally. The patient gives a history of slowly progressive hearing loss without middle ear infection.

The diagnosis is evident from the findings of the audiometer test. Tuning-fork sound transmission by air is markedly reduced, while intensification of sound is noted by placing the tuning-fork handle over the mastoid and recording the marked difference in hearing between air and bone. The bone conduction is far better than air conduction, which is the reverse of normal. There is no known treatment for this form of deafness other than the help offered by amplification with an electric hearing aid or preferably, a stapedectomy.

Surgery. History of surgery for otosclerosis has been fascinating. Although stapes surgery was attempted three quarters of a century ago, the results were poor because of ineffective lighting, inadequate magnification and infection. In 1925 Sourdille in France developed a 2-stage operation involving the creation of a small window in the horizontal semicircular canal. Through this window, sound was transmitted to the cochlea, thereby improving hearing. In 1938, Lembert in New York perfected the popular *fenestration operation.*

In this operation, a new window for passage of sound waves into the labyrinth is created, after a partial mastoidectomy. The newly created window reroutes sound, and an artificial covering for the newly created window, or fenestra, is made from the skin of the external canal. The surgical procedure is delicate and is performed by those specially trained in the techniques. The high-speed, motor-driven dental drill and cutting bur are essential to the operation. Optical aids, such as a loupe worn by the operating surgeon or a dissecting binocular microscope, make details of the operation safe.

Rosen in 1957 advanced a new technique in the treatment of otosclerosis. A portion of the foot-plate at its center was extracted by a special hooklike excavator and the defect covered with a strip of Gelfoam. In the performance of this technique, carried out at that time with the use of 2½ magnification of the binocular loupe and using the illumination of a head lamp, it is most reasonable to assume that the few lasting hearing improvements that resulted were due to mobilization of the foot-plate as a whole or to fragmentation of the thin portion of the foot-plate with subsequent motility that persisted. However, in most cases the hearing improvement was short-lived, and in many, the hearing remained acute only in the operating room until the tympanomeatal flap was reflected back in position; the hearing then regressed.

Later, John J. Shea, Jr., began his search for a tech-

Fig. 33-4. Techniques of stapedectomy. (1) Partial stapedectomy by cutting anterior crus and bisecting footplate. The posterior crus and remaining footplate are mobile (Hough). (2) Stapes removed and replaced with a vein graft. Polyethylene strut provides continuity (Shea). (3) Wire-fat prostheses replacing the stapes (Schuknecht). (4) Oval window covered with Gelfoam (House). Preformed wire placed on Gelfoam. (5) Footplate not removed. Footplate drilled and preformed wire-Teflon piston placed through hole in footplate (Shea; Guilford). Note otosclerotic fixation of the anterior footplate margin shown in (1) and (5). (DeWeese and Saunders: Textbook of Otolaryngology, St. Louis, Mosby)

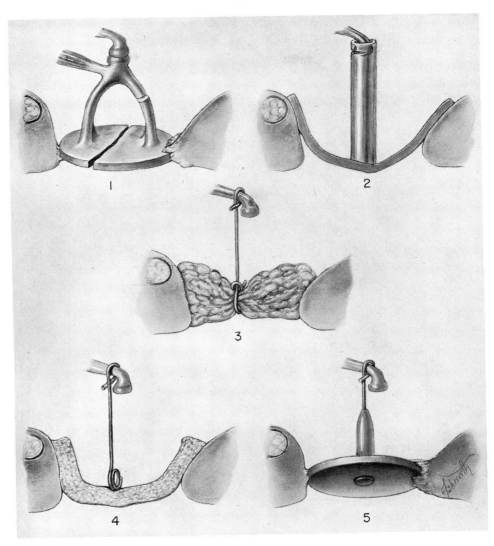

nique to remove the stapes in toto and to fashion a suitable prosthesis to restore this part of the conductive mechanism in otosclerotic patients. Otologic surgeons also have pioneered in the techniques of *stapedectomy*—the removal of the otosclerotic lesion at the foot-plate of the stapes and the creation of a suitable tissue implant with a prosthesis to replace this portion of the conductive mechanism.

Stapedectomy

Indications. Stapedectomy at first was reserved for patients with otosclerotic lesions diffuse enough to involve the entire foot-plate of the stapes, making it impossible to employ stapes mobilization, and for advanced cases of otosclerosis requiring either a chisel or the motor-driven bur to excavate or fenestrate the oval window. As a consequence of the increasing numbers of regressions that occurred after stapes mobilization, stapedectomy was employed as a secondary operative technique to salvage the failures of initial mobilization attempts. With the initial success of this operation, the indications have extended to all classes of otosclerosis; and in clinics where this technique is carried out, virtually all patients with otosclerosis are treated by a routine stapedectomy.

Micro-Surgery. The otologic binocular microscope is of distinct value in this operation. After the exposure of the middle ear with adequate removal of the bony annulus to expose the incudostapedial joint, the incus, and its major portion of the lenticular process, the facial canal, and the adjoining foot-plate of the stapes should be well delineated. Hemostasis control is important and is achieved by Gelfoam soaked in epinephrine, or by the coagulating current in minute amperage. The removal of the stapes proceeds delicately. The mucosa of the foot-plate and its margins are left undisturbed. A strip of Gelfoam then is placed over the foot-plate, and the prosthesis is fashioned after the distance is measured accurately from the level of the foot-plate to the underside of the lenticular process.

To bridge the gap between the incus and the inner ear, a prosthesis is fashioned. Schuknecht's type is the steel wire and fat implant whereas House's technique employs Gelfoam and prefabricated stainless steel wire (two most popular procedures). Kos uses wire and a segment of vein as a plug in the oval window, and Shea advocates a vein graft with polyethylene tubing (Fig. 33-4). In any case, the prosthetic device should be fashioned and ready preliminary to the removal of the stapedial foot-plate.

Today stapedectomy is the operation of choice in the surgical treatment of otosclerosis. This operation has largely supplanted the stapes mobilization and fenestration operation.

Nursing Management. The nursing care in this extremely delicate operation is essential for consistently successful end-results. Microscopic instruments and the detailed steps of the operation makes the experienced help of the nurse an important phase of this newer surgery of the deaf.

In the postoperative care the nurse should record unusual symptoms such as fever, headache, vertigo or ear pain. External otitis and otitis media have occurred as complications and require treatment with antibiotics. Vertigo initiated by this operation may protract the patient's hospital stay. Although the patient becomes ambulant in 24 hours, the nurse should be alert for the occasional patient who has vertigo and gait disturbance that may mean labyrinthitis or inner ear reaction requiring further observation and treatment. The initial hearing gain at the time of operation is masked by the ear packing and subsequent swelling of the tissues, so reassurance should be offered by the nurse that hearing gain may be noted from one to several weeks after operation. Reports from various observers doing this work indicate that a high percentage of patients can obtain useful hearing levels by this relatively simple operation.

PATIENTS WITH PROBLEMS OF THE INNER EAR

Balance of the body is maintained by the cooperation of muscle, joint, tendon, visceral senses, the eyes and the inner ear or vestibular apparatus. The last is the most important in this function. This inner apparatus informs the individual regarding the movements and the position of the head in space, coordinates all body muscles and positions the eyes in rapid motion or head movement. This apparatus consists of the utricle, the saccule and the semicircular canals, of which there are 3 in each ear. Each canal lies in a plane at right angles to the others, and they are grouped in working pairs for this complex function. The mechanism of action of the semicircular canals may be likened to the cochlea or organ of hearing. Here, also, fluids are set in motion by head or body movement which, in turn, stimulate extremely delicate nerve fibers which transmit messages as electric impulses along the nerve to centers in the brain for interpretation.

Endolymphatic Hydrops (Meniere's Syndrome)

Although there is almost general agreement that the symptoms of Meniere's syndrome stem from labyrinthine dysfunction, the cause has not been definitely established. Many theories have been advanced, such as an increase in pressure in the endolymph, vasomotor changes causing a spasm of the internal auditory artery, emotional or endocrine disturbance or an allergic manifestation.

Symptoms are primarily vertigo, tinnitus and reduced hearing. Some patients also complain of headache, nausea, vomiting and incoordination.

Attacks are sudden and the patient complains of the room appearing to spin around him. Any sudden motion of the head may induce vomiting. This symptom complex usually occurs in persons who have had previous ear trouble and allergic symptoms, especially vasomotor rhinitis. When vasospasm of the blood vessels occurs, the mucous membrane of the cochlea becomes swollen and congested, the fluid increases in quantity, and the resultant pressure on the labyrinth produces the symptoms of Meniere's syndrome.

The patient's most comfortable position is lying down, and he probably favors one side. He may be irritable and withdrawn and reject food. Every effort must be exerted to prevent noise and sudden jarring. He should be fed; bathing and turning should be done gently.

Vertigo, the outstanding symptom of Meniere's disease, occurs as a sudden attack and at irregular intervals of hours, days or months. Each attack lasts several hours or all day. Between attacks, the patient works or proceeds normally and complains only of tinnitus or hearing impairment. The patient does not complain of pain nor does he lose consciousness.

The *caloric test* may be done to differentiate this syndrome from an intracranial lesion. Fluid above or below body temperature is instilled into the auditory canal. The normal person complains of dizziness; the patient with an acoustic neuroma has no reaction; and a severe attack is produced in the patient with Meniere's syndrome. A few patients react to this caloric test by vomiting, hence the nurse anticipates this possibility and has an emesis basin and towel available. Following the test, the patient may still feel a bit dizzy and need assistance in walking.

Medical Management. Usually the patient is placed on a low sodium diet to aid in edema control. Vasodilators are given to control vasospasm. For this reason also, no smoking may be recommended. Fairly successful symptomatic treatment is reported from a combination (Antivert) of 2 medications: meclizine, which eases vestibular tension, and nicotinic acid, which acts as a vasodilator. Vitamin therapy (vitamins A, C, thiamine, nicotinic acid, riboflavin, and pyridoxine) appears to help older patients. An allergy search is conducted on patients whose signs and symptoms warrant this type of clinical investigation.

Symptoms may be relieved, but hearing does not improve.

Surgical Management. For the patient who has had progressive hearing loss and experiences severe vertigo attacks, the destruction of the membranous labyrinth (inner ear) is probably the most helpful technique. For those who have a reasonable amount of hearing, *ultrasonic surgery* may be helpful. This requires a mastoidectomy incision to gain access to the horizontal semicircular canal. By means of a probe, ultrasonic energy is applied directly to the bone in the canal. Proponents claim that hearing is preserved while vertigo is eliminated.

Recently, the use of cryosurgery by way of a mastoid approach has been reported.

Nursing Measures. The nursing approach to the individual who has vertigo attacks is two-pronged. First, the patient needs understanding and encouragement, because many find it difficult to define a problem that has subjective symptoms. The patient looks well enough to work, but he does not feel well. Secondly, he needs assistance in slowing down his movements so that he does not precipitate an attack. This need for self-protection is extended when an attack takes place; his best place is lying in a bed equipped with side-rails, but, if he is standing, he needs help to avoid injuring himself from falling.

Postoperatively, the patient who has had a surgical destruction of the labyrinth may experience vertigo for up to 48 hours, when it gradually subsides and permits him to get out of bed. Some unsteadiness and vertigo may persist as long as 3 to 6 weeks, but this may be controlled by moving easily.

The individual who has had ultrasonic surgery continues to have destructive effects of ultrasonic vibrations for 3 to 5 days. Usually he is able to be up and about in 2 to 3 days, leave the hospital in a week and return to work in 3 weeks. Bell's palsy* may be a postoperative complication, but this clears between 2 weeks and 3 months. The possibility of this occurring might be explained to the patient.

A variety of medical and surgical treatments exist for Meniere's disease, one of which may give a particular patient the relief he needs. Research continues in an effort to find the cause of this syndrome, which will more clearly suggest definitive therapy.

CLASSIFICATION OF HEARING LOSS

Conductive Loss

Such loss results from an impairment of the outer ear, middle ear or both. The inner ear is not involved in this type of loss; it can analyze clearly the sounds that come to it. Correction of the problem (see pp. 746-754) may be all that is necessary to treat and correct this type of impairment. If the problem cannot be corrected, these individuals benefit greatly from hearing aids because in most instances they require only amplification of sounds.

Sensorineural Loss

A disease of the inner ear or nerve pathways produces a type of hearing loss in which sensitivity to and discrimination of sounds are impaired. Sounds may be conducted properly through the external and middle ear but are not analyzed correctly in the inner ear. Because of poor sensitivity to sound, hearing aids are not as helpful as they are to those with conductive loss.

Combined Hearing Loss

This is a common problem in which a patient has both a conductive and a sensorineural loss.

Psychogenic Hearing Loss (Nonorganic, Functional)

This loss is unrelated to detectable structural change in the hearing mechanism. Usually it is a manifestation of an emotional disturbance and the loss is frequently total.

---

* Bell's palsy is a peripheral facial weakness attended by aching pain near the angle of the jaw or behind the ear.

REHABILITATION

It is important to classify the kinds of hearing impairment so that rehabilitative efforts are more likely to meet a particular need. The Conference of Executives of American Schools for the Deaf* proposed the following classification based on (1) time of onset of hearing loss, and (2) functional status of hearing:

1. The deaf—those in whom the sense of hearing is nonfunctional for ordinary purposes of life. This general group is made up of two distinct classes:
   (a) The congenitally deaf
   (b) The adventitiously deaf—those born with normal hearing in whom the sense of hearing became nonfunctional through illness or accident.
2. The hard of hearing—those in whom hearing, although defective, is serviceable with or without a hearing aid.

Hearing Aids

A hearing aid is an instrument through which sounds, both speech and environmental, are received by a microphone, converted into electrical signals, amplified and reconverted to acoustical signals.

Whether an individual would benefit by a hearing aid can best be determined by an otologist. When the hearing loss is more than 30 decibels in the range of 500 to 2,000 cycles per second in the better ear, a patient can benefit from a hearing aid used with this ear. A variety of aids are available; the problem is to select the best aid for the individual patient. He or a salesman cannot make the decision alone; it should be made with the advice of an otologist. Even this does not ensure optimal benefit from such an instrument. Psychological factors such as vanity may be involved, as well as other types of sensitivity.

The patient needs to know that the aid will not restore his hearing to the level of the person with normal hearing but will improve it in the range of 300 to 3,500 cycles per second (range of primary speech). (See Fig. 33-1.)

A problem with most hearing aids is that background noise is also amplified, which may be distressing to the wearer; examples of such noises are apparent when one speaks to a friend and there is passing traffic or other persons in the group are talking at the same time. Binaural aids, that is one for each ear, may be indicated. Such aids can be concealed in the arms of specially made eyeglasses.

In caring for a hearing aid, the ear mold is the only part of the instrument that may be washed. It should be washed in soap and water every day and the cannula cleansed with a small applicator or pipe cleaner. Before snapping it into the receiver, the mold must be dry. The transmitter usually is worn by men in the shirt pocket and by women in a special pocket just under the dress as on the outer side of a slip. Children may wear the transmitter in a cloth pocket as a harness over the outer clothing. A spare battery and cord should be carried by the wearer at all times.

When a hearing aid is not functioning properly, these several steps should be followed as listed below: (1) note whether the on-off switch is on; (2) check the positioning of the batteries; (3) try a new battery; (4) examine the cord for breaks and whether it is plugged in correctly; (5) examine the ear mold for cleanliness. If the aid still will not work, notify the local service agency. Meanwhile, if the unit requires days to repair, the agency from whom it was purchased may lend an aid, or one may be borrowed from the local Chapter of the American Hearing Society.

A hearing aid makes speech louder but it does not always make it clear enough for the deaf person to understand what is said. The wearer must experiment and adjust the controls for optimal results. He needs to recognize that he will never hear what others cannot hear, nor will he hear as well as one who has no hearing impairment. It may be necessary for him to have auditory training and speech reading (lip reading) in order to make the new hearing aid effective. With such assistance, this person can learn to interpret sounds and use advantageously whatever hearing remains. Speech reading can help fill in the gaps of those words that might be missed.* The otologist or the hearing center can direct the patient to such classes.

Communicating With a Person Who Has a Hearing Impairment

Terry *et al.*† offer the following suggestions for better communication with deaf persons whose speech is difficult to understand:

1. Devote full attention to what he is saying. Look and listen—do not try to give attention to another task while listening to him.
2. Engage him in conversation where it is possible for you to anticipate his replies. This will enable you to become accustomed to the peculiarities of his pattern of speech.

---

* Saunders, W. H., *et al.*: Nursing Care in Eye, Ear, Nose, and Throat Disorders. p. 339. St. Louis, C. V. Mosby, 1968.

* In auditory training, speech discrimination and listening skills are emphasized.

† Terry, F. J., *et al.*: Rehabilitation Nursing, p. 310. St. Louis, C. V. Mosby.

3. Try to catch the essential context of what he is saying; you can often fill in the details from context.

4. Do not try to appear as if you understand him when you do not.

5. If you cannot understand him at all or have serious doubt about your ability to understand him, have him write his message rather than risk misunderstanding. Having him repeat the message in speech, after you know its content, will also aid you in becoming accustomed to his pattern of speech.

Suggestions for better communication with deaf persons who lip-read:

1. When speaking, always face the person as directly as possible.

2. Make sure your face is as clearly visible as possible; locate yourself so that your face is well-lighted; avoid being silhouetted against strong light; do not obscure that person's view of your mouth in any way; avoid talking with any object held in your mouth.

3. Be sure the patient knows the topic or subject of your verbal expression before going ahead with what you plan to say—this will enable him to use contextual clues in his lip-reading.

4. Speak slowly and distinctly, pausing more frequently than you would normally.

5. If you question whether the patient has understood some important direction or instruction, check to be certain that he has the full meaning of your message.

6. If for any reason your mouth must be covered (as with a mask) and you must direct or instruct the patient, there is no alternative but to write the message for him.

BIBLIOGRAPHY

Books

DeWeese, D. D., and Saunders, W. H.: Textbook of Otolaryngology, ed. 3, St. Louis, C. V. Mosby, 1968.

O'Neill, J. J.: The Hard of Hearing, Englewood Cliffs, N. J., Prentice-Hall, Inc., 1965.

Quigley, S. P.: The Vocational Rehabilitation of Deaf People, Washington, D.C. 20201 (Rehabilitation Services Adm., 330 Independence Ave., S.W.)

Saunders, W. H., *et al.*: Nursing Care in Eye, Ear, Nose, and Throat Disorders, ed. 2, St. Louis, C. V. Mosby, 1968.

Shambaugh, G.: Surgery of the Ear, ed. 2, Phila., W. B. Saunders, 1967.

General Articles

Brown, L. A.: Newer types of ear surgery. Nurs. Forum, *4*:(No. 3) 95-98, 1965.

DiBiasio, A. G.: Postoperative care of patients having ear surgery. Nurs. Forum, *4*:(No. 3) 104-108, 1965.

McCurdy, H. W.: Preoperative care of patients having ear surgery. Nurs. Forum, *4*:(No. 3) 99-103, 1965.

Myers, D., Schlosser, W. D., and Winchester, R. A.: Otologic diagnoses and the treatment of deafness. Clinical Symposia, *2*:39-73, Apr., May, June, 1962.

Hearing Impairment

Bender, R. E.: Communicating with the deaf. Amer. J. Nurs., *66*:757-760, April, 1966.

Klotz, R. E., and Robinson, M.: Hard-of-hearing patients have special problems. Amer. J. Nurs., *3*:88-89, May, 1963.

External Ear

Goldman, L., and Kitzmiller, K. W.: Earlobe piercing with needles and wires. Arch. Derm., *92*:305-306, Sept., 1965.

Middle Ear

Compere, W. E., Jr.: Hearing restoration through stapes surgery. AORN Jour., *5*:61-65, June, 1967.

Delaney, R. E.: Stapedectomy. Amer. J. Nurs., *69*:2406-2409, Nov., 1969.

Ingerman, M.: Current trends in surgery of the middle ear. AORN Jour., *7*:50-57, May, 1968.

Myers, D.: Permanent restoration of hearing. AORN Jour., *6*: 61-63, Dec., 1967.

Sanches, R. T.: Microsurgery of the middle ear for otosclerosis. AORN Jour., *2*:59-70, July, 1965.

Wilson, M. R.: The role of the operating room nurse in microsurgery of the ear. AORN Jour., *2*:64-67, July, 1964.

Inner Ear

Ariagno, R. P.: Ultrasonic surgery for Meniere's disease. Amer. J. Nurs., *60*:1778-1780, Dec., 1960.

Pulec, J. L. (ed.): Symposium on Meniere's disease. Otolaryngologic Clin. N. Amer., Oct., 1968.

Wolfson, R. J., *et al.*: Cryosurgery for Meniere's disease. Laryngoscope, *78*:632-642, Apr., 1968.

———: Vertigo. Clinical Symposia. *17*:99-103, Oct.-Nov.-Dec., 1965.

Wood, C. D.: Medications for vertigo and motion sickness. Amer. J. Nurs., *66*:1764-1767, Aug., 1966.

PATIENT EDUCATION

Canfield, N.: Hearing, a Handbook for Laymen. Garden City, Doubleday, 1959.

O'Neill, J. J.: The Hard of Hearing. Englewood Cliffs, N.J., Prentice-Hall, 1965.

Superintendent of Documents
Government Printing Office
Washington, D.C. 20402
  U.S. Dept. of H.E.W.: Hearing Loss; Hope Through Research. P.H.S. Publication No. 207, 1965.

U.S. Public Heath Service
National Medical Audiovisual Center
Atlanta, Georgia 30333
  "Silent World, Muffled World." 28-min. 16-mm. sound and color documentary, produced by Deafness Research Foundation and the American Academy of Ophthalmology and Otolaryngology. Available on free loan.

NATIONAL ORGANIZATIONS

Alexander Graham Bell Assoc. for the Deaf, Inc.
  Volta Bureau
  1535 35th St., N.W.
  Washington, D.C. 20007
    Volta Review (monthly journal)

American Hearing Society
  919 18th St., N.W.
  Washington, D.C. 20006
    Hearing News (bimonthly periodical)

The American Speech and Hearing Association
  1001 Connecticut Ave., N.W.
  Washington, D.C. 20036
    The Journal of Speech and Hearing Disorders, The Journal of Speech and Hearing Research

The Deafness Research Foundation
  366 Madison Ave.
  New York, N.Y. 10017

The National Assoc. for the Deaf
  2025 Eye Street, N.W.
  Washington, D.C. 20006
    The *Silent Worker* (monthly publication)

American Academy of Ophthalmology and Otolaryngology of the American Medical Associaiton
  535 Dearborn Street
  Chicago, Illinois 60610

CHAPTER **34**

Patients with Neurologic and Neurosurgical Problems

- *Normal and Altered Anatomy and Physiology*
- *Assisting with the Neurologic Examination*
- *Special Problems of Neurologic and Neurosurgical Patients*
- *The Patient with a Headache*
- *The Patient with Increasing Intracranial Pressure*
- *Febrile and Hypothermic Patients*
- *The Unconscious Patient*
- *Patients with Cranial, Spinal and Peripheral Neuropathies*
- *Cerebrovascular Disease*
- *Patients with Brain Tumors and Aneurysms*
- *The Patient with Multiple Sclerosis*
- *Patients with Extrapyramidal Disease*
- *Patients with Cerebral Infection*
- *The Patient with a Convulsive Disorder*
- *Patients with Injuries of the Central Nervous System*
- *The Patient with Intractable Pain*

SCOPE OF NEUROLOGIC NURSING

The field of neurologic nursing is a fascinating one. Within its scope the nurse has an opportunity to utilize all her powers of observation. She is a vital source of information in assisting with the diagnosis and in planning the therapeutic management of the patient.

Recovery from organic disease of the nervous system is not always followed by complete restoration of function. The rehabilitation needs of these patients are unusually complex, their solution requiring occupational therapy and guidance, recreational opportunities, physical therapy and re-education of the most difficult sort. The most important of the neurologic disorders and the principal problems of neurologic nursing are considered in this chapter.

By her optimism, nursing ability and concern for the patient as a person, the nurse can help to ease many of the difficult experiences of her patient and his family. When she realizes that the behavior and the personality of a person can be affected markedly by organic lesions of the brain, she is less inclined to think of an individual as an uncooperative patient with a foul disposition; instead he becomes one who needs help and understanding. His reactions may be beyond his control; the nurse must realize this.

The many interesting diagnostic tests in which the nurse participates are much like solving a puzzle. But the diagnosis is not the end; it is merely a stepping-stone to the removal of the cause. Surgery must be done accurately, for otherwise the penalty may be the death of the patient or the reduction of his mental and/or physical abilities to the level of mere existence. Although surgery has many successful cases, there are instances in which an injury is too great to repair, or a tumor too extensive to remove, and the patient's prognosis is hopeless. It is important that even in these

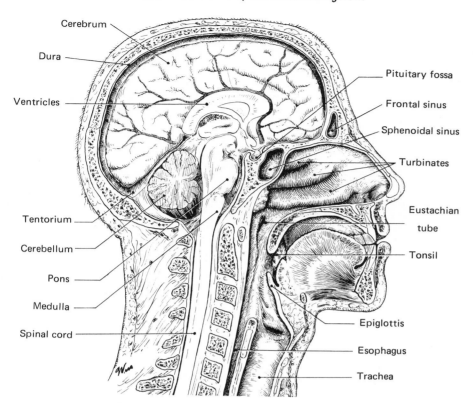

Cerebrum
Dura
Ventricles
Tentorium
Cerebellum
Pons
Medulla
Spinal cord

Pituitary fossa
Frontal sinus
Sphenoidal sinus
Turbinates
Eustachian tube
Tonsil
Epiglottis
Esophagus
Trachea

FIG. 34-1. Cross-sectional view, showing the anatomic position and the relation of structures of the head and the neck.

instances the nurse exercise as much concern for the comfort and the feelings of her patient as she does in situations in which the prognosis is more encouraging. This kind of care is significant, not only from the point of view of the individual patient but also from that of his family.

The nurse has an opportunity to use many procedures in giving sound, conscientious bedside care. It is important to apply the principles of good body mechanics, since the position of the patient must be changed frequently. From the moment the patient shows response after his operation, the nurse is on the alert to help him in his rehabilitation. Often every activity may have to be relearned, such as using his fingers to hold a spoon, learning to say words and sentences, acquiring the ability to write, etc. In addition, he needs psychological assistance in the form of encouragement. The nurse is a key person in that she is with him day and night and therefore is responsible for much of his future progress.

NORMAL AND ALTERED ANATOMY AND PHYSIOLOGY

Cerebrospinal Components and Connections

The nervous system comprises the brain and the spinal cord, together with all extensions therefrom and neural connections thereto. Its function is to control and to coordinate cellular activities throughout the body. The signaling device that it employs involves the transmission of electrical impulses, a system which permits each stimulus to be placed accurately in the area that is intended to receive it. These impulses are routed by way of nerve fibers, pathways that are direct and continuous, and the responses that these elicit are practically instantaneous, because changes in electrical potential transmit the signals.

The brain is divided into cerebrum, brain stem and rigid, bony box—the skull or cranium. At the base of this box is a foramen magnum, an opening through which the spinal cord is continuous with the brain (Fig. 34-1) and the spinal cord. The brain has 3 coverings. These are (1) the dura, the outer covering of dense fibrous tissue that closely hugs the inner wall of the skull, (2) the arachnoid, and (3) the pia mater, which adheres closely to the brain and the spinal cord.

The brain is divided into cerebrum, brain stem and cerebellum. The brain stem consists, from top down, of midbrain, pons and medulla oblongata (Fig. 34-1).

The *cerebrum* is divided into 2 hemispheres and consists of 5 lobes: frontal, parietal, temporal, occipital and insular (Fig. 34-2). The cerebrum is the largest part of the brain, and on its surface or cortex are located the "centers" from which motor impulses are

Fig. 34-2. (*Top*) Diagrammatic representation of the cerebrum, showing relative locations of various lobes of the brain and the principal fissures. (*Bottom*) Diagrammatic representation of cerebral localization for motor movements of various portions of the body.

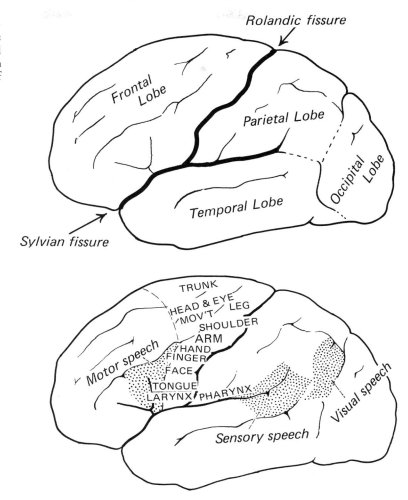

carried to the muscles, and to which sensory impulses come from the various sensory nerves.

The *midbrain* connects the pons and the cerebellum with the cerebral hemispheres. The *cerebellum* or "little brain" is located below and behind the cerebrum. Its function is the control or the coordination of muscles and equilibration.

The *pons* is situated in front of the cerebellum between the midbrain and the medulla and is a bridge between the two halves of the cerebellum as well as between the medulla and the cerebrum.

The *medulla oblongata* transmits motor fibers from the brain to the spinal cord and sensory fibers from the spinal cord to the brain. The majority of these fibers decussate at this level. The pons also contains important centers controlling heart, respiration and blood pressure and gives origin to the fifth, sixth, seventh and eighth cranial nerves.

There are 2 glands present in the brain: the pituitary and the pineal. The pituitary gland is frequently approached surgically. It lies at the base of the brain in a bony fossa termed the sella turcica, just posterior to the optic chiasm, upon which it may press when the gland is enlarged.

Spinal Cord. The spinal cord, surrounded by the vertebral column, extends from the foramen magnum of the skull, where it is continuous with the medulla oblongata, to the first lumbar vertebra, where it tapers off into a fine thread of tissue (Fig. 34-3). The spinal cord is an important center of reflex action for the body and contains the conducting pathways to and from the higher centers in the cord and the brain.

Cerebrospinal Fluid. Within each cerebral hemisphere is a central cavity, the lateral ventricle. This is filled with clear *cerebrospinal fluid*, which forms at this site by a process of extraction from the blood as the latter circulates through the capillaries of the choroid plexus by well-defined channels from the lateral ventricles through narrow tubular openings to the third and the fourth ventricles. From this narrow cav-

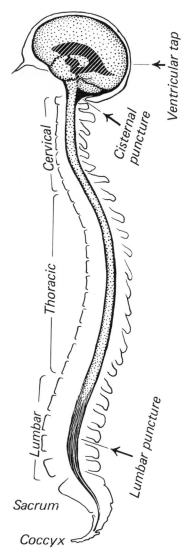

FIG. 34-3. Diagrammatic representation of the cerebrospinal system, showing the brain, the cord and the spaces occupied by cerebrospinal fluid, ventricles and dural sac. The sites for the introduction of needles for ventricular tap, cisternal puncture and lumbar puncture are indicated.

ity it escapes to the subarachnoid space to bathe the entire surface of the brain and the spinal cord. The cerebrospinal fluid normally is absorbed by the large venous channels of the skull and along the spinal and the cranial nerves.

The spinal fluid is clear and colorless, having a specific gravity of 1.007. The average patient's ventricular and subarachnoid systems contain about 150 ml. of this fluid. The organic and inorganic contents of the cerebrospinal fluid is very similar to that of the plasma; however their concentration is somewhat different.

Disease produces changes in the composition of this fluid. Determinations of the protein content and the quantity of glucose and chloride present constitute the chief chemical examinations. In a state of health there are a minimal number of white cells and no red cells in the spinal fluid; thus the examination for cells is important. Other diagnostic examinations include the Wassermann reaction for syphilis and the colloidal-gold reaction, which is a colloidal precipitation test based on the protein content in the spinal fluid.

By replacing cerebrospinal fluid with air, the radiologist is able to visualize with x-rays the size, shape and position of the ventricles. Any interference or distortion may be suggestive of a space-occupying lesion.

Cerebral Cortex. The cells in the cortex are quite similar in appearance; their functions, however, vary widely, depending on their geographic location. Figure 34-2 depicts the topography of the cortex in relation to certain of its specific functions. The posterior portion of each hemisphere, i.e., the occipital lobe, is devoted to all aspects of visual perception; the lateral region, or temporal lobe, incorporates the hearing center. The mid-central zone, or parietal zone, posterior to the fissure of Rolandi, is concerned with sensation; the anterior portion is concerned with voluntary muscle movements. The large uncharted area beneath the forehead, i.e., the frontal lobes, contain the association pathways that determine emotional attitudes and responses and contribute to the formation of thought processes. Damage to the frontal lobes as a result of trauma or disease is by no means incapacitating from the standpoint of muscular control or coordination, but has decided effect on the personality of the individual, as reflected by his basic attitudes, sense of humor and propriety, self-restraint and motivations. Surgical division of frontal lobe tracts has been carried out as a therapeutic measure in patients with major psychoses.

Internal Capsule, Pons and Medulla. Nerve fibers from all portions of the cortex converge in each hemisphere and make their exit in the form of tight bundles known as the "internal capsule." Having entered the pons and the medulla, each bundle crosses the corresponding bundle from the opposite side. Some of these axons make connections with axons from the cerebellum, basal ganglia, thalamus and hypothalamus; some connect with the cranial nerve cells. Other fibers from the cortex and the subcortical centers are channeled through the pons and the medulla into the spinal cord.

Vision and Cortical Blindness. There is a definite area in the rear of each hemisphere where the fibers of the corresponding optic nerve end. It is by means of these receiving cells that we see. The eyes may be normal and the optic nerve perfect, but if these cells in one hemisphere are diseased, the person is half-blind. In such a case he has *cortical blindness*. He cannot see to one side of the midline. He sees only half of any object. This is *hemianopsia* (half-blindness).

Cortical blindness of one optic area (that is, of the

posterior tip of one cerebral hemisphere) always affects both eyes equally. Total blindness in one eye may be due to disease of that eye itself or to disease of its optic nerve. Just behind the two eyes, however, the two optic nerves become confluent (the chiasm), then again become separate and continue to the brain as the two optic tracts.

In each of these tracts is just half of each optic nerve, so that if one tract is injured, there is complete blindness of exactly one half of each retina. For example, if the right tract is injured, the patient is blind on the right half of each retina, so that with either eye he can see nothing to his left but will see perfectly to his right. Destroy the cortical optical area of the hemisphere to which that tract runs and we have this same form of hemianopsia. The pituitary gland is located just beneath the chiasm; a tumor of this gland often disturbs the chiasm and produces blindness of both inner halves of the retinas, since it is only the fibers in the nasal halves of the optic nerves that cross. In many cases of blindness it is thus possible to locate the disorder.

Aphasia

Aphasia is a disturbance of langauge function. In the majority of patients with aphasia, there is no impairment of intellect or disintegration of personality. The cortical area that is responsible for integrating the myriad association pathways required for the mere understanding of words and for controlling the countless motor activities that are entailed in the process of verbalizing measures little more than a square inch in extent (marked Motor speech in Fig. 34-2, *bottom*). The principal speech center, called *Broca's area*, is located in a convolution adjoining the motor cortex on the left side in the case of right-handed individuals, or on the right in left-handed persons. Here are stored the combinations of muscular movements necessary to speak each word. They are not the cells that govern the muscles of speech; these cells are in the motor area itself. Each word requires for its utterance a combination or sequence of combinations of muscular contractions. Not only must the muscles of the vocal cords contract, but also those of the throat, the tongue, the soft palate, the lips and the chest wall. These combinations are stored in the cells of Broca's convolution. They direct the cells of the motor area, which make the muscles contract at the proper time and with the proper force.

Broca's area is so near the left motor area that disease of the latter often affects the former. This is the reason that so many persons who are paralyzed on the right side (due to a lesion of the left hemisphere) are unable to speak, whereas those paralyzed on the left side almost never have speech disturbances. Some patients do, but these usually are left-handed persons whose speech area is located on the right hemisphere.

Motor Aphasia. The destruction of Broca's convolution by hemorrhage, thrombosis or tumor results in motor aphasia. The patient understands all that is said to him; he knows the words he wants to say; he may be able to write them and read them; but, although he has absolutely no paralysis of the vocal cords, he cannot produce the sequence of movements necessary to utter them, and, if he tries, he makes an unintelligible noise. He is conscious of this defect, and it distresses him. To cause a permanent motor aphasia, however, the lesion must (and usually does) affect the white matter beneath this convolution where the fibers are going to and coming from other parts of the brain. When only the gray matter of Broca's convolution is destroyed, the aphasia may be transitory. The inability to write (agraphia), often lost in motor aphasia, probably is due to the involvement of the posterior end of the second frontal convolution.

Cortical Sensory Aphasia. Auditory aphasia is the inability of a person to understand and to repeat words spoken to him. Often he talks jargon, but he is unaware that he is not talking correctly. This defect is the result of lesions in the posterior part of the left superior temporal convolution, where the memory of sounds is stored. This type also is called *receptive aphasia*. The patient has difficulty in naming objects set before him, and yet he understands their use. Pure word blindness (*alexia*) is due to lesions in the angular gyrus (marked Visual speech in Fig. 34-2, *bottom*).

The most common type of aphasia is the result of cerebral hemorrhage that injures the left internal capsule and the surrounding fibers and also produces marked hemiplegia without loss of sensation. This is the mixed type, with loss of voluntary speech, impaired ability to read and difficulty in the comprehension of spoken words.

In some cases it would seem as though another part of the cortex can take over the work of the destroyed area, for through careful training a person with motor aphasia may learn to talk again.

Nursing Management. Give the patient as much psychological security as possible. A young child learning to speak is dealt with in a kindly and nonhurried manner. So also, the adult patient with aphasia who is basically starting over again needs encouragement, patience and *time*. Relearning of vocal skills may take several years. The goal is to help the patient communicate, and recovery of language is only part of his total rehabilitation.

In working with the aphasic patient, the nurse must remember to *talk* to the patient while she is caring for him. This keeps the patient in a social world. Requests and directions should be simple. When he at-

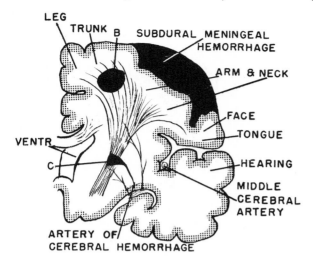

FIG. 34-4. A cross section of the left hemisphere of the brain through the motor area. The subdural meningeal hemorrhage compresses the brain over the arm-neck area. There is no real destruction of brain substance, but paralysis would result from pressure. (B) Subcortical hemorrhage. This hemorrhage does destroy brain substance. Although a smaller hemorrhage than the subdural, it possibly produces more paralysis, since it cuts fibers that have converged somewhat. (C) Hemorrhage into the internal capsule. This explains the common stroke of paralysis. Although the hemorrhage is small, it causes total paralysis of the right side of the body, since it cuts all the fibers in the internal capsule.

tempts to communicate, the nurse should make a real effort to understand him. The patient is treated as an intelligent adult. He never should be forced to correct his mistakes, as this merely adds to his tension. During periods of emotional lability, employ a calm, accepting and deliberate manner.

The patient may react with frustration and depression when he is unable to communicate. The nurse accepts his behavior, relieves his embarrassment, and gives support by assuring him that there is nothing wrong with his intelligence, and that she realizes he knows what he wants to say. The environment should be relaxed and permissive, and the socialization of the patient with his family and friends should be encouraged. The language retraining program is carried out by a speech pathologist, if one is available, or by a speech therapist.

The Spinal Cord and Its Connections

The spinal cord, a direct continuation of the medulla oblongata, is that part of the nervous system contained within the vertebral column. It is a cord about 18 in.* long and approximately the thickness of a man's finger. Like the brain, it consists of gray and white matter, but, although in the brain the gray matter is external and the white internal, in the cord the gray matter is in the center and is surrounded on all sides by the white fibers, both those of sensory tracts running up to the brain and those of motor fibers coming down from the brain (Fig. 34-3).

Gray Matter. The gray matter is shaped like two pairs of horns, the anterior horn and the posterior horn. The cord gives off 31 pairs of spinal nerves. Each is formed by the union of two roots, an anterior or motor root and a posterior or sensory root on which is the sensory ganglion. These two roots unite to form one spinal nerve. As a result, all the spinal nerves are mixed. Those leaving the right side of the cord supply the muscles, the skin and the organs on the right side of the body; those of the left side supply the corresponding muscles on that side of the body.

Motor Controls: Paralysis and Dyskinesia

A vertical band of cortex on each cerebral hemisphere governs the voluntary movements of the body. This region, known as the "motor cortex," can be located accurately.

We know the exact location of the cells in which originate the voluntary movements of the muscles of the face, the thumb, the hands, the arm, the trunk or the leg. Before a person can move a muscle, these particular cells must send the stimulus down along their fibers. If these cells are stimulated with an electric current, the muscles that they control will contract.

En route to the pons, as described previously, the motor fibers converge into a tight bundle known as the capsule. A comparatively small injury to this bundle causes paralysis in more muscles than does a much larger injury to the cortex itself. The brain is like a telephone station, in which one blow of an axe can sever all the wires at the point where they leave the building, but a similar blow on the switchboard would sever only a few.

The ordinary cause of a stroke, followed by paralysis of one half of the body (hemiplegia), is usually a small hemorrhage from a blood vessel in this capsule (see Figs. 34-4 and 34-5). A much larger hemorrhage nearer to or in the cortex might paralyze one limb, but hardly half of the body. Hemiplegia may be due to the rupture of a miliary aneurysm of a tiny artery running to the internal capsule or to the plugging of this artery by a thrombus or an embolus, and the sub-

* 45.72 cm.

sequent death of the fibers which it supplies with blood.

Immediately after a stroke, one half of the body, as a rule, is paralyzed. Then, gradually, the person recovers the use of certain muscles, usually those of the leg, often those of the upper arm, least often those of the hand. Although the hemorrhage actually destroys the fibers of only a few nerves, it temporarily injures all those in its neighborhood, perhaps by the pressure of the escaped blood or by the edema that surrounds it. As the swelling from the hemorrhage diminishes, these latter fibers resume their function, but those actually destroyed never do.

Within the medulla the motor axons from the cortex form two well-defined bands known as the *corticospinal* or *pyramidal tracts*. Here the majority of these fibers cross (or decussate) to the opposite side, continuing thereafter as the "crossed pyramidal tract." The remaining fibers then enter the cord on the original side as the "direct pyramidal tract," each fiber in this tract finally crossing to the opposite side of the cord near the point of termination and coming to an end within the gray matter comprising the anterior horn on that side, in close proximity to a motor nerve cell. Fibers of the crossed pyramidal tract terminate within the anterior horn and make connections with anterior horn cells on the same side. All of the motor fibers of the spinal nerves represent extensions of these anterior horn cells, with each of these fibers communicating with only one particular muscle fiber. Thus each muscle fiber is under voluntary control through a combination of two nerve cells. One is located in the motor cortex, its fiber in the direct or crossed pyramidal tract, and the other is located in the anterior horn of the spinal cord, its fiber running to the muscle. The former is referred to as the upper motor neuron; the latter, as the lower motor neuron. Every motor nerve serving a muscle is a bundle comprised of several thousand lower motor neurons.

Several motor nerve tracts, other than the corticospinal, are contained in the spinal cord. Some represent the pathways of the so-called "extrapyramidal system," establishing connections between the anterior horn cells and the automatic control centers located in the basal ganglia and the cerebellum. Others are components of reflex arcs, forming synaptic connections between anterior horn cells and sensory fibers that have entered adjacent or neighboring segments of the cord.

Motor Paralysis. Paralysis of a muscle may be due to pathologic changes in either the upper or the lower motor neuron. If a motor nerve were cut somewhere between the muscle and the spinal cord, the muscle becomes paralyzed, and the individual is not able to

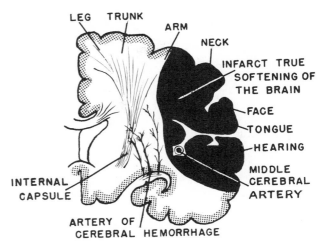

Fig. 34-5. A cross section of the left hemisphere of the cerebrum through the motor area. The middle cerebral artery is represented as plugged by a thrombus. That part of the brain (black area) supplied with food by this artery has died (infarction or softening). This patient would have paralysis of the right side of the face, the tongue and the neck and part of the right arm; he would be unable to talk or to understand what was said to him.

move it. Furthermore, it takes no part in reflex movements. Moreover, this muscle becomes limp and wastes away; that is, it atrophies owing to disuse. The injury to the spinal nerve trunk may heal, and the patient may regain the use of the muscles that it supplies. But if the anterior horn motor nerve cells are destroyed, the nerve cannot regenerate, and that muscle never will be useful again. This is exactly what occurs in anterior poliomyelitis.

If the upper motor neuron is destroyed, a different condition exists in the muscle. It is paralyzed as far as voluntary movement is concerned, but not necessarily for reflex (involuntary) movements, because these originate in the nerve cells in the cord or the medulla. The muscle does not atrophy, and it will not become limp; on the contrary, it remains permanently more tense than normal. This paralysis seldom affects a part of one muscle, one single muscle or only a few muscles; it usually affects a whole limb, both limbs or an entire half of the body (hemiplegia).

A good illustration of this form of paralysis is the spastic (stiff) paralysis of those infants who during birth receive some mechanical injury that may have caused the rupture of a blood vessel in the meninges of the brain. The long-continued pressure of the escaped blood may injure large areas of cortex; hence these children are frequently mentally deficient. Many have convulsions. When such a child begins to walk, it is noted that the legs and the arms are stiff. During life his movements are awkward, stiff and weak. Since those muscles that draw the feet and the knees toward each other (the adductor muscles) are naturally stronger than those that spread those limbs apart (the abductor muscles), these persons walk by a cross-legged progression, called also the *scissors gait;* that is, in each step the leg is moved not only forward but is swung round across the front of the other. When both legs and both arms, or both arms only, are paralyzed, the disease is called *diplegia;* when both legs alone, *paraplegia;* and when the arm and the leg on the same side are paralyzed, *hemiplegia.* Paralysis of all four extremities is *quadriplegia.*

A more common illustration of upper motor neuron paralysis is the hemiplegia of adults. If a hemorrhage, an embolus or a thrombus destroys the fibers from the motor area in the internal capsule, the arm and the leg of the opposite side promptly become stiff and more or less paralyzed, and the reflexes are exaggerated. Another illustration of upper neuron disease is seen in adults with spastic paraplegia, a chronic stiffness of both legs due to a gradual degeneration of the fibers in the pyramidal tract. The person so afflicted walks stiffly, as though wading through water, the knees always touching each other, and scarcely raising his feet from the ground (the spastic gait).

Both an upper and a lower motor neuron paralysis may result from an injury that crushes the spinal cord, a type of injury that is all too common. A boy diving into too-shallow water, for example, strikes his head and "breaks" his neck. That is, at one point the vertebrae are no longer in line, and the cord is badly crushed at the point of the dislocation. Knuckling of the backbone due to tuberculosis may accomplish the same thing, only more slowly. The result of such crushing of the cord leads to a rigid paralysis on both sides of all muscles whose nerves leave the cord below the crushed spot, the limp paralysis of the muscles whose motor nerve fibers come from cells in the crushed area. There also will be insensibility of the skin below the crush, since the sensory fibers from below the injury no longer reach the brain. Tumors of the cord ultimately cause this same picture. At first, only that part of the cord directly involved is disturbed, but as the tumor grows, it may completely crush the cord.

Extrapyramidal Motor Controls. The smoothness, the accuracy and the strength that characterize the muscular movements of a normal individual are attributable to the influence of the cerebellum and the basal ganglia.

The cerebellum (Fig. 34-1), nestled beneath the posterior lobe of the cerebrum, chief assistant to the higher motor centers in the cerebral cortex, is responsible for coordinating, balancing, timing and synergizing with precision all muscular movements that originate in those centers. Through the agency of the cerebellum, the contractions of opposing muscle groups are adjusted in relation to each other to maximal mechanical advantage; muscular contractions can be sustained evenly at the desired tension and without significant fluctuation, and reciprocal movements can be reproduced at high and constant speed, in stereotyped fashion and with relatively little effort.

The basal ganglia are masses of gray matter in the midbrain beneath the cerebral hemispheres. These border or project into the lateral ventricles and lie in close apposition to the internal capsule. It is their function to control habitual or automatic acts and to maintain a "postural background" against which voluntary movements are performed. These ganglia, aided by their connections with the organs of special sense, keep the contractile tone of every muscle in the trunk and the extremities in a constant state of adjustment, so that an individual is able to keep his balance regardless of the posture of his body, in darkness as well as in light and irrespective of the status underfoot. Moreover, thanks to this control station, the individual is equipped to react swiftly, appropriately and automatically to any smell, sight or sound that demands an immediate response.

Dyskinesias. Loss of cerebellar function, which may occur as a result of intracranial injury, hemorrhage, abscess or tumor, results in muscular flabbiness, weakness and fatigue. The patient exhibits a coarse involuntary tremor that increases in intensity in association with voluntary movements. He is unable to control his movements accurately or to coordinate his muscles efficiently or smoothly, every act being performed in disjointed fashion, according to stages, or "by the numbers." He is incapable of performing alternating movements with speed or uniformity, a characteristic of cerebellar disease called "adiadochokinesis." When he walks, he staggers, lurching from side to side as though intoxicated, feet wide apart but steps short and not stamping, i.e., with the vertiginous, reeling gait of cerebellar ataxia.

Destruction or dysfunction of the basal ganglia does not lead to paralysis but to muscular rigidity, with consequent disturbances of posture and movement. Such patients are afflicted by a tendency to display involuntary movements. These may take the form of coarse tremors, characterized by approximately 6 oscillations per second; athetosis, namely, movements of a slow, squirming, writhing, twisting type; or chorea, marked by spasmodic, purposeless and grotesque motions of the trunk and the extremities and facial grimacing. Clinical syndromes based on lesions involving the basal ganglia include Parkinsonism (p. 806), Sydenham's chorea, Huntington's chorea (p. 808), Wilson's disease, or "hepatolenticular degeneration," and spasmodic torticollis.

Sensory Pathways and Disturbances

The transmission of sensory impulses from their points of origin to their cerebral destinations involves 3 neuron relays; moreover, there are 3 major pathways by which they may be routed, depending on the type of sensation that is registered. Specific knowledge regarding these paths is of great importance from the standpoint of neurologic diagnoses, being indispensable for the accurate localization of brain and cord lesions in many patients.

The axon of the nerve in which the sensory impulse originates enters the spinal cord by way of the posterior root. Axons conveying sensations of heat, cold and pain immediately enter the posterior gray column of the cord, where they make connections with the cells of secondary neurons. Pain and temperature fibers cross immediately to the opposite side of the cord and course upward to the thalamus. Fibers carrying sensations of touch, light pressure and localization do not connect immediately with the second neuron but ascend the cord for a variable distance before entering the gray matter and completing this connection. The axon of the secondary neuron crosses the cord and proceeds upward to the thalamus.

The third category of sensation, produced by stimuli arising from muscles, joints and bones, includes position sense and vibratory sense. These stimuli are conveyed, uncrossed, all the way to the brain stem by the axon of the primary neuron. In the medulla, synaptic connections are made with cells of the secondary neurons, whose axons then cross to the opposite side and proceed to the thalamus.

Sensory Losses. Severance of a sensory nerve results in total loss of sensation in its area of distribution. Transection of the spinal cord yields complete anesthesia below the level of injury. Selective destruction or degeneration of the posterior columns of the spinal cord, a characteristic of combined system disease, is responsible for a loss of position sense in segments distal to the lesion, unaccompanied by loss of touch, pain or temperature perception. Such individuals, unless they look, cannot tell where their feet are, or in what direction they are pointing. Moreover, they cannot perceive vibrations in the affected area. A lesion such as a cyst in the center of the cord causes dissociation of sensation, that is, loss of pain at the level of the lesion. This is explainable on the basis of the fact that the fibers carrying pain and temperature cross the cord immediately upon entering; thus, any lesion that divides the cord longitudinally divides these fibers likewise. Other sensory fibers

TABLE 34-1. Comparison of parasympathetic and sympathetic effects on specific organs and tissues*

Organ or Tissue	Parasympathetic Effects	Sympathetic Effects
Vessels:		
Cutaneous	—	Constriction
Muscular	—	Variable
Coronary	Constriction	Dilatation
Salivary gland	Dilatation	Constriction
Buccal mucosa	—	Dilatation
Pulmonary	Variable	Variable
Cerebral	Dilatation	Constriction
Of abdominal and pelvic viscera	—	Constriction
Of external genitalia	Dilatation	Constriction
Heart:	Inhibition	Acceleration
Eye:		
Iris	Constriction	Dilatation
Ciliary muscle	Contraction	Relaxation
Smooth muscle of orbit and upper lid	—	Contraction
Bronchi	Constriction	Dilatation
Glands:		
Sweat	—	Secretion
Salivary	Secretion	Secretion
Gastric	Secretion	Inhibition? Secretion of mucus
Pancreatic		
Acini	Secretion	—
Islets	Secretion	—
Liver	—	Glycogenolysis
Adrenal medulla	—	Secretion
Smooth muscle:		
Of skin	—	Contraction
Of stomach wall	Contraction (predominantly)	Inhibition (predominantly)
Of small intestine	Increased tone and motility	Inhibition
Of large intestine	Increased tone and motility	Inhibition
Of bladder wall (detrusor muscle)	Contraction	Inhibition
Of trigone and sphincter	Inhibition	Contraction
Of uterus, pregnant	None	Contraction
Of uterus, nonpregnant	None	Inhibition

* Best, C. H., and Taylor, N. B.: Physiological Basis of Medical Practice. ed. 6. Baltimore, Williams and Wilkins.

ascend the cord for variable distances, some even to the medulla itself, before crossing, thereby bypassing the lesion and avoiding destruction.

Dysesthesias. Irritative lesions affecting the posterior spinal nerve roots may cause intermittent severe pains that are referred to their areas of distribution. This phenomenon explains the pains of tabes dorsalis. The sensation of tingling of the fingers and the toes constitutes a prominent symptom of combined system disease, presumably due to degenerative changes in the sensory fibers that extend to the thalamus, i.e., belonging to the spinothalamic tract.

The Thalamus. The thalamus, major receiving and communication center for the afferent sensory nerves, is a large and complicated structure located in the midbrain. It lies in close relation to the third ventricle, forming its lateral wall, and to the lateral ventricle, forming its floor, and is in close proximity to the basal ganglia and adjacent to the internal capsule. To the thalamus may be attributed the vague awareness of sensations described as "feelings" of pleasure, discomfort or pain. Moreover, it is responsible for the routing of all sensory stimuli to their many destinations, including the cerebral cortex, which receives them and translates them automatically into appropriate responses.

Autonomic Systems and Syndromes. The contractions of muscles that are not under voluntary control, including the heart muscle, the secretions of all digestive and sweat glands and the activity of certain endocrine organs as well, are controlled by a major component of the nervous system known as the *autonomic nervous system.* The term "autonomic" refers to the fact that the operations of this system are independent of the desires and the intentions of the individual. It is not subject to his will; i.e., it is in a sense autonomous.

To the extent that it is not subject to regulation by the cerebral cortex, the autonomic nervous system resembles the extrapyramidal systems that are centered in the cerebellum and the basal ganglia. However, in other respects it is unique. First, its regulatory effects are exerted not on individual cells but on large expanses of tissue and on entire organs. Second, the responses that it elicits do not appear instantaneously, but only after a lag period, and they are sustained far longer than other neurogenic responses, a type of response that is calculated to ensure maximal functional efficiency on the part of receptor organs, such as the blood vessels and the hollow viscera.

The quality of these responses is explained by the fact that the autonomic nervous system transmits its impulses only partly by way of nerve pathways, the remainder of the route being serviced by chemical mediators, resembling in this respect the endocrine system. Electrical impulses, conducted through nerve fibers, stimulate the formation of specific chemical agents at strategic locations within the muscle mass, the diffusion of these chemicals being responsible for the contraction.

The autonomic nervous system comprises two divisions that are anatomically and functionally distinct, referred to as the sympathetic and the parasympathetic nervous systems. The majority of the tissues and the organs under autonomic control are innervated by both systems. Sympathetic stimuli are mediated by norepinephrine; parasympathetic impulses, by acetylcholine. These chemicals produce opposing and mutually antagonistic effects, as indicated in Table 34-1.

Sympathetic Nervous System. Sympathetic neurons are located in the thoracic and the lumbar segments of the spinal cord; their axons, called *preganglionic fibers*, emerge by way of all anterior nerve roots from the eighth cervical or first thoracic segment to the second or third lumbar segment, inclusive. A short distance from the cord these fibers diverge to join a chain composed of 22 linked ganglia that extends the entire length of the spinal column, flanking the vertebral bodies on both sides. Some form multiple synapses with nerve cells within the chain. Others traverse the chain without making connections or losing continuity to join large "prevertebral" ganglia in the thorax, the abdomen or the pelvis, or one of the "terminal" ganglia in the vicinity of an organ, such as the bladder or the rectum. Postganglionic nerve fibers originating in the sympathetic chain rejoin the spinal nerves that supply the extremities and are distributed to blood vessels, sweat glands and smooth muscle tissue in the skin. Postganglionic fibers from the prevertebral plexuses, i.e., the cardiac, the pulmonary splanchnic and the pelvic plexuses, supply structures in the head and the neck, the thorax, the abdomen and the pelvis, respectively, having been joined in these plexuses by fibers from the parasympathetic division.

The adrenals, the kidneys, the liver, the spleen, the stomach and the duodenum are under the control of the giant celiac plexus, familiarly known as the "solar plexus." This receives its sympathetic nerve components by way of the 3 splanchnic nerves, composed of preganglionic fibers from 9 segments of the spinal cord (i.e., T-4 to L-1), and is joined by the vagus nerve, representing the parasympathetic division. From the celiac plexus, fibers of both divisions travel along the course of blood vessels to their target organs.

Parasympathetic System. The preganglionic nerve cells of the sympathetic division, as described above, are consolidated in consecutive segments of the cord, from C-7 to L-1 or L-2. Those of the parasympathetic system, on the other hand, are located in two sections, one in the brain stem and the other from spinal segments below L-2. On this account the parasympathetic system is referred to as the "craniosacral" division, as distinct from the "thoracolumbar" division of the autonomic nervous system.

The cranial parasympathetics arise from the midbrain and the medulla oblongata. Fibers from cells in the midbrain travel with the third oculomotor nerve to the ciliary ganglia, whence postganglionic fibers of this division are joined by those of the sympathetic system. Forming the ciliary nerve, these channel to the ciliary muscles of the eye to control the caliber of the pupil. Parasympathetic fibers from the medulla travel with the seventh (facial), ninth (glossopharyngeal) and tenth (vagus) cranial nerves. Those from the facial nerve end in the splenopalatine ganglion, whence emanate the fibers that innervate the lacrimal glands, the ciliary muscle and the sphincter of the pupil. Those from the glossopharyngeal nerve innervate the parotid gland. The vagus nerve carries preganglionic parasympathetic fibers without interruption to the organs that it innervates, joining ganglion cells within the myocardium and within the walls of the esophagus, the stomach and the intestine.

Preganglionic parasympathetic fibers from the anterior roots of the sacral nerves coalesce to become the pelvic nerves, consolidate and regroup in the pelvic plexus, and terminate around ganglion cells in the musculature of the pelvic organs. These innervate the colon, the rectum and the bladder, inhibiting the muscular tone of the anal and the bladder sphincters and dilating the blood vessels of the bladder, the rectum and the genitalia.

The vagus, the splanchnic, pelvic and the other autonomic nerves carry impulses generated in the viscera to the dorsal nucleus of the vagus, where connections are made with efferent parasympathetic neurons, forming a series of reflex arcs. These provide the basis for self-regulation, a cardinal feature of the autonomic nervous system, and one reason for "autonomy."

Autonomic Functions and Dysfunctions. A detailed listing of the effects produced by the 2 divisions of the autonomic nervous system is supplied in Table 34-1. This listing provides impressive evidence of the scope and the importance of autonomic activity in relation to all bodily functions and from the standpoint of survival itself. Both sympathetic and parasympathetic divisions are in a constant state of activity, the activity of each relative to the other being one of controlled opposition, with a delicate balance maintained between the two at all times.

The Hypothalamus. Overall supervision of the autonomic nervous system is considered a function of the hypothalamus. The hypothalamus is a portion of the diencephalon (interbrain) located immediately beneath and lateral to the lower portion of the wall of the third ventricle. It includes among its components the optic chiasm, the tuber cinereum, the pituitary stalk, which originates from the latter, and the pituitary gland itself. Large cell groups in adjacent portions of the hypothalamus have been assigned the role of the probable centers of autonomic regulation. These centers are richly endowed with connections linking the autonomic systems with the thalamus, the cortex, the olfactory apparatus and the pituitary gland. Here reside the mechanisms for the control of visceral and somatic reactions that were designed originally for defense or attack, but in man these are associated with his emotional states, i.e., his fears, anger, anxiety, etc.; for the control of metabolic processes, including fat, carbohydrate and water metabolism; for the regulation of body temperature, arterial pressure and all muscular and glandular activities of the gastrointestinal tract; the genital functions; and the sleep rhythm. The close proximity, histologic similarity and multiple connections between the pituitary gland, master gland of the endocrines, and this portion of the brain suggest that here may be located the supreme headquarters of the endocrine and autonomic nervous systems, commanding all vital processes.

Sympathetic Syndromes. Certain syndromes are distinctive of diseases of the sympathetic nerve trunks. Among these are dilatation of the pupil of the eye on the same side as a penetrating wound of the neck (evidence of disturbance of the cervical sympathetic cord); temporary paralysis of the bowel (indicated by the absence of peristaltic waves and the distention of the intestine by gas) following fracture of any one of the lower dorsal or upper lumbar vertebrae, with hemorrhage into the base of the mesentery; and the marked variations in pulse rate and rhythm that often follow compression fractures of the upper 6 thoracic vertebrae. Certain diseases, few in number, including Raynaud's disease, acroparesthesia, erythromelalgia, scleroderma and giant colon, also are considered to be autonomic nervous disturbances.

ASSISTING WITH THE NEUROLOGIC EXAMINATION

Cranial Nerve Tests

In addition to the usual complete physical examination, every patient suspected of having a neurologic disorder and every neurosurgical patient is subjected to a systematic and detailed neurologic examination. This involves the testing of each cranial nerve in the manner specified in Table 34-2. Maximal cooperation of the patient is essential for the proper conduct of this diagnostic routine and can be elicited only if he understands what he is expected to do. All equipment for these tests should be available in one place.

Examination of the peripheral motor and the sensory systems also is done. Motor tests include observation of posture and gait, reflex tests, coordination observations, etc. Sensory tests determine skin sensa-

TABLE 34-2. Neurologic examination for testing cranial nerves

Nerve	Equipment	Procedure
1. Olfactory	Four small bottles of volatile oils, such as (1) turpentine, (2) oil of cloves, (3) oil of wintergreen, (4) vanilla	Instruct the patient to sniff and to identify the odors. Each nostril is tested separately.
2. Optic	Ophthalmoscope	In darkened room the patient is examined with this instrument. More detailed examination with special equipment is used for accurate determination of visual fields.
3. Oculomotor 4. Trochlear 6. Abducens	Flashlight	Because of close association these nerves are examined collectively. They innervate pupil and upper eyelid and are responsible for extraocular muscle movements.
5. Trigeminal	Test tube of hot water Test tube of ice water Cotton wisp from cotton applicator stick Pin	*Sensory* branch—Vertex to chin tested for sensations of pain, touch and temperature. This includes reflex reaction of cornea to wisp of cotton. *Motor* branch—Ability to bite is tested.
7. Facial	Four small bottles with solutions which are salty, sweet, sour, and bitter (Four clean medicine droppers)	Observe symmetry of face and ability to contract facial muscles. Instruct patient to taste and to identify substance used. He should rinse his mouth well between each drop of solution. This is a test for the anterior ⅔ of tongue.
8. Acoustic	Tuning fork	Tests for hearing, air and bone conduction.
9. Glossopharyngeal	Cotton applicator stick	Test for taste posterior ⅓ of tongue and check gag reflex.
10. Vagus	Tongue depressor	Checking voice sounds, observing symmetry of soft palate will give suggestion of function of vagus.
11. Spinal Accessory		Since this innervates the sternocleidomastoid and the trapezius muscles, the patient will be instructed to turn and to move his head and to elevate shoulders with and without resistance.
12. Hypoglossal		Observe tongue movements.

tion and deeper tissue sensation, as well as the ability to recognize objects by the sense of touch.

The nurse should know the results of the findings of the neurologic and the physical examination, be-cause only then is she able to observe intelligently the symptoms and aberrant reactions of her patient. These deviations must be charted accurately if they are to be meaningful to the physician or the neuro-surgeon.

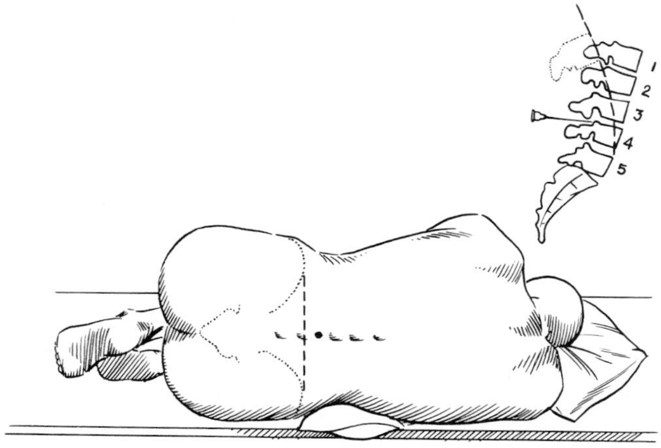

Lumbar and Cisternal Punctures

Frequently it is necessary to insert a needle into the spinal subarachnoid space to determine the pressure of the fluid and to obtain fluid for examination. In the majority of patients this is done by inserting the needle into the subarachnoid space between the third and the fourth lumbar spinous processes (*lumbar or spinal puncture*) (Fig. 34-3). For technical or other reasons it may be necessary to introduce the needle between the rim of the foramen magnum and the first cervical lamina into the cisterna magna (*cisternal puncture*) (Fig. 34-3). For both procedures the patient must be relaxed, since straining produces a false increase in the pressure reading. Normal pressures in the recumbent position range between 80 and 180 mm. of water (6 to 13 mm. Hg.). Pressures over 200 mm. of water are considered abnormal. Pressures with the patient in the sitting position are much higher and not reliable.

FIG. 34-6. Lateral position for lumbar puncture. The back is flexed and the knees drawn toward the chin as far as possible to obtain maximal widening between the interspinous spaces.

Before a lumbar puncture, the bladder and the bowels should be emptied. The patient is placed on his side at the edge of the bed, with his back toward the operator. The thighs and the head are flexed acutely and the body is curved forward as much as possible to increase the space between the spinous processes of the vertebrae. A small pillow is placed under the head, so that the patient's spine is horizontal (Fig. 34-6). It may be necessary for the nurse to hold the patient in this position, especially in the case of children and nervous adults. The patient is encouraged to breathe normally and to relax during the procedure.

For a cisternal puncture the neck must be shaved up to the external occipital protuberance in the midline. The patient is placed on his side, with his head on a sandbag to keep the head in a straight line with the thoracic spine; at the same time he flexes his head forward on his chest. It is very important that the patient refrain from moving during the procedure.

Queckenstedt Test. This test determines the presence of any obstruction between the cranial cavity and the lumbar puncture needle. Pressure is made firmly upon the jugular veins on each side of the neck simultaneously for 10 seconds. The increase in intracranial pressure caused by the compression is noted, and if the pressure does not return to its original position in 10 seconds, the pressure is recorded at 10-second intervals until it has returned to its original level. If there is any obstruction in the spinal subarachnoid space, the rise and the fall of pressure is slow and gradual or does not occur at all. A blood pressure cuff may be used to apply compression about the neck at intervals of 20, 30, 40 and 50 mm. of pressure, the cerebrospinal fluid pressure being measured simultaneously.

Usually, specimens are sent to the laboratory for cell count, culture and chemical analysis. These should be sent immediately, since changes take place that alter the result if the specimens are allowed to stand.

Following the lumbar puncture, the patient should lie quietly for several hours.

Postpuncture Headache. Within a period of a few hours or days following a lumbar puncture there frequently develops a throbbing occipital headache that is particularly severe when the patient sits or stands upright, and that tends to disappear when he lies horizontal. The cause of this unpleasant complication is the leakage of spinal fluid at the puncture site, the fluid continuing to escape by way of the needle tract from the spinal canal into the tissues, whence it is absorbed promptly by the lymphatics, never having accumulated in sufficient volume to be detected. Depletion of cerebrospinal fluid as a result of this leak causes the supply remaining in the cranium to be insufficient for proper mechanical stabilization of the brain. The latter becomes displaced caudally, exerting traction on the dural attachments to the venous sinuses and causing headache. Traction on these pain-sensitive structures is maximal, and the pain is most severe when the patient is in a vertical position; both traction and pain are lessened by recumbency, which also reduces the leak. The lumbar puncture headache is avoidable to a large extent by using the smallest needle practical and by insistence that patients remain recumbent for 12 to 24 hours following lumbar puncture.

Pneumoencephalography and Ventriculography

The cerebrospinal fluid spaces in and around the brain may be seen in x-ray examination when the fluid is replaced with a gas. Withdrawal of fluid and injection of a gas directly into the ventricles through openings in the back of the skull is called *ventriculography.* A similar injection made by the spinal subarachnoid route is called *pneumoencephalography.* The latter procedure is done as a general rule in patients without evidence of increased intracranial pressure.

Preparation of Patient. The night before encephalography or ventriculography the patient should have a good rest. On the morning of operation the breakfast is withheld to avoid vomiting. Appropriate sedatives and analgesics should be administered prior to departure for the operating room or x-ray department. The back of the head should be shaved before ventriculography, or all of the head if craniotomy is to follow. All hairpins should be removed, and long hair should not be braided before pneumoencephalography, since braids cast shadows on the x-ray films. As with other surgical procedures, dentures are removed.

Pneumoencephalography. This is done under local or general anesthesia. Because of the severe reaction of headache, retching, shock and sometimes unconsciousness when done under local anesthesia, general anesthesia is preferred. A lumbar puncture is performed with the patient in the sitting position— usually in a special chair with casters to allow easy movement of the patient while taking x-ray pictures. Ten ml. of fluid is removed, and 10 ml. of air or gas is injected until all of the fluid has been removed. The vital signs of pulse, respiratory rate and blood pressure are evaluated throughout the procedure. If the procedure is done under local anesthesia, it is important to have adequate personnel to treat the complications. At no time should the patient be left alone, even when the roentgenograms are being taken.

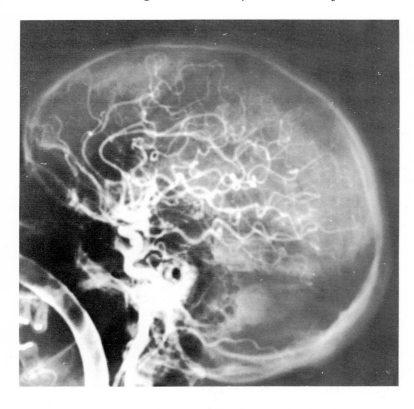

Fig. 34-7. Normal arteriogram of the brain.

Ventriculography. This is usually done under local anesthesia with the patient sitting in a special chair. The posterior half of the head is prepared and draped. Through scalp incisions trephines (burr holes) are made, and the ventricles are punctured by a special needle. The fluid is replaced with air, the cannulae are withdrawn, and the scalp wounds are closed. If a lesion is present, there is a change in size, shape or position of the ventricular, subarachnoid or cisternal spaces. During the procedure of ventriculography the patient develops a mild headache, may become nauseated, may retch and very rarely may have a convulsive seizure. The reaction to this procedure is usually milder than that attending pneumoencephalography.

Nursing Care. Following the above procedures the nurse must observe the patient for signs of increased intracranial pressure (see p. 777) or shock reaction. Special care must be taken to see that the patient does not aspirate any vomitus. Vital signs are taken frequently until they are stabilized. Parenteral fluids may be necessary for the first 24 hours.

Since headache is the major complaint, an icecap to the head and adequate analgesics must be given for the duration of the headache, which usually lasts for 2 to 4 days, depending on the speed with which the intracranial air is absorbed and replaced once more with fluid. Occasionally, especially following

pneumoencephalography, headache persists much longer.

Fractional Pneumoencephalography. In this test small amounts of fluid are withdrawn, and small amounts of air are injected. During the procedure the patient is placed in different positions so that specific areas of the ventricles and the subarachnoid system are filled and visualized. With smaller amounts of air injected into the ventricles, more subtle lesions can be demonstrated, and the attention is directed to the specific area rather than the whole ventricular system. The patient does not have to be under general anesthesia and is able to cooperate in assuming the various positions. There is less incidence of headache following this diagnostic test. Fractional pneumoencephalography is used to diagnose space-occupying lesions and atrophy or blockage of the ventricular system.

Electroencephalography

This procedure is the recording of the electrical activity passing through the surface of the brain by applying electrodes to the unshaved scalp. Tumors, abscesses, brain scars, blood clots and infection may cause electric changes that are different from the normal pattern or rhythm. Thus, this test sometimes helps not only in diagnosis but also in localization.

FIG. 34-8. Compare the normal lumbar myelogram (*left*) with the abnormal myelogram (*right*).

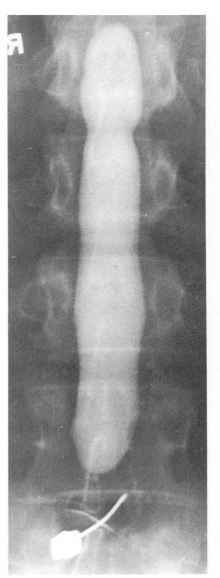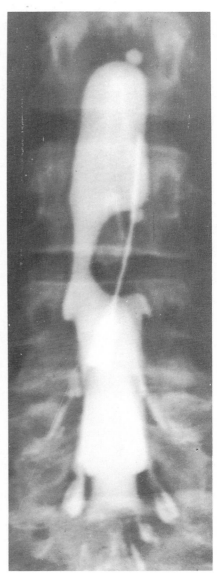

Arteriography

Following the injection of a radiopaque substance into the common carotid artery or into the vertebral artery, it is possible to visualize by means of x-rays the cerebral arterial system. Through abnormal positions and configurations of the blood vessels it is possible to detect aneurysms, occlusions of major vessels, abscesses, tumors and other lesions. The dye is injected through a No. 18 spinal needle that has been inserted into the artery. The procedure can be done under local or general anesthesia and either by the "open" or the "closed" method. In the open method the artery is exposed, whereas in the closed method the artery is palpated, and the needle is inserted through the skin into the artery. As the dye is injected into the artery, roentgenograms are taken (Fig. 34-7).

Following the procedure the site of injection must be observed for hematoma formation. The region usually is somewhat swollen, painful and tender. An icebag helps to relieve swelling and discomfort. In a small percentage of patients, either during the actual injection or following the procedure, the irritant dye in the blood vessels may produce a reaction. Symptoms include alterations in the state of consciousness, weakness on one side and speech disturbances. It is necessary for the nurse to make repeated observations of the patient for these signs and to report them immediately.

Radioisotope Scanning

Some intracranial lesions may be detected by intravenous injection of certain radioactive compounds such as RISA or mercurial preparations and the application of a scintillation scanner. This technique is based on the preferential uptake of radioactive material at the site of pathology. The preferential uptake may be due to a breakdown in the blood brain barrier or increased vascularity. Lesions commonly detectable by this method are cerebral neoplasm, hematoma, abscess and arteriovenous malformation.

Echoencephalography

The ultrasound echo has been used to measure midline structures in the cranial vault. The source of the midline echo has not been established with certainty. The septum pellucidum and/or wall of the third ventricle have been considered as the source of the echo by some investigators, while the pineal body has been favored by the others.

Echoencephalography is a rapid and useful technique for detecting a shift of the cerebral midline structures precipitated by a subdural hematoma, intracerebral hemorrhage, massive cerebral infarction and cerebral neoplasms. Although echoencephalography may show shifts from the midline, it does not have the diagnostic accuracy of the other neurosurgical studies such as carotid angiography or ventriculography.

Myelography and Discography

In a *myelogram* a radiopaque oil is injected into the spinal subarachnoid space through a lumbar puncture needle. The subarachnoid space surrounding the spinal cord is visualized by x-ray pictures, and abnormalities of the oil column may indicate spinal cord tumors, herniated intervertebral disks or other lesions (Fig. 34-8). After the x-ray examination is completed, the oil is then withdrawn because the continued presence of oil may cause inflammation of the arachnoid membrane. To withdraw the oil, the needle has to be manipulated. By this maneuver the needle frequently touches the nerve roots and causes pain. Sedation prior to the procedure and informing the patient just before the pain is initiated helps the patient to accept a myelogram better. Following the procedure the patient should be treated like a patient who has had a lumbar puncture.

Discography is the injection of a radiopaque substance directly into the intervertebral disk. The pathology of the disk then may be seen by taking AP and lateral views of the spine. This study is very useful in patients suspected of having a herniated nucleus ˙pulposus that is undiagnosed by myelography. Discography is confined primarily to the lumbar disks of L-3, -4 and -5.

SPECIAL PROBLEMS OF NEUROLOGIC AND NEUROSURGICAL PATIENTS

Nursing Priorities

Nursing Observations. The nurse's observations relative to all systems of the body may be of great assistance in establishing the diagnosis of many neurologic disorders. Of utmost importance are changes in muscle strength and disturbances of sensation. The appearance of pain, its type and location, should be noted with care. Oliguria and incontinence should be reported; also any episode of vomiting should be reported, with a full description of it (whether or not accompanied with nausea, its relationship to the preceding meal and the nature of the vomitus). Mental and nervous symptoms should be observed and studied analytically, because their complete description is likely to be of value in the diagnosis and the therapeutic management of the patient. The general attitude of the patient may reveal depression or euphoria; the mood swings may run the gamut of irritability, apprehension, anger and elation. Disturbances of vision, hearing, speech, smell, taste, touch, pressure or pain may be elicited in the course of routine care, possibly indicating a new development in the patient's neurologic status. In other words, the nurse should practice observation as she cares for the neurologic patient, because the diagnostic value of her findings, completely and accurately described, can be very significant.

Special Problems

Skin Care. Special nursing problems arise from paralyses, sensory disturbances, psychosis and coma. If hyperesthesia is present, superficial pain may be aroused through slight stimulation of the terminals of the affected nerve branches by simple drafts or gentle friction, causing marked discomforts.

Disturbances in the skin innervation may cause anesthesia, thereby favoring the development of decubitus ulcers. Since pressure is one of the major causes of decubiti, the patient's position should be changed frequently. Small foam rubber pads under pressure areas are beneficial. The skin must be kept scrupulously clean and dry. Provision should be made on the nursing care plan for frequent nursing inspection of areas susceptible to decubiti. Special skin care (bathing and massage in a circular motion) should be done at specified intervals. Unusual care is indicated in the use of hot-water bottles, the temperature of which should not exceed 46°C. (115°F.) to prevent the development of skin burns. (See pp. 168-170.)

Nutritional Needs. Nutritional problems arise if there is any disturbance connected with the swallowing reflex. They may be overcome by homogenizing the patient's meals in a food blender and feeding him through a tube. Vitamin preparations usually are added to the feeding. The blenderized meal is tolerated well, since the patient's gastrointestinal tract is accustomed to this type of diet, and there is less incidence of diarrhea. Plastic drinking tubes should be used by patients who are subject to convulsions, and dentures, of course are removed from the mouths of such patients, as well as from those in coma.

Oral Hygiene. The condition of the patient's mouth should be checked often, because the buccal structures are prone to become exceedingly dry after a short period of mouth breathing if this process is sustained without interruption, as is likely to be the case. The lips, the tongue and the gums should be lubricated systematically, and the hydration of the patient should be maintained at an adequate level.

Eye Care. Patients with facial palsy on any basis, who are incapable of shutting their eyes, need special eye care in the form of irrigations with sterile saline and lubrication of the outer lids with trace amounts of mineral oil to prevent drying and ulceration of the cornea. These procedures should be carried out several times each day, and the eyes should be inspected regularly for signs of inflammation. Patients who are conscious and cooperative can administer their own eye care with proper instruction and supervision.

The Incontinent Patient. Many patients with diseases of the central nervous system initially or eventually, temporarily or permanently, exhibit urinary and fecal incontinence. The hygienic care of patients with incontinence is an important nursing priority, because it is essential that the patient be kept clean and dry.

Urinary incontinence may be an indication for tidal drainage. This method permits continuous rhythmic lavage of the bladder, thereby simulating and stimulating the reflex control of normal bladder activity. The number of catheterizations required lessens gradually. The bladder is irrigated continuously with any antibacterial solution (1% Neosporin) and residual urine is eliminated by this technique (see p. 828). Urinary tract infections are thus prevented to a large extent.

Placing the patient on a regular bowel program will avoid the occurrence of spontaneous defecation. A regular routine is developed in which prune juice is given nightly. A glycerine suppository is inserted above the patient's internal sphincter at the same time every morning. The patient is encouraged to wait for an interval before attempting to have a bowel movement. Then he is given the bedpan. If the nurse sees that this routine is carried out regularly every day, the patient will form a habit pattern that is the basis for bowel training.

Prevention of Deformities. Any paralyzed extremity deserves careful attention on the part of the nurse. Care must be taken lest a patient lie on it, or its circulation in any way becomes impeded. Footboards or cradles prevent pressure from weighty linen.

To prevent contractures, the nurse must see that the patient is positioned correctly, and that the joints are moved, either actively or passively, through their range of motion several times daily. When the condition of the patient permits, active exercises (bathing, walking, therapeutic exercises) are desirable. Massage may be instituted and perhaps later supplemented by electrical stimulation. Passive exercises and, as soon as possible, active motions are prescribed for the purpose of developing strength.

Psychological Aspects. Various psychic disturbances appear in neurologic patients and complicate their care in hospital and home; and some patients present diagnostic problems with mild symptoms that strongly suggest neuroses. A sincere attempt should be made to accept the complaints in good faith, and the patient never should be made to feel that he is not believed. The consulting psychiatrist will guide the medical therapy and give suggestions regarding the proper approach for meeting the personality requirements of the individual. The family attitude may be unsympathetic, and a feeling of reserve and tension and a general lack of understanding may develop. The physician must give the family a point of view that is helpful, and the medical social worker must help to plan for future care.

Occasionally patients are admitted to the nursing units with a manic psychosis. They obviously require treatment in the psychiatric division of the hospital where the environment is better suited for their care, and they should be transferred there as soon as feasible. Meanwhile, good nursing practice requires that adequate protection and care be given.

THE PATIENT WITH A HEADACHE

Possibly the commonest of all human afflictions and a symptom that virtually no man is spared wholly is headache or *cephalgia* ("condition of head pain"), as it is known in technical parlance. Headache may arise from a variety of sources through different mechanisms and its basic cause may reside inside or outside the skull.

Tension Headache

Emotional or physical stress may cause spasm of the neck and scalp muscles and produce tension headache. The headache may be characterized by a steady, pressing ache, which usually begins in the forehead, the temple or the nape of the neck. It then spreads to one side of the head or the entire head. Its severity may be slight or great, and its duration may be a matter of minutes, hours or days.

Various pharmacologic agents are useful in the treatment of severe tension headache, including analgesics, such as aspirin, phenacetin and codeine, muscle relaxants, and tranquillizing agents.

Eyestrain Headache

Refractory errors or prolonged use of the eyes under unfavorable lighting conditions may stimulate sustained contractions of the extraocular muscles, with spasm spreading to the frontal, the temporal and even the occipital muscles, producing a special variant of the tension headache described above. It is a steady, not a throbbing, pain that predominantly resides in the orbit or the temple and may include the occiput. Relief depends on the acquisition of glasses that compensate for the refractory error and on the improvement of illumination or body posture while the patient is reading. Analgesic medications, such as aspirin, are useful as a temporary expedient.

Sinus Headache

Inflammation of the mucosal lining of the sinuses and reduction of the atmospheric pressure in their cavities due to blockage of the small draining channels are the cause of sinus headaches. Frontal sinusitis produces pain in the periorbital area and the involvement of the sphenoid sinus in the vertex, the occiput or elsewhere. The pain of sinusitis tends to be most severe as the patient awakens in the morning, and to improve after he has arisen, is in a vertical position, and the sinus blockade has been relieved.

Sinus headache is alleviated by salicylates and similar analgesics, and complete relief may be anticipated with subsidence of the inflammatory process.

Temporal Arteritis

Inflammation of the temporal artery is characterized by a unilateral or bilateral temporal and frontal headache lasting for weeks or months. Sometimes a thickened artery is visible and palpable, and loss of vision may occur due to thrombosis of the central retinal artery.

Treatment consists of early administration of a corticosteroid drug to prevent the possibility of loss of vision, and analgesic agents are given for comfort. The temporal artery is sometimes excised to relieve the pain.

Histamine Headache

This kind of headache was formerly thought to be due to a sensitivity to histamine, but it is now considered to be a variant of migraine. The pain is localized to one side of the forehead and is accompanied by tearing of the eye and a feeling of congestion of the nose on the side of the pain. The duration of the pain is quite short, lasting only a few minutes or ½ hour at the most, but it may recur several or many times daily.

Desensitization with histamine has been recommended for relief of pain. However the evaluation of therapy is difficult because of the short duration of the attacks and the tendency for spontaneous occurrence of long remissions.

Headache in Meningitis

Inflammation and stretching of the meninges and blood vessels are the cause of headache in meningitis. The headache is usually generalized and is accompanied by stiff neck. A slight movement of the head may markedly aggravate the headache. A septic picture plus headache and stiff neck are highly suggestive of meningitis.

Headache in Subarachnoid Hemorrhage

This headache may be localized in the back of the eye, in the occipital region or on one side of the head at its onset, but in later stages it is usually generalized. It is uncertain whether the headache is caused by the stretching of the perivascular tissue or irritation of the meninges. Analgesics may be of value in relieving the pain.

Headache in Brain Tumor

The headache that occurs in patients with a brain tumor cannot be differentiated either by its nature or its location from headaches due to any other causes. It is commonly generalized, but it may be localized or more intense in the frontal or occipital region, regardless of the location of the tumor. The headache is usually intermittent, lasting for several minutes or hours. It may be increased by change of posture, coughing or straining. The cause of the headache is not known; it is not directly related to the degree of intracranial pressure. Irritation of the dura, perivascular tissue or nerves probably plays a role in the production of pain.

Hypertensive Headache

This type may take any form, but typically is a dull, pounding occipital headache, which is present upon awakening in the morning and tends to wear off during the day. The precise mechanism of the headache is not certain, but it is thought to emanate from overly-stretched extra- and intracranial arteries. The headache is relieved by antihypertensive therapy.

Febrile Headache

The pain may be throbbing or steady, and may be frontal, occipital or generalized. It is thought to be

F IG. 34-9. Chart showing changes in mental state, pupils, blood pressure, pulse rate, respiration rate and temperature before and after the onset of fatal increase of intracranial pressure. (Penfield: Canadian Army Manual of Military Neurosurgery, Ottawa, Government Distribution Office)

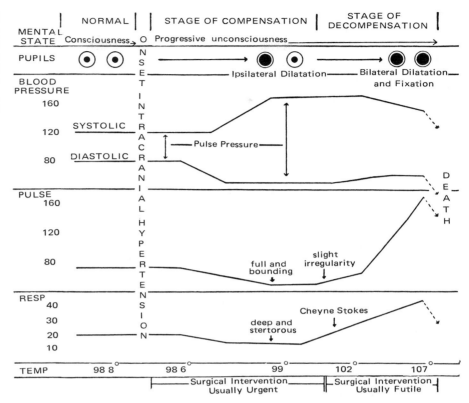

caused by stretched extra- and intracranial arteries. Relief is usually achieved with aspirin and similar analgesic medication.

Migraine

Migraine is a symptom complex characterized by unilateral or generalized periodic attacks of severe or mild headaches, with or without associated visual, gastrointestinal or other symptoms, in an individual who is in good health in the interval between attacks. The cause of migraine has not been clearly demonstrated. At the present the most accepted theory is that the headache results from dilatation of the dural and scalp arteries. The commonly used analgesics such as aspirin and codeine may be effective in relieving the symptoms. However, in severe attacks, these drugs are usually of no avail and ergot preparations are the only recourse.

THE PATIENT WITH INCREASING INTRACRANIAL PRESSURE

The usual causes of increased intracranial pressure are head injury, cerebral edema, abscess, infection, hemorrhage or brain tumor. In the majority of patients having cranial surgery, varying degrees of cerebral edema occur, or, rarely, bleeding causing increased intracranial pressure. Therefore, it is important to know the following signs:

1. Changes in the Levels of Responsiveness. The level of responsiveness is the most important measure of the patient's condition. The earliest sign of increasing intracranial pressure is *lethargy*. Watch for slowing of speech and delay in response to verbal suggestions. Any sudden changes in condition, such as shifting from quietness to restlessness (without apparent cause), from orientation to confusion, or increasing drowsiness, have neurologic significance. These signs may result from compression of the brain due to either swelling or hemorrhage or a combination of both. As pressure increases, the patient may react only to loud auditory or painful stimuli. At this stage, serious impairment of brain circulation is probably taking place and immediate surgical intervention may be required. If the stupor deepens, the patient responds to painful stimuli by moaning but may not attempt to withdraw. As the condition worsens, the extremities are flaccid and reflexes are absent. The jaw sags and the tongue becomes flaccid, producing inadequate respiratory exchange. When the coma is profound, there is no response and a fatal outcome is usually inevitable.

Nursing Assessment for Determining the Patient's Level of Responsiveness. The nursing assessment for determining the patient's level of responsiveness can be organized on these levels: (1) response to commands, (2) assessment of spinal motor reflexes, and (3) observation of spontaneous activities. The first two levels involve purposeful nursing action or interference to which the patient reacts. In order that everyone caring for him knows the baseline condition and the present status of the patient, a neurologic observation record is kept (Fig. 34-29).

1. Response to commands:

   A. Answers questions readily and correctly
   B. Can perform a complex maneuver
   C. Responds to simple command
   D. Delayed or unequal response
   E. Reacts only to loud voice
   F. Does not respond

2. Assessment of spinal motor reflexes (pinch Achilles tendon, arm or other body site):

   A. Prompt purposeful withdrawal
   B. Sluggish or nonpurposeful movement of extremities
   C. Facial grimace
   D. Voiding involuntarily
   E. No response

3. Observation of patient's spontaneous activity:

   A. Verbal or other communication
   B. Changes in posture (frequency)
   C. Breathing pattern
   D. Retching, vomiting
   E. Restlessness, twitching, tremors, convulsions.

2. Changes in Vital Signs. As intracranial pressure increases, the pulse rate and respiratory rate are slowed and the blood pressure and temperature rise. The body signs compensate in this way as long as the major circulation of the brain is preserved. If, as a result of brain compression, the major circulation begins to fail, the pulse and respirations become rapid and the temperature usually rises but does not follow a consistent pattern. The pulse pressure (the difference between the systolic and diastolic pressure) widens; this is considered a serious development. Immediately preceding this reversal of clinical responses, there is usually a period of rapid fluctuations in pulse, varying from a slow rate to a rapid one. Surgical intervention is indicated or death will ensue (Fig. 34-9). The vital signs may not always be altered, even in the event of increased intracranial pressure. However, these signs are assessed in relation to changes in the level of the patient's responsiveness to give a clearer picture of the patient's condition.

3. Headache. The headache is constant, increasing in intensity and aggravated by movement or straining.

4. Vomiting. Vomiting is recurrent and may be projectile, but not necessarily.

5. Pupillary Changes. The pupils should be periodically inspected with a flashlight. Note the size and configuration of the pupils and test their reaction to light. Any progressive changes are recorded and reported.

6. Tense Bulging Decompression. In most patients, part or all of the temporal bone is removed during craniotomy for the purpose of relieving postoperative brain edema. This area is located in front of the ear on the side of operation, and its tension is an indication of the degree of intracranial pressure. The nurse should palpate the area periodically and note the degree of tension without contaminating the wound.

Treatment. The treatment of increased intracranial pressure consists of administering steroids and/or intravenous urea and mannitol. With this therapy, urinary output is recorded hourly; vital signs and level of consciousness are evaluated frequently. Fluid intake is maintained up to 2,500 ml., with special consideration given to the proper electrolyte balance.

FEBRILE AND HYPOTHERMIC PATIENTS

Because of severe intracranial infection or damage to the heat-regulating center in the brain, neurologic and neurosurgical patients often develop very high temperatures. Such temperature elevations must be controlled, because the increased metabolic demands by the brain will overburden brain circulation and deterioration will result.

With the persistent use of proper therapy, there is seldom a patient in whom the temperature cannot be lowered in a matter of a few hours. It has been shown that body temperatures well below normal decrease cerebral edema and lower the metabolic rate of the brain. Also, there is a collateral circulation in the brain that may be adequate if the body metabolism can be lowered. Occasionally, it is desirable to lower the body temperature to a level ranging between 30°C. (86°F.) and 32°C. (90°F.).

The induction and maintenance of hypothermia is a major clinical procedure and requires knowledge and skilled nursing surveillance and action. Measures to induce hypothermia in the order of increasing effectiveness are:

1. Aspirin medication and sponging of the trunk and the extremities with alcohol.
2. Icebags applied to groin and axilla.
3. Aspirin, alcohol sponging and an electric fan blowing directly on the patient to increase surface cooling.

4. All clothes, except a loin cloth, are removed from the patient. A bath towel saturated with cold water is placed over the trunk. An electric fan, placed at the foot of the bed is directed toward the saturated towel. When the towel becomes almost dry, it is resaturated with cold water. Rectal temperatures should be taken every 15 minutes during this treatment to prevent lowering the temperature too rapidly.

5. The use of a hypothermia blanket connected to a temperature-regulating apparatus.

6. Another method is to suppress the heat-regulating center in the brain by the use of drugs, whether alone or in combination with the above methods. The usual combination is Thorazine, Demerol and Phenergan, commonly called the "lytic cocktail." It is used practically always to reduce temperatures to a below-normal level.

THE UNCONSCIOUS PATIENT

Unconsciousness is a condition in which there is a depression of cerebral function. It may range from stupor to coma. In stupor the patient shows symptoms of annoyance when stimulated by something unpleasant, such as a pinprick, loud clapping of hands, etc., by drawing back, facial grimacing and making unintelligible sounds. In coma, there is no response.

The quality of nursing care given an unconscious patient may literally mean the difference between his life and death. His protective reflexes are impaired. The nurse assumes responsibility for the patient until he can once again cough, blink, swallow and is oriented to himself and his environment.

The most important consideration in the management of the unconscious patient is to establish and maintain the airway. The accumulation of secretions in the pharynx presents a serious problem that demands intelligent and conscientious treatment. Since he is unable to swallow and lacks pharyngeal reflexes, these secretions must be removed to eliminate the danger of aspiration. The patient is positioned in a lateral or semiprone position to facilitate drainage of respiratory secretions. (Never allow an unconscious patient to remain on his back.) Suction is employed to remove secretions from the posterior pharynx and upper trachea. With the suction turned *off*, a whistle-tip catheter is lubricated with a water-soluble lubricant and maneuvered to the desired level. Then the suction is turned on (negative pressure) while the aspirating catheter is withdrawn with a twisting motion of the thumb and forefinger. This twisting maneuver prevents the suctioning end of the catheter from irritating the tracheal or pharyngeal mucosa, since irritation merely increases secretions and produces mucosal bleeding. The suction catheter should be kept meticulously clean. (If the patient has a tracheostomy,

it should be kept sterile.) The frequency of suctioning is determined by the amount of secretions present.

The mouth of the unconscious patient is an area that also needs conscientious care. The mouth should be swabbed carefully and rinsed thoroughly. The tongue as well as the space underneath must be included. A soothing lubricant within the mouth and on the lips prevents drying and the formation of encrustations.

The nutritional needs of this patient are met by giving the required fluids intravenously. Intravenous solutions and blood transfusions for patients with intracranial conditions must run in slowly. If given too rapidly, they may increase the intracranial pressure. Sixty drops per minute is the average rate of flow. In addition, a nasogastric tube may be passed, and the patient can be given liquid and blenderized feedings. The procedure is much the same as for gastrostomy feedings (see p. 469). One way of testing to see whether the patient is able to swallow without choking is to give him a swab wet with water to suck. *Never give fluids by mouth to the patient who cannot swallow.*

Urinary incontinence may be managed by inserting a 3-way catheter attached to continuous drainage or by instituting tidal drainage (see p. 828). This is important if diuretics are used. Clamping the catheter at intervals helps to prevent contracture of the bladder, as this procedure more closely approximates normal functioning. A full bladder, on the other hand, may be the overlooked cause of incontinence. Colonic irrigations administered every second or third day eliminate fecal incontinence or reduce the frequency of involuntary stools. Frequent loose stools are an indication of fecal impaction.

Special attention is given to these patients because they are insensitive to external stimuli. They must be turned frequently and positioned properly. To effectively prevent decubiti, attention should be given to those areas where pressure is greatest. Sheets must be free of wrinkles, crumbs and moisture. A lotion with lanolin may be used to keep the skin lubricated.

Maintaining good body position is important; equally important is passive exercise of the extremities, so that contractures are prevented. The use of a footboard aids in the prevention of footdrop and eliminates the pressure of bedding on the toes. Trochanter rolls supporting the hip joints keep the legs in good position. The arm should be in abduction, the fingers lightly flexed, and the hand in a position of slight supination.

The temperature of the patient's environment is determined by his condition. If he has a temperature elevation, he should have a sheet or perhaps only a loin cloth covering him. The room may be cooled to

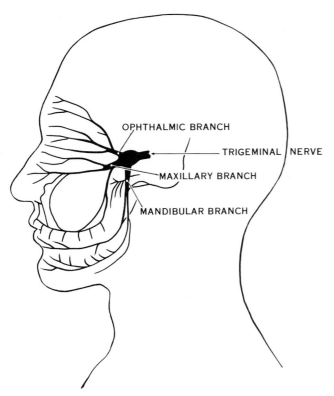

Fig. 34-10. Diagram showing nerves affected by trigeminal neuralgia.

18.3° C.* However, if the patient is older and does not have an elevation of temperature, he needs a warmer atmosphere. Regardless of the temperature, the air should be fresh and free from odors. The body temperature of these patients never is taken by mouth. Rectal temperature is preferred to the less-accurate axillary temperature.

Because there are occasions when the corneal reflex is absent, the cornea is likely to become irritated or scratched. It may be necessary to irrigate the eyes with normal saline solution and to lubricate them with mineral oil. Often, a patient has periocular edema following head surgery. Cold compresses may be used, and care must be exerted to avoid contact with the cornea.

If there is ear or nasal bleeding, or oozing of cerebrospinal fluid, the physician should be notified immediately. A small sterile cotton pledget may be placed loosely in the nostril or ears, but no attempt to clean them should be made until the patient is further evaluated.

If the patient is restless, side-rails should be provided. If it is possible for him to sustain injury

* 65° F.

against the side attachments, they should be padded satisfactorily. Every measure that is available and appropriate for the calming and quieting of the disturbed patient should be carried out. Any form of restraint is likely to be countered by rebellion, whether the patient is fully conscious or not, and fury so incited may lead to self-injury or to a dangerous increase in intracranial pressure.

A summary of the nursing management of the unconscious patient is found on pages 781-783.

PATIENTS WITH CRANIAL, SPINAL AND PERIPHERAL NEUROPATHIES

First Cranial (Olfactory) Nerve

Disturbances of the olfactory bulbs by intracranial diseases reveal themselves by either loss of smell sensation (anosmia) or alterations in it (perversions).

Anosmia. This follows fractures of the base of the skull which lacerate the olfactory nerves (fine filaments that pass from the bulb to the olfactory mucous membrane through small holes in the cribriform plate of the ethmoid bone). Falls or blows on the back of the head that merely jar the skull by contusing these filaments also may produce temporary anosmia.

Second Cranial (Optic) Nerve

Diseases of and injuries to the optic nerves, whatever their nature, cause reduction in the acuity of vision and contraction of the visual fields, symptoms that may progress to complete blindness.

Choked Disk. Edematous swelling of the head of the optic nerve appears in all conditions that increase the intracranial pressure, such as tumor and abscess of, and acute hemorrhage into, the brain.

Secondary Optic Atrophy. This is the outcome of prolonged severe choking of the disk, neuritis of the optic nerve, closure of its central artery, pressure against it by brain tumors and fractures of the base of the skull that involve the optic foramen (through which the optic nerve leaves the skull). Optic atrophy is an important early sign of multiple sclerosis. It is one of the manifestations of central nervous system syphilis and a product of methanol poisoning.

Third, Fourth and Sixth Cranial Nerves (Oculomotor, Trochlear and Abducens)

The oculomotor nerve supplies all but two of the muscles that move the eyeball. Of these two, one, the superior oblique, is innervated by the 4th cranial (trochlear) nerve; the other, the external rectus muscle, which rotates the eyeball outward, is innervated by the 6th cranial (abducens) nerve. Paralysis of any one of these three nerves produces strabismus (squint), the type of which depends on the muscle

NURSING MANAGEMENT OF THE UNCONSCIOUS PATIENT
Objectives, Principles and Rationale of Care

The basic nursing principles underlying the care of an unconscious patient are applicable to any unconscious patient regardless of the clinical cause. There are 2 major threats to the patient: (1) the disease or trauma that produced unconsciousness and (2) the threat of the unconscious state. The primary problem is that the patient's normal protective reflexes are impaired. The nursing goal is to assume these protective mechanisms for the patient until he is aware of himself and can function in his environment.

Nursing Action	Rationale
I. To establish and maintain an adequate airway	Inadequate respiratory exchange promotes CO_2 retention, which can produce diffuse cerebral edema.
A. Place the patient in a lateral recumbent position with his face dependent	A dependent position prevents the tongue from obstructing the airway, encourages drainage of respiratory secretions and promotes respiratory exchange.
B. Insert oral airway if tongue is paralyzed or is obstructing airway	*A noisy airway is an obstructed airway.* (An obstructed airway increases intracranial pressure.) The use of an oropharyngeal airway is considered a short-term measure.
C. Prepare for insertion of cuffed endotracheal tube if patient's condition requires	Endotracheal intubation is more effective in permitting positive-pressure ventilation. The cuffed tube seals off the digestive tract, thus preventing aspiration, and allows efficient removal of tracheobronchial secretions.
D. Utilize oxygen therapy, positive pressure assisted breathing techniques or artificial ventilation with a respirator when there is indication of impending respiratory failure	When arterial blood gas measurements reveal the patient has insufficient ventilation and gas exchange, respiratory failure may ensue.
E. Keep the airway free of secretions with efficient suctioning	With the absence of the cough and swallowing reflexes, secretions rapidly accumulate in the posterior pharynx and upper trachea, and can pave the way to fatal respiratory complications.
1. Attach open-end catheter to Y-tube	
2. Keep one end of Y-tube open while inserting the catheter	
3. When catheter is at desired level, close the open-end of Y with finger	
4. Turn the suction *on* and slowly withdraw catheter with a twisting motion of the thumb and forefinger	Negative pressure (suction on) is applied only as the catheter is withdrawn. The twisting motion of the suction catheter reduces prolonged contact with pharyngeal mucosa. Forceful suction irritates the mucosa, increases the amount of secretions, produces mucosal bleeding and can precipitate infection.

5. Gently turn the head from side to side while suctioning
         a. Limit tracheal aspiration to intervals of a few seconds
         b. Allow patient to rest between aspirations	

F. Prepare for tracheostomy if coma is deepening and there are evidences of inadequate respiratory exchange	

1. Keep tracheostomy tube meticulously clean
         a. Carefully inject 3 to 5 ml. saline solution through trachea stoma and then suction
         b. Spray saline solution in mouth and nasopharynx and suction at periodic intervals
	The dryness of the respiratory tract produces rapid formation of mucus plugs, which are difficult to remove. The careful washing (3 to 5 ml. of saline) of the trachea also stimulates the cough reflex, which helps clear the tracheobronchial tree.

NURSING MANAGEMENT OF THE UNCONSCIOUS PATIENT (*Continued*)

Nursing Action (*Continued*)   **Rationale (*Continued*)**

2. Wear sterile gloves and use a sterile catheter each time the tracheostomy is aspirated
3. Suction trachea around cannula and through tube
4. Have adequate humidification

Keeping the upper respiratory tract clean and free of mucus plugs and dried secretions lessens subsequent pulmonary complications.

G. Give antibiotics as per schedule

A screen of broad spectrum antibiotics is maintained in the unconscious patient to prevent infectious and pulmonary complications.

II. To assess the level of responsiveness

A. Maintain a constant assessment of the patient's level of consciousness and changes in responsiveness

The level of consciousness is the most important measure of the patient's condition. Unconscious patients may deteriorate rapidly from numerous clinical causes.

B. Record the patient's *exact reactions,* movements, and quality of speech
1. Request the patient to speak
2. Ask the patient to perform some activity (raise arm, protrude tongue, etc.)
3. Apply painful stimuli if there is no response (pinching skin of arms, thighs, etc.) and assess patient's perception of pain

No response or a delayed or unequal response is an unfavorable clinical sign.

III. To evaluate the progression of vital signs

A. Know the patient's baseline (initial) vital signs and alert the physician if there are significant fluctuations of blood pressure and instability of the pulse and respiratory cycles

Fluctuations of vital signs indicate a change in intracranial homeostasis. Monitoring of vital signs is also essential to alert personnel for hidden bleeding.

B. Take blood pressure readings, pulse and respiratory rate and temperature at frequently specified intervals until there is clinical evidence of stabilization

Taking and recording of temperature is mandatory since temperature-regulating mechanisms may be disturbed. Hyperthermia is an unfavorable prognostic sign.

IV. To maintain fluid and electrolyte balance

A. Give intravenous fluids as indicated (use vein in hand)

Laboratory electrolyte evaluations are made when the patient is maintained on intravenous fluids to ensure proper balance.

B. Initiate nasogastric feedings

Feeding through a gastric tube ensures better nutrition than does intravenous feeding. Electrolyte and protein balance is maintained by selective absorption. Also, paralytic ileus is fairly frequent in the unconscious and a nasogastric tube assists in gastric decompression.

1. Insert small plastic gastric tube through nose into stomach
2. Aspirate stomach before each feeding

If aspirated residual exceeds 50 ml., the patient may be developing an ileus. Gastric distention and vomiting may result.

3. Elevate patient's head and thorax and give 100 to 150 ml. blenderized formula slowly. Give small amount at first and gradually increase until 400 to 500 ml. are given at each feeding

Elevation of the patient's head before, during and after feeding reduces likelihood of regurgitation and aspiration.

4. Give 2,000 to 2,500 ml. of fluid through tube daily

An unconscious patient requires at least 2,500 ml. of fluid daily. High protein feedings can produce a solute diuresis which will produce dehydration unless an adequate fluid intake is ensured. Fever, excessive sweating or fluid loss elsewhere in the body increase the fluid requirements.

5. Rinse the tube with water after each feeding

NURSING MANAGEMENT OF THE UNCONSCIOUS PATIENT (*Continued*)

Nursing Action (*Continued*)	Rationale (*Continued*)
V. To give nursing support as the patient's changing condition indicates	
A. Be aware of the varying phases of restlessness	A certain degree of restlessness may be favorable, as it may indicate the patient is regaining consciousness. However, restlessness is quite common in cerebral anoxia or when there is a partially obstructed airway, distended bladder, overlooked bleeding or fracture; it may be a manifestation of brain injury.
1. Have adequate lighting in the room to prevent hallucinations in the patient who is regaining consciousness	
2. Pad side-rails, wrap mitts or boxing gloves on hands or use other devices to protect patient	
3. Avoid oversedating the patient	
B. Keep the skin clean, dry and free of pressure	
1. Lubricate skin with emollient lotions to prevent sheet irritation, dryness, chafing and cracking	All these activities are to prevent the formation of decubiti on pressure-sensitive areas.
2. Inspect pressure areas for evidences of skin redness and breakdown	
C. Put all extremities through range-of-motion exercises 4 times daily	Contracture deformities develop early in unconscious patients.
D. Turn the patient from side to side at regular intervals	Turning relieves pressure areas and helps keep lungs clear by mobilizing secretions. Prolonged pressure on extremities produces nerve palsies.
E. Observe the patient for indications of an overdistended bladder	
1. Utilize external sheath catheter for male patient	Involuntary voiding indicates an impaired state of consciousness.
2. If patient is unable to' void, insert 3-way indwelling catheter with continuous drainage	Infection invariably follows prolonged use of an indwelling catheter that is attached to straight drainage.
3. Tape the catheter to the lower abdomen of the male patient and the inner thigh of the female to prevent traction on the urethra	
F. Protect the eyes from corneal irritation	
1. Routinely inspect size of pupils and condition of eyes using a flashlight	The cornea functions as a shield. If the eyes remain open for long periods, corneal drying, irritation and ulceration are apt to result.
2. Remove contact lens if worn	
3. Irrigate eyes with sterile saline solution and instill sterile mineral oil drops in each eye	
4. Prepare for temporary tarsorrhaphy (suturing of eyelids in closed position) if unconscious state is prolonged	
G. Protect the patient during convulsive seizures (see p. 813)	A patient with head trauma is a potential candidate for convulsive seizures.
1. Protect the patient from self-injury	
2. Observe the patient during the seizure and record observations	
3. Give prescribed anticonvulsant medications through the nasogastric tube	

paralyzed, but paralysis of the 3rd nerve produces ptosis and dilation of the pupils as well. Such paralysis follows poisoning by alcohol, lead or carbon monoxide; infections, such as those of botulism, measles and encephalitis. Much more often, the cause is related to syphilis, multiple sclerosis, fractures of the base of the skull, and middle ear infections, both most apt to injure the 6th nerve.

Fifth Cranial (Trigeminal) Nerve

The trigeminal nerve supplies all the sensory fibers to the skin of the face (except the angle of the jaw and the anterior half of the scalp), to the teeth, the conjunctivae, the mucous membrane covering the inside of the mouth, the nose, the paranasal sinuses and the greater part of the tongue. The lowest branch of this nerve also contains the motor fibers that control the muscles of mastication (see Fig. 34-10).

One, two or all three branches (the ophthalmic, the maxillary and the mandibular) of this nerve may be affected by diseases and by trauma, and the disturbances that follow always correspond exactly to the areas of distribution of the branch affected. Severe injury to one of these nerves, such as contusions over the supraorbital notch or the infraorbital foramen, may be followed by anesthesia of the area it supplies, but is followed by pain if the trauma merely irritates or compresses it. If, however, the trauma causes bleeding into the tissue about the nerve, the scar tissue that forms afterward may so compress its fibers that months later localized pain appears in the forehead or the cheek. This pain may continue indefinitely.

Herpes. The pustular rash and burning neuralgic pains of ocular herpes, one form of herpes zoster, are limited to the area of distribution of the upper branch of one trigeminal nerve and therefore are likely to involve the lid, the conjunctiva and the cornea. The healing of pustules on the cornea may leave it scarred, resulting in impairment of vision. Herpes simplex (cold sores) about the nose and the mouth, also attributed to irritation of the trifacial ganglion, appears in all sorts of acute infections, ranging from common colds to cerebrospinal meningitis.

Symptomatic Trigeminal Neuralgia. This is due both to lesions that directly irritate the trigeminal nerve or its ganglion and to diseases of other organs that refer their pains to its area of distribution. Among such lesions are inflammatory processes and neoplasms in the soft tissues and the bones of the face; paranasal sinus infections; infected teeth; unerupted third molar teeth; tumors and aneurysms about the base of the skull; venous sinus thrombosis; basilar meningitis; tumors of the gasserian ganglion; diseases of the sphenopalatine ganglion, the middle ear and the orbit of the eye; such conditions as eyestrain, migraine and multiple sclerosis; and, occasionally, syphilis, diabetes, nephritis and malaria.

Trigeminal Neuralgia (*Tic Douloureux*). This is a malady characterized by paroxysms of lancinating or burning pain limited in its radiation to the area of distribution of one, two or all three branches of one trigeminal nerve and separated by periods of complete comfort. Its early attacks, which appear most often during the 5th decade of life, usually are infrequent, mild and brief; but with advancing years they tend to become more and more frequent and agonizing. This, the commonest of all primary neuralgias, is a disease whose cause is unknown. Sclerosis of the vessels and degeneration of the gasserian ganglion may be responsible for a few cases; however, disturbances in the subthalamic vasomotor nuclei now are thought to be more important.

The pain of this neuralgia is felt in the skin, not in the deeper structures, but it is more severe at the periphery of the areas of distribution of the affected nerve, hence, notably over the lip, the chin, the ala nasi and in the teeth. Paroxysms are aroused by any stimulation of the terminals of the affected branches, such as washing the face, brushing the hair or the teeth, eating, drinking, a draft of cold air and direct pressure against the nerve trunk. Certain areas are called *trigger points*, since the slightest touch over one of them at once starts a paroxysm. In severe cases of this neuralgia, called *tic douloureux*, the paroxysms are accompanied by quick contractions of some of the facial muscles, such as a sudden closing of the eye or a twitch of the mouth.

Treatment. Recently, antiepileptic drugs (sodium diphenylhydantoin or Dilantin) in daily doses of 100 mg. to 400 mg. have been used for pain relief. Vitamin B_{12} administered parenterally in daily doses has been beneficial to some patients. Injections of alcohol or phenol are used to anesthetize the trigger zone and to prevent recurrence of pain. This may bring about relief for 6 to 18 months.

Surgical Treatment. The operative procedure most commonly used at the present time to relieve the pains of trigeminal neuralgia is sectioning of the second and third division of the nerve in the middle fossa. Thus ulceration of the cornea is avoided because the fibers of the first division are spared. The operation is performed under general anesthesia in the sitting position. An opening is made in the temporal region and after elevating the dura, the nerve fibers are cut behind the semilunar ganglion.

Following the operation the patient has a complete loss of sensation in the distribution of the divided nerve fibers. Complications that may occur in a small percentage of the operations include transient facial paralysis, herpetic lesions of the face, keratitis and corneal ulceration.

A supraorbital neurectomy can be carried out in the patients whose pain is in the distribution of the first division of the nerve. Other surgical procedures such as simple decompression of the root, manipulation of the semilunar ganglion and division of the descending tract of the fifth nerve in medulla (tractotomy) are seldom performed today.

Nursing Emphasis. Preoperative care of a patient with trigeminal neuralgia includes a recognition on the part of the nurse that certain factors may aggravate excruciating facial pain. Food that is too hot or too cold may initiate this pain; careless handling, such as jarring a bed, also may precipitate discomfort. Even washing the face, combing the hair or brushing the teeth may produce acute discomfort. The nurse can lessen these discomforts by using cotton pads to wash the face, substituting a blunt-tooth comb to comb the hair, etc.

Among the most serious of the complications that may follow a trigeminal nerve operation is a corneal infection (keratitis). Sensations in and about the eye are mediated by a branch of this nerve. Destruction of the latter renders the cornea insensitive to injury and to the presence of foreign bodies, thus opening the gates to infection. To protect the eye from this danger it should be irrigated 3 times daily with warm saline solution and sometimes kept covered with an eye shield. The patient later is provided with a special form of protective glasses for a time. He should be instructed to carry a pocket mirror and to inspect his eye for foreign bodies several times a day. He is taught to do his own eye irrigations, using an eye cup. (If sensation of the eye has not been destroyed, these precautions are unnecessary.)

As the patient with trigeminal neuralgia usually is an older individual, every precaution should be taken to prevent pulmonary complications. Turning, deep breathing and early ambulation are the usual preventive measures.

The stay of this patient in the hospital is usually less than a week. His chief adjustment is to become accustomed to the lack of sensation in the area involved and to recognize and to avoid anything that might irritate his face or eyes without his feeling it. A specific teaching point to remember is that he should visit his dentist regularly, since he may not have a toothache in the presence of dental caries.

Seventh Cranial (Facial) Nerve

The facial nerve is the chief motor nerve of the muscles of the face. Its few sensory fibers are disregarded in this discussion.

Facial Paralysis. There are 3 types of facial paralysis: the peripheral, the nuclear and the upper motor neuron type. The peripheral type is produced by interruption or dysfunction of the facial nerve due to involvement of its trunk distal to its exit from the skull or within the temporal bone through which it courses. External lesions are usually the result of direct trauma or a suppurative infection of the parotid gland, whereas those occurring within the skull are encountered as complications of mastoiditis, mastoid surgery or fractures of the skull that involve the temporal bone.

Peripheral facial neuritis is manifested by complete paralysis of the face on the same side as the lesion. Because if it, the mouth is drawn toward the normal side, whereas on the paralyzed side the wrinkles of the forehead and the nasolabial fold are obliterated, and the eye remains open, its upper lid drooping and its lower lid slightly everted, allowing the tears to escape over the cheek. The patient cannot puff out the cheek, close the mouth or show the teeth on the paralyzed side.

Bell's Palsy. The most common type of peripheral facial paralysis is the so-called Bell's palsy. This has its onset following local chilling of the face and is considered by some to represent a type of pressure palsy, the inflamed, edematous nerve becomes compressed to the point of damage, or its nutrient vessel occluded to the point of producing ischemic necrosis of the nerve within its long canal—a channel in which the fit at best is very snug.

The treatment of peripheral palsies of the facial muscles, including Bell's palsy, is to keep these muscles in as good condition as possible by repeated galvanic stimulation, heat to the face and, eventually, by massage.

Frequently, the patient's eye does not close completely and his blink reflex is diminished. Then he may develop conjunctivitis or keratitis from exposure of the eye to air and irritants. Lessened lacrimation may produce corneal irritation and ulceration. Instruct the patient to use eye drops at prescribed intervals to moisten and protect the cornea. The eye should be covered with a protective shield at night.

The nuclear type of facial palsy is caused by destruction of the nuclei from which the fibers of the 7th nerve originate by luetic, neoplastic, vascular or degenerative lesions in the pons.

In upper motor neuron facial paralysis due to lesions (such as tumors, abscesses, depressed skull fractures, etc.) which injure the motor cortical area governing the face, there is paralysis of the muscles of the lower half of the face only (those about the eyes and of the forehead escape), but the paralysis occurs on the side opposite to that of the lesion. Patients with facial palsy of the upper motor neuron type cannot force a smile, no matter how hard they try, but they do smile involuntarily when amused. Their 7th nerve connections to the cortex are severed, but the 7th nerve itself is intact, and the subcortical centers are in sole control.

Eighth Cranial (Auditory-Vestibular) Nerve

Each 8th nerve has two divisions: the auditory (cochlear) and the vestibular portions (the nerve to the semicircular canal system). Disturbances of the auditory nerve impair hearing; disturbances of the vestibular nerve produce vertigo (sensations of turning or falling) and nystagmus. Meniere's disease, a disease of the 8th cranial nerve, is discussed in Chapter 33.

9th Cranial (Glossopharyngeal) Nerve

Glossopharyngeal Paralysis. This (usually in association with disturbances of the vagus nerve) causes difficulty in swallowing, anesthesia of the upper portion of the pharynx and loss of taste over the posterior third of the tongue on the same side as the lesion. It most often is due to brain diseases—for example, tumors.

Glossopharyngeal Neuralgia. Due to neuritis of this nerve, this is characterized by severe pain radiating from the base of the tongue to deep in the ear and also by increased salivation. It may be cured by resection of this nerve.

10th Cranial (Vagus) Nerve

The vagus nerve is the motor nerve of the voluntary muscles of the throat and the larynx, and is the nerve that slows the rate of heartbeat and supplies the parasympathetic nerves to the lungs, the stomach, the esophagus and other abdominal organs.

Neuritis. Neuritis of this nerve occasionally occurs in such acute infections as pneumonia and influenza and results from the action of such poisons as alcohol, lead and arsenic. The vagus nerve (usually in association with the glossopharyngeal) frequently becomes injured by lesions of the pons and the base of the skull.

Paralysis. Paralysis of one vagus causes unilateral paralysis of the larynx, with resultant impairment of speech, difficulty in swallowing, temporary changes in the heart rate and rhythm and, occasionally, vomiting, abdominal pain and anorexia. Complete paralysis of both vagi is followed by permanent tachycardia, since the accelerator nerves of the heart (sympathetic fibers) then lack the normal inhibition of the vagi.

The recurrent laryngeal branch of this nerve, because of its position, is injured easily. The result is paralysis of the larynx and, therefore, hoarseness. This may be caused by the pressure of mediastinal tumors, masses of enlarged lymph nodes in the mediastinum or the neck, aneurysms of the aorta or the subclavian artery and malignant growths of the thyroid gland or adjacent structures. This nerve occasionally is cut by wounds and operations on the neck, such as thyroidectomy.

11th Cranial (Spinal Accessory) Nerve

The spinal accessory nerve, entirely motor in nature, supplies the sternomastoid muscle and the upper portion of the trapezius muscles. Injuries to and diseases of this nerve, therefore, weaken the power to rotate the head to the side opposite the lesion and cause a slight drooping of the shoulder on the side of the lesion. Such paralysis may result from penetrating wounds and operations on the neck, fracture of the skull, injuries to and diseases of the cervical vertebrae, rickets, unilateral poliomyelitis and all diseases that involve the upper portion of the cervical cord.

12th Cranial (Hypoglossal) Nerve

The hypoglossal nerves, entirely motor in character, innervate the muscles of the tongue only. It is rarely that one of these nerves is injured, with resultant paralysis of that side of the tongue, by deep penetrating wounds, abscesses and tumors of the neck, and by trauma to and tuberculosis of the first cervical vertebra; much more often this paralysis is evidence of brain disease.

The tongue, paralyzed on one side, when protruded deviates toward the weak side. When both hypoglossal nerves are paralyzed, the tongue cannot be moved; hence, speech, mastication and swallowing cannot be performed properly.

The Brachial Plexus

Paralysis of the brachial plexus and the nerves arising from it occasionally follows violent movements of the shoulder, the head and the arm, which overstretch or even tear the root of this plexus. (Erb's palsy of the infant results from dislocation during birth of the humerus, which forcibly pushes the head of the bone against this plexus.) The brachial plexus (also its roots) occasionally suffers from the pressure of local tumors, aneurysms and masses of enlarged lymph nodes in the neck or the axilla.

Cervical Ribs. A cervical rib is one or a pair of extra ribs attached usually to the 7th cervical vertebra. If a pair is present, one only may produce symptoms. They are found more frequently in women than in men, occasionally in several members of the same family, and usually in association with other anatomic anomalies.

A cervical rib is a lifelong hazard to the brachial plexus. Because of its presence, the plexus may be crushed by accidents that suddenly force or pull the shoulder down; this trauma is followed by pain and numbness, felt first in the fingers and gradually extending up the forearm, and later by weakness, followed by atrophy of the muscles of that hand and arm. The continuous pressure of a cervical rib on the brachial plexus (the symptoms of which seldom appear before middle life) affects first its sympathetic nerve fibers, as shown by such vasomotor signs as cyanosis, coldness, paleness and edema (a syndrome that early may suggest Raynaud's disease, p. 352). Later this pressure causes disturbances of sensation and finally atrophy of the muscles of the arm and the hand.

Since the presence of a cervical rib frequently produces developmental abnormalities in the pattern of the brachial plexus, the findings on physical examinations often are puzzling. Thus, various muscles and skin areas of the arm and the hand seem to be supplied by the wrong nerves; the arteries of the shoulder region may lie in an unusual position or be abnormal in their relative size; and often the pulse volume of the radial artery of that arm is unusually small and the blood pressure low. Cervical ribs are not always visible on x-ray films, since some constitute merely fibrous bands. However, they exert pressures just as serious as those composed of bone.

The Nerves of the Arms

Fleeting Neuralgic Pains. Pains referred to the shoulder and the upper arm are common following exposure to cold, in chronic and often latent general infections, in cases of spondylitis and of chronic subdeltoid bursitis. To this region, particularly on the left side, are referred the pains of aortitis and coronary artery disease (for example, angina pectoris); and to both sides, those of acute pleuritis. More constant pains, with or without accompanying muscular weakness, result from pressure against the roots of the brachial plexus by spinal tumors, a herniated cervical disk and occasionally by the scalenus anticus neck muscles, between which these nerves course. A true toxic neuritis, which affects the radial nerve in particular, is one of the features of lead poisoning.

Radial Nerve Paralysis. This paralysis, causing *wristdrop*, may be the result of pressure against the trunk of this nerve as it lies in the axilla, as by a crutch or the back of a bench over which the arm is thrown. It also follows blows against the outer aspect of the upper arm, where this nerve lies in an unprotected position. The same type of paralysis likewise may be caused by a tourniquet applied to the arm too tightly or allowed to remain on for too long a time. Late radial paralysis, appearing in 3 to 4 weeks following fracture of the humerus, is due to the gradual compression of this nerve by either excessive callus formation or—and more often—by contracting scar tissue formed in tissues infiltrated by blood.

Ulnar Nerve. The ulnar nerve is often traumatized at the elbow, where it lies in an exposed position. "To hit the crazy bone" really is to strike the ulnar nerve. Even the simple act of reclining on the elbow may cause a pressure paralysis of several weeks' duration of the muscles that this nerve supplies. Dislocation of the elbow and fracture of the bones near this joint, by stretching or compressing this nerve, may cause immediate paralysis of the same muscles or weakness due to delayed neuritis.

The Intercostal Nerves

The intercostal nerves may be injured by trauma to the chest wall and fracture of the ribs, causing pain in their areas of distribution. Anesthesia never results if only a single nerve is injured because of the overlapping of the areas supplied by the two adjacent nerves.

Neuritis. Neuritis of the intercostal nerves is often part of a general neuritis; but neuralgic pains referred to but a few nerves occur as symptoms of diseases of the spinal cord, such as tabes dorsalis (the "lightning pains" of this disease occasionally are almost limited to this radiation), thoracic herpes zoster, in which case they may precede as well as accompany the herpetic skin eruption, both precisely limited to the area of distribution of the intercostal nerve; malignant tumors or exostoses of the vertebrae (as in hypertrophic spondylitis); and spinal tuberculosis, all diseases that irritate the roots of these nerves.

The Lumbar Plexus

Tumors of the vertebrae, retroperitoneal neoplasms, enlarged inflamed pelvic lymph nodes and psoas abscesses occasionally press on the lumbar plexus sufficiently to cause weakness or paralysis of the anterior thigh muscles that are supplied by the femoral nerve.

The Sacral Plexus

The sacral plexus may be torn by fractures of the lower lumbar vertebrae and the sacrum, may be pressed on by large fibroid tumors of the uterus and malignant growths within the pelvis, and may be traumatized during difficult labor.

The chief symptom produced is spasmodic or continuous pain, often called *sciatica*, which extends down the back of the leg, even to the ankle. The trunk of the sciatic nerve is subject to all forms of neuritis that affect other nerves, with, if all its fibers are involved, resultant motor and sensory disturbances of the leg.

Sciatica. The term *sciatica* refers to any condition in which the most prominent symptom is pain along the course of the sciatic nerve. Its etiology in the great majority of cases is uncertain. Some patients give a past history of sprain of the lumbosacral or the sacroiliac joints; for other cases, spondylitis, spondylolisthesis or a ruptured intervertebral disk pressing on the cauda equina may be responsible. In some instances primary neuritis is assumed. It is believed that the usual cause of sciatica is mechanical compression or irritation of the 5th lumbar spinal root, the one from which it receives the majority of its fibers. This root not only is the largest trunk that enters into the formation of the sacral plexus, but also it emerges from the spine through the smallest of the foramina accommodating these roots. Therefore, it easily would be compressed by the slightest amount of edema or exudate that might result from minor traumata, such as strains, contusions or arthritis of the lower lumbar spine.

Peripheral Neuropathies

Neuritis. This is the term applied to both demonstrable inflammatory or degenerative changes in peripheral nerves and (less scientifically) to symptoms that suggest these changes. Although, of the latter, pain is often a prominent feature, and such distress may correctly be called *neuralgic,* yet the use of the term *neuralgia,* usually applied to pains referred over normal sensory nerves to normal regions of the body, implies ignorance of their cause.

Neuritis may involve one nerve only (mononeuritis), or many, this condition being called *polyneuritis* or *multiple neuritis.* In all cases of the latter, the same nerves on the two sides of the body are involved similarly. The symptoms of all types of neuritis, according to the character of the nerves involved, are sensory, motor and vasomotor, these always being limited to the structures that the affected nerves supply. Mononeuritis and polyneuritis, however, differ much in their etiology, course and treatment.

Neuritis of a sensory nerve causes pain and disturbances of sensation, provided that the nerve is able to function in some degree. Anesthesia occurs if the process is severe. In the case of nerves partly or wholly motor, the result of neuritis is either weakness or complete paralysis of the muscles that they control, depending on the severity.

Mononeuritis. This is neuritis limited to a single peripheral nerve and its branches. It arises when the trunk of the nerve is traumatized, as when bruised by a blow; overstretched, as in cases of dislocation of a joint; pressed upon, as by a tumor, a cervical rib, bony exostoses (e.g., in that type of arthritis that narrows the apertures between adjacent vertebrae through which the spinal nerves pass) or the use of a crutch; punctured by the needle used to inject a drug or poisoned by the drugs thus injected; or inflamed because of the extension to its trunk of an adjacent infectious process.

One type of mononeuritis appears many months after injuries that caused considerable bleeding into the tissues surrounding a nerve. In tissues thus infiltrated with blood, considerable scar tissue forms, and this, contracting, slowly compresses the nerve. Similarly, delayed nerve paralyses follow the healing of an abscess, the encapsulation of a foreign body or sequestra of bone and the knitting of fractured bone. In this last case, however, the nerve trunk is caught in the callus.

Pain is seldom a conspicuous symptom of mononeuritis due to trauma, but in patients with complicating inflammatory conditions, such as arthritis, this feature is prominent. Such pain is increased by all body movements that tend to stretch, strain or cause pressure on the injured nerve, and by all sudden jars of the body, such as those incident to coughing and sneezing. The skin in the areas supplied by nerves that are injured or diseased may become reddened and glossy; its subcutaneous tissue may become edematous, and the nutrition of the nails and the hair in this area, defective. Chemical injuries to a nerve trunk, as by drugs injected into or near it, often are permanent.

Treatment. The treatment of mononeuritis, if possible, is to remove the cause, such as by freezing the enmeshed nerve. The pain may be relieved by aspirin or codeine, and the function of the muscles may be maintained by weak galvanic currents.

Causalgia. This is the term applied to a painful posttraumatic condition that begins weeks or months after injury to a nerve trunk. This condition resembles both neuralgia and neuritis, but in fact it is neither. The nerves most often affected, and in order of frequency, are the median, the ulnar, the radial and the internal and the external popliteals.

The chief symptom of causalgia is severe burning pain along the course of the traumatized nerve. This is more or less persistent, but becomes severe following such physical stimuli as the contact of clothes. The skin over the affected limb becomes hot, shiny and, at times, swollen; it shows abnormalities in sweating and, eventually, atrophic changes involving also the nails. The patient holds the limb quiet, since each movement tends to increase the pain. Sympathectomy may be effective in relieving the severe pain of this patient.

Polyneuritis. This is a disease that involves many nerves, particularly those of the legs and the arms, but always the same nerves on both sides of the body. Although the symptoms of this disease suggest that the terminal branches of the affected nerves alone are involved, yet multiple peripheral neuritis involves entire nervous pathways—that is, terminal branches, trunks, related fibers in the spinal cord and possibly in the brain.

Causes. The causes of polyneuritis include poisons and toxins circulating in the bloodstream and a dietary deficiency involving the B complex, notably thiamine. Among exogenous poisons important in the causation of this disease are methyl alcohol, lead, bismuth, mercury, arsenic, sulfonamides, carbon disulfide, aniline and other coal-tar products, emetine, apiol, thallium and several less common drugs and poisons. Peripheral neuritis may occur in the course of various infectious diseases.

A deficiency of thiamine causes disturbances in the metabolism of nerve tissue, as a result of which this tissue is unable to utilize carbohydrates normally. This inability gives rise to symptoms of muscle pains, tenderness and weakness after use, which clear up rapidly after the oral administration of thiamine.

Anatomic polyneuritis is much slower to heal and involves reflex changes, skin hyperesthesias, or hypesthesias, motor weakness or diminution or loss of the deep-tendon reflexes. It is probably due to deficiencies involving other components of the water-soluble vitamin group. This accounts for the polyneuritis formerly called *alcoholic neuritis*, since it was supposedly due to the direct action of ethyl alcohol on the nerves. The deficient diet of habitual drinkers now is considered to be altogether responsible. Similar are the polyneuritides of beriberi, diabetes, pregnancy and malnutrition (particularly if there is a preponderance of carbohydrate in the diet).

Although in cases of multiple neuritis all the peripheral nerves have an equal opportunity to become affected, yet each poison and toxin attacks certain nerves in particular. Thus, botulinus toxin injures the nerves to the muscles of the eyes and the throat, and lead poisoning, those to the muscles of the hands and the feet.

Symptoms. Polyneuritis, whatever its cause, when well-developed presents a fairly uniform clinical picture. The symptoms may be sensory only, but they are never exclusively motor; sensory changes always accompany any muscular weakness or paralysis that appears. The hands and the feet are most affected. Sensations of numbness, hyperesthesia and diminution of heat perception and cold perception appear early and may last for weeks. Sometimes there is a slight fever.

The initial symptoms are followed by anesthesia of the fingers and the toes, which gradually extends toward the trunk. Associated with this is marked tenderness of the affected nerve trunks and of the skin overlying their branches. Pain is a marked early feature in some patients. There is more or less loss of the deep sensations; hence the pseudotabetic

(ataxic) gait occasionally present, observed particularly in the cases of complicating diabetes mellitus and chronic alcoholism.

Muscular weakness then follows, either suddenly or over a period of days. Since the fibers to the extensor muscles of the feet and the hands are more susceptible to the effects of toxins than are those to the flexor muscles, the first motor symptom to appear is an ankledrop or a wristdrop; but after a week or two, paralysis of the entire limb may become complete. Convulsions may occur, frequently in children, because (as stated above) the pathology is not limited solely to the peripheral nerves.

In the majority of patients the symptoms of polyneuritis are superimposed on those of the more primary disease, but in a few patients they so overshadow all others that it is difficult to determine the cause.

Treatment. The treatment of polyneuritis is first to treat the cause—for example, to eliminate all exposure to lead, to supply thiamine in the diet and by parenteral injection, and to treat any infection present. In all cases the patient should rest in bed and receive general supportive treatments. Since the nerves require months to recover, during which time the muscles they control may become so weak and atrophied as to become permanently useless, the latter should be kept in good condition by daily massage, passive movements, or galvanic stimulation. Often splints are indicated to prevent footdrop and wristdrop. Analgesic drugs are often necessary.

CEREBROVASCULAR DISEASE

Scope of the Problem

There are over 200,000 deaths in the U.S. yearly from cerebrovascular disease which comprises 11 per cent of all deaths. The cost of cerebrovascular disorders amounts to 100 million dollars annually. Over half a million Americans suffer from a stroke each year and there are at least 2 million persons who have had a stroke and face the possibility of recurrent vascular accidents. Approximately 8 of 10 stroke victims survive the initial phase but require intensive care and rehabilitation to prevent dependency and a mere vegetative existence. Much knowledge has been gained in the past decade in stroke prevention as well as in rehabilitating the large majority of patients to attain their maximal potential for independent living.

Classification

A committee of the Public Health Service* classified the principal types of cerebrovascular diseases as follows:

* U.S. Public Health Service: A classification and outline of cerebrovascular disease. *Neurology,* 8:1, 1958.

TABLE 34-3. The nurse as a case finder
It is now recognized that the incidence of strokes can be decreased if the stroke-prone individual is identified early and preventive measures started promptly. The following conditions predispose the patient to a cerebral vascular accident: 1. Hypertension (increases stroke risk 4 times) 2. Presence of atherosclerosis in other parts of the body 3. Hypercholesterolemia 4. History of heart disease (angina pectoris, myocardial infarction) 5. Diabetes 6. Obesity 7. Cigarette smoking (in males) 8. Sudden decrease in total blood volume in elderly persons

1. Cerebral infarction
   A. Thrombosis with atherosclerosis
   B. Cerebral embolism
   C. Other conditions (arteritis, hematologic disorders, syphilis)

2. Transient cerebral ischemia without infarction
   A. Recurrent focal cerebral ischemic attacks
   B. Systemic hypotension (syncope)

3. Intracranial hemorrhage
   A. Hypertensive intracerebral hemorrhage
   B. Ruptured saccular aneurysm
   C. Angioma
   D. Hemorrhagic disorders (leukemia, aplastic anemia, thrombopenic purpura, complication of anticoagulent therapy, etc.)

4. Hypertensive encephalopathy
   A. Malignant hypertension
   B. Acute glomerulonephritis
   C. Eclampsia

5. Dural sinus and cerebral venous thrombosis
   A. Secondary to infections of cranial structures (otitis, sinusitis, etc.)
   B. Secondary to meningitis or subdural empyema

The Patient with Cerebrovascular Disease

Cerebrovascular disease refers to any functional abnormality of the central nervous system caused by a pathologic condition of the individual cerebral vessels or of the cerebral vascular system. The vascular pathology may involve the artery or the vein or both. It either causes hemorrhage from a tear in the vessel wall, or impairs the cerebral circulation by a partial or complete occlusion of the lumen of the vessel.

Hemorrhage may occur outside the dura mater (extradural hemorrhage), beneath the dura mater (subdural hemorrhage), or in the subarachnoid space (subarachnoid hemorrhage), or within the brain substance (intracerebral hemorrhage).

Impairment of cerebral circulation may be (1) arterial, causing transient ischemic attacks, cerebral thrombosis or cerebral embolism; (2) venous, producing cavernous sinus thrombosis, cortical vein thrombosis, or sagittal sinus thrombosis; (3) both arterial and venous, such as cerebral arteriovenous malformation and carotid cavernous fistula.

Cerebrovascular Disease from Hemorrhage. *Extradural Hemorrhage.* Extradural hemorrhage (epidural hemorrhage) is a neurosurgical emergency that requires urgent care. If the patient is not treated within hours following the accident, he has very little chance of survival. This is discussed under head injuries on pp. 817-821.

Subdural Hemorrhage. The subdural hematoma (excluding the acute subdural) is basically the same as an epidural hemorrhage, except that in subdural hematoma usually a bridging vein is torn. Thus, a longer period of time (longer lucid interval) is required for the hematoma to form and cause pressure on the brain. This is discussed under head injuries on pp. 817-821.

Subarachnoid Hemorrhage. The most common cause of subarachnoid hemorrhage is a leaking congenital aneurysm about the circle of Willis and congenital arteriovenous malformation of the brain.

An unruptured congenital cerebral aneurysm is usually silent and causes no functional abnormality. Neurologic disturbances start at the time of rupture. The rupture is usually preceded by some degree of physical strain and is associated with a sudden shoot-

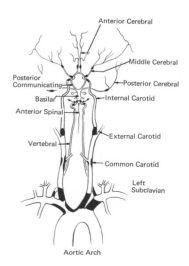

FIG. 34-11. Common sites of atherosclerotic obstruction in the major arterial system of the head. (Beeson, P. B., and McDermott, W.: Textbook of Medicine, Philadelphia, W. B. Saunders, p. 1547)

ing pain in the back of one eye or a very severe headache, nausea, fainting and sometimes immediate loss of consciousness. Physical examination reveals a rigid neck and sometimes cranial nerves, motor or sensory disturbances. A spinal tap shows blood in the cerebrospinal fluid.

Some patients with leaking congenital cerebral aneurysm undergo surgical procedures following demonstration of the aneurysm by angiography; others may be treated by medical measures. Either group requires special care. Absolute bed rest and avoidance of any physical strain are most important in the early stage of the disease. Rerupture of the aneurysm and sudden death may occur while the patient is trying to sit up in bed or while straining on a bed pan.

Intracerebral hemorrhage. Hemorrhage in the substance of the brain is most common in persons with high arterial blood pressure and cerebral atherosclerosis. The bleeding is usually arterial and occurs particularly about the basal ganglia. Intracerebral hemorrhage is occasionally due to hemorrhagic disorders, such as leukemia, thrombocytopenia, or is a complication of anticoagulent therapy. The clinical picture and the prognosis depend mainly on the degree of hemorrhage and brain damage. Occasionally the bleeding ruptures the wall of the lateral ventricle and causes intraventricular hemorrhage, which is frequently fatal.

At the time of hemorrhage the patient may experience a severe headache, nausea, a feeling of fainting and loss of consciousness. Abnormalities in the vital signs and neurologic impairment vary, depending on the severity of hemorrhage. In less severe cases with relatively good recovery, the vital signs remain stable. The neurologic examination may show some degree of unilateral weakness or complete hemiplegia, with or without aphasia. Usually, right-handed patients with a right hemiplegia also exhibit aphasia. Distension of the urinary bladder may also be present.

The treatment of intracerebral hemorrhage is generally based on medical and nursing care. The majority of these patients are not able to swallow for some time, and anything given by mouth may cause either asphyxia or pneumonia. After the first 2 or 3 days of intravenous fluid therapy, it is best to feed these patients through a nasogastric tube with a diet adequate in volume and in calories.

Three major and sometimes fatal complications may develop if the patient's care is not adequate: pressure sores, pulmonary infection and urinary infection. Pressure sores may be avoided if the patient is turned on his side every 2 hours day and night, and is given frequent skin care. Pulmonary infection is also best prevented by frequently changing the patient's position, encouraging him to cough, careful suctioning of the upper respiratory tract in comatose and semico-

matose patients, chest exercise, and nasopharyngeal and mouth care. Urinary infection may be prevented either by sterile catheterization performed 3 times a day or the placement of an indwelling 3-way catheter with continuous irrigation. A complete urinalysis is indicated every other day.

As soon as the patient has passed the acute stage of the disease, rehabilitation measures should be started. Intensive nursing care and rehabilitation have tremendously improved the prognosis of these neurologic patients; without them, results are most discouraging.

Cerebrovascular Disease from Impairment of Cerebral Circulation. *Transient ischemic attacks.* These are characterized by transient attacks of dysfunction of the central nervous system, lasting one or several minutes, and the absence of neurologic disturbance between the attacks. The cause of this clinical entity is a transient impairment of the cerebral blood flow to a specific region, owing to atherosclerotic involvement of the vessels supplying the brain.

The most common sites of atherosclerosis in the extracranial arteries occur at the bifurcation of the common carotid and the origin of vertebral arteries. Among the intracranial arteries, the middle cerebral artery is the most common location of atherosclerosis (Fig. 34-11). If the ischemia arises in the carotid system, the patient may experience hemiparesis, blind-

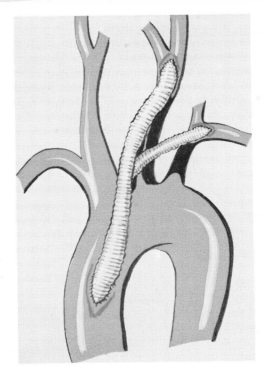

Fig. 34-12. The use of shunt in the treatment of vascular block of the carotid, used in some types of "strokes."

ness in one eye, aphasia or confusion. If the ischemia occurs in the vertebral basilar system, there may be vertigo, blindness, disturbances of consciousness and various signs of motor and sensory impairments.

Following angiographic evaluation of the diseased vessels, some patients are treated by reconstructive vascular procedures, such as endarterectomy or shunting procedures (Fig. 34-12). Patients who are not good candidates for surgical intervention are usually placed on anticoagulant therapy (Coumadin), in order to prevent future attacks and the development of a massive cerebral infarction.

Cerebral Thrombosis. Cerebral arteriosclerosis and slowness of the cerebral circulation are major causes of cerebral thrombosis.

Headache is rather uncommon at the onset of cerebral thrombosis. Some patients may experience dizziness, mental disturbances or convulsions, and some may have an onset indistinguishable from that of intracerebral hemorrhage or cerebral embolism. In general cerebral thrombosis does not develop abruptly and a transient loss of speech, hemiplegia or paresthesias in one-half of the body may precede the onset of a severe paralysis by a few hours or days.

Cerebral Embolism. Pathologic abnormalities of the left heart, such as subacute bacterial endocarditis, rheumatic heart disease, and myocardial infarction, as well as pulmonary infections, are the sites where emboli originate. The embolus usually lodges in the middle cerebral artery or its branches, where it disrupts the cerebral circulation. Sudden onset of hemiparesis or hemiplegia with or without aphasia or loss of consciousness in a patient with cardiac or pulmonary disease is very characteristic of cerebral embolism. Although endarterectomies of the intracranial arteries have been occasionally tried, either by gross or microsurgical procedures, the treatment of the cerebral thrombosis and embolism chiefly consists of medical and nursing care similar to that given in intracerebral hemorrhage.

Cavernous Sinus Thrombosis. Infections of the upper half of the face, orbit and nasal sinuses may extend into the cavernous sinus, and by causing thrombosis interrupt the venous drainage of the eye and other draining veins. Initially, edema, congestion, proptosis* and pain occur in the homolateral eye, and later in the contralateral eye as well because of extension of the infection to the other cavernous sinus. These patients are treated by antibiotic and anticoagulant medications and occasionaly by surgical intervention.

Sagittal sinus thrombosis. Infective processes involving the frontal or nasal sinuses and osteomyelitis

of the skull may extend into the sagittal sinus and disturb the cerebral venous drainage, producing cerebral congestion and edema. Usually, there are no localizing signs, but symptoms and signs of increased intracranial pressure may develop.

Cerebral Arteriovenous Malformation. There are two types of congenital cerebral arteriovenous malformation: (1) the cryptic type, which usually occurs mainly in the brain stem, and (2) the large type, which is usually located on or near the surface of the cerebral hemisphere, particularly in the parietal region. They commonly produce either spontaneous subarachnoid hemorrhage or focal seizures. The treatment consists of anticonvulsive medications or surgical removal of the A-V malformation.

Carotid cavernous fistula. This condition is usually posttraumatic, occurring either from a small tear in the intracavernous portion of the internal carotid artery, or from disruption of one of its branches in this location. Through this abnormal communication, the high pressure carotid flow enters the cavernous sinus and disturbs the sinus drainage. The clinical picture consists of headaches, noise in the head, congestion, proptosis, papilledema and bruit in the homolateral eye. Carotid angiography demonstrates the arterial flow into the cavernous sinus. If spontaneous regression does not occur, ligation of the internal or common carotid artery may be necessary.

Nursing the Patient with a Cerebral Vascular Accident

Nursing During the Acute Phase. Skillful nursing is required during the period that the patient is unconscious.* One of the primary nursing objectives is the maintenance of the airway. The patient should be placed in a lateral or semiprone position with the bed flat. If stertorous respirations are present, an artificial airway should be inserted. The negative pressure produced by the stertorous respirations causes an increased amount of secretions.

If oropharyngeal suctioning is indicated, the nurse should lubricate the catheter with water, "pinch it off," and then pass the catheter through the nose to the epiglottis. This initiates the cough reflex and serves to make the suctioning procedure more efficient. Repeated irritation to the mucous membrane by suctioning produces an increase of secretions, which is the direct opposite of its purpose. Oxygenation should be provided if there is any indication of a decreased blood flow, insufficient pulmonary ventilation, or impending heart failure.

A rectal temperature should be taken frequently,

---

* Bulging of the eyeball.

* The principles which underlie the management of the unconscious patient are summarized on pages 781-783.

FIG. 34-13. Hemiplegic deformities. The involved leg immediately falls into external rotation. The knee almost invariably flexes. As soon as knee flexion occurs, abduction of the upper leg follows. The foot falls into plantar flexion, so there is always a footdrop and a shortening of the Achilles tendon. This position of the leg is assumed whether the leg is flaccid or spastic.

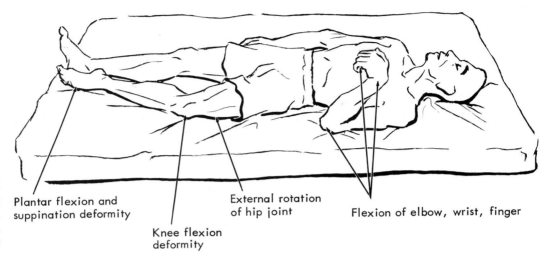

Plantar flexion and suppination deformity

Knee flexion deformity

External rotation of hip joint

Flexion of elbow, wrist, finger

The arm on the affected side is held against the body. Often, a flail arm is placed across the body for convenience in handling the patient, but if spastic, the elbow flexes to about 90°. With the arm across the body, the wrist is dropped. If the arm is spastic, the fingers curl into a fist, with the thumb adducted and flexed under the fingers. (Covalt, N. K.: Preventive technics of rehabilitation for hemiplegic patients, G.P. *17*:131)

as a patient with cerebral hemorrhage may readily develop hyperthermia. The temperature of the skin may not necessarily reflect the degree of body heat. If the hypothalamus has lost control, the skin may be cold while the thermometer records a high temperature. To reduce this type of central nervous fever, warm sponges are administered to "bring the blood to the surface." When this is accomplished, cool sponges are given to promote superficial cooling. The nursing management of hyperthermia is discussed on pages 778-779.

Nursing Assessment. Nursing observations are of the utmost importance in diagnosis, and therefore they should be recorded in detail. The following observations are especially significant:

1. A change in the level of responsiveness as evidenced by movement, resistance to changes of position, and response to stimulation

2. Presence or absence of voluntary or involuntary movements of the extremities; the tone of the muscles; the body posture and the position of the head

3. Stiffness or flaccidity of the neck

4. The equality and the size of the pupils and pupillary reactions to light

5. The color of the face and the extremities; the temperature and the moisture of the skin

6. The quality and the rates of pulse and respiration; the body temperature and the arterial pressure

7. The volume of fluids ingested or administered, and the volume of urine excreted each 24 hours

While the patient is unconscious, an indwelling catheter with a closed drainage system and a continuous antibacterial drip is used. The problem of incontinence is resolved by initiating a program that simulates normal bladder functioning as soon as the patient shows that he is aware of his environment. The program should include offering the patient the urinal or bedpan at scheduled short intervals and increasing the time intervals as more control is gained.

When the patient begins to regain consciousness, he will be confused because there is some degree of cerebral edema following a C.V.A. If his right side is affected, some degree of aphasia probably will be present. The patient should be informed that he has "trouble" with his speech, will be taught to communicate, and reassured that he has not lost his mind. (See pp. 763-764).

Rehabilitation Phase. The patient with hemiplegia has a unilateral paralysis and requires intensive rehabilitation nursing. The *immediate nursing goals* are (1) to prevent deformities, (2) to retrain the affected arm and leg, and (3) to help the patient gain independence in personal hygiene and dressing activities.

When control of the voluntary muscles is lost, the strong flexor muscles exert control over the extensors. The arm tends to adduct (adductor muscles are stronger than abductors) and to rotate internally. The elbow and the wrist tend to flex. The affected leg tends to rotate externally at the hip joint, flex at the knee, and plantar flex and supinate at the ankle joint (Fig. 34-13).

Positioning. Correct positioning in bed is of prime importance. By the use of proper positioning the nurse can help to prevent contractures, relieve pressure, and

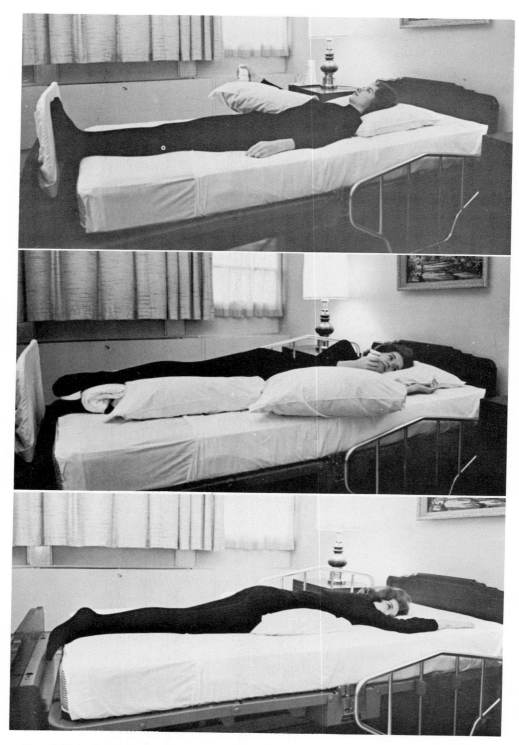

Fig. 34-14. Positioning the patient following a cerebrovascular accident. (*Top*) Dorsal supine position. Note that the heels are suspended in the interspace between the mattress and the footboard. (*Center*) Lateral or side-lying position. (*Bottom*) Prone position.

assist in maintaining good body alignment. A bed board under the mattress gives the body firm support. The patient should remain flat in bed except when he is engaged in his activities of daily living. Maintaining the upright position in bed for extended periods of time is one of the greatest contributors to hip flexion deformity. A footboard is used to keep the feet at right angles to the legs when the patient is in a supine (dorsal) position (Fig. 34-14). This prevents footdrop and heel cord shortening, caused by contracture of the gastrocnemius muscle. The footboard also prevents the weight of the bed linen from pushing the feet into plantar flexion.

Because flexor muscles are stronger than extensor muscles, it may be necessary to apply a posterior splint at night to prevent flexion of the affected extremity. If such a splint is not available, it may be improvised by applying a cast to the affected extremity and bivalving it. The posterior portion is padded. The heel portion should be well padded with foam rubber or lamb's wool. The leg is positioned in it and wrapped with an elastic bandage to keep it in an extended position. The posterior splint is used only at night to maintain correct positioning while the patient is sleeping.

To prevent external rotation at the hip joint, a trochanter roll (Fig. 10-2) is used. The trochanter roll should extend from the crest of the ilium to the mid-thigh, as the hip joint lies between these two points. Sandbags applied laterally to the leg do not prevent external rotation. This motion originates in the ball and socket joint of the hip. The knee has no such rotating function. The trochanter roll acts as a mechanical wedge under the projection of the greater trochanter and prevents the femur from rolling.

To prevent adduction of the affected shoulder, a pillow is placed in the axilla. This keeps the arm away from the chest. A pillow is placed under the arm, and the arm is placed in a neutral (slightly flexed) position, with each joint positioned higher than the preceding one. Thus the elbow is higher than the shoulder, and the wrist is higher than the elbow. The elevation of the arm helps to prevent edema and the resultant fibrosis that will prevent future use if control returns. The fingers are positioned so that they are barely flexed. A small hand roll helps to maintain this position and keeps the thumb away from the hand in the position of opposition. The hand is placed in slight supination, which is its most functional (i.e., useful) position.

The patient's position should be changed every 2 hours. To place a patient in a lateral (side-lying) position, put a pillow between his legs before turning him. The patient should be turned on his unaffected side. His upper thigh should not be acutely flexed (Fig. 34-14).

It is desirable to assist the patient to a prone position for 15 minutes to a half hour several times a day. Place a small pillow or a support under the pelvis and extend it from the level of the umbilicus to the upper third of the thigh (Fig. 34-14). This helps to promote hyperextension of the hip joints, which is essential for normal gait.

Exercise. The affected extremities are exercised passively and put through a full range of motion 4 to 5 times a day. Repetition of an activity forms new pathways in the central nervous system and therefore encourages new patterns of motion.

Frequent short periods of exercise always are preferred to longer periods at infrequent intervals. *Regularity* in exercise is most important. Improvement in muscle strength and maintenance of range of motion can be achieved only through daily exercise.

The patient is encouraged and reminded to exercise his unaffected side at intervals throughout the day. It is well to work out a written time schedule that can be used to remind the patient of his exercise activities. The nurse has the responsibility of supervising and supporting the patient during these activities. The patient can be taught to put his unaffected leg under his affected one to move it when he is turning and exercising. Bed exercises prepare the patient for ambulation and give the patient a goal. Quadriceps muscle setting and gluteal setting exercises are started early to improve the muscle strength needed for walking. These are done at least 5 times daily for 10 minutes at a time.

QUADRICEPS SETTING. Instruct the patient to contract the quadriceps muscle (on the anterior portion of the thigh) while he raises the heel and attempts to push the popliteal space against the mattress. Hold the muscle contracture until the count of 5. Then relax until the count of 5. Repeat. This exercise is performed by each extremity.

GLUTEAL SETTING. Contract or "pinch" the buttocks together until the count of 5. Then relax until the count of 5. Repeat.

GETTING OUT OF BED. A patient who is hemiplegic from a thrombosis usually is started on an active rehabilitation program as soon as he regains consciousness, whereas a patient who has had a cerebral hemorrhage cannot participate actively until cessation of all evidences of bleeding. If this means waiting a number of weeks or months, as it may, all precautions should be taken to ensure function when the patient is permitted to start activities.

SITTING BALANCE. As soon as the physician permits, the patient may be out of bed. A patient with this

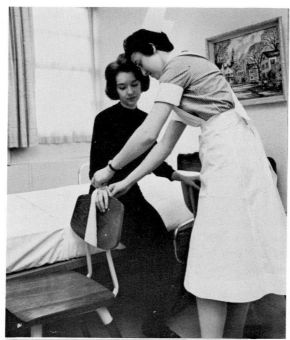

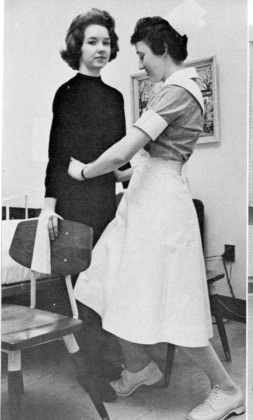

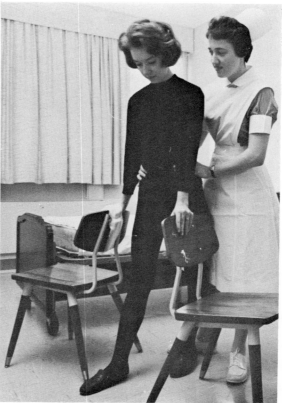

FIG. 34-15. Preparing the patient following a cerebrovascular accident. (*Left*) Assisting the patient to a standing position. First, the nurse makes sure that the patient's hands are firmly secured to the back of a chair to prevent slipping when the body weight is supported on them. (*Bottom, left*) Note the nurse stabilizing the patient's knee. (*Bottom, right*) Standing position.

condition tends to lose his sense of balance rapidly. He needs to learn to balance himself in the sitting position before he can be expected to balance in the standing position. The bed should be in a low position, so that his feet can rest on the floor. (Place a chair under his feet if an adjustable bed is not available.) Extend the patient's unaffected arm with his hand flat on the bed behind him to assist in balancing him. The nurse stands in front of the patient to observe and, if necessary, to help him to maintain this posture. A change in color, shortness of breath, increasing pulse rate or profuse perspiration is an indication that he should be placed in bed again. The sitting time is increased as rapidly as the patient's condition permits.

STANDING BALANCE. As soon as he is able to balance while sitting, he is taught standing balance. He should wear walking shoes with a strong shank for all ambulation activities. Seat the patient on the edge of the bed, and place a straight-back chair on each side of him (Fig. 34-15). If the patient lacks strength to grasp and to push the chair with his affected hand, the hand can be tied to the top of the chair. This stabilization gives the patient greater support. The nurse may help the patient to come to a standing position by grasping him around the waist and supporting his affected knee with the side of her knee. This support will prevent the patient's affected knee from buckling (Fig. 34-15). The patient should be reminded to lean forward when he comes from a sitting to a standing position. The patient's arms must be left free for balance and support. The nurse stands behind the patient and stabilizes him at his waist (Fig. 34-15). It is well to put a waistband or a belt (a scultetus binder can serve as a waistband) around the patient's waist, so that the nurse can grasp it for patient support. Dizziness, pallor and an increasing pulse rate indicate that the patient should be permitted to rest in a sitting position, and if the symptoms continue, the patient should be put back in bed. With repeated effort the patient will tolerate this activity for longer periods.

If the patient has difficulty in achieving standing balance, a tilt table will help him assume an upright position. There should be frequent periods of standing and walking throughout the day.

SUPPORTS AND SPECIAL EXERCISES. If the patient has a weakened or absent quadriceps muscle, support for the knee joint with a posterior knee splint may be advisable. Reflex contractures of the muscles of stance are brought into play by putting on a posterior knee brace (temporary fiber glass splints may be used) and standing the patient. Splinting of the extremity and early standing accomplish the following: (1) they keep muscles in good tonus through reflex action, (2) they give the patient a better command of balance,

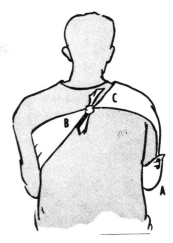

FIG. 34-16. Sling support to prevent subluxation of the shoulder. The sling should support the wrist and the hand; there should be no pull at the shoulder. (Strike Back at Stroke, Publication No. 596, p. 33, Public Health Service, Washington, D.C., U.S. Dept. Health, Education and Welfare)

and (3) they prevent loss of position sense. After a period of time has elapsed, the physician determines whether the patient needs to be fitted with a short or a long leg brace. As the patient gains in strength, he can begin to walk alone, using an adjustable aluminum cane. In the beginning a three- or four-prong cane provides the patient with a more stable support.

If the patient's arm is paralyzed completely, subluxation (incomplete dislocation) can occur. The weight of the paralyzed arm causes the incomplete dislocation at the shoulder. A sling (Fig. 34-16) prevents subluxation when the patient is ambulating and a pillow support or an arm chair will aid its prevention when he is seated.

Another painful and difficult condition to reverse is frozen shoulder, which comes as a result of lack of motion. The sling must be taken off at intervals to permit the patient to exercise. He may exercise his affected arm by raising and lowering it with his unaffected one. A clothesline may be strung through a pulley attached to a door jamb (or over a shower rod) and tied on the affected hand. The patient pulls the rope up and down with his unaffected hand and so exercises his own affected arm and shoulder. The combination of sling support and range-of-motion exercises will prevent the painful frozen, subluxated shoulder.

By changing the position of the chair, other shoulder motions may be achieved. When the patient is seated, the arm should not remain limply in his lap but should be elevated on a support. The patient is instructed to flex his affected wrist at frequent intervals and to move all the joints of his affected fingers.

The patient is taught to assist in his personal hygiene as soon as he is able to sit up. *Have the patient immediately transfer all self-care activities to the unaffected side.* Grooming activities may be done with one hand. He should be encouraged to brush his teeth, comb his hair, and bathe and feed himself. The unaffected side is thereby strengthened with use.

Dressing Activities. The morale of the patient will improve if he can do his ambulatory activities while he is fully dressed. The family is instructed to bring in clothing that is preferably a size larger than that normally worn. Clothing fitted with front fasteners is the most suitable. The patient has better balance if he does most of his dressing activities while he is seated. In the early stages the patient needs to be helped or supported by the nurse. He should not be permitted to become overfatigued and discouraged.

The following procedure for dressing has been found to be workable for many patients. However, the nurse must use judgment in assisting the patient to work out individual modifications.

UNDERCLOTHING. Use a flare leg or boxer-type shorts with an elastic waistband. With the unaffected hand bring the affected ankle to rest on the top of the unaffected knee. Place the unaffected hand through the outside opening of the shorts. With the hand through the shorts, grasp the affected foot firmly and shake the garment off the unaffected hand and well over the affected foot. While holding the garment, allow the affected foot to rest on the floor. Draw the shorts up the affected leg. Then put the unaffected extremity into the shorts, and pull them up as far as possible. To complete the procedure of bringing the shorts up over the buttocks, roll to each side, and pull up the shorts on the opposite side.

UNDERSHIRT. Place the undershirt in the lap, back up. Thread the paralyzed arm through the appropriate armhole to above the elbow. Introduce the normal arm through its armhole. With the good arm pull the garment on the affected side up to the shoulder and over the head, and adjust the garment with the normal hand.

BRASSIERE. Stabilize one end of the garment with the affected arm while fastening it in the front with the unaffected hand. Slide the garment around the body, so that the fastener is in the back. With the unaffected hand, pull the affected arm through the strap and place the strap over the shoulder. Then place the unaffected arm through the other strap.

SHIRT, BLOUSE OF FRONT-FASTENING DRESS. Button the cuff on the normal side. Thread the sleeve over the paralyzed arm to the shoulder. Place the hand and the arm through the other sleeve. Button the sleeve on the affected side. It is wise to wear collars a size larger than normal, because buttoning a tight neckband is difficult. Snap-on ties may be worn, or four-in-hand ties may be loosened and removed over the head without untying.

TROUSERS. The use of suspenders makes it easier to pull up the trousers. Trousers are put on in the same manner as shorts. If the patient prefers, he can pull the shorts and the trousers up over the buttocks at the same time. When more balance has been achieved, an over-the-head type of garment (dress, slip, sweater) is put on in the same manner as is the undershirt. It is suggested that stretchable clothing be used.

Preparing the Patient and the Family for Discharge. The patient's family plays an important role in his recovery. They may have difficulty in accepting the patient's disability and be unrealistic in their expectations. Help the family to feel that the patient can care for himself. Assure them that their loving and warm interest in the patient is part of his therapy. The family needs to be informed that the rehabilitation of the hemiplegic patient requires many months and progress may be slow. All should approach the patient with an optimistic and encouraging attitude.

The patient is apt to have some brain damage, and he may be emotionally labile. The family should be prepared to expect occasional episodes of emotional instability. The patient may laugh or cry easily, and he is likely to become depressed. Explain to the family that his laughing does not necessarily mean the patient is glad nor does crying mean that he is sad. The family can help by supporting the patient and praising him for the progress that is being made. The pamphlet *Strike Back At Stroke*** has pictorial and written instruction that may be useful to the patient and his family.

A shower is more convenient than a tub for the hemiplegic patient. Sitting on a stool of medium height with rubber suction tips will permit him to wash with greater ease. A long-handled bath brush with a soap container is helpful to the patient who has only one functional hand. If a shower is not available, a stool may be placed in the tub and a portable shower hose attached to the faucet. Handrails may be attached by the bathtub and the toilet. There are numerous self-help devices on the market that can assist the patient in his activities of daily living.

When feasible, it is best if the patient can return to work or some modification of his former job. The local or the regional branch of the State Office of Vocational Rehabilitation provides individual evaluation and retraining services, depending on the needs of the patient.

All nurses coming in contact with the patient, whether as members of the hospital health team, public health nurses, office or industrial nurses, should encourage the patient *to keep active*, faithfully adhere to his exercise program, accept his limitations, and yet, confidently continue to remain as self-sufficient as possible.

* Write the Superintendent of Documents, U. S. Government Printing Office, Washington, D. C. 20402.

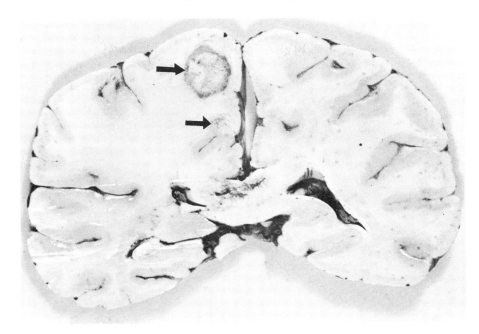

Fig. 34-17. Twin nodules in the brain, representing cerebral metastases from a carcinoma of the lung. (Rudolph Osgood, M.D., Boston)

PATIENTS WITH BRAIN TUMORS AND ANEURYSMS

Tumors of the brain, which appear at all ages of life, originate in the brain (including the roots of the cranial nerves and the meninges) in about 95 per cent of all patients. The remaining 5 per cent are either metastases from primary growths elsewhere in the body (Fig. 34-17) or malignancies of the skull that have ulcerated through into the cranial cavity.

Tumors

Classification

Brain tumors may be classified into three groups: (1) those arising from the coverings of the brain, such as the dural meningioma; (2) those developing in or on the cranial nerves, best exemplified by the acoustic neurinoma and the optic-nerve spongioblastoma polare and (3) those originating in the brain tissue, such as the various gliomas, sarcoma, tuberculoma, gumma and metastatic lesions. Tumors may be benign or malignant. However, because it may be in a vital area, a benign tumor may have effects as serious as a malignant tumor.

Cerebellar Tumors

These are the most common brain tumors found in children. Vomiting, staggering gait and headaches gradually become very severe unless operation is performed. Because tumors in the cerebellum lie very near the medulla oblongata, death may occur very suddenly.

Pituitary Gland Tumors

The pituitary gland is a small, olive-shaped body located in a small pocket just below the optic nerves. The functions of this gland may be increased or decreased by the presence of a tumor in it (see p. 712). Increased function (hyperpituitarism) accelerates growth, which in children results in gigantism. In adults the face becomes coarse and the hands large, a condition called *acromegaly.*

A decrease in function leads to hypopituitarism, characterized by marked adiposity and loss of sexual characteristics. In addition to these disturbances of function, the tumor, by exerting pressure on the optic nerves, causes increasing loss of vision resulting in blindness. Roentgenograms are an important aid in the diagnosis, showing an enlargement or deformity of the bony shell surrounding the pituitary gland.

Angiomas

Brain angiomas, masses composed largely of abnormal blood vessels, are found either in or on the surface of the brain. Some persist throughout life without causing symptoms, others give rise to symptoms of brain tumor. Occasionally, the diagnosis is suggested by the presence of another angioma somewhere on the head or by a bruit audible over the skull. Since the walls of the blood vessels in angiomas are thin, a cerebral vascular accident frequently occurs. In fact, cerebral hemorrhage in persons under 40 years of age always should suggest the possibility of this diagnosis.

TABLE 34-4. Classification of the most common brain tumors

Benign:
1. Meningioma
2. Pituitary adenoma
3. Dermoids
4. Craniopharyngioma
5. Cystic astrocytomas
6. Hemangioblastomas
7. Acoustic neuromas, neurofibroma

Malignant primary tumors:
1. Gliomas

Malignant secondary tumors:
1. Breast
2. Lung
3. Thyroid
4. Kidney
5. Melanoma

(From G.P., *34*:93, August, 1966.)

Symptoms

The symptoms of brain and meningeal tumors may be divided into general and local.

General Symptoms

These are caused by a gradual compression of the brain due to the tumor growth. The pressure of the cerebrospinal fluid usually is increased when evaluated by lumbar puncture. The most common symptoms produced by increased intracranial pressure are headache, vomiting, choked disk and stupor. Headache is most common in the early morning and increases in severity and frequency. Often it is generalized, but even when the pain is local, it gives no clue to the position of the neoplasm. Vomiting occurs often without preceding nausea and without relation to meals. It is of the forceful type described as "projectile" vomiting. Papilledema or choking of the disk is present in 70 to 75 per cent of the patients.

Localizing Symptoms

These are the neurologic signs produced by the tumor and depend on the location of the tumor. The *progression* of the signs and symptoms is important, because it indicates tumor growth and expansion. Because the physician knows the functions of the different parts of the brain, he is able to diagnose the location of the tumor from disturbances of function brought about by its presence. For example, a tumor of the motor cortex manifests itself by causing convulsive movements localized to one side of the body, spoken of as "jacksonian epilepsy." Tumors of the occipital lobe cause blindness of half of each eye (hemianopsia) by involving the centers or the tracts for vision of one side of the brain. Tumors of the cerebellum cause dizziness and a staggering gait, with a tendency to fall toward the side of the lesion, and marked muscle incoordination and nystagmus (rhythmical vibration of the eyeballs). Tumors of the frontal lobe frequently produce personality disorders and a disinterested mental attitude. The patient often becomes extremely untidy and careless and may use obscene speech.

Tumors of the cerebellopontine angle usually originate in the sheath of the acoustic nerve and give rise to a sequence of symptoms that is the most characteristic of all brain tumors. First, tinnitus and vertigo appear, soon followed by progressive nerve deafness (eighth nerve dysfunctions); next, numbness and tingling of the face and the tongue (due to involvement of the fifth nerve); still later, weakness or paralysis of the face (seventh nerve involvement); and, finally, since the enlarging tumor presses on the cerebellum, the cerebellar syndrome mentioned above.

Many tumors are not so easily localized, because they lie in the so-called silent areas of the brain (i.e., areas whose functions are not definitely determined).

Since definite localization of the tumor must be ascertained before an operation for its removal can be attempted, the surgeon frequently resorts to encephalography, isotopic localization, arteriograms, echoencephalograms and ventriculograms (see pp. 771-774).

Treatment

An untreated brain tumor inevitably leads to death, either from progressively increasing intracranial pressure or from primary brain damage. Patients with possible brain tumor should be investigated and treated as soon as possible before irreversible damage sets in.

The treatment of brain tumor is surgical extirpation, when possible, followed by radiation therapy when indicated. In general, patients with meningiomas, acoustic neuromas, cystic astrocytomas of the cerebellum, colloid cyst of the third ventricle, congenital tumors such as dermoid cyst, and some of the granulomas can be cured by surgical removal of the tumor. A complete extirpation of the infiltrating gliomas is not possible. In these patients, biopsy for the establishment of the diagnosis, partial removal, if necessary, and radiation therapy is the accepted treatment. The results of chemotherapy in malignant gliomas have not been encouraging.

Craniotomy is an operation carried out for the extirpation of tumors in or about the cerebral hemisphere. A large flap of scalp and bone is turned down, the dura is incised, and the tumor is removed. After bleeding is controlled, the bone flap is replaced and the muscle and the scalp are sutured.

THE NEUROSURGICAL PATIENT
Objectives and Principles of Nursing Management

When there is a disturbance in the neurohumorophysiologic mechanism, whether caused by operative intervention for an intracranial lesion or trauma, the resultant signs and symptoms are similar. Therefore, certain nursing principles apply to the management of all such patients.

I. To assess the level of the patient's response
   A. Ascertain the patient's level of responsiveness and record in detail on the neurologic observation record (see p. 820)
   B. Assess for variability in levels of responsiveness
   C. Record the vital signs, color and palpable skin temperature every 15 minutes until well-stabilized and according to orders thereafter
   D. Stimulate the patient
      1. Use verbal and painful stimuli (see p. 778)
      2. Request the patient to perform a simple maneuver
      3. Move the extremities

II. To establish and maintain a clear airway
   A. Keep patient in a lateral or semiprone position to facilitate respiratory exchange
   B. Aspirate secretions as needs of patient indicate
   C. Employ assisted ventilatory measures as condition indicates (see pp. 282-287)

III. To monitor body temperature and institute hypothermia measures when necessary
   A. Take rectal temperature at specified intervals
   B. During hypothermia
      1. Control shivering with prescribed medications
      2. Utilize ECG monitoring to detect arrhythmias

IV. To evaluate for signs and symptoms of increasing intracranial pressure
   A. Assess patient for
      1. Decrease in response to stimuli
      2. Fluctuations of vital signs
      3. Restlessness
      4. Weakness and paralysis to extremity
      5. Increasing headache
      6. Changes or disturbances of vision
   B. Control postoperative cerebral edema
      1. Give prescribed adrenalcortical steroids I.V. and I.M. as ordered in postoperative period
      2. Prepare for I.V. hypertonic urea
      3. Institute hypothermia procedures to decrease brain metabolism

V. To perform supportive nursing measures until the patient is able to care for himself
   A. Change the position frequently as pain and pressure responses are variable
   B. Support the patient if convulsive seizures occur (see p. 813)
   C. Relieve signs of periocular edema
      1. Lubricate eyelids and around eyes with petrolatum
      2. Apply light ice compresses in pliofilm (taped over eye) at specified intervals
   D. Put extremities through range-of-motion exercises
   E. Use aseptic measures in management of indwelling urethral catheter

Cerebellar tumors, and tumors of the adjacent structures are extirpated by an operation called **suboccipital craniectomy.** The scalp and the muscles are dissected away from the suboccipital region, and the bone is removed by rongeur. After removal of the tumor, the soft tissues are closed, leaving a defect in the bone.

The Patient With an Intracranial Operation

Preoperative Care. The nurse should become familiar with the symptoms of the patient, so that she can make comparisons postoperatively. These should include observations of paralysis, vision, personality, speech and incontinence. Paralysis of the hand can be tested by the hand grip. Observations of leg movement should be specially noted if the patient is not ambulatory.

If there is paralysis of the extremities, the nurse should apply trochanter rolls to both extremities and position the feet against a footboard. Patients who have speech difficulties, failing vision and hearing loss challenge the nurse's ingenuity. If the patient is aphasic, writing materials or picture and word cards showing the bedpan, glass of water, blanket, etc., may be supplied to help him to communicate. The emotional preparation of the patient is important. Many times he does not realize that he is about to undergo surgery. Even so, encouragement and attention to his needs usually will make him amenable to any form of treatment. The patient is encouraged to ambulate if he is able to do so. The environment should be one that is conducive to rest, and the nurse's approach should be quiet and unhurried. Reassurance

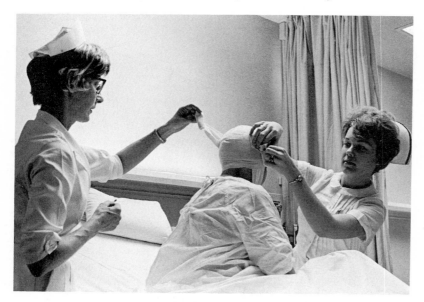

FIG. 34-18. Nurses securing the dressings of a neurosurgical patient in preparing to assist her to ambulate. (Clinical Center, National Institutes of Health)

and consideration for the family is extremely important, because they recognize the seriousness of a brain operation.

Preparation for Operation. The preparation for an operation on the brain or the skull consists first in shaving the entire scalp. Usually, a shampoo of the scalp on the day before operation is advisable. Any infection found on the scalp should be reported. All evacuations of the rectum should be made without causing straining by the patient, as death may occur due to the increased intracranial pressure.

Morphine sulfate usually is not given to neurosurgical patients because of its action as a respiratory depressant and its masking of pupillary signs. Other preoperative *anticipatory* measures include giving preoperative steroids to decrease brain volume and inserting an indwelling urethral catheter to assess urinary volume during the dehydrating operative period. An indwelling spinal catheter may also be used. Surgery may be done under hypothermia.

Postoperative Nursing Management. The nursing surveillance and quality of care in the postoperative period frequently decide the outcome for the patient who has had an intracranial operation. The bed should permit easy access to the patient's head. A turning sheet, placed from the head to the midthigh level, will facilitate moving the patient. The nursing management of the unconscious patient is outlined on pp. 781-783. The equipment needed for the patient is as follows:

Suction set with aspiration catheters
Airway
Oxygen
Respirator
Sphygmomanometer and stethoscope

Rectal thermometer
Flashlight
Hypothermia mattress (or blanket)
Tracheotomy tray (for patients with anticipated respiratory problems)
Neurologic observation record

Postoperative Positioning. Following operation, the patient should never be left in supine position as long as he is unconscious. Such a position poses two major hazards: (1) hypoxia and cerebral edema may result from posterior displacement of the tongue and blockage of the respiratory pathway; (2) pulmonary infection may develop from the aspiration of nasopharyngeal secretion owing to loss of function of the glossopharyngeal nerve.

The patient should be placed on his side in a natural and comfortable position with the lower leg extended and the upper leg partially flexed. He is supported by pillows to the back, between the legs and under the arm. The patient's position is changed every 2 hours, day and night, and skin care given frequently.

Dressings. The dressing is often stained with blood shortly following operation. It is important to reinforce the dressing with sterile pads so that contamination and infection may be avoided. If the dressing is heavily stained or displaced, it should be reported immediately. A rubber drain is sometimes placed in the craniotomy wound to facilitate drainage. This is usually removed by the surgical staff within 24 hours. The wound is usually dressed on the third to the fifth postoperative day and sutures are removed.

Especially in wounds following suboccipital craniectomy, cerebrospinal fluid may leak through the wound. This complication is dangerous because of the possibility of meningitis. Any sudden discharge of fluid from a cranial or spinal wound should be reported at once.

Patients with suboccipital craniectomy are sometimes dressed with firm adhesive strappings to prevent movement of the head and the neck. In turning the patient, it is important to turn the body and the head as a unit to prevent any strain on the wound that may result in tearing of sutures.

Postoperative Complications. Complications that may develop within hours following surgery include changes in respiration, pulse, blood pressure, pupils and level of consciousness.

A drop in blood pressure, fast pulse and respiration, pale and cold body are usually manifestations of a hypovolemic shock following long operations. This type of shock is best treated by blood transfusion.

Inversely, an increase in blood pressure and decrease in pulse with respiratory failure may indicate increased intracranial pressure. The pressure can be reduced temporarily by tapping the lateral ventricle and removing several milliliters of cerebrospinal fluid. The ventricular tap is done with sterile brain cannula that is attached to the head of the bed at all times. More effective methods to reduce the intracranial pressure include intravenous administration of mannitol and, if the patient is unconscious, hyperventilation.

Aside from the immediate postoperative complications, other complications may occur during the first 2 weeks or later that may endanger the patient's recovery. The most important of these are pulmonary infection, pressure sores, urinary infection and thrombophlebitis. The majority of these complications may be avoided by frequent change of position, nasopharyngeal suction, observation and auscultation for pulmonary complications and urinary bladder and skin care as is described in the care of patients with cerebrovascular disease.

Rehabilitation and Convalescence

The convalescence of a neurosurgical patient depends on the extent of trauma and the success with which treatment was carried out. When a benign tumor is removed successfully, it is most gratifying to help the patient to make his recovery. Good nursing eliminates untoward complications and permits the major emphasis to be placed on regaining function. Gradual exercising of extremities, getting out of bed, and learning to feed himself are devices by which the nurse can help the patient to help himself. Doing everything for the patient hinders his successful rehabilitation.

Close cooperation between the nurse and the physical therapist helps the patient to achieve good muscle function. He should be accompanied when he is walking, because sudden attacks of dizziness or unconsciousness may occur. If aphasic, the patient may have to relearn to talk. This is likely to become a long-term and time-consuming project—one demanding great patience and continual encouragement on the part of the nurse (see p. 763).

With regard to the appearance of the head in the convalescence following surgery, men usually have no problem because of short hair. Women who still have very short hair may wear attractive turbans, scarfs, or a wig. The family must be aware of the limitations of the patient, but should be informed of his progress and how they can help to promote his recovery.

When tumor, injury, or disease is of such a nature that the prognosis is poor, convalescence is geared to making the patient comfortable and as happy as possible. Perhaps he is left with a paralysis, is blind or suffers from seizures. The family is kept informed of the progress of the patient by the surgeon; however, many times the real expression of their emotions takes place after the physician leaves. It is then that the nurse must help them to accept their responsibility. Often the care of this patient is transferred to some member of the family. Whoever is responsible must have proper instruction regarding the physical and the emotional care of the patient. If a family member is not able to give this care, perhaps some adjustment can be made with a visiting nurse to assume part care as needed. The medical social worker may be called in to assist in making financial arrangements or to help in placing this individual in good hands.

Intracranial Aneurysms

An aneurysm is an outpouching, a "blister or bubble" on the wall of an artery. In most cases they are due to a congenital defect in the arterial structure. Aneurysms produce symptoms by enlarging and compressing nearby cranial nerves or by rupturing and causing intracranial hemorrhage. Diagnosis depends largely upon arteriography. The object of any treatment is to stop or to diminish the flow of the blood in the aneurysmal sac. If there is a stalk connecting the aneurysm to the parent artery, it may be possible to do a craniotomy, isolate the aneurysm and place a small clip on the stalk. This would stop all blood flow to the aneurysm. Occasionally, it is possible to put clips on the parent artery above and below the aneurysm. It may be necessary to ligate the carotid artery in the neck or to wrap muscle around the aneurysm. In the latter instance, the muscle forms scar tissue on the wall and possibly prevents rupture.

Nursing Care

A patient admitted to the hospital when he is drowsy, stuporous or in coma with a history of the sudden onset of severe headache a few hours or 1 or

2 days previously is suspected of having a leaking aneurysm. The patient in coma is treated like any unconscious patient. The patient who is alert or partially cooperative must be kept in bed, and to prevent fatal bleeding, he must be prevented from doing anything that requires exertion, such as straining during an enema. Periodic observations should be made for decrease in mental alertness, increase in headache and alteration in size of pupils, and any changes should be reported to the physician immediately. These changes usually signify additional bleeding, and speed of action is necessary if a fatal hemorrhage is to be prevented. The crucial time for a second episode is during the second or the third week after the first hemorrhage.

THE PATIENT WITH MULTIPLE SCLEROSIS

Multiple (disseminated) sclerosis is a chronic, progressive disease of unknown cause that appears in early adult life. In this disease, scattered irregularly throughout the central nervous system, degeneration of the myelin nerve axon sheaths occurs; subsequently, the axons themselves degenerate. The areas of involvement are distributed in patches which are without consistency or regularity, so that the resultant

Affect: Emotional instability

Eyes: Nystagmus; Visual changes (scotomas, blurring); Extraocular muscle paresis (diplopia)

Speech scanning

Motor weakness; incoordination (ataxia, spasticity, intention tremor)

Deep tendon hyperreflexia
Absent abdominals
Ankle clonus
Babinski sign

Chewing and swallowing difficulties

Sensory aberrations: Paresthesias (numbness, tingling)

Sphincteric and sexual impairment

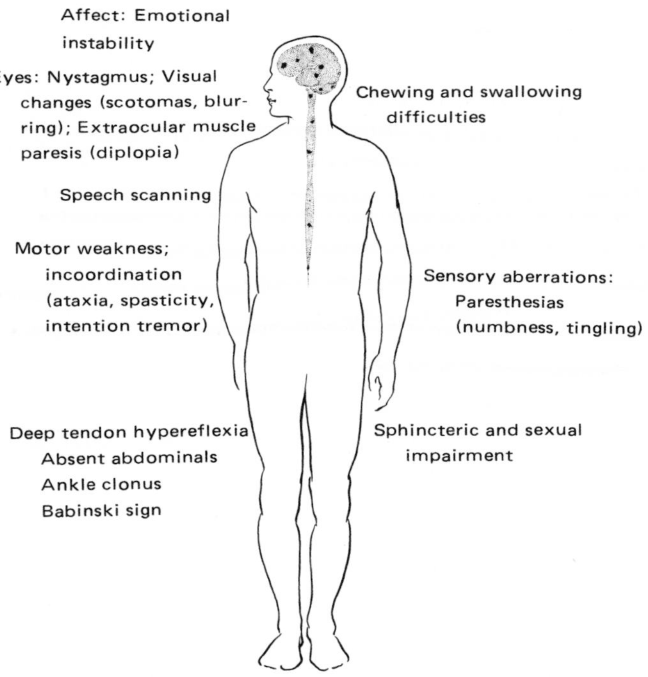

FIG. 34-19. Characteristic signs and symptoms of multiple sclerosis.

symptoms and signs, when nerve conduction along the unsheathed and diseased axons finally is interrupted, are most varied in character.

Multiple sclerosis means "many scars." It is one of the most common neurologic disorders and affects over a quarter of a million persons in this country.

Varied Manifestations of Multiple Sclerosis

This disease is marked by long remissions and exacerbations of several neurologic symptoms (Fig. 34-19). These symptoms are multiple and variable due to the multiple neural lesions. Early symptoms of multiple sclerosis can be easily mistaken for neurosis, peripheral neuritis or spinal lesions since many systems or parts of the body are involved.

Symptoms include visual disturbances, due to lesions in the optic nerves or their connections; nystagmus; "scanning" speech, of slow, monotonous and slurred character; muscular intention tremor and loss of tonicity, due to cerebellar lesions. Spastic weakness of the extremities and loss of the abdominal reflexes are due to involvement of the main motor pathways (pyramidal tracts) of the spinal cord. Euphoria and emotional hyperexcitability result from loss of cortical control connections to the basal ganglia. There may be vertigo, with nausea and vomiting if the vestibular nuclei or their connections are diseased; bladder, rectal and genital disturbances, if the process involves the cord pathways connected with the sacral plexus. The most common group of symptoms includes spastic paraplegia with slight speech disturbance, nystagmus and muscular tremor.

The prognosis for a fairly prolonged life is good. Symptoms abate and recur with increasing frequency and severity each time for many years, death usually resulting from an intercurrent infection, most often of the urinary tract.

Epidemiology

Multiple sclerosis is characteristically a disease of cold, damp climates; it is aggravated by exposure to cold, damp weather and improves when and where the climate is mild and dry. Fatigue, malnutrition and acute febrile infections have been shown to predispose to the occurrence of exacerbations, if not the initial onset of multiple sclerosis. Many investigators believe that allergic hypersensitivity and autoimmunity are factors in the development of the disease.

Treatment

There is no specific treatment for multiple sclerosis. During acute exacerbations, high dosages of corticosteroids may be beneficial. The patient is informed

Fig. 34-20. Evaluating the efficacy of the parkinsonism patient's medication has been a problem, as there are many variables such as concurrent infections and the individual's emotional state that can influence his condition. An electronic device (variable reluctance accelerometer) can be attached to the finger and measure the degree of tremor. After the patient takes an antispasmodic, improvement or lack of improvement may be measured on a more scientific basis. (U.S. Department of Health, Education and Welfare)

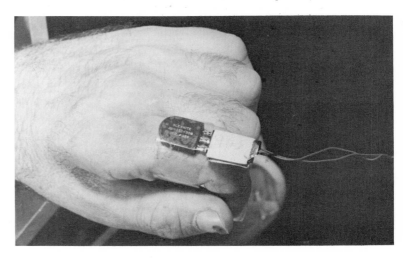

that this drug suppresses the symptoms but does not cure the disease. He must take a maintenance dose to diminish the possibilities of a relapse. The objectives of treatment are *to keep the patient active* and in as good physical condition as possible, and to prevent the complications of urinary infections, decubitus ulcers and contracture deformities.

Nursing Management and Rehabilitation of the Patient With Multiple Sclerosis

Although rehabilitation measures will not alter the disease process, it is the aim of the rehabilitation program to bring about functional improvement, so that the patient can perform his activities of daily living whether he is ambulatory, in a wheelchair or confined to bed. If the patient's disease is not progressing too rapidly, the goal is to return the patient to satisfying employment or to keep him happily engaged in his present employment. He is placed on an individualized therapeutic program that is determined after an appraisal has been made of the extent of his disability and muscle strength. Relaxation and coordination exercises promote muscle efficiency, and progressive resistive exercises are used to strengthen weak muscles. The nurse can encourage the patient to work up to the point of fatigue without becoming exhausted. If certain muscle groups are irreversibly affected, other muscles can be trained to take over their action. Warm baths, packs and muscle relaxants may be beneficial if painful muscle spasm is present. Sometimes the patient presents the clinical picture of hemiplegia, although more commonly he may have the same disabilities as does the patient with paraplegia. Any one extremity or combination of extremities may be involved. Therefore, the principles of rehabilitation of these conditions can be used for the patient who has

similar problems due to multiple sclerosis (see pp. 793-798).

Occupational therapy is prescribed as part of the muscle education program, and it also serves to keep the patient motivated. Hobbies help the patient's morale and give him satisfying interests when he reaches the stage in which he is unable to participate in normal activities.

Management of bladder and bowel control are among the patient's most difficult problems, because there may be sphincter impairment. The sensation to void must be heeded immediately, and the bedpan or the urinal should be readily accessible. If urinary incontinence develops, pads and protective pants or a catheter draining into a collecting bag attached to the thigh will help the patient to feel more socially acceptable. A bowel-training program is effective if there is loss of bowel control (see p. 176).

As the patient's disease progresses, self-help devices that include feeding devices, handrails, canes, braces, wheelchairs and ramps are utilized to maintain independency as long as possible. When vision begins to fail, painting the cane tip and the shoe tips with fluorescent paint helps.

The National Multiple Sclerosis Society conducts a research and educational program. Local Multiple Sclerosis units give direct services to patients. Through group participation the patient has an opportunity to learn of self-help methods in a social environment.

The nurse has the responsibility of emphasizing to the patient and his family the importance of a regular program of work, exercise and recreation. The patient should stay under constant medical supervision. Reassurance and encouragement by those who come in contact with the patient are necessary in helping the patient to maintain a good adjustment to his disease, therapeutic program and environment.

PATIENTS WITH EXTRAPYRAMIDAL DISEASE

Parkinson's Disease

Parkinson's disease is a disease of the basal ganglia, the chief symptoms of which include muscular rigidity, tremor and weakness. The cause of the disease is not always known. It usually is due to cerebrovascular disease, but it also may follow encephalitis, carbon-monoxide or manganese poisoning and electrical shock. Family history is also a factor.

The anatomic lesion found at necropsy consists of atrophy and destruction of the cells of the basal ganglia, especially the globus pallidus, at the base of the brain and the thalamus. Parkinson's disease is America's third most crippling illness, and it affects over 300,000 persons.

Characteristics

In this disease the mental faculties are unimpaired. Early, the patient notices that his limbs are getting stiff, a wax-like rigidity in the performance of all movements develops, and later the tremor begins, often first of one hand and arm (Fig. 34-20), then of the other and later of the head.

The tremor is characteristic. It is a slow, turning motion (pronation-supination) of the forearm and the hand, and a motion of the thumb against the fingers, as of a man rolling a pill. If the patient gets excited, the tremor becomes worse; when he makes a voluntary motion, it ceases, allowing him to perform the most delicate acts, such as picking up a pin. At the same time the rigid limbs become definitely weaker. His facies, station and gait are characteristic. Since his muscles move but little, the face has so little expression that it is said to be *mask-like*, a feature that can be recognized at a glance. The patient stands with head bent a little forward and walks as if in danger of falling on his face. Push him a little forward, and he tends to go forward faster and faster (propulsion); pull him back, and he tends to run backward faster and faster (retropulsion).

Classification

The Parkinson's Disease Information and Research Center classifies the disease into these categories:

1. Parkinson's disease (paralysis agitans or idiopathic parkinsonism)
2. Postencephalitic parkinsonism
3. Other central nervous system disease with some parkinsonian features
4. Symptomatic pseudoparkinsonism
5. Essential tremor (of unknown cause)

The aim of treatment of the patient with parkinson- ism is to keep the patient functionally useful and productive as long as possible. *This is done with appropriate medications, physical therapy and rehabilitation techniques, and patient and family education.

Medication

Symptomatic improvement is afforded in the majority of patients by the long-term use of an appropriate drug or combination of drugs. These are prescribed on the basis of 3 or 4 doses daily, and the dosage is adjusted primarily in accordance with the patient's age, patients over 50 years of age receiving ½ to ⅔ the amount prescribed for individuals in a younger age group.

As the basic medication for control of the majority of symptoms, including rigidity, tremor, akinesia (muscular weakness) and mental depression, the physician may prescribe Artane or Pagitane. If muscle cramps persist, Cogentin may be prescribed. Severe tremor may yield to Parsidol or hyoscine (1-scopolamine). Nervousness or hallucinations may be controlled by Rauwolfia, lethargy by Dexedrine, and insomnia by Thorazine. A promising new drug, L-dopa, has brought about significant improvement in many patients.

Patient and Family Education

It is important that the patient be oriented correctly with respect to the ailment that he is destined to live with. Its nature must be explained to him in detail. The disease may be described as one that affects a small motor control station at the base of the brain— but not the brain itself; It is neither inherited nor contagious, and progresses in severity, but very slowly, the periods of progression alternating with periods lasting from 5 to 15 years or more when there is little or no progress. The disease does not impair intellect, sight or hearing and does not shorten life; it causes rigidity and tremor, but does not lead to paralysis and is painful only if neglected.

Problems of Patients With Parkinsonism

A patient with parkinsonism has severe problems with constipation. Among the factors causing this condition are weakness of the muscles used in defecation, lack of saliva (lost from drooling), lack of exercise, and an inadequate fluid intake. The drugs used for the treatment of the disease also inhibit normal intestinal secretions. The nurse assists the patient in establishing a bowel routine by seeing that he follows a regular habit time, consciously increases the fluid intake, and eats high-residue foods. A raised toilet seat is a useful device to facilitate toilet activities, since the patient has difficulty in changing from a standing to a sitting position.

The patient also has a problem in maintaining

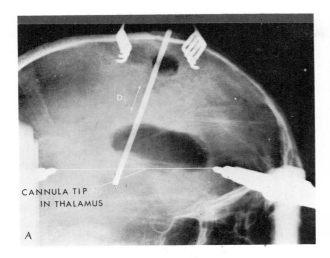

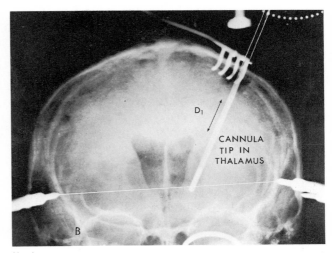

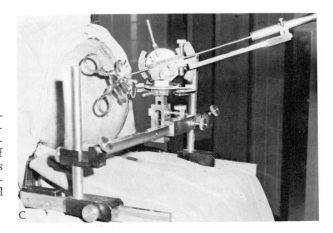

Fig. 34-21. A and B. Radiographs obtained during the cryo-thalamectomy show the cannula in place within the ventro-lateral nucleus of the thalamus, following placement of a permanent lesion, which completely alleviated the symptoms of tremor and rigidity in this parkinsonian patient. C. This shows the cryocannula held in position in the basal ganglia guide during the preliminary aiming procedure. (Cooper, I. S.: Surgical alleviation of the dyskinesias, AORN Jour., 4:70, 1966)

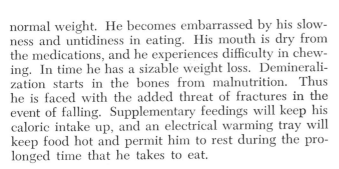

normal weight. He becomes embarrassed by his slowness and untidiness in eating. His mouth is dry from the medications, and he experiences difficulty in chewing. In time he has a sizable weight loss. Demineralization starts in the bones from malnutrition. Thus he is faced with the added threat of fractures in the event of falling. Supplementary feedings will keep his caloric intake up, and an electrical warming tray will keep food hot and permit him to rest during the prolonged time that he takes to eat.

Rehabilitation

Physical therapy is useful in the treatment of the rigid musculature and in the prevention of contractures that occur when affected muscles are not in use. Warm baths with massage and active and passive motion help to relax muscles. Stretching exercises loosen the joint structures. Postural exercises are important, as the patient's head and neck are drawn forward and downward if measures are not taken to prevent this

posture. The gait becomes shuffling and propulsive. The patient also may walk off balance due to the rigidity of the arms. (Arm swinging is necessary in normal walking.) The patient is taught early in the course of the disease to concentrate on walking erect, using a broad base, i.e., walking with the feet widely separated. Instruct him to raise his feet consciously and to walk with a heel-toe, heel-toe gait. He must think while *deliberately* swinging his arms in a reciprocal back and forth motion. A small electronic amplifier (such as used by the laryngectomized person) is useful for the patient with a weak voice from parkinsonism.

The nurse should seek every way possible to encourage the patient to care for his own daily needs. Placing an adjustable mirror on the lavatory and providing a chair for the patient to be seated enables a man with parkinsonism to shave himself. This is just one example of the modifications that may be made by an imaginative nurse.

Faithful adherence to an exercise and walking program helps to delay the progress of the disease. Encouragement and reassurance can be given by all who care for the patient and all those about him by praising him for his perseverance and pointing out that his activities are being maintained through his active participation. A combination of physiotherapy, psychotherapy and sociotherapy may be necessary to help combat the depression that so often accompanies this condition.

Surgery for Parkinsonism

The unsatisfactory results of medical therapy in some patients with Parkinson's disease have led to the introduction of various surgical procedures. The operations utilized in the past include section of the pyramidal tract in the spinal cord or cerebral peduncle, removal of the precentral cortex, ablation of parts of the caudate nucleus and ligation of the anterior choroidal artery.

The procedure most frequently utilized at the present time is the production of a lesion in the ventrolateral, posteroventrolateral and posteroventromedial nuclei of the thalamus. Best results have been obtained in patients whose symptoms are confined to one side of the body and who are under the age of 60 years. Contraindications to the operation include serious cardiovascular disease, mental deterioration and disability produced by akinesia or oculogyric crises.

The operation is carried out under local anesthesia. Pneumoencephalography is done previously, and a cannula or electrode is placed in the desired region through a small opening made in the skull. A skull x-ray at this time shows the location of the cannula in relation to the air in the lateral ventricle. When the tip of the cannula is in the desired location an injection of procaine temporarily relieves the patient's tremor. Following this test a permanent lesion is then made either by freezing (cryosurgery), electrocoagulation or alcohol.

Nursing Care. The manifold types of neurologic, psychological, medical and nursing problems demonstrated by patients with Parkinson's disease almost demand a team approach in finding some solutions. Even the careful selection of patients for surgery is done by a group of specialists, with the result that only a portion of Parkinson patients meet the criteria.

Depending on the overall condition of the patient postoperatively, some type of rehabilitation program is initiated. Transient speech difficulties and psychological difficulties often are apparent. The needs of the patient must be evaluated and met on an individual basis.

In addition to observing the vital signs postoperatively, the nurse notes the muscle strength of the upper and the lower extremities, the presence or the absence of tremor, the quality of speech, and the state of consciousness. A catheter usually is in place and this must be protected from being dislodged. The patient continues to be observed for unilateral weakness. The rehabilitation program and follow-up care continue beyond the patient's discharge from the hospital.

Hereditary (Huntington's) Chorea

Huntington's chorea is a chronic, incurable, fatal disease of hereditary origin, the basic pathology of which is unexplained atrophy of the basal ganglia and portions of the cerebral cortex. The most prominent clinical feature of the disease is the onset in early adult life of uncontrolled, spasmodic jerking movements of the extremities and the trunk. These motions are completely devoid of purpose and lacking in direction; their rhythm is totally irregular, their rate, approximately 80 per minute. All of the body musculature is involved. Facial movements produce grimacing of the most grotesque sort. Speech is affected; it is sometimes hesitant and again explosive in character, and eventually it is incoherent. The gait is similarly disorganized, to the point that locomotion becomes impossible. The sensorium likewise is involved, and in particular the special senses. Equanimity gives way to uncontrollable fits of anger; judgment and memory are lost; deterioration of the intellect, marked by delusions and disorientation, finally leads to complete dementia, and death supervenes.

No treatment has yet been discovered that succeeds in halting or reversing the underlying process. Recent evidence, however, suggests that variable degrees of symptomatic improvement may follow the administration of procaine, e.g., in the form of procaine amide (Pronestyl), given orally in doses of approximately 1 gm. 4 times each day.

PATIENTS WITH CEREBRAL INFECTION

Brain Abscess

True brain abscesses are collections of pus within the substance of the brain itself. From 33 to 50 per cent of them are secondary to middle ear infections. Others are due to septic thrombosis of a dural venous sinus, penetrating wounds and compound fractures of the skull that perforate the dura mater, cerebrospinal meningitis, and infections of the face and the scalp, whereas a few are caused by septic emboli to the brain, often from the lungs and the bones.

Symptoms. The patient has general symptoms similar to those of all mild chronic infections, wherever located: malaise, slight fever, anorexia and loss of

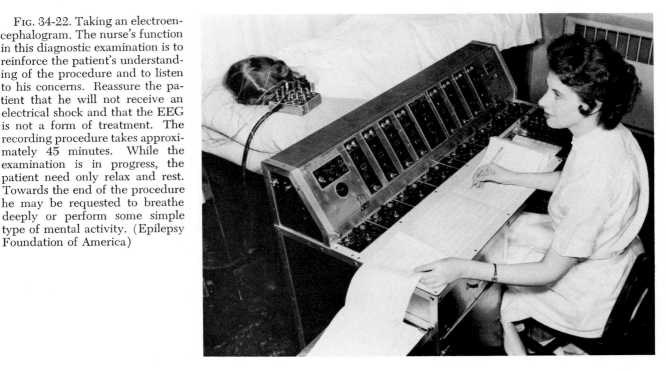

Fig. 34-22. Taking an electroencephalogram. The nurse's function in this diagnostic examination is to reinforce the patient's understanding of the procedure and to listen to his concerns. Reassure the patient that he will not receive an electrical shock and that the EEG is not a form of treatment. The recording procedure takes approximately 45 minutes. While the examination is in progress, the patient need only relax and rest. Towards the end of the procedure he may be requested to breathe deeply or perform some simple type of mental activity. (Epilepsy Foundation of America)

weight. The signs of increased intracerebral pressure usually are slight, since a brain abscess is an area of liquefied brain tissue infiltrated by pus which, unlike a tumor, unless surrounded by a zone of edema, adds little to the contents in the cranial cavity. Headache is the patient's most constant symptom; vomiting is common, but seldom is it projectile in type, whereas choked disks appear rather late. Such localizing symptoms as occur are most inconstant and less complete than in cases of brain tumor and, when present, they usually indicate pathology in either a temporal lobe or the cerebellum, since so many abscesses are aural in origin.

Treatment. Brain abscesses, depending on the character of the infection, may subside and heal completely in response to antibacterial chemotherapy, precisely as expected had the infection localized elsewhere in the body. When they fail to give a satisfactory response to conservative measures, surgical drainage of pus with chemotherapy as an adjunctive measure, then is undertaken.

Postoperative Nursing Care. A single abscess may be cured by incision and drainage. After operation the drainage may be copious. Dressings should be reinforced as soon as they become moist and strict aseptic technique is maintained. The patient should lie on his operative side to promote drainage. The chemotherapeutic agents are administered on an exact time schedule because meningitis is an ever-present danger. The nurse should watch these patients carefully for retraction of the head, stiffness of the neck, headache, chills, sweats, etc., symptoms suggestive of a postoperative meningitis.

It is important that the patient be maintained on a high-caloric diet. Palatable forms of carbohydrates and proteins should be administered at 3-hour intervals in addition to the usual diet.

THE PATIENT WITH A CONVULSIVE DISORDER

The Patient With Epilepsy

Epilepsy is a symptom complex characterized by attacks of unconsciousness that may or may not be associated with convulsions, sensory phenomena or abnormalities in behavior. An epileptic seizure is a state produced by an abnormal excessive neuronal discharge within the central nervous system. The basic problem is thought to be due to an electrical disturbance (dysrhythmia) in the nerve cells in one section of the brain. The characteristic epileptic seizure is a manifestation of this excessive neuronal discharge.

Scope of the Problem

There are almost 4 million known persons with epilepsy in this country. It is estimated that 1 in every 100 persons in the U.S. has epileptic seizures and there is an increasing incidence of this condition, probably because of a number of factors. Improved obstetrical and pediatric care salvages babies who previously would have succumbed from cerebral birth defects but who are predisposed to intermittent seizures. The improved medical, surgical and nursing management of patients with head injuries, brain tumors, meningitis and encephalitis saves those whose conditions may produce cerebral changes with resultant seizures. Also, advances in electroencephalography have aided in the identification of patients with epilepsy. Education has served to enlighten the general public and has lessened the stigmata associated with the condition, so that more persons admit that they have epilepsy.

Types

Epilepsy is classified as "genetic" or "essential" if it is based on an hereditary defect rather than an organic lesion in the brain, and as "acquired" or "symptomatic" if it is attributable to organic brain pathology. The genetic type, which usually begins in childhood and persists throughout life, is the presumptive diagnosis in all patients with epilepsy without evidence of organic brain disease prior to the onset of convulsive seizures. Symptomatic epilepsy may result from a traumatic injury to the brain before or during birth or at any time thereafter; it also may appear as a complication of cerebral tumors, vascular lesions or infections of the central nervous system. Convulsive seizures that are not epileptic in origin, and must be distinguished with care from epilepsy, include hysterical convulsions, syncopal or convulsive attacks due to carotid sinus sensitivity, low-calcium and alkalotic tetany, hypoglycemic convulsions and malingering.

Of all the tests now available, the most illuminating is the electroencephalogram, which furnishes positive diagnostic evidence in a substantial proportion of epileptic patients, aids in their classification and serves as a guide in establishing their prognosis (Fig. 34-22). Abnormalities in the electroencephalogram usually continue to be apparent between attacks, or, if concealed, may be brought out by hyperventilation, by sleep or by the slow intravenous injection of Metrazol.

Classification of Seizures

Six major types of convulsive seizure are observed in epileptics: jacksonian, grand mal, focal, psychomotor (psychic equivalent), petit mal and autonomic (diencephalic) types.

Jacksonian Seizures. These are characterized by clonic convulsive movements, or abnormal sensations, which begin in one hand or foot and spread centrally in an orderly "march" to other muscle groups, the manner of progression always being the same. Convulsions may be limited to one extremity and consciousness may be retained, so that the patient may be able to observe the entire episode; or it may be generalized, developing into a grand mal seizure, with complete loss of consciousness.

Grand Mal Seizures. These usually are preceded by an "aura," a sense of dreamy detachment, warning of the impending attack. The signal may be a hallucinatory flash of light or sound. But these warnings are of little or no help to the patient, since the convulsion follows so promptly that he has no time to save himself. Other individuals, however, have no aura, and the first they know of their attack is after it is all over. The convulsion begins with a cry, possibly a scream, and the patient falls as if shot, making no effort whatever to protect himself, and, therefore, he often is injured. At first the body is perfectly rigid, jaws fixed, hands clenched and legs extended (the tonic stage). The muscles of respiration likewise are in spasm; hence the patient becomes cyanotic.

In about 15 seconds the convulsive movements begin. These are slight at first, then become increasingly severe and soon involve practically every muscle in the body (the clonic stage). Often the tongue is chewed; stools and urine may be passed involuntarily. After 1 or 2 minutes the convulsive movements become less violent, the body relaxes, and the patient lies in deep coma, breathing noisily. The respirations at this point are chiefly abdominal. For a few minutes or even hours the patient cannot be aroused, then he begins by degrees to regain consciousness, and finally he awakens, sometimes alert, but usually confused, suffering from headache, malaise and nausea.

Focal Seizures. This type is most often observed in patients with post-traumatic epilepsy and may be characterized by either motor or sensory phenomena. As in the jacksonian type, the symptoms of focal epilepsy are localized on one side of the body or in one portion of an extremity; the characteristic "march," however, that typifies the former is lacking. These patients may exhibit clonic movements of an extremity, a twitching of the face or a turning of the head and the eyes to one side. Following the seizure, the muscles on the affected side may be very weak for a time. Focal seizures may consist entirely of paroxysmal, unilateral sensations of numbness, tingling or, rarely, pain in the distal portion of an extremity. The patient may experience hallucinations of odor, sound, taste or sight that develop and disappear very suddenly and without warning, whereas others describe merely a sense of unreality.

Psychomotor Seizures (Temporal Lobe). These seizures are marked by periods of amnesia, occasionally accompanied by tonic spasm or contortion of the trunk muscles. These patients sometimes perform movements in automatic fashion, appearing dazed or stupid and quite out of touch with their surroundings.

Some sit quietly, muttering or ruminating. Others have "running fits," becoming violent if restrained. Nothing of these events, however, is remembered afterward, the patient being totally unaware of any unusual occurrence.

Petit Mal Seizures. Called also "pyknoepilepsy," these are manifested solely by repeated transient loss or impairment of consciousness. Attacks last only from 5 to 30 seconds and may be scarcely noticeable. The patient, as though momentarily dazed, stops talking, walking or whatever he is doing, and then he resumes, as though no interruption had occurred; to him, the attack was just a blank moment. A rhythmic twitching of the eyelids or the head may be observed during an attack; the patient may jerk his head or make some other automatic motion, sometimes a violent one; a sudden muscular collapse may allow the head to nod, or the patient to crumple, suddenly helpless, to the ground. Whatever its manifestations, petit mal epilepsy is distinguished by its rarity in adults and by the frequency of its attacks, which may recur several times each day.

Autonomic Seizures. An uncommon variant of the disease, these seizures are featured by sudden episodes of extreme flushing or pallor of the skin, sweating, tachycardia, gagging, fluctuations in blood pressure, fever, hyperperistalsis and fear, or some other emotion, which cannot be explained, usually appearing in patients who exhibit other manifestations of epilepsy.

Status Epilepticus. This term denotes a rapid succession of epileptic seizures, which may be grand mal or petit mal in type. If they are of the former type, the patient continues to convulse violently, with only short pauses and without return of consciousness between attacks, heroic sedation occasionally being required to prevent exhaustion. Status epilepticus of the petit mal variety is characterized chiefly by mental confusion, which may persist for many hours.

Treatment

The medical management of epilepsy is planned according to a long-range program, one that will cover a period of many years, and is tailored to meet the special needs of each individual patient. One of the salient features of all such programs is the encouragement to practice regularity: in the matter of the diet, the quantity of fluids ingested, the amount of exercise indulged in, the duration of rest each day, and the timing of all activities, i.e., regularity of schedule.

The aim of medical and nursing management is to prevent a recurrence of seizures. The patient must learn to adapt to his disease and control its manifestations. Encourage him to study himself and also his environment to determine whether certain factors precipitate his seizures (emotional disturbance, fever, new environmental stresses, onset of menstruation). Assure him that activity is good therapy. Above all he must follow his therapeutic regimen explicitly. The exact amount of anticonvulsant medication must be taken at the prescribed time. The medication cannot be stopped or "tapered off" without medical surveillance, because such an action may bring on severe seizures. The drug and dosage depend on the type of seizures the patient is having.

Table 34-5 summarizes the anticonvulsant drugs currently in use.

TABLE 34-5. Drugs used in epilepsy

Drug	Indications	Average Daily Dose	Toxicity and Precautions	Remarks
Diphenylhydantoin sodium (Dilantin)	Grand mal, some cases of psychomotor epilepsy	0.4-0.6 gm. in divided doses	Gum hypertrophy (dental hygiene); nervousness, rash, ataxia, drowsiness, nystagmus (reduce dosage)	Safest for grand mal and psychomotor epilepsy. May accentuate petit mal
Mephenytoin (methylphenylethylhydantoin, Mesantoin)	Grand mal, some cases of psychomotor epilepsy. Effective when grand mal and petit mal coexist	0.3-0.5 gm. in divided doses	Nervousness, ataxia, nystagmus (reduce dose); pancytopenia (frequent blood counts); exfoliative dermatitis (stop drug if severe skin eruption develops)	Does not cause gum hypertrophy
Ethotoin (Peganone)	Grand mal	2-3 gm.	Dizziness, fatigue, skin rash (decrease dose or discontinue)	
Trimethadione (Tridione)	Drug of choice in petit mal	0.3-2 gm. in divided doses	Bone marrow depression, pancytopenia, exfoliative dermatitis (as above); photophobia (usually disappears; dark glasses); nephrosis (frequent urinalysis; discontinue if renal lesion develops)	Do not use alone for grand mal; may aggravate this condition

(Continued on page 812)

TABLE 34-5. Drugs used in epilepsy (*Continued*)

Drug	Indications	Average Daily Dose	Toxicity and Precautions	Remarks
Paramethadione (Paradione)	Petit mal	0.3-2 gm. in divided doses	As for trimethadione	Toxic reactions stated to be less than with trimethadione. Other remarks as for trimethadione
Phenacemide (Phenurone)	Psychomotor epilepsy	0.5-5 gm. in divided doses	Hepatitis (liver function tests at onset; follow urinary urobilinogen at regular intervals); benign proteinuria (stop drug; may continue if patient is having marked relief); dermatitis (stop drug); headache and personality changes (stop drug if severe)	
Phenobarbital	All epilepsies, especially as adjunct	0.1-0.4 gm. in divided doses	Drowsiness (decrease dose); dermatitis (stop drug and resume later; if dermatitis recurs, stop drug entirely)	One of safest drugs. May sometimes aggravate psychomotor seizures. Toxic reactions rare
Mephobarbital (Mebaral)	As phenobarbital	0.2-0.9 gm. in divided doses	As for phenobarbital. Usually has no advantage over phenobarbital and must be used in twice the dosage	
Metharbital (Gemonil)	Grand mal	0.1-0.8 gm. in divided doses	Drowsiness (decrease dose)	Especially effective in seizures associated with organic brain damage and infantile myoclonic epilepsy
Primidone (Mysoline)	Grand mal	0.5-2 gm.	Drowsiness (decrease dose); ataxia (decrease dose or stop drug)	Useful in conjunction with other anticonvulsants
Bromides (potassium bromide or sodium bromide)	All epilepsies, especially as adjuncts	3-6 gm. in divided doses	Psychoses, mental dullness; acneiform rash (stop drug; may resume at lower dose)	Rarely used now. Effective at times when all else fails
Phensuximide (Milontin)	Petit mal	0.5-2.5 gm. in divided doses	Nausea, ataxia, dizziness (reduce dose or discontinue); hematuria (discontinue)	
Methsuximide (Celotin)	Petit mal, psychomotor epilepsy	1.2 gm. in divided doses	Ataxia, drowsiness (decrease dose or discontinue)	
Ethosuximide (Zarontin)	Absence, akinetic, and myoclonic attacks	750-1500 mg.	Drowsiness, nausea, vomiting	Useful in minor attacks in children
Acetazolamide (Diamox)	Grand mal	1-3 gm. in divided doses (0.25 gm. t.i.d. initially). Drowsiness and paresthesias may occur (reduce dose)		
Chlordiazepoxide (Librium)	Mixed epilepsies	15-60 mg.	Drowsiness, ataxia	Useful in patients with behavior disorders
Diazepam (Valium)	Mixed epilepsies	8-30 mg.	Drowsiness, ataxia	Useful in patients with behavior disorders; also in status epilepticus (5-10 mg. I.V. infusion)
Meprobamate (Equanil, Miltown)	Absence attacks, myoclonic seizures	1200-2000 mg.	Drowsiness	
Dextroamphetamine (Dexedrine)	Absence and akinetic attacks	20-50 mg.	Anorexia, irritability, insomnia	Counteracts sleepiness. Useful in narcolepsy
Methamphetamine (Desoxyn)	Absence and akinetic attacks	2.5-10 mg.		

From Chusid, J. G., and McDonald, J. J.: Correlative Neuroanatomy and Functional Neurology. ed. 13, pp. 370-371. Lange, 1967.

Treatment of Status Epilepticus. Treatment of status epilepticus of the grand mal type obviously entails constant observation of the patient and the employment of whatever measures are required to protect him from exhaustion and self-injury. Convulsions, if extremely violent and uncontrolled by other measures, may be treated by rectal instillations of Avertin with amylene hydrate, an effective dosage being 70 mg. per kilogram of body weight, or by intramuscular injections of sodium phenobarbital (0.2 gm.) or paraldehyde (2 to 8 ml.), given at 8-hour intervals. Failure of the seizures to subside, despite these medications, is an indication for the induction of general anesthesia with ethyl ether and oxygen mixtures, supplemented, perhaps, with injections of curare to produce muscular relaxation.

Surgical Treatment for Epilepsy. Surgery is indicated in cases of symptomatic epilepsy due to intracranial neoplasm, abscess or cysts. In addition to the removal of the space-occupying lesions, favorable results have been obtained by the removal of cortical scars due to cerebral trauma or birth injuries and block excision of a localized area of the brain involved with a congenital arteriovenous malformation. The rationale of this kind of therapy is that such lesions, or the brain adjacent to them, act as a trigger mechanism for the production of epilepsy.

The anterior portion of the temporal lobe has been removed in patients with psychomotor epilepsy with encouraging results. Hemispherectomy has been carried out in children with intractable convulsive attacks with hemiplegia due to birth injury or developmental defect. Good results have been obtained with regard to relief of seizures, without increasing neurologic deficit.

Nursing Support During Convulsive Seizure. During a convulsive seizure the nursing objective is to prevent injury to the patient. This includes not only physical support but psychological support as well. Give him privacy and protect him from curious onlookers. The patient who has an aura may have time to seek a safe place. The head should be protected with a pad to prevent injury from striking a hard surface. Loosen constrictive clothing. Push aside any furniture that he may strike during a seizure. If he is in bed, remove the pillows. If an aura precedes the seizure and it is noticed in time, a handkerchief can be inserted between the teeth to reduce the possibility of tongue and cheek biting. *Do not attempt to pry open jaws that are clenched in spasm to insert a mouth gag.* Broken teeth and injury to the lips and tongue may result from such an action. No attempt should be made to restrain the patient during the seizure. If possible, place the patient on his side because he is unable to swallow during a convulsive epi-

sode and a lateral position facilitates drainage of mucus and saliva. After the seizure, keep him turned on his side to prevent aspiration. Make sure he has an adequate airway. When the patient awakens, reorient him to his environment.

Nursing Assessment During a Seizure. A major responsibility of the nurse is to observe and to record the march of symptoms. Note should be made of:

1. The first thing the patient does in an attack, where the movements or the stiffness starts, and the position of the eyeballs and the head at the beginning. (In recording, always state whether or not the beginning of the attack was observed.)
2. The type of movements of the part involved.
3. The parts involved. (Turn back bed covers and expose patient.)
4. The size of both pupils
5. Incontinence of urine or feces
6. Duration of each phase of the attack
7. Unconsciousness, if present, and its duration
8. Any obvious paralysis or weakness of arms or legs after the attack
9. Inability to speak after the attack
10. Whether or not the patient sleeps afterward

Most seizures are controlled by anticonvulsant medication. Status epilepticus is an emergency disorder and may require general anesthesia to control. The focus of uncontrolled jacksonian seizures may be localized by electroencephalography and the area excised with reasonable success. Removal of the anterior part of the temporal lobe is the present therapy for psychomotor seizures.

Patient and Family Education

The complete cooperation of the patient and his family is of the utmost importance. They must have confidence in the value of the regimen that is prescribed and must be taught that eventual freedom from seizures, with or without the continued use of an anticonvulsant drug, definitely is to be expected. It also should be emphasized to those receiving continuous medication that the medicine they are taking is not a habit-forming "dope," but may be taken without fear for many years, if necessary, no harm resulting from its use when it is supervised by the physician, provided that the latter's instructions are followed faithfully.

Of all the services that are contributed by the nurse to the care of the epileptic, perhaps the most valuable are her efforts to reorient the attitude of the patient and of his family to the disease itself. Concepts that reflect all of the ignorance and the brutality that might be associated with the Middle Ages still prevail regarding epilepsy. For other patients there are public

SPACES   LAYERS

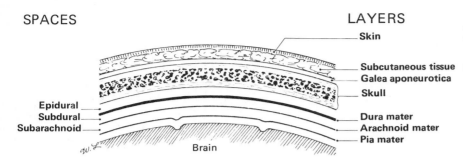

- Skin
- Subcutaneous tissue
- Galea aponeurotica
- Skull
Epidural
Subdural
Subarachnoid
- Dura mater
- Arachnoid mater
- Pia mater

Brain

FIG. 34-23. Diagram showing the various layers from skin to brain. (*Left*) The intracranial spaces are indicated. (*Right*) The various layers of tissue structure.

sympathy and support in abundance; for the epileptic, abhorrence, rejection, ostracism and legal shackles.

For the average person an epileptic seizure is a terrifying or a repulsive spectacle; for the individual who experiences them, every seizure, therefore, is inevitably a source of humiliation and shame, which in turn breeds anxiety, depression, hostility, secrecy and deceit, to which the public reacts with abhorrence, etc., and the vicious cycle is complete. The reaction of shame and the recourse to deceit is not confined merely to the epileptics themselves but extends to their families as well.

In order to escape from this vicious cycle, patients with epilepsy, their families and the public at large need facts. These are the facts:

Epilepsy is not a mysterious disease; it does not reflect the supernatural. The usual case is due to a metabolic disorder, like diabetes. It is not a stigma. Epilepsy is no more disgraceful than diabetes, pernicious anemia or hyperthyroidism. It is not a form of insanity. It does not tend to get worse with time. It can be controlled effectively. It should not prevent the child from completing his schooling or keep the adult from work. *Activity tends to inhibit, not stimulate, epileptic seizures.* Epilepsy is abhorrent to most

people because it frightens them; it frightens them because they do not understand it. Understanding of epilepsy is increasing rapidly, and the public is becoming better informed. As knowledge improves, attitudes change, and complete social acceptance of this disease is only a matter of time. Once social acceptance is achieved, epilepsy in the great majority of patients is no barrier to a normal life.*

The hereditary transmission of epilepsy has not been proved. The matter of marriage and children must be decided on an individual basis but this right should not be denied to the person with epilepsy merely because he has the disease.

Services to Patients. Since epilepsy is a long term disorder, the continuous use of expensive medications may present a sizeable burden to the patient and his family. The National Epilepsy League† provides epilepsy medicine for its members for at least 25 per cent below the retail price. The patient's physician authorizes and signs the prescription, and it is filled by registered pharmacists at the League Headquarters. This important service is most beneficial in enabling patients to take their medications regularly and thus control their seizures. Patients with epilepsy should carry a Emergency Medical Identification card in their wallet or wear an Emergency Medical Signal Device around the neck, wrist or ankle. The American Medical Association lists companies selling these devices.

For many, employment problems still remain the greatest handicap of epilepsy. Studies have demonstrated that the epileptic who is properly placed in his work has a satisfactory job performance. The director of each State Vocational Rehabilitation agency can provide information about vocational rehabilitation. If the individual's seizures are not well-controlled, information about workshop opportunities may be obtained from Epi-Hab U.S.A., Inc.† Counseling and job training is provided for qualified persons through the Veterans' Administration. The U.S. Civil Service Commission now grants government jobs to individuals if

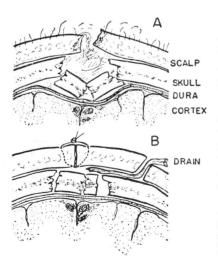

A

SCALP
SKULL
DURA
CORTEX

B

DRAIN

FIG. 34-24. Diagram showing a depressed fracture of the skull. (A) The fracture has not punctured the dura, but it has caused contusion of the underlying cerebral cortex. (B) Shows the relation of the structures after operation and elevation of the depressed fragment. (Penfield: Canadian Army Manual of Military Neurosurgery, Ottawa, Government Distribution Office)

* Paraphrased from Lennox, W. G., and Markhorn, C. H.: J.A.M.A., *152*:1690-1694, 1953.

† Address at end of chapter.

seizures are controlled and the person is otherwise qualified. Private firms are becoming enlightened and the number of employers are increasing who knowingly hire epileptics.

PATIENTS WITH INJURIES OF THE CENTRAL NERVOUS SYSTEM

Injuries to the head are among the most frequent and serious neurologic disorders. We live in an age of unprecedented speed, resulting in accidents that have profound results. The most important consideration in any head injury is whether or not the brain has been injured. The brain dies when its blood supply is interrupted for only a few minutes; there is no regeneration of damaged neurons.

In transporting the patient from the scene of the accident, he should be rolled "log fashion" on a board or stretcher while the extremities are kept in alignment and slight traction is maintained on the head (see p. 959). Injuries to the cervical spine frequently coexist with head injuries. The patient may also be in shock from other body injuries.

Scalp Injury

Because of the many blood vessels, the scalp bleeds readily when injured. Trauma may be an abrasion ("brush wound"), contusion, laceration or avulsion. Before such a wound can be cared for properly, an area about 2 inches should be shaved around the wound. The injection of procaine makes it easier for the wound to be cleaned and treated. If the patient is unconscious, showing evidence of shock, this type of wound is the last to receive attention except for the application of a sterile dressing.

Skull Injury

If there is a depression of cranial bones, the likelihood of increased intracranial pressure is great and must be watched for. When the fracture is compound, the area must be cleansed, débrided and closed as early as possible, because there is the added danger of infection (see Fig. 34-24). Antibiotic therapy is immediately instituted and blood for transfusion is made available.

Fracture of the skull is treated as a neurosurgical condition, because the fracture in itself is of less importance than the injury to the brain that may be produced. For this reason, every patient with head injury, even though it appears to be slight, should be under constant observation for several days.

In fractures of the vault an operation always is necessary if the fracture is compound, or if fragments are so depressed as to press upon or be driven into the brain. After shaving the scalp, the wound is cleaned by cutting away the infected and the de-vitalized tissue. Bone fragments are removed or elevated. A metal or a polyethylene plate can be shaped to fit the opening at a later time.

Fractures of the base are much more serious because of the danger of grave cranial complications and meningitis. The nasopharynx and the external ear should be kept clean, and usually a plug of sterile cotton is placed in the latter channel to absorb discharges. At times repeated lumbar punctures are performed to remove the bloody fluid in an attempt to lessen adhesion formation between the spinal cord and its membranes, which would otherwise occur.

All fractures of the skull should be suspected of brain injury until proved otherwise. The nurse must bear in mind that the patient may have other injuries that are masked by his head injury. The successful treatment of this condition falls largely to the nurse.

Symptoms

The symptoms, besides those of the local injury, depend on the amount and the distribution of brain injury. Fractures of the vault produce swelling in the region of the fracture, and for this reason an accurate diagnosis cannot be made without a roentgenogram. Fractures of the base of the skull frequently produce hemorrhage from the nose, the pharynx, or the ears, and blood may appear under the conjunctiva. The escape of cerebrospinal fluid from the ears and the nose is a diagnostic sign of importance. Bloody spinal fluid, if present, suggests brain laceration or contusion.

Treatment

Depressed skull fractures are treated by operating, after recovery from shock, to reduce the incidence of infection and further brain damage. Foreign bodies and loose pieces of bone are removed.

Bony defects that may result from extensive fractures, from osteomyelitis of the skull or following the removal of tumors involving the skull may be repaired by *cranioplasty*. This consists of the insertion of a substitute material to protect the brain and for cosmetic reasons. Such a substitute may be bone (calf skull), Vitallium, tantalum, acrylate or polyethylene sheeting. There are advantages and disadvantages to each.

Brain Injury

Serious brain injury may occur following blows or injuries to the head, with or without fracture of the skull. When the lesions produced are microscopic, and the immediate symptoms are mild and not of long duration, the condition is spoken of as a *concussion*. The jar of the brain may be so slight as to cause only dizziness and spots before the eyes (spoken of as "seeing stars"), or there may be complete loss of consciousness for a time.

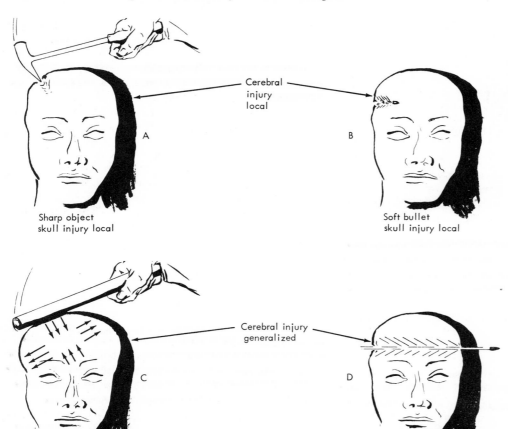

`Fig. 34-25. Compression injury. (A, B) Local cerebral injury—prognosis good. (C, D) Generalized cerebral injury — prognosis grave. (Mullan, S.: Essentials of Neurosurgery, p. 139, New York, Springer)

Cerebral injury local

A

Sharp object skull injury local

B

Soft bullet skull injury local

Cerebral injury generalized

C

Compression skull molding generalized

D

Hard bullet high velocity skull injury local or fragmented

In more marked cerebral injuries (Figs. 34-25, 34-26), with bruising of the brain or hemorrhage on its surface, unconsciousness is present for a considerable period. These are spoken of as *cerebral contusions,* and the symptoms, as would be expected, are more marked. The patient lies motionless with feeble pulse, shallow respiration and pale, cold skin. Often there is involuntary evacuation of the bowels and the bladder. He may be aroused with effort but soon slips back into unconsciousness. The blood pressure and the temperature are subnormal, and the picture is somewhat similar to that of shock. The patient may never recover from this primary state. On the other hand, however, he may recover completely and perhaps pass into a second stage of cerebral irritability. Vomiting is commonly the first symptom indicative of recovery from the stage of primary shock.

In the stage of cerebral irritability the patient is no longer unconscious. On the contrary, he is easily disturbed by any form of stimulation, noises, light and voices, and he may even become maniacal at times. Gradually, the pulse, the respiration, the temperature and the other body functions return to normal. However, recovery is not complete at once. There are commonly residual headache and vertigo and often impaired mentality or epilepsy as a result of irreparable cerebral damage.

Epidural, Subdural and Intracranial Hemorrhage

The most serious injuries are caused by the development within the cranial vault of a hematoma, which may be epidural, subdural or intracerebral depending upon the location. The signs and symptoms of brain ischemia resulting from clot compression are variable and depend upon the speed with which vital areas are encroached upon. In general, a small hematoma that develops rapidly may be fatal, whereas the patient may adapt to a more massive hematoma if it develops slowly.

Epidural Hematoma
(Extradural Hematoma or Hemorrhage)

Following a head injury, bleeding may occur in the epidural (extradural) space. This may result from rupture of the middle meningeal artery, which runs between the dura and the skull; hemorrhage from it causes pressure on the brain. More frequently, bleeding sites along the fracture line produce acute hematomas. Epidural hematomas most frequently occur in the temporal area.

The symptoms are caused by the expanding hematoma. There is usually a momentary loss of consciousness at the time of injury followed by an interval of apparent recovery. Then, often suddenly, signs of compression appear, usually with muscular twitchings or convulsions, because the clot presses on the region of the cortex that sends impulses to the muscles (the motor cortex). There may be focal neurologic signs such as dilatation and fixation of a pupil and weakness and paralysis of an extremity.

Treatment. This is considered an extreme emergency, since marked neurologic deficit or even cessation of breathing may occur within minutes. The treatment consists in making openings through the skull, removing the clot and controlling the bleeding point.

Subdural Hematoma

Not infrequently, either with or without injury, hemorrhage may take place over the brain underneath the dura (Fig. 34-26, right). A subdural hemorrhage is more frequently venous in origin and the blood spreads over the brain surface. A subdural hematoma may be either acute, subacute or chronic, depending on the size of the involved vessel and the amount of bleeding present. Usually the patient is comatose and his clinical signs are similar to those of epidural hematoma. A rising blood pressure with slowing of pulse and respirations indicates a rapidly increasing hematoma. The survival rate for patients with acute subdural hematomas is still less than 50 per cent, although the condition is amenable to early surgical intervention. The clot may be evacuated and the hemorrhage controlled. Postoperative cerebral edema is treated by drugs such as mannitol, urea and steroids.

Chronic subdural hematoma imitates other conditions and may be mistaken for a stroke. In fact, it has been termed "the great imitator." The bleeding is less profuse and there is compression of the intracranial contents. The blood within the brain changes in character in 2 to 4 days, becoming thicker and darker. In a few weeks the clot breaks down and has the color and consistency of motor oil. Eventually calcification or ossification of the clot takes place (Fig. 34-27). The brain adapts to this foreign body invasion and the pa-

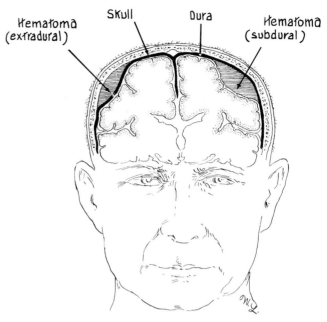

FIG. 34-26. Diagrammatic views showing the difference in the relations of an extradural hematoma (*left*) and a subdural hematoma (*right*).

tient's clinical signs and symptoms fluctuate. There may be severe headache which tends to come and go, alternating focal neurologic signs, personality changes,

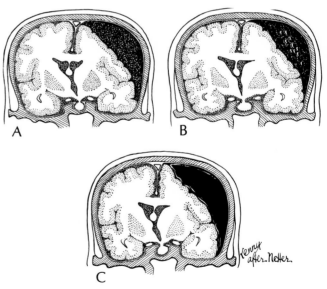

FIG. 34-27. Progressive stages of chronic subdural hematomas. (A) Dark blood spreads widely over brain surface beneath dura. (B) (2 to 4 days) Blood changes, becoming thicker and darker. (C) In a few weeks, the clot breaks down and has the consistency of motor oil. (Adapted from Netter, Frank H.: Clinical Symposia. Summit, N.J., CIBA Pharmaceutical Co.)

TABLE 34-6.

	The Patient With Increasing Intracranial Pressure	The Patient With Shock
Levels of Responsiveness	Variable: Alert and active Lethargic → drowsy Stuporous → comatose	Alert → coma
Pulse	Slowing rate to 60 or below, Increasing rate to 100 or above	Rapid
Respiration	Slowing of rate with lengthening periods of apnea Irregular respirations may occur, with Cheyne-Stokes or Kussmaul breathing	Rapid and shallow
Blood Pressure	Falling diastolic pressure Widening pulse pressure	Falling
Temperature	Moderately elevated Does not usually rise until brain compression is quite extensive	Subnormal
Skin Temperature (by palpation)	Normal until hyperthermia develops	Cold, moist and clammy, unless hyperthermia develops

mental deterioration and focal convulsions. Unfortunately, the patient may be labeled as "neurotic" or "psychotic" if the cause of the symptoms is overlooked.

The treatment of the patient with chronic subdural hematoma consists of surgical evacuation by suction and irrigation of the defibrinated blood through multiple burr holes, or opening of the dura and evacuating the blood.

Intracerebral Hematoma

Intracerebral hemorrhages are more frequently seen in the elderly and occur after a fall. In severe injuries to the brain, scattered petechial hemorrhages or a large parenchymal hematoma may occur. The neurologic signs and symptoms may be masked by coma and confusion. The clot may be evacuated following a craniotomy but the associated mortality rate is high.

Outline of Treatment of Severe Head Injuries

1. Place the patient flat in the bed in a semiprone or prone position with the head to the side.

2. Oxygen therapy—if rhinorrhea, use oxygen tent; if no rhinorrhea, use oropharyngeal oxygen.

3. Keep nasal and tracheal passageways clear of secretions by aspiration as often as necessary.

4. Turn patient from one side to the other every 2 hours.

5. Temperature (by rectum), blood pressure, pulse and respirations every 15 minutes to ½ hour until signs become stabilized.

6. For rectal temperatures of 38.9° C.* or over, start treatment for hyperthermia (see pp. 778-779).

7. Insert indwelling catheter for assessment of urinary volume.

8. Nasogastric tube feedings (300 ml.) every 3 hours when peristaltic sounds are heard.

9. Do not give sedation or morphine deriavtives.

10. Frequent neurologic evaluations to be made and recorded. (See Fig. 34-29.)

11. For convulsions, give 120 mg. (2 grains) of sodium phenobarbital intramuscularly (on physician's order).

The Nursing Management of a Patient With a Head Injury

Upon admission of the patient to the Emergency Room, obtain a complete history as possible. Don't let the observer get away. The following questions have significance:

1. What caused the injury? A high velocity missile? An object striking the head? A fall?

2. Was there a loss of consciousness? What was the duration of the unconscious period? Could the patient be aroused?

3. Was there bleeding from the orifices? Eyes? Ears? Nose? Mouth?

4. Was there paralysis or flaccidity of the extremities?

Among the most important nursing objectives in the management of the patient with a head injury is the establishment and maintenance of an adequate airway. Following head injury, cerebral anoxia from inadequate airway or injury to the brain by contusion, laceration or compression is a frequent cause of death. Therapeutic and nursing activities to ensure that the patient is adequately exchanging air are summarized on pages 781-783. These include keeping the unconscious patient in a semiprone or prone position, providing for endotracheal intubation, establishing effective suctioning procedures, guarding against aspiration and instituting intermittent positive pressure breathing or other ventilatory procedures for respiratory insufficiency.

An equally important nursing objective is constant assessment of the level of responsiveness, since irre-

* 102° F.

versible changes occur rapidly. This nursing priority is discussed in detail on pages 777-778. It includes determining the orientation of the patient, his reaction to auditory and painful stimuli, response to command, presence or absence of paralysis as well as observations of his spontaneous activity. *The nurse is concerned with any change or variation, no matter how subtle, in the patient's level of responsiveness.*

Although the presence of shock is rarely the result of a head injury, it is apt to occur in the patient who has associated injuries. Fracture of the extremities, fractured vertebrae, chest wounds, ruptured internal organs, etc. may be extracranial causes of shock in the patient with multiple injuries. Since the presence of shock is life-threatening, its immediate treatment has first priority. Table 34-6 gives comparative data to assist in the clinical assessment of the patient.

A brain-injured patient who is in shock is not placed in a head-low position because this would increase the likelihood of cerebral edema and hemorrhage. The extremities may be elevated to increase return of blood to the heart. Shock is treated with intravenous fluids, plasma, or dextran until blood transfusions can be started. An indwelling catheter is inserted to measure hourly urinary volume, which indicates adequacy of perfusion.

An intake and output record is maintained to keep the patient in fluid and electrolyte balance. Usually 2,000 ml. of fluids are given daily, but the amount is increased with fever, diuresis, vomiting or other conditions causing fluid loss. After 3 to 4 days on parenteral fluids, nasogastric feedings may be started. Small frequent feedings lessen the possibility of diarrhea and vomiting. Elevating the head of the bed and aspirating the tube before feeding for evidences of residual feeding in the stomach are measures used to prevent distention, regurgitation and aspiration pneumonia. (The principles and technique of nasogastric feeding are discussed on p. 469.)

Although deterioration of the patient's level of consciousness is the most sensitive neurologic indication of impending danger, vital signs are monitored at frequent intervals to assess the intracranial state. The pulse and respirations are slowed and the blood pressure and temperature increases rapidly when intracranial pressure is raised rapidly. If brain compression encroaches upon cerebral circulation, the vital signs tend to be reversed—the pulse and respiration become rapid, and the blood pressure may fall. This is an ominous development, as is a rapid fluctuation of vital signs. A rapid rise in body temperature is regarded unfavorably because hyperthermia increases the metabolic demands of the brain. (The nursing management of the patient with hyperthermia is discussed on pp. 778-779.)

The size of the pupils and their reaction to light is evaluated. Motor function is checked frequently by observing the patient's spontaneous movements, requesting him to raise and lower the extremities, and comparing the power of his hand grip. Notice whether he moves one extremity less frequently than the other. Also determine the patient's ability to speak and note the quality of the speech.

The orifices (eyes, ears, nose, mouth) require careful scrutiny. To determine whether the patient has spinal fluid otorrhea or rhinorrhea, blot the area with sterile gauze. If the discharge is bloody (which is readily observed), a red spot forms on the gauze, but if the discharge also contains cerebrospinal fluid, a clear wet halo encircles the bloody spot. Persistence of spinal fluid otorrhea or rhinorrhea usually requires surgical exploration.

Restlessness may indicate injury to the brain, but it is also a sign that the unconscious patient is regaining consciousness. (Some restlessness may be beneficial.) Make sure that the patient's airway is adequate and his bladder is not distended. Likewise, bandages and casts should be checked for constriction. It is not wise to treat restlessness with opiates and narcotics, because these depress the respiration, constrict the pupils and alter the level of the patient's responsiveness. Chlorpromazine and paraldehyde may be given for restlessness. To keep the patient from hurting himself and dislodging body tubes, side-rails are padded and his hands may be wrapped in mitts or even encased in boxing gloves. Restraints are to be avoided, because straining against them can increase intracranial pressure. Lubricate the skin with oil to prevent sheet irritation. An air mattress is useful. If incontinency is a problem, an external sheath catheter may be used on the male patient. Since prolonged use of an indwelling catheter inevitably produces infection, a catheter employing a continuous antibacterial drip and attached to a closed drainage system is used.

Convulsions following head injury may occur from bruising of the cortex or may be associated with intracranial hemorrhage. Intravenous phenobarbital is used to control seizures and intramuscular Dilantin is employed after control is obtained. (The nursing management of the patient during convulsive seizures is on p. 813.)

Keep the patient oriented to time, place and person, especially if he is emerging from an unconscious state. Adequate lighting may prevent visual hallucinations. The head of the bed may be elevated (20°) unless the patient has associated injuries. Complications following a traumatic head injury include pneumonia, epilepsy, cerebral edema and infection and vascular complications.

The care of these patients encompasses every phase

OBSERVATION RECORD FOR PATIENTS WITH NEUROLOGIC CONDITIONS

Mr. John M. Mallory, a 29-year-old accountant, was recovering from an acute middle ear infection. While taking his antibiotic one morning, a sudden episode of dizziness caused him to fall and strike his right temple on the bathroom washbasin. He was found lying on the floor unconscious. He gradually recovered over a period of 15 to 20 minutes. After being seen in the Emergency Room, he was sent to the Neurologic Unit for observation for a possible subdural hematoma. Upon admission he complained of severe headache but was able to answer questions intelligently.

Date and time	Spontaneous behavior	Levels of response to stimulation	Pupils	Pulse	Resp.	B.P.	Temp.	Intake Output	Remarks
6/8									
8:00 A.M.	Undressed without assistance. Lying quietly in bed.	Gave name, address and telephone number correctly.	Equal	80	20 (eupneic)	120/80	98		
8:15 A.M.	Drowsy.	Roused when name was called.	Equal	82	22 (eupneic)	110/60			
8:25 A.M.	Sleeping.	Mutters when shaken.	Equal	94	26 (rapid and shallow)	140/90	98		Neurosurgeon notified of changing in state of responsiveness.
8:35 A.M.	Sleeping. No spontaneous movements noted.	When pinched on right Achilles tendon, withdrew right leg promptly and muttered. Withdrew left leg feebly.	Right pupil dilated and fixed.	88	16 (thoracic breathing)	140/9			To operating room.

Name of patient:	Mallory, Mr. John M.		*Location of injury:*	Observation for possible subdural hematoma

The neurologic observation record (filled out by nurse) shows the patient's baseline condition and can help personnel caring for him to interpret and evaluate changes. It also serves as a guide in planning care.

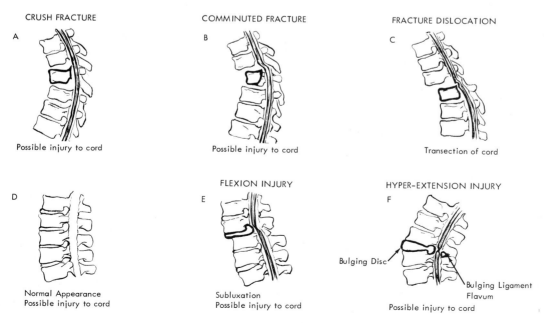

CRUSH FRACTURE

A

Possible injury to cord

COMMINUTED FRACTURE

B

Possible injury to cord

FRACTURE DISLOCATION

C

Transection of cord

D

Normal Appearance
Possible injury to cord

FLEXION INJURY

E

Subluxation
Possible injury to cord

HYPER-EXTENSION INJURY

F

Bulging Disc

Bulging Ligament Flavum

Possible injury to cord

Fig. 34-28. Vertebral trauma. The radiograph may show: (A) a crush fracture; (B) a comminuted fracture; (C) a fracture dislocation; or (D) a normal appearance. The patient whose radiography looks normal may have had (E) a hyperflexion injury or (F) a hyperextension injury which caused severe cord damage at the moment of the accident. (Mullan, S.: Essentials of Neurosurgery, p. 160, New York, Springer)

TURNING THE PATIENT WITH CRUTCHFIELD TONGS WHO IS NOT ON A STRYKER FRAME

If a patient has Crutchfield tongs and is not on a Stryker frame, an order from the physician must be obtained before turning him. The patient's head *never should be flexed*, neither forward nor laterally, and at all times should be kept in a direct line with the axis of the cervical spine.

To Turn the Patient:

The nurse supporting the head gives the commands for turning. Place a pillow between the legs of the patient to prevent the upper leg from slipping forward and jarring the patient's head.

Place a pillow longitudinally on the chest, with the patient's upper arm resting on it. The pillow prevents the shoulder from sagging and pulling on the neck as the patient is turned.

Three persons should turn the patient in a log-rolling fashion, making sure that the shoulder turns with the head and the neck. One nurse should support the head; the second nurse or attendant, the shoulders; and the third person, the hips and the legs.

As the patient is turned, the traction should be moved carefully to keep it in direct line with the cervical spine. The patient's position should be adjusted so that the traction, the patient's head and the cervical spine are in correct alignment.

While the nurse still supports the head in the lateral position, a small pillow is placed under the head to maintain cervical alignment.

and facet of nursing. It may be said without qualification that no group of patients presents greater opportunities for the exercise of clinical judgment and nursing competency and in no category of disease does therapeutic success depend more on excellence in nursing care.

Spinal Fractures and Dislocations

Fractures and dislocations of the spine are serious injuries because of the danger of injury to the spinal cord (Fig. 34-28). They appear most frequently in the fifth, sixth and seventh cervical (neck) the twelfth thoracic and the first lumbar vertebrae because there is a greater range of mobility of the vertebral column in these areas.

Fractures of the Cervical Vertebrae

In fractures of the cervical vertebrae, usually the body is crushed due to hyperflexion of the neck (Fig. 6-1). Such injuries occur in diving accidents, auto accidents and from being struck on the head by a heavy object. During war, gunshot injuries in this area are not uncommon. The danger from cervical vertebral fractures is injury to the spinal cord, which in this area is relatively large, and injury to the spinal cord may produce paralysis of the entire lower body. Because the injury usually results from crushing the cord by acute hyperflexion of the neck, the neck must be extended and the head held well back in the position of extension even in the medical emergency management of these patients. It is desirable to reduce the

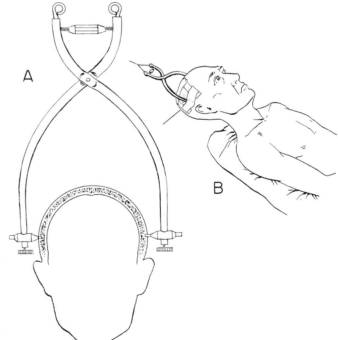

Fig. 34-29. (A) Diagrammatic drawing shows method of application of skull traction. Note that the pegs extend through the outer layer of the skull and thus produce direct skeletal traction. (B) Drawing shows method of protection of tong when applied to the skull. Traction rope extends over pulley at the head of the bed. The head of the bed usually is elevated.

fracture as soon as possible to prevent cord damage.

In the treatment of fractures lower down in the spine, hyperextension can be obtained by the use of a Bradford frame or other appliances. In cervical fractures, however, this is not as easy, and some form of weight extension often is used. Leather-covered slings under the chin and the occiput have been used, but they are uncomfortable. More positive traction can be obtained by the use of Crutchfield, Barton or Vinki tongs apparatus. Through small incisions, the short pins of the tongs are inserted through the outer table of the skull (Fig. 34-29). Traction then can be provided by weight and pulleys. A small longitudinal support is placed between the scapulae, and the head is maintained in a position of extension. With the chest slightly elevated on pillows and the head low, extension can be maintained easily. Extension of the neck is more effective if the head of the bed is raised (counter traction). Usually, 15 to 20 pounds of weight are applied at first, and gradually the weights are built up to 30 pounds. The period of traction is about 4 to 6 weeks. Patients with subluxation may have to wear a plaster or a plastic cast for some weeks after the skeletal traction is removed.

Nursing Care of a Patient With a Cervical Vertebral Fracture. In a compression fracture of the vertebral body an attempt is made to restore the normal contour of the spine by a head halter or tongs, to which traction is applied. The head halter is made of heavy canvas or leather and can cause considerable pressure on the skin. Thin, soft padding inside the halter may make it more comfortable for the chin and the ears. For the male patient, it is sometimes possible to obtain the consent of the physician to remove the halter long enough to shave him. (Traction can be maintained by exerting manual pull on the same parts as the halter, e.g., the chin and the occiput.) Care to the back is achieved by pressing down on the mattress with one hand and washing or massaging with the other. Other pressure areas that especially need attention are shoulders, sacrum and heels. Pieces of foam rubber padding placed under the pressure areas are helpful. If possible, the patient should be turned on his side while he is being fed to minimize the possibility of aspiration of food and fluids. More leeway is permitted in the turning of the patient who has Crutchfield tongs. During this process, the patient must be observed carefully for signs of respiratory impairment.

The foot end of the bed (the patient's head) can be elevated on shock blocks to provide counter traction. The nurse must watch for drainage from the stab wounds and for other signs of infection. The back of the head must be checked periodically for signs of pressure; massage will help. All extremities should be put through the normal range of motion several times daily on order of the physician.

The use of the Stryker frame for this patient is an added advantage, inasmuch as the nurse can turn him more easily and administer care more satisfactorily.

Diversional activity provided by the radio, television, visitors, etc., may be helpful. A frame can be made to hold a book conveniently for this kind of patient. Reassurance and patience are essential. The period of time an individual is thus incapacitated varies with the nature of the problem. Often a plastic collar or a Thomas collar is used to replace traction, and greater freedom is permissible.

The Patient With a Spinal Cord Injury

Nursing During the Acute Phase. *The first aid and later handling of these patients is extremely important, because much damage can be done to the spinal cord by inexpert care.*

At the scene of the accident the patient should be placed in a neutral position (head, back, legs, knees and arms straight). If he is lying in a twisted position, his extremities should be straightened with extreme caution. At least 4 persons should slide him carefully on a board for transfer to the hospital (see p. 959). Any twisting movement may irreversibly damage the spinal cord by causing a bony fragment of the vertebrae to cut into, crush, or sever the cord completely.

As soon as possible, the patient should be evaluated for motor and sensory changes. Motor ability is tested by requesting the patient to move his toes or to turn his feet. Sensation is evaluated by pinching the skin, starting at the shoulder level and working down both sides of the extremities. He is asked where he feels the pinching sensation. It is necessary to record these findings immediately, so that changes can be evaluated accurately. Edema of the spinal cord may occur with any severe cord injury. The patient must be watched constantly for any indications of motor or sensory loss, and these should be reported immediately.

Emergency Medical Management. During the emergency treatment the patient is kept on the board, and he should remain on it while the x-ray pictures are being taken. The transfer of the patient to a bed presents a definite nursing problem. The patient always must be maintained in an extended position. No part of the body should be twisted or turned; nor should the patient be allowed to assume a sitting position. He should be placed on a Stryker frame when he is ready to be transferred to bed. Later, if it is proved that there is no cord injury, the patient always can be moved to a conventional bed without harm; the re-

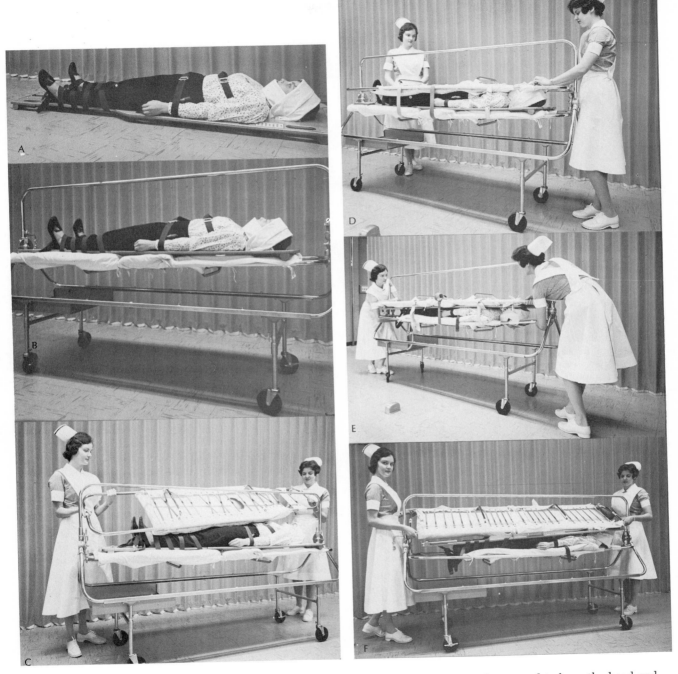

FIG. 34-30. (A) Position of the patient on a transfer board. Note the bandage that is used to keep the head and the neck in a neutral position. (B) The board is placed on top of the posterior frame. (C) The anterior frame is placed in position. (D) The anterior frame is secured with the frame straps. (E) The frame is turned. Observe the position of the nurses' hands while turning the Stryker frame. (F) The posterior frame is removed; then the transfer board is removed.

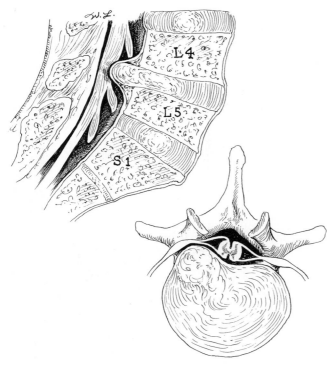

Fig. 34-31. Diagram shows herniation of the nucleus pulposus. The upper drawing shows how such herniation presses upon the structures of the spinal cord. The lower drawing shows how such herniation may press upon the exit of the spinal nerve and produce pain and other symptoms.

verse, however, is not true. If a Stryker frame is not available, the patient should be placed on a firm mattress (preferably foam rubber) with a bedboard under it.

Figure 34-30 A to F shows how a patient should be transferred from a board to a Stryker frame. Place the patient who is strapped to the board directly on the posterior frame. Unstrap the patient from the board. Do not remove the head strappings. Place a blanket roll between the legs. Place the anterior frame in position, and secure the frame straps. Turn the frame so that the patient is in the prone position. Remove the frame straps and the posterior frame. Remove the head strapping with care. Then remove the transfer board.

The patient is watched for symptoms of progressive neurologic damage. Symptoms of cord compression depend on the level at which the compression occurs. It may be impossible in the early stages of injury to determine if there has been an anatomic transection of the cord, since the clinical symptoms of cord transection are indistinguishable from those of cord edema. There is a loss of sensation, with complete paralysis of all muscles supplied by the nerves arising from the

cord at the level of the lesion and below. Therefore, if the patient has no feeling and is unable to move an extremity, cord compression should be suspected. Some neurosurgeons advocate that a laminectomy be done if this paralysis occurs, as this procedure permits direct exploration and decompression of the cord.

Every patient with a spinal cord injury must be watched for symptoms of *spinal shock.* In this condition there is a depression of all the reflexes. The blood pressure falls, and the parts of the body below the level of the cord are paralyzed and without sensation. The reflexes that initiate bladder and bowel function likewise are affected. The patient does not perspire on the paralyzed portions of his body, as sympathetic activity is blocked. Therefore, he must be watched carefully for an abrupt onset of fever. Hyperthermia is treated as outlined on pages 778-779. Usually, the acute period of spinal shock is transient, but residual results may linger for a much longer time.

The patient should be watched closely for bladder and bowel distention. Since the patient has no sensation of bladder distention, urinary tract damage may occur at this time. An indwelling catheter is inserted early in the acute phase. The catheter is removed as soon as possible, so that a bladder-training regimen can be started. If the bowel distention is severe, the use of neostigmine methylsulfate (0.5 mg.) and intestinal decompression sometimes is indicated.

Prevention of Decubitus Ulcers. There is an ever-present, life-endangering threat of decubitus ulcers to the patient with a cord injury. In areas of local tissue ischemia where there is continuous pressure, and where the peripheral circulation is inadequate as a result of the spinal shock and recumbency, decubitus ulcers have been known to develop within 6 hours.

Turning not only aids in the prevention of decubiti but also prevents the pooling of blood and tissue fluid in the dependent areas. The patient should be turned every 2 hours. (If the patient is not on a Stryker frame, a doctor's order is necessary before the patient may be turned.) Every few hours the patient's skin should be washed with a mild soap, rinsed well, and *blotted* dry. Sacrum, trochanters, ischia, iliac spines, knees and heels are especially susceptible to pressure. These areas should be kept soft and well-lubricated with an emollient lotion. Massage should be done gently with a circular motion. The linen under the patient must be kept dry. (See pp. 168-170.)

Prevention of Deformities. The patient must be maintained in proper alignment at all times. It is a nursing function to improvise ways to support paralyzed parts of the body.

The patient is placed in *the dorsal or the supine position* as follows:

The feet are positioned against a padded footboard to prevent footdrop. There should be a space between the end of the mattress and the footboard to allow free suspension of the heels. A wooden block on either end of the mattress prevents the mattress from pushing against the footboard. Trochanter rolls are applied from the crest of the ilium to the midthigh of both extremities to prevent external rotation of the hip joints.

Owing to disuse, the patient will undergo atrophy of the extremities. If ordered by the physician, passive range-of-motion exercises can be started to the affected extremities within 48 to 72 hours after injury. These exercises preserve joint motion and stimulate circulation. A joint that is immobilized too long becomes fixed as a result of tendon and capsule contracture. Toes, metatarsals, ankles, knees and hips should be put through a full range of motion at least 4 and ideally 5 times daily. Range-of-motion exercises can prevent many complications.

If the neurologic examination reveals that the patient has partial cord function, indicating that some nerve units are intact, the patient is not permitted to get up. Activity may produce further injury to the cord. Ambulation activities are scheduled by the neurosurgeon.

Herniation of an Intervertebral Disk (Herniation of the Nucleus Pulposus)

One very distressing complaint is pain in the back. This may arise from various muscular strains or ligamentous sprains, but these usually improve rapidly. Lumbar back pain that persists, is severe, and radiates into the buttock and down the sciatic nerve often is due to pressure on a spinal nerve from a ruptured intervertebral disk.

The intervertebral disk is a cartilaginous plate that forms a cushion between the vertebral bodies. This tough gristlelike material is incorporated in a capsule. A ball-like condensation in the disk is called the *nucleus pulposus*. Incidental to back injury, falls, automobile accidents, lifting strains, etc., the cartilage may be injured. In most patients the immediate symptoms of trauma are shortlived, and those resulting from injury to the disk do not appear for months or years. Then with degeneration in the disk, the capsule pushes back into the spinal canal, or it may rupture and allow the nucleus pulposus to be pushed back against the dural sac or against a spinal nerve as it emerges from the spinal column (Fig. 34-31). This sequence produces pain due to pressure in the area of distribution of the involved nerve. The pain is intensified when the pressure is increased by coughing, sneezing, bending or lifting. Continued pressure may produce degenerative changes in the involved nerve, such as changes in sensation and reflex action. A myelogram usually demonstrates the area of pressure.

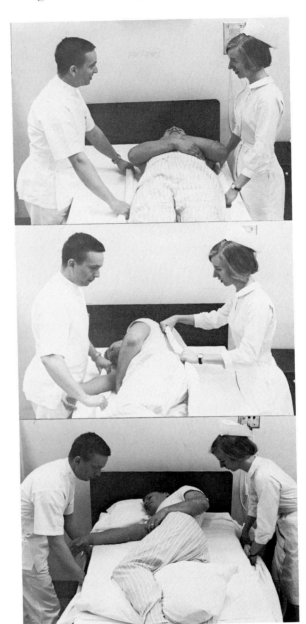

FIG. 34-32. Turning the patient who has had a laminectomy. Two nurses are required. This procedure is known as logrolling, because the patient is turned as a whole. A turning sheet or a drawsheet is kept under the patient to facilitate the rolling. (*Top*) The pillow is removed from beneath the patient's head. Each nurse grasps a side of the drawsheet and the patient is moved to the side of the bed. His arms are folded across his chest. (*Center*) The patient has been rolled like a log by pulling the sheet upward on his left side. (*Bottom*) The turning sheet is straightened and anchored. The patient is made comfortable, with his body put in good alignment by the use of pillows.

Treatment. This injury may be treated by conservative means, rest in bed, heat and massage, reconditioning exercises, traction, fitted back braces, etc. If this does not give relief, a more direct attack is decided upon, removing the basic pathology. Surgery is usually preceded by a myelography and definite localization of the herniated disk. The operation consists of a partial hemilaminectomy, exposure of the compressed root and removal of the herniated disk. Sometimes, an additional stabilizing procedure is added, in which a bone graft from the tibia or the fibula is used to fuse the spinous processes. The spinal fusion has the purpose of bridging over the defective disk to prevent a recurrence of pain or deformity.

Nursing Care. Preoperative preparation is a shave and a hexachlorophene soap scrub of the back, from the midthorax to the middle of the buttocks. In addition, a leg should be prepared if spinal fusion also is to be done. Most patients possess a fear of surgery of any part of the spine and therefore need assurance and explanations all along the way. The patient should be taught how to turn himself as a unit (log-rolling) in order to facilitate postoperative turning. Learning muscle setting exercises will help him to maintain muscle tone postoperatively. The usual preanesthetic drugs are given as ordered.

Postoperatively, the patient's bed is kept flat. There need be no restriction of diet. Frequent turning from side to side relieves pressure, and the change of position is welcomed by the patient (Fig. 34-32). He must be reassured that no injury will result from such turning.

The vital signs are frequently checked, and the wound is inspected for evidences of hemorrhage. The sensation and motor power of the extremities are evaluated at specified intervals.

Sometimes immediately after operation or more often after removal of the sutures, a body cast is applied from the axilla to the groin. This must be inspected for areas of pressure. The patient wears the cast from 6 to 8 weeks and then is fitted for a brace to be worn for an additional 3 to 6 months. Some surgeons keep patients in bed from 6 to 8 weeks in the cast; others allow them to be up and about, their activities limited only by the cast.

Spinal fusion involves the added danger of a longer procedure carrying the potential of greater shock. The patient has an additional wound and cast of the leg, and it may be several days before he is alert and relatively pain-free. Postoperative care also includes attention to moving the operated leg. Pillows must be adjusted for support and comfort, and care must be taken to avoid sudden flexion and extension at the knee, which cause pain. The recovery period is somewhat slower than in those patients with simple re-

moval of the ruptured portion of the disk, because bony union must take place, which requires 6 to 8 weeks.

Other details of nursing care are similar to those mentioned in the care of patients with spinal cord injuries and tumors.

Spinal Cord Tumors

Tumors within or pressing on the spinal cord cause symptoms that are in effect the same as those caused by fracture of the spine, except that they are slower in development. There is usually sharp pain in the distribution of the spinal roots arising from the cord in the region of the tumor, associated with increasing paralysis below the level of the lesion. The level of the tumor usually may be determined by a neurologic examination; however, myelography is necessary for exact localization.

Operation. The treatment consists of a laminectomy with the removal of the tumor. This operation, in which the spinal cord is exposed, is performed with the patient in the prone position. A median incision is made over the spinous processes, and the soft tissues are separated on each side. These bony projections are removed with large bone-cutting forceps, and the posterior part of the vertebral arch is removed to expose the dura. After obtaining a bloodless field, the dura is incised, and the tumor or clot is removed. The dura then is closed, the soft tissues are sutured over it, and an adhesive dressing is applied.

The Paraplegic Patient*

Paraplegia (loss of motion and sensation to lower extremities) most frequently follows trauma from accidents and gunshot wounds but may follow poliomyelitis, multiple sclerosis and cerebral palsy. The patient requires extensive rehabilitation, which will be less difficult if the appropriate nursing measures have been carried out (pp. 822-825). Nursing care is one of the determining factors in the success of the rehabilitation program.

It is usually some time before the patient comprehends the magnitude of the disability. He may be successively depressed and withdrawn or even hostile and anxious. He is involved in a struggle with himself, and in addition he must meet the strenuous physical demands of the rehabilitation program (psychological implications of a disability are further

---

* Quadriplegia (tetraplegia) is loss of motion and sensation involving both upper and lower extremities. These patients require the same meticulous nursing management to prevent complications that are given patients with paraplegia. Their rehabilitation problems and procedures are more complex. Therefore patients with quadriplegia are treated in rehabilitation centers with personnel and facilities that can meet their special needs.

SUMMARY AND PREVENTION OF COMPLICATION OF PARAPLEGIC DISORDERS*

The complications of paraplegic disorders that can be avoided or minimized by general nursing and therapeutic measures are:

1. *Infection of the genitourinary tract. Formation of urinary calculi. Urethrocutaneous fistula.*

   Measures:
   a. Prevention of bladder overdistention.
   b. Observation of sterile precautions in catheterization.
   c. Use of indwelling catheter.
   d. Adequate maintenance of indwelling catheter: twice-daily irrigation of catheter with prescribed solution. Change of catheter twice a week.
   e. Frequent evaluation of patency of bladder drainage.
   f. Frequent urinalysis.
   g. Maintained acidity of urine.
   h. Institution of tidal drainage in accordance with Munro's principles at the earliest feasible time, but not later than 1 week after onset of paraplegia.
   i. Adequate fluid balance with a minimal output of 2,000 ml. every 24 hours, usually necessitating a minimal intake of 4,000 ml.
   j. Earliest possible *regular* ambulation to prevent formation of calculi.
   k. Early recognition of existence of urinary calculi by roentgenograms: flat plate of abdomen once a month. Microscopic examination of urine.
   l. Periurethral abscess formation and resulting urethrocutaneous fistula can be prevented by taping the penis loosely to the abdominal wall to prevent kinking of the urethra on the catheter at the penoscrotal junction.

2. *Development of decubital ulcers.*

   Measures:
   a. Positioning and turning: use of Stryker, Foster, or CircOlectric frame for turning. Turning every 2 hours day and night.
   b. Proper positioning to prevent pressure on heels and other bony prominences. Padding between inner surfaces of knees and between inner malleoli.
   c. Smooth, soft pillows placed transversely on the frame.
   d. Maintenance of dry, clean skin. Skin care every 2 hours immediately after turning. Special attention to perineal area.
   e. Prevention of hypoproteinemia.
   f. High vitamin, high protein, high caloric diet. High protein formula as "between meal" feeding.
   g. Maintenance of normal hemoglobin and normal red cell count.

3. *Fecal impaction. Abdominal distention. Reflex ileus.*

   Measures:
   a. Carefully supervised enema every other day with total evacuation of all fecal material from lower bowels by use of high colonic irrigations.
   b. Repeated, regularly performed digital examinations of rectum with digital removal of impacted fecal material.
   c. Frequent use of rectal tube.
   d. Use of rectal tube and Wangensteen drainage in patients with high thoracic and cervical cord lesions.
   e. Occasional use of Prostigmine Methylsulfate (neostigmine methylsulfate).
   f. Omission of gas-forming foods and liquids.

4. *Ankylosis of joints. Tendon contractures.*

   Measures:
   a. Early physiotherapeutic measures with passive (and active) exercises.
   b. Positioning of joints: use of footboard in supine position. Fifteen-degree flexion of knee joints in supine position. Feet perpendicularly to the floor in supine position, with lower pillow and canvas reaching to the ankles only. Use of orthopedic supports and appliances for finger and wrist joints even prior to ambulatory status.

* Adapted from Coates, J. B., Jr., and Meirowsky, A. M.: Neurological Surgery of Trauma. pp. 303-304. Washington, D.C., Office of the Surgeon General, Department of the Army, 1965.

discussed on p. 160). Moreover, he may become afflicted with decubitus ulcers, genitourinary infections and calculi, joint pains and muscle spasm. Most of these complications are preventable, and every effort should be made to prevent them, because if they occur, they will delay the patient's rehabilitation.

Weight-bearing Activities

A patient with complete severance of the cord should begin weight-bearing activities early, because no further damage can be incurred. Early standing lessens the opportunity for osteoporotic changes to take place in the long bones. Weight-bearing also diminishes urinary infections and the formation of renal calculi and enhances many other metabolic processes. A tilt table helps the patient to overcome vasomotor instability and to gain tolerance of the upright posture. Wearing elastic hose and the application of an abdominal binder may alleviate the pooling of blood in the abdominal area.

At first the patient may be able to tolerate only an elevation of 45° (or less), but gradually the angle of elevation is increased. The patient should be observed closely for signs of intolerance. These include nausea, perspiration, pallor, dizziness and syncope. The patient's blood pressure is taken before getting him up and as soon as he is positioned on the tilt table, since periods of recumbency favor the development of orthostatic hypotension.

Bladder Training

Immediately after a spinal cord injury the patient is unable to recognize the desire to void because of the interruption of the sensory pathways to the brain. Therefore, the care of the bladder is a major problem to the patient and a challenge to the nurse. There are two major objectives to attain: (1) the prevention of infection of the urinary tract and (2) the preservation of the normal bladder capacity and musculature. There should be meticulous management of the indwelling catheter. Sterile irrigations with an antiseptic solution are done daily to ensure patency of the drainage system and to minimize bladder infections. Supportive treatment is given with antibiotics or chemotherapy.

It is desirable that a urologic evaluation be obtained before a bladder program is started. Tidal drainage usually is instituted early, as the periodic filling and the emptying of the bladder simulates normal bladder functioning.

The apparatus shown in Figure 34-33 alternately fills the bladder to a predetermined degree of intravesical pressure and then empties it by a combination of siphonage and gravity flow, the siphonage being interrupted when evacuation is complete. Dr. Donald Munro, of Boston, describes this method as follows:

The solution in the 1,000-ml. container flows about 40 to 60 drops per minute into the reservoir. During this filling, air escapes through the air vent. When the reservoir is filled to the level of the horizontal arm of the T tubes, the solution flows through the tubing to the bladder and rises simultaneously in the glass manometer and tubing (34-33). This continues until the solution, filling both the bladder and tubing, reaches the desired intravesical pressure determined by the height of the curved tubing (34-33). When the liquid reaches the apex of the curved tube, it begins to flow down into the waste bottle, thereby creating suction, the loop acting as a siphon to empty the reservoir of solution and to drain the bladder of its contents. Since the glass tube in the reservoir is one half the size, or less, of that of the bladder connection, the reservoir empties only one half as rapidly. When the reservoir is emptied, air enters the system through the manometer, thus breaking the siphonage system and starting a new cycle. It will be recognized that the size of the reservoir and the rate of the flow of the solution influence the length of the cycle. The complete cycle is usually regulated to last 2 to 3 hours. The distance of the loop above the bladder determines the maximum pressure to which the bladder is subjected.[*]

As the patient begins weight-bearing activities, the tidal drainage is clamped off to permit the patient greater freedom. At this time the patient is observed for signs of leakage around the catheter. When the catheter is removed, the patient is cautioned to be alert for any signs that might indicate that his bladder is full, such as perspiration, coldness of hands or feet, feelings of anxiety, a sensation of fullness. He must develop an awareness of this sensation, as it is an indication that he should void. A position that will increase intra-abdominal pressure is necessary to help the patient to void. It is preferable that the patient's feet rest on a flat surface to allow for acute flexion of the hips and the knees. Instruct him to do several "sit-ups" and then to bend forward. This exercise can be followed by light pressure over the bladder. Thinking about the act of voiding while sipping water may be part of the conditioning routine. The bladder should be emptied as completely as possible. This routine should be followed whenever the patient has the sensation to void or according to a schedule set up by the patient. The fluid intake should be at least 3,000 ml. daily, and the patient should be instructed to chart his fluid intake and voiding times, so that the pattern of bladder function can be determined. Regularity of routine is the key to the establishment of this habit

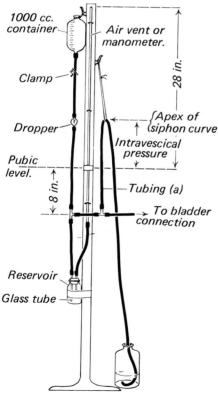

Fig. 34-33. Munro apparatus for irrigating and emptying the "cord bladder." For instructions as to working of apparatus, see this page.

1000 cc. container

Air vent or manometer.

Clamp

28 in.

Dropper

Apex of siphon curve

Intravescical pressure

Pubic level.

8 in.

Tubing (a)

To bladder connection

Reservoir

Glass tube

[*] Munro, Donald: New Eng. J. Med., *212*:229-239.

FIG. 34-34. Sites of neurosurgical procedures for relief of pain. The 9th, the 10th and the 11th nerves leave the brain stem along a line dorsal to which lies the descending trigeminal tract (incision 5) and ventral to which lies the crossed pain pathway from the limbs and the torso (incision 4). (Rhoads, J. E., *et al.*: Surgery: Principles and Practice, Fig. 54-21, Philadelphia, Lippincott, 1970)

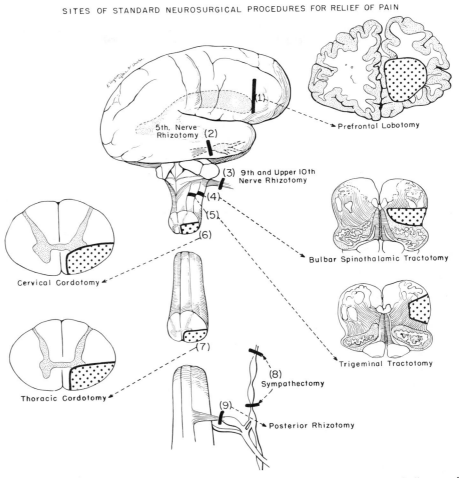

SITES OF STANDARD NEUROSURGICAL PROCEDURES FOR RELIEF OF PAIN

5th. Nerve Rhizotomy (2)

(3) 9th and Upper 10th Nerve Rhizotomy

(4)

(5)

(6)

(7)

(8) Sympathectomy

(9)

Prefrontal Lobotomy

Bulbar Spinothalamic Tractotomy

Trigeminal Tractotomy

Cervical Cordotomy

Thoracic Cordotomy

Posterior Rhizotomy

pattern. The motivation of the patient also determines the success of bladder training. It will be reassuring and encouraging to the patient if the nurse informs him that others have successfully accomplished automatic bladder control. If a reflexly functioning bladder is not attainable, surgical establishment of an automatic bladder is carried out.

Gaining Strength for Ambulation

The diet usually is high in protein, vitamins and calories. The unaffected parts of the body are built up to optimal strength, as ambulating with braces and crutches is the ultimate goal for the patient. This requires better-than-normal strength. The muscles of the hands, the arms, the shoulders, the chest, the spine, the abdomen and the neck must be strengthened, since the patient must bear full weight on these muscles. The triceps and the latissimus dorsi are important muscles used in crutch-walking. The muscles of the abdomen and the back also are necessary for balance and the maintenance of the upright position. To strengthen these muscles, the patient can do "push-ups" when he is in a prone position and "sit-ups" while he is in a sitting position. Extending the arms while he holds weights (traction weights can be used) also develops muscle strength. Squeezing rubber balls or crumpling newspaper promotes hand strength. Through the encouragement of all the members of the rehabilitation team, the patient develops an increased exercise tolerance that is needed for gait training and ambulation activities.

By the application of braces, and with the aid of crutches, these patients can learn to become completely ambulatory and even drive manually operated automobiles. To help the patient to give up his sense of futility and to encourage him in the emotional adjustment that must be made before he is willing to venture into the "outside world" is a role that an intelligent and informed nurse can fill better probably than any other person. She must realize that a too sympathetic attitude may develop a dependence that defeats the purpose of the entire program. She should teach, help when necessary, but not take over activities that the patient can do for himself with a little effort. This type of nursing care more than re-pays itself in the satisfaction of seeing a completely demoralized and helpless patient begin again to live a happy and a useful life.

THE PATIENT WITH INTRACTABLE PAIN

Intractable pain refers to pain that cannot be re-lieved satisfactorily by drugs short of drug addiction or incapacitating sedation. Such pain usually is the result of malignancy, but it does occur in many other conditions, such as postherpetic neuralgia, tic dou-loureux and spinal cord arachnoiditis. Surgery for intractable pain and mental disease involves destroy-ing tissue; therefore, it is resorted to only as a last measure.

Lobotomy

In certain painful states that cannot be relieved by cutting specific nerves or nerve tracts in the spinal cord, it may be necessary to destroy certain pathways in the frontal lobe. These pathways have to do with the patient's interpretation of the pain. After such a procedure the patient still feels the pain, but the emo-tional component of pain is eliminated. The pain is there, but it does not bother the patient. The opera-tion is much less popular than it was a decade ago. The problems of rehabilitation are usually very diffi-cult and require almost constant supervision. Some mental deterioration usually results.

The procedure consists of making an opening in the frontal bone and destroying certain areas of the frontal lobe with an instrument, boiling water, or alcohol.

A simple and effective method of relieving pain while still preserving the intellect is a *percutaneous lobotomy*. Frontal burr holes are made and lesions pro-duced by radio frequency currents. Much of the men-tal anguish of pain may be relieved by this procedure.

Rhizotomy and Cordotomy

These procedures are used in most instances to re-lieve intractable pain. In *rhizotomy* the sensory roots of the spinal nerves are cut before they join the motor root. This operation may be done at any spinal level. This procedure is used frequently in controlling the severe chest pain that may be experienced in lung cancer and is used to give pain relief in head and neck malignancies.

Patients with metastatic malignancies may not be in condition to tolerate a rhizotomy, because this is a major procedure. It is now possible to perform a *chemical rhizotomy* in which Pantopaque is injected into the subarachnoid space. The medication is ma-neuvered over the affected nerve roots by tilting the patient. This renders the sensory nerve roots function-less. The patient's perception of pain is absent but the motor nerve roots are usually not affected.

Cordotomy is a more complicated procedure. The spinal pain fibers are severed in the high thoracic or cervical region. This procedure interrupts or destroys conduction of pain and temperature sense while touch and position sense are preserved. Cordotomy is used most frequently in controlling severe pain of terminal cancer. The surgical approach for cordotomy is the same as for a laminectomy.

More recently, radio frequency currents or radio-active isotopes are used to produce lesions in the anterolateral spinal cord. This is the percutaneous approach and is a simplified form of surgical cordot-omy. Under local anesthesia, a needle is inserted into the neck below and behind the mastoid process. It is guided into the spinal cord under x-ray control and then an electrode is inserted through it. Using radio frequency currents, a lesion is made at the desired spinal cord level.

Nursing Care. Nursing activities described on page 825 for laminectomy would apply to the postopera-tive and the rehabilitative requirements of this patient.

It is important for the patient to know what changes in sensation will take place as a result of surgery. The length of the incision for rhizotomy varies directly with the number of nerves to be cut; the incision for cordotomy is relatively small.

Following a cordotomy the patient is kept flat for the prescribed time period, because there is less ten-sion on the incision and hemostasis is facilitated by this position. A patient with a thoracic cordotomy may be turned in the prone position. The patient with a cervical incision should not have a pillow in the supine position. Trauma to the surgical site is eliminated when the neck is kept in extension. The patient is turned as a unit ("log" fashion) by two persons using a turning sheet to prevent twisting of the body and pressure on the incision.

Test the motion, strength and sensation of each ex-tremity every few hours (or more frequently if neces-sary) during the first 48 hours postoperatively. Hem-orrhage may produce motor and sensory loss and im-mediate surgical intervention is indicated. Feel the patient's skin at intervals to ascertain temperature changes, since the patient is unable to detect them. Pressure sores may develop without the patient realiz-ing it. If there is permanent loss of motor control from a high cervical procedure a bladder training program is carried out (p. 828).

After operation, the nurse must be alert for signs of shock, respiratory distress, bladder disturbances, pa-ralyses and constipation.

Patient Education Emphasis. Since temperature sense is permanently lost, the patient is instructed concerning external temperature changes. Bath water should be tested by a family member before the patient gets into the tub. Because the individual can become frostbitten or sunburned without experiencing any discomfort, protection must be taken against inclement weather. Warn the patient of the danger of impaired circulation and to avoid using constricting clothing, such as tightly tied shoes.

BIBLIOGRAPHY

Books

Alvarez, W. C.: Little Strokes. Philadelphia, J. B. Lippincott, 1966.

Agranowitz, A., and McKeown, M.: Aphasia Handbook for Adults and Children. Springfield, Ill., Charles C Thomas, 1964.

Bendixen, H. H., *et al.*: Respiratory Care. St. Louis, C. V. Mosby, 1965.

Boyarsky, S. (ed.): The Neurogenic Bladder. Baltimore, Williams & Wilkins, 1967.

Caveness, W. F., and Walker, A. E.: Head Injury (Conference Proceedings). Philadelphia, J. B. Lippincott, 1966.

Chusid, J. G., and McDonald, J. J.: Correlative Neuroanatomy and Functional Neourology. ed. 13, Los Altos, Lange, 1967.

Coates, J. B., Jr., and Meirowsky, A. M. (eds.): Neurological Surgery of Trauma, Washington, D.C., Office of the Surgeon General, Department of the Army, 1965.

Davis, M. G., *et al.*: Rehabilitation Nursing: A Source Guide for Instructors. Sister Elizabeth Kenny Foundation, Inc., 1964.

Carini, E., and Owens, G.: Neurological and Neurosurgical Nursing. ed. 5, St. Louis, C. V. Mosby, 1970.

Elson, R.: Practical Management of Spinal Injuries for Nurses. Baltimore, Williams & Wilkins, 1966.

Forster, F. M.: Synopsis of Neurology. St. Louis, C. V. Mosby, 1966.

Gardner, E.: Fundamentals of Neurology. Philadelphia, W. B. Saunders, 1968.

Gurdjian, E. S.: Operative Neurosurgery. Baltimore, Williams & Wilkins, 1964.

Guyton, A. C.: Textbook of Physiology. pp. 651-708 and 758-871. Philadelphia, W. B. Saunders, 1966.

Hooper, R.: Neurosurgical Nursing. Springfield, Ill., Charles C Thomas, 1964.

Kenny Rehabilitation Institute. A Handbook of Rehabilitative Nursing Techniques in Hemiplegia. Minneapolis, American Rehabilitation Foundation, 1964.

Krenzel, J. R., and Rohrer, L. M.: Paraplegic and Quadriplegic Individuals (Handbook for Nurses). Chicago, The National Paraplegia Foundation, 1966.

Lennox, W. G., and Lennox, M. A.: Epilepsy and Related Disorders. vol. 1 and 2. Boston, Little, Brown, 1960.

Lewin, W.: The Management of Head Injuries. Baltimore, Williams & Wilkins, 1967.

Livingston, S.: Living with Epileptic Seizures. Springfield, Ill., Charles C Thomas, 1963.

Mayo Clinic and Mayo Foundation: Clinical Examinations in Neurology. Philadelphia, W. B. Saunders, 1963.

Merritt, H. H.: A Textbook of Neurology. ed. 4. Philadelphia, Lea and Febiger, 1967.

McAlpine, D., *et al.*: Multiple Sclerosis. Edinburgh, Livingstone, 1965.

Rhoads, J. E., *et al.*: Surgery: Principles and Practice. Chap. 54. Philadelphia, J. B. Lippincott, 1970.

Smith, G. W.: Care of the Patient with a Stroke. New York, Springer, 1967.

Toole, J. F., and Patel, A. N.: Cerebrovascular Disorders. New York, McGraw-Hill, 1967.

Articles

Aldes, H. J.: Rehabilitation of multiple sclerosis patients. J. Rehab., 33:10-12, March-April, 1967.

Baxter, C. R.: Three days with Mrs. M. Amer. J. Nurs., 67: 774-778, April, 1967.

Bonner, C. D., *et al.*: The team approach to hemiplegia. Postgrad. Med., 40:708-714, Dec., 1966.

Butts, C. L., and Canney, V. E.: The unresponsive patient. Amer. J. Nurs., 67:1886-1888, Sept., 1967.

Cerebrovascular disease epidemiology. Public Health Service Monograph No. 76, 1966.

Cooper, I. S.: Cryogenic neurosurgery. G.P., 39:96-109, Feb., 1969.

Cotzias, G. C., *et al.*: Modification of parkinsonism-chronic treatment with L-dopa. New Eng. J. Med., 280:337-345, Feb., 13, 1969.

Culp, P.: Nursing care of the patient with a spinal cord injury. Nurs. Clin. N. Amer., 2:447-457, Sept., 1967.

DeJong, R. N.: Treatment of epilepsy. Mod. Treatment, 1:1047-1165, Sept., 1964.

Fangman, A., and O'Malley, W. E.: L-dopa and the patient with Parkinson's disease. Amer. J. Nurs., 69:1455-1457, July, 1969.

Gage, E. L.: Diagnosis of brain tumors in middle age. Geriatrics, 22:150-167, Oct., 1967.

Gardner, M. A. M.: Responsiveness as a measure of consciousness. Amer. J. Nurs., 68:1035-1038, May, 1968.

Greenhouse, A. H.: Modern concepts in cerebral vascular disease. G.P., 35:99-105, May, 1967.

Holliday, J.: Bowel programs of patients with spinal cord injury: a clinical study. Nurs. Res., 16:4-15, Winter, 1967.

Hope-Simpson, R. E.: Herpes zoster in the elderly. Geriatrics, 22:151-159, Sept., 1967.

Hunkele, E., *et al.*: A patient with a fractured cervical vertebrae. Amer. J. Nurs., 65:82-84, Sept., 1965.

Jennings, C. R.: The stroke patient—his rehabilitation. Amer. J. Nurs., 67:118-121, Jan., 1967.

Kast, E. C.: A limited discussion of the treatment of Parkinson's disease. Dis. Nervous Sys., 28:684-685, Oct., 1967.

Kirgis, H. D., *et al.*: Strokes and their treatment. Geriatrics, 23: 144-159, Feb., 1968.

Knapp, M. E.: Spinal cord injuries. Postgrad. Med., 42:A95-A99, Aug., 1967.

LaRoche, L. P.: Head injuries at Cape Kennedy. Amer. J. Nurs., 65:102-105, June, 1965.

Lang, E. F.: Neurosurgical management of intracranial metastatic malignancy. Surg. Clin. N. Amer., 47:737-742, June, 1967.

Large, H., *et al.*: In the first stroke intensive care unit. Amer. J. Nurs., 69:76-80, Jan., 1969.

Livingston, S.: The epilepsies. Disease-A-Month, 3-45, July, 1967.

Locke, S.: The neurological aspects of coma. Surg. Clin. N. Amer., *48*:251-257, April, 1968.

Marshall, A. M.: Neurosurgical nursing with relation to rehabilitation. Rehab. Lit., *11*:342-344, Nov., 1967.

Matheney, R. V.: Cerebrovascular accident and personality organization. Nurs. Clin. N. Amer., *1*:443-449, Sept., 1966.

McDowell, F. H.: Treatment of stroke. Mod. Treatment, *2*:15-114, Jan., 1965.

McHenry, L. C., Jr., and Jaffe, M. E.: Cerebrovascular disease. G.P., *37*:88-101, March, 1968.

Miller, B. E.: "Assisting aphasic patients with speech rehabilitation. Amer. J. Nurs., *69*:983-995, May, 1969.

Musick, D. T., and MacKenzie, M.: Nursing care of the patient with a laminectomy. Nurs. Clin. N. Amer., *2*:437-445, Sept., 1967.

Newman, L.: Physical medicine and rehabilitation for stroke patients. Amer. Geriatrics Soc., *15*:111-128, Feb., 1967.

Owens, G.: Brain tumors. G.P., *34*:93-100, Aug., 1966.

Piskor, B. K., and Paleos, S.: The group way to banish after-stroke blues. Amer. J. Nurs., *68*:1500-1503, July, 1968.

Plummer, E. M.: The MS patient. Amer. J. Nurs., *68*:2161-2167, Oct., 1968.

Ramey, I. G.: The stroke patient is interesting. Nurs. Forum, *6*:273-279, 1967.

Rovit, R. L.: Surgical treatment of epilepsy. Postgrad. Med., *41*:355-365, April, 1967.

Sarno, J. E., Jr.: New concepts on the rehabilitation of the stroke patient. Rehab. Lit., *28*:177-179, June, 1967.

Schwartz, M. L., and Dennerll, R. D.: The employable epileptic: fact, fiction, and contradiction. J. Rehab., *33*:36, Jan.-Feb., 1967.

Selby, G.: Stereotactic surgery for relief of Parkinson's disease. J. Neurol. Sci., *5*:315-342; 343-375, Sept.-Oct., 1967.

Shillito, J.: Head injuries in adults. Hosp. Med., *2*:65-73, Oct., 1966.

Siekert, R. E.: Symposium on neurologic disorders. Med. Clin. N. Amer., *52*, July, 1968.

Stanton, J. H., *et al.*: Care of the patient with infectious neuronitis. Nurs. Clin. N. Amer., *1*:503-510, Sept., 1966.

Stern, W. E.: Tumors of the brain. Calif. Med., *102*:40-44, Jan., 1965.

Symposium: Management of Meniere's Disease. Laryngoscope, *75*:1491-1557, Oct., 1965.

Symposium on Neurologic and Neurosurgical Nursing. Nurs. Cl. N. Amer., *4*:199-300, June, 1969.

Therrien, B., and Salmon, J. H.: Percutaneous cordotomy for relief of intractable pain. Amer. J. Nurs., *68*:2594-2597, Dec., 1968.

The stroke spectrum. (Entire issue) J. Rehab., *29*, Nov.-Dec., 1963.

Tweed, G. G.: Guillain-Barre syndrome. The illness. Amer. J. Nurs., *66*:2222-2224, Oct., 1966.

Victor, M.: Dizziness and vertigo: their neurologic significance. Hosp. Med., *2*:74-83, Oct., 1966.

Webber, M. M., *et al.*: The use of radioisotope scanning in medical diagnosis. Ann. Int. Med., *67*:1059-1083, Nov., 1967.

Wilcoxson, H. L., Cerebrovascular accident: the role of the public health nurse. Nurs. Clin. N. Amer., *1*:63-72, March, 1966.

Wilkinson, H. A.: Neurosurgical management of systemic malignancy. G.P., *36*:90-94, Dec., 1967.

Zohn, D. A., *et al.*: Bell's palsy: management based on prognosis. G.P., *36*:99-103, Oct., 1967.

AGENCIES

Governmental

National Institute of Neurological Diseases and Blindness
National Institutes of Health
Bethesda, Maryland 20014

The President's Committee on Employment of the Handicapped
Washington, D.C. 20210

The Rehabilitation Services Administration
Dept. of Health, Education and Welfare
Washington, D.C. 20201

Voluntary

American Rehabilitation Foundation
1800 Chicago Avenue
Minneapolis, Minnesota 55404

Institute of Rehabilitation Medicine
400 East 34th Street
New York, New York 10016

Epi-Hab U.S.A., Inc.
1200 South Figueroa Street
Los Angeles, Calif. 90015

Epilepsy Foundation of America
Suite 1116, 733 N.W. 15th Street
Washington, D.C. 20005

National Epilepsy League, Inc.
203 North Wabash Avenue
Room 2200
Chicago, Illinois 60601

National Multiple Sclerosis Society
257 Park Avenue
New York, New York 10010

National Paraplegic Foundation
333 North Michigan Avenue
Chicago, Illinois 60601

National Parkinson Foundation and Its Allied Diseases
1501 West 9th Avenue
Miami, Florida 33136

Parkinson's Disease Foundation, Inc.
710 West 168th Street
New York, New York 10032

National Society for Crippled Children and Adults
2023 West Ogden Avenue
Chicago, Illinois 60612

PATIENT EDUCATION

General

Public Health Service
U.S. Dept. of Health, Education and Welfare
Washington, D.C. 20003

Dizziness. Publication No. 1651
Headache. Publication No. 905
Multiple Sclerosis. Publication No. 621
Parkinson's Disease. Publication No. 811
Shingles (Herpes Zoster). Publication No. 1308
Spinal Cord Injuries. Publication No. 1747

Other information available from agencies listed previously.

Aphasia

Public Affairs Press
  419 New Jersey Ave.
  Washington, D.C. 20003
    Houchin, T. D., and DeLanoa, P. J.: How to Help Adults
    With Aphasia.

McGraw Hill Book Co.
  330 W. 42nd St.
  New York, New York 10036
    Taylor, M. L., and Marks, M. M.: Aphasia Rehabilitation
    Manual and Therapy Kit.

Interstate Printers and Publishers, Inc.
  19 N. Jackson St.
  Danville, Illinois 61832
    Boone, D. R.: An Adult Has Aphasia.

American Heart Association
  (Local Chapter)
    Aphasia and the Family.

National Society for Crippled Children and Adults
  2023 West Ogden Ave.
  Chicago, Illinois 60612
    Horwitz, B.: An Open Letter to the Family of an Adult Pa-
    tient With Aphasia. (Reprint from Rehabilitation Litera-
    ture, 23:141-144, May, 1962.)

Institute of Physical Medicine
  New York University Medical Center
  400 East 34th Street
  New York, New York 10016
    Taylor, M. L.: Understanding Aphasia.

Cerebral Vascular Accident

Federation for the Handicapped
  211 West 14th Street
  New York, New York 10011
    Danzig, A. L.: Handbook for One-Handers; A Practical
    Guide for Those Who Have Lost the Functional Use of an
    Arm or Hand.

Public Affairs Pamphlets
  381 Park Avenue South
  New York, New York 10016
    Good News for Stroke Victims. No. 259.

Public Health Service
  U.S. Dept. of Health, Education and Welfare
  Washington, D.C. 20201
    Little Strokes. Publication No. 689
    Strike Back at Stroke. Publication No. 596
    Up and Around: A Booklet to Aid the Stroke Patient in the
    Activities of Daily Living. Publication No. 1120

Springer Publishing Company
  200 Park Avenue South
  New York, New York 10016
    Smith, G. W.: Care of the Patient With a Stroke; A Hand-
    book for the Patient's Family and the Nurse.

American Heart Association
  (Local Chapter)
    Do It Yourself Again.
    Strokes, A Guide for the Family.

Epilepsy

National Epilepsy League, Inc.
  203 North Wabash Ave., Room 2200
  Chicago, Illinois 60601
    Exploring the Brain of Man.
    Epilepsy, The Ghost is Out of the Closet.
    Horizon. (Newspaper)
    The Patient With Epilepsy.

Epilepsy Foundation of America
  Suite 1116, 733 15th Street NW
  Washington, D.C. 20005
    A Patient's Guide to EEG.

Public Health Service
  U.S. Dept. of Health, Education and Welfare
  Washington, D.C. 20201
    Epilepsy. Publication No. 938

Public Affairs Pamphlets
  381 Park Avenue South
  New York, New York 10016
    Epilepsy—Today's Encouraging Outlook. No. 387.

Paraplegia

Paralyzed Veterans of America and
    National Paraplegic Foundation
  935 Coastline Drive
  Seal Beach, California
    Paraplegia News. (Monthly publication)

CHAPTER **35**

Patients with Musculoskeletal Conditions

- *Musculoskeletal Structures and Functions*
- *Patient Problems and Nursing Solutions*
- *Patients with Musculoskeletal Trauma*
- *Fractures of Specific Sites*
- *The Patient with an Amputation*
- *Patients with Bone and Joint Infections*
- *Patients with Arthritis*
- *The Patient with a Bone Tumor*
- *The Patient with Low Back Pain*
- *Deformities of the Feet*
- *Dupuytren's Contracture, Osteomalacia, Osteoporosis, Osteitis Deformans*
- *The Primary Muscular Dystrophies*
- *Myasthenia Gravis*

MUSCULOSKELETAL STRUCTURES AND FUNCTIONS

The musculoskeletal system, composed of bones, muscles, cartilage, ligaments and fascia, provides the body with its structural framework, its protective casing, its power plant, its power tools, its weapons of combat, its static stability, its means of locomotion and a great deal else besides. It is made up of many bones, attached to each other by strong ligaments at the joints. The ends of the bones are provided with smooth coverings of cartilage where they articulate with each other. At other sites, where flexibility instead of rigidity is desirable, cartilage is found instead of bone. Thus, cartilage is found as part of the framework of the nose and the rib cage and as a cushion between the vertebral bodies.

The bony framework acts as a support and a protective mechanism for body organs; also, it moves, because the bones have attached to them a system of muscles that are fastened by strong fibrous cables

called *tendons.* The muscles act as motors by reason of their ability to contract (shorten) and to relax (lengthen) under the control of nerve impulses arising in the cerebral cortex. The power of muscles permits the bones to act as levers with the joint as a fulcrum, to rotate with the joint as an axis, or to remain in a fixed position. In most places in the body the muscles are so placed as to have one set acting as antagonists to the other set; thus, the biceps flexes the forearm on the upper arm, whereas the triceps extends it. The muscles are divided and surrounded by strong fibrous envelopes called *fascia.* In the extremities they surround and give support to the main blood vessels and nerves.

The joints have a smooth lining called *synovium;* this secretes a synovial fluid that lubricates the joints to prevent friction. At points where muscles glide over bony prominences, e.g., the greater trochanter of the femur, or where one bone glides under another, as at the shoulder, or where skin glides over a bony point, as at the elbow, nature develops a gliding mechanism called a *bursa*, a closed cavity in the *areolar tissue*.

The smooth working of this complex system depends on all parts functioning normally and together.

PATIENT PROBLEMS AND NURSING SOLUTIONS

Psychosocial Problems

The patient with a musculoskeletal condition faces not only physical problems but also psychological and social problems. The nurse must be able to meet the needs and to help to solve the problems of patients who cannot engage in normal activities. Orthopedic patients are of all ages; economic problems usually are present. Protracted periods of disability are especially threatening to the wage earner, and the patient may develop a hopeless attitude toward his illness. Many patients faced with long disability are in need of physical, emotional and spiritual rehabilitation.

To help meet the patient's emotional needs, it is desirable to keep him busy. "Action absorbs anxiety" is a rehabilitation axiom that is doubly true in orthopedic nursing. A patient receives security and a sense of purpose when he is participating in a regularly scheduled program of activity. This schedule should be written on the nursing care plan so that all nursing personnel know the patient's program. If possible, the patient should engage in an exercise regimen. Occupational therapy designed with the patient's problems in mind is beneficial. During rest periods the patient may read, watch television or listen to the radio. If the patient is completely immobilized, he still should be consulted about his preferences and encouraged to make some decisions relative to his activities of daily living.

The primary objective in preventive therapy, however, is the avoidance of ischemia through the application of appropriate nursing principles and not merely the abolition by chemical means of its manifestations.

Pain

Most patients with diseases and traumatic conditions of muscles, bones and joints experience pain. Bone pain is characteristically described as aching and boring in nature, whereas the patient suffering from muscular pain states that he is "sore and aching." Because orthopedic conditions require long periods of treatment, the management of the patient with pain is important.

Prolonged pain consumes energy, and the patient in pain has a tendency to become self-centered and dependent. The patient should sense that he is important as a person, and that his problems are understood by the members of the health team. The nurse should observe the patient carefully to evaluate the effect of the physical, emotional and social factors that may be present. Pain is variable and its assessment and nursing management must be individualized.

Nursing Assessment of Pain. What was the patient doing before he complained of pain? Is his body in proper alignment? Is there pressure from traction, bed linen, a cast or other appliances? Is he overly tired from lack of sleep, exciting stimuli or too much activity? Can he localize the pain? How does he describe it? What was the manner of onset? Is there radiation of pain? If so, in what direction does it occur? Is there pain in any other part of the body? What is the character of the pain? Is it constant? What relieves it? What makes it worse?

Regardless of the cause, the presence of pain is exhausting, and every nursing measure should be directed toward its relief. The patient should be positioned skillfully in correct alignment. Painful parts of the body should be supported, and the patient should be moved gently with coordinated movements.

Sharp or sudden movements are painful. Slow, steady movement may be tolerated. Use of a turning sheet can prevent uneven painful pulling on the patient. Care should be exercised not to bump the bed, as this greatly increases discomfort. Provision is to be made for the patient to have regular periods of rest, as this is important in the control of pain.

Heat may be beneficial in relieving muscle spasm, joint and bone pain. Cold applications, especially in inflammatory conditions, may give comfort. Analgesics are given when necessary, but symptoms of physical or psychological tolerance should be watched for and evaluated. Since pain always is worse at night, sedatives, soporifics and ataractic drugs are of value. Of course, the administration of backrubs and warm drinks, and the presence of a sympathetic, understanding nurse are all adjunctive measures in the management of pain. See pages 142-143 for a summary of the nursing management of the patient with pain.

Prevention of Contracture Deformities

It is the aim of orthopedic nursing to prevent contracture deformities and to maintain as much normal function as possible. Pain and muscle spasm produce limitation of motion. Inflammation also limits the motion of a joint and causes the formation of fibrous tissue that in turn may produce fibrous or bony ankylosis. Any weight-bearing joint that has its normal motion restricted for a prolonged period loses motion.

Muscle spasm occurring in the strong flexor muscles causes these muscles to shorten, as flexor muscles are stronger than extensors. The patient is unable to extend his extremities, and thus crippling flexion deformities result.

Positioning. To prevent muscle contractures and loss of joint function the nurse must position the patient in accordance with correct principles of body alignment. His mattress should be firm or placed on a bed board. The bed should be flat, unless otherwise ordered. To keep the patient in a semi-upright position for prolonged periods of time is highly undesirable; this position promotes flexion deformities of the hip. The nurse should exercise ingenuity in the use of supportive devices, such as pillows and sandbags. (Correct positioning in bed is exemplified in Fig. 34-14.)

Muscle Exercises. If a patient becomes inactive as a result of trauma, infection, paralysis or any other cause, the musculature loses strength, joint mobility becomes restricted, and deformities are likely to ensue. To avoid these complications the physician prescribes therapeutic exercises that may be performed under the guidance and with the assistance of the physical therapist or the nurse. The nature and the objectives of the exercise program are dictated by the patient's disease and his general condition. Exercises, properly performed, help (1) to maintain or to improve muscle strength, (2) to maintain or to restore optimal joint function, (3) to prevent deformities, (4) to stimulate circulation and (5) to build endurance. (See pp. 161-167).

Muscle Spasm

These cramps commonly interrupt the sleep of bedfast patients who are elderly and arteriosclerotic. Pain, often intense, is the result of strong involuntary muscular contractions that may be sustained for several seconds or several minutes. The calf muscles are involved most frequently, the effect of their contraction being a forcible extension and inversion of the foot and the plantar flexion of the toes. There is no certainty regarding the precise mechanism responsible for these abnormal contractions; the phenomenon apparently is attributable to an impairment of the blood supply to the lower extremity owing to the mechanical compression of the popliteal or the posterior tibial artery or a major branch of those vessels supplying arterial blood to the affected muscles. As a result of deficient oxygenation, these muscles become abnormally susceptible to nerve stimuli and contract with maximal vigor in response to the weak discharge that is received constantly by way of the motor nerves, a discharge that normally excites a steady but minimal contractile response described as muscle "tone." If such is the case, the cramp represents a terrifically exaggerated muscle tone.

The development of this complication is favored by any posture that permits pressure to be exerted in the region of the popliteal space, behind, immediately proximal or distal to the knee. The prolonged application of such pressure normally provokes sufficient discomfort in the calf muscles to compel an individual, unless deeply asleep, to shift position and thereby to relieve the compression, but individuals with sensory disturbances may be incapable of perceiving this premonitory discomfort. The patients most susceptible to repeated muscle cramps are those with advanced arteriosclerosis whose leg muscles are weak, flaccid and reduced in volume following prolonged immobilization in bed rest, and in whom ischemia of the calf muscles is produced readily as a result of external compression, particularly following sedation, when ischemic pain is not perceived quickly. Pregnancy frequently causes leg cramps.

Treatment. Prompt relaxation of a muscle cramp is achieved through "reflex inhibition," i.e., by vigorously contracting the opposing muscle group. If, for example, the cramp involves the muscles of the calf, relief is obtained by forcibly elevating the foot and the toes into a position of dorsiflexion, simultaneously pressing downward on the dorsum of the foot with the heel of the opposite foot, so that the ankle on the affected side is held at an angle of approximately 90°, a procedure that automatically inhibits the transmission of all motor nerve impulses to the spastic muscle. Massage of the cramped muscles helps to restore the circulation of blood to these anoxic tissues; massage should be performed in conjunction with the maneuver just described or as an alternative measure when reflex inhibition is impossible.

Nursing Care and Prevention. Preventive measures to be undertaken for patients exhibiting an abnormal susceptibility to leg cramps include frequent changing of the patient's position and adjustment of the bed in such a manner as to ensure an even distribution of pressure on the undersurface of the leg, compression of the popliteal space being avoided by slight flexion of the knee. Sedatives and soporifics should be curtailed to a minimum, or if their use is necessary, their dosage should be barely sufficient to induce sleep. Protective bed clothing should be adequate to prevent chilling without imposing excessive weight on the legs, a bed cradle being employed, if necessary, to eliminate its pressure and immobilizing effect on the lower extremities.

Benign muscular cramps usually are prevented by the ingestion of 0.2 gm. of quinine sulfate on retiring. Myanesin, 250 mg. at bedtime, is reportedly as effective as quinine and is without known hazard, whereas sensitivity to quinine is not uncommon. Moreover, quinine is contraindicated during pregnancy, when susceptibility to cramps is notoriously great. Benadryl (50 mgm.) in capsule form is probably the best and safest way to prevent and treat muscular cramps. In addition it has a mild sedative effect.

ORTHOPEDIC SURGICAL NURSING PRIORITIES

Preoperative Care

In general, the principles of preoperative care are the same as in the care of any surgical patient (see Chapter 9). Only the differences are stressed here.

Psychological Support. Many orthopedic patients experience a curious mixture of fear and anticipation before surgery. Will I be able to walk again, or is this too much to hope for? If an individual has been handicapped and dependent for most of his life, he faces reconstructive surgery with added concern. Some patients have faced repeated operations; patience and hope are almost gone. These are the people who need much help from an understanding nurse.

Following surgery, if the patient is to be placed in a different type of bed with special apparatus such as traction or a plaster cast, he should have some preparation for this preoperatively.

Physical Care. Whatever the method used in preparing the skin of the orthopedic patient for surgery, the principles remain the same. The procedure usually is more painstaking because of the difficulty in controlling infection in the bone, should that occur. A meticulous nontraumatizing cleansing of the skin with soap and water, followed by careful shaving, is done first. Then, soap-and-water washing is repeated, and a fat solvent can be used, followed by a mild antiseptic.

It is known that the number of the bacteria of the skin can be reduced by daily washing with a product containing hexachlorophene. If the operation is an elective one, the orthopedist may advise the patient to use a hexachlorophene preparation for skin cleansing for a period of time before hospital admission.

Disability can result should infection occur within a bone or a joint. In no instance should one rely on the antibiotics to control infection and thereby justify slipshod preoperative preparation.

It is well to remember that, when a cleansing enema is ordered, it should be given before the skin preparation is begun. Many orthopedic surgeons do not require a preoperative enema for surgery on the extremities.

Adequate hydration is always an essential objective in orthopedic patients, particularly those immobilized for a long period of time. This prevents the occurrence of stones, infection and kidney complications. Notice should be taken of the urinary output.

Postoperative Care

Patients who have bone and joint surgery experience real *pain*. Many times, the person who has had surgery to correct a foot condition is much more uncomfortable than one who has had intensive abdominal surgery. Narcotics and other pain-relieving measures should be administered liberally. However, in the long-term patient it is well to remember that habit-forming possibilities may pose a considerable problem. Even though a patient has had an orthopedic operation, pain may not result from the wound and the operative trauma. Swelling frequently follows, and when it occurs under tight bandages or casts, there may be interference with the blood supply, which also produces excruciating pain. This type of pain may be suspected when there is blueness and swelling beyond the limits of the cast, and it may be relieved by relieving the pressure (cutting the cast or bandages).

Another type of pain occurs in orthopedic patients when there is prolonged pressure over bony prominences such as areas of the heel, the head of the fibula on the lateral side of the leg just below the knee and the tuberosity of the tibia. Even though they have been well padded before the cast has been applied, these areas eventually may become painful. The pain is characteristically of a burning type. It is wise not to treat this with narcotics but to call it to the attention of the surgeon, who may wish to cut away areas of the cast to relieve the pressure. In major orthopedic surgery, *shock* also is a common problem, and the nurse must be on the alert for its symptoms.

Bone does not mend as readily as soft tissues. Therefore, even though the skin incision is well-healed, bony structures underneath still need time to repair. This is especially important to remember in surgery of the lower extremities, for in addition to normal movement, bone must be able to bear weight in ambulation.

Other complications that may occur are similar to those of general surgical patients. They are oozing and bleeding, abdominal distention, wound infection and pulmonary and circulatory problems.

Rehabilitation

An important nursing principle in the management of orthopedic patients is to *mobilize the patient*. Keep the patient moving even though he must remain in bed. Keep all parts moving that are not restricted by the surgeon. When encouraging the patient to help himself, be sure he is taught the proper way.

The physical therapist working with the physician and the nurse can guide the patient in the proper use of his muscles and joints. Emphasis is placed on activities of daily living so that he will be able to perform those functions which allow him independence. He needs patience and constant encouragement. He may want to perform a certain activity but fear that self-inflicted injury may result. The extent to which a patient may progress safely must be understood clearly by him as well as all who care for him.

When he goes home, the patient should have explicit

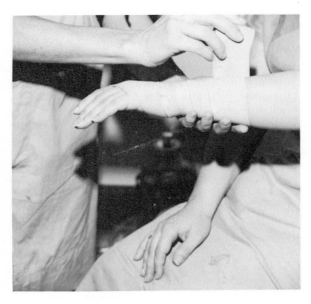

Fig. 35-1. Wrapping a sprained wrist with elastic compression bandage.

instructions that he understands, indicating those activities which he may and may not perform. It is not enough to bid him "good-bye, and take it easy." The patient must know any untoward signs and symptoms that should be reported to his physician. He must be aware of the importance of follow-up visits. If he has any difficulties, he ought to know where and how to get help. The nurse has a major part of the responsibility for educating her patient before he leaves the hospital. (See also Principles and Practices of Rehabilitation Nursing, Chapter 10.)

PATIENTS WITH MUSCULOSKELETAL TRAUMA

Basic Problems and Objectives

Injury to one part of the system usually produces injury to other parts and to the structures enclosed or supported by them. If the bones are broken, the muscles cannot function; if the nerves do not send impulses to the muscles, as in paralysis, the bones cannot move; if the joint surfaces do not articulate normally, neither the bones nor the muscles can function properly. Thus, a fracture also produces injury to the muscles surrounding the injured bone and to the blood vessels and the nerves in its vicinity.

Treatment of Injury

In the treatment of injury to the musculoskeletal system, support is provided the injured part until nature has time to heal it. Support may be accomplished by bandages, adhesive strapping, splints or plaster casts, applied externally. In some patients, support may be applied directly to the bone in the form of pins or plates. In others, it may be necessary to correct deformity and to overcome overlapping by weighted traction.

After the immediate and the painful effects of the injury have passed, consideration must be given to the prevention of fibrosis and the resulting stiffness in the injured muscles and the joint structures. *Active function by the patient is the best form of treatment to guard against this disability.* In some cases the support applied may permit active function almost from the start. In other cases, the nature of the injury may not permit function, and even in those cases in which partial function is possible, we may aid nature in the healing process and hasten recovery of function by various forms of physical therapy.

Contusions, Sprains and Dislocations

Contusions

A *contusion* is an injury to the soft tissues, produced by blunt force (a blow, kick, fall, etc.). There is always some hemorrhage into the injured part (ecchymosis), due to the rupture of many small vessels. This produces the well-known discoloration of the skin (black-and-blue spot), which gradually turns to brown and then to yellow, until it finally disappears as absorption becomes complete. When the hemorrhage is sufficient to cause an appreciable collection of blood, it is called *hematoma*. The local symptoms (pain, swelling and discoloration) are easily explained.

Treatment consists of elevating the affected part and applying moist or dry cold for the first 8 or 10 hours. Pressure in the form of an elastic or an elastic adhesive bandage also is of distinct value in reducing contusion, hemorrhage and swelling. When the hemorrhage has stopped, moist or dry heat and massage promote absorption, thus hastening the cure.

Sprains

A *sprain* is an injury to the ligamentous structures surrounding a joint, caused by a wrench or a twist. As is the case with contusions, ruptures of blood vessels occur, with a resultant rapid swelling due to the extravasation of blood within the tissues. The movement of the joint becomes painful. To be certain that there is no bone injury, all these patients should have an x-ray examination.

The treatment of a sprain consists of cold compresses, rest, elevation and support with either a temporary splint or wrapping with elastic compression bandages (Fig. 35-1).

Dislocations

A *dislocation* of a joint is a condition in which the articular surfaces of the bones forming the joint are

Fig. 35-2. Types of fractures. (Ethicon, Inc.)

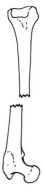

Simple (closed) fracture
—No open wound

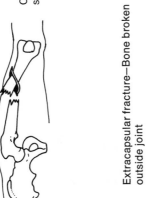

Compound (open) fracture—Wound in
skin communicates with fracture

Extracapsular fracture—Bone broken
outside joint

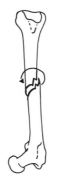

Transverse fracture—Break runs
across bone

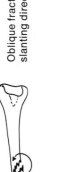

Oblique fracture—Break runs in
slanting direction on bone

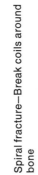

Intracapsular fracture—Bone broken
inside joint

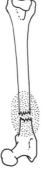

Spiral fracture—Break coils around
bone

Comminuted fracture—Bone
splintered into fragments

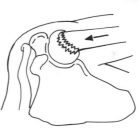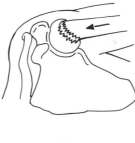

Pathologic fracture—Break is at site
of bone disease

Impacted fracture—Bone broken and
wedged into other break

Greenstick fracture—Bone broken,
bent but still securely hinged at one
side

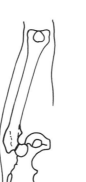

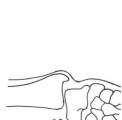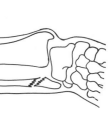

Depressed fracture—Broken skull
bone driven inward

Fracture dislocation—Break
complicated by bone out of joint

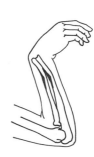

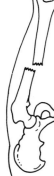

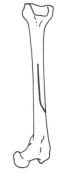

Longitudinal fracture—Break runs
parallel with bone

no longer in anatomic contact. Dislocations may be (1) congenital (present at birth, due to some maldevelopment, most often noted at the hip); (2) spontaneous or pathologic, owing to disease of the articular or the periarticular structures and (3) traumatic, owing to injury, such as the application of force in such a manner to produce disruption of the joint.

Symptoms. The cardinal symptoms of a dislocation are: (1) change in contour of the joint, (2) change in the length of the extremity, (3) loss of normal mobility, (4) change in the axis of the dislocated bones. Roentgenograms confirm the diagnosis and should be made in every case, because not infrequently there is an associated fracture.

Treatment and Nursing Management. Irreparable damage may result when someone who is not trained attempts to reduce a dislocation. Immobilization of the part is the best first-aid procedure before medical aid is obtained. Reduction of a dislocation usually is performed under general anesthesia. The head of the dislocated bone is manipulated back into the joint cavity, and the joint is immobilized by bandages and splints for 3 or 4 weeks.

The nursing care following reduction of dislocations is essentially the same as that following the reduction of fractures. The part must be kept immobilized for a sufficient time to permit the ligamentous structures about the joint to heal. Therefore, splints and casts are the usual dressings. The nurse must watch for the complications that are common to such appliances, such as constriction due to tight dressings producing venous and, sometimes, even arterial obstruction. Cyanosis, pain and the disturbance or the loss of sensation should be familiar signs to the nurse, who should immediately notify the surgeon. Attention must be paid to the slightest complaint of the patient. The nurse must watch for signs of pressure, both within and outside the immobilization dressing.

The Patient with a Fracture

Orientation

Any break in the continuity of a bone is called a *fracture*. The break may be *incomplete*, only a line or fissure in the bone, as frequently found in fractures of the skull. It may extend only part way through the bone, splintering the fibers on one side and bending them on the other. This latter form is spoken of as a *greenstick* fracture, and it occurs in children at an age when the bones are soft and pliable. On the other hand, the bone may be *completely* broken, transversely or in a spiral direction, and very frequently it is broken into several (more than two) fragments, when the fracture is said to be *comminuted*.

When the fractured surfaces are protected from contamination with the outside air, that is, when the skin remains intact, it is said to be a *closed* or *simple* fracture, but if a wound occurs at the time of the fracture, so that air and therefore bacteria may be admitted, the fracture is spoken of as being *open* or *compound*. Such a fracture is more difficult to treat than a simple fracture, because the wound and possibility of infection must be considered as well as the fracture itself. At times, soft-tissue injury may cause a greater problem than the fractured bone.

Not infrequently other structures such as nerves, blood vessels, joints, lungs, bladder and other organs are injured by the force causing the fracture or by the fracture fragments. When such injuries occur, the fracture is called a *complicated* one.

Growth in long bones in early life takes place from two lines of cartilage, called epiphyseal lines, which separate the main shaft of the bone (the diaphysis) from the articular extremities (the epiphyses). As full growth is attained, these lines of cartilage disappear, being transformed into dense bone.

In childhood and in early youth, an accident frequently occurs that is in effect a fracture, but actually involves a separation of the epiphysis from the rest of the bone. These injuries, which are called *epiphyseal separations*, frequently pass undiagnosed or are diagnosed as sprains. They are important because an accurate reposition of the epiphysis must be secured and maintained, otherwise the bone may not attain its normal growth. Therefore, such separations are looked upon and treated as fractures.

Most fractures are the result of trauma, but some fractures occur because the bone itself becomes weakened and cannot bear the weight of the patient's body. This occurs frequently in older people, due to osteoporosis (increased porosity of bone). Similar fractures occur as a result of tumors—either primary tumors of the bones or metastatic tumors. When these tumors invade the bone, the bone becomes decalcified to the point that it is no longer strong enough to maintain its integrity under stress and thus sustains a fracture.

Physiology of Bone Healing

A fracture of bone, the result of deceleration forces, initiates all of the physiologic responses of inflammation and wound healing. In addition, there is new bone formation to reconstruct rather than patch the area together with scar.

As in wound healing in every other part of the body, fracture repair begins with the clotting of extravasated blood. The organization of the blood clot begins within 24 hours on all surfaces, and is replaced by granulation tissue, in part of hematogenous origin, within a few days. The torn ends of fracture periosteum, endosteum and bone fragments at the fracture line supply cells. These proliferate and differentiate into fibrous connective tissue, fibrocartilage and hyaline cartilage. At this stage, except for the predominance of cartilage, the process resembles the repair of any tissue following injury. In long bones, this mass of differentiated, preliminary tissue bridges across the fracture area and acts as a model or template of connective tissue and cartilage, through which osteogenesis is drawn into and across the fracture gap from each side. The fibrous connective tissue and cartilage form a complex structure termed *callus.*

The external callus of the healing fracture develops in great part from the periosteum. The contribution of the periosteum to the repair of bone is of major importance. The vascular network of the callus is a new growth of small arteries, capillaries and veins arising from the vascular supply of surrounding muscle, periosteum and bone marrow.

The bridging of a fracture by bone starts from the periosteal cuff adjacent to the fracture, growing over the surface of the callus model and enveloping the fibrocartilagenous callus. It then grows inward through the model toward the fracture gap. Finally, it grows between the bone ends. With the passage of time, there is resorption of some or all of the new bone surrounding the fracture such that the exact site may be hard to determine.

The shape of the callus and the volume of tissue required to bridge the defect is directly proportional to the amount of bone damage and displacement. The healing time depends on the total volume of damaged tissue, the area of the fracture as well as the regional condition of blood supply and the age of the patient.

The growing callus is calcified in the same way as bone or cartilage in other parts of the skeleton. The calcium phosphate crystal or "apatite" is deposited on and in collagen fibers that make up the connective tissue of the callus. Collagen is a long-chain protein with a specific amino acid content and x-ray diffraction pattern. The spaces between the collagen fibers are filled with "ground substance" or the amorphous component of connective tissue. These substances are known as mucopolysaccharides. Collagen makes up 95 per cent of the organic matter of bone (approximately 35 per cent of bone weight); the crystals are the inorganic fraction. The ground substance in bone is quite small. Collagen and ground substance are produced by the bone forming cells called *osteoblasts.* The collagen and ground substance are called *osteoid.* It is this osteoid that is "calcified" and appears on the x-ray demonstrating evidence of progressive healing at the fracture site.

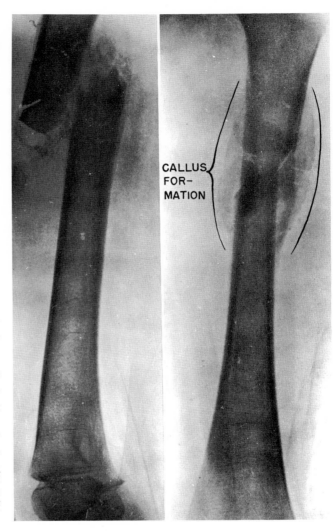

CALLUS FOR- MATION

Fig. 35-3. A fractured femur of 4 weeks' duration. (*Left*) Lateral view. Note overlapping. (*Right*) Anteroposterior view. Note deposition of callus.

Symptoms

The symptoms of a fracture may be learned easily by picturing what happens when a bone is broken. The break follows unnatural movement in a position that is normally rigid. The displacement of the fragments causes a deformity of the limb when compared with the sound member of the opposite side of the body. The limb cannot function properly because normal function of the muscles depends upon the integrity of the bones to which they are attached.

Upon examination of the limb, a grating sensation, called *crepitus,* is imparted to the examining fingers, owing to the rubbing of the fragments one upon the other. In fractures of long bones there is actually shortening of the limb because of the contraction of the muscles that are attached above and below the site of the fracture. The fragments may often overlap as much as an inch or two. Finally, there are pain, tenderness, false motion, swelling and discoloration of the skin owing to the trauma causing the fracture and the hemorrhage that follows it.

All of these symptoms are not necessarily present in every fracture. When there is a linear or fissure fracture, or in cases where the fractured surfaces are driven together (called *impacted* fractures), many of these symptoms may be lacking.

Diagnosis

In modern practice, the diagnosis and the treatment of fractures are not thought to be complete without at least one and often many x-ray examinations. By this means the position of the fragments may be determined accurately, and the indications for further treatment confirmed.

The *fluoroscope* is an apparatus by means of which the position of anything opaque to the x-rays may be visualized on a screen. The newer *image intensifiers* reduce the amount of x-ray exposure. By the aid of this apparatus the bone fragments may be brought into position with considerable ease and accuracy, but a roentgenogram always should follow to serve as a permanent record of the reduction.

Emergency Management

For transportation, the fractured extremity should be rendered as immobile as possible *before the patient is moved.* This is done by the temporary application of such makeshift splints as well-padded pieces of wood, cane, etc., firmly bandaged over the clothing. Adequate splinting is essential for the prevention of soft tissue damage by bony fragments. It must be remembered that the pain associated with a fractured bone is severe, and the surest way to decrease the discomfort of the patient and prevent possible shock is by fixing the bone so that the joints above and below the fracture are immobilized. Before transportation is attempted, morphine should be given if available.

In a compound fracture, the wound should be covered with a clean (sterile) dressing, no attempt being made to reduce the fracture, even if one of the bone fragments is protruding through the wound. Splints should be applied as described above. Immediately following injury, a patient who is in a state of confusion may not be aware of the possibility of a fracture, i.e., he may walk on a fractured extremity. Therefore, it is important to immobilize that part of the body immediately when a fracture is suspected.

Immediate Hospital Treatment and Nursing Care

When a patient comes to a hospital suffering from a fracture, he should be given morphine or Demerol sufficient to relieve his pain. The intravenous route allows smaller dosage, prompt action and is effective in the "shock patient."

Then with care and gentleness his clothes are removed, first from the uninjured side of his body, and then from the injured side. The fractured extremity must be moved as little as possible to avoid disturbing it; sometimes the patient's clothing must be cut away on the injured side.

As a rule, patients with fractures should not be moved until the injured part has been supported by temporary splints. However, there are times when moving is necessary. In those cases, the extremity should be supported both above and below the site of the fracture, and traction should be made in the line of the long axis of the bone in order to prevent rotation as well as angular motion.

Fracture Reduction

Reduction of a fracture ("setting" the bone) refers to restoration of the fracture fragments into anatomic rotation and alignment as nearly as possible. This is accomplished by manipulation, or by surgery when manipulation fails.

Before reduction of the fracture, time enough usually elapses for the patient to be undressed, washed and made comfortable. A limb that is to be manipulated and dressed in a splint or a cast should not be dirty.

In treating a fracture, the most important objectives are: (1) to regain correct alignment through reduction, (2) to maintain the alignment, and (3) to regain the function of the involved part.

Methods Employed to Obtain Fracture Reduction

Several methods may be used to obtain reduction of a fracture; the method selected depends on the nature of the fracture. Variations of these methods are carried out, but the underlying principles are the same. Usually fractures should be reduced as soon as possible because tissues may lose their elasticity because of infiltration by edema or hemorrhage. In most cases, fracture reduction becomes more difficult as the hemorrhage at the fracture site becomes organized.

Closed Reduction. In most instances, closed reduction is accomplished by bringing the bone fragments into apposition by manipulation and manual traction. Anesthesia is generally given to relieve the patient's pain and relax the muscles. Following the manipulation, x-ray films are taken to determine that the bone fragments are in correct alignment. A cast is usually

TABLE 35-1. The Treatment of Fractures

Principles of Care in Treating Fractures
1. Obtain reduction of the fracture
2. Maintain reduction in place until healing occurs (immobilization)
3. Regain normal function of the affected part (rehabilitation)

Methods Used to *Obtain* Fracture Reduction
1. Closed reduction
2. Traction
3. Open reduction

Methods Used to *Maintain* Fracture Reduction
1. Plaster cast
2. Splints
3. Continuous traction
4. Pin and plaster technique
5. Internal fixation devices
   a. Nails
   b. Plates
   c. Screws
   d. Wires
   e. Rods

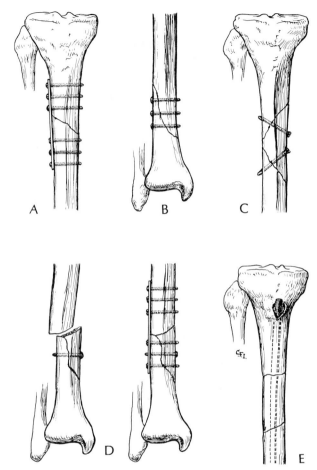

FIG. 35-4. Techniques of internal fixation. (A) Plate and six screws for a transverse or short oblique fracture. (B) Screws for a long oblique or spiral fracture. (C) Screws for a long butterfly fragment. (D) Plate and six screws for a short butterfly fragment. (E) Medullary nail for a segmental fracture. (From Smith, H.: Fractures. *In* Crenshaw, A. H. (ed.): Campbell's Operative Orthopaedics. vol. 1, ed. 4. St. Louis, C. V. Mosby, 1963)

applied to immobilize the extremity and maintain reduction. The nurse may be asked to maintain traction on the affected extremity while it is being encased in plaster.

Use of Traction to Obtain Reduction. Traction is force in 2 directions. This method may be employed for fractures of all long bones. The purpose of traction is to regain normal length and alignment. It may be applied to an extremity by *skin traction,* using adhesive or moleskin strips, or by *skeletal traction,* using wires, pins or tongs placed through bone. To apply the needed force a system of ropes, pulleys and weights is used. The nursing management of a patient in traction is discussed more fully on pages 850-853.

Open Reduction or Open Operation. Many fractures require open operation or open reduction; this necessitates a formal incision. The bone fragments are replaced under direct visualization. Internal fixation devices in the form of metallic pins, wires, screws, plates, nails or rods may be used to hold the bone fragments in position until solid bone healing occurs. Internal fixation devices may be attached to the sides of bone, put through bony fragments or inserted directly into the medullary cavity of the bone (Fig. 35-4). These devices assure the patient better maintenance of alignment of the fracture fragment. After closure of the wound, external immobilization of the fracture is often employed by the application of splints or casts. The internal fixation device may be removed after bony union has taken place, but for the majority of patients it is not removed unless it produces symptoms.

Nursing Management Following Open Reduction. During the immediate postoperative period following open reduction, the nursing management is the same as for any other major surgical procedure (Chapter 9). Before the patient leaves the recovery room, his bed on the unit should be made ready with traction apparatus appropriate to his needs. The circulation of the affected part should be evaluated at frequent intervals. Compare the affected extremity with the unaffected one for color and skin temperature. Symptoms of pain, pallor, pulselessness, paralysis (the four P's), rubor or coolness indicate abnormal circulatory changes and consequent neurovascular disturbances.

Notify the orthopedist immediately so that necessary loosening of dressings or bivalving of casts to relieve pressure may be done. Dressings should be inspected at regular intervals.

The assessment and management of postoperative pain is an individualized problem. Remember that upon awakening, the patient is susceptible to suggestion. Reassure him that the operative procedure is over and that someone is with him. During the immediate postoperative period narcotics may be necessary. In general, an elderly patient requires less narcotic than a younger patient. As soon as possible, oral non-narcotic analgesics should be given, since patients who have undergone orthopedic operations may have prolonged musculoskeletal complaints. Restlessness, anxiety and general discomfort may be relieved by ap-

Fig. 35-5. Preparing plaster of Paris bandages. Plaster may come in a plastic bag encasement. This can be used as the "bucket" for the plaster by filling the bag with water and standing it on end until the plaster is saturated. Other forms of plaster bandages are wrapped in individual rolls.

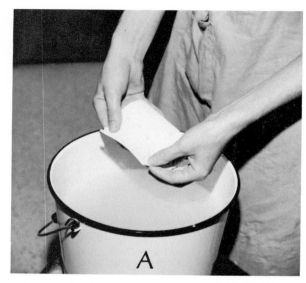

(A) Unwind the end of the bandage for a few inches so it will be easily grasped when the bandage is wet. Some manufacturers indicate the end of the plaster with a colored paper tab.

Submerge the plaster *vertically* in warm water. (70-75° F.)

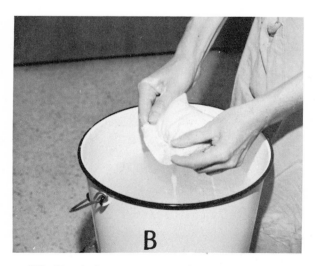

(B) Expel the excess water by gently squeezing the ends with the palms of the hands. The end "pinch" prevents the center of the wet roll from falling out during application.

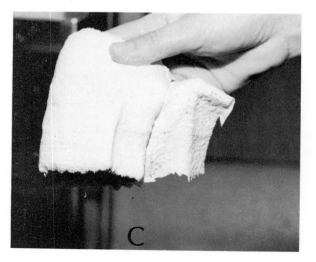

(C) Pass the plaster bandage to the surgeon so that the starting end is easily grasped.

propriate nursing measures, reassurance, physical therapy, tranquilizers and other forms of treatment.

Orthopedic wounds have a tendency to ooze more than other surgical wounds. External muscle dissection frequently produces wounds in which hemostasis is poor. Wounds closed while under tourniquet control may bleed upon release of the tourniquet in the postoperative period.

Redressings are required for many fractures dressed with splints, especially those that involve or are near

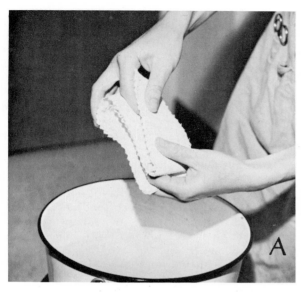

(A) Splints are prepared by loosely fan folding the plaster bandage in the hand before they are dipped.

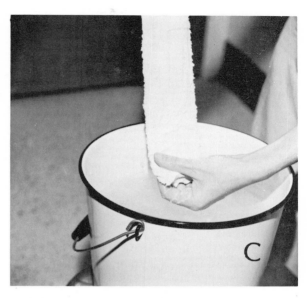

(C) Excess water is removed by rubbing the splint carefully on the side of the bucket or by passing it between the index and long finger in a "squeeze" action to remove excess water.

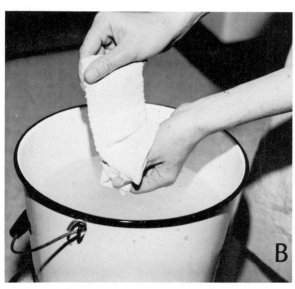

(B) Dip the splints in a vertical position in warm water.

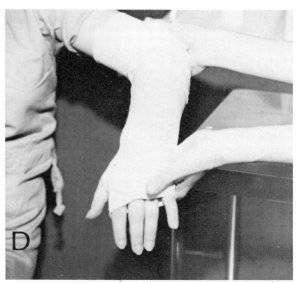

(D) Posterior plaster splint in place.

Fig. 35-6. Preparing plaster splints.

the joints. Fractures complicated by joint involvement, or those treated by the application of a cast, are often benefited by a regimen of heat and massage after union is firm enough for external support to be discontinued. Under ordinary conditions with proper treatment, the fragments of the broken bone unite by the formation of a soft callus in which are deposited calcium salts, so that in time a patch of bone results that is as strong as the original part (Fig. 35-4).

Fracture Immobilization. After the fracture has been reduced, bone fragments must be held in position until union has had time to take place. This immobilization may be accomplished by bandages, adhesive, splints or by traction. If the fragments have been properly reduced and immobilized, swelling should disappear rapidly, and the part should become less and less painful. If pain persists or increases, the nurse should suspect that something is wrong and call the surgeon at once. Increasing pain usually means an ill-fitting cast or splint. Early remedy is necessary to prevent necrosis.

Bandages

Bandages of muslin or felt elastic weave are used commonly to immobilize certain fractures. The Velpeau bandage dressing is applied by many surgeons for fractures about the shoulder. The Barton bandage is applied for fractures of the jaw. Minor fractures of the fibula may be treated with elastic adhesive tape. Wooden or plastic splints are useful as temporary dressings and occasionally as permanent dressings for many fractures, especially those of the upper extremity. Air splints are quite commonly used by rescue squads and ambulance crews. Any splint that does not fit the curve of the extremity should be well-padded to prevent pressure.

Plaster Casts

Plaster of Paris is the most common form of fracture immobilization. Plaster of Paris bandages are rolls of crinoline impregnated with a solid crystalline material known as gypsum or calcium sulfate dihydrate. Gypsum is reduced to a powder to break up the crystals and then subjected to intense heat to drive off the water in the crystal. The product of this action is plaster of Paris.

$$2CaSO_4 \cdot 2H_2O \xrightarrow{\triangle} (CaSO_4)_2 \cdot H_2O + 3H_2O\uparrow$$
(Gypsum) (Plaster of Paris)

When water is added to the plaster, the calcium sulfate dihydrate absorbs the water and recrystallizes or "sets" as calcium sulfate or gypsum. This process of recrystallization gives off heat (exothermic reaction) and is equal to the heat required to decompose the original gypsum. For this reason, a freshly applied cast should not be placed on a pillow or mattress or covered with a blanket. Such actions insulate the cast from free access to air and cause a sharp temperature rise, that could give the patient a burn. Most casts begin to cool 5 to 15 minutes after application. (Fig. 35-5 show how plaster bandages are saturated with water for application.)

Before applying a plaster cast, the skin and soft tissue must be protected. Bandages of sheet wadding or other commercial equivalents usually are employed, and if considerable pressure is likely to result, felt pads are used. (Felt can be fixed to the plaster to prevent movement beneath the cast.) Elastic tubular jersey sleeving (stockinette) with cotton batting may be applied.

The plaster bandage is then applied turn upon turn, exerting moderate pressure to each layer with the open hand in order to make it unite with the one beneath it. Places where strain will take place, like the groin, back of the knee, etc., may be reinforced with plaster splints. These are pre-cut and packaged in a variety of sizes. Figure 35-6 show how splints are saturated and prepared for use.

Before the cast is dry the operator should smooth it by rubbing with the open hand, at the same time making sure that it fits the limb. If the first few bandages have been applied firmly and smoothly, the cast usually will be well-molded and without wrinkles.

When the plaster has set, but before it is dry, incisions are made with a plaster knife through all the layers of the cast. When such incisions are made on each side of the cast, it may be removed with comparative ease or easily spread to relieve pressure should signs of constriction appear (cyanosis, coldness, or loss of sensation in fingers or toes). *Any complaints by the patient of painful areas under the plaster should be reported or investigated.*

Plaster Splints

Plaster of Paris is also used in the form of splints that are available commercially. The extremity is wrapped with sheet wadding before the plaster splint is applied. The plaster reaches its maximal temperature 5 to 15 minutes after application; therefore, the splint is usually not overwrapped with an elastic bandage until after this time. Figure 35-6A show how plaster splints are prepared. Figure 35-6D shows a posterior splint in place on an extremity. The nurse is supporting the splint with her fingers extended to avoid possible distortion of the cast while it is still "green."

Application of Cast. When plaster is being used, the hands may be protected by disposable gloves. A thin coating of petroleum jelly on the hands may be preferred to rubber gloves. The room in which plaster is applied should be one having a minimum of furnishings to facilitate cleaning. Some form of lubricant applied to the orthopedic table makes it easier to remove plaster and prevents rust formation. Plaster knives and shears are the only instruments needed. They must be cleaned thoroughly and oiled after use.

The plaster-laden water in which the bandages are soaked should not be poured into the ordinary drain basin, because a clogged pipe is almost sure to result. It is better to allow the plaster to settle in the bucket, then the water may be poured off, and the remaining plaster emptied into the waste can. Plastic liners placed in the bucket also help ease the cleaning problem. In most modern hospitals, plaster traps are installed in the drain pipes of sinks in rooms where plaster is used. The trap catches most of the plaster poured into the sink, but it must be cleaned frequently if it is to work efficiently.

As soon as the cast is applied, clean the plaster off the patient's skin with a damp towel. Small pieces of plaster remaining on the skin will crumble and slide down under the cast, causing the patient a great deal of discomfort.

The Patient in a Cast. The purpose of a cast is to immobilize and support the injured part and protect it during the healing process.

Experience has taught that any complaint of discomfort must not go unheeded. Two types of complications occur. One is due to pressure of the cast on tissues, especially on bony points. Pain may be the first indication of local pressure which, if allowed to go untended, may produce necrosis (pressure sores) or paralysis, due to pressure on a nerve over a bony point. The latter is seen most commonly to produce peroneal palsy with footdrop, resulting from pressure on the peroneal nerve.

The second complication is caused by swelling underneath the cast, which produces a circulatory impairment. Toes and fingers of extremities recently encased in plaster must be inspected frequently to note any signs of circulatory impairment. *Swelling, blanching or discoloration, tingling, numbness, inability to move fingers and toes, or any temperature change must be reported immediately*, because serious results such as paralysis and necrosis may occur. Conscientious observations should continue as long as the patient is in the cast; if there is swelling, the cast will seem tighter. Elevation of the part helps to control swelling. If the patient continues to have pain, pressure within the cast on a nerve, a blood vessel, or a bony prominence should be suspected. The cast will have to be bivalved to relieve the pressure. This action does not disturb the alignment of the fracture. Elevate the extremity after the cast is bivalved until the circulation is restored and the swelling diminishes.

When a large cast is applied, such as a body or hip spica, the bed must be prepared before the patient is received. A board under the mattress gives the necessary firmness to the bed. To make allowances for the contour of the cast, 3 pillows placed crosswise on the bed will suffice for the body cast. For a hip spica, one pillow placed crosswise at the waist and 2 pillows placed lengthwise for the affected leg are necessary. If both legs are involved, 2 additional pillows are necessary. It is important that the pillows be next to each other, because any spaces in between will allow the damp cast to sag, become weak and possibly break.

In moving a patient from side to side in a large cast, at least 3 people are necessary. Only the palms of the hands are used to lift the cast; fingers make indentations in soft plaster. Support should be given to the entire cast and most particularly at such vulnerable points as the hip and the knee.

The nurse must remember that the patient receives first consideration and his cast is secondary in importance.

Drying the Cast. A freshly applied cast should be exposed to circulating air so that it will dry.

Covers are not necessary because they restrict the escape of moisture. As the moisture evaporates and the cast hardens, heat is generated. In a warm room it may be necessary to use an electric fan to keep the patient comfortable. When a large cast is dried, it is often desirable to use mechanical aids, such as a heat lamp or hair dryer, to facilitate the process. This should not be placed closer than 45.7 cm (18 inches), and then it should be moved frequently from one area to another so that drying is achieved evenly. It is to be remembered that burns may occur under the cast from overexposure even though the skin is not exposed directly.

If the patient is cold, those parts of the body not encased in plaster should be covered and kept warm. When the patient is in shock, the cast can be exposed piecemeal. It takes about 24 hours for a cast to become dry, depending upon the size of the cast and the moisture in the air; a dry cast is white and shiny, resonant and odorless as well as firm; a wet cast is gray and dull in appearance, dull to percussion, feels damp and has a musty odor.

Turning the Patient. While the cast is still in the process of drying, the patient should be turned at least every 6 hours to promote even drying of the cast and to prevent fatigue of the patient (this may vary with the physician or the hospital policy). The initial turning of a large cast is usually done on the evening of the day it is applied so that the posterior surface may be dried. This should be done with sufficient help. The patient is first moved to the side of the bed toward the leg encased in plaster. At this time fresh pillows and sheets may be placed on the vacant side so that it is ready to receive the turned patient. The patient with a hip spica should be turned as one piece on the leg *not involved* and adequate support must be given to the uppermost leg, which is encased, especially at the groin. His arms may be placed above his head or kept at his sides, whichever is most comfortable. Two persons on the side of the bed to which the patient is closest and one person on the opposite side can turn a patient effectively without lifting him. When he is lying prone, a pillow placed crosswise under the dorsum of the feet will prevent the toes from being forced into the mattress. Sometimes allowing the toes to hang over the edge of the mattress is more comfortable.

After the cast is thoroughly dry, pillows are used as necessary to maintain comfort and good body alignment. They are used also to bring the level of the cast up to that of the bed pan when the latter is used. A pillow under the abdomen often adds to the comfort of the patient.

A comfort measure that will be appreciated by the patient in a body cast is the "back scratcher." This may be a length of 3-inch flannel inserted inside the back of the cast by a long alligator forceps. (A thoughtful nurse might suggest this to the surgeon immediately before the application of the cast.) By holding each end of the flannel, the nurse can give the patient a friction rub.

Protection of the Skin and Hygienic Care of the Patient. Pressure areas may develop over any bony prominence. A common site of pressure from a large cast is the buttocks. When the patient is turned on his abdomen, the exposed skin can be washed carefully and massaged. The rough edges of the cast here as well as elsewhere must be padded. Often pulling stockinette inside the cast over the rough edge and fixing it to the outside with plaster will eliminate cast crumbs and make the edge smooth. The nurse should reach up under the cast edges as far as possible with her fingers to remove plaster crumbs and to massage the skin area.

Around the perineal area, it is often necessary to protect the cast against excretions. If the opening is inadequate for hygienic care, the nurse should report this. When the cast is dry, the perineum is covered with a towel and the perineal area of the cast may be sprayed with aerosol plastic spray. Four-inch strips of thin polyethylene sheeting may be tucked under the cast and fastened to the exterior, allowing for adequate coverage of the outside of the cast. These may be replaced as necessary.

The skin around the edges of the cast must be inspected frequently for signs of irritation. All accessible skin should be massaged gently with an emollient lotion. When there is irritation, the area must be treated as a potential decubitus.

Exercising the Patient in a Cast. While the patient is in a cast he should be taught to tense or to contract his muscles without moving the joints. The patient may actually forget how to "will" a motion through the central nervous system pathways to the immobilized muscle. Therefore by isometric muscle contractions (contracting the muscle without moving the part), atrophy is prevented and muscle strength maintained.

If the patient is in a leg cast, place your hand under the knee and instruct the patient to "push down." If the patient has an arm cast, instruct him to "make a fist." Isometric muscle contractions should be done at least hourly while the patient is awake. He is taught to exercise his fingers and his toes frequently and actively.

Removal of the Patient from the Cast. A cast is removed by using an electric cast cutter or by making an incision with a plaster knife and cutting the cast with heavy shears. One of the most important things to remember when a cast has been removed is that the part or parts involved have been immobilized for a considerable period of time. When the support and protection of the cast have been removed, stresses and strains are placed on tissue that has been resting. The patient complains of pain and stiffness, often much different from the original injury, and he is depressed and discouraged, because the anticipated release from the cast has only added further to his problems.

The responsibility of the nurse is to help make the adjustment of the patient easier. This can be accomplished by supporting the part to maintain the same position as existed in the cast, with small pillow supports under the knee, the lumbar spine, etc., allowing for gradual removal of support. In moving an extremity, the nurse must provide adequate support and move the limb gently. After the cast has been removed, exercises are prescribed to redevelop and to increase strength. If the patient has been doing isometric muscle contractions, he will not have to relearn to contract his muscles and will progress more rapidly with his rehabilitation program.

After a long leg cast is removed, edema of the foot and leg frequently occurs. Elevation of the extremity, massage and the use of an elastic compression bandage when the patient is ambulatory are useful in prevention of edema. If possible the patient should wear his shoes. If edema persists, permanent swelling may produce chronic disability.

Following the removal of a cast, the skin is washed with mild soap followed by the application of oil or lanolin. If a new cast is to be applied, the skin is thoroughly washed and dried carefully. The skin and the

Fig. 35-7. Method of applying adhesive strips for traction.

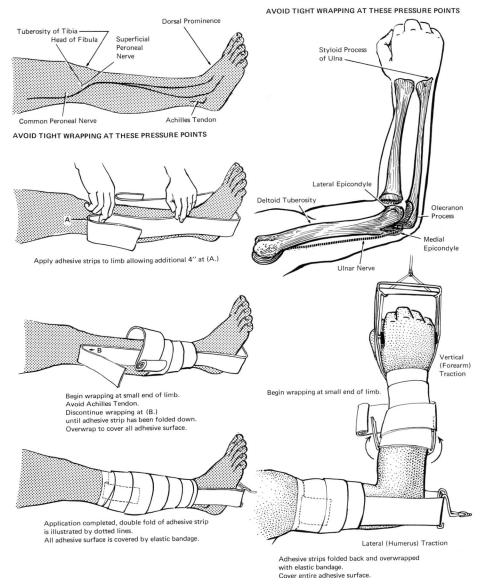

AVOID TIGHT WRAPPING AT THESE PRESSURE POINTS

Tuberosity of Tibia
Head of Fibula
Superficial Peroneal Nerve
Dorsal Prominence
Common Peroneal Nerve
Achilles Tendon

AVOID TIGHT WRAPPING AT THESE PRESSURE POINTS

Styloid Process of Ulna
Lateral Epicondyle
Deltoid Tuberosity
Olecranon Process
Medial Epicondyle
Ulnar Nerve

Apply adhesive strips to limb allowing additional 4″ at (A.)

Begin wrapping at small end of limb.
Avoid Achilles Tendon.
Discontinue wrapping at (B.)
until adhesive strip has been folded down.
Overwrap to cover all adhesive surface.

Begin wrapping at small end of limb.

Vertical (Forearm) Traction

Application completed, double fold of adhesive strip is illustrated by dotted lines.
All adhesive surface is covered by elastic bandage.

Lateral (Humerus) Traction

Adhesive strips folded back and overwrapped with elastic bandage.
Cover entire adhesive surface.

underlying tissues must be handled carefully until gradual restoration of normal function is achieved. Atrophy of the part may be noted but this disappears gradually with the return of muscle function. Should the patient go home with a cast, he must be instructed as to the care of his cast. If the cast has been removed, the principles of skin care must be understood. He must know also the signs of impaired circulation and evidence of infection or skin breakdown. The nurse should stress the importance of his returning to his physician or clinic for follow-up care.

Turnbuckle Cast. In some instances casts are applied not only for immobilization but also for the purposes of overcoming bony deformities and mus-cular contractures. Traction with weight pulleys is sometimes used for this purpose, but for many patients casts are applied that may be cut and the contracture overcome gradually by changing the angle of the cast. In such cases a gradual change may be brought about by incorporating a turnbuckle in the cast, usually across a joint. The part may be straightened by gradually turning the turnbuckle. The nurse must be extremely careful when turning the patient so that this extra appliance is not pulled on and displaced so as to break the cast and interrupt the patient's treatment. She also must be alert *constantly* for new signs of pressure with each manipulation of the turnbuckle.

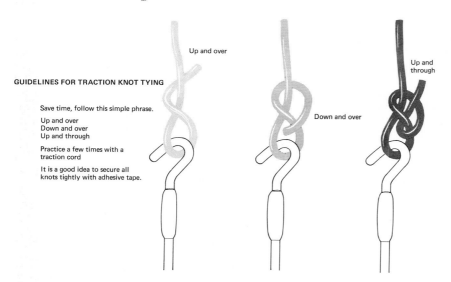

GUIDELINES FOR TRACTION KNOT TYING

Save time, follow this simple phrase.

Up and over
Down and over
Up and through

Practice a few times with a traction cord

It is a good idea to secure all knots tightly with adhesive tape.

Up and over

Down and over

Up and over

Up and through

FIG. 35-8. Tying knots correctly is an orthopedic nursing activity essential for the safety of the patient in traction. (Zimmer manufacturing Company)

The Patient in Traction

The purposes of traction have been discussed on page 842. Traction may be applied directly to the skin (skin traction) or to the bone (skeletal traction).

Skin Traction. Skin traction is accomplished by a weight that pulls on tape, sponge rubber or plastic materials attached to the skin; traction on the skin transmits traction to the musculoskeletal structures. Skin traction is used in the form of Buck's extension or Russell's traction in adults when the pull is exerted in one plane and partial or temporary immobilization is desirable. In Buck's extension, strips of adhesive, moleskin or perforated flexafoam are applied smoothly to each side of the affected extremity and attached to a spreader block at the foot. The spreader prevents pressure along the side of the foot. The extremity is wrapped with elastic bandage to improve adherence of the tape to the skin and prevent slipping. A traction rope is attached to the spreader block and then over a pulley, thence to a weight hung over the side of the bed (Fig. 35-9).

Shaving the part and applying tincture of benzoin to the skin makes the traction strip adhere better if adhesive is used. Benzoin tincture also acts as a skin disinfectant and is said to prevent an itching skin and to be more comfortable. When skin traction is

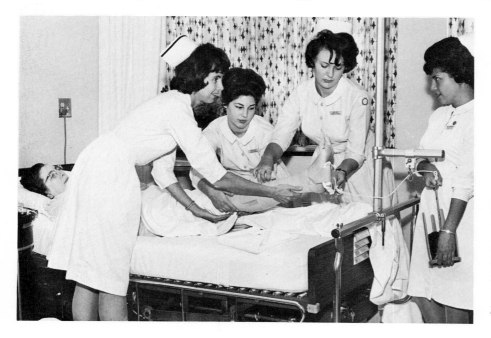

FIG. 35-9. Nursing instructor assisting students to care for a patient in Buck's extension. The extremity is supported while the elastic compression bandage is applied. Then the traction weight will be lowered slowly and carefully and allowed to hang free. (Southern Missionary College, Division of Nursing, Madison, Tenn.)

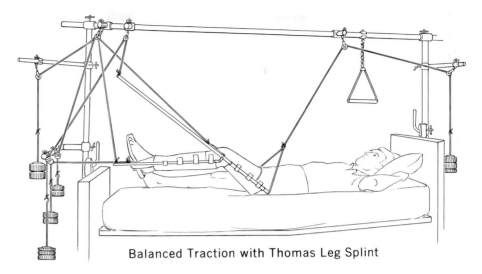

FIG. 35-10. Principles of balanced suspension traction. Force means to push or pull. Force, as used in traction, means push or pull in a given direction. In the nursing management of the patient in traction one has to understand the direction in which the force is operating. Study the line drawing carefully. Notice that the force produced by the weights is changed in direction by the pulleys.

Balanced Traction with Thomas Leg Splint

applied to the leg, pressure not infrequently develops over the Achilles tendon about the heel. This area should be inspected several times daily (Fig. 35-7). Care must be taken to avoid pressure on the peroneal nerve as it passes around the neck of the fibula just below the knee. Pressure here will produce footdrop. A pillow is used to support the lower leg and to reduce friction of the heel against the bed linen.

Patients with lower extremity traction have a tendency to slide down toward the foot of the bed. This may be counteracted by elevation of the foot of the bed 30.5-38 cm (12 or 15 inches).

When skin traction is applied to the arm, tight wrapping of the ulnar nerve at the elbow and other pressure points should be avoided (Fig. 35-7).

Skin traction can produce irritation of the skin and the elastic bandage can cause pressure on peripheral nerves (Fig. 35-7). The chief limitation of skin traction is that no more than 8-10 pounds* of traction may be used on a part. Therefore, skeletal traction is more commonly used when prolonged or heavy traction weight is necessary.

Skeletal Traction. This method of traction is used most frequently in the treatment of fractures of the femur, the humerus and the tibia. The traction is applied directly to the bones by the use of a metal pin or wire inserted into or through a bone distal to the fracture. Instead of the tongs or pin, many surgeons use the Kirschner steel wire, which is drilled through the bone with a hand- or electric-driven drill. Usually the tongs, pin or Kirschner wire may be inserted through a small opening in the skin made under local anesthesia. They are sterilized and inserted with all the sterile precautions of an operation.

* 3.6 to 4.5 kg.

Following insertion of the pins, the wound is covered with a small gauze square. If the wire or pin extends beyond the caliper, a cork placed over the end of the pin prevents the tearing of linen and other more serious accidents.

Traction is applied by weights and pulleys as described for skin traction. The Thomas splint with the Pearson attachment is usually used with skeletal traction in fractures of the femur (Fig. 35-10). It may be used with skin traction and other balanced suspension apparatus. Because upward traction is required for these fractures, the patient is placed on a fracture bed.

When the apparatus has been properly adjusted, the fracture should become constantly more comfortable. Occasionally, one part of the tongs may slip from its bony anchorage and exert its traction on the soft tissues. As might be expected, considerable pain is caused by this accident. The surgeon should be notified at once.

The main problem with skeletal traction is infection, which may develop in or around the pin tract. The site must be inspected by the nurse daily. Daily cleaning of the tract is necessary to clear the tract and pin of the slight drainage that always occurs. The drainage dries at the mouth of the tract and about the pin and forms a plug, setting up conditions for bacterial invasion of the tract and bone.

Inasmuch as fractures occur under varying circumstances and involve individuals of different ages, weights, and body builds, no two fractures are alike, and every fracture patient requires individualized treatment. By the same token, traction procedures may be modified in many ways to meet a variety of special requirements, as exemplified by the so-called "balanced suspension traction," and the "running trac-

THE PATIENT IN TRACTION
Nursing Principles and Implications

The purpose of traction, regardless of how it is achieved, is (1) to reduce and to immobilize a fracture, (2) to lessen or to eliminate muscle spasm, and (3) to prevent fracture deformity. Nursing implications underlying all traction procedures include the following:

1. The patient is placed on a firm mattress with a hinged bed board beneath it.
2. The ropes and the pulleys should be in straight alignment.
3. The pull should be in line with the long axis of the bone.
4. Any factor that might reduce the pull or alter its direction must be eliminated.
   (a) Weights should hang free.
   (b) Ropes should be unobstructed.
5. The amount of weight applied in skin traction must not exceed the tolerance of the skin. The condition of the latter must be inspected frequently.
6. A possibility always to be kept in mind in connection with skeletal traction is the risk of a complicating bone infection. The nurse must be alert to detect odors, signs of local inflammation or other evidence of osteomyelitis.
7. The patient's skin should be examined frequently for evidence of pressure or friction over bony prominences.
8. Provision should be made for supplying additional countertraction by increasing the pull in the opposite direction, i.e., by raising the bed in such a manner that the weight of the patient's body tends to oppose the pull of the traction.
9. Active motion of all unaffected joints should be encouraged.
10. Every complaint of the patient in traction should be investigated.

Principles of Balanced Suspension Traction

Definition: Balanced suspension traction is produced by a counterforce other than the patient's body weight. The extremity balances or floats in the traction apparatus. The line of traction on the extremity remains fairly constant despite changes in position of the patient.

Example: Russell's leg traction for treating fractures of femoral shaft.

Activities permitted patient:

1. The patient may sit, turn slightly and move as desired.
2. The affected heel must remain free of the bed to maintain the traction.

Nursing implications:

1. The angle of hip flexion is 20°. (This is the angle between the thigh and the bed.)
2. A pillow may be used under the thigh to maintain this angle, and a second pillow placed under the calf to support the lower leg.
3. The ropes and the pulleys should be freely movable, and the traction should be applied securely to the leg.
4. Observe for skin irritation around the traction bandage.
5. Check the patient for signs of odor and infection.
6. Observe for pressure under the sling at the popliteal space.
7. The patient should have foot supports to prevent foot drop.
8. The traction must be continuous to be effective.

Principles of Running Traction

Definition: Running traction is a form of traction in which the pull is exerted in one plane. It may utilize skin or skeletal traction, and it may be either unilateral or bilateral.

Example: Buck's extension (Fig. 359).

Activities permitted patient:

1. The head of the bed may be elevated to the point of countertraction (e.g., if the countertraction is 20.3 cm. (8 inches), the head of the bed may be elevated 20.3 cm.).
2. The patient may not turn from side to side, because the position of the leg on the bed will cause the bony fragments to move against each other.

Nursing implications:

1. The foot should be inspected for circulatory difficulties within a few minutes and then periodically after the elastic bandage has been applied.
2. Special care must be given to the back at regular intervals, because the patient maintains a supine position.
3. Any complaint or burning sensation under the traction bandage should be reported immediately.
4. Observe for wrinkling or slipping of the traction bandage.
5. The patient should have foot supports to prevent foot drop.

tion" procedures. These procedures, and the special nursing implications involved with them, are outlined on page 852. The basic nursing principles for traction procedures in general, as set forth on page 852, apply equally to these and all other modified forms of traction.

Nursing Priorities for Patients in Traction. The importance of frequent inspection of the fracture dressing in the first 24 hours after application cannot be impressed too strongly on the nurse responsible for the care of the patient. A bandage that appears sufficiently loose when applied may in a very few hours cause serious constriction which, if not relieved, may lead to gangrene of the extremity.

Dressings always should be applied in such a way as to leave the tips of the fingers and toes exposed. Any cyanosis, loss of temperature, tingling, or loss of sensation in these parts should warn the nurse that the dressings are too tight. If the condition is caused by a single turn of the bandage, the turn may be divided with the scissors, but it is usually advisable to notify the surgeon who has charge of the patient. After the first 24 hours, the fracture dressing should be inspected by the nurse at least 3 or 4 times daily. She should inquire whether there are any painful areas, look for evidences of constriction and see that there are no pressure points, e.g., heel is not on the bed, bedclothes do not rest on toes, there is no pressure on the Achilles tendon, etc.

If traction is being used, the nurse should inspect the apparatus to see that the ropes are in the wheel groove of the pulleys, that the supporting apparatus is free of the pulleys, that the weights hang free, and that the patient has not slipped down in bed. The foot must be in a natural position; rotation outward or inward should be reported. Footdrop is to be avoided, and the patient's foot must be maintained in a neutral position supported by appropriate orthopedic devices. The rope sometimes frays; therefore, it too must be inspected at least daily. An alert nurse will examine the skin around the traction for evidence of circulatory impairment.

Weights are necessary to provide constant force and may be ordinary metal traction weights or bags of water, shot or sand. Enough weight is applied at first to overcome the shortening tendency of the injured limb, but it is gradually lessened as the fracture becomes more fixed. *A nurse never should remove weights from a patient with a fracture under any consideration.* Weight and pulley traction is applied to secure constant corrective extension. If, then, the weights are removed to move the patient from one department to another, the whole purpose of their use has been defeated.

When there is a pull in one direction, there must

be an equal pull in the opposite direction. (For every action there is an equal and opposite reaction—this is Newton's third law of motion.) Countertraction is supplied by either the patient's body weight and friction against the bed (fracture of an upper extremity) or by elevating the foot of the bed (fracture of a lower extremity).

When traction frames are used, a trapeze may be suspended overhead within easy reach of the patient. This apparatus is of great help in assisting the patient to move about in bed, on and off bedpans, etc. It is also a help to the nurse in caring for these patients. When a patient is not permitted to turn on one side or the other or on his abdomen, the nurse must make a special effort to give him good back care and to keep the bed dry and free of crumbs and wrinkles. This can be accomplished without her straining her back, because the patient may raise his hips from the bed by holding onto the overhead trapeze. Often a patient uses the heel of his good leg to act as a brace when he raises himself. This digging of the heel into the mattress may be injurious to the tissues; hence, it must be massaged with lanolin and inspected for pressure areas. Some physicians wrap both legs of traction patients in elastic bandage in an attempt to decrease the incidence of thrombophlebitis. If the patient is unable to raise himself, the nurse can push down on the mattress with one hand, leaving space for the other hand to massage the skin.

FRACTURES OF SPECIFIC SITES

In caring for a patient with a fracture, the nurse needs to know the extent of the fracture, the therapeutic aim, the management to accomplish this aim as well as the care required through convalescence. An injury to the skeletal structure may vary from a simple linear fracture to a severe crushing one. The therapeutic program is determined by the type and location of the fracture and the degree of involvement of parosseous structures.

Skull and Cervical Spine

These have been considered in Chapter 34 on the nursing of neurosurgical patients.

Mandible

Fracture of the mandible is discussed in Chapter 21 in conditions of the mouth, neck and esophagus.

Clavicle (Collar Bone)

This is one of the most common fractures. The clavicle helps to hold the shoulder upward, outward and backward from the thorax. Therefore, in a fracture of the clavicle, the therapeutic aim is to hold the shoulder in the same position. This is accomplished by closed reduction and immobilization with external splinting. A clavicular strap (Fig. 35-11) holds the shoulders in the desired position. The axilla is padded; pressure in the axilla must be avoided, because serious neurologic damage can occur. In addition, pressure on the vascular structures at this site poses a hazard. Other forms of immobilization include the figure-of-8 bandage, the figure-of-8 plaster cast and the T-splint. The fracture is immobilized until union takes place (5 to 6 weeks). As soon as healing occurs, active exercise of the shoulder joint is carried out to prevent pain and stiffness. In severely displaced fractures in adults, open reduction may be necessary.

Ribs

Uncomplicated fractures of the ribs are common and usually unite with no resultant impairment of function. However, fractures of the ribs produce painful respirations. The patient tends to decrease his respiratory excursions and refrains from coughing. Tracheobronchial secretions are not coughed up, aeration of the lung is diminished and a predisposition to pneumonia

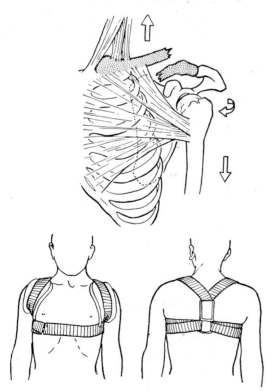

Fig. 35-11. Fracture of the clavicle. (*Top*) Anteroposterior view, showing typical displacement of midclavicle fracture. (*Bottom*) Method of immobilization with a clavicular strap. (From Rhoads, *et al.*: Surgery—Principles and Practice, p. 479, ed. 4, Lippincott, 1970)

and atelectasis is created. Intercostal nerve blocks with procaine are done to relieve respiratory pain and permit productive coughing.

Adhesive strapping of the ribs may alleviate the pain. Before adhesive straps are applied, it is well to shave the hairy region to make removal of the adhesive less painful. Elastic rib belts also provide rib cage control while allowing the patient slight chest expansion. Patients with adhesive strapping or rib belts should be watched for symptoms of pulmonary complications.

Multiple rib fractures may lead to a flail chest, which is a serious problem (p. 270). Severe rib fractures may result in puncture of the lung with the escape of air into the pleural space (pneumothorax).

Humerus

Surgical Neck. The commonest fracture in the upper arm and the shoulder is that of the surgical neck of the humerus. It occurs most often in adults, and the patient comes for aid with the affected arm hanging limp at the side, supported with the uninjured hand.

Many of the impacted fractures of the surgical neck of the humerus do not require reduction. The arm is supported by a sling and swathed for the patient's comfort. In any fracture of the arm, limitation of motion and stiffness of the shoulder occurs from disuse. Therefore pendulum exercises are begun as soon as tolerated by the patient. (In pendulum or circumduction exercises, the patient is instructed to lean forward and to allow the affected arm to abduct and rotate.) Early motion of the joint does not displace the fragments if motion is carried out within the limits imposed by pain.

If there is a displaced fracture at the neck of the humerus, reduction is accomplished under x-ray control. After the fragments are in apposition, they are maintained by an appropriate dressing and sling. These fractures may require open reduction and internal fixation.

Shaft. These fractures are among the most difficult of all fractures to treat. The bone is surrounded by thick muscles that often become interposed between the fragments and make reduction difficult. The musculospiral nerve lies posterior to the bone, in the musculospiral groove, and not infrequently it is involved in shaft fractures or in the callus formed by their healing. It is important, therefore, to make frequent inspection for wrist drop, the sign of paralysis of this nerve, both before and after reduction of the fracture.

Many dressings are used for this fracture: the shoulder cap, axillary pad and sling; many forms of traction with splints; the airplane splint.

A form of dressing known as the "hanging cast" is

Fig. 35-12. Patient in a pelvic sling.

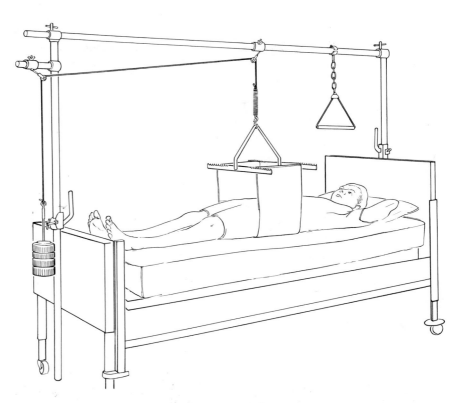

used. A plaster cast is applied to the forearm and the arm, holding the elbow flexed to a right angle. The cast is slung at the wrist, the weight of the cast producing traction upon the lower fragment. Movement of the arm at the shoulder is encouraged. Union occurs without the usual immobilization of the fragments.

Above the Elbow. These fractures are very common in childhood and adolescence. There are many varieties, the most common being the supracondylar type. They are usually attended with considerable swelling, and, because the lower fragment is displaced posteriorly in most cases, the forearm appears to be shortened. The fragments are best maintained in position by holding the elbow acutely flexed. The usual dressings are applied with the arm in this position. A sling from the wrist draws the hand close to the neck.

A very important nursing measure in caring for a patient with an elbow fracture treated by acute flexion of the arm is to observe the hand for swelling and blueness of the nails. These signs may indicate a disturbance of blood supply and should be reported immediately.

Forearm

Both Bones of Forearm. These fractures are most common in the middle third of the forearm. It is almost impossible to tell which dressings are indicated

until the fracture reduction has been completed.

Above the Wrist. These fractures result very often from falls on the out-stretched hand. The Colles (suprastyloid) type is the most common. This is a fracture of the radius from ½ to 1 inch above the wrist, with a posterior displacement of the lower fragment. The hand is deviated to the thumb side. The position is often spoken of as the "silver-fork deformity." These fractures are dressed in many ways, most often by the use of casts.

The Vertebral Body

Injuries to the vertebrae of the dorsal and lumbar spine may involve (1) the vertebral body, (2) lamina and articulating processes and (3) spinous processes or transverse processes. Fractures of the vertebral body are compression fractures. They are often multiple and comprise the most common type of fractures of the spine.

A person with a fracture of a vertebral body complains of severe pain in the back, which may radiate down the legs or to the abdomen and chest. *The most important consideration is to determine if there is injury to the spinal cord.* This may occur if any of the vertebra has been dislocated. Assessment and treatment of patients with spinal cord injury is discussed on pages 822-830.

Frequently, after compression fracture of the lower

TABLE 35-2. Comparative study of patients with two types of hip fractures

Age of patient	Intracapsular (Neck) Usually 60-75 years	Extracapsular (Trochanteric) Usually 70-85 years
Operative technique	Internal fixation, using 3-flanged nail, collapsing nail-plate or multiple pins, or excision of head and insertion of hip-endoprosthesis	Internal fixation, using nail-plate with screws, such as Jewett, McLaughlin, Neufeld, etc.
Nonoperative technique	Ineffective	Continuous traction effective, but dangerous and inferior to operative treatment
Nonunion	Common	Very rare
Avascular necrosis of head	Common	Very rare
Mortality before weight-bearing is resumed	15-20%	30-35%
Expected period for union	4-12 months	3-4 months

(From Rhoads, J., *et al.: Surgery   Principles and Practice*, ed. 4, Lippincott, 1970)

dorsal or lumbar spine, the patient experiences paralytic ileus and difficulty in voiding the first few days. Undoubtably, this is the major nursing problem for several days. The treatment and nursing aspects of the patient with paralytic ileus are found on page 494. If the fracture of the lower dorsal or lumbar spine is without complication, the patient is placed on a firm mattress and kept at bed rest until the pain subsides. When ready for ambulation he may be fitted with a back support or a full-length back brace to support the region of the fracture. Exercises are prescribed to increase and maintain the strength of the back muscles. Recently, patients with injuries to the anterior portion of the vertebrae have been treated symptomatically for pain and encouraged to ambulate immediately. Extension exercises for the back are prescribed as soon as tolerated.

For severe compression fractures, the patient may be placed in a position of hyperextension of the spine and a plaster of Paris jacket applied. This position reduces the compression of the affected vertebral bodies. However, this treatment is not now often used because it causes considerable discomfort and may produce prolonged back pain and stiffness of the spine.

The Pelvis

Pelvic fractures are commonly found following automobile accident crush injuries and falls from buildings and scaffolds. They are serious injuries, because frequently they are associated with injuries to the intrapelvic structures. In fact, the associated mortality with fractures of the pelvis is 10 to 30 per cent. The bladder, the urethra, or the intestines may be ruptured, and prove to be of more serious import than the fracture itself.

Treatment and Nursing Care. If the patient cannot void immediately upon admission to the unit, he should be catheterized to determine whether the bladder has been damaged or ruptured. (This should be done by a physician.) The urine and stools should be examined daily for several days for evidences of blood, and the patient must be watched carefully for signs of intra-abdominal trouble. Palpate the peripheral pulses of both lower extremities, because absence of these pulses may indicate the possibility of a damage to the major vascular supply.

Most pelvic fractures can be treated by the closed method. For many patients with fracture of the pelvis with little or no displacement, rest in bed is all that is required. Of course, a bed board should be placed under the mattress. If anterior displacement of the pelvic ring has occurred (Fig. 35-12), the *pelvic sling* serves to exert a compression force against the iliac bones, which help mold the fracture back in place. Pressure is adjusted by moving the ropes of the sling closer together or farther apart. The pelvic sling lifts the weight of the pelvis very slightly from the mattress. The sling may be folded back over the buttocks for the patient to use the bed pan. (Some orthopedists

Sites of Fractures of the Femur

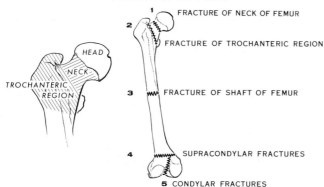

1 FRACTURE OF NECK OF FEMUR

2 FRACTURE OF TROCHANTERIC REGION

3 FRACTURE OF SHAFT OF FEMUR

4 SUPRACONDYLAR FRACTURES

5 CONDYLAR FRACTURES

HEAD

NECK

TROCHANTERIC REGION

FIG. 35-13A. Sites of fracture of the femur.

Fig. 35-13B. Smith-Peterson nail inserted for fracture of the neck of the femur.

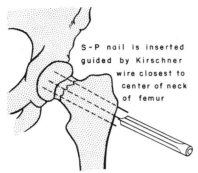

S-P nail is inserted
guided by Kirschner
wire closest to
center of neck
of femur

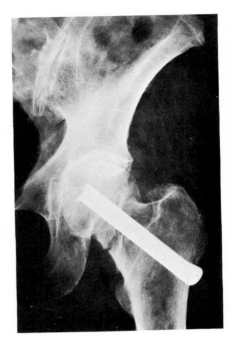

permit the sling to be loosened for certain nursing care activities if the patient's condition permits.) Skin care is a problem. The nurse's ingenuity will be taxed as she reaches under the sling to massage the skin.

In some instances the fracture may be treated with weight traction applied to one or both hips. The nurse must frequently inspect all traction apparatus and watch carefully for signs of pressure. Good care of the skin and gentle handling of the patient do much to prevent complications and to allow him to bear his difficulties more easily.

The Femur

The Patient With a Hip Fracture. Elderly patients have a high incidence of hip fractures because of fragility of bone from osteoporosis caused by endo-skeletal factors, sedentary existence and disuse, poor nutrition and periodic disturbances of balance. Their therapeutic and nursing management is further complicated by associated medical diseases (diabetes, renal and cardiovascular disorders) many of which afflict the majority of elderly patients. Hip fractures are more common in women and often follow insignificant injuries. The affected leg has a characteristic position of shortening, adduction and external rotation. In most instances the patient is unable to move the leg because of pain.

Several types of hip fractures may occur. When the bone is broken inside the joint, it is an *intracapsular fracture*. A fracture outside the joint is classified as an *extracapsular fracture*. This type includes all fractures between the base of the neck and lesser trochanter. Fractures of the neck of the femur heal with more difficulty than those of the trochanteric region, because the head and neck of the femur has a blood supply that may be easily damaged with the fracture. For this reason, nonunion or aseptic necrosis are common in these patients. (See Table 35-2.)

Operative and Nursing Management. Surgeons usually treat fractures of the neck of the femur by the use of pins or nails (Fig. 35-13). The open method may

be used in which the fracture is reduced and nailed under direct vision. The nails are introduced through the trochanter along the neck of the femur into the head. Patients so treated may be up and in a chair within a few days. It is desirable that they be taught to use a walker, bearing weight on the unaffected leg only, as soon as possible.

In a trochanteric fracture of the femur, the operative method is carried out utilizing a nail-plate type of fixation. This patient may also be out of bed using a nonweight-bearing technique (see p. 858). Although there is an excellent blood supply and fractures at this site almost always unite, there is a fairly high mortality rate. These patients are generally older (70 to 85) and are poorer operative risks. Usually, more soft tissue damage occurs at the time of injury and greater blood loss during the operation. The fracture is frequently comminuted and unstable.

In some fractures, the fragments of the head of the femur cannot be replaced. In such a case, the femoral head is removed and a femoral head prosthesis inserted. Many orthopedists prefer this method because nonunion and avascular necrosis of the head are common complications of the subcapital nailing technique.

These patients, because of their age, are particularly prone to develop complications that may become more important with regard to treatment than the fracture itself. The shock of the injury may be fatal. Shock also has been known to cause bladder incontinence, although control is gradually regained later. Other complications include disorientation in the elderly patient, pneumonia, thrombophlebitis and pulmonary

THE ELDERLY PATIENT WITH A HIP FRACTURE
(Treated by an Internal Fixation Device)
Objectives, Principles and Rationale of Nursing Management

Primary objectives: 1. To prolong the patient's life
2. To prevent physical, psychological and social dependence
3. To restore the function of the hip joint

Nursing Action	Rationale
Preoperative Management	
I. To attain mobilization of the patient	Elderly patients tolerate inactivity poorly. Inactivity predisposes to decubitus ulcers, thromboembolism, pneumonia and senile dementia.
A. Alleviate the pain	
1. Handle the affected extremity gently	
2. Give anaglesics as patient's condition indicates	
3. Utilize proper positioning techniques	
4. Assist with the application of Buck's extension as indicated (see p. 850-852)	Buck's extension is used to afford patient mobilization and relieve pain until the operative procedure is performed.
5. Keep the skin dry and relieve pressure areas	Decubitus ulcers develop rapidly in the preoperative period from immobilization.
B. Ensure that the patient is in as favorable condition as possible preoperatively	Elderly patients in poor condition with prefracture disabilities and associated diseases are considered poor risks.
1. Coordinate ECG, blood chemistry studies and x-ray evaluation procedures preoperatively	Mental alertness, bright facial expression and good skin turgor are considered favorable prognostic indications.
2. Give intravenous infusions (if ordered) *slowly*	Patients with limited cardiac reserve cannot stand additional circulatory loading.
Postoperative Nursing Management	
II. To maintain physical and mental capabilities	
A. Encourage the patient to move by himself as much as possible	
1. Teach the patient to assist with turning by grasping the bedrails for support	
2. Support the affected extremity in a position of adduction when the patient turns on his side	
B. Get the patient out of bed as soon as possible	
1. Wrap the lower extremities with elastic compression bandages	Wrapping the extremities supports venous circulation and helps minimize dependent edema. Active motion is an effective method of relieving edema.
2. Use the tilt table as soon as patient's condition permits	With the use of the tilt table the patient becomes accustomed to the upright position. Circulatory and respiratory functioning improve.
3. Assist the patient into a wheelchair several times daily as ordered	
a. With the aid of the overhead trapeze, encourage the patient to move himself into the dangle position (use a Hi-low bed)	
b. Assist him to stand on the *unaffected extremity* and to transfer to a chair	
c. Allow the patient to get up at his own pace and avoid hurrying him	
4. Encourage the patient to participate in activities of daily living (eating, bathing, hair care, etc.)	Participation in A.D.L. helps condition the patient for future ambulation activities and assists him to maintain a degree of independence.

THE ELDERLY PATIENT WITH A HIP FRACTURE (*Continued*)

Nursing Action (*Continued*)	Rationale (*Continued*)
III. To be alert for and prevent complications	Complications have a serious prognostic significance leading to death in the elderly. Anticipation of complications may prevent them.
A. Watch for signs and symptoms of	
1. Pneumonia. Have patient breathe deeply and cough to clear tracheobronchial tree of secretions	Elderly patients who are immobilized are prone to develop hypostatic pneumonia.
2. Fat embolism (characterized by fever, tachycardia, dyspnea, cough. See p. 863.)	Fat embolism sometimes occurs after fractures of the long bones, particularly in elderly patients.
3. Heart failure	
B. Prevent knee contractures	There is a functional inter-relationship of the knee joint with the hip joint that is essential for ambulation. There is a tendency to flex the knee when hip joint pain is present.
1. *Maintain the knee in a position of extension while in bed*	Do not place a pillow under the knee or raise the knee gatch, because this encourages flexion contraction.
2. *Flex the knee in a 90° angle while the patient is in the chair*	Avoid extending the knee when the patient is in a sitting position, because extension produces undue strain on the fractured hip.
3. Move the knee through assisted range-of-motion exercises	
C. Evaluate for urinary tract infection	
1. Avoid the routine use of an indwelling catheter	Infection almost always follows the presence of an indwelling catheter. A urinary tract infection can cause a prolonged period of morbidity and incontinence in the elderly.
2. Watch the color, odor and volume of urinary output	
3. Maintain a liberal fluid intake (within limits of cardio-renal function)	
D. Maintain constant vigilance for signs of decubitus ulcers	Peripheral arterial insufficiency, poor nutrition and lack of movement from pain contribute to skin breakdown.
1. Encourage the patient to move about freely using the overhead trapeze as an assistive device	
2. Use protective heel padding and massage reddened skin areas (see p. 852 for nursing prevention)	
IV. To prepare the patient to walk	
A. Start active exercises as soon as pain and soreness subside	
1. Encourage quadriceps setting exercises hourly	The quadriceps femoris muscle extends the leg and is one of the major muscles necessary for ambulation.
2. Do heel-cord stretching of both legs and abdominal and gluteal contractions (isometric contractions)	Isometric muscle contractions strengthen the muscle but do not move the joint.
3. Assist the patient to perform arm strengthening exercises (flexion and extension of the arms)	The muscles in the shoulder girdle and upper extremities must be strong enough to bear the patient's weight while he is using the walker.
4. Assist the patient to learn to use the walker—ambulating with a nonweight-bearing technique	Most elderly patients lack the muscle strength and balance to participate in nonweight-bearing crutch-walking. Using a walker promotes the feeling of security and independence.
B. Remind the patient *not* to bear weight on the affected extremity until the orthopedist gives permission and x-rays reveal complete healing.	Early weight-bearing before bony union occurs exerts too much stress and may cause bending or fracture of the pin or crushing of the bone.

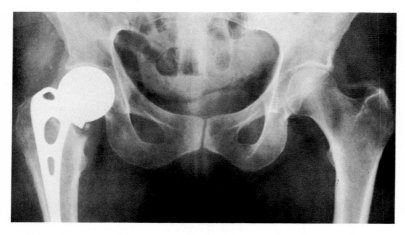

FIG. 35-14. Intramedullary prosthesis, Moore type.

emboli. Because these patients have a tendency to remain in one position and the peripheral circulation is poor, bedsores frequently develop. The nurse may do much to avert the occurrence of decubiti by giving attention to the skin on the back, especially under the hips and the shoulders, and to the heels, and by relieving constant pressure by turning and the use of airfoam pillows, etc. A trapeze suspended from the fracture bed permits the patient to lift himself; this is a great boon to nursing care. *Despite the use of the trapeze, triceps and shoulder exercises should be continued preparatory to ambulatory activities.*

The patient may be turned on his unaffected extremity. A pillow is placed between the legs to keep the affected leg in an abducted position. Then the patient is pulled over gently on his side. After initial soreness has gone and the incision is healed, the patient usually may be turned in the same manner on the affected hip.

Renal calculi and kidney and bladder infections may arise. Pulmonary complications, such as hypostatic congestion of the lungs and bronchopneumonia, may occur and may be fatal. Deep-breathing exercises and changing the position at least every 2 hours help to prevent the development of these complications. The nurse should be familiar with the precautions to be observed in treating patients in traction or casts. The nursing management of the patient with a hip fracture is summarized on page 858-859.

Hip Arthroplasty. Arthroplasty of the hip is undertaken for a painful, degenerative joint. The degeneration is found most often within the head of the femur and finds its source in general metabolic disease, systemic cortisone treatments, chronic alcoholism, the consequence of trauma and, in a vast number of people, for no known cause or idiopathic. The treatment consists either of interposing a membrane or a metal cup, following refashioning of the pelvic and the femoral portions of the joint, or the endoprosthetic replacement of the femoral head portion of the joint.

Additionally, total replacement devices for the hip joint are in somewhat limited use in the United States. The postoperative care of an "arthroplastic hip" requires an intensive and rather prolonged period of rehabilitation with the emphasis on maintenance and the acquisition of motion, as well as muscle power. The early postoperative care is similar to that of the hip fracture (see p. 858-860). The later postoperative care consists of an intense period of re-education of the musculature.

Shaft of Femur. These fractures occur most commonly in youth and middle age. There is marked swelling of the thigh and shortening. The use of intramedullary pins has become increasingly popular. Frequently, reduction is accomplished by traction, using a Thomas splint and Buck's extension, or by the use of a Thomas splint with a Pearson attachment, applying traction to the lower fragment by means of a Kirschner wire, a Steinmann pin, or tongs. Some surgeons apply upward as well as horizontal traction on the lower fragment. A spica cast may also be used.

In the treatment of most patients with a fractured femur, a traction frame is necessary to which the pulleys for traction may be attached. The fracture must be immobilized for 10 to 12 weeks, at the end of which time the patient may be allowed to get up and to walk with the aid of crutches. Full weight-bearing must not be allowed for at least 6 months. To preserve muscle strength, remind the patient to exercise the lower leg, foot and toes on a regular regimen.

Medullary Nailing. The medullary pin is used in some clinics to align fractures of the shaft of the femur. The patient may be placed in skeletal traction for a week preoperatively, which allows time for systemic studies and for the reduction of any swelling.

The medullary nail may be introduced by the open or the closed method. The chief advantage of such nailing is that the patient can be up and out of bed. Prior to this time, he has opportunity to move his leg,

Fig. 35-15. Unilateral leg traction using Bohler Braun splint.

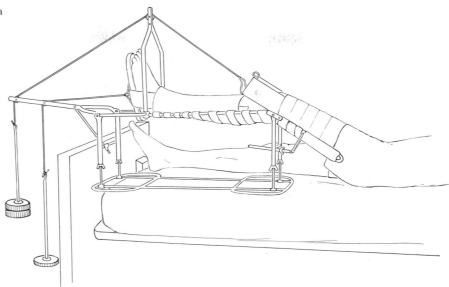

thereby preventing stiffening and muscular atrophy. Disadvantages are (1) there is a possibility of producing bone infection, and (2) there is a chance for the formation of a fat embolism in the closed method.

After the operative procedure, the extremity is usually placed in balanced suspension for 7 to 10 days. Encourage the patient to perform active flexion and extension of the knee. Usually the patient is out of bed on crutches without weight-bearing at the end of 10 to 14 days. After about a year, the stainless steel nail is removed through a small incision.

Tibia and Fibula

Fractures of the shafts of these bones often occur in association with each other. Considerable swelling usually occurs, which disappears readily if reduction and immobilization are accomplished early. The most common fracture below the knee is a fracture of the lower 2 or 3 inches of the fibula due to "twisting the ankle." Frequently associated with such a fracture is fracture of the internal malleolus and of the posterior portion of the articular surface of the tibia. Swelling and discoloration about the ankle are marked.

Reduction is best done under x-ray guidance by traction and manipulation. An intramedullary pin may be used. The leg is dressed in a plaster cast or lateral plaster splints, extending from toe to thigh. Elevation of the leg for several days reduces the swelling very rapidly. Function may be renewed in 6 weeks to 3 months, depending on the amount of involvement. Encourage active flexion of the toes hourly. Quadriceps setting exercises should be continued throughout convalescence.

Assistive Devices for Lower Extremity Fractures

Crutches. Practically all fractures of the lower extremity require the use of crutches during convalescence. Adjustable crutches should be secured for the patient. They should be about 1 inch longer than the distance from the axilla to the heel and should be fitted with rubber suction tips as well as axillary and hand cushions. Gaits used in crutch walking are discussed in chapter 10.

Walking Heel. In many clinics, these fractures are treated by the application of a cast in which is incorporated a walking heel or iron. This treatment cannot be employed until after the early pain and swelling have subsided. By the use of the walking heel, the patient may be able to walk fairly easily without any support or with the aid of a cane.

Internal Derangement of the Knee

Injury to most joints consists of a tear of its supporting ligaments. In the knee joint, however, there may be also a displacement or tear of the semilunar cartilages. These are two crescent-shaped cartilages attached to the edge of the shallow articulating surface of the head of the tibia. They normally move slightly backward and forward to accommodate the change in the shape of the condyles of the femur when the leg is in flexion or extension. In sports and falls, the body is often twisted with the foot fixed. Since little torsion movement is normally permitted in the knee joint, an injury results that very often is either a tear of the cartilage from its attachment to the head of the tibia or an actual tear or fracture of the cartilage itself.

TABLE 35-3. Approximate immobilization time
necessary for union

Fracture Site	Number of Weeks
Phalanx	3-5
Metacarpal	6
Carpal	6
Scaphoid	10
	(or until x-ray shows union)
Radius and ulna	10-12
Humerus:	
Supracondylar	8
Midshaft	8-12
Proximal (impacted)	3
Proximal (displaced)	6-8
Clavicle	6-10
Vertebra	16
Pelvis	6
Femur:	
Intracapsular	24
Intratrochanteric	10-12
Shaft	18
Supracondylar	12-15
Tibia:	
Proximal	8-10
Shaft	14-20
Malleolus	6
Calcaneus	12-16
Metatarsal	6
Toes	3

(From Compere, E. L. *et al.*: Pictorial Handbook of Fracture Treatment. ed. 5, p. 72. Chicago, Yearbook Medical Publishers, 1963).

These injuries leave a loose cartilage in the knee joint that may slip between the femur and the tibia and may prevent full extension of the leg. If this happens when the patient is walking or running, he often describes his disability as his "leg giving way" under him, and there are times when the cartilage gets caught between the articulating surfaces so that the knee "locks." The patient may hear or feel a click in his knee when he walks, especially when he extends his leg bearing his weight, as in going upstairs. When the cartilage is attached front and back, but torn loose laterally (bucket-handle tear), it may slide between the bones to lie between the condyles and prevent full flexion or extension.

These various types of injury arising from a common cause are spoken of as internal derangements of the knee joint, and they produce a disturbing disability because the patient never knows when the knee will give him trouble. The treatment of this disability is removal of the injured cartilage. This can be done with relative ease through an incision into the knee joint. The joint function is thereby returned to normal, and no apparent disability results from the loss of the cartilage.

Preparation for operation consists of shaving the entire leg. Some surgeons desire a "sterile prep" in addition.

Postoperative Nursing Care. After suture of the wound, a pressure dressing is applied, and at times a posterior splint. The leg should be elevated on pillows with a slight bend at the knee. The most common complication is an effusion into the knee joint which produces marked pain. The physician should be called. Relief can be obtained by cutting the pressure dressing and reapplying it more loosely. Frequently, the joint may be aspirated under local anesthesia and pressure relieved by withdrawing the fluid in the joint.

To prevent atrophy of the thigh muscles, these patients are instructed to contract their muscles while in bed. After 1 or 2 days the patient may be up with crutches bearing his weight. In a short time (1 to 2 weeks), full unsupported weight-bearing is possible. The knee usually is supported for another few weeks by an elastic bandage. Full and normal function may be expected in 6 to 8 weeks from the time of operation.

Compound Fractures

Compound fractures may be associated with so much damage to the soft tissue that amputation of the member is necessary. If it is possible, however, that a useful limb may result, the surgeon will thoroughly débride the wound. After débriding or excising devitalized tissue and removing foreign material, he places the fragments in position and repairs the soft tissues (muscles, nerves and tendons). These wounds may be closed under favorable circumstances; otherwise, they are left open, loosely packed with petrolatum gauze and a compression dressing applied. Tetanus prophylaxis is given.

In these days of antibiotic therapy, compound fractures may be expected to heal primarily with primary closure if they have been treated early. When the wounds are grossly contaminated or when treatment has been delayed, débridement and immobilization are carried out, with secondary closure done in 5 to 7 days. If much tissue has been lost, skin grafting may be necessary.

Healing Time of Fractures

The rapidity with which healing occurs varies with many factors. The reduction of the displaced fracture fragments must be accurate and successfully maintained to assure healing. The affected bone must have an adequate blood supply. In addition the age of the patient and the type of fracture affect healing time. In general, fractures of flat bones (pelvis, scapula) heal quite rapidly. Fractures at the ends of long bones where the bone is more vascular and cancellous heal more quickly than do fractures in areas where the bone is dense and less vascular (midshaft). Table 35-3 shows the approximate immobilization times necessary for union of the most common types of fractures.

Complications of Fractures

Immediate Complications. The immediate complications following a fracture are *shock*, which may be fatal within a few hours after injury; *fat embolism*, which may occur within a week; and *thromboembolism* (pulmonary embolism), which may cause death several weeks after injury.

Hypovolemic or traumatic shock as a result of hemorrhage and loss of extracellular fluid into damaged tissues occurs in fractures of the extremities, thorax, pelvis and spine. Treatment consists of replacing the depleted blood volume, relieving the patient's pain, adequate splinting and protecting the patient from further injury.

Fat embolism occurs usually after severe multiple injuries, particularly in the long bones. A day or two following injury, innumerable fat globules may appear in the bloodstream. Serious complications may occur in the brain, heart or lung. The patient so affected may have an increasing pulse and respiratory rate without apparent cause. Petechiae from the fat embolism may be seen on the skin or in the retinae. If fat emboli lodge in the brain, mental confusion occurs and the patient may become comatose and die. Adequate oxygenation of the brain and heart must be preserved when fat embolism is suspected. The administration of Heparin appears to be beneficial in treating this serious complication.

The problem of thromboembolism is discussed on page 332.

Delayed Complications. *Delayed Union and Nonunion.* *Delayed union* occurs when healing is not advanced at the average rate for the location and type of fracture. *Nonunion* is failure of the ends of a fractured bone to unite. Delayed union and nonunion are caused by infection at the fracture site, interposed tissue between the bone ends, motion that converts healing callus to fibrous tissue and a combination of limited bone contact and restricted blood supply. If union does not result by adequate immobilization, the fracture is said to be *ununited.*

Bone fragments have between them only fibrous tissue; no bone salts have been deposited. Such patients often develop a false joint (pseudoarthrosis) at the site of the fracture. When such an unfortunate result occurs, braces may be used to give the patient a useful limb. An operation may be performed by which the ends of the bone are freshened, and an attempt is made to unite them by means of a graft removed from another bone, which is placed in position spanning the fragments. Fractures of the middle of the humerus, of the neck of the femur in elderly people, and of the lower third of the tibia most frequently result in nonunion.

Avascular Necrosis of Bone. Avascular necrosis may occur when the bone loses its blood supply following fracture or dislocation, notably in the hip. The head and neck of the femur have a blood supply that is subject to injury and thus cause severe damage to the bone. The dead bone may be reabsorbed and replaced by new bone. If revascularization takes place, the structure may collapse. Healing can occur in the presence of avascular necrosis, but the patient may develop a painful arthritis. Usually the interruption of the blood supply is an unpreventable complication that occurs at the time of injury.

THE PATIENT WITH AN AMPUTATION

Amputation of extremities is frequently necessary in the treatment of gangrene, tumors, deformities, septic wounds, compound fractures and severe crushing injuries, gas gangrene, etc. In severe trauma, an amputation is done to save a patient's life.

Psychological Considerations

The nurse will be aware that amputation forces the patient to make a major adjustment. One day he may be a perfectly normal individual, and the next day he must accept his loss. An individual who has a long-standing disease that causes him pain and restricts his ability to get around may find it less difficult to accept an amputation.

The patient's adaptation to the disability produced by an amputation depends not only on his physical condition and the usefulness of his prosthetic device but also on his *perception* of his disability. An amputation produces a permanent physical handicap that certainly thwarts some physiological, psychological and social needs. The patient must accept his limitations realistically. Physicians, nurses, prosthetists and physical therapists share the task of helping the patient to accept himself and make necessary changes in his life pattern with minimal interference in his life activities.

Nursing Management

Preoperative Care. Often before surgery, the physician performs tests to determine the patency of circulation. These include surface temperature, color changes when the limb is elevated or dependent, oscillometric readings and arteriography. The patient's state of nutrition must be determined and improved if necessary. Psychological preparation cannot be neglected. The physician and the nurse can help to build a healthy optimism in this patient by making him realize that he can overcome his handicap and be independent.

Preparation for the operation when possible should consist in shaving of the part and thorough cleansing with soap and water. Intravenous fluids are administered to combat dehydration; blood is made available. Before the operation the extremity should be elevated continuously for at least 5 minutes to allow the venous blood to drain as completely as possible from the part. This procedure is aided in many clinics by the application of a pneumatic tourniquet or an Esmarch bandage, an elastic bandage of 2-inch rubber applied in the direction of the trunk, to compress the extremity. A tourniquet of heavy rubber then is applied and drawn tight enough to compress the blood vessels.

If the amputation is not an emergency procedure, efforts should be made to strengthen the upper extremities as well as the trunk and the abdominal muscles. It is ideal to teach the patient to crutch-walk before the surgical procedure. The patient can be given traction weights and encouraged to flex and to extend his arms while he is holding the weights. Doing push-ups while he is in a prone position and sit-ups while he is seated will strengthen the tricep muscles, which are so important in crutch-walking.

Postoperative Care. Amputations are usually performed by making soft-tissue flaps, which are used to cover the bone end. The site of the amputation is determined by two factors: circulation in the part and the requirements of an artificial limb (prosthesis). In many amputations of the leg, when performed for gangrene of the foot due to vascular impairment, a high amputation (midthigh) must be done because the circulation of the leg below is insufficient to bring about healing of an amputation site at a lower level.

Experience with artificial limbs has shown that stumps of some certain length function best in these appliances. If the stump is too long, it may be awkward and hard to fit; if it is too short, the adjacent joint cannot function well. When they are made below the knee and the elbow joints, it is well to splint the part for a time to prevent contractures.

These patients should be watched carefully for any signs or symptoms of hemorrhage. As a precaution, a tourniquet should be in plain sight at the foot of the bed, and, if bleeding occurs, should be applied to the stump and pulled sufficiently tight to stop the bleeding. It should be left in place until the surgeon can be notified. The stump should be elevated for the first few days on a pillow protected with a rubber or plastic pillow case. Such a pillow should support the entire stump from the hip down, in order that knee flexion be prevented. *This pillow is removed as soon as possible by physician's order to avoid hip joint flexion contracture.* Oozing usually appears at the bottom of the dressing; linen may be spared by placing the stump upon a sterile cellucotton pad. The dressings should be reinforced rather than changed. A foot board should be used to keep the remaining foot in dorsiflexion.

During the first 24 hours, especially in older patients, a shocklike state is frequently present, and the patient does not fully realize that he has had an amputation. Often the realization may come as a shock to him, even though he knew before his operation that an amputation was to be performed. Frequently, complications arise by the production of pulmonary emboli and the patient must be watched carefully for such findings as cough, chest pains, hemoptysis, severe sudden collapse, cyanosis, or even sudden death. On occasion, especially when the amputation has been done for infection, a guillotine-type operation may be performed without any attempt to suture the skin. In such cases, to prevent the retraction of the skin, traction may be applied and eventual healing brought about. The principles given under Nursing Care of the Patient in Traction (p. 852) apply here.

Rehabilitation

Effective preprosthetic care is important to prosthetic fitting. The major problems that are preventable during this period are (1) flexion deformities, (2) nonshrinkage of the stump, and (3) abduction deformities of the hip. These deformities will delay the prosthetic fitting.

After the first 24 to 48 hours, depending on the physician's orders, the patient should be encouraged to turn from side to side and to be in the prone position to prevent flexion contracture of the hip. A pillow can be placed under the abdomen and the stump; the forefoot can be placed over the edge of the mattress. The legs should remain close together while the patient is in the prone position to prevent an abduction deformity. He must learn to recognize the value of moving the stump so that contractures are avoided.

Sometimes patients use an overhead trapeze when changing their position in bed; this strengthens the biceps. However, this set of muscles is not as necessary in crutch-walking as are the triceps. The triceps can be strengthened by pressing with the palms against the bed while moving the body and continuing the push-up exercises. Exercises under the supervision of the physical therapist, such as hyperextension of the stump, also aid in strengthening muscles as well

FIG. 35-16. Bandaging an above-the-knee amputation stump. (See guide on p. 866)

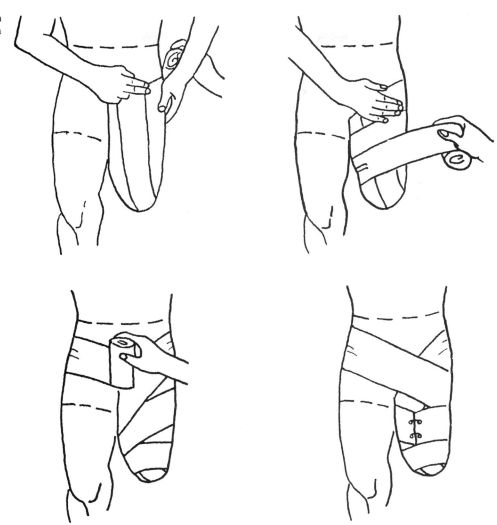

as increasing circulation, reducing edema and preventing atrophy. In getting the patient out of bed, regard must be given to maintaining good posture.

The patient should be fairly adept at balancing himself on one leg and walking with crutches before he leaves the hospital. Several weeks or many months may elapse before the patient is fitted with a prosthesis.

Exercises that assist in developing balance are:

1. Arising from a chair and standing
2. Standing on toes while holding on to a chair
3. Bending the knees while holding on to a chair
4. Balancing on one leg without support
5. Hopping on one foot while holding on to a chair

The nurse may stand behind the patient and stabilize him by his waist while he is learning to perform these exercises. While crutch-walking, the patient should learn to use a reciprocal gait. The stump should move back and forth while the patient is walking with his crutches. The stump should not be held up in a flexed position to prevent a permanent flexion deformity from occurring.

Stump Conditioning. After the wound has healed, the nurse should learn from the surgeon how he wishes the stump to be bandaged. Thereafter the nurse can teach the patient or some member of his family the correct method of bandaging.

The stump has to be conditioned if a prosthesis is to be fitted properly. (However, the nurse must bear in mind that not every patient can be fitted for a prosthetic device.) To shrink and to shape the stump, the stump must be bandaged correctly. Bandaging supports the soft tissue and minimizes the formation of edematous fluid while the stump is in a dependent position. The bandage is applied in such a manner

GUIDE TO BANDAGING AN ABOVE-THE-KNEE AMPUTATION STUMP*

Purpose: The purpose for bandaging a stump is to shrink and to shape the stump for the application of an artificial leg.

Problems: Improper bandaging will produce:

a. Constriction of the stump

b. Delayed healing

c. Skin abrasions

d. Formation of creases or adipose tissue at distal end

Basic Principles: The bandage is applied before the patient gets out of bed after periods of recumbency. The bandage should be maintained continuously and reapplied when tension is lost. Pressure should be applied under moderate tension to the entire stump, guarding against any tourniquetlike action at the proximal portion of the stump. The stump is kept in *hyperextension* while the bandage is applied.

Technique of Applying Bandage:

1. Begin the recurrent, vertical turns on the anterior surface of the stump just inferior to the level of the inguinal ligament (Fig. 35-16 A).

    Pass the bandage over the distal end of the stump posteriorly to the gluteal fold. The patient assists by holding the recurrents in place.

    Make two additional recurrents over the medial and the lateral aspects of the end of the stump.

2. Anchor the recurrents by several horizontal circular turns of the bandage (Fig. 35-16 B).

    When anchoring the recurrents, the circular turns begin at the lateral side and run posteriorly to the medial side.

    When the recurrents are firmly secured, bring the bandage down and around the stump and up again using oblique turns or a modified figure-8.

    Keep the pressure away, up and out from the distal portion of the stump to eliminate creases. Do not use circular turns which are not oblique, as they tend to constrict circulation.

3. Start the hip spica from the anterior medial aspect of the stump and bring it laterally across the anterior surface of the stump in the inguinal region (Fig. 35-16 C). (The hip spica anchors the bandage and covers the tissue high in the groin and the lateral surfaces of the hip, thus eliminating the formation of bulges in this area.)

    Bring the bandage around the body on a level with the iliac crest.

4. Return around the stump making a figure-8, and bring the bandage around the pelvis again. Finish the bandaging by making oblique turns on the stump.

    Anchor the bandage with safety pins at the lateral or the anterior surface of the stump. Fasten where bandage ends and at crossing of spica at the hip (Fig. 35-16 D).

* From Nattress, L. W., Jr.: Orthopedic and Prosthetic Appliance Journal, pp. 1 to 55, June, 1957.

that the remaining muscles required to operate the prosthesis are as firm as possible, while those muscles that are no longer useful will atrophy. See figure 35-16.

In order to "toughen" the stump in preparation for using a prosthesis, the doctor usually orders stump-conditioning activities. The patient is taught to push his stump into a soft pillow. Progressively he increases the resistance, pushing the stump against a firmer pillow and then against a hard surface.

When amputations of the leg have been performed on elderly, debilitated patients, especially those with diabetes and arteriosclerosis, particular care is taken to protect the stump against external infection. Such patients frequently become incontinent of urine and feces, and not infrequently the dressing and the wound of the stump may become soiled. Plastic material secured by a wide adhesive strip about the leg above the dressing has proved to be a good prophylactic measure.

Often during the convalescence while the muscle stumps are adjusting themselves, twitching and spasms occur. Heat, massage, change of position to procure relaxation, a light sandbag on a thigh stump to counteract the psoas action—all will help. During this stage, and often for an indefinite period to follow, the patient may complain as though the pain were in the amputated limb—the "phantom limb" complication so often very difficult to treat.

The complete rehabilitation of an amputee requires a rehabilitation team. The orthopedic surgeon, the physiatrist, the limb maker, the physical therapist, and the occupational therapist all unite their efforts to condition and train the patient to make a satisfactory adjustment to his prosthesis. With vocational counseling and job-retraining where necessary, many of these patients can return to work. If it is not possible for the patient to use a prosthesis, he can be taught to participate in self-care activities in a wheelchair. The pamphlet *Step Into Action** is a teaching booklet designed for the amputee; it has illustrations and descriptions concerning stump hygiene, bandaging, and other activities that are important to the patient.

* Superintendent of Documents, U. S. Government Printing Office, Washington, D. C. 20402.

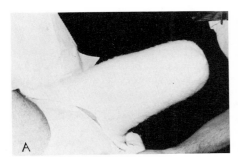

(A) The sterilized stocking is pulled into place.

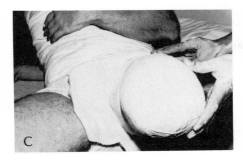

(C) The hardened cast after removal of the casting fixture.

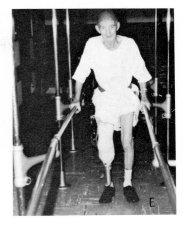

(E) A typical patient 24 hours after a below-the-knee amputation. This patient was 83 years old at the time of surgery.

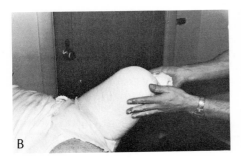

(B) The wrap is begun by applying elastic plaster bandage beginning at the distal end.

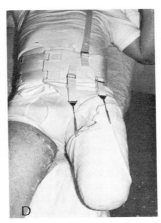

(D) A suspension harness is in place to maintain the plaster cast in place at all times.

FIG. 35-17. Bandaging a below-the-knee amputation stump that will be immediately fitted with a prosthesis.

Immediate Postsurgical Prosthesis Fitted on the Lower Extremity

A milestone has been reached recently in the management of the lower extremity amputee patient. As a result of a federally supported Prosthetics Research Study,* patients are being fitted with prostheses immediately after surgery. With this technique there has been a reduction of postsurgical pain and discomfort and more rapid stump healing. Early crutch ambulation with partial weight-bearing can usually be accomplished on the first postoperative day. The patient ambulates and returns to his family and work in a much shorter period of time.

Following the amputation, a sterilized stump sock is applied to the stump. Felt pads are placed over pressure-sensitive areas. Starting from the distal end, the stump is wrapped with elastic plaster of Paris bandages while firm, even pressure is maintained. Care is taken not to constrict circulation. As soon as the rigid dressing has dried, the prosthetic unit, consisting of a prosthetic extension and foot, can be

* Since 1964, the Prosthetic and Sensory Aids Service of the Veterans' Administration has been supporting this study.

applied. The length of the prosthesis is tailored to the individual patient in the operating room after the amputation is performed (Fig. 35-17).

Nursing Emphasis. The patient returns from the recovery room with the special plaster cast on the stump and his prosthetic extension and foot attached or nearby. *A most important consideration is that the amputation stump remain in the plaster cast socket during the patient's entire hospitalization.* If the cast inadvertently comes off, the stump must be immediately wrapped tightly with an elastic compression bandage and the surgeon notified so that another cast can be applied. Excessive edema can develop within a short period of time and may prevent early weight-bearing, which is so essential.

After 24 hours the patient is permitted to stand and bear some weight on the prosthesis. This activity produces surprisingly little pain. In fact, these patients do not complain of the severe pain and phantom limb discomfort that is experienced by patients who are treated by the more conventional method. Usually, only mild opiates are needed for pain relief during the immediate postoperative phase.

According to the individual patient's condition, he is encouraged to increase his activity daily, utilizing parallel bars, a walker, crutches and canes as assistive devices. Ambulation is always carried out with the prosthesis on and is done under the supervision and encouragement of a nurse or physical therapist.

The original cast may be left on for 8 to 14 days unless contraindicated by elevated body temperature, loose fitting cast, etc. A second cast is then applied, and removed 15 to 20 days postoperatively. At this time the patient may be measured for a more permanent prosthesis. A light plaster cast is provided to limit edema during the times the patient is not wearing his permanent prosthesis. Gait training is continued under the direction of a physical therapist until optimal gait is achieved.

If the patient has coexisting vascular disease, the immediate fitting of a prosthesis after an amputation may not be feasible.

PATIENTS WITH BONE AND JOINT INFECTIONS

Osteomyelitis

Acute hematogenous osteomyelitis is an acute infection of the endosteal bone that rapidly involves other bony structures. It affects the long bones most frequently and is caused most commonly by the *Staphylococcus aureus*. The infection usually is blood-borne from other foci of infection, but it may follow slight trauma or exposure to cold and wet. It is essentially a disease of childhood and adolescence. However, osteomyelitis may occur by direct infection of the bone resulting from compound fractures.

The onset of the hematogenous disease usually is sudden, occurring often with a chill, high fever, rapid pulse and general malaise. In children, in whom the disease usually begins as an acute epiphysitis, these constitutional symptoms at first may overshadow the local signs completely. As the infection extends from the marrow cavity through the cortex of the bone, it involves the periosteum and the soft tissues, and the limb becomes painful, swollen and extremely tender. Thus an abscess of bone is formed.

In the natural course of events, the abscess may point and drain but, more often, incision and drainage are done by the surgeon. The resulting abscess cavity has in its walls areas of dead tissue, as in any abscess cavity; however, in this case the dead tissue is bone, which cannot liquefy easily and be discharged as pus. This dead bone is called a *sequestrum*. Healing in a bone abscess is more difficult than in an abscess in soft tissue, because the cavity cannot collapse and heal. New bone, the *involucrum*, forms as the body's attempt at repair. Often it grows so as to surround a sequestrum. Thus, even though healing appears to take place, a chronically infected sequestrum remains that is prone to produce recurring abscesses throughout the life of the individual. This is the so-called chronic type of osteomyelitis.

Treatment. Acute osteomyelitis begins as a staphylococcic septicemia, and formerly the acute toxemia frequently was fatal. Since antibiotics became available, early and intensive treatment usually produces a rapid recovery. The development of an abscess of the bone with the resulting marked and prolonged morbidity, thus can be avoided.

The antibiotic to which the causative organism has demonstrated sensitivity is the drug treatment of choice. Usually the antibiotic is given intravenously or intramuscularly to maintain a sustained therapeutic level.

In neglected or untreated cases, aspiration or incision and drainage of an abscess may be necessary.

In chronic osteomyelitis, all dead, infected bone and cartilage must be removed before permanent healing takes place. This operation, which is called a *sequestrectomy*, consists of the removal of enough involucrum with mallet and chisel to enable the surgeon to remove the sequestrum. Often sufficient bone is removed to convert a deep cavity into a shallow saucer (saucerization). Muscle sometimes is used to help to obliterate the resulting wound. These operations are becoming increasingly rare since the advent of effective antimicrobial chemotherapy. Primary healing may be obtained frequently by the use of an appropriate antibiotic (e.g., methicillin or oxacillin), if the cavity can be closed and the skin approximated. Sometimes the granulating wound may be covered by a split-thickness skin graft.

When osteomyelitis occurs in a compound fracture by direct implantation of the offending organism, there is no preceding septicemia, but the treatment generally follows that outlined above, except that the fracture must be treated in addition.

Nursing Management. Osteomyelitis is a disease that demands good nursing care. The wounds themselves frequently are very painful and require great care and gentleness in their handling. The affected part may be immobilized with a splint until the wound has healed. Immobilization decreases pain and muscle spasm as well as the exudate.

Pillow support to the adjoining joints and maintenance of good alignment are comfort measures. Careful handling also is essential because of the possibilities of cross-infection and pathologic fracture. Hot packs may be prescribed for indurated areas. Less pain is experienced if petrolatum gauze is used in the dressing. Scrupulous care of the skin is required to prevent bedsores. Fresh air, sunlight and a high caloric diet rich in vitamins will hasten the convalescence of these patients. They should be watched carefully for any development of painful areas or sudden rises in temperature, as these symptoms usually indicate the formation of a secondary abscess.

A frequent problem encountered is an unpleasant odor due to the foul drainage. (A deodorizer near the patient's unit may help.) Explaining that this is a usual result of bone infection may reassure the patient somewhat. Because of the long period of hospitalization and frequent readmissions sometimes necessary in the treatment of these patients, their morale often is low and they need stimulation and diversion.

Bone and Joint Tuberculosis

A common form of nonpulmonary tuberculosis is that involving the bones and the joints. Tuberculous arthritis usually is monarticular, involving most often a vertebra, a hip, a knee or an elbow. It occurs predominantly in children and is characterized by pain of variable severity, wasting of surrounding muscles, weight loss and fever. During its acute stage this disease produces the well-known *cold abscesses*, so named to distinguish them from the acute inflammatory abscesses that are associated with acute infectious processes, and which are hot or warm to palpation. Sinuses from a tuberculous joint may burrow their way for long distances; those from the spine, for example, opening through the skin of the thigh. Destruction of the joint, with permanent ankylosis and eventual deformity—the results—explain hip disease and hunchback. More than one half of these patients show signs of pulmonary tuberculosis.

The diagnosis is suggested by a positive family history of tuberculosis, signs of tuberculosis elsewhere in the body and the monarticular character of the joint involvement.

Tuberculous Tenosynovitis and Bursitis. *Tuberculous tenosynovitis* most often develops in association with tuberculosis of nearby bones and joints. The tendons most frequently affected are those about the wrists—either the flexor or the extensor group, seldom both. Rarely are those about the ankles similarly affected.

Tuberculous bursitis may be the only demonstrable focus of this infection in the body. This type of bursitis develops very slowly, distending the sac with a serous fluid, in which, later, great numbers of rice bodies appear. Such swelling generally is painless, but it may interfere with the motions of the part which the bursa is intended to aid.

Treatment. These periarticular infections, as in the case of other tuberculous lesions, respond quite readily to vigorous chemotherapy conducted as specified earlier.

PATIENTS WITH ARTHRITIS

Public Health Aspects of Arthritis

Excluding mental illness, joint disease causes more disability than all other chronic diseases combined. It has been estimated that 1 out of every 10 persons in the United States over the age of 14 years is afflicted with some form of arthritis. Twelve million Americans have arthritis. The U.S. Public Health Service reports that each year more than 300,000 individuals are barred from employment because of chronic joint disease, 50 per cent of these persons becoming complete invalids. Thus, arthritis incapacitates 10 times as many persons as do diabetes and tuberculosis, 7 times as many as all cancers and twice as many as heart disease. Considered from the economic standpoint, arthritis regularly is responsible for the loss of more than 90 million workdays per year, which is equivalent to a financial loss of half a billion dollars—more than is forfeited as a result of any other illness, with the exception of nervous and mental disease. The financial burden alone entailed in providing medical care for arthritic patients exceeds $100,000,000 every year, a figure that does not take into account the tremendous drain on the productivity of persons affected with the disease.

It must be recognized, of course, that for every patient who is hospitalized for arthritis, there are scores of others, equally incapacitated, who are receiving treatment in nursing homes or in their own homes. This being the case, it behooves the nurse to study the application of therapeutic principles she learns in the hospital to the care of the patient in the home, bearing in mind that her advice will be sought by the families of her arthritic patients regarding the treatment for which they will ultimately be responsible.

Definition and Classification of Arthritis

The term "arthritis" implies joint inflammation, although it frequently is used to describe any disorder involving the joints. "Rheumatism" is used to denote pain, stiffness or deformity of joints, muscles and related structures, while the term "rheumatic diseases" refers to musculoskeletal disorders in which changes take place in the tissues comprising or surrounding the joints. (One can readily understand how these terms have come to be used interchangeably!) The two main types of arthritis are rheumatoid arthritis and osteoarthritis. Table 35-4 gives a tentative classification of arthritis and rheumatism.

The Patient With Rheumatoid Arthritis

Rheumatoid arthritis is a chronic systemic disease of unknown cause, characterized most prominently by recurrent inflammation involving the synovium or lining of the joints.

Clinical Course

The disease usually begins acutely as a recurring polyarthritis with fever, the first attacks of which may closely resemble acute rheumatic fever. Following one or several such attacks, some of the joints involved never quite return to normal, but remain stiff and sore. During subsequent acute exacerbations, other joints likewise become chronically injured, and each attack leaves the joints involved more damaged than before.

The disease affects primarily the joint cartilages and the articular surfaces of the bones, destroying

TABLE 35-4. Primer on rheumatic diseases
ARA Nomenclature and Classification of Arthritis and Rheumatism (Tentative)

I. Polyarthritis of unknown etiology
 A. Rheumatoid arthritis
 B. Juvenile rheumatoid arthritis (Still's disease)
 C. Ankylosing spondylitis
 D. Psoriatic arthritis
 E. Reiter's syndrome
 F. Others

II. "Connective tissue" disorders
 A. Systemic lupus erythematosus
 B. Polyarteritis nodosa
 C. Scleroderma (progressive systemic sclerosis)
 D. Polymyositis and dermatomyositis
 E. Others

III. Rheumatic fever

IV. Degenerative joint disease (osteoarthritis, osteoarthrosis)
 A. Primary
 B. Secondary

V. Nonarticular rheumatism
 A. Fibrositis
 B. Intervertebral disc and low back syndromes
 C. Myositis and myalgia
 D. Tendinitis and peritendinitis (bursitis)
 E. Tenosynovitis
 F. Fasciitis
 G. Carpal tunnel syndrome
 H. Others
 (See also shoulder-hand syndrome, VIII. E.)

VI. Diseases with which arthritis is frequently associated
 A. Sarcoidosis
 B. Relapsing polychondritis
 C. Henoch-Schönlein syndrome
 D. Ulcerative colitis
 E. Regional ileitis
 F. Whipple's disease
 G. Sjögren's syndrome
 H. Familial Mediterranean fever
 I. Others
 (See also psoriatic arthritis, I.D.)

VII. Associated with known infectious agents
 A. Bacterial
 1. Brucella
 2. Gonococcus
 3. Mycobacterium tuberculosis
 4. Pneumococcus
 5. Salmonella
 6. Staphylococcus
 7. Streptobacillus moniliformis (Haverhill fever)
 8. Treponema pallidum (syphilis)
 9. Treponema pertenue (yaws)
 10. Others
 B. Rickettsial
 C. Viral
 D. Fungal
 E. Parasitic
 (See also rheumatic fever, III.)

VIII. Traumatic and/or neurogenic disorders
 A. Traumatic arthritis (viz., the result of direct trauma)
 B. Lues (tertiary syphilis)
 C. Diabetes
 D. Syringomyelia
 E. Shoulder-hand syndrome
 F. Mechanical derangement of joints
 G. Others
 (See also degenerative joint disease, IV.; carpal tunnel syndrome, V.G.)

IX. Associated with known biochemical or endocrine abnormalities
 A. Gout
 B. Ochronosis
 C. Hemophilia
 D. Hemoglobinopathies (e.g., sickle cell disease)
 E. Agammaglobulinemia
 F. Gaucher's disease
 G. Hyperparathyroidism
 H. Acromegaly
 I. Hypothyroidism
 J. Scurvy (hypovitaminosis C)

 K. Xanthoma tuberosum
 L. Others
 (See also multiple myeloma, X.G.; Hurler's syndrome, XII.C.)

X. Tumor and tumor-like conditions
 A. Synovioma
 B. Pigmented villonodular synovitis
 C. Giant cell tumor of tendon sheath
 D. Primary juxta-articular bone tumors
 E. Metastatic
 F. Leukemia
 G. Multiple myeloma
 H. Benign tumors of articular tissue
 I. Others
 (See also hypertrophic, osteo-arthropathy, XIII.G.)

XI. Allergy and drug reactions
 A. Arthritis due to specific allergens (e.g., serum sickness)
 B. Arthritis due to drugs (e.g., hydralazine syndrome)
 C. Others

XII. Inherited and congenital disorders
 A. Marfan's syndrome
 B. Ehlers-Danlos syndrome
 C. Hurler's syndrome
 D. Congenital hip dysplasia
 E. Morquio's disease
 F. Others

XIII. Miscellaneous disorders
 A. Amyloidosis
 B. Aseptic necrosis of bone
 C. Behcet's syndrome
 D. Chondrocalcinosis (pseudogout)
 E. Erythema multiforme (Stevens-Johnson syndrome)
 F. Erythema nodosum
 G. Hypertrophic osteoarthropathy
 H. Juvenile osteochondritis
 I. Osteochondritis dissecans
 J. Reticulohistiocytosis of joints (lipoid dermato-arthritis)
 K. Tietze's disease
 L. Others

(From the Committee of the American Rheumatism Association: Primer On Rheumatic Diseases. The Arthritis Foundation.)

the joint cavity, which becomes filled with adhesions. Marked joint crepitation can be obtained; dislocations are common; ankyloses follow; and muscular contractures may become marked—hence the descriptive name *arthritis deformans*. Atrophic changes appear early, involving the soft tissues about the affected joints. The disease occurs more commonly in women and rarely in children.

The clinical course is variable, ranging from a mild episode to a severe unremitting disorder. Usually mild deformities develop slowly and the patient at first experiences only mild discomfort.

The clinical picture presented in a well-marked case of this condition is typical. The patient appears chronically ill; the muscles of his extremities, especially of their distal segments, are apt to be wasted; the subcutaneous fat often is greatly decreased. The joints become deformed—some of them dislocated. If the condition is extreme, the patient can scarcely move a single joint in the body. The early immobility of the joints, however, does not result from bony ankylosis but from tense muscular spasm.

The deformities of the hands are characteristic. The distal phalanges are hyperextended, the proximal flexed, and there is ulnar deviation of the fingers. The skin covering the fingertips is thin, pale, smooth and shiny, the nails are rough and brittle, and the intrinsic muscles of the hand are wasted. The spine may be stiff and the jaw partly fixed. This typifies the most advanced grade of rheumatoid arthritis, the severity of which may vary from this marked degree to a mild stiffening and swelling of the finger joints.

Although joint pain and destruction are the most apparent problems, rheumatoid arthritis is a systemic disease. There may be associated inflammation of connective tissue. The skin, eyes and nervous system may be affected by vasculitis, which may produce thrombosis and ischemia. The rheumatoid process may affect changes on the serosal surfaces of the heart and lungs. Any or every organ or system may be involved by the rheumatic disease.

Other clinical phenomena observed in addition to the joint involvement include subcutaneous nodules which in many respects are indistinguishable from those of rheumatic fever; frequent generalized lymphadenopathy and splenomegaly; fever, which may be high and prolonged; anemia, leukocytosis and elevation of the sedimentation rate.

The etiology of rheumatoid arthritis is unknown, and its relation to rheumatic fever is not clear. The disease is coming to be regarded as a disorder of immunity. In support of this concept is the presence in the serum of most of these patients of the so-called "rheumatoid factor," a plasma protein with properties akin to those of an immune antibody which is capable of reacting specifically with human (and/or rabbit) gamma globulin (i.e., conceivably an anti-antibody). However, the origin and the significance of this "factor" remain to be discovered.

Therapeutic and Nursing Objectives

The primary objective of treatment in the acute stage of rheumatoid arthritis is the *prevention of crippling deformities*. Other therapeutic goals are (1) to maintain joint mobility and muscle power; (2) to promote comfort; (3) to halt the activity of the disease; (4) to help the patient and his family to adjust to his chronic disability; and (5) to assist the patient to become functionally independent as soon and as completely as possible.

Maintenance of Joint Mobility and Muscle Power. Inflammation, scarring or other mechanical damage to joint structures result in pain and disability. The patient, in an effort to avoid pain, tends to immobilize the affected joints, and muscular spasm further limits their motion. If acutely inflamed, these joints should be rested by the application of splints, sandbags, bivalved casts or any other mechanical device that will maintain them in functional positions. Above all, they should not be permitted to "freeze" in positions of flexion, which is their natural tendency because of the predominant strength of the flexor muscles. While he is in bed, the patient should lie flat on a firm mattress with only one pillow under his head because of the risk of dorsal kyphosis. (At no time should a pillow be placed under his knees, as this promotes flexion contractures of those joints.)

Joints may lose their normal range of motion due to deformity and atrophy. This loss can be prevented to a large extent by systematic range-of-motion exercises (p. 164-167). If activity is painful, the nurse may help the patient (with active-assisted exercises) to perform the required motions. The nurse must emphasize constantly that the daily performance of these therapeutic exercises increases muscle strength, which is essential for the restoration of joint mobility.

Chairs that are too low may produce considerable pain for patients with involvement of knees or hips. The height of chairs can be increased by extending their legs or by raising their elevation with sponge rubber seat cushions. Toilet seats can be raised by attaching built up seats to standard toilet fixtures.

Rheumatoid arthritis is a long-term disease, and its management is a long-term project, which must include a program of systematic exercises in the home. The pamphlet *Strike Back At Arthritis!** explains and

* Superintendent of Documents, U. S. Dept. of Health, Education and Welfare, U. S. Government Printing Office, Washington, D. C. 20402.

THE PATIENT WITH RHEUMATOID ARTHRITIS
Objectives and Principles of Patient Education

I. To understand the disease in order to learn to live with it

    A. Learn the nature of the disease and its treatment

    B. Have confidence in your physician and individualized treatment program

    C. Avoid "miracle cures"—drugs not prescribed by your physician and other forms of "quackery"

    D. Report to the physician or clinic *regularly* for evaluation

    E. Accept the *realities* of the disease and live within the limits imposed by it

    F. Maintain your independence

        1. Rely on your own capabilities

        2. Participate in as many activities as possible without producing fatigue

        3. Use self-help devices and "gadgets" to conserve energy and expand efficiency

        4. Study and use methods of work simplification

        5. Build up muscle strength and endurance by participating in exercise program

    G. Try to avoid anxiety, worry and emotional crises

II. To relieve pain and reduce inflammation

    A. Achieve a balance between rest and activity

    B. Have scheduled rest periods in bed to reduce joint stresses

        1. Use a bed board under the mattress to prevent sagging

        2. Use a bed cradle when the joints of ankles and feet are involved

        3. Rest in positions of extension maintaining good posture (see p. 161)

        4. Place only one pillow under the head

        5. Avoid putting pillows under painful joints, to prevent contracture deformities

        6. Turn in prone position twice daily to prevent hip flexion and knee contractures

        7. Modify rest time gradually as improvement is seen

        8. Secure a long period of sleep at night

    C. Rest and support inflamed joints

        1. Use prescribed splints and supports to relieve pain and muscle spasm

        2. Wear splints during sleeping hours

        3. Keep in mind that the splint may need to be altered every week or two

        4. Avoid stroking and rubbing joints that are swollen and painful

        5. Avoid overactivity that produces fatigue

    D. Use heat treatments for muscle relaxation and relief of pain

        1. Take a warm shower or tub bath upon arising to relieve morning stiffness

            a. Rest in bed 20 to 30 minutes if possible after warm bath

        2. Apply hot moist compresses to especially painful joints *as directed* several times daily

            a. Leave hot application on only for prescribed length of time

            b. Cover moist compresses with hot water bottle, plastic wrap and a heavy towel to prevent a rapid loss of heat

        3. Use paraffin dips as prescribed

            a. Melt paraffin in a double boiler

            b. Use a candy thermometer to determine exact temperature (52-54° C. or 126-130° F.)

            c. Immerse part in warm paraffin, withdraw and immerse again (Fig. 35-20)

               (1) Repeat procedure 8 to 10 times

               (2) Cover with plastic bag and towel to retain heat

               (3) Leave in place for ½ to 1½ hours

               (4) Peel off paraffin and re-use at next treatment time

               (5) Do finger and hand exercises immediately after treatment

        4. Use contrast baths (hot and cold) as prescribed

            a. Immerse part in hot water 43° C. (110° F.) followed by immersion in cold water 16° C. (60° F.) for length of time prescribed by physician

            b. End the treatment with hot immersion

        5. If heat intensifies pain, discontinue heat treatments and notify physician

        6. Try an electric blanket to ascertain its usefulness in relieving morning stiffness

    E. Take prescribed drugs for pain relief on a regular schedule

        1. Develop an awareness of the *amount* of aspirin or sodium salicylates necessary to provide individual pain relief

        2. Report symptoms of ringing in the ears, as this is a guide to adequate dosage

        3. Watch for symptoms of gastric irritation and diminished hearing

---

THE PATIENT WITH RHEUMATOID ARTHRITIS (*Continued*)

III. To preserve joint function and prevent deformities

    A. Do the prescribed exercises to preserve joint motion and to gain muscular strength and endurance

        1. Know the purpose of each exercise

        2. Perform the exercise slowly

        3. Perform one set of exercises after using systemic heat (shower/bath)

    B. Carry out range-of-motion exercises several times daily

        1. Do muscle setting and deep breathing exercises at 1 or 2 hour intervals

        2. Start active exercises and progress to resistive exercises when condition permits

    C. Increase gradually the frequency and duration of the exercise period

        1. Do the exercises 2 to 4 times daily

        2. Decrease the time if pain persists more than 2 hours following exercise

    D. Use swimming pool for exercise periods when available

    E. Avoid prolonged sitting, which produces stiffness and flexion adduction deformities

    F. Wear proper shoes (not slippers) and arch supports when necessary

    G. Use supports (crutches, braces) during periods of exacerbation of disease of the weight-bearing joints

    H. Protect the joints from further injury

        1. Sit in chairs with higher seats to avoid "collapsing" into chair with resultant knee and hip joint trauma

        2. Avoid continued standing and walking when fatigued

        3. Refrain from sudden, jerky movements

---

illustrates how these exercises and other therapeutic measures may be carried out.

Control of Pain. To promote the patient's comfort, pain must be alleviated. Salicylates are given in doses that are individualized in accordance with the patient's responses. It is desirable that the first dose be given immediately on arising in the morning, and the last at bedtime. The remaining doses should be spaced evenly throughout the day.

Heat relieves muscle spasm and joint soreness. It may be supplied in the form of water tub baths, hot compresses, homemade bakers, paraffin baths for hands and wrists, and radiant heat. Therapeutic exercises can be carried out more comfortably and effectively after heat has been applied.

Rest helps to allay pain. Since arthritis is a systemic disease, the whole patient—not merely his joints—must be treated. Frequent periods of bed rest during the day take the weight off the joints and relieve fatigue. If joint inflammation is severe, the patient should, of course, be placed on complete bed rest. (Nevertheless, range-of-motion exercises should still be carried out.) At bed rest, the patient should lie flat, with his feet propped against a footboard. Trochanter rolls are utilized when he is lying in the dorsal position for prolonged periods (p. 167). As joint stiffness and tenderness diminish and function improves, the patient is permitted to increase his out-of-bed activities. He may anticipate pain in the knees and hips on arising from a chair. The nurse should select a straight-back chair with a seat that is high enough to permit the patient to keep his feet flat on the floor (or stool) while his hips and shoulders are resting against the back of the chair.

Drug Therapy. Aspirin (or other forms of salicylates), when used in sufficient amounts, has an anti-inflammatory as well as an analgesic action in the treatment of rheumatoid arthritis. Instruct the patient to take the medication after meals and at bedtime. Other anti-inflammatory drugs used are indomethacin, and phenylbutazone; these drugs are capable of producing severe toxic side-effects.

Systemic hormonal therapy by the oral administration of one of the corticosteroids, such as prednisone or dexamethasone, while temporarily palliative in effect, is not considered curative in any sense at all. Steroid chemotherapy carries with it all of the undesirable complications previously described, including sodium and water retention, potassium depletion, hypertension, glycosuria, menstrual irregularities and other features of the Cushing syndrome, and at the same time exposes the patient to a demoralizing dependence on a treatment that offers no hope of permanent benefit.

To halt the disease process, joints that are severely inflamed and fail to respond promptly to the measures outlined above may be treated by the local instillation of 25 to 50 mg. of hydrocortisone acetate. Quiescence of activity may be anticipated almost immediately following this maneuver, and its beneficial effect may be expected to last for several days or even several weeks.

Table 35-5 summarizes the drugs used in the treatment of rheumatoid arthritis. The nurse, especially the visiting nurse and the nurse in the out-patient clinic, should be familiar with the side-effects and potential toxicity of all these drugs.

Surgical Intervention for Rheumatoid Arthritis. More and more, surgery is giving renewed hope to patients with rheumatoid arthritis. In its early stages, the disease is localized in the joints and affects mainly the thin layer of synovial tissue. Therefore, it is in the synovium that joint damage begins. As the synovium thickens and enlarges, proliferation and invasion into surrounding cartilage, ligaments and tendons occurs. Surgical intervention (*synovectomy*) is performed to remove the hypertrophied eroding synovium within the joint. This also helps to prevent the recurrence of the inflammatory process. Gratifying results have been demonstrated in synovectomy in the knees,

TABLE 35-5. Drugs used in rheumatoid arthritis

Generic Name, Trade Name, and Usual Dose	Possible Side-Effects	Generic Name, Trade Name, and Usual Dose	Possible Side-Effects
Salicylates (Aspirin, Empirin, Ascriptin, Vanquish, and the sustained release preparations, Measurin, Persistin.) 0.3 Gm. (5 gr.) approximately 12 tablets per day.	Gastrointestinal bleeding, nausea, tinnitus, hearing loss, hyperpnea.	*Adrenocorticosteroids:* The following drugs and doses are approximately equivalent and are administered 3-4 times per day: Dexamethasone (Decadron) 0.75 mg. Methylprednisolone (Medrol, Depo-Medrol, Wyacort) 4 mg.	
Acetaminophen (Tylenol) 5-10 gr. 3-4 times per day.	Rare	Triamcinolone (Aristocort, Kenacort) 4 mg.	*Minor:* moonface, acne vulgaris, hirsutism, fat deposition, weight gain, dyspepsia, sleeplessness.
Propoxyphene hydrochloride (Darvon) or with aspirin (Darvon Compound) up to 65 mg. 4 times per day.	Dizziness, sedation, rash, gastrointestinal disturbance.	Prednisolone (Cotolone, Delta-Cortef, Fernisolone, Hydeltra, Meti-Derm, Meticortelone, Paracortol, Predne-Dome, Prednis, Sterane, Sterolone, Ulacort) 5 mg.	*Major:* peptic ulcer, osteoporosis, edema due to sodium and water retention, frank psychosis, ecchymosis, hypertension, muscle weakness, abdominal bleeding, hypopotassemia, glycosuria, hypoglycemia, kidney stones.
Indomethacin (Indocin) up to 200 mg. per day.	Headache, dizziness, nausea, anorexia, vomiting, diarrhea, GI bleeding, tinnitus.	Prednisone (Cotone, Deltasone, Deltra, Liscort, Metasone, Meticorten, Paracort) 5 mg.	
Oxyphenbutazone (Tandearil) up to 400 mg. per day.	Generalized fatigue, anemia, nausea, edema, rash.	Hydrocortisone (Cort-Dome, Cortef, Cortifan, Cortispray, Cortril, Domolene-HC, Heb-Cort, Hycortole, Hydrocortone, Hytone Lotion, Optef, Otosone-F, Tarcortin, Texacort Lotion 25, Topicort) 20 mg.	
Phenylbutazone (Butazolidin) up to 400 mg. per day.	Edema, allergic skin reactions, hypertension, GI bleeding, suppression of bone marrow, fever, sore throat, symptoms of blood dyscrasia.	Cortisone Acetate (Cortisone Acetate Cortogen, Cortivite, Isopto- Cortisone) 25 mg.	
Antimalarial compounds:		*Articular injectables:* Neomycin sulfate- hydrocortisone acetate (Neocortef) 0.2 to 1.0 ml	Mild hormonal systemic effects due to cortisone, local reactions, infection.
Chloroquine phosphate (Aralen Phosphate) 250 mg. per day.	Reduced visual acuity (irreversible), skin lesions, GI symptoms, headache, dizziness, leukopenia.	Lidocaine hydrochloride (Xylocaine Hydrochloride) up to 500 mg.	Dizziness, blurred vision, nausea, cardiovascular depression, respiratory arrest, local reactions or infection.
Hydroxychloroquine (Plaquenil Sulfate) 200-400 mg. per day.			
Gold sodium thiosulfate, gold thioglucose (Gold Sodium Thiosulfate with Sodium Thiosulfate Solution) 50 mg. injected weekly or less frequently.	Dermatitis, stomatitis, hepatitis, colitis, hematuria, blood dyscrasias.		

(From Amer. J. Nurs., July, 1967.)

elbows, wrists and fingers. It is desirable to perform the surgery in the early stage of the disease before bone and cartilage destruction takes place.

Naturally, the surgical technique may differ somewhat for each joint. For example, in the knee, part of the synovium above the patellar area may be left intact while the remaining synovial tissue is removed. This permits better knee motion after surgery. Quadriceps exercises are instituted preoperatively and continued for a prolonged period postoperatively. Following a synovectomy in any joint, exercises are prescribed for the affected joint as well as daily range-of-motion exercises for all joints. The nurse must encourage and help the patient to mobilize his resources to strengthen the muscles affected by the disease and subsequent surgical intervention. Fig. 35-18 shows a synovectomy in a rheumatoid knee.

If the patient has been on steroid preparations, he

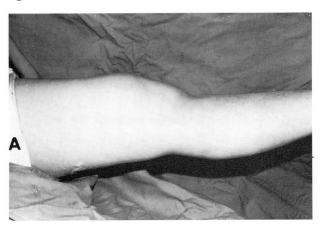
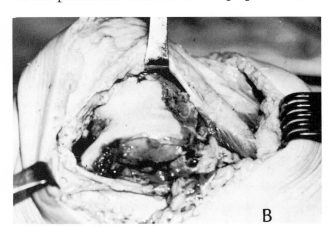
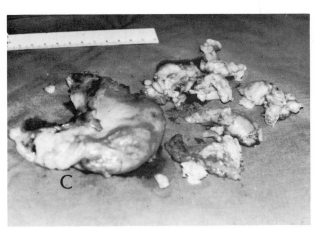
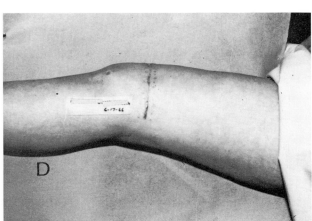
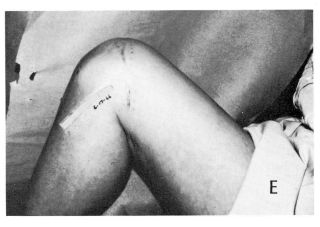

FIG. 35-18. Synovectomy for rheumatoid knee. (A) Boggy swollen knee joint of patient before surgical removal of diseased synovium. (B) Operative exposure of knee after removal of synovial tissue. As much of the rheumatoid synovium as possible was removed at operation. (C) Gross appearance of tremendously hypertrophied synovial tissue removed at operation. (D and E) Range of extension and flexion several weeks after elective knee synovectomy. (Ralph C. Williams, Jr.: G.P., 36:131, 1967)

will require extra steroid dosage immediately prior to surgery and during the postoperative period to prevent severe surgical shock.

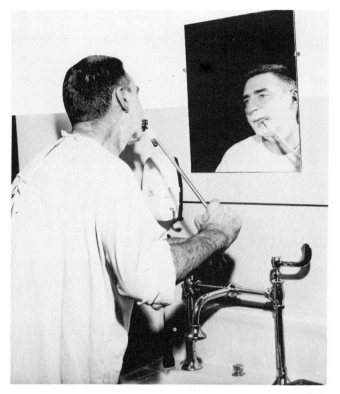

A variety of corrective procedures can be performed on patients with other crippling deformities. Finger and hand deformities can be repaired. Wrists immobilized by the disease in poor position can be ankylosed (fixed) in more effective positions of function. Several surgical procedures may be performed for the very painful hip of arthritis; arthroplasty, arthrodesis (fusion) and resection of the head and neck of the femur with replacement by a prosthesis. Resection of the bony prominences of the feet can correct claw toes and dislocation of the metatarsal-phalangeal joints. Thus, surgery is a valuable approach in relieving pain and improving function.

Psychological Support. To help the patient and his family to adjust satisfactorily to his chronic illness is an important and a challenging responsibility. The nurse must be prepared psychologically to cope with the formidable problems of emotional adjustment that so commonly beset patients with chronic arthritis, reminding herself that a trying personality often is a sign of despair in a person who has had a long and painful illness that has rendered him completely helpless, and to which no end is in sight. For most persons a state of dependency is an unhappy state, especially when they are reduced to it as a result of disease. Fear of being disliked and of becoming an unwanted burden often proceeds to the conviction that such, indeed, actually is the case. In other words, the chronic invalid is highly susceptible to a form of paranoia, manifested by a show of immature hostility

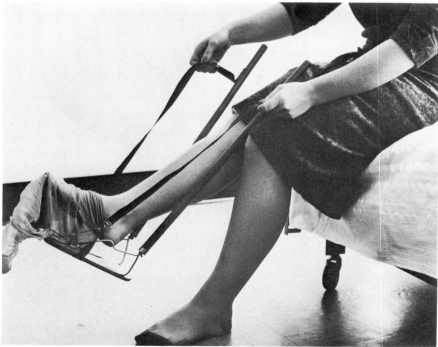

Fig. 35-19. The purpose of self-help devices is to conserve energy and help the patient maintain his independence. There are many such devices available. Ingenious nurses working with patients can invent "gadgets" to solve individual problems. (The Arthritis Foundation)

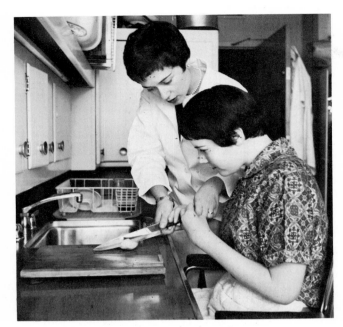

FIG. 35-20. An occupational therapist visits the home and teaches a patient work-simplification methods. This will amplify the patient's efficiency and conserve her energy. (The Arthritis Foundation)

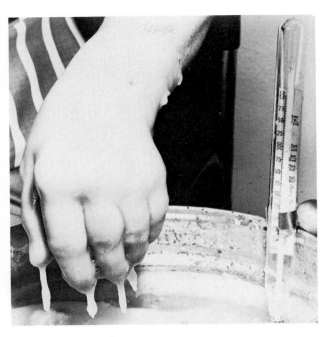

FIG. 35-21. Hot paraffin applications are useful for the patient with arthritis because they provide uniform heat. Paraffin dips are particularly effective for painful hands and wrists. See p. 872 for instructions to the patient for the use of paraffin applications. (The Arthritis Foundation)

toward those who are devoting themselves to his care.

The nurse may assume, as a working hypothesis, that when a patient displays recalcitrance, irritability, inexplicable surliness or unprovoked anger, he is reacting to the imaginary hostility of others toward him. Assuming this to be the case, the role of the nurse in the mental hygiene of her chronically ill patients is clearly to convince the patient that he is accepted, trusted and wanted. She should be sure to educate the family to realize that this sick member is desperately and constantly in need of reassurance, and teach them to reinterpret his show of hostility in terms of anxiety, i.e., viewing it as an indication that he is afraid of their hostility. If they are willing to adopt this interpretation and govern their responsibility accordingly, the prognosis of the patient, from the standpoint of sound mental health, is vastly improved.

The patient must be convinced that, while no quick cure is available, he can stay ahead of his disease and get the better of it by following faithfully his rest and exercise program, by taking the medications and the treatments that have been prescribed, and by continuing to cooperate fully with the physician in whom he has placed his confidence.

Patient Education and Rehabilitation. To assist him to become functionally independent, the patient should be instructed and trained by the nurse and others of the rehabilitation team in activities of daily living. There are many self-help devices available to assist with dressing, bathing, and eating. Corrective shoes are helpful in treating and preventing foot deformities and will make walking easier. Canes or crutches may be prescribed as assistive devices. As the patient gains more independence, vocational counseling and job placement services may be used to help the patient to secure employment.

To correct pre-existing deformities, progressive resistive exercises that have been individually prescribed for the patient are carried out by the physical therapist.

Although there is no specific "cure" for rheumatoid arthritis, much can be done to alleviate suffering and prevent crippling by applying specific therapeutic measures. The patient must be wholeheartedly involved in his therapeutic program. The following summary includes the major aspects of patient education and rehabilitation.

Osteoarthritis

Osteoarthritis, otherwise known as "hypertrophic arthritis" or "degenerative arthritis," is the most common of all joint diseases, the result of "wearing out" of the articular structures. It is characterized by spur formation at the edges of the joint surfaces and thickening of the capsule and the synovial membrane. The joint cartilages degenerate and atrophy, the bones harden at their articular surfaces, and the ligaments calcify. Nevertheless, the joint spaces themselves remain preserved; no adhesions form in them. Sterile joint effusions not infrequently develop, particularly in the knees.

Osteoarthritis may be limited to the spine, affecting most markedly its cervical and lumbar regions. Minor grades of this condition are so common that many clinicians consider them to be almost normal; but this spinal arthritis is responsible for much of the backache so common in persons of middle age and older. Films of the spine demonstrate spur formation and gross irregularities involving the margins and the articular surfaces of the vertebral bodies, which greatly restrict their freedom of movement. In extreme cases, ossification of the spinal ligaments may be observed.

Heberden's nodes, a manifestation of osteoarthritis, are nodular bony excrescences that grow in pairs, symmetrically placed, on the distal joints of a few, several or all of the fingers. They appear most often among middle-aged women, particularly those who work hard, and whose hands are much exposed to wet and cold. While forming, these nodes may be sore; but when fully developed, they cause no pain and very little limitation of joint motion. No known treatment modifies their development.

Osteoarthritis is to be regarded essentially as a senescent process—the result of prolonged wear and tear of the joint surfaces which has produced changes, not only in the bony structures but also in the cartilaginous and soft tissue components of the joints. Precipitating factors include repeated trauma, faulty body posture and mechanics, strenuous physical labor and obesity, which subject the weight-bearing joints to unusual strain. Habitual use of vibrating tools, such as pneumatic hammers, predisposes to the development of degenerative arthritis.

The disease progresses slowly, with early stiffness, and later pain and swelling of the joints. The hips, the knees, the vertebrae and the fingers are the joints particularly affected.

Treatment

The treatment of all types of hypertrophic arthritis is largely symptomatic. Also, it involves measures designed to protect the joints from undue strain and trauma; that is, an obese patient must lose weight, and a physically active patient must learn to adhere to a more sedentary mode of life.

Inasmuch as osteoarthritis in some form or another afflicts almost everyone over the age of 50, opportunities for patient teaching are rife and should not be neglected by the nurse. Irrespective of their basic diagnoses or presenting complaints, many of her patients will be suffering from this condition.

The following is a summary of nursing principles and teaching points that are applicable in relation to osteoarthritis.

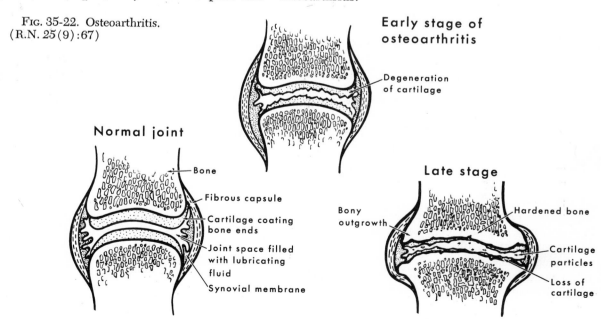

FIG. 35-22. Osteoarthritis. (R.N. 25(9):67)

Early stage of osteoarthritis

Degeneration of cartilage

Normal joint

Bone

Fibrous capsule

Cartilage coating bone ends

Joint space filled with lubricating fluid

Synovial membrane

Late stage

Bony outgrowth

Hardened bone

Cartilage particles

Loss of cartilage

THE PATIENT WITH OSTEOARTHRITIS
Objectives and Principles of Nursing Management

I. To relieve strain on the affected joints

    A. Rest involved parts with splints, braces, cervical collars, etc.

    B. Avoid pain-precipitating factors

    C. Relieve stiffness with prescribed forms of physical therapy

    D. Give analgesics for pain control

    E. Use correct body mechanics

    F. Avoid emotional strain, which increases muscle tension and joint strain

    G. Use crutches or braces, when indicated, to reduce weight on the joints

II. To avoid trauma and further wearing of the weight-bearing joints

    A. Use postural exercises to correct poor posture

    B. Wear corrective shoes for foot disorders

    C. Carry out weight reduction under medical supervision

    D. Stop excessive weight-bearing activities, such as lifting, carrying heavy loads, excessive vigorous overhead reaching, etc.

III. To restore function to the maximal extent

    A. Use range-of-motion exercises to prevent capsular and tendon tightening

    B. Avoid flexion deformities

    C. Use corrective and graded exercises to improve muscle strength around the involved joint

    D. Hip arthroplasty, if hip joint motion is seriously restricted

    E. Orthopedic surgery, when indicated, for severely disabling arthritis of knee joints, etc.

Arthritis Due to Rheumatic Fever

The most prominent clinical manifestations of acute rheumatic fever are fever and arthritis. The latter is an acute nonsuppurative polyarthritis, the onset of which is abrupt and usually is preceded 1 or 2 weeks earlier by a sore throat. It is characterized by excruciating migratory joint pain, accompanied by joint swelling, redness and tenderness, which responds remarkably well to salicylates. The temperature rises rapidly as one or two joints become red, hot, swollen and exquisitely painful; within 24 hours the process is well-developed. The pain in the joints typically is excruciating; the slightest weight of the bedclothes and any jolting of the bed are unbearable.

The fever is usually high, the pulse rapid and prostration profound. With the fever there is a polymorphonuclear leukocytosis, elevation of the sedimentation rate and a progressive secondary anemia, often reaching marked grades.

In most patients with rheumatic fever during the acute stage, signs of cardiac involvement may be detected, with findings indicative of acute myocarditis, valvular leakage signifying endocarditis, and occasionally pericarditis. The ECG usually shows signs of delayed conduction of the impulses between the atrium and the ventricle. With clearing of the acute polyarthritis these complications usually terminate. The joints revert to normal, thereafter exhibiting no trace of residual damage. The endocardium, on the other hand, if it has been involved, remains permanently scarred. Moreover, with each successive bout of rheumatic activity more damage is inflicted, with the result that one or more heart valves become deformed to the point of obstruction, leakage, or both, and cardiac function is permanently impaired, as described on page 377.

Management and Nursing Care

The most important aspects of therapy in cases of acute rheumatic fever include: (1) the eradication of group A streptococcus from the patient's tissues; (2) control of inflammatory reactions throughout the body by the administration of salicylates or corticosteroid drugs; and (3) rest.

Antistreptococcal therapy may take the form of daily injections of crystalline penicillin G for 10 days or a single intramuscular injection of 1.2 million units (720 mg.) of benzathine penicillin G.

Anti-inflammatory treatment can be accomplished with equal efficacy by means of salicylates and corticosteroid drugs, such as prednisone or dexamethasone. Both types of agents may be employed simultaneously. The sore joints may be rubbed gently with oil of wintergreen, wrapped in cotton and, with the aid of pillows or even splints, kept in the most functional position. The application of moist heat to the affected joints may be welcomed by the patient during the initial phase of therapy before the salicylates have become fully effective.

Rest is mandatory during the acute phase of this illness; i.e., complete and continuous rest is the rule as long as rheumatic activity is apparent. On the other hand, as soon as the patient becomes afebrile, the leukocytosis has disappeared, and the electrocardiographic signs have returned to normal, bed rest is no longer mandatory. Each increase in effort is controlled on the basis of its influence on the pulse rate. The patient's family should be instructed with regard to the patient's medical and nursing requirements at home, and he should be given specific directions concerning his activity. Medical supervision should be exercised for a period of months if signs of heart damage have developed in the course of the illness. The long-range prospects for the patient with rheumatic fever and the preventive aspects of this condition are discussed elsewhere (p. 377).

Arthritis Due to Infection

Pyogenic arthritis is the result of bacterial penetration and growth within a joint cavity. It is most often caused by *Staphylococcus aureus* or the hemolytic streptococcus, and less frequently by the pneumococcus, the meningococcus or the gonococcus. Usually, it occurs as a complication of a bacteremia, in the course of which the infecting organism becomes localized in a joint, especially a joint previously damaged by trauma. It also may result from the extension of an osteomyelitis that involves some bone in the vicinity of a joint; and it may be produced by a wound that penetrates the joint.

Symptoms

The symptoms of purulent arthritis are redness, swelling, edema and tenderness of the joint; fluctuation, if the amount of pus is considerable; pain, increased by pressure and by motion; chills, fever, leukocytosis and other general symptoms of sepsis. The pus in joints infected by staphylococci is thick and creamy; that in streptococcal cases is thin and contains only a few pus cells, but the general symptoms of sepsis are severe, out of all proportion to the local signs.

Treatment

Occasionally, it is necessary to drain the joint cavity, either by repeated needle aspiration or by the institution of incision and open drainage, restoration of movement being afforded as soon as possible after subsidence of the infection. The objectives of therapy are to halt the infection by chemotherapy before the joint cartilage is destroyed and to mobilize the joint before adhesions have formed and muscle atrophy has progressed too far—i.e., to destroy the organism and to protect the joint.

A bacteriologic diagnosis is established as soon as possible, and chemotherapy is instituted without delay. Instillation of the drug directly into the cavity of the infected joint may prove to be necessary.

Ankylosing Spondylitis

Ankylosing spondylitis is a systemic disease, which as a result of inflammatory involvement causes pain and stiffness of the sacroiliac, the intervertebral and the costovertebral joints. If the disease progresses, there is ossification and ankylosis of these joints, and the entire spine and the thorax become extensively ankylosed.

Poker spine, one that is perfectly rigid, may develop slowly without pain, and the patient may be quite unconscious of its presence, or it may appear with severe root pains. This disease, which may be akin to rheumatoid arthritis, predominates in males. Its usual starting point is the sacroiliac joint and lumbar spine.

Treatment

The goal of therapy is to help the patient to maintain an erect posture, so that if spinal ankylosis does occur, the patient will be in a functional upright position. The greatest deformity occurs in the cervical and thoracic spine.

The treatment is similar to that of rheumatoid arthritis, with emphasis on periodically resting on a flat surface, avoidance of strain and fatigue, and the administration of analgesics. Indomethacin has an analgesic and anti-inflammatory action and appears useful in this condition. Phenylbutazone is effective in minimizing painful attacks. If a significant deformity develops, removal of a portion of the vertebra (*modified wedge osteotomy*) to allow straightening of the spine may be indicated.

The nurse has the responsibility of reinforcing the physician's health teaching and encouraging the patient to carry out his prescribed remedial exercises.

Traumatic Arthritis

Of all joints, those most susceptible to injury resulting in arthritis are the knee, the lumbosacral and the sacroiliac joints. Following a sprain, inflammation of the interior joint lining (the synovial membrane) may develop, and, later, in the course of a few weeks, degenerative changes may occur in the cartilaginous articular surfaces and in underlying bones. These changes resemble those found in the hypertrophic arthritis of elderly persons. Joint movements may be limited permanently by scar tissue formed in capsules which have been torn by dislocations, while subluxations (near dislocations) often leave the joints loose and weak. If dislocated pieces of cartilage (for example, the semilunar cartilage of the knee), chipped off into the joint cavity as the result of injury are not removed by operation, the joint remains painful, and its movements are limited.

Lumbosacral and Sacroiliac Strain

Backache due to strain of the lumbosacral joint (the joint that articulates the spine with the pelvis) is a fairly common complaint and often leads to prolonged and painful disability. The only objective finding in cases of this condition may be spasm of the deep muscles of the lower back, which hold the spine erect. That the marked abnormalities in the shape of the fifth lumbar vertebra, often seen on roentgenograms (some of them developmental defects and others due to the fusion of one of the transverse processes with the sacrum), ever cause backache is not certain; but in some patients this would seem to be the case.

Sacroiliac strain, though uncommon, is a most painful and disabling condition that may follow lifting, contusion to the back, or a slight misstep; it may appear to develop spontaneously. The wonder is that it is not a more common disorder, since mere standing and walking subject the ligaments of this articulation to great tension. Sacroiliac strain develops also as the result of inequality in the length of the two legs, ankylosis of one hip and, occasionally, from scoliosis of the spine. Relief may be afforded by the wearing of a tight supporting belt or elevation of a heel when inequality of legs is found, but at times it requires surgically induced bone ankylosis of the joint.

Nonarticular Rheumatism

The term *muscular rheumatism* is conveniently applied to all painful conditions of the limbs not definitely localized in the joints. Certain forms, which the laity designate as *lumbago* and *stiff neck*, are due to ruptured intervertebral disks and other abnormalities of the spine that can exert mechanical pressure on the spinal nerve roots, producing pains which radiate to the terminals of the peripheral sensory nerves. The pathology of many cases never is properly elucidated; some are presumed to be due to acute or chronic strain of the supporting muscles of the trunk, as a result of faulty posture or unaccustomed exertion. However, the vast majority of patients in this category can be shown to be suffering from an inflammatory disorder involving one of the periarticular structures—i.e., a structure that is located in close proximity to a joint, although not always an integral part of the joint itself. Three such conditions account for almost the entire group: namely, fibrositis, bursitis and synovitis or tenosynovitis.

Fibrositis

This is a subacute inflammatory disease, usually of unknown etiology, which involves the subcutaneous tissue and other fibrous structures of the extremities (fasciae, sheaths of muscles and nerves, tendons and periosteum).

The onset of this malady follows, within a few hours, exposure to cold and dampness, muscular strain or trauma. Its chief symptom is pain, which is increased by movement, seldom lasts more than 3 or 4 days and is followed by the development in the subcutaneous tissue of brawny inelastic areas. The latter may take the form of nodules varying in size from that of a pea to that of an almond, thick cords of induration or circumscribed tender spots—all due to infiltration of the connective tissue by a serofibrinous exudate rich in small round cells—later replaced by scar tissue. This condition explains the so-called *indurative* or *nodular* headaches, some cases of stiff neck or torticollis, one type of lumbago and some cases of pleurodynia. When chronic, this disease often is called *muscular rheumatism*, since it is characterized by a sense of muscular fatigue, pain in the extremities and stiffness of the joints.

Treatment. Since the causes of fibrositis (other than trauma) are not known, the treatment is symptomatic. The affected part should be kept quite warm and immobilized. Salicylates relieve the acute pain. For the more chronic cases, warm moist heat and massage is indicated. All chronic infections in the body, of course, should be treated adequately.

Bursitis

A *bursa* is a small space between muscles, tendons and bones that is lined with synovium and contains a small amount of synovial fluid. Its function is to promote muscular movement with the least possible amount of friction.

These sacs frequently are the seat of inflammation due to trauma, infection or calcareous deposits that form in their walls, and the bursa fills up with fluid, with the result that muscular movement becomes painful. Common examples are those involving the olecranon bursa (which lies over the point of the elbow), which explains "miners' elbow," and the prepatellar bursa (superficial to the patella), causing "housemaids' knee"; "hod carriers' shoulder" is due to subacromial bursitis. Other bursae often affected are the tibial (which overlies the tibial tuberosity, to which the patella ligament is attached) and the subdeltoid in the shoulder.

Rest for the part, removal of focal infection and physical therapy frequently effect a cure. If the inflammation becomes acute or is not relieved by conservative treatment, operation with drainage or incision of the bursa is necessary.

Subdeltoid Bursitis. The bursa most commonly giving symptoms is the one that lies between the

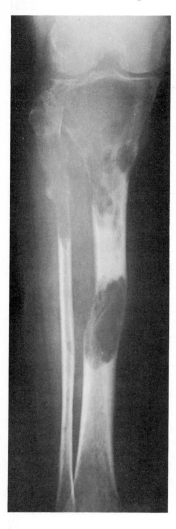

Fig. 35-23. Roentgenogram showing marked destruction of tibia by metastatic carcinoma. The carcinoma in this patient occurred primarily in the breast.

The acute form of bursitis may be relieved by immobilization of the part, local injections of procaine or hydrocortisone and analgesic drugs. If pain and disability persist, operative removal of the calcium deposit or joint aspiration may be indicated. Some forms of the chronic type may respond to conservative therapy and injected hydrocortone.

Synovitis and Tenosynovitis

Synovitis. This term is given to an inflammation of the synovial membrane of the joint. It may be due to trauma—*traumatic synovitis.* It is characterized by a swelling and pain in the affected joint. The knee is the joint injured most commonly, and "water on the knee" is the descriptive term applied to it by the laity. The pain is caused in most part by distention of the joint capsule and may be relieved by aspiration of the joint. If the fluid is bloody, an associated fracture or other injury is suspected. As a rule, restriction of motion, pressure bandages and application of heat result in a rapid recovery.

Tenosynovitis. Inflammatory conditions that involve tendons invariably involve their synovial sheaths as well; therefore, in each case the condition is one of tenosynovitis.

Pyogenic Tenosynovitis. This frequently follows infected wounds, develops secondary to infection of adjacent structures, as in cases of osteomyelitis, and, occasionally, is a bloodstream infection. The wrists and ankles are peculiarly vulnerable to tenosynovitis of bacteremic origin. The infected structures appear swollen, owing to a seropurulent exudate within these sheaths and to edema of the surrounding tissue. The superficial evidences of this condition may be slight, but the pain and the disability it causes are extreme.

The treatment is heat and chemotherapy.

Noninfectious Tenosynovitis. This follows direct blows over the tendons themselves, strains that overstretch them and trauma from overuse. Repeated movements continued over long periods of time—for example, those incident to playing the piano or the violin or typing—may give rise to this disorder. Its symptoms are slight swelling and local tenderness on pressure over the injured tendon sheaths and marked pain on motion of the related joints. The proper treatment is rest, change of activities and warmth. Local injection of corticosteroids may be of value. Surgical excision of the sheath may be necessary for persisting pain.

Ganglion. A ganglion is a round, firm projection, usually near the wrist. It is a collection of gelatinous-like material near tendon sheaths and joints. It is caused by strains, contusions or a series of repeated minor strains, as a result of which the tissues of the sheath or sac involved have gradually become weakened and

deltoid muscle and the greater tuberosity of the humerus. This bursa may be injured by falls on the outstretched hand, so that the bursa is pinched between the head of the humerus and the overlying acromium process of the scapula. However, most commonly, the bursa becomes painful as a result of degeneration. Often a calcium deposit appears in the tendons that lie underneath it over the head of the humerus. The calcified area may be the seat of an inflammation producing tension in the dense supraspinatus tendon. This produces acute pain when the shoulder is moved and is spoken of as *acute bursitis*. The chronic form of bursitis often follows repeated use of the arm above the head. Pain is produced by certain abduction movements of the arm, as in putting on a coat, and often at night when the patient rolls over on the arm of the affected side. These affections really involve the bursa secondarily but produce marked disability in shoulder motion.

distended. As a rule, the ganglion is painless, but the affected joint often is weak and moderately painful. A ganglion has a tendency to rupture and disappear; it can be made to do so by a sharp blow purposely delivered, or may be removed by operation. Not infrequently it recurs.

THE PATIENT WITH A BONE TUMOR

Tumors involving the skeleton are by no means rare and represent a particularly malignant form of neoplastic disease. Such tumors may be primary, arising from bone tissue cells or bone marrow elements, or they may be secondary, having metastasized from primary sites of malignancy elsewhere in the body. A benign tumor arising from bone cells is known as an osteoma; tumors that are malignant are grouped under the term *osteogenic sarcoma*. To one neoplasm derived from bone marrow tissue, the term *myeloma* is applied (Fig. 35-23).

Osteogenic Sarcoma

The term "osteogenic sarcoma" refers to several varieties of malignant tumors arising from the bone cells. As a rule, they appear in individuals under 30 years of age, and they classically produce signs of local swelling and pain, fever and cachexia. The primary lesion may involve any bone; the most common sites are the femora, the tibiae and the humeri. Metastases very early involve the lungs, to which these abnormal cells are transported by way of the bloodstream.

The diagnosis is made on the basis of the clinical features noted above, together with the radiologic findings before and after x-ray irradiation of the site. Biopsy is always indicated because it is difficult to determine a malignant tumor solely by x-ray.

The prognosis is poor despite prompt and radical amputation, because these tumors metastasize so early.

Giant-Cell Tumor

This lesion classically affects the epiphyses of the long bones. Its growth is protracted but progressive, locally producing much bone destruction with cystic excavation and widening of the bone shaft. Tumors of this type do not metastasize, nor are they likely to recur after irradiation therapy. Therefore, they are classified as benign. Many cases, particularly of the multiple type, definitely have been ascribed to hyperparathyroidism.

Clinically, the patient presents signs of swelling and pain at the site of the lesion, but a spontaneous fracture may be the earliest evidence of the disease. The prompt and usually entirely satisfactory response to x-ray irradiation is of great diagnostic, as well as therapeutic, value in this condition. Other evidences of hyperparathyroidism should be sought. If found, cure can be accomplished through the removal of the hyperfunctioning parathyroid tissue (see p. 692).

Myeloma

Myeloma (multiple myeloma; myelomatosis; plasma cell leukemia) is a disorder based on a malignant overgrowth of plasma cells and is characterized by the development of multiple tumors of bone. The tissue primarily and predominantly affected is the bone marrow, and the earliest manifestations of the disease usually are those produced by bone destruction.

Clinical and radiologic signs of bone involvement, which may be in the form of localized areas of lysis or diffuse osteoporosis, appear almost simultaneously at several sites. The first and the most profoundly affected areas usually are the "flat" bones, i.e., the ribs, the sternum, the skull, the vertebrae and the pelvic bones. Bone absorption is most pronounced where the proliferation of plasma cells is most active, giving rise to the so-called "punched-out" areas of rarefaction seen on x-ray examination, which are so suggestive of myeloma. Organs and tissues other than the bones and the bone marrow likewise become the site of malignant plasmacytosis, notably the spleen, the liver, the lymph nodes and the kidneys.

The disease occurs most characteristically in middle-aged males, and its presence is revealed clinically through the signs of bone pain, the electrophoretic pattern of the plasma protein, and the bone changes seen on x-ray examination. Anemia, splenomegaly, cachexia and pathologic bone fractures (those occurring as a result of apparently trivial trauma) are features commonly observed in the course of this disease.

The plasma globulins (which are manufactured by plasma cells) increase markedly, and if this increase involves a globulin of large molecular size, the patient exhibits the syndrome of *macroglobulinemia*, of which there are several important complications, including Raynaud's phenomena (p. 352) and excessive bleeding. A pathologic tendency to bleed is characteristic of myeloma for two major reasons: (1) a numerical deficiency of platelets (thrombocytopenia), due to destruction of the megakaryocytes, their parent cells, in the marrow; and (2) platelet dysfunction, the macroglobulins tending to coat these formed elements and to interfere with their hemostatic functions.

The major objective of therapy is to suppress the plasma cell growth. Melphalan (Alkeran) is the antitumor drug of choice. It may be combined with androgen therapy, but leukopenia and marrow suppression may be a limiting factor. Adrenocorticosteroids and androgens have been used to promote bony remineralization. Adrenocortical steroids also may help reverse the hypercalcemia. The nurse should encourage a

Fig. 35-24. (A) Second hammer toe. (B) Pronated flatfeet. (C) Clawfoot. (D) Congenital hammer toe. (E) Congenital talipes equinovarus—clubfoot. (F) Hallux valgus.

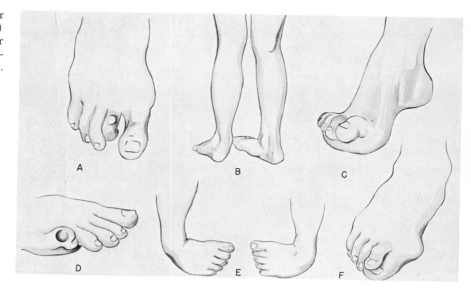

liberal fluid intake because hydration is important when hypercalcemia is present.

A major problem of the patient is usually bone pain. During acute stages, bed rest is advocated as well as various forms of physical therapy. X-ray therapy is utilized for localized bone pain. Analgesics and narcotics may be necessary. (See p. 142 for the principles of nursing management of patients with pain.) A discussion of this disease as it relates to the blood-forming organs may be found on page 320.

The course of myeloma may be prolonged for several years, but most patients succumb to renal failure.

Metastatic Bone Cancer

Tumors arising from tissues other than the bone may invade the bone, producing localized bone destruction with results that are clinically quite analogous to those occurring in primary bone tumors. Those most frequently metastasizing to bone include carcinomas of the kidney, the prostate, the lung, the breast, the ovary and the thyroid. A sign of diagnostic importance in patients with metastatic carcinoma of the prostate is an elevation of the serum acid phosphatase. The first indication of disease in such cases may be a pathologic bone fracture; in later stages, the peripheral blood may show evidences of bone marrow interference. If the bone marrow becomes seriously crowded by the invading malignancy, a myelophthisic anemia is produced.

THE PATIENT WITH LOW BACK PAIN

Low back pain is one of the most ubiquitous complaints of man. The sources of the complaint are multiple. In the young and vigorous, it not infrequently represents muscular or ligamentous strains and,

possibly, pericapsular strains of the joints of the spine. With the passage of time and aging, the complaints are more chronic, of lower grade, and relate to the degenerative processes in the disks and the joints of the distal back. A small portion of the total spectra of backaches is represented by the ruptured disk (p. 825).

Treatment is purely symptomatic. It is based on the dual approach of rest and anti-inflammatory agents. In the acute stages, the treatment regimen consists of rest, mild, intermittent heat, antispasmodic drugs, analgesics and, where necessary, narcotics. Physical therapeutic modalities are employed for the production of subjective comfort. With subsidence of the acute symptomatology, supportive devices where necessary plus attempts at rehabilitation of the musculature and the re-acquisition of the mobility of the spine is the approach utilized by the orthopedist.

Care of the Back

An important consideration in the prevention and treatment of low back pain is the correction of faulty posture. Correct body position produces no strain upon muscles, joints, bones and ligaments. The body should be in correct alignment while lying, sitting, standing, walking, working and exercising.

DEFORMITIES OF THE FEET*

Hallux valgus is a medial deviation of the first metatarsal and an outward deviation of the toe. This is associated with an exostosis on the head of the first metatarsal and a bursa overlying the exostosis, which is called a *bunion*. Bunions may be acquired or congenital. Properly fitting shoes and support of the

* Fig. 35-24.

metatarsal arch usually relieve pain and discomfort, but in severe cases operative correction of the deformity is required.

Flatfoot deformity in children frequently is found with bowlegs or knock-knees. Usually, prescribed shoes with heel lifts are recommended; these are changed as the child grows. Flat feet are common also in adults. Supportive arches in shoes usually give relief.

Hammer toes may be congenital or acquired and result from the spasmodic contracture of the extensors of the toes. The first interphalangeal joint is usually prominent; it is flexed and often has a corn on top. The treatment is any measure to release the contracture of the muscle and often requires operation.

Clawfoot is a contracture of the muscles and the ligaments of the plantar arch and is seen following infantile paralysis. Treatment may involve arch supports and probably a tenotomy of the extensor tendons to the toes.

Nursing responsibility in relation to foot conditions is primarily a teaching one. It is for the nurse to relay important information to her patients regarding foot exercises, the proper selection and care of shoes, the care and the use of foot pads and plates, the care of boot casts and the significance of symptoms of circulatory constriction. The socio-economic factors must not be ignored.

ORTHOPEDIC PROBLEMS FOLLOWING POLIOMYELITIS

Paralytic deformities frequently appear following infantile paralysis. The widespread use of Sabin vaccine has reduced greatly the incidence of the paralytic form of poliomyelitis. This disease affects children and adults and results in a destruction of anterior horn cells of the spinal cord. Paralysis appears in the muscle groups innervated by the destroyed cells. It involves most commonly the muscles of the extremities and often is bilateral; but any part may be affected, including the muscles of the spine and the abdomen. The paralysis is of the flaccid type, leaving the limb flail-like. Contractures of the unparalyzed muscles may cause increasing deformities.

As soon as the paralysis becomes evident, it is necessary to prevent, so far as possible, the development of deformity and protect weak musculature. The usual method of accomplishing this is by means of splints or molded plaster casts that maintain the affected extremities in the neutral position (e.g., the foot should be at right angles to the leg). The bedclothes are supported with pillows or a cradle.

Sister Kenny's method of treatment consists of the periodic application of hot packs to the affected parts and painstaking re-education of the involved muscles as soon as the patient's condition permits it. For its

proper use this treatment requires specially trained nurses and physiotherapists. Physiotherapy measures should be used to maintain the range of motion in the joints.

After the acute symptoms subside, carefully supervised physiotherapy (bathing, massage, electrical treatments, hydrotherapy and exercises) may be beneficial. Swimming exercise in a pool or otherwise is still a most valuable adjunct of the rehabilitation treatment in many cases of paralysis when muscle action is to be restored. Often some form of supportive brace or appliance is indicated, and the nurse should see to it that these are in the proper position at all times. Considerable improvement may be observed under this treatment. Usually, after the lapse of a year or two, no further improvement will be evident.

Operation is indicated for many of these patients for the relief of deformities that develop from neglect of, or in spite of, proper supporting apparatus and to attain optimal functional return. Tendons may be transplanted so that functioning muscles may act in place of paralyzed ones or, when paralysis is extensive, the flail-jointed "dangle foot" may be converted into a much more useful member by producing an artificial union of the bones forming the joint. This is done by an operation called an *arthrodesis*. The leg must be encased in a plaster cast for a time (usually 12 weeks) to give the bones a chance to form a solid union.

After operation, the leg should be elevated to prevent undue swelling. Even with this precaution, the toes must be watched carefully for signs of interference with the circulation, i.e., swelling, cyanosis and numbness. Often it is necessary to bivalve the cast enough to permit an adequate circulation.

DUPUYTREN'S CONTRACTURE

Dupuytren's deformity is an unyielding flexion of the little, ring and, often, middle fingers, rendering them more or less useless. It is a fairly common abnormality, its cause unknown. It starts as a thickening of the palmar fascia. The fibrous thickening extends to involve the skin in the distal palm, and produces a contracture of the fingers to which the palmar fascia is inserted. This condition always starts in one hand, but eventually both become symmetrically deformed. Plastic surgery offers excellent relief; the operation consists of total excision of the involved palmar fascia.

OSTEOMALACIA

This is a disease of the skeleton, the essential feature of which is widespread softening and weakness of the skeleton resulting from decalcification or failure of calcium salts to become deposited in the bone matrix. Depending on the age at which this defect occurs,

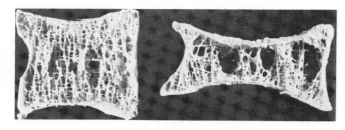

Fig. 35-25. Normal (*left*) and osteoporotic (*right*) vertebrae illustrate the difference in total bone volume. (Schinz, H. R., *et al.*: Lehrbuch der Röntgendiagnostik. ed. 5, Thieme, Stuttgart, 1952)

characteristic deformities are produced. The decalcification of the bones is evident from their faint outlines, and absorption is indicated by the thinness of their cortex, both observed on roentgenograms. Bone softness is shown by the bowing of bones owing to body weight and muscle pull; their brittleness, by the numerous fractures that occur. Associated with this process are severe pains and tenderness over the affected bones and muscular weakness.

Etiology

Osteomalacia may occur as a result of inadequate dietary intake of calcium or phosphate ions, failure of these ions to be absorbed from the food, or excessive loss of these materials from the body. The juvenile type, or rickets, is attributable to a deficiency of vitamin D and consequent failure of calcium absorption, in addition to a dietary deficiency involving calcium and phosphorus, or either one. The malnutrition type is apt to occur in destitute populations particularly. The majority of cases among adults, however, occur in women between the ages of 20 and 30 years, two thirds of whom have had frequently repeated pregnancies and lactation. During pregnancy, 2 factors may operate to produce this disease: the fetal demand for calcium and phosphorus and the loss of these minerals in the breast milk.

Gastrointestinal disorders in which fats are inadequately absorbed are prone to produce osteomalacia through loss of vitamin D (among other fat-soluble vitamins) and calcium, the latter being excreted in the feces in combination with fatty acids. Such disorders include sprue, celiac disease, chronic biliary tract obstruction, chronic pancreatitis and small bowel resections or operative shunts that involve the small intestine.

Renal disorders that cause excessive retention of acids or favor the urinary secretion of calcium or phosphorus are responsible for a type of osteomalacia known as "renal rickets." Finally, hyperparathyroidism (p. 692) leads to skeletal decalcification, i.e., osteo-

malacia, through the promotion of phosphorus excretion in the urine.

Symptoms

Osteomalacia in adults may begin so insidiously that bone deformities are the first signs of its presence. Its most common subjective symptom is pain in the affected bones, which may be acutely tender on pressure. Because of body weight and muscle pull, the legs become markedly bowed, and the softened vertebrae compressed, thus shortening the patient's trunk and deforming the thorax. The sacrum is forced down and forward and the pelvis is compressed laterally; these two deformities explain the characteristic shape of the pelvis that often necessitates caesarean section in afflicted pregnant women.

Treatment

If osteomalacia occurs as a manifestation of calcium or phosphate deficiency, treatment prescribed for classic rickets should be pursued vigorously. This includes a full diet, including milk, eggs, fish and vegetables, supplemented with calcium salts, phosphates and large amounts of vitamin D.

OSTEOPOROSIS

Osteoporosis (decreased density of bone) is a bone disorder in which there is an imbalance between bone formation and bone reabsorption. It is characterized by generalized loss of density and tensile strength throughout the skeleton, and is similarly responsible for an abnormal susceptibility to fractures in response to relatively slight trauma. The basis of osteoporosis is not failure of calcium phosphate to become or to remain deposited in the bones, but a deficiency of the organic matrix of bone. The matrix either fails to form, atrophies or is destroyed. Familiar examples of osteoporosis are presented by cases of scurvy, which is due to vitamin C deficiency; senile osteoporosis; atrophy of disuse; endocrine disorders, such as Cushing's syndrome, hyperthyroidism and hypothyroidism, acromegaly, Simmond's cachexia, eunuchoidism and estrogen deficiency. In fact, it has been estimated that approximately one third of all postmenopausal women develop osteoporosis.

Treatment with calcium or sex hormones (estrogen) has shown good clinical results. Physical activity is most essential in preventing further bone destruction.

OSTEITIS DEFORMANS (PAGET'S DISEASE)

Osteitis deformans is a malady that develops slowly and chiefly affects men beyond middle life. Eventually it produces marked hypertrophy and bowing of the long bones and great thickening and irregular deformities of the flat bones. It may start in any part of the skeleton, but usually begins in the skull, the tibia or the vertebral column. The entire skeleton may become involved—least often the bones of the face, the hands and the feet.

This disease begins insidiously, in many cases with pain and tenderness on pressure in the bones, usually first noticed in the shins. Such pain, which often is attributed to old age, neuritis, rheumatism, etc., may precede the gross skeletal changes by years. In the majority of patients, however, decreasing height and an increasing size of the head are the first symptoms noticed. For years the disease may seem limited to one bone.

In well-marked cases of Paget's disease the cranium is much enlarged, but not the face, which therefore appears small and triangular in shape. The spine is bent forward and is rigid; the chin rests on the chest. The thorax is compressed and immobile on respiration. The trunk is flexed on the legs to maintain equilibrium; the arms, which are bent outward and forward and appear long in relation to the shortened trunk, give to the patient an apelike appearance; and the legs are greatly bowed, hence the gait is labored and waddling. As a result of the kyphosis and the bowing of the legs, the patient's height may be reduced as much as 30.48 cm (12 inches). Since the bones involved, though massive, are brittle, fractures occur frequently.

Associated features include general weakness, chronic cardiovascular and pulmonary diseases (such as emphysema and bronchitis) and, occasionally, symptoms indicative of cerebral damage (impairment of sight and hearing, and muscular atrophy or spasticity). Nevertheless, the patient's general health is little disturbed. After advancing for 20 to 30 or more years, the disease often becomes quiescent. Death usually is due to complications of generalized arteriosclerosis (i.e., cerebral accident, cardiac or renal disease). A fatal complication of this disease is the development of bone sarcoma.

Patient Evaluation

Early cases usually can be recognized on roentgenograms, which reveal changes developing simultaneously in both the skull and the tibia. Serum alkaline phosphatase, the level of which serves as an index of bone absorption, usually is elevated markedly in this condition, occasionally attaining a figure of 300 Bodansky units (normal, 3 to 5).

Treatment

There is no specific treatment for Paget's disease. Irradiation of the painful extremities has been reported to afford occasional symptomatic relief, as well as the use of fluoride.

TABLE 35-6. Characteristics of clinical types of muscular dystrophy

1. *Childhood Dystrophy* (Pseudohypertrophic, Duchenne, severe generalized)
   A. *Mechanism of hereditary transmission:* Sex-linked recessive trait with high mutation rate. Found almost exclusively in the male.
   B. *Age of onset:* 2-10 years.
   C. *Sequence of muscle involvement:* Glutei, abdominals, anterior tibial, peroneals, erector spinae. Late and minor face involvement. Muscles of respiration.
   D. *Prognosis:* Poor. Great majority die before age 20.

2. *Facioscapulohumeral Dystrophy* (Landouzy-Déjerine, mild restrictive)
   A. *Mechanism of hereditary transmission:* Somatic dominant. No sex predilection.
   B. *Age of onset:* 10-18 years.
   C. *Sequence of muscle involvement:* Face, pectoralis major, lower trapezius, deltoid and other scapular muscles, erector spinae, abdominals, glutei, peroneal, and anterior tibial.
   D. *Prognosis:* Fair—slow but variable. Some patients with disability live virtually a normal life expectancy.

3. *Myotonic Dystrophy* (Dystrophia myotonica, distal dystrophy)
   A. *Mechanism of hereditary transmission:* Somatic dominant. Onset earlier in child than parent.
   B. *Age of onset:* 15-80 years.
   C. *Sequence of muscle involvement:* Small hand muscles, forearms, anterior tibial. Masseters and sternocleidomastoid nearly always involved. Levator palpebrae superioris (ptosis), facial muscles.
   D. *Muscle reactivity:* Prolonged contraction of muscles following electrical or mechanical stimulation. Delayed relaxation after strong voluntary contraction.
   E. *Associated defects:* Gonadal atrophy, reduced libido, cortical cataracts.
   F. *Prognosis:* Poor. Slowly progressive with involvement of muscles of deglutition and mastication.

4. *Ophthalmoplegic Dystrophy* (Progressive dystrophic ophthalmoplegia)
   A. *Mechanism of hereditary transmission:* Somatic dominant. Hereditary history in one half the cases.
   B. *Age of onset:* 1-40 years.
   C. *Sequence of muscle involvement:* Levator palpebrae superioris (ptosis), extrinsic ocular muscles (ophthalmoplegia), facial muscles, occasionally sternocleidomastoid and other neck muscles.
   D. *Prognosis:* Good. Disabling but not ordinarily fatal.

(From Swinyard, C. A., and Deaver, G. C.: Rehabilitation of Patients With Progressive Muscular Dystrophy and Atrophy. Rehab. Lit., *29*: 271, 1960)

THE PRIMARY MUSCULAR DYSTROPHIES

Pseudohypertrophic Muscular Dystrophy

This is a disease characterized by the progressive weakness and final atrophy of groups of muscles. It is thought to arise from a genetic abnormality. This disease is more common in males and usually appears during childhood.

The first evidences of this disease are the increased size of certain muscles, a marked lordosis and a waddling gait. Early the calf muscles, the deltoids and those attached to the scapula may become markedly hypertrophied, yet are very weak. The patient falls frequently, has difficulty in climbing stairs and is unable to rise from the ground without "climbing up his legs" with the use of the arms. Gradually all the affected muscles atrophy until the patient is helpless.

Landouzy-Déjerine Type

In this condition the muscles of the face, the shoulder girdle and the arm become markedly atrophied without preceding hypertrophy. Those of the forearms, the hands, the legs and the back seldom are affected. The atrophy of the facial muscles usually begins early in life, producing the peculiar myopathic facies (the lips are thick, and the lower lip, because of atrophy of the orbicularis oris, curves downward, hence the so-called *tapir mouth*).

Treatment

The primary myopathies are not different diseases, since patients with any one of them are likely to present features of other types. In none of them can any lesion in the central nervous system be found at autopsy—the primary lesion appears to involve the muscle. Treatment is not very satisfactory and is limited to general and supportive management.

The patient should be encouraged to live as normally and as fully as possible. Self-help devices can assist him to achieve a greater degree of independence. The necessity for new self-help devices becomes apparent as new muscle groups become involved. As the muscle weakness progresses, a wheelchair, braces and other assistive devices may prolong independence in performing the activities of daily living. A therapeutic exercise program is prescribed for the individual patient to prevent muscle tightness, contractures and disuse atrophy. Because of the genetic nature of this disease, parents and siblings of the patient may be advised to seek genetic counseling.

MYASTHENIA GRAVIS

Myasthenia gravis is a chronic disease of unknown etiology, affecting young adults particularly. Its one symptom is great muscular fatigue, quickly produced by repeated movements, which soon disappears following rest. Patients with this disease tire on such slight exertion as combing the hair, chewing and talking, and quickly must stop for rest. Symmetrical muscles always are involved, first and foremost those innervated by the cranial nerves. No sensory disturbances are apparent.

Because of the involvement of the ocular muscles, diplopia is a common early symptom. The facies, a sad, sleepy, masklike expression with ptosis of the eyelids, early becomes characteristic. Sudden attacks of dyspnea and collapse frequently occur and are sometimes fatal, but the disease usually runs on, even for years, and some patients improve spontaneously.

No significant lesion is found at autopsy. The muscles show no atrophy and give no reaction of degeneration, but do give the characteristic myasthenic reaction. (When stimulated at intervals of seconds by a faradic current, the muscular contractions become progressively weaker and soon cease, but return after a short rest.)

The diagnosis is confirmed by means of a therapeutic test employing neostigmine: 1.5 mg. of neostigmine methylsulfate, combined with 0.6 mg. of atropine sulfate, are injected intramuscularly, or 1 ml. of a 1:2,000 dilution (0.5 mg.) of neostigmine, intravenously, alone, a positive result being evidenced by a striking increase in muscular strength within a period of 5 to 10 minutes.

The basic abnormality in myasthenia gravis is a defect in the transmission of impulses from nerve to muscle cells. Conduction of these impulses is presumably mediated by acetylcholine. In view of the observation that the intra-arterial injection of acetylcholine corrects the defect, briefly at least, it is quite possible that the principal difficulty in these cases resides in the inadequate synthesis or release of acetylcholine at the neuromuscular junction. Support for this view is provided by the fact that chemicals that delay the enzymatic destruction of acetylcholine in the body (i.e., compounds with anticholinesterase activity) such as neostigmine, tetraethylpyrophosphate (TEPP) or octamethyl pyrophosphoramide (OMPA), produce temporary remissions of the disease, as evidenced by transient gains in muscle strength.

Treatment

Treatment of myasthenia gravis during its acute stages includes rest in bed and, later, the limitation of all unnecessary efforts. Neostigmine bromide, supplied at frequent intervals according to a fixed, permanent schedule, generally is effective in the control of symptoms, at least to the extent that life is protected. Most patients require from 15 to 45 mg. of the drug orally at 2-hour to 4-hour intervals. Severely affected patients must be provided with this agent during their sleeping hours. Those unable to swallow must receive neostigmine by intramuscular injection, the usual dose by this route varying from 1 to 2 mg. every 1 to 3 hours.

Two other anticholinesterase compounds which are equally effective in myasthenia gravis are pyridostigmine (Mestinon) and ambenomium (Mytelase), given orally in 4-hourly doses of 240 and 20 mg., respectively. The action of these agents is sufficiently long to eliminate the necessity of interrupting sleep for medication.

The administration of antibiotic drugs and the application of suction are indicated in the event of an intercurrent pulmonary infection. The use of a respirator and performance of tracheotomy may be life-saving procedures when the muscles of respiration and swallowing become severely involved. Whereas the prognosis is extremely grave for the majority of patients who reach this stage, some have exhibited very gratifying and sustained remissions, enabling them to relinquish the respirator and even to resume normal lives thereafter.

Prognosis

The life expectancy for about one third of all patients with myasthenia gravis is less than 6 years from the onset of symptoms. On the other hand, approximately one quarter of all patients exhibit complete or nearly complete remissions in the course of their disease, the average duration of which has been 4 to 5 years.

Precaution

A note of warning is indicated, which the nurse should heed with care, because she may be in a position to prevent a death armed with the following facts. Morphine, intrinsically a respiratory depressant, is made more potent in its effects by anticholinesterase compounds, such as are customarily received by patients with myasthenia gravis. Its use, therefore, is extremely dangerous in these patients. Even small doses have proved to be fatal. Demerol is tolerated well enough in the average case, but should be given in no more than one half the usual dosage. *No sedative, even the mildest, should be employed in any case of myasthenia gravis in which there is difficulty in breathing or in swallowing. The use of morphine should be regarded as being strictly contraindicated.*

AGENCIES

American Podiatry Association
3301 16th Street, N.W.
Washington, D.C. 20010

American Orthotics & Prosthetics Association
Suite 130, 919 18th Street, N.W.
Washington, D.C. 20006

The Arthritis Foundation
1212 Avenue of the Americas
New York, New York 10036

Muscular Dystrophy Associations
of America, Inc.
1790 Broadway
New York, New York 10019

The National Foundation
800 Second Avenue
New York, New York 10017

National Society for Crippled
Children and Adults
2023 West Ogden Avenue
Chicago, Illinois 60612

BIBLIOGRAPHY

Books

American College of Surgeons, Committee on Trauma: An Outline of the Treatment of Fractures and Soft Tissue Injuries. Philadelphia, W. B. Saunders, 1965.

Brunnstrom, S.: Clinical Kinesiology. Philadelphia, F. A. Davis, 1966.

Compere, E. L., *et al.*: Pictorial Handbook of Fracture Treatment. Chicago, Yearbook Medical Publishers, 1963.

Cozen, L.: An Atlas of Orthopedic Surgery. Philadelphia, Lea and Febiger, 1966.

Crenshaw, A. H. (ed.): Campbell's Operative Orthopaedics. St. Louis, C. V. Mosby, 1963.

Gartland, J. J.: Fundamentals of Orthopaedics. Philadelphia, W. B. Saunders, 1965.

Harrison, T. R. (ed.): Principles of Internal Medicine. Pp. 1316-1366. New York, McGraw-Hill, 1966.

Herfort, R. A.: The Surgical Relief of Pain in Arthritic Disease. Springfield, Ill., Charles C Thomas, 1967.

Hollander, J. L.: Arthritis. Philadelphia, Lea and Febiger, 1966.

Hoppenfeld, S.: Scoliosis. Philadelphia, J. B. Lippincott, 1967.

Humm, W.: Rehabilitation of the Lower Limb Amputee. Baltimore, Williams & Wilkins, 1965.

Larson, C. B., and Gould, M.: Calderwood's Orthopedic Nursing. St. Louis, C. V. Mosby, 1965.

Marmor, L.: Surgery of Rheumatoid Arthritis. Philadelphia, Lea and Febiger, 1967.

Moyer, C. A., *et al.*: Surgery. Principles and Practice. Pp. 415-539. Philadelphia, J. B. Lippincott, 1965.

Powell, M.: Orthopaedic Nursing. Baltimore, Williams & Wilkins, 1966.

Prosthetic and Sensory Aids Service, Veterans Administration: Immediate Postsurgical Prosthetics in the Management of Lower Extremity Amputees. Washington, D.C., 1967.

Ricci, B.: Physiological Basis of Human Performance. Philadelphia, Lea and Febiger, 1967.

Rowe, J. W., and Wheble, V. H. A.: Concise Textbook of Anatomy and Physiology Applied for Orthopedic Nurses. Baltimore, Williams & Wilkins, 1967.

Schmeisser, G.: A Clinical Manual of Orthopedic Traction Techniques. Philadelphia, W. B. Saunders, 1963.

Shands, A. R., *et al.*: Handbook of Orthopaedic Surgery. St. Louis, C. V. Mosby, 1967.

Turek, S. L.: Orthopaedics. Philadelphia, J. B. Lippincott, 1967.

Articles

American Journal of Orthopedics: Hygiene and the full body cast. 9:141, July, 1967.

Brodsky, I., *et al.*: Treatment of multiple myeloma. Geriatrics, 22:140-148, March, 1967.

Engel, A., and Burch, T. A.: Chronic arthritis in the U.S. Health Examination Survey. Arth. Rheum. *10*:61-62, Feb., 1967.

Furey, J. G.: Complications following hip fractures. J. Chron. Dis. *20*:103-113, Feb., 1967.

Haas, H. G.: Osteoporosis. Geriatrics, *22*:100-111, Dec., 1967.

Howard, F. M. (ed.): Treatment of neuromuscular disorders. Vol. 2, Mod. Treatment, *2*:231-235, March, 1966.

Jones, J. P. (ed.): Care of orthopedic patients. Nurs. Clin. N. Amer. *2*:383-471, Sept., 1967.

Katz, S., *et al.*: Long term course of 147 patients with fracture of the hip. Surg. Gynec. Obstet., *124*:1219-1230, June, 1967.

Kellgren, J. H.: Epidemiology of rheumatoid arthritis. Arth. Rheum. *9*:720-724, Oct., 1966.

Kirkpatrick, S.: Battle casualty: Amputee. Amer. J. Nurs., *68:* 998-1005, May, 1968.

Laine, V. A.: Early synovectomy in rheumatoid arthritis. Ann. Rev. Med. *18*:173-184, 1967.

Lowman, E. W.: Clinical management of disability due to rheumatoid arthritis. Arch. Phys. Med. Rehab., *48*:136-141, March, 1967.

Marmor, L., *et al.*: Rheumatoid arthritis. Surgical intervention. Amer. J. Nurs., *67*:1430-1433, July, 1967.

Michele, A. A.: Principles of fracture care. Amer. J. Orthop., *9*:34-37, Feb., 1967; 54-59, March, 1967.

Pearson, C. M., *et al.*: Rheumatoid arthritis and its systemic manifestations. Ann. Intern. Med., *65*:1101-1130, Nov., 1966.

Sullivan, C. R.: Fractures of the pelvis: fundamentals of management. Postgrad. Med., *39*:45-55., Jan., 1966.

Thomas, B. J.: Nursing care of patients with cancer of the bone. Nurs. Clin. N. Amer., *2*:459-471, Sept., 1967.

Walike, B. C.: Rheumatoid arthritis. Personality factors. Amer. J. Nurs., *67*:1427-1430, July, 1967.

Walike, B. C., *et al.*: Rheumatoid arthritis. Amer. J. Nurs., *67:* 1420-1426, July, 1967.

Warren, J. D.: The early management of fractures. App. Therap. *8*:614-616, July, 1966.

Williams, R. C.: Osteoarthritis and rheumatic disease. Postgrad. Med., *42*:334-338, Oct., 1967.

————: Recent concepts in the treatment of arthritis and the rheumatic disorders. G.P., *36*:129-132, Nov., 1967.

PATIENT EDUCATION

The Arthritis Foundation
1212 Avenue of the Americas
New York, New York 10036

Gout, A Handbook for Patients.

Arthritis and Modern Woman.

Osteoarthritis.

Rheumatoid Arthritis.

Today's Facts About Arthritis.

Home Care Programs in Arthritis.

Inquiries Branch,
Public Health Service
U.S. Department of Health, Education and Welfare
Washington, D.C. 20201

Cancer of the Bone. (HIS-110)

Muscular Dystrophy. (P.H.S. 996)

Osteoporosis, Facts About. (HIS-118)

U.S. Public Health Service
Superintendent of Documents
Government Printing Office
Washington, D.C. 20402

Report, Surgeon General's Workshop on Prevention of Disease from Arthritis. Publication No. 1444.

Arthritis Source Book. Publication No. 1431.

Step Into Action. Guidebook for Above-Knee Amputee. Publication No. 980.

Strike Back At Arthritis. Publication No. 1747.

American Orthotics and Prosthetics Association
Suite 130, 919 18th Street, N.W.
Washington, D.C. 20006

Hygienic Problems of the Amputee.

Ismael and Shorbe: Care of the Back. Philadelphia, J. B. Lippincott, 1969.

CHAPTER **36**

Principles of Communicable Disease Nursing

- *Reporting of Disease*
- *The Nurse as a Case Finder*
- *Principles of Communicable Disease Nursing*
- *The Nurse's Role in Immunization*
- *Immune Therapy*

Communicable diseases are still the major health problem of the vast majority of people inhabiting the earth. In the industrialized countries, nearly 70 per cent of all deaths are attributable to degenerative diseases and accidents. However, in the developing countries the principal causes of death are infectious and parasitic diseases. These diseases drain the capabilities of humans to work and to learn. Thus the conquering of these diseases is necessary for economic self-sufficiency and national development.

The Infectious Process

Epidemiology is the science concerned with the study of the history and occurrence of a disease. It includes techniques whereby factors that may directly or indirectly favor the development of a disease are studied.

A chain of events is necessary for the continuance of an infectious disease. These events may be likened to links in a chain (Fig. 36-1). The *causative agent,* or invading organism, may be bacterial, viral, rickettsial, protozoal, fungal or helminthic. Infection by each type of organism gives rise to specific reactions in the infected organism. These invading organisms need a place to live and multiply; i.e., a reservoir. The *reservoir* is the environment in which the agent is found. The reservoir may be human, animal or non-

animal, e.g., humans are the reservoir for syphilis, soil is the reservoir for tetanus, and animals are the reservoir for brucellosis. Most infectious diseases of humans arise from other infected persons.

The next link is the *mode of escape* from the reservoir. These avenues of escape are the respiratory tract (most common when the reservoir is a human), intestinal tract, genitourinary tract, open lesions or through mechanical escape, which includes the bite of insects.

After the infectious organism has escaped from its reservoir, it is dangerous only if it finds a way of reaching a host. This *mode of transmission* (the next link) may be by direct transmission (direct contact) or indirect transmission (transfer without close contact). An example of indirect transmission would be the typhoid bacillus which is able to survive for a long period of time outside the body.

The fifth link in the chain is the *mode of entry* of organisms into the human body. These correspond somewhat to the mode of escape and include the respiratory tract, gastrointestinal tract, direct infection of mucous membranes or infection through a break in the skin. The sixth link in the chain is a *susceptible host.* The presence of an infectious agent does not inevitably produce disease. Whether or not the person becomes ill following the entrance of infectious organisms into his body depends on the organism

TABLE 36-1. Epidemiology, therapy and control of communicable infections

Disease	Infective Organism	Infectious Sources	Entry Site	Method of Spread	Incubation Period	Chemotherapy*	Prophylaxis
Amebiasis	Endamoeba histolytica	Contaminated water and food	Gastrointestinal tract	Patients and carriers; fecal-oral route	Variable	Emetine; chloroquine; diiodohydroxyquin; chlortetracycline	Detection of carriers and their removal from food handling; plumbing safeguards
Bacillary Dysentery	Shigella group	Contaminated water and food	Gastrointestinal tract	Patients and carriers; fecal-oral route	24–48 hours	Ampicillin; sulfadiazine; chloramphenicol	Detection and control of carriers; inspection of food handlers; decontamination of water supplies
Brucellosis	Brucella melitensis and related organisms	Milk or meat from infected cattle, goats and pigs	Gastrointestinal tract	Oral ingestion of infective material	6–14 days	Tetracycline and streptomycin	Milk pasteurization; control of infection in animals
Chancroid	Ducrey bacillus	Human cases and carriers	Genitalia	Sexual intercourse	2–5 days	Sulfadiazine; streptomycin; chloramphenicol; tetracycline	Effective case-finding and treatment of infection
Chickenpox (Varicella)	Virus	Human cases	Probably nasopharynx	Probably respiratory droplets	14–16 days	None	Patient isolation
Diphtheria	Corynebacterium diphtheriae	Human cases and carriers; food; fomites	Nasopharynx	Nasal and oral secretions; respiratory droplets	2–5 days	Diphtheria antitoxin; penicillin	Active immunization with diphtheria toxoid or toxin-antitoxin mixture; case quarantine; disinfection of carriers
Encephalitis, epidemic (Eastern and Western Equine)	Viruses	Chicken and wild-bird mites; horses; hibernating garter snakes	Skin	Mosquitoes	Variable	None	Formolized virus vaccines
German Measles (Rubella)	Virus	Human cases (early)	Probably nasopharynx	Probably respiratory droplets	10–22 (aver. 18) days	None	Patient isolation when pregnant woman is in household. Rubella virus vaccine
Gonorrhea	Neisseria gonorrhoeae	Urethral and vaginal secretions	Urethral or vaginal mucosa	Sexual intercourse	3–8 days	Penicillin	Chemotherapy of carriers and potential contacts; case-finding and treatment of patients
Granuloma Inguinale	Donovan body (bacillus)	Infectious exudate	External genitalia; cervix	Sexual intercourse	3–40 days	Chloramphenicol; tetracyclines; streptomycin	Chemotherapy of carriers and potential contacts; case-finding and treatment of patients
Hepatitis, epidemic	Virus (I.H.)	Contaminated food or water; parenteral inoculum	Gastrointestinal tract; skin	Fecal-oral route; parenteral injection	2–6 weeks	None	Enteric precautions applied to infected cases; passive immunization with gamma globulin
Hepatitis, serum	Virus (S.H.)	Infected blood donor; contaminated injection equipment	Skin	Parenteral injection	6 weeks to 6 months	None	Screening of blood donors; avoidance of unnecessary use of blood and blood derivatives; passive immunization of blood recipients with course of gamma globulin injections

TABLE 36-1. Epidemiology, therapy and control of communicable infections (continued)

Disease	Infective Organism	Infectious Sources	Entry Site	Method of Spread	Incubation Period	Chemotherapy*	Prophylaxis
Infectious Mononucleosis	Virus	Human cases and carriers	Mouth	Uncertain	30–50 days	None	None
Influenza	Virus (types A and B)	Human cases; animal reservoir	Respiratory tract	Respiratory	18–36 hours	None	Specific virus vaccine
Lymphogranuloma Venereum	Virus	Human cases	External genitalia; urethral or vaginal mucosa	Sexual intercourse	2–30 days	Sulfadiazine; tetracyclines	Case finding and treatment of infection
Malaria	Plasmodium, vivax, falciparum, malariae and ovale	Human cases	Skin	Mosquitoes (Anopheles).	2 weeks	Chloroquine; primaquine; paludrine; atabrine	Coordinated measures for wide-scale mosquito control; prompt detection and effective treatment of cases
Measles	Virus	Human cases	Respiratory mucosa	Nasopharyngeal secretions	11–14 days	None	Measles vaccine
Meningococcal Meningitis	Neisseria meningitidis	Human cases and carriers	Nasopharynx; tonsils	Respiratory droplets	Variable	Penicillin	Group chemotherapy with sulfadiazine (when strain is sensitive to sulfonamide)
Mumps	Virus	Human cases (early)	Upper respiratory tract	Respiratory droplets	8–30 (aver. 18) days	None	Live mumps vaccine
Paratyphoid Fever	Salmonella paratyphi A and B; S. typhimurium; S. choleraesius and related organisms	Contaminated food and water, rectal tubes and barium enemas	Gastrointestinal tract	Infected urine and feces	7–24 days	Chloramphenicol; tetracycline; ampicillin	Control of public water sources, food vendors and food handlers; treatment of carriers; individual vaccination with S. paratyphi A and B vaccine
Pneumococcal Pneumonia	Pneumococcus	Human carriers; patient's own pharynx	Respiratory mucosa	Respiratory droplets	Variable	Penicillin	Control of upper respiratory infections; avoidance of alcoholic intoxication; communicable disease precautions applied to cases
Poliomyelitis	Polioviruses (Types I, II, III)	Human cases and carriers	Gastrointestinal tract	Infected feces and pharyngeal secretions	4–7 days	None	Wide-scale application of parenteral (Salk) and oral (Sabin) poliovirus vaccines; case isolation
Rocky Mountain Spotted Fever	Rickettsia rickettsii	Infected wild rodents, dogs, wood ticks and dog ticks	Skin	Tick bites	3–12 days	Tetracyclines; chloramphenicol	Avoidance of tick-infected areas, or wearing of protective clothing in such areas; frequent search for, and prompt removal of, ticks from body; specific vaccination of exposed persons

TABLE 36-1. Epidemiology, therapy and control of communicable infections (continued)

Disease	Infective Organism	Infectious Sources	Entry Site	Method of Spread	Incubation Period	Chemotherapy*	Prophylaxis
Scarlet Fever	Streptococcus hemolyticus	Human cases; infected food	Pharynx	Nasal and oral secretions	3–5 days	Penicillin	Case isolation; prophylactic chemotherapy with penicillin; asepsis during obstetrical procedures; specific chemoprophylaxis for persons with recurrent streptococcal infections
Syphilis	Treponema pallidum	Infected exudate or blood	External genitalia; cervix; mucosal surfaces; placenta	Sexual intercourse; contact with open lesions; blood transfusion; transplacental inoculation	10–90 days	Penicillin; Furadantin; tetracycline	Case-finding by means of routine serologic testing and other methods, and adequate treatment of infected individuals
Tetanus	Clostridium tetani	Contaminated soil	Penetrating and crush wounds	Horse and cattle feces	5 days to 5 weeks (aver. 10 days)	Tetanus antitoxin; penicillin	Wound debridement; toxoid booster injections for patients previously immunized and tetanus antitoxin plus penicillin for nonimmune persons
Trichinosis	Trichinella spiralis	Infected pigs	Gastrointestinal tract	Ingestion of infected pork, undercooked	3–7 days	Thiobendazole	Regulation of hog breeders; adequate meat inspection; thorough cooking of pork
Tuberculosis	Mycobacterium tuberculosis	Sputum from human cases; milk from infected cows	Respiratory or gastrointestinal mucosa	Sputum; respiratory droplets; infected milk	Variable	Isoniazid; streptomycin; para-aminosalicylic acid	Early discovery and adequate treatment of active cases; milk pasteurization
Tularemia	Pasteurella tularensis	Wild rodents	Eyes; skin; gastrointestinal tract	Insect parasites of infected rodents; ingestion of undercooked infected meat	3–5 days	Streptomycin; tetracyclines	Avoidance of contact with potentially infected rodents; adequate cooking of wild rabbit dishes; vaccination of hunters, butchers and laboratory workers risking heavy exposure
Typhoid Fever	Salmonella typhi	Contaminated food and water	Gastrointestinal tract	Infected urine and feces	5–14 days	Chloramphenicol; ampicillin	Decontamination of water sources; milk pasteurization; individual vaccination; control of carriers
Typhus, endemic	Rickettsia mooseri	Infected rodents	Skin	Flea bites	5–21 days	Tetracyclines; chloramphenicol	Delousing procedures; specific vaccination; case quarantine
Whooping Cough (Pertussis)	Hemophilus pertussis	Human cases	Respiratory tract	Infected bronchial secretions	12–20 days	Ampicillin; tetracycline	Active immunization with H. pertussis vaccine; case isolation

* Research developments produce changes in drug therapy. The reader is referred to drug brochures and digests to keep abreast of changing dosages and uses.

dosage, duration of exposure, the person's general physical, mental and emotional state, his hemopoietic system and other factors. A healthy body has the ability to combat invading organisms. However, if the level of resistance is not sufficient to combat a given dose of infecting organisms at a given time, the host is susceptible.

Removing one link in the chain of the infectious process controls infections which is the purpose of all public health measures. The reader is referred to a microbiology textbook for a more complete discussion of the infectious process. Table 36-1 shows the epidemiology, therapy and control of the most common communicable infections.

REPORTING OF DISEASE

When a communicable disease occurs in the community, the practicing physician has the legal responsibility of reporting its occurrence to the local health department. The method of this reporting is unique for each state. The report may be telephoned, telegraphed or written on a special form provided for the purpose. The local health department forwards this information to the state health department, which sends weekly reports to the National Communicable Disease Center in Atlanta, Georgia. There data about communicable and chronic disease are compiled and published in the *Morbidity and Mortality Weekly Report.* This publication is fed back to all local health departments and practicing physicians. Thus, the occurrence of any local communicable disease becomes part of a huge network of health surveillance.

The World Health Organization receives data about communicable diseases from all countries. Regional epidemiologists keep a careful watch on regional disease trends and disseminate this information to the appropriate individuals and services within the various countries. Computers are being used to help in this rapid dissemination of information. Six internationally quarantinable diseases are now reported world-wide: cholera, plague, louse-borne relapsing fever, smallpox, louse-borne typhus fever and yellow fever.

Other diseases currently receiving emphasis in global surveillance include influenza, poliomyelitis, measles, venereal diseases and malaria. Health problems vary from country to country, as do the available medical personnel and financial resources necessary to carry out effective surveillance programs. In Europe, salmonellosis, poliomyelitis and rabies are receiving epidemiologic attention, while in Southeast Asia, cholera, malaria and hemorrhagic fever vie for attention. Cerebrospinal meningitis, yellow fever and sleeping sickness have great importance in Central Africa. In the Americas, viral encephalitis, vampire bat rabies and Chaga's disease have given impetus to inter-

The Infectious Process
of Acute Communicable Diseases

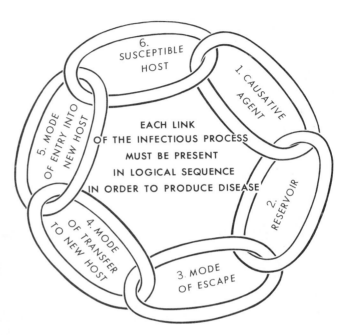

FIG. 36-1. The public health nurse assists in discovering and removing the weak link. If one link of an infectious process is removed, a disease is controlled. (From Communicable Disease Section of Public Health Nursing Guide, State Health Department of Virginia)

national surveillance activities. Only through unrelenting vigilance will it be possible to predict outbreaks of disease and take countermeasures for their control.

The nurse has an individual responsibility. She should know the method of reporting disease in her immediate locality and state, as well as have a knowledge of the most common health problems of the area, in which she is practicing.

THE NURSE AS A CASE FINDER

Nurses, especially those in public health, are frequently called upon to "look at this rash." A rash may be an indication that the patient has an infectious disease. Table 36-2 lists the diseases that produce exanthems (rashes) and describes the nature of the eruption as well as other clinical features of the disease. This material should be helpful to the nurse in assessing patients and recording and reporting their conditions.

PRINCIPLES OF COMMUNICABLE DISEASE NURSING

The nurse who is caring for a patient with any of the communicable diseases should be able to answer all of the following questions:

1. What is the nature of the infecting organism?
2. Where is this organism harbored in the host (i.e., the carrier or patient)?
3. How is the pathogen disseminated by the host?
4. What is the principal portal of entry for this organism?

5. How does the infective agent survive outside the host (i.e., under what circumstances and how long is it likely to survive)?
6. How is immunity to this agent acquired or conferred, and how long is it effective?
7. What communicable disease precautions are indicated in caring for a patient with this infection?

Details regarding the identity and the properties of the causative organism and the epidemiology of each infection are contained in Chapter 37 (see also Table 36-1). The following paragraphs are concerned with communicable disease precautions implicit in the nursing care of infected patients in general.

TABLE 36-2. Clinical features of some acute exanthems*

Disease	Prodromal Signs and Symptoms	Nature of Eruption	Other Diagnostic Features
Measles (rubeola)	3-4 days of fever, coryza, conjunctivitis and cough	Maculopapular, brick-red; begins on head and neck; spreads downward. In 5-6 days rash brownish, desquamating	Koplik's spots on buccal mucosa
German measles (rubella)	Little or no prodrome	Maculopapular, pink; begins on head and neck, spreads downward, fades in 3 days; no desquamation	Lymphadenopathy, postauricular or occipital
Chickenpox (varicella)	0-1 day of fever, anorexia, headache	Rapid evolution of macules to papules, vesicles, crusts; all stages simultaneously present; lesions superficial, distribution centripetal	Lesions on scalp and mucous membranes
Smallpox (variola)	3 days of fever, severe headache, malaise, chills	Slow evolution of macules to papules, vesicles, pustules, crusts; all lesions in any area in same stage; lesions deep-seated, distribution centrifugal	
Scarlet fever	½-2 days of malaise, sore throat, fever, vomiting	Generalized, punctate, red; prominent on neck, in axilla, groin, skinfolds; circumoral pallor; fine desquamation involves hands and feet	Strawberry tongue, exudative tonsillitis
Exanthem subitum (roseola infantum)	3-4 days of high fever	As fever falls by crisis, pink maculopapules appear on chest and trunk; fade in 1-3 days	
"Fifth disease"	None	Red, flushed cheeks; circumoral pallor; maculopapules on extremities	"Slapped face" appearance
Meningococcemia	Hours of fever, vomiting	Maculopapules, petechiae	Meningeal signs
Rocky Mountain spotted fever	3-4 days of fever, chills, severe headaches	Maculopapules, petechiae, distribution centrifugal	History of tick bite
Typhus fevers	3-4 days of fever, chills, severe headaches	Maculopapules, petechiae, distribution centripetal	Endemic area, lice
Infectious mononucleosis	Fever, adenopathy, sore throat	Maculopapular rash resembling rubella, rarely papulovesicular	Splenomegaly
Enterovirus infections (ECHO, Coxsackie)	1-2 days of fever, malaise	Maculopapular rash resembling rubella, rarely papulovesicular or petechial	Aseptic meningitis
Drug eruptions	Occasionally fever	Maculopapular rash resembling rubella, rarely papulovesicular	
Exzema herpeticum	None	Vesiculopustular lesions in area of eczema	

* Courtesy of Ernest Jawetz; M.D. (From Brainer, H., Margen, S., and Chalton, M. J.: Current Diagnosis and Treatment, p. 739. Los Altos, Lange, 1968)

The basic purpose of communicable disease nursing is to halt all communication between infectious sources and their targets. Varying degrees of isolation are imposed on the infectious patient, depending on the character of the infective organism and the manner of its spread. Direct contact with the patient is limited exclusively to those persons who are responsible for his immediate care, and steps are taken to prevent such a person or any object that has become contaminated through direct contact with the patient from becoming a vehicle for the transmission of the infection.

These objectives can be achieved only through strict adherence to a rigid routine on the part of all who are personally engaged, directly or indirectly, in the care of the patient.

Nursing the Patient in Isolation

The purpose of isolation technique is to protect patients and personnel from infection. Although the details of isolation technique vary depending upon the nature of the infection, the following considerations are generally applicable.

Handwashing

For those coming in contact or caring for patients with communicable disease, handwashing is the foundation of control. Effective handwashing consists of wetting the hands, working up a lather, using friction, rinsing and repeating this process a second time. The hands should be washed thoroughly after each contact with the patient or with an object that is potentially contaminated. Ideal facilities for handwashing include a sink with foot or knee controls, hot and cold water, hexachlorophene soap or a detergent dispenser and paper towels. If running water is not available, a basin and pitcher may be used. It is desirable to have a second person pour the water from the pitcher. For the protection of her skin (which is a source of entry for infectious organisms), the nurse should take pains to remove all traces of soap or detergent and then dry her hands with a paper towel. Roughened hands may carry an infection; it is advisable to use a hand lotion after handwashing.

Gowns

Gowns should be worn by all persons who make direct contact with a patient on complete isolation. Each direct contact with the patient involves the donning of a clean gown, which then is discarded in the appropriate container. In the home the attendant may wear a large apron which is changed daily (or more often if soiled) and left in the patient's room.

Glossary of communicable disease terms

Antigen—agent that when introduced into body of susceptible person is capable of producing antibodies

Antiserum—a serum containing antibodies given to provide immunity against a specific disease. Usually regarded as temporary protection

Attenuation—the weakening of the toxicity or virulence of an infectious agent

Bacteremia—presence of bacteria in the circulating blood

Bactericidal—lethal or killing to bacteria

Carrier—one who harbors and eliminates organisms causing a specific disease although he gives no evidence of having the disease

Case—a particular instance of disease

Communicable—transmissable from person to person, directly or indirectly

Contact—a person known or believed to have been exposed to an infectious disease

Contaminated—persons or objects that have come in contact with infectious agents or materials

Disinfection—destruction of pathogenic organisms by chemical or physical means

Endemic—a disease occurring habitually within a given geographic area

Epidemic—a disease attacking many people in a community simultaneously

Exanthem—an eruption on the skin

Fomites—inanimate vehicles other than food, milk, water and air that may harbor or be the means of transmission of organisms

Immune—protected against disease

Incubation period—the development of an infection from the time it gains entry into the body until the appearance of the first signs and symptoms

Infectious—capable of causing infection or disease

Infestation—invasion of body by arthropods; including insects, mites, mosquitoes and ticks, and by helminths

In vitro—within the test tube

In vivo—within a living body

Isolation—procedures directed toward separating one patient from others

Morbidity rate—the number of illnesses compared to the population. The rate may be measured in *incidence* or *prevalence: incidence*—the number of cases occurring in the population in a year; *prevalence*—the average number of cases existing in the population

Mortality rate—the number of deaths compared to the population

Pandemic—disease affecting large portion of population; extensive epidemic

Pathogenic—disease producing

Prodromal—symptoms occurring at the beginning stage of the disease

Prophylaxis—measures taken to prevent disease

Quarantine—separation of contacts of the patient from others for the incubation period of the disease

Toxin—a poison elaborated by a microorganism

Toxoid—a modified toxin capable of stimulating the production of antibodies

Vaccine—a suspension of attenuated or killed microorganisms given to build up an active immunity against an infectious disease

Masks

The wearing of a mask is a requirement in some institutions but not in others, there being no general unanimity in opinion concerning the effectiveness of masks. If masks are to be worn, they should be applied in such a manner as to cover the mouth and the nose completely. If contact is to be prolonged, masks are discarded and replaced frequently. A wet mask should not be worn. As soon as a mask is removed it should be discarded into a receptacle that is covered and clearly labeled.

Environmental Control

Rooms occupied by infectious patients, including floors, walls and contents, are considered contaminated, as are the interiors of all sinks and hoppers. On the other hand, corridors, kitchens and utility rooms are considered clean and cross-contamination should not be allowed to occur. In the patient's room, the window (preferably with a ventilator) should be kept open as much as possible. The door to the room should be closed. The room is cleaned daily by damp mopping and damp dusting to control the spread of air-borne bacteria.

Decontamination of objects that have been in direct contact with the patient is referred to as *concurrent disinfection.* Items requiring concurrent disinfection, depending on the nature of the disease, include oral and nasal discharges, sputum, urine, vomitus, exudates, contaminated dressings, solid and liquid food wastes, dishes, utensils, drinking cups, trays, water carafes, towels, beddings, linens, mattresses, pillows, hypodermic needles, syringes, therapeutic instruments and diagnostic equipment, including clinical thermometers.

For the safe disposal of oral and nasal discharges the patient is supplied with paper tissues and a receptacle in the form of a paper bag of ample capacity, which should be placed in a convenient location within reach of the patient. Disposable sputum cups with tops should be provided by the bedside and the patient instructed in their proper use. All disposable receptacles, including used tissues, sputum cups and contaminated dressings, together with their paper containers, as well as disposable drinking cups, dishes and utensils, should be collected at frequent intervals and placed in special containers for burning; burning is the most effective method of destroying organisms. Table waste may be wrapped in newspaper and burned.

In most institutions the sanitary facilities permit disposal of all excreta by the public sewage system that serves the hospital. However, if such facilities are not available, then all stools, urine, vomitus and liquid food waste should be pooled in a covered can containing a disinfectant solution, such as 5 per cent chlorinated lime or 5 per cent creosol, and allowed to stand for 1 hour before they are emptied into the sewage system. Feces should be broken up into fine particles so that the lime comes in contact with all parts. Bedpans, of course, must be sterilized after each use.

Contaminated bed linen from infectious patients should be collected and enclosed securely in special bags. Packaged in this manner, the laundry chute may be used for the transportation of these goods. All contaminated clothing and linens should be sterilized by autoclaving before they are laundered with noninfectious goods. In the home, linens should be thoroughly washed with soap or detergent and *hot* water.

Heat is a practical and the safest form of sterilization. All instruments and items used on the patient should be cleaned with detergent, rinsed and dried before sterilization. The following are suggested methods and recommended time intervals necessary to inactivate the virus of hepatitis, which is among the most difficult to destroy:

Dry heat—160° C. for one hour
Autoclave—121° C. at 15 pounds pressure for 30 minutes
Boiling—30 minutes
(Principles of asepsis are discussed on pp. 991-992.)

As soon as the patient is discharged from the hospital, the room in which he was isolated should be subjected to *terminal disinfection.* In most instances this involves merely the thorough scrubbing of the floors, open ventilation and exposure to sunlight, if possible, for 12 to 24 hours. Each side of the mattress should be exposed to direct sunlight for at least 6 hours.

Other aspects of communicable disease control in the hospital are discussed in the chapters to follow. It is important to emphasize that optimal isolation technique and nursing care in a communicable disease involve much more than merely skill and knowledge; the essential need is a conscientious attitude and a sense of responsibility on the part of the nurse, without which the entire routine of nursing protection becomes a sham and a pretense.

THE NURSE'S ROLE IN IMMUNIZATION

Active immunization is the introduction into the body of killed or attenuated microorganisms or their products for the purpose of stimulating the body's defense mechanism. Recently, great advances have been made in the control of poliomyelitis and measles, and new vaccines for other infectious diseases are being developed. There are 19 active immunizing agents now available that are listed in Table 36-3.

The first 6 agents listed in Table 36-3 are recommended for all healthy infants. The others are given in special situations in which there is apparent risk of infection. Since May, 1963, a national immunization program has been supported by federal legislation (Vaccination Assistance Act) to assist states and communities in carrying out intensive vaccination programs against poliomyelitis, diphtheria, pertussis, tetanus, measles and other infectious diseases of public health importance for which a preventive agent might become available. Studies show that the socially deprived and low income groups do not receive the protection of immunization programs; this is a challenge to all medical personnel. Nurses, using gentle persuasion, can reach out and listen to the fears of people and teach them the benefits of immunization.

Immune Prophylaxis

Principles of Active and Passive Immunity

Specific immunity to a particular organism implies that an individual either has generated the appropriate antibody in his own body or has received ready-made antibody from another source. A child is born temporarily immune to certain infections by virtue of the fact that the mother's antibodies are able to diffuse through the placenta into the fetus. An individual can be rendered temporarily immune by the injection of blood or serum from an immune animal or person, but such "passive immunity" is short-lived and usually effective for only a few weeks. It offers a useful method of protecting, for a limited period, persons known to be susceptible to a particular infection (e.g., the administration of human gamma globulin to prevent or lessen the severity of hepatitis or measles after exposure to these diseases).

For more permanent protection, a person must continuously manufacture his own antibodies, and before his reticuloendothelial cells can be stimulated to undertake this task, they require some immediate experience with the organisms in question—not necessarily the whole live organism, but at any rate some constituent of the organism that is antigenic. Having had such contact, the cells manufacture the proper antibodies to combat the antigen and continue to do so for some time after the stimulus has departed, often for years or for the duration of that individual's life.

One way of obtaining the necessary contact, of course, is to become infected with the living organism. However, it is precisely to avoid the necessity for such contact that preventive immune therapy is used.

Exposure to a living pathogenic organism is not an obligatory step in the acquisition of a specific, protective immunity: the same immune response can be produced by exposing the reticuloendothelial system to

TABLE 36-3. Active immunizing antigens available*

1. Diphtheria—toxoid	11. Influenza
2. Tetanus—toxoid	12. Mumps
3. Pertussis—antigen	13. Tularemia
4. Poliomyelitis	14. Typhus
5. Measles	15. Rocky Mountain Spotted
6. Vaccinia	Fever
7. BCG—tuberculosis	16. Cholera
8. Yellow fever	17. Plague
9. Rabies	18. Adenovirus
10. Typhoid	19. German Measles (Rubella)

* Adapted from Coriell, L. L.: Active immunization in the pediatric age group. Med. Clin. N. Amer., *51*:582, May, 1967.

organisms that have been killed by heating (such as typhoid), or by chemical inactivation. (Similarly, infection by organisms altered in some way may explain the phenomenon of "natural immunity," i.e., resistance to a particular infection on the part of an individual who has never exhibited signs of that infection in the past.) Moreover, this mechanism is the basis of one of the most important prophylactic measures ever devised for the control of an infectious disease, namely, the induction of a relatively benign infection, cowpox, in order to stimulate the production of antibodies against a very dangerous infection, smallpox. This type of vaccination is described in detail on page 901.

Other examples of vaccinations include the injection of heat-killed *H. pertussis* to protect against whooping cough; mixtures of killed *E. typhosa* and *S. paratyphi* A and B to prevent typhoid and paratyphoid fevers; chemically inactivated viruses of yellow fever, rabies and poliomyelitis for the prevention of those infections; and the killed *Rickettsia prowazekii* for protection against typhus fever. In some instances, especially with some viruses, living microorganisms whose virulence has been attenuated by serial passage in the laboratory have been found to produce better and more prolonged immunity than dead agents. Immunization with living attenuated measles and polio viruses is superior to immunization with killed virus.

Immunization techniques involve the administration of the infective agent in one form or another, and the type of immunity obtained relates to the organism itself. The nature of the antibodies so produced is such as to interfere with the ability of the organism to grow and spread in the body. But there are some organisms—for example, the diphtheria bacillus—whose toxins are much more dangerous than their invasive qualities. The latter, in fact, may play a very small role as the cause of symptoms or of death in the infected individual. In order to induce the body to produce antibodies against toxins, these must be injected—but before administration they either are altered chemically or mixed with antitoxin prepared from the serum of immunized animals, which lessens or altogether prevents their toxic effect when injected. Thus, in both the cases of diphtheria and tetanus immunization, one uses toxins from the tetanus or diphtheria bacillus after chemically treating it with formaldehyde ("toxoid"). These procedures neutralize the toxic effects but do not prevent the person injected from manufacturing his own neutralizing antibodies.

By such means, prolonged immunity against organisms and their toxins can be induced artificially, and the body of the immunized individual can be stimulated to protect itself against particular types of infections without having to experience the infection.

Standard Immunization Procedures

Diphtheria-Tetanus-Pertussis Prophylaxis (DTP). Simultaneous immunization against diphtheria, tetanus and pertussis, or "DTP," has become a routine procedure in pediatric practice. This measure involves multiple injections of a mixture containing diphtheria toxoid, tetanus toxoid and heat-killed *Hemophilus pertussis*, together with alum, which serves to delay the absorption of these antigens. Three 0.5-ml. doses are given at monthly intervals, followed by a "booster" injection at a later date. If the first injection is received at the age of 3 months, 3 monthly injections plus 1 booster injection 1 year after the first dose comprise the series. If the first dose is given at 6 months of age or later, 3 monthly doses are administered in succession, with the first recall dose scheduled several years later.

Children under 3 years of age should receive these injections deep in the gluteal muscles, laterally, on the left and right sides alternately, starting on the left. Children over 3 years may be injected in the deltoid muscles, the right and the left being selected alternately, the left first. For deltoid injections the needle should be directed distally (toward the hand); after its withdrawal the injection site should be covered with sterile gauze and stroked manually 3 or 4 times in a distal direction. Irrespective of the injection site, the following precautions are applicable:

1. Individual syringes and needles should be employed for each recipient of vaccine, both portions of the equipment being sterilized by autoclaving prior to use; or sterile disposable needles and syringes should be used.

2. Sterile precautions should be observed meticulously in the transfer of vaccine from vial to syringes and in the protection of the injection site after its preparation.

3. The course of the needle should be guided straight, and its direction not changed after its insertion.

4. Approximately 0.1 ml. of air should be injected following the 0.5 ml. of vaccine in order to clear the needle before it is withdrawn.

Complications of DTP. *Febrile reactions* of mild or moderate severity may follow these injections in a significant percentage of cases. When febrile reactions are severe, convulsions may occur in some children. Such children are prone to have seizures ("febrile convulsions") in association with fever of any cause, as well as immunizations. It is probable that these phenomena represent a precursor of idiopathic epilepsy, since many of these children prove to be so afflicted in later life. To minimize the severity of febrile reactions mothers of immunized infants should be advised to keep their children as inactive as possible during the 24-hour period after injection, and, if they appear to be restless or feverish, to give them aspirin, increase their fluids, reduce their solid foods, decrease their coverings and protect them from the sun. Anticonvulsant drugs may be administered to children who have had previous febrile convulsions.

Postinoculation encephalopathy, marked by fever, convulsions and irreversible nervous system changes, occurs rarely after DTP and after other vaccination procedures as well. This phenomenon has been ascribed to the familial occurrence of neurologic disorders, and, by implication, an inherited "instability" of the nervous system. However, its actual cause is unknown.

Alum cysts are avoided by adhering to the technique outlined above for injecting the vaccine, the objective of which is to avoid tracking the alum-containing material along the course of the puncture wound.

Nursing Responsibilities in DTP Programs. Mass immunization of DTP to preschool children often are located at well-baby clinics, primary schools or mobile units, holding sessions at regular intervals of 1, 2 or 4 weeks. Infants may be referred to the clinic through the public health nurse or some other agency with responsibilities in the area of child welfare.

Ideally, very soon after birth in the community, a public health nurse should contact the mother, informing her when and where to bring her infant (at age 3 to 4 months) for immunization. Each appointment should be confirmed routinely by a visiting nurse in order to remind the mother of the date on which the first injection is scheduled.

A team of 4 persons, including a physician and at least one nurse, can handle 50 children an hour with perfect efficiency and safety. Nursing assistants may keep the records, teach the mothers how to expose the injection sites and hold their infants, give out cards scheduling appointments for second and third injec-

FIG. 36-2. Public health officer using a vaccine jet injector. (World Health Organization)

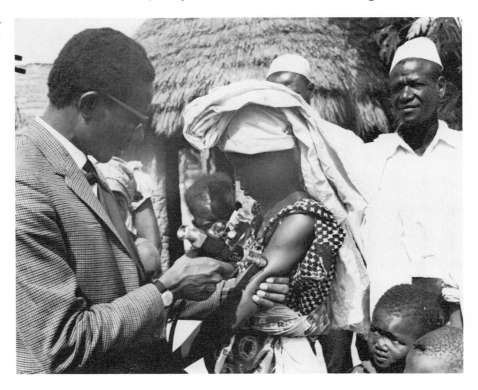

tions, etc., and instruct them in procedures to follow in event of febrile reactions. A registered nurse is responsible for ensuring that syringes and needles are sterile, for custody of the antigen and for the activities of the nursing assistants.

The technique of injection is as follows: the physician washes his hands under running water, drying them on clean, individually dispensed towels or tissues, thereafter avoiding all contact with individuals other than the respective recipient until the injection is completed. The infant is held prone on the mother's lap with only the injection site exposed. Her left hand clasps the infant's knees, her right hand pressing downward above the level of the hips to prevent squirming during inoculation. A 0.5-ml. solution of alum-containing DTP (plus 0.1 ml. of air) is loaded into a 1.0- or 2.0-ml. syringe and injected through a 1-in. No. 23 (approx.) gauge needle deep in the lateral aspect of the gluteal region, the injection terminating with the introduction of the air bubble. After a few seconds the needle is quickly withdrawn, and the site, covered with sterile gauze, is massaged gently.

Smallpox Vaccination. *Vaccinia* is the mild, relatively noncontagious, pustular reaction induced by vaccination with lymph from a vesicle of cowpox; this procedure protects the individual against smallpox.

Technique of Vaccination and Course of Vaccinia. The region to be vaccinated is cleaned with ether or acetone. A drop of vaccine is placed on the dry clean skin. A sharp, sterile needle, held parallel to the surface of the skin, is pressed through the vaccine a dozen or more times, penetrating only the superficial layers of epidermis. The site is left undisturbed for 5 to 10 minutes, after which any residual vaccine is absorbed with dry sterile gauze. No dressing is necessary.

About the 4th day after the vaccination a papule appears, surrounded by a red zone. By the 5th or 6th day this has become an umbilicated vesicle, which on the 10th day has developed into a pustule surrounded by an areola of swollen red skin. Often the arm and the glands in the axilla are sore. On the 11th or the 12th day the areola disappears. On the 14th day, the pustule has dried to a brown scab, which, during the following week, gradually separates and falls off, leaving a superficial pitted scar.

Accelerated reactions are those in which the papule appears on the 4th day, but the pustule reaches its height between the 4th and the 9th days. This indicates a partial immunity, conveyed by a previous vaccination. An immediate reaction is the macule or papule that appears about 12 hours after vaccination, persists for 48 to 72 hours, then disappears. This signifies the presence of a strong immunity.

Complications. *Postvaccinal encephalitis* is an infrequent but dangerous complication of vaccinia. Its development is exceptionally rare during the summer months. It is also rare among children under the age

PRINCIPLES AND OBJECTIVES OF COMMUNICABLE DISEASE PRACTICES

I. To assist in identifying the etiologic agent and establishing the diagnosis

    A. Obtain specimens of blood, urine, stools, sputum, throat swabbings, nasal secretions and pyogenic exudates for bacteriologic study

    B. Assist in securing smears of blood and other materials for microscopic examination

    C. Assist with aspirations of spinal fluid, bone marrow and other body fluids or tissues for cytologic, serologic and bacteriologic tests

    D. Carry out appropriate skin tests for specific diagnostic reactions as directed

II. To control the infection

    A. Administer the appropriate antimicrobial agents as ordered

    B. Assist in administering specific immune therapy, if available, employing immune antiserum, gamma globulin, antitoxin, toxoid, vaccine or an appropriate mixture of antigen and antibody, depending on the circumstances

    C. Observe patient carefully for evidences of drug or serum sensitivity

III. To prevent spread of the infection

    A. Carry out isolation technique as required

    B. Observe asepsis as indicated

    C. Use mask technique effectively

        1. Change mask frequently

        2. Refrain from handling mask while in use

    D. Wash hands immediately after each patient contact and after every contact with material that may be contaminated and is potentially infectious

    E. Disinfect and handle wastes with all due precautions

    F. Handle bed linens and fomites with care

    G. Carry out concurrent disinfection of fomites

    H. Control dissemination of infectious droplets

        1. Encourage patient to cover nose and mouth when coughing or sneezing

        2. Wrap contaminated tissues and articles in paper before disposal

    I. Control dust

        1. Require damp dusting of furniture and wet vacuum cleaning of floors

        2. Reduce to a minimum the activity of personnel in the patient's room

        3. Maintain cleanliness of surroundings

    J. Ventilate patient's room well

    K. Keep door to room closed

    L. Disinfect room air with ultraviolet light, if indicated

IV. To provide physiologic support

    A. Ensure adequate hydration in the face of excessive fluid loss through vomiting, diarrhea or excessive sweating

        1. Encourage the ingestion of fluids

        2. Prepare for the administration of intravenous fluids as required

    B. Reduce the fever

        1. Administer antipyretic drugs, as prescribed

        2. Employ cool sponges cautiously, as indicated

    C. Measure and record body temperature, pulse and respiratory rates frequently

    D. Measure arterial pressure at regular intervals if patient exhibits a tendency to vascular collapse

    E. Weigh patient periodically

V. To provide symptomatic relief

    A. Combat generalized aching and malaise

        1. Utilize warm applications and massage, as indicated

        2. Apply cold compresses for headache

        3. Administer analgesic medications as ordered

        4. Attend to oral hygiene

        5. Restrict physical activity

    B. Relieve cough

        1. Humidify inspired air

        2. Administer hot gargles and throat irrigations

        3. Supply expectorants or cough depressants as indicated and prescribed

    C. Relieve anxiety and depression

        1. Recognize loneliness of the isolated patient

        2. Lend strong encouragement to patient faced with prospect of prolonged convalescence

VI. To protect exposed individuals and public at large against infectious illness

    A. Make available, facilitate or perform whatever vaccination procedures are known to be effective and are indicated for the stimulation of active immunity in exposed and susceptible individuals

PRINCIPLES AND OBJECTIVES OF COMMUNICABLE DISEASE PRACTICES (*Continued*)

B. Furnish specific immune serum (heterologous or human convalescent) or human gamma globulin, if indicated, to provide passive immunity and temporary protection to contacts who are particularly vulnerable

C. Quarantine patients with communicable infections, as well as known carriers and contacts, when required

D. Educate the public with respect to:

1. The availability and importance of prophylactic immunizations

2. The manner in which infectious illnesses are spread and methods of avoiding spread

3. The importance of seeking medical advice in the event of a febrile illness or skin eruption

4. The importance of environmental cleanliness and personal hygiene

5. Means of preventing the contamination of food and water supplies

    a. Discipline, cleanliness and inspection of food handlers

    b. The dangers of "perishable" foods; the identity of foods that tend to promote bacterial growth; and methods of food preservation

    c. The significance of milk pasteurization

    d. The indications for, and methods of, sterilizing food by means of heat

6. Knowledge of insect, rodent and other animal vectors and reservoirs of human infections and importance of their elimination

---

of 2 years and following a revaccination. Therefore, it is recommended that vaccination be performed during the first year of life, and that the child be revaccinated at school age, both inoculations being accomplished during the summer season.

Secondary vaccinia (vaccinia innoculata) consists of secondary pocks at various sites resulting from scratching the primary site of vaccination. *Generalized vaccinia* and *eczema vaccinatum*, fortunately very rare, follow widespread distribution of the vaccina virus over the skin, with resultant development of multiple pustular lesions and a profound systemic reaction. These reactions tend to occur in patients with chronic itching skin disorders, particularly eczema; spread of the virus is accomplished in the process of scratching. In such patients, vaccination should be deferred until any skin disease present has been controlled, and during this period they should be protected from contact with recently vaccinated persons. Children with eczema should not be vaccinated. Moreover they should be protected from contact with any sibling or playmate who has just been vaccinated, so susceptible are they to the development of eczema vaccinata.

Secondary infections may cause ulceration, sloughing, a boil or erysipelas at the vaccinated point.

Vaccination protects a person for only about 10 years, at the end of which time he should be revaccinated. Vaccinated persons occasionally do contract smallpox, but the attack as a rule is mild (varioloid).

Poliomyelitis Vaccination. Polio immunization may be given as inactivated polio vaccine in 3 parenteral doses, the first 2 doses 1 month apart and the third dose 7 months later, with a booster dose every 2 years. The combined oral attenuated virus vaccine containing types I, II, and III consists of a course of 2 doses 1 month apart and a third dose within a year. Also used is the monovalent attenuated vaccine for oral use. Type I is given, followed in a month by Type III, and in another month by Type II with a filler dose of the combined vaccine in 1 year.

Measles Vaccination. Measles vaccine consists of attenuated live virus propagated in chick embryo tissue culture. It is supplied in dry single dose units with a diluent and disposable syringe. It is given to infants at 12 months of age and to older individuals who have not had measles. The dose is 0.5 ml. subcutaneously.

Mumps Vaccination. A new mumps vaccine composed of attenuated live virus propagated in chick embryo tissue is now available. It is given in a single 0.5 ml. subcutaneous dose and confers immunity for at least 2 years, possibly longer.

German Measles (Rubella) Vaccination. There is now available a live virus vaccine for immunization against German measles. It is indicated for boys and girls from age one to puberty. Women of child-bearing age should not be considered for vaccination unless there is no possibility of pregnancy in the next three months after receiving the vaccine.

IMMUNE THERAPY

Specific Antisera. A nonimmune patient who has acquired an infection may be aided in his struggle against it, because immune substances prefabricated in other bodies can be furnished to him during the period (usually lasting several days) required for his own antibody production to get under way. Thus, patients with tetanus or diphtheria-bacillus infections are injected with serum from animals immunized against tetanus or diphtheria toxin. Antitoxins also are available against toxins of certain anaerobic bacilli causing gas gangrene and one type of food poisoning (botulism) and also snake venoms. These antibodies ordinarily are obtained from serums of animals artificially immunized against the organisms themselves or their toxins.

Gamma Globulin (γ **globulin**). This is the fraction of plasma that contains most or all, of the antibodies found in the circulating blood. When prepared from vast pools of human plasma obtained from representative groups of adult population, as is the case with Red Cross gamma globulin, the material might be expected to contain, in high concentration, antibodies against most of the infections that are endemic in the population at large, those to which children are principally heir and to which adults generally are immune.

The validity of this assumption has been proved in the case of 3 viral infections: measles, poliomyelitis and epidemic hepatitis. Given sufficiently early in the incubation period of measles, i.e., within 1 week following exposure, and in adequate dosage (0.1 ml. per pound of body weight), gamma globulin prevents this infection altogether. In a lesser amount (0.02 ml. per pound of body weight) it modifies this infection in such a manner that the clinical course is relatively mild, and the incidence of important complications is reduced practically to nil. Similarly gamma globulin has been shown to protect against polio virus. However, since active immunization is so much more effective, gamma globulin is little used today for measles or polio prophylaxis. Individuals exposed to infectious hepatitis also may be passively protected by the administration of 0.01 to 0.02 ml. per Kg. body weight of gamma globulin.

Gamma globulin is given by intramuscular injection. No complications are anticipated following its administration in the vast majority of cases, since the only ingredient of the material is homologous protein, i.e., globulins of human origin. Exceedingly rare instances of homologous serum jaundice have been reported in recipients of gamma globulin, but the incidence of that complication is so low as to render it of negligible importance as a contraindication to immunization. Gamma globulin is given now as a preventive of homologous serum hepatitis following blood transfusion.

BIBLIOGRAPHY

The student is referred to the bibliography following Chapter 37.

CHAPTER **37**

Patients with Specific Communicable Disease Problems

- *Patients with Specific Bacterial Infections*
- *Patients with Rickettsial Infections*
- *Patients with Protozoan Infections*
- *Patients with Systemic Mycoses*
- *Patients with Helminthic Infestations*

PATIENTS WITH SPECIFIC BACTERIAL INFECTIONS

Types of Bacteria

Bacteria include the round *cocci* (berries), and the rodlike *bacilli*. Some cocci exist in pairs, for example, those causing pneumococcal pneumonia, meningococcal meningitis and gonorrhea, and are called *diplococci*. Some, the "staphylococci," grow in clusters and are responsible for skin abscesses, certain abscesses of bone and a variety of other infections. Others, found in chains resembling strings of beads, are the "streptococci," which cause, many infections including scarlet fever, erysipelas and puerperal sepsis. Bacilli are responsible for diphtheria, typhoid fever and gas gangrene, among other diseases.

Another type of bacterium is the spirochete, of which there are several types or genera:

1. *Spirochaete* is a threadlike, corkscrew-shaped organism which moves about by rotation on its long axis, propelling itself with the aid of flagella:

2. *Leptospira*, one species of which causes Weil's disease, curves at one end to form a hook.

3. *Borrelia*, the agent causing relapsing fever, has large wavy spirals and a long filamentous end.

4. *Spirilla*, responsible for rat-bite fever, has a motile flagellum at each end.

5. *Treponema*, which include the organisms causing syphilis and yaws, have flagella and small spirals.

Tetanus (Lockjaw)

Etiology

Tetanus is a disease caused by *Bacillus tetani (Clostridium tetani)*. The bacillus is an anaerobe, i.e., it cannot live in the presence of oxygen (air). It is found most commonly in wounds with small external openings. It may occur in any deep wound that is contaminated with soil or harbors foreign bodies. Not infrequently, the wound of entrance is so insignificant that it cannot be found.

Signs and Symptoms

The toxins formed in this disease have an especial affinity for nervous tissue. They are absorbed by the peripheral nerves and carried to the spinal cord, where they produce a reaction that amounts to a stimulation of the nervous tissue. The sensory nerves become sensitive to the slightest stimuli, and the hypersensitive motor nerves carry impulses that produce spasms of the muscles that they supply.

The muscle group first affected is that of the jaws, and the patient is unable to open his mouth. This characteristic symptom has given the disease the name of *lockjaw* (trismus), which is used commonly by the laity.

Other groups of muscles are involved rapidly in the spasms, until the whole body is affected. The spasm of groups of muscles is continuous, but the least stimulus—a door banging or a loud voice—may cause a generalized convulsion, with every muscle in violent contraction. Because the extensor muscles are stronger than the flexors, the head is retracted, the feet are extended fully, and the back is arched, so that during a convulsion the whole body may be supported on the back of the head and the feet. This condition is called *opisthotonos*.

The spasms of the facial muscles produce a so-called sardonic grin, which is quite characteristic for this disease and persists even during convalescence.

Death may occur from asphyxia due to spasms of the respiratory muscles, and, more frequently, from exhaustion resulting from loss of sleep, lack of nourishment, and excessive fatigue due to the constant muscle spasms.

Preventive Measures

Routine immunization with tetanus toxoid is recommended in all child health, industrial or other immunization programs, especially in an environment, situation or occupation in which the incidence of the disease or exposure is increased. Booster doses are given preferably every 4 or 5 years.

Primarily, infected wounds, especially puncture wounds, should routinely be treated as though they were infected with tetanus bacilli. Thorough débridement with removal of all foreign material and washing of the wound is the most important step in the prevention of tetanus. A booster injection of tetanus toxoid is administered if the patient has received tetanus immunization or has had a booster injection of tetanus toxoid within the past 10 years. If not, a prophylactic dose of 1,500 to 5,000 units of tetanus antitoxin should be given. Penicillin (600,000 units I.M.) is often administered as well.

Reactions to tetanus antitoxins (horse serum) may occur in a significant proportion of patients. For this reason, it is preferable to administer a booster injection of toxoid to previously immunized patients. It also is important to ensure that injured patients, previously unimmunized, receive tetanus immunization shortly after receiving antitoxin injections to avoid the necessity for further antitoxin in the event of future injuries. Because of the problem of sensitivity reactions to tetanus antitoxin (horse serum), antitoxin obtained from humans immunized with tetanus toxoid has recently been made available. In as much as antitoxin does not represent foreign protein, allergic reactions do not occur in response to its administration. Moreover, it is eliminated from the body less rapidly than is a foreign protein such as horse serum, so that less of it is required for effective tetanus prophylaxis.

Treatment and Nursing Management

If the disease already has developed when the patient is first seen, the same care of the wound is indicated. To neutralize the toxins that have formed, large doses (as much as 100,000 units daily) of the antitoxin are given around the wound, by intramuscular and by intravenous injection. Usually, penicillin is given intramuscularly in a dosage of 600,000 units or more each day.

These measures are to be supported by most careful nursing of the patient. Since the slightest stimulation may excite convulsions, absolute silence must be enforced. Even such apparently insignificant disturbances as a draught of cold air, the jarring of the bed, bright lights, squeaky doors and cold hands are to be avoided.

One of the important problems of tetanus is the maintenance of an adequate airway. Convulsive spasms, especially those involving the respiratory muscles, interfere with normal breathing, so that in many hospitals tracheotomy is done routinely in these patients. This makes the nursing care the most important aspect of the patient's treatment. (See Tracheotomy Care, pp. 222-226.)

Efforts are made to control the muscular spasms with various drugs, sedatives, anticonvulsants, and muscle relaxants. Some of these may be given by mouth or intramuscularly. Meprobamate (Miltown), secobarbital (Seconal), pentobarbital (Nembutal), methocarbomal (Robaxin) and chlorpromazine (Thorazine) seem to be the best of these drugs.

Clostridial Myonecrosis (Gas Gangrene)

Gas gangrene is a rare but often lethal infection that may complicate compound fractures or contused or lacerated wounds. Occasionally, it may follow surgical procedures such as cholecystectomy or amputations for gangrene. Several different species of *Clostridia* (*Cl. welchii* or *perfringens, Cl. septicum, Cl. novyi, Cl. histolyticum, Cl. sporogenes* and others) may produce gas gangrene. These organisms resemble tetanus bacillus in being strict anaerobes as well as spore-formers. Their growth occurs primarily in deep wounds where the oxygen supply is reduced, a situation enhanced by the presence of foreign bodies or necrotic tissue, which leads to further reduction of oxygen tension in wounds. Spores formed by anaerobic bacilli are extremely resistant to drying and to variations in temperature; they may remain viable in soil for many years.

Signs and Symptoms

The onset of gas gangrene is usually attended by sudden severe pain at the site of injury occurring 1 to 4 days following the injury. The wound is exquisitely tender and bronzed discoloration of the surrounding skin may be seen. Crackling (crepitus) produced by gas in the tissue may be felt. Frothy fluid with a foul sweetish odor may escape from the wound. The involved muscles are black or reddish purple. The areas of involvement may spread rapidly and systemic manifestations become prominent. The patient is pale, prostrated and apprehensive, but usually quite alert. Pulse and respirations are rapid but the temperature usually does not exceed 38.3° C.° Anorexia, diarrhea, vomiting and vascular collapse may occur. Death from toxemia is frequent.

Another, more benign, form of clostridial infection (clostridial cellulitis) may involve the skin and subcutaneous tissue. It may be differentiated from gas gangrene by the absence of muscle involvement and relatively less severe systemic manifestations.

Treatment and Nursing Emphasis

The prophylactic treatment here, as in tetanus, is most important. Early excision (débridement) of all devitalized and infected tissue with wide incisions will prevent the disease in most traumatic cases. Once the infection has developed, extensive incisions are made in the affected part to allow air to inhibit the growth of the anaerobic organisms. This, plus excision of gangrenous tissue, and the use of antitoxin and antibiotics (particularly penicillin and the tetracyclines) may help prevent the spread of infection. Amputation of an affected extremity often is necessary. Supportive therapy is essential to maintain fluid and electrolyte balance.

In recent years, the use of hyperbaric oxygen (oxygen administered under pressure greater than atmospheric in specially designed chambers) has proven extremely effective. This method of therapy may prevent the necessity for amputations and decrease the extent of surgical débridement required.

Because the gas bacillus is an inhabitant of the human intestinal tract, it is likely to be the infecting organism in wounds of thigh amputations, especially if the patient is incontinent. Gangrene, incontinence and debility often are combined in patients with diabetes, and it is in the amputation stump of diabetic patients in which gas gangrene is most prone to occur.

The disease is important from the nursing point of view because of the extreme care that is necessary. The danger, of course, is the spread of the infection to other wounds. To guard against this, strict aseptic

° 101° F.

technique is practiced and all dressings are disposed of by incineration. It is advisable to isolate the patient and to keep a single dressing tray for that patient alone.

Gas bacillus infection produces an intense toxemia. Other essentials in nursing care are the adequate administration of fluids, either by mouth or intravenously, and an easily assimilated high caloric diet.

Staphylococcosis (Staphylococcus Infections)

Staphylococci are responsible for most human skin infections. The furuncle, or common boil, is almost always a staphylococcal abscess, and the familiar carbuncle on the back of the neck represents a coalition of staphylococcal abscesses. Most staphylococcal abscesses are located in superficial subcutaneous tissues and do not extend beyond the original site. Eventually, their purulent contents, under mounting pressure, perforate the overlying skin and are evacuated externally, leaving the empty cavities to fill in with granulation tissue, close over and heal.

This common, usually benign, sequence of events might be misconstrued as evidence that the staphylococcus is a relatively innocuous microbe. Far from it! From the standpoint of aggressiveness, destructiveness, tenacity and talent for survival, this organism has few equals. The prevalence of the common boil is a tribute to its ability to penetrate the body's first line of defense and a reflection of its ubiquitous presence. The tendency of the organism to localize in superficial areas of the body merely establishes its potency as an antigen that rouses the defense mechanisms to feverish activity; and the voluminous pus that typifies its lesions demonstrates the lethal effect that it has on tissue cells and defending leukocytes.

Systemic Staphylococcal Infections

If the peripheral defenses are unable to contain the staphylococcus, extensive spread of the infection or bloodstream invasion may occur, attended by profound toxemia. Invasion of the lymphatics may result in axillary, cervical, mediastinal, retroperitoneal or subdiaphragmatic abscesses. Bloodstream invasion may produce acute ulcerative endocarditis, staphylococcal pneumonia, empyema, perinephric abscess, hepatic abscess, staphylococcal enteritis, pyogenic arthritis, meningitis, osteomyelitis or generalized sepsis. Constitutional symptoms are extremely severe. Irrespective of location, staphylococcal lesions possess many characteristics in common, including extreme degrees of necrosis, a tendency to localize and a tendency to persist, despite intensive chemotherapy, until the exudate finds an escape route or is evacuated. Its resistance to therapy is explained in part by the extraordinary ability of the staphylococcus to adapt itself to an unfavorable environment. Resistance to the commonly used antibiotics is frequently observed in strains of staphylococci. Thus, responsiveness to antibiotic chemotherapy, however gratifying at the outset, may diminish to the point of true refractoriness. The ability of staphylococci to produce antibiotic resistant mutants becomes apparent when one compares strains of staphylococci recovered from patients who acquired an infection in the hospital with strains isolated elsewhere. Staphylococci acquired in a hospital are almost always resistant to the 3 antibiotics most used in hospitals—namely, penicillin, streptomycin and tetracycline—while strains from the community at large often are sensitive to these particular agents.

Hospital Staphylococcal Infections

During recent years many hospitals throughout the world have experienced serious outbreaks of staphylococcus infections that have been responsible for a number of fatalities, especially among infants. The problem is not diminishing in magnitude, but growing, and is the source of immense concern. Many factors have conspired to produce this situation, among them the capacity of the staphylococcus to develop resistance to most antibiotics, the ability of this organism to penetrate skin and destroy tissue and the prevalence of the staphylococcus, especially in hospitals, where its presence is ubiquitous.

Control Measures. The prevention of hospital staphylococcosis requires the combined and coordinated efforts of many individuals, from all departments of the hospital. Housekeeping practices that need special review, since they are potential vectors of infection, include all operations tending to disperse dust. Vacuum cleaning and the use of rotary buffs must not be permitted. Dry mopping and dry sweeping, if practiced, likewise must be discontinued and supplanted by wet mopping. Germicidal solutions should be applied to the floors, and the mops used should be autoclaved regularly. Containers for the disposal of waste should be equipped with disposable liners, and the receptacles themselves should be autoclaved frequently. Bedpans likewise should be equipped with disposable covers and should be sterilized frequently. Garbage removal carts should be covered with a sterile cover. Soiled linens should be packaged with a special bag that is kept separate from other hospital linen until autoclaved. Mattresses should be protected by a plastic cover. Intensive antiseptic scrubdowns should be carried out in the nurseries, the operating room and the recovery room. Effective measures for controlling flies and other pests should be adopted as needed.

The major source of staphylococci within the hospital is by way of person-to-person transmission. It is vitally important that all personnel with staphylococcal lesions, even those as insignificant as paronychia, report these infections so that they may be relieved of duty until healing has occurred or cultures have become negative after treatment. In addition, all patients with staphylococcal infections, including pneumonia and enterocolitis, must be placed under strict isolation precautions until antibiotic therapy has rendered cultures negative for staphylococci. Patients with hematologic disorders and malignancies receiving irradiation or cancer chemotherapy are especially susceptible to staphylococcal infections. In such cases, protective ("reverse") isolation procedures often are instituted to help prevent acquisition of staphylococci. Newborn infants likewise are vulnerable targets and potential sources of infection. Occupants of the nursery must be protected from all unnecessary contacts. Those in contact with infants in the nursery should observe meticulously all the precautions that are entailed in communicable disease nursing.

Nursing Policies and Practices. Cross-traffic between hospital areas housing infected patients and those in which noninfected patients are quartered should be reduced to a minimum. None but authorized personnel should be allowed entry into isolation units. Devices that permit the immediate detection of persons who are "off-limits" should be worn by all personnel. For example, personnel attached to the operating room, the obstetric department and the nursery might be distinguished by the color of their scrub clothes. Visitors from outside should be allowed only limited, infrequent and carefully supervised access to isolation areas. Visits between patients are likewise to be discouraged. Isolation techniques should be reviewed and demonstrated for the benefit of the nursing staff and rehearsed by every nurse in the institution.

Chemotherapy of Hospital Staphylococcal Infections. Treatment is selected that is most apt to eradicate the infection rapidly. Oxacillin, methicillin, nafcillin, cephalothin and vancomycin are among the most efficacious of the antistaphylococcal drugs currently available. Parenteral, rather than oral, therapy is preferred in almost all serious staphylococcal infections. Because of the large doses required, intravenous administration is usually selected. Methicillin customarily is given in a dose of 200 mg. per Kg. of body weight per day in 6 divided doses, administered at 4-hour intervals. The usual dosage for cephalothin, nafcillin and oxacillin is 100 mg. per Kg. per day, given every 4 hours. Nafcillin and oxacillin may be given by mouth in the milder staphylococcal infections. Vancomycin (Vancocin) is administered by intravenous injection in 2 to 4 divided doses totaling 2 gm. each day.

Gram-Negative Bacteremia

Gram-negative bacilli (*Escherichia coli, Klebsiella pneumoniae, Aerobacter aerogenes, Proteus* species and *Pseudomonas aeruginosa*) have become increasingly important as the cause of hospital acquired infections. During the past 2 decades, bloodstream infections (bacteremia) caused by these organisms have become even more frequent than staphylococcal bacteremia in hospitalized patients. These bacteria normally are found in the gastrointestinal tract. Thus, such infections may arise from the patient's own bacterial flora, or may be acquired from other sources. Gram-negative bacilli frequently are responsible for wound infections, infections of decubitus ulcers, bladder infections and kidney infections complicated by bloodstream invasion. Such infections are especially hazardous in patients with impaired body defenses. Patients with diabetes, leukemia and cancer are particularly susceptible to gram-negative bacteremia.

Signs and Symptoms

Bloodstream infection with gram-negative bacilli generally produces a characteristic set of symptoms. There is usually an abrupt onset with chills, followed by temperature elevations often as high as 40.6° to 41.1° C.* Nausea, vomiting and diarrhea generally occur shortly after the onset of bacteremia. Vascular collapse and shock develop in about a quarter of the patients. Death may ensue as a result of vascular collapse.

Preventive Measures

Prevention of gram-negative infections is difficult to achieve, since these often originate from the patient's own bacterial flora. Bacteremia often develops from infections induced by indwelling bladder catheters, intravenous catheters, decubitus ulcers and wound infections. Meticulous care in the use of closed drainage systems of the bladder, as well as frequent irrigations with antibiotic or antiseptic solutions, help decrease the frequency of urinary tract infections complicating bladder catheterization. Similarly, limiting the duration of indwelling intravenous catheterization to 48 to 72 hours and the daily application of antibiotic ointments decrease the frequency of bacteremia arising from this source.

Treatment and Nursing Management

Treatment of gram-negative bacteremia includes the following: (1) administration of appropriate antimicrobial agents; (2) drainage of any localized infections; (3) removal of any foreign bodies, such as venous or bladder catheters when possible; and (4) prevention or treatment of shock. Careful nursing of

* 105° to 106° F.

the patients plays an important role in management. The temperature, pulse and respiratory rate, and especially the blood pressure, should be monitored at frequent intervals. The patient should be kept warm and quiet. An antibiotic, such as tetracycline, chloramphenicol, ampicillin, kanamycin, polymyxin or colistin is administered, preferably by the intramuscular or intravenous route.

Intravenous fluids are usually administered. Complete and accurate recording of fluid intake and output is obviously important. An intravenous catheter is frequently placed in a brachial or jugular vein and advanced into the superior vena cava to measure central venous pressure. This is used to estimate the amount of intravenous fluids, plasma or whole blood required to combat vascular collapse. In addition, such determinations help safeguard against circulatory overload and heart failure. The central venous pressure should be maintained between 70 and 120 mm. water pressure.

Other agents may be employed for the treatment of shock. These include drugs that cause vasoconstriction, e.g., norepinephrine (Levophed) and metaraminol (Aramine), or increase the output of the heart, like isoproterenol (Isuprel). Large doses of adrenocorticosteroids are given to some patients.

Streptococcal Pharyngitis

There are many strains of the hemolytic streptococci but Group A accounts for the majority of pathogenic infections in humans. Streptococci may invade any organ or tissue. There are some avirulent strains as well as those that produce epidemics of acute throat infections. The organism establishes itself in the lymphoid tissues and produces an abrupt onset of illness with sore throat, fever, 38.2° C (101° F), chills and headache. The patient may complain bitterly of throat pain which is aggravated by swallowing or even turning his head. He may have nasal discharge, cough and earache. Upon inspection the pharynx shows varying degrees of redness and edema and may be covered with an exudate. In some patients a rash appears starting over the neck and chest and spreading over the skin of the abdomen and extremities. If the rash becomes pronounced the patient has scarlet fever. Although these are the usual symptoms associated with streptococcal pharyngitis, most patients have some but not all of these symptoms. It is important that a throat culture be done to confirm the presence of streptococci.

Penicillin is the drug of choice as streptococci are very sensitive to the action of this drug. Erythromycin may be given to patients who are allergic to penicillin. Adequate penicillin treatment of streptococcal pharyngitis can prevent the development of complications of this infection; namely, acute rheumatic fever and acute glomerulonephritis.

In addition to penicillin therapy the therapeutic regimen and nursing support are directed at the relief of the patient's symptoms.

Typhoid Fever

Typhoid fever is caused by a bacillus called *Salmonella typhi,* its characteristic lesions being ulcer formation in the ileum and in the colon, and its distinctive clinical features consisting of long-continued fever, rose-spot rash, enlarged spleen, slow pulse and leukopenia.

This bacillus produces no spores. Under suitable conditions, however, it can live for months outside the body, and, since it is eliminated in the stools and the urine of patients, it is very likely to find its way into food and water through sewage, flies and dirty fingers. Unfortunately, the typhoid bacillus changes neither the appearance nor the taste of milk, cream or butter which it contaminates, as harmless saprophytes often do. Today it is spread chiefly by carriers, patients who have recovered from this fever, but whose stools, urine or both may for years spread these bacilli. Another common source is the ingestion of oysters and shellfish infected from offshore sewage disposal depots.

Pathology

The organism enters the body by the gastrointestinal tract, the walls of which it invades. There, multiplying rapidly, it gives rise to a massive bacteremia which continues for about 10 days. Its chief localization is in the mesenteric lymph nodes and the masses of lymphatic tissue in the mucous membrane of the intestinal wall, which are called *Peyer's patches,* and in small solitary lymph follicles, numerous in the ileum and the colon. The blood vessels of the Peyer's patches become thrombosed, and the swollen mass of lymphatic tissue dies and sloughs away, leaving clean ulcers in the mucous membrane, the floor of which may be the muscularis or even the peritoneum. If the latter, they may perforate, causing peritonitis. The solitary follicles may or may not ulcerate, but they are so tiny that they do little harm. Healing then begins, and soon no trace of these deep ulcers is left.

The spleen is enlarged from the outset.

Clinical Course

The incubation period of typhoid fever lasts from 5 to 14 days. Then there develop symptoms of generalized malaise, weakness, headache, muscle pains and fever. Early in the disease, chills and fever may be the predominant symptoms.

Fever. The temperature rises by a stepladder ascent, reaching its highest level—usually from 40° C.-41° C. (104° to 106° F.)—in from 3 to 7 days. During this period of rising temperature the headache is severe, sometimes excruciating.

Usually the patient is constipated. Often the abdomen becomes distended with gas. During the 2nd week of the fever the temperature remains consistently high. During the 3rd week, however, it becomes more and more remittent, a little lower each morning and not quite so elevated each afternoon, the curve, therefore, resembling a snake fence, until in a week or so the highest record is at or below normal.

Nursing Observations

The pulse in typhoid fever at its height is usually remarkably slow (between 80 and 90). Also, one often feels the dicrotic wave so distinctly that there is danger of mistaking it for a separate beat.

The rose spots characteristic of typhoid fever, few or many in number, usually appear at the end of the first week, often in successive crops. These are low papules, rose-red in color, which disappear entirely on pressure. They are most common over the abdomen.

Laboratory Studies

The white blood cell count usually declines below 5,000, sometimes to a level as low as 1,500 cells per cu. mm. A progressive anemia is characteristic of typhoid fever. During the first week of the fever, the typhoid bacillus can be grown from the blood in practically every case. After the first week, blood cultures occasionally are positive, but more often the germ can be grown from the urine and the stools. The easiest method of diagnosis, then, is the Widal agglutination test, which is negative at first but becomes increasingly positive as the disease progresses.

Complications

Many structures may become infected in the course of typhoid fever. These include the lungs, the pleura, the pericardium, the heart, the kidneys and the bones. However, the most common of the dangerous complications, are intestinal hemorrhage and perforation of the bowel with resultant peritonitis.

Hemorrhages from the bowel occur in at least 5 per cent of all patients and cause about 10 per cent of all deaths from typhoid fever. They occur most frequently during the 3rd week. Some patients have many. Evidently, they come from ulcerating Peyer's patches, the slough of which opens a small artery as it separates.

Intestinal perforation, the most dreaded complication of typhoid fever, occurs in 5 per cent of all cases and explains almost a third of all fatalities. It may occur at any time, but most often it happens during the 3rd week. It arises when the ulcer causing the slough involves the entire thickness of the bowel wall. The intestinal contents pour into the abdominal cavity, at once producing peritonitis.

Late complications, appearing from the 3rd to the 6th weeks, are not infrequent. As is liable to happen to severely ill, bedfast patients, phlebitis often develops. This is evidenced by long-continued fever and painful swelling of an extremity, usually a leg, which should be immobilized and protected with a cradle. Cholecystitis, marked by the development of crampy right upper quadrant pain accompanied by tenderness, nausea, vomiting and jaundice, may occur from direct infection of the gallbladder by the typhoid bacillus. This is treated conservatively with sedatives, antispasmodics and parenteral fluids. Urinary tract infection, favored by the enforced bed rest with its attendant feature of mechanically difficult urinary drainage, complicates many a typhoid convalescence. Its treatment depends, of course, on the degree and the bacteriologic type of infection. Typhoid spine, giving rise to severe low back pain, may be due to an arthritic process or to a typhoid abscess in a vertebra. The spine should be immobilized mechanically during the acute stage.

Chemotherapy and Nursing Management

Chemotherapy now available for the treatment of typhoid fever is efficacious in a high proportion of cases. Chloramphenicol (Chloromycetin) is the drug of choice. The recommended dose of Chloromycetin is 50 mg. per Kg. of body weight initially, followed by 0.25-Gm. doses at 2-hour to 3-hour intervals, this schedule being continued for 5 days after complete subsidence of the fever. Ampicillin also has some effect in typhoid and is ranked as the drug of second choice. Defervescence* may be expected within 3 to 5 days from the time of the initial dose, paralleled by disappearance of clinical signs and subjective improvement. However, bacteriologic cure is not obtained in all cases, relapses having occurred and positive stool cultures having been obtained after one course and even after repeated courses of antibiotic therapy. Thus, while chloramphenicol has reduced the fatality rate of typhoid fever significantly and has curtailed the excretion of typhoid bacilli during convalescence, it has not reduced the frequency of complications or the incidence of the chronic carrier state following typhoid fever. Ampicillin 6 Gm. daily is an alternative to Chloramphenicol in milder cases of typhoid but less certain of success.

Nursing Care. With or without specific chemother-

apy, typhoid fever is largely a nursing problem. In planning the care of each patient, certain features of this disease should be borne in mind.

First, typhoid fever is distinctly dangerous from the standpoint of contagion, since both urine and stools from these patients are apt to be heavily laden with typhoid bacilli.

Second, the mental state of the patient during the active febrile stage is one of drowsiness, indifference to his surroundings or physical hypesthesia, accompanied by a partial incontinence of urine and feces. In other words, a patient in a "typhoidal state" is prone to be careless and noncooperative in matters of personal hygiene.

Isolation technic must be carried out in full, and no precaution may be relaxed until the patient's stools are free of *S. typhi.* Wearing of a gown is obligatory. Every necessary step must be taken to exclude flies from the patient's room and its environs. All excreta from the patient and food wastes on his tray must be disposed of, and their containers sterilized, without delay. His garments, linens, dishes and utensils, as well as his clinical thermometer and any other items with which he has had contact, must be handled carefully until they have been disinfected.

The temperature should be taken by rectum, since the patient cannot be trusted to keep his mouth closed while holding the thermometer. At first it should be taken every 2 hours day and night. Fever sponges are given at frequent intervals for temperatures of 40° C. (104° F.) or more.

This is one of the few diseases in which it is desirable to arouse the patient for the purpose of recording his body temperature on schedule. Also, it may be necessary to arouse him for each feeding and for the administration of fluids. It is important that he be turned methodically from side to side in order to avoid the formation of decubiti due to prolonged pressure over bony prominences. Many patients are so toxic that they lose the urge to void, with the result that the bladder becomes distended; the nurse should not be deceived by frequent involuntary voidings which often accompany urinary retention and bladder distention, but should measure and record the urinary output daily in order to obtain quantitative data concerning the state of the water balance. Special mouth care is necessary for the avoidance of stomatitis and parotitis, as well as for the comfort of the patient.

Retention of feces, as well as of urine, may pose a problem in patients with typhoid fever. In order to avert constipation, repeated low-saline enemas (500 ml.) may be employed, the fluid reservoir being elevated no higher than the level of the hips, to diminish the chances of intestinal perforation caused by an

---

* Fever reduction.

increase in the pressure or the volume of the fluid within the colon.

Distention may be reduced by the insertion, for short intervals (20 minutes), of a rectal tube. Constipation should be relieved not by drugs but by enemas, as indicated above.

Perforation is the most important of all complications from the standpoint of risk and the necessity for early recognition. Every hour, after the appearance of the first symptom is of great importance, for the earlier the operation is performed the more successful it will be. Therefore, the nurse should know the danger signals and report them at once to the doctor in charge. The initial pain may be located anywhere in the abdomen. It occurs suddenly and is different from any previously experienced by the patient. This pain lasts for a few seconds, then stops, and in a few minutes the patient may be sound asleep. This last point is deceiving, for the nurse hardly can believe that such a pain can be important.

When hemorrhage has occurred or is suspected, the patient is kept quiet and moved as little as possible, and nothing is given by mouth except sips of tap water.

Decubiti, unless skillful precautions are taken to forestall this complication, can be severe. They occur with the greatest frequency if the patient is not kept clean and dry, or if steady pressure on the back, the sacrum, the buttocks or the heels is not prevented by pillows, pieces of sheep skin, and frequent changes of position.

The mouth should be rinsed repeatedly and swabbed to prevent mouth infections and parotitis. Maintenance of adequate general hydration is most important from this point of view.

The diet is a therapy of major importance. A bland diet with at least 3000 calories is given. Solid foods may be taken when the patient's appetite and condition improves.

Hydrotherapy (cold sponges, cold packs or alcohol rubs) is useful in reducing the fever and has an excellent tonic effect. As a result, the delirium disappears, the patient feels better, his mind is keener, and the condition of the skin is better.

Convalescence

Typhoid fever is a self-limiting disease; that is, the body cures itself by developing an adequate immunity against the invading organism. In this fever, however, the process is a slow one. The convalescence of typhoid fever, therefore, is long and tedious; it even may take months, and during this time the various sequelae may arise. The temperature often remains continuously subnormal and the pulse rate slow, possibly 50 or less to the minute.

The patient convalescing from typhoid fever must be kept under observation until urine and stool cultures are consistently negative. This may take from three months to a year. The patient is taught correct hand washing procedures. He should not engage in food handling occupations until he has been cleared by the local health authority.

Discovery and Supervision of Carriers

All typhoid patients must be reported to the local health authority who immediately endeavors to find the source of infection. All of the patient's contacts are investigated. Approximately 2 to 5 per cent of typhoid patients become permanent carriers, continuing to harbor the organism and to excrete it in urine and stools. It may be impossible to cure this carrier state without removing the focus of infection, which most commonly is the gallbladder. Usually carriers are advised to have a cholecystectomy. A carrier should not handle food or milk except for his own consumption or for members of his immediate family who have been immunized against typhoid fever. Meticulous handwashing techniques should be carried out.

Prevention and Control

Typhoid fever in large degree can be prevented by prophylactic vaccination with the dead organisms of this disease. One milliliter of the triple vaccine usually used contains 1 billion typhoid bacilli inactivated by phenol or merthiolate. The first and second injection for an adult is one half a milliliter. These injections are given subcutaneously, at intervals of from 3 to 4 weeks. This measure should be enforced in hospitals, schools, armies and throughout the community. However, it is no substitute for good sanitation, for the immunity produced can be broken down by massive infection.

At the turn of the century typhoid was the fourth leading cause of death. Since then the annual incidence of typhoid in the U.S. has declined steadily as the disease has been brought under epidemiological control. A very important factor in the success of this achievement has been the widespread adoption of typhoid vaccination as a routine prophylactic measure. Of equal, and possibly greater, importance has been the decontamination of drinking water, which has become standard practice throughout the country.

The infection confers an immunity presumed to last for at least 3 years. After this interval of time, whether after vaccination or after convalescence from the disease itself, a booster dose of vaccine is advisable, and this is certainly true if one contemplates traveling in an area where health standards are uncertain.

Salmonella Infections (Paratyphoid Fever)

Paratyphoid fever is a name applied to numerous intestinal infections caused by bacilli of the salmonella group, which were not differentiated from the typhoid bacillus or from each other until precise bacteriologic techniques became available. The organisms most commonly producing salmonella infections include *Salmonella paratyphi, S. schottmülleri, S. typhimurium, S. hirschfeldii* and *S. enteritidis.* The diseases resulting from these infections are quite similar clinically, and the infecting organisms are spread in exactly the same manner as the typhoid bacillus. The patient is usually infected by the oral route from contaminated food or drink. Meat or egg products from animals harboring salmonellas or water contaminated with excreta can produce the infection. In fact, any food product is a potential source of human infection.

Symptoms and Course

Generally, the salmonella infections run a briefer course than typhoid and their complications are milder and their mortality lower. The incubation period varies from 7 to 24 days, and the duration of the acute disease from 3 to 10 days. The onset is usually more acute than that of typhoid, often with a chill, malaise, generalized aching and marked apathy. The initial headache, bronchitis, vomiting, diarrhea and abdominal cramps are more pronounced than in typhoid fever.

The temperature curve usually reaches its peak, not by a slow, stepladder climb, but within 48 hours or less. As a rule, it is markedly irregular, the remissions occurring frequently, accompanied by profuse sweating, and the patient is usually afebrile within 2 weeks. The pulse rate, while relatively slow, seldom can be described as a true bradycardia. Petechiae, splenomegaly and leukopenia are features of paratyphoid as well as typhoid fever.

Complications

Intestinal perforation and hemorrhage are unusual complications of salmonella infection, and relapses are rare in this disease. The mortality rate varies between 1 and 10 per cent.

Diagnosis

Early in the disease, every attempt should be made to recover and identify the infecting organism from stools, blood, vomitus and urine. Later, after subsidence of the acute infection, serologic agglutination tests are useful in establishing the diagnosis.

Treatment and Nursing Care

Patients with salmonella infections of all types present essentially the same problems as those described in typhoid fever and are managed in the same way (p. 910). Tetracycline, ampicillin and chloramphenicol are usually effective antibiotics.

The mode of transmission is by way of the ingestion of food and fluids in most cases, and, to the extent that it is a food infection, its control is a community problem, involving detection and control of carriers, decontamination of water supplies, checking of food handlers, etc. However, there are other possible routes of infection, including infected barium enemas and contaminated rectal tubes, the elimination of which clearly is the responsibility of the nurse and other members of the medical team.

Shigellosis (Bacillary Dysentery)

Shigellosis includes a group of enteric infections caused by bacilli of the shigella group, of which there are 4 types: *Sh. dysenteriae, Sh. flexneri, Sh. boydii* and *Sh. sonnei.* The source of infection is feces from an infected person. The route of spread is fecal-oral.

While encountered in all countries, bacillary dysentery is endemic in the tropics, where serious epidemics are frequent. It was the scourge of armies before proper methods of guarding food and water supplies became general. Bacillary dysentery continues to pose a very substantial problem for the civilian population of the United States.

The pathology of shigellosis in severe cases consists of necrosis involving large areas of the intestinal mucous membrane; indeed, the entire colon wall may be destroyed by the invasion of these bacilli. In milder cases, the denuding of epithelium gives rise to superficial ulcers.

Course

The onset of shigellosis is abrupt, with fever, abdominal pain and the passage of small amounts of blood, mucus and pus. At the height of the active infection, the symptoms are severe and the prostration profound. The patient has a constant desire to defecate, and the straining is severe during the attempts. Death in severe cases may ensue in a few days. The mild cases recover in 8 to 10 days; others last 2 or 3 weeks, and the chronic cases last several months, or even years, unless adequately treated.

Treatment and Nursing Care

It is essential to maintain the fluid and electrolyte balance of the patient and to prevent profound dehydration owing to an excessively great loss of water and salts in the diarrheic stools. Adequate amounts of physiologic saline solution are administered intravenously, and large doses of paregoric are given to quiet the inflamed bowel. Morphine may be required to control pain and tenesmus.

The chemotherapeutic agent of choice in shigellosis is ampicillin. One of the soluble sulfonamide drugs or tetracyclines may also be effective, but bacterial resistance to these drugs is becoming widespread.

Prevention

Dysentery bacilli are spread by drinking water polluted by infected human excreta and by food handled carelessly by shigella carriers, some of whom have the active disease, others being entirely asymptomatic. Thus, the same precautions must be observed, and the same control of water sources and food handling enforced, in the prevention of dysentery as of typhoid fever.

Botulism

Botulism, caused by the toxin of the anaerobic bacillus *Clostridium botulinum,* is a serious condition, the chief symptoms of which are cranial nerve palsies. The germ itself introduced into the body is not pathogenic; it liberates its toxin while growing under strictly anaerobic conditions in nitrogenous foods. So poisonous is this toxin that death has followed the mere tasting of infected food—it was not swallowed.

Preserved Foods

Home-preserved foods pose a serious danger of *Cl. botulinum,* because this germ is a spore-bearer, hence is not killed rapidly at boiling temperature. (Reliable commercial packing houses sterilize their products at 120° C.,* which kills all the spores.) Preserved foods in which this germ has been growing look soft, contain gas bubbles and give off an odor of decay. Since the toxin is destroyed rapidly by heat (within a few seconds at temperatures over 82.2° C.†), foods containing it are safe if heated to the boiling point before being eaten; but if allowed to cool and stand for a while, the organism will immediately proceed to form more toxin. Home-canned vegetables should be boiled 3 minutes and stirred thoroughly before serving.

Clinical Symptoms and Course

The symptoms of botulism begin in 4 hours to 6 days, but usually in 18 to 36 hours after the ingestion of the contaminated food. Although the toxin enters the body by way of the gastrointestinal canal, nevertheless gastrointestinal symptoms seldom develop. Early, there are malaise, headache, dizziness, a pro-

* 248° F.
† 180° F.

gressive and profound muscular weakness and incoordination which result in an unsteady gait. Incontinence of urine is common. Eye signs, very important in diagnosis, appear early. These include photophobia, ptosis, paralysis of the eye muscles and sometimes blindness. Progressive weakness of the muscles of speech, of swallowing and finally of respiration also appears early. The clinical picture, when fully developed, is quite characteristic. The patient is cyanotic, helplessly weak, his pulse is rapid, he cannot swallow, cannot talk, struggles more and more to breathe and finally dies of asphyxia. The deep reflexes remain normal. There are no sensory disturbances and no pain. The mind remains clear.

Botulism may continue for 48 hours to 26 days, but the majority of cases terminate fatally before the 5th day of cardiac or respiratory failure. In each of its epidemics, some cases of botulism have been very mild.

Convalescence may be slow and tedious, with months of weakness and disturbed vision.

The mortality from botulism in general ranges between 45 and 60 per cent.

Treatment

Antitoxins for 2 pathogenic strains of this organism have been prepared. They are protective and, if injected early, curative. While waiting for the antitoxin to take effect, artificial respiration should be continued as long as the heartbeat can be felt.

In any case of suspected botulism, telephone the United States Public Health Service in Atlanta, Georgia (Phone: 404-634-2561) for immediate information regarding use and source of antitoxin.

Gonorrhea

Gonorrhea is a venereal infection noted for its chronicity, its latency and multiplicity of localization. Next to measles, it is the most prevalent of all the notifiable communicable diseases. The incidence of gonorrhea is by no means on the wane; on the contrary, it is increasing steadily. There has been a 74 per cent increase in the last decade.

The gonococcus is transmitted almost wholly by sexual intercourse; it affects both sexes. In this era of social unrest there appears to be a cultural change in sexual behavior. Sexual activity is increasing at earlier ages, thus increasing the incidence of venereal disease. The age group 15 through 29 accounts for over three-fourths of all cases of gonorrhea in recent years. Another factor contributing to the problem of VD control is that gonorrhea has a short incubation period, which promotes its rapid spread. Also, the disease may be relatively asymptomatic in females, making case finding more difficult.

The gonococcus (*Neisseria gonorrhoeae*) causes a surface infection, ascending in almost all cases by way of the lower genital tract. The primary infection, following an incubation period of 3 to 8 days, takes place in or near the urethra. If drainage is good, it subsides spontaneously and clears in the course of a few days or weeks. However, infection of the prostatic urethra in the male and also of the female urethral and vaginal glands predisposes to chronic infection, with occasionally very serious sequelae. Females are apt to contract secondarily a mixed infection of the endometrium and, thereafter, of the tubes, constituting *pelvic inflammatory disease,* with resultant pelvic peritonitis. The ascent of infection is precipitated by such factors as menstruation, douches and the trauma associated with sexual intercourse or instrumentation.

Symptoms

The initial symptoms of gonorrhea, in both sexes, are urinary frequency, dysuria and the discharge of a yellowish exudate from the urethra or the vagina. In the female, tubal infection (salpingitis) may ensue in 2 to 3 weeks, usually manifested by symptoms of low abdominal and back pain, which is aggravated by defecation, and by dysmenorrhea or menorrhagia. Gonorrheal salpingitis is typically self-limited, and pelvic inflammatory disease of the chronic variety generally is considered to be the result of a mixed infection (that is, caused by other organisms in association with the gonococcus) or of recurrent infection from a chronic gonorrheal focus in the lower genital tract.

Complications

The commonest complications of gonorrhea in the female include chronic inflammation of the glands about the urethra and the vagina, chronic cervicitis and salpingitis. Associated with the salpingitis may be severe peritoneal inflammation followed by adhesions about the pelvic organs, including the rectum, and about the liver. Strictures of the cervix and the fallopian tubes are responsible for many cases of sterility.

Chronic gonorrhea in the male usually involves the prostate, constituting a common cause of chronic prostatitis. Occasionally the seminal vesicles likewise are infected. Urethral stricture is a complication of the disease in males particularly. Males and females alike may be victims of gonorrheal arthritis and endocarditis.

Treatment

The treatment of gonorrhea is in a state of uncertainty although penicillin still remains the drug of choice. Some strains of the gonococcus are developing increasing resistance to penicillin, but this resistance is relative and not absolute. Treatment schedules presently recommended are as follows: [*]

> Uncomplicated gonorrhea in men: Aqueous procaine penicillin G, 2,400,000 units in one IM injection.

> Uncomplicated gonorrhea in women: Aqueous procaine penicillin G, 4,800,000 units IM in two injection sites at one visit, or the combination of aqueous procaine penicillin G and procaine penicillin G in oil with 2 per cent aluminum monostearate for two separate IM injections of 2,400,000 units in each site given at one visit.

Prophylactic or epidemiologic treatment for gonorrhea (male and female) is accomplished with the same treatment schedules as for uncomplicated gonorrhea. Treatment of gonorrhea with severe complications must be individualized, using large amounts of short-acting penicillin. Gonorrhea patients sensitive to penicillin may be treated effectively with tetracycline, erythromycin or oleandomycin.

Acute pelvic inflammatory disease due to gonococcal infection is treated conservatively, the important elements of therapy being bed rest and the administration of penicillin, tetracycline or erythromycin chemotherapy. Surgical intervention sometimes is indicated for persistent tubo-ovarian abscesses and other late complications of neglected gonorrhea, such as chronic urethral stricture, which is not amenable to dilatation with sounds, and for some cases of cervicitis or chronic inflammation of the vaginal glands.

The nurse must exercise caution in handling pads or other objects potentially contaminated by drainage from the genital tract. Handwashing is indicated after every contact with the patient. The patient should be instructed thoroughly regarding the importance of protecting the eyes and of maintaining adequate cleanliness in general.

Meningococcal Meningitis

Meningococcal meningitis is an infectious disease caused by the meningococcus (*Neisseria meningitidis*). This malady, if it goes through its entire course, starts as an acute infection of the nasopharynx or the tonsils, followed by a meningococcal septicemia, ending as a localized infection of the meninges of the brain and the upper regions of the spinal cord.

The meningococcus is a tiny diplococcus, the two cocci of the pair flattened against each other, usually found engulfed in leukocytes. Over 20 types of this organism are recognized.

Widespread epidemics of this disease have occurred. However, the majority of them are limited, occurring

[*] U. S. Dept. of Health, Education and Welfare: VD Fact Sheet, pp. 17-18, Washington, D. C., Public Health Service, 1967.

notably in cities, crowded institutions, army camps or jails, but also in country regions—in which children in particular are attacked. The germ is spread by the droplet method, the portals of entry being the mucous membrane of the nose and the tonsils. Of those exposed to it, the great majority do not develop the infection but become carriers, harboring this organism in the nasopharynx for months. In only a few does the organism enter the bloodstream.

Pathology

At autopsy the pia mater (the delicate membrane that immediately covers the brain and the cord and in which are the tiny vessels that provide the cortex with food) is found to be congested and infiltrated with a purulent exudate; the pus is most abundant over the base of the brain and the posterior surface of the cord. The inflammation spreads also to the membrane lining the cerebral ventricles. In acute cases, however, the patient dies from the toxin of the germ before pus has had time to collect.

Symptoms and Course

During each epidemic some patients are scarcely ill; others, at once overwhelmed by the toxemia, develop either a high or a subnormal temperature, the skin is covered by purpura, and the patient dies within a few hours of the onset (the fulminant type).

The typical disease begins as a cold in the head or an attack of paranasal sinusitis, which is soon followed by the stage of septicemia. During the septicemic stage the patient is dull, immobile, refuses to talk, aches all over and desires to be undisturbed. His fever is high and irregular; he may chill. A petechial rash appears on the skin and fever blisters on the lips; joint and lung complications may develop. This stage may last for hours, days or weeks; then the meningeal stage begins. Often, however, there is no definite second stage. In such, the disease begins suddenly with fever, a chill and meningeal symptoms: vomiting, headache, fever, stiffness of the neck and drowsiness.

The meningitis having developed, the patient for most of the time is dull and apathetic, but at intervals he is irritable and restless and, if disturbed, delirious or even maniacal. Later there is stupor or possibly coma. The headache, which is excruciating, comes in spasms; exquisite pains are felt in the back and the limbs; convulsions are not uncommon. The neck is rigid: to raise the head, one must lift the shoulders and, occasionally, the entire body as well from the bed. In some patients, especially in infants, internal hydrocephalus results, evidenced by severe headaches, cyanosis, engorged veins of the forehead, delirium, vomiting, choked disks and sudden death.

The diagnosis is made by lumbar puncture. The cerebrospinal fluid, instead of being perfectly clear, contains so much pus that it looks like thin milk; it is under high pressure and the germ can be isolated from it. Blood cultures are likewise often positive for the meningococcus.

Meningococcemia

A certain proportion of patients with meningococcal infection do not develop meningitis, their disease instead being characterized by persistent or transient bloodstream invasion by the organism. In these cases the meningococcus spares the meninges but localizes in the skin or in the joint synovia. These patients have fever, which may be high and irregular or mild, low-grade, and intermittent. A macular rash commonly appears, often giving the best clue to the clinical diagnosis. Pains in the joints typically are present, and occasionally an acute infection of one of the large joints develops. A leukocytosis may or may not be present. The diagnosis is established by the isolation of the meningococcus from the blood.

Treatment

In general, the mortality of untreated meningococcal infections is 50 to 80 per cent. Since the development of the sulfonamides and penicillin, however, it has been possible to control meningococcal meningitis, and other meningococcal infections likewise, with gratifying regularity.

A large loading dose of penicillin is usually given intravenously. The dosage usually is 15 million units per day of penicillin G or ampicillin 150 mg. per Kg. of body weight per 24 hours. Therapy is continued for 7 to 10 days after the patient has become afebrile. Many sulfa-resistant meningococci have evolved in recent years. Penicillin is the drug of choice, and tetracycline and cephalothin are alternative drugs for the patient with penicillin allergy.

Nursing Aspects

The course of the body temperature must be followed at 2-hour or 4-hour intervals by rectal recordings until the acute phase has subsided. A blood pressure record is maintained. During this period the patient should be protected from injury by placing side rails on his bed. Of utmost importance is the hydration of the patient, particularly during the administration of sulfadiazine therapy. The intake by all routes, oral and parenteral, must be measured as accurately as possible and recorded. The urinary output likewise must be measured and volumes recorded for time intervals corresponding to those on which the intake volumes are based.

The patient with meningitis is likely to be uncomfortable for 3 to 5 days after therapy is begun, complaining of headache, nausea and general malaise. Mouth and skin care should be meticulous. Until full consciousness has returned the patient should be turned frequently. Comfort is afforded by darkening the room, applying tepid sponges and an icecap to the head. Salicylates, codeine and small doses of Demerol, if necessary, are used to control headache. However, depression of vasomotor and respiratory function may ensue and minimal sedation should be employed.

Precautions against communicable disease should be taken in caring for patients with meningococcal infection, at least until the acute stage of the illness has passed.

Influenzal Meningitis

Hemophilus influenzae is responsible for a type of meningitis that primarily affects children between the ages of 6 months and 6 years—a type that is uniformly fatal, unless treated, and one that cripples permanently unless treatment is prompt, vigorous and correct. Few adults have contracted the disease. Of these, the majority have been individuals with cerebrospinal rhinorrhea, hence unduly vulnerable to bacterial invasion of the central nervous system. (The discharge of spinal fluid through the nose indicates that an individual has previously sustained a fracture of his cribriform plate, the thin bone forming the roof of the nose, as a result of which there is an open communication between his cranial and nasal cavities.)

The prodromal period of influenzal meningitis may be featured by symptoms of an upper respiratory infection, often with additional signs of otitis media or pneumonia. Extension of the infection to the meninges is marked by the appearance of nausea and vomiting, headache and high fever. Convulsions are common, ranging from episodes of generalized twitching to tonic-clonic seizures. The patient may be drowsy, stuporous or deeply comatose. Laboratory studies demonstrate anemia, depressed concentrations of sugar in the spinal fluid and the presence of *H. influenzae* in the blood.

Complications that occur as a consequence of delayed or inadequate therapy and take the form of motor or sensory paralyses, diffuse cerebral dysfunction or a convulsive disorder are attributable to blockage of cerebrospinal fluid circulation or injury to the cranial or spinal nerves at their exit points, by tissue swelling and exudate associated with the infection, or to cerebral hemorrhage or thrombosis caused by direct involvement of the cranial vessels themselves during the acute stages.

Treatment

Ampicillin, 150 mg. per Kg. of body weight per 24 hours intravenously for 4 or 5 days followed by intramuscular dosage thereafter is given. Tetracycline, 2 Gm. a day intravenously, and chloramphenicol, 100 mg. per Kg. of body weight per 24 hours, are alternative drugs. Nursing problems and details of nursing care are similar to those encountered in meningococcal meningitis (p. 915).

Pneumococcal Meningitis

Pneumococcal infection is another fairly common form of meningitis with signs and symptoms similar to other bacterial meningitides. Penicillin 10 to 20 million units per day parenterally is the drug of choice. Keflin is an alternative for patients who are sensitive to penicillin. Nursing problems and details of nursing management are similar to those encountered in meningococcal meningitis.

Leprosy (Hansen's Disease)

Leprosy is a granulomatous disease caused by *Mycobacterium leprae*. The characteristic features of the disease are its life-long course, waves of acute exacerbations separated by long periods of remission and destructive granulomatous lesions that develop in the skin and along the nerves.

Mycobacterium leprae is an organism which, in its appearance and acid-fast staining characteristics, resembles the tubercle bacillus. It differs from the latter, however, in that it does not infect animals and cannot be cultivated. The infectious granulomata of leprosy are larger and more diffuse than those of lues and tuberculosis, are painless, contain surprisingly large numbers of the bacilli and do not caseate.

Incidence

Leprosy is common in Asia, Hawaii, Iceland and Scandinavia; in America there are approximately 2000 patients with this disease.

Leprosy is transmitted by direct penetration of normal skin (particularly, and perhaps specifically, the skin of a child) by *Mycobacterium leprae*. The invading organism then finds its way into the axis cylinders of nerves by way of the axon-plasma filaments, i.e., the ultimate terminals of the nerves supplying the skin. Next begins a gradual ascent, organisms breaking out of these nerves at various points in the corium to produce macules and papules. These are painless, of course, since the germs that caused them to form had already destroyed the nerve supply.

Clinical Symptoms and Course

There are two varieties of leprosy, the tubercular and the anesthetic (neural). In the early stages, the tubercular variety is characterized by the appearance of crops of dusky-red patches on the skin—the "leper spots." These may either disappear or develop into slightly raised, flat, infiltrated, anesthetic plaques of all sizes. A single plaque may cover the entire back. Later, losing their pigment, the plaques may become pale. These nodules appear on the prominences of the body and at points of trauma. Those on the face, together with the loss of the eyebrows and the eyelashes, give the face a typical leonine appearance. These nodules, since anesthetic, easily become infected, ulcerate deeply and heal slowly, leaving deforming scars. This process often dissects fingers and toes, possibly a whole hand or foot. The sight is often lost. Acute exacerbations, characterized by fever and the appearance of a fresh crop of lesions, occur at irregular intervals.

In the anesthetic variety the granulomatous infiltration involves nerve trunks particularly; those under the skin are felt quite easily as nodular cords. As a result of these nerve lesions, anesthetic spots appear in the skin, red at first but later white, while the muscles and other tissues supplied by these nerves atrophy. The muscular contractures that result may be extreme. Patients with this variety of leprosy may show no conspicuous signs of their disease for years.

Diagnosis

The appearance of the anesthetic lesions described above is distinctive. Diagnosis often is made first by the discovery of leprosy organisms, usually abundant in the nasal secretion or in a biopsy specimen cut from a nodule.

Treatment

Most promising of all the chemotherapeutic agents presently used in leprosy are the sulfones. The sulfone, Diaminophenylsulfone (DDS, avlosulfone, Dapsone) is the major drug at present and is given in increasing doses, starting with 25 mg. per week and increasing by 25 mg. weekly increments to a maximum of 100 mg. daily. The duration of therapy depends on clinical response and may last 1 to 2 years. Maintenance therapy of long duration may be needed.

Some subjective improvement often is evident within 6 months; improvement is described by the majority of patients after 1 year and by nearly all after 3 years of sulfone therapy. Mucosal lesions respond most rapidly, oral nodules and infiltrations disappearing within a few months, paralleled with relief of nasal obstruction and clearing of laryngeal lesions.

The smaller nodullary lesions in the skin shrink and absorb, leaving only pigment spots, and larger lesions disperse, with eventual scar formation.

Toxic complications of sulfone therapy include hemolytic anemia, leukopenia, allergic dermatitis, nausea, vomiting and headache.

The U.S. Public Health Service maintains a leprosarium at Carville, La., where excellent facilities and nursing care are made available to these patients by the Sisters of Charity, and where intensive therapeutic investigations have long been in progress, culminating in the recent developments outlined above, which are the most promising reported to date.

Spirochetal Infections

Syphilis

Syphilis, or lues (the "great pox"), is an infectious disease acquired through venereal contact and induced by the spirochete *Treponema pallidum,* which, if untreated, runs a characteristic course. A single initial lesion appears at the point where the treponemata entered the body; widespread transitory cutaneous and visceral manifestations then appear and, years later, scattered destructive granulomatous lesions.

Treponema pallidum is a threadlike, actively motile spirochete 6 to 20 micra long, twisted into a corkscrew spiral. It always produces its effects locally—never at a distance, as through toxins. It is killed quickly by a few minutes' exposure to cold or drying.

Community and Epidemiologic Aspects

Following the development of penicillin therapy in the 1940's, the incidence of reported cases of syphilis fell dramatically. Relaxation of concern has led to a rising incidence again in recent years, leaving no doubt that the disease is far from being eradicated and that the need for mass testing and strong public health epidemiologic measures remains. New cases today are seen particularly among teenage groups, homosexuals, certain racial groups and the lower socioeconomic classes. However, this is *not* to say that any group is immune to the disease; there appears to be no natural immunity of man to contracting syphilis.

Open, untreated lesions contain spirochetes. These and infected material are capable of transmitting the disease. The fetus is infected by the mother by way of the placenta. The vast majority of cases are contracted through sexual intercourse; the danger of transmission by direct contact is greatest in the first 4 years of the disease.

Syphilitic infection arouses powerful forces of resistance in the recipient and temporary immunity to further infection develops early in the course of the disease. Probably 10 to 15 per cent of untreated cases of syphilis go on to develop manifestations many years later in the central nervous system, heart, bone, skin and viscera.

Course and Symptoms

Some of the manifestations of lues are designated as early and others as late. The time interval between early and late syphilis is about 4 years, during which period the patient has developed a partial immunity and an altered tissue response to the spirochete.

Early Syphilis. The manifestations of early lues include the chancre, generalized skin eruptions, enlargement of the lymph nodes and widespread visceral involvements that are more or less transitory.

The Chancre. The chancre, or primary sore, typically single, usually appears in 10 to 28 days following the infection and always at the point where the treponemata entered the body. In about 10 per cent of all cases, it is located on one lip, the tongue, a finger, an eyelid or a nipple. The primary sore usually is painless; although ulcerated, there is no discharge; there is induration of the underlying tissues. Invariably the regional lymph nodes become enlarged. In some cases, however, no primary sore can be found.

Chancres on the lip often appear as a painless crack in the mucous membrane which for weeks refuses to heal; one on the eyelid may be mistaken for a sty; those on the fingertips often constitute an insignificant persistent fissure at the edge of the fingernail.

In untreated cases, the chancre disappears in 4 or more weeks, usually leaving a permanent scar.

The General Infection. Even before the chancre appears, and while it is present, the treponemata have begun to spread throughout the entire body by way of the lymph and the bloodstream. In many cases this period of general dissemination is symptomless; in others there are lassitude, a slight fever, loss of weight and anemia, which in some patients is marked.

Secondaries. In 6 weeks to 6 months following the healing of the chancre, the so-called *secondaries* appear. These include: skin eruptions; a general lymphadenitis (enlargement of the epitrochlear and posterior cervical nodes especially characteristic); acute leutic arthritis, which may resemble closely acute rheumatic polyarthritis; pain in the bones, which is worse at night, caused by luetic osteitis and periosteitis; enlargement of the spleen and the liver, sometimes with jaundice; acute iritis, in some cases the first and only symptom of this disease; otitis media, usually bilateral; various neuralgias, neuritis of various nerves, especially of the optic and auditory; and, on rare occasions, an acute luetic meningitis.

Early Luetic Skin Eruptions. The rashes, which may fail to appear altogether, present so many variations that they may simulate practically every known skin

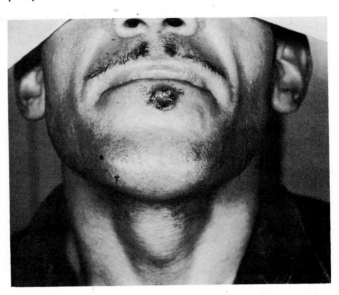

Fig. 37-1. Primary syphilis. Typical Hunterian chancre on lower lip. (From Syphilis—A Synopsis. U.S. Department of Health, Education and Welfare, Public Health Service, 1968)

disease. However, certain features are more or less common to all variations: the lesions are bilaterally symmetrical in distribution and the distribution is generalized; the eruptions are almost invariably polymorphous (that is, almost never are the skin lesions of any one type only, as macules alone, or papules alone); they cause no itching and no pain; they persist for weeks; even untreated, they gradually fade entirely, leaving no scars; and, finally, they quickly disappear under treatment. Concomitantly, the hair often drops out, sometimes in patches, giving the scalp a motheaten appearance.

The macular eruption (the roseola), which usually appears early, may cover the entire trunk, sparing the face. It may be merely a diffuse rosy blush, rose-colored spots, or an eruption of slightly elevated copper-colored macules. Papular luetic lesions, covered with scales, may appear on the body surface. These papules are prone to become secondarily infected, and the resultant pustular eruption may resemble acne vulgaris, impetigo or even smallpox. Nodular skin lesions, small, bluish-red or brown in color, also may develop. These nodules may persist for years and, on disappearing, leave areas of pigmentation.

The luetic lesions that develop on moist skin surfaces, for example, about the anus, take the form of broad wartlike plaques (the so-called *condylomata*), which tend to crack and ulcerate. Those that appear on the mucous membranes of the mouth and the tongue are glistening, slightly elevated flat circumscribed patches, usually covered with a white or yellowish exudate. These papules, the so-called *mucous patches,* are the most characteristic, persistent and infectious of all luetic lesions. Other papules, dry and scaly in character, develop on the palms and the soles. Those on the fingertips occasionally destroy the bed of the nails, which become brittle and fissured. This luetic onychia is most refractory to treatment.

Late Syphilis. After the disappearance of the early luetic manifestations in untreated or inadequately treated cases there follows a period of apparent good health; more than half the patients have no further trouble, with or without treatment. But, after about 4 years, those less fortunate begin to show signs of the late (formerly called *tertiary*) luetic lesions. The most distinctive form that these lesions take is the gumma, a discrete tumor, but the much more common diffuse luetic infiltrations have the same significance. Any organ of the body may be attacked.

Late Luetic Skin Lesions. No sharp line can be drawn between the skin and the mucous membrane lesions of early and late lues, but those of late lues are few in number, not symmetrically distributed, contain few treponemata, are more infiltrated, chronic and destructive. Such lesions produce the large, deep punched-out ulcers on the lower legs, which leave characteristic scars with sinuous borders, pigmented areolae and atrophied bases upon healing; the rupia lesions seen around the elbow, with peculiar many-layered crusts; the lesions in the mouth, the throat and the nose, which ulcerate and perforate the soft palate or the septum and explain the saddle nose; the diffuse thickenings on the tongue, which may either ulcerate or become cancerous.

Late Bone and Joint Syphilis. Among the important late luetic bone lesions are necrosis of the cranial bones and bony overgrowths or exostoses owing to periostitis, which make the shins, the clavicles, the sternum and the cranial bones nodular. Gumma of bone occur, which are destructive and occasionally cause deformities of the spine and other bones.

Late luetic arthritis, usually monoarticular, is a gummatous thickening of the synovial membrane and the joint capsule, because of which the joint is swollen and fluctuates. This condition is remedied quickly by antiluetic treatment. The Charcot joint, a feature of locomotor ataxia, is a special type of arthritis, notably affecting the knee. It is characterized by the gradual and extensive painless disintegration of all joint tissues, which results in great joint deformity. Because of the tabetic spinal cord changes, all joint pain is lost and traumatic changes become extreme. The patient continues to use the disintegrating joint as long as it will support any weight.

Late Vascular or Visceral Syphilis. Lues can affect nearly all the organs of the body. The most marked effects are usually those of the vascular system, but there are hardly any organs or systems of the body that escape.

Congenital Lues

Women with active syphilis give birth to luetic children. Luetic children, born late in the course of the maternal infection, at birth may or may not present evidences of the disease. If they do, the most common symptoms are snuffles, various distinctive skin eruptions, rhagades (scars at the corners of the mouth), fissures of the skin, onychia, alopecia, enlarged liver and spleen and emaciation.

Other infants with congenital lues show no signs of this disease until they are 10 or 12 years old, or even later. At this time, the following may appear: Hutchinson's teeth (notched and usually peg-shaped upper middle permanent incisors); luetic lesions of the liver, which occasionally result in cirrhosis at puberty; enlarged spleen; tender enlargements of the bones and the epiphyses, particularly of the femur and the tibia; and saber shins. Still later may appear an almost pathognomonic bilateral interstitial keratitis, which if inadequately treated results in permanent cloudiness of the cornea, optic neuritis and deafness. The simultaneous presence of Hutchinson's teeth, interstitial keratitis and deafness (Hutchinson's triad) is diagnostic of congenital lues.

Diagnostic Features of Syphilis in General

The chancre, if typical, can be recognized without difficulty; in any case, treponemata should be sought in serum expressed from the suspected sore or aspirated from a neighboring lymph node. Throughout life the presence of the scar of the chancre is of great aid in diagnosis.

Most important to exclude is the chancroidal ulcer (soft chancre), a deep, characteristically punched-out ulcer, often multiple, with elevated undermined edges, an inflammatory areola and a dirty, moth-eaten soft floor that exudes an abundant purulent fluid containing Ducrey's bacillus.

Diagnostic Serum Reactions. The Wassermann reaction is one of the most consistent of laboratory tests for lues, but today most clinics use, in addition, one of several precipitin reactions, such as the Kahn, Klein, Hinton, VDRL or Kolmer tests.

A positive serologic reaction in the great majority of cases indicates that the patient has, or has had, active syphilis. A falsely positive test may appear in systemic lupus erythematosus, leprosy, infectious mononucleosis, following smallpox vaccination and in other spirochetal diseases such as yaws. A negative

Wassermann in the presence of active lues may occur in cardiovascular syphilis and in several varieties of central nervous system syphilis. More specific serologic tests for syphilis now are undergoing world-wide trial. These include the *Treponema pallidum* immobilization test (TPI) of Nelson and Mayer, the *T. pallidum* immune adherence (TPIA) test, the *T. pallidum* complement-fixation (TPCF) test, and the *T. pallidum* fluorescent antibody (TPFA) tests, one or more of which may well be adopted generally as a supplement to the simpler, standard serologic tests in order to identify or exclude biologic false-positive (BFP) reactions.

Treatment

Penicillin alone is effective against all forms of syphilis. Early syphilis, in almost all cases, responds to a single treatment with 2,400,000 units of benzathine penicillin G (Bicillin, Permapen), 4 ml., containing 300,000 units per ml., being injected into each buttock. Alternatively, procaine penicillin G in oil and aluminum monostearate (PAM) may be injected intramuscularly in divided doses of 1,200,000 units at intervals of 2 to 4 days. Recommended treatment for all forms of late syphilis is intramuscular PAM in a total dose of 6,000,000 to 10,000,000 units, individual doses of 1,200,000 units being given 2 or 3 times a week. The existence of pregnancy does not appear to alter the therapeutic requirements. Congenital syphilis is treated in the same manner as acquired syphilis, except that smaller doses of penicillin may be administered to children weighing less than 32 Kg. (70 lbs.). The total dose in such cases may be 75,000 to 100,000 units per Kg. of body weight. This may be administered in the form of procaine penicillin in oil and aluminum monostearate, given intramuscularly in doses of from 0.5 to 1 ml. (150,000 to 300,000 units) every 2 to 4 days until the course is completed.

Penicillin-sensitive individuals, or penicillin-resistant syphilis, require the substitution of another antibiotic. Early syphilis responds satisfactorily to 3 or 4 gm. of tetracycline daily by mouth for 10 days. For late syphilis, 2 gm. of erythromycin daily by mouth for 15 to 20 days is recommended.

Congenital syphilitic interstitial keratitis should be treated with the topical administration of cortisone (5 mg. of cortisone acetate to 1 ml. of istonic sodium chloride solution), 1 drop instilled every 3 hours, as a supplement to antisyphilitic penicillin therapy.

Public Health Education

Information regarding syphilis should be disseminated widely; education of physicians, nurses as well as of the general public must be undertaken. Syphilis

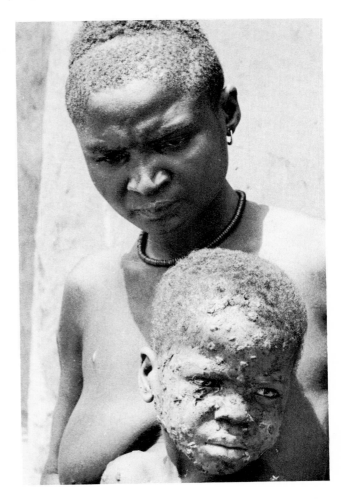

FIG. 37-2. These ugly sores can mean a lifetime of pain. Yaws is a disease that is widespread throughout tropical areas. In Africa alone, some 25 million suffer from this unsightly and painful disease. Usually contracted in childhood, it can last a lifetime if not treated, destroying the skin and attacking the bones. This little boy, Ede Nwaebgo, is 5 years old. He lives in a bush village in Nigeria. The misery of yaws is clearly reflected in the unsmiling faces of Ede and his mother. That was before the visit of a WHO-assisted yaws team. (World Health Organization)

must be regarded as a disease, not a stigma. The treatment must be initiated as early as possible. Congenital syphilis can be prevented readily by prenatal blood tests and prompt therapy.

Public funds are available to ensure adequate treatment. Most states finance blood tests and antiluetic medications with the assistance of the U.S. Public Health Service. The public health nurse has a responsibility in interpreting the doctor's instructions to patients and impressing them with the importance of treatment and the value of premarital and prenatal blood tests. Her attitude must be understanding and her approach skillful in order to secure the confidence of her patients, for whose guidance she is in part responsible.

Yaws (Frambesia)

Yaws is a highly contagious disease of the tropics. It is caused by an organism quite similar to that of syphilis, although the disease is nonvenereal. The two chief features of yaws are anemia and an eruption of granulomata scattered over the body surface (Fig. 37-2).

The source of infection is exudate of the skin lesions of infected persons; it is spread principally by direct contact. The disease affects children most frequently but does occur in adults.

The primary lesion, "mother yaw," appears at the site of inoculation (most often on the face or the neck) as a tubercle or group of tubercles. This lesion grows in size, becomes conical and confluent and discharges a yellow exudate that dries to form a crust.

In 4 to 6 weeks following the initial lesion *the secondary stage* begins, with fever, mild constitutional symptoms and a rash of minute reddish papules (yaws) that appear in crops on the face and the extremities especially. These papules grow to become raspberrylike lesions, 1 or 2 cm. in diameter, the majority of which become crusted. The crust covers a red pulpy tubercle that resembles a raspberry and exudes a serum with a disagreeable odor. Those lesions occurring on moist surfaces become condylomatous; those on the dorsa of the feet, warty; those on the palms and the soles, painful ulcers. After a few weeks the lesions disappear, leaving white areas that later become pigmented.

A tertiary stage may follow, the characteristic lesions of which are indolent deep-skin ulcers which may also involve underlying bones. Upon healing, these ulcers leave disfiguring scars.

The blood serum of patients with yaws almost invariably gives a positive Wassermann reaction. Nevertheless, the organism causing yaws is *not Treponema pallidum:* this disease is extragenital and noncongenital, the mucous membranes are not involved, and the skin eruption, unlike that of lues, is uniform. Yaws responds readily and rapidly to penicillin therapy.

The tertiary stage of yaws evidently explains *gangosa,* a mutilating nasopharyngitis seen in the West Indies, and *goundou* (of Africa and South America), an ulcerating process that attacks the nose, often entirely destroying it.

Leptospirosis

Leptospirosis is a broad term that includes all leptospiral infections. Serologic studies show that a given type of leptospira may cause several different syndromes. Twenty-two serotypes of leptospirae are found in the United States in a wide variety of animals. The leptospirae cannot grow outside a host. Human infections occur by contact with infected urine or animal tissue or contaminated water and soil; transmission from person to person is rare.

Leptospirosis is an occupational disease among farmers, sewer workers, veterinarians and abattoir workers. The important leptospiral infections include Weil's disease (*L. icterohemorrhagicae*), swineherd's disease (*L. pomona*), canicola fever (*L. canicola*) and pretibial fever (*L. autumnalis*). Weil's disease is a severe form of leptospirosis associated with fever, jaundice, hemorrhages, hepatic and renal failure and is usually caused by *L. icterohemorrhagicae*. However, it is now known that this species can produce less severe states of Weil's disease and that other leptospirae can produce severe forms of it; therefore, the term leptospirosis is a better term than Weil's disease. In some instances of leptospirosis, the clinical picture of aseptic meningitis predominates.

The disease is characterized by the sudden onset of chills and fever, ocular injection, muscle aching and tenderness, headache and stiff neck occurring between 4 and 20 days after exposure. During this initial phase, which may last for a period of 3 to 9 days, the leptospira can be demonstrated in the patient's blood by means of cultures or animal inoculations. The white blood cells are increased, and the spinal fluid contains leukocytes and often leptospira as well.

The second stage is marked by variable degrees of jaundice, hemorrhagic phenomena, symptoms of meningitis and signs of renal infection, including hematuria and albuminuria. The liver may enlarge and a skin rash may appear. Leptospira may be recovered from the urine at this time and for a period of from 2 to 5 weeks hence. Serum agglutinins specific for leptospiral antigen can be demonstrated, and muscle biopsy might show characteristic lesions. Fever and symptoms usually begin to subside during the course of the second or third week of the disease. Convalescence is apt to be slow and characterized by depression, weakness and anemia. Relapse may occur. The mortality of the disease has approached 50 per cent in some reports.

Treatment, given early in the course of the disease, consists in the administration of penicillin, still the drug of choice in all spirochetal infections. Tetracycline, streptomycin and chloramphenicol have also been reported useful, but have little effect in leptospirosis unless begun in the first 1 to 2 days of the illness.

Rat-Bite Fever

Rat-bite fever, caused by *Spirillum minus,* is introduced into the body by the bite of an infected rat. It is characterized by a series of febrile paroxysms that may continue for months or years, a skin rash of large, sharply defined, red macules, weakness, and polyarthritis. The period of incubation may last for months. The original wound caused by the rat bite, and perhaps had healed, then becomes swollen, red and ulcerated, and the regional lymph nodes are enlarged.

The attack begins with a chill and a fever which last 3 or 4 days. Then the skin eruption appears, with pain in the muscles and joints, and sometimes delirium. Each paroxysm lasts for 7 or 8 days, and each 2 are separated by 1 or 2 weeks of apyrexia. A false positive serologic test for syphilis may appear.

Treatment consists of cleansing the wound and administering an intensive course of penicillin.

PATIENTS WITH VIRAL INFECTIONS

Nature of Viruses

Viruses are submicroscopic particles that pass through bacterial filters. They are known as filtrable particles or filtrable viruses and can be visualized only by electron microscopy. The viruses range in size from the 30-μ yellow fever virus to the 205-μ smallpox virus. Viruses may be made of RNA or DNA. They cannot propagate outside living tissue; they require tissue cells of the host or tissue culture preparations (in contrast to bacteria, which will grow on artificial culture media). Viruses infect cells and cause disease by subverting the cellular metabolism to their own needs for growth. The infected cell is often killed in the process. Like bacteria, viruses are antigenic and stimulate the host to produce antibodies. This fact is useful both as an aid to diagnosis and in conferring immunity to recurrence of the same disease. It is not known why one virus will infect the respiratory tract and another the central nervous system; they tend to be specific in the type of cells they invade. Viruses may infect the human being from embryo stage throughout life, though particularly during childhood. The severity of the initial virus infection tends to increase with increasing age (except for the neonatal period). For example, poliomyelitis and viral hepatitis have more severe sequellae in adults than in children. Some viruses, like that of herpes simplex, maintain a persistent presence in the host and recur from time to time, especially in the presence of other illness (e.g., the fever blisters in pneumonia are reactivations of latent herpes simplex infection and are activated by the febrile illness of pneumonia). Currently, viruses are not susceptible to antibiotics or chemotherapy, but prophylactic vaccines are available for many of them.

Smallpox (Variola)

Smallpox (variola vera) is an acute virus disease with a characteristic skin rash that evolves according to a remarkably regular schedule. The principal natural reservoir is man.

The virus is present in the skin lesions. The disease may be transmitted by direct contact at all stages and, for a long time, by exposed clothes or furniture. Lifelong immunity follows an attack.

Smallpox once was the most dreaded of epidemic diseases, and few exposed persons escaped it; today epidemics arise only in unvaccinated communities. About 100,000 cases are reported yearly to the World Health Organization.

Clinical Course

The incubation period varies from 5 to 21 days. The onset is sudden—in adults, often with a chill; in children, with a convulsion. Headache and pain in the back and the limbs appear, and the patient vomits; the temperature quickly rises to 40.6° C.* or higher, the pulse becomes rapid, and sweats are common. At this time a confusing prodromal rash, often slightly petechial, may develop.

On the fourth day of the fever, the typical smallpox rash appears as an eruption of bright red macules from 2 to 3 mm. in diameter, which soon covers the body. These macules within a few hours become shotty papules that develop into vesicles with depressed centers containing pus and blood. These pustules, always most abundant on the face, the hands and the feet, have a characteristic greenish or grayish-yellow color. Each is surrounded by a narrow areola of inflamed skin. With the pustular stage the temperature, which may have subsided temporarily, again rises. This fever abates after 1 or 2 more days, and then the patient usually remains afebrile. The pustules, after the 14th day, dry and form crusts, which, beginning on the face, gradually drop off, often leaving a slight scar. Pitting, however, is made worse if the pustules and the scabs are scratched or picked.

The rash in severe cases may appear within 3 days after the onset of fever, and the total duration of the acute stage may far exceed the usual 3 weeks. The mortality is high in the severe forms of the disease.

* 104° F.

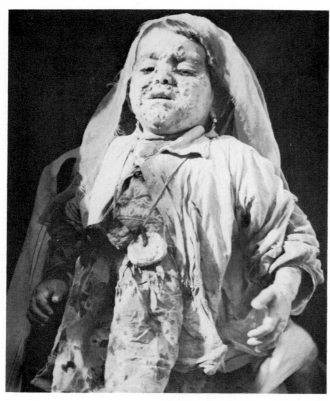

Fig. 37-3. Young Afghan girl struck by smallpox. Her parents have dressed her in her finest clothes as if to protect her from evil. Since 1962 WHO has been assisting the government of Afghanistan with its smallpox eradication campaign—part of the eradication program of the South East Asia region of WHO. Apart from the services of a medical officer and sanitarian, WHO has provided over a million doses of freeze-dried vaccine. (World Health Organization photo by W. Wilkie)

In those who recover, all the crusts may not have separated at the end of a month, and in this case the face is always left badly pitted.

Hemorrhagic Smallpox. More severe cases assume hemorrhagic features. On the 2nd or 3rd day of the fever in true hemorrhagic smallpox (black smallpox), subcutaneous hemorrhages cover the entire body, subconjunctival hemorrhages appear, and there is bleeding from the mouth, the nose, the lungs, the rectum and the kidneys. While a few patients recover, the majority die—some even before the smallpox eruption has had time to appear.

Complications

The complications of smallpox include laryngitis with edema of the larynx, bronchitis, bronchopneumonia and acute nephritis. Usually, secondary infec-

tion of the lesions occurs, which may result in residual pitting.

Prognosis

The general mortality of epidemics formerly was between 25 and 35 per cent. It now is between 6 and 8 per cent. Over 80 per cent of all fatal cases are children under 10 years of age. In each outbreak, cases of all grades of severity occur, including those so mild that the patient remains up and about with an eruption consisting only of a dozen or so pustules.

Nursing Care

Any patient who has been acutely ill for less than 4 days with severe headache, backache and vomiting who presents papules, vesicles, pustules or crusts on the forehead and the wrists, all eruptions being at about the same stage of development, should be quarantined as a possible case of smallpox, regardless of how comfortable he may feel. Mild ambulatory cases dismissed as cases of chickenpox are responsible for the spread of epidemics.

The patient with smallpox must be cared for in a suitable hospital. The treatment is chiefly symptomatic. The severe pains of onset may be relieved by phenacetin, acetylsalicylate or morphine. Hydrotherapy is the best measure to control the fever. Paregoric will check the diarrhea. Good oral hygiene is essential.

Early in the attack the patient should be kept at bed rest despite the benign character of his symptoms, since complications are most apt to rise during this stage. The room is darkened, for the eruption is less severe if the skin is protected from bright light. During the vesicular and pustular stages the affected areas should be covered with an antibacterial agent such as tyrothricin or penicillin. Later the crusts are kept moist with petrolatum.

The amount of pitting is reduced by relieving the intense itching through use of calamine zinc lotion with phenol (2%), so that the patient will not pick at his skin lesions. The eyes should be irrigated frequently with boric acid solution. If signs of conjunctivitis are detected, an ophthalmic ointment should be applied that contains an antibiotic, such as tetracycline (Achromycin), 1 per cent, and hydrocortisone, 1.5 to 2 per cent. A liquid diet is indicated.

The patient should be kept in isolation until every scab has separated, at which time precautions may be relaxed.

Prevention

A cross-immunity exists between smallpox and another viral infection, which is relatively mild and harmless, called "cowpox." By inducing the latter through the inoculation of the active virus, as described on page 901, a permanent active immunity against smallpox is conferred.

The World Health Organization has as its goal the world-wide eradication of smallpox by 1977. This must be a world-wide enterprise, because international travel may produce an outbreak in any country. The disease can spread among the unvaccinated and those whose vaccine-induced immunity has worn off. Freeze-dried vaccine has come into widespread use and can be painlessly injected under pressure through the skin by a jet injector. As many as 500 people can be immunized in an hour. In areas with little or no smallpox, routine vaccination is recommended at the age of 6 to 18 months with continuing maintenance vaccination every 5 years. (See page 901 for vaccination technique.) In endemic areas, vaccination should be repeated every 3 to 5 years.

Infectious Mononucleosis

Infectious mononucleosis, or glandular fever, is an acute infectious fever, characterized predominantly by sore throat, painful enlargement of cervical lymph nodes, and prostration. This disease is presumed to be of viral origin, although this has not been proved.

This disease is encountered almost exclusively in individuals between the ages of approximately 14 and 30 years. The distribution of incidence between sexes is almost precisely equal. The term "mononucleosis" is derived from the appearance of the blood leukocytes at the height of the infection, when the majority appear to be young histiocytes, which bear a superficial resemblance to monocytes, or hybrid forms, combining the features of monocytes and lymphocytes (i.e., "atypical lymphocytes").

Epidemiology

Infectious mononucleosis, although very common indeed among individuals in the age group specified above, is not a highly contagious infection. Transmission from one member of a family to another, or from one roommate to another, is rare. Hospital patients with this disease appear to pose no hazard to other patients on the ward. Neither nurses nor other hospital personnel seem to acquire the infection from these patients. Transmission from blood donor to transfusion recipient, however, probably has occurred. The most satisfactory explanation for the vast majority of cases proposes that the infectious agent is an extremely fragile virus that is excreted in the saliva of patients with the active disease and of individuals who are convalescent following the infection, or whose convalescence is complete, but who are carriers of the virus. Passage of the virus from one individual to another appears to require salivary interchange. The incubation period ranges from 30 to 50 days.

A typical attack begins with fever, chills and sweating, sore throat, cough and abdominal pain. On the second or third day, the lymph nodes begin to swell and become tender, usually the posterior cervical group first, then the anterior groups, later, sometimes, those of the axillae, and, on rare occasions, those over the entire body. These lymph nodes remain firm and later return to normal size. Occasionally the spleen also is enlarged. A morbilliform (measleslike) rash may appear transiently. The fever which is high and markedly intermittent, continues for 2 to 3 weeks.

The leukocytosis, with an absolute decrease in the number of granular cells, is the most characteristic sign. The morphology of the leukocytes may be so atypical that a diagnosis of acute leukemia may be entertained and an unwarranted bad prognosis tendered. The total white cell count reaches its height (usually from 20,000 to 30,000 per cu. mm.) from the 10th to the 14th day of the fever. A valuable test for diagnosis is the heterophilic antibody agglutination test. It is positive if the serum or the plasma, after preliminary heating, in dilutions of more than 1:16, causes a suspension of sheep erythrocytes to agglutinate.

Complications

The enlarged spleen of infectious mononucleosis is unusually vulnerable to injury and may fracture if subjected to relatively mild trauma. Inasmuch as the consequences of splenic fracture are potentially serious, because of the substantial volume of blood that may be lost into the peritoneal cavity, patients with splenomegaly in the course of infectious mononucleosis must abstain temporarily from all exertional activities. A small percentage of patients (0.7 to 1.0) develop signs of encephalitis; a larger number may acquire the symptoms and signs of viral hepatitis (see p. 515); and rarely there may appear acquired hemolytic anemia, thrombocytopenic purpura, self-limited cardiac complication or evidences of renal inflammation.

Practically all patients recover. The treatment is to keep the patient in bed and as comfortable as possible during the acute, febrile stage of the disease.

Influenza

Influenza is a viral infection that has swept through the entire civilized world approximately every 20 years, attacking as many as 40 per cent of individuals in affected areas. The striking features of these epidemics have been the rapidity of their spread and an extremely high attack rate.

Typical epidemics of influenza have been characterized by 3 successive waves, separated by brief intermissions. The first wave lasts from 3 to 6 weeks, is explosive in outbreak, is widespread, and the majority of cases are mild and with few complications. The second wave also is widespread, but lasts longer; the cases are more severe, and the complications are serious. The third wave lasts still longer (from 8 to 10 weeks), involves fewer persons, but the complications are quite severe. During the years succeeding a major epidemic there follow scattered local waves of decreasing severity, with sporadic cases of influenza occurring during the intervals.

Etiology

The primary factor in the etiology of influenza is a filtrable virus, of which two major strains have been isolated, designated Types A and B. Recent pandemic outbreaks have been caused by an antigenic variant of Type A (Asian, or Far East strain). Complications are due to secondary invaders, such as *Hemophilus influenzae,* various streptococci, pneumococci and other organisms.

Symptoms

True influenza, in the majority of cases, after a short incubation period of about 2 or 3 days, begins as an acute coryza, but one that presents several characteristic clinical features: suddenness of onset with high fever, a fiery redness of the upper respiratory mucous membrane, profound prostration, severe aching pains in the back and the extremities, injection of the conjunctivae and leukopenia.

Other cases start as acute sinusitis, bronchitis, pleurisy or bronchopneumonia. These always are abrupt in onset and prostrating. In another group of cases, nervous features—headache, profound depression and prostration—predominate from the first; in still another group there are gastrointestinal symptoms of nausea, vomiting, abdominal pain, diarrhea, jaundice and collapse ("intestinal flu"); and, finally, in each epidemic, cases develop without local symptoms but with chills almost typical of malaria or with a continuous fever suggesting typhoid. The acute fever of the influenza itself lasts 1 to 4 days, and convalescence is rapid.

Influenzal bronchopneumonia, usually due to the pneumococcus, the staphylococcus or the streptococcus, is the most common serious complication of influenza. The most dreaded type of this complication is streptococcal or staphylococcal pneumonia, which during severe epidemics develops early and may prove to be fatal within 24 hours from the onset of the influenza.

Late in an epidemic the cases develop serious complications, probably caused by organisms for which the influenza virus seems to have prepared the way. Among these are pericarditis, endocarditis, septicemia, peritonitis, appendicitis, nephritis, chronic bronchitis, bronchiectasis, otitis media and infections of the central nervous system.

The immediate mortality of uncomplicated cases of influenza is only 0.5 per cent, but its complications, such as acute pneumonias and empyemas, are exceedingly serious. Other sequelae, of a chronic nature, include paranasal sinusitis, bronchitis and pneumonitis.

Prophylaxis

It has been recommended by the Surgeon General's Advisory Committee on Influenza that individuals over 65 years of age, pregnant women, and persons who have chronic cardiovascular, pulmonary, renal, or metabolic diseases be immunized against influenza.

Vaccines have been prepared from certain strains of influenza A and B. Ample evidence was obtained during the epidemic of Asian influenza in 1957 to indicate that individuals immunized against the Denver strain of Type A were not protected against the Asian strain of the same type. Any vaccine which could be expected to check an epidemic would have to be in readiness and on hand well in advance, long enough, in fact, to have been inoculated into a sizable proportion of the population at least 2 or 3 weeks ahead of the outbreak.

Nursing Considerations

There is no specific treatment for influenza. Phenacetin or aspirin may relieve the general aching. The nurse should be instructed as to proper local treatments to keep the nasal passages clear. Secondary pulmonary infections with streptococci or pneumococci may be expected to respond to penicillin therapy. Any empyema that develops should be aspirated, or surgically drained if the effusion is large.

The greatest danger in cases of influenzal bronchopneumonia is that of vasomotor lapse, for which vasopressor drugs are indicated. Dehydration must be combated by the intravenous administration of saline solutions and blood, as indicated.

The patient with influenza should be kept in bed until convalescence is well established, in hope of preventing complications and sequelae. It is doubtful whether there is any virtue in isolating him or in disinfecting his sputum, since this disease seems to be communicated to others immediately before its onset. The patient should receive from 3,000 to 5,000 ml. of fluid daily and the fullest diet that can be retained. Because of his great physical and mental depression, he should receive every encouragement and his surroundings should be made as pleasant and comfortable as possible.

Because of the frequency with which paranasal sinusitis complicates this disease, the nurse should see that medications in the form of nose drops or inhalants, prescribed to keep the nasal passages clear, are applied regularly.

The patient with influenzal pneumonia demands particularly careful attention. Should the slightest cyanosis appear, she should report this to the physician at once and be prepared to administer oxygen.

Weeks or months may pass after an attack of influenza before the patient is truly well. For many patients a change in climate, when possible, is of great aid.

Enteroviral Infections

Members of the enteroviral family are poliomyelitis, the Coxsackie and the ECHO viruses, which have been implicated as the cause of several epidemic infections.

Poliomyelitis

Since the advent of the Salk and Sabin vaccines, the problem of poliomyelitis has decreased considerably and is not discussed here.

Coxsackie Viruses

"Coxsackie" viruses are named after the town in New York State where the initial epidemiologic studies were carried out in connection with these agents. Two major types of Coxsackie virus are recognized, designated "A" and "B." Nineteen Type A and 5 Type B Coxsackie viruses have been distinguished so far. Type A has been responsible for aseptic meningitis, such cases having been precisely similar to nonparalytic cases of polioviral infection, or to lymphocytic choriomeningitis. Type A also is the cause of a mild infectious illness of children called "herpangina," a disease of summer which is characterized by the abrupt onset of fever and sore throat, the appearance of a vesicular eruption on the buccal mucosa and the pharynx and gastrointestinal disturbances, all of which subside completely within a period of a week or less. A rather nonspecific summer illness marked by fever, headache, stiff neck or back, an occasional rash and variable muscle aches also has been ascribed to Type A Coxsackie virus.

Type B has been known to cause all of the illnesses enumerated above, including aseptic meningitis, which has been complicated by a transient and mild motor weakness comparable with that occurring in mild paralytic poliomyelitis. Type B also has produced a nonspecific febrile illness, with and without skin rash, as well as one variety of epidemic pharyngitis. It is the etiologic agent in epidemic pleurodynia, and it is also responsible for a dangerous type of myocarditis that occurs during the neonatal period and in early childhood and carries a high mortality.

ECHO Viruses

The term "ECHO," designating another group of enteroviruses, is composed of the first letters of the words "enteric" (indicating their intestinal location), "cytopathogenic" (producing damage to the cells supporting their growth in tissue culture), "human orphan." Orphan refers to the fact that this viral species was discovered before it was known with what, if any, disease it might be associated. Approximately 31 strains of ECHO viruses are recognized, some of which have been responsible for an aseptic meningitis comparable with nonparalytic poliomyelitis. Paralytic cases of ECHO viral infection have been reported also. Other forms of ECHO infection include a nonspecific febrile illness, occasionally complicated by a skin rash; febrile illnesses accompanied by upper respiratory and gastrointestinal symptoms; and "summer diarrhea" of infants and young children. Most of the enteroviral infections are confined to the summer months. Two notable exceptions are caused by ECHO Types 10 and 20, both illnesses marked by a combination of respiratory and gastrointestinal symptoms.

Treatment

None of the enteroviruses is susceptible to any chemotherapeutic agent now available. Nursing measures are indicated, depending on the nature and the severity of the symptoms in each individual patient.

Viral Encephalitis

Encephalitis (inflammation of the brain) may be caused by a number of agents, including viruses, bacteria, chemicals, etc. The viral encephalitides comprise a group of acute infections that affect predominantly the central nervous system. Each variety is caused by a specific virus. For each of these viruses there exists a particular animal reservoir, and each finds its access to man through the bite of a particular species of blood-sucking arthropod. Von Economo encephalitis (encephalitis lethargica, or "sleeping sickness"), first of the pandemic encephalitides to be recognized as such, has not recurred since 1926, in other words, since virologic techniques have developed to the stage that permits the identification of its causative organism, its vector or its animal reservoir. With respect to the viruses responsible for other forms of epidemic encephalitis, such identification has been possible and these data are available.

The clinical features of epidemic encephalitis are extremely variable and depend less on the type of virus that causes the infection than on the age of the patient who contracts it. Two forms of the disease, namely, the von Economo and the St. Louis types, have been characterized unusually well and are described jointly as being representative of the group as a whole.

Von Economo Encephalitis

This type of encephalitis, commonly known as "sleeping sickness," is characterized by its mild and gradual onset, with headache, insomnia and diplopia due to early paralysis of the eye muscles. Symptoms of meningeal and spinal cord involvement are not prominent. This stage is followed by one of pronounced lethargy. There is a marked tendency to permanent sequelae.

The first (acute) stage, which lasts from 1 to 7 days, often beginning as an upper respiratory infection with slight fever, headache, malaise and general muscle soreness, often is interpreted as influenza, but there also is marked insomnia and often diplopia. Following this stage some patients recover. Others progress to a stage of lethargy, during which, with consciousness clear, they lie motionless in bed or sit for hours staring ahead, incontinent and apparently oblivious to their surroundings. They eat nothing unless it is placed in the mouth; they never speak unless they are asked a question, when they respond briefly but clearly. Many other features, however, may dominate: paralyses, ataxia and symptoms suggesting paresis or dementia praecox. The patient may recover at this point, but usually with one or more permanent sequelae, such as paralysis of one of the cranial nerves, deafness or vertigo.

The second stage of this disease, of variable duration, is characterized by easy fatigability, headaches, insomnia or alterations in character suggesting psychoneurosis.

The third (parkinsonian) stage, almost characteristic of the von Economo type, presents slowness of thought (bradyphrenia), slowness of muscular movements (bradykinesia), tremor resembling that of paralysis agitans and other possible sequelae, including tics, disturbances of sleep and characteristic personality changes. Such patients may become actively aggressive, unruly, destructive, cruel, yet without any sense of responsibility for their occasionally murderous acts, and they are not at all deterred by punishment. Young children may suffer permanent arrest of intellectual development.

St. Louis Encephalitis

This type of encephalitis is characterized at the onset by symptoms that suggest an acute infectious disease much more than do cases of the Economo type. Usually it begins suddenly with high fever, severe headache, a leukocytosis of 12,000 to 20,000 per cu. mm., mental confusion or delirium, often with pronounced signs of meningitis and spinal cord irritation, but seldom with paralyses of the eye muscles. The course of this disease usually is stormy. However, after 2 or 3 weeks improvement starts, and this often is the beginning of rapid and complete recovery. A chronic stage seldom develops.

The spinal fluid in all types of epidemic encephalitis is clear, its pressure moderately raised (from 60 to 120 mm.), its cell count fairly high (from 50 to 200 mononuclear cells per cu. mm.); there is only a slight pellicle or none at all, globulin is not increased, and the glucose level is normal.

The prognosis is varied. In outbreaks of epidemic encephalitis recoveries have ranged from 20 to over 60 per cent.

Secondary (Sporadic) Encephalitis

Secondary or "sporadic" encephalitis, clinically somewhat similar to the more primary types, occasionally follows various acute infectious diseases, particularly influenza, smallpox, chickenpox, vaccination, whooping cough, measles and mumps. It appears at a fairly definite period in the course of the primary disease, that is, after the disease has subsided and the patient is ambulatory. In cases following measles and other of the acute exanthemas the meningeal features are quite prominent (hence the term *meningoencephalitis*).

Nursing Aspects

In general, the treatment of acute encephalitis of all types is unsatisfactory. Elevation of the cerebrospinal fluid pressure is an indication for frequently repeated lumbar punctures and perhaps the administration of hypertonic sucrose intravenously. Respiratory paralysis necessitates the use of a mechanical respirator. For high fever, alcohol sponge baths and antipyretics are administered; sedatives are used to advantage for discomfort and restlessness.

Therapy in the chronic stages likewise is symptomatic. Stramonium, atropine and belladonna are of some value in the treatment of the spasticity of parkinsonism. Patients with postencephalitic narcolepsy and myasthenia are benefited by the administration of Prostigmin and amphetamine. Behavior disorders require rehabilitation and patient and family education. The patient should be isolated, kept quiet in bed in a darkened room, fed an adequate liquid diet, through a nasogastric tube if necessary, and given fluids in abundance. Because incontinence is so common, the urinary bladder and the rectum should be watched carefully for retention or fecal impaction, and scrupulous attention should be paid to the protection of the skin. To quiet the patient, hydrotherapy, paraldehyde and the barbiturates are recommended;

however, if cerebral edema is present, morphine is never given, since this drug tends to depress the respiratory center further.

Rabies

Rabies (hydrophobia) is an acute and almost invariably fatal disease communicated to man through the saliva of a rabid animal, usually dogs, foxes, squirrels and bats. Dogs, fortunately, always present evidence of the disease before becoming infective. The etiologic agent is an ultramicroscopic virus present in the saliva and the central nervous system. Negri bodies (round objects about one quarter the size of red blood corpuscles) are found in the brain tissues so constantly in this disease that their presence is sufficient for diagnosis.

The course of rabies in dogs is characterized by an incubation period of 20 to 30 days. This is followed by a period of excitement, when the animal becomes vicious. The excitement stage may not be evident at all (dumb rabies) or may be entirely absent. Paralysis then develops, first involving the hind legs and thereafter becoming general. Death occurs within 10 days following the first symptom.

Clinical Course in Man

In humans the incubation period varies from 2 weeks to 1 year, depending on the location of the wound and the extent of the bite. After infection from a wound, the average period of incubation is 40 days. This period is shorter following bites on the face.

The attack starts with a premonitory stage, during which the flesh around the point bitten becomes inflamed, and the patient is mentally depressed and irritable. Then follows the stage of excitement, during which even the slightest sensations produce violent spasms, particularly of the throat. The very sight of water induces such spasms of the muscles of the pharynx and larynx that the patient writhes (therefore, the name *hydrophobia*). Maniacal attacks occasionally occur but are rare. This stage lasts from 1 to 3 days and is followed by the paralytic stage, which lasts from 6 to 18 hours, terminating in coma and death. The disease is fatal and there is no treatment for it.

Diagnosis

If a dog is suspected of being rabid, the animal should not be killed, but instead should be captured and closely watched. If within 2 weeks no signs of disease have developed, rabies is ruled out. If the above-described symptoms develop, the animal is killed at once and the brain is examined for the characteristic Negri bodies. If the dog escapes observation (as is usually the case), should rabies be suspected in the slightest degree, the person bitten must be vaccinated.

Prophylaxis

The bite should be subjected to thorough lavage at once, and as soon as it can be procured, antirabic serum should be infused into, and injected under, the wound. Rabies vaccination (Pasteur treatment) should be started immediately, since, by virtue of the long incubation period in this disease, it may be possible to stimulate an active immunity in the patient before the virus takes effect.

Pasteur found that by inoculating one rabbit after another, each with an emulsion of the spinal cord of the former of the series, the virulence of the rabies virus so increased that its incubation period shortened from 15 or more to only 7 days. Preparations made from spinal cords of rabbits infected with this "7-day virus," attenuated by drying for various periods of time, are injected subcutaneously into the patient in ascending doses for 21 consecutive days. The result of Pasteur treatment, when properly applied, is occasionally satisfactory.

The Semple vaccine now is used most commonly. The virus, obtained as described above, is weakened with formalin. Its injection daily over a period of 2 weeks affords a measure of protection which hopefully lasts for several months. Another vaccine prepared in duck embryos is also available. Sensitivity to rabies vaccine can occur. It may cause encephalomyelitis and paralysis.

Nursing Care

If the disease does develop, the patient is placed in a quiet dark room, sedated heavily and given hypnotics, analgesics and antispasmodics without stint. Curare, administered under expert supervision, occasionally is beneficial. Nevertheless, a fatal outcome is the rule.

Nursing Precautions. It is to be borne in mind that the rabies virus is contained in the saliva of patients with this disease, constituting a distinct hazard to nurses and attendants who are responsible for their care. All personnel must be on guard against being bitten by such a patient or allowing saliva from the patient to contaminate a skin abrasion. If this occurs, personnel must receive the same treatment as the patient, including antirabic serum and rabies vaccine.

Psittacosis

Psittacosis is a specific acute virus disease of parrots and birds of the parrot family, highly contagious for exposed persons. The virus may be demonstrated in the droppings of sick birds. It withstands prolonged drying and enters man through the mucous mem-

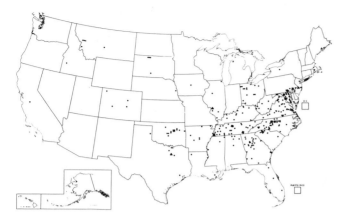

Fig. 37-4. Geographic distribution of Rocky Mountain Spotted Fever, United States, 1967. (U.S. Dept. H.E.W. Morbidity and Mortality. Vol. XVI. Summary, 1967)

branes of the upper respiratory tract. It is disseminated from infected persons by way of the excreta and the sputum. However, these patients cough very little, and transmission from man to man, therefore, is not a serious problem.

Symptoms and Course

The illness may appear as a transient influenza-like illness, as a severe pneumonia, or it may be asymptomatic. After an incubation period lasting 7 to 15 days (it may be as long as 6 weeks in man, 6 months in a parrot), the disease begins abruptly with malaise, headache, photophobia and chills. Its course is characterized by high fever, great weakness, marked depression and delirium, with surprisingly slow pulse and respiration. Typhoid-like rose spots may appear on the skin. The respiratory complications of bronchitis and bronchopneumonia characteristically are present. This pneumonia is central and, therefore, difficult to discover except by x-rays. In patients who recover, the temperature falls by lysis during the 2nd or the 3rd week. Convalescence is slow, and relapses are common.

The mortality of psittacosis is approximately 20 per cent, although it has been reported as high as 40 per cent. Among older individuals, death in the early stages is most apt to be due to heart failure; in the late stages, as a result of pneumonia.

Psittacosis responds to antibiotic therapy with the tetracyclines, the administration of which ordinarily is followed by a rapid and uneventful convalescence. Active immunity is acquired as a result of the infection; artificial immunization, therefore, theoretically is possible, but its value has not as yet been demonstrated.

Respiratory Infections

See Unit VII, *Patients With Conditions of the Respiratory Tract,* for further discussion of virus infections of the respiratory tract.

PATIENTS WITH RICKETTSIAL INFECTIONS

Rickettsiae

The rickettsial diseases, of which the 3 most common on this continent are typhus fever, Rocky Mountain spotted fever, and trench fever, are named after Dr. H. T. Ricketts in honor of his pioneering work in this field. They are vermin-spread infections caused by tiny organisms found in the patient's tissues and in the bodies of their insect vectors, the latter, for the most part, being ticks, fleas, and lice. As in the case of viruses, these organisms make their habitat, thrive and produce their effect within the tissue cells, as contrasted with the bacteria whose activities are extracellular. Like viruses, the rickettsiae cannot live apart from animal cells, and their culture, to date, has proved impossible in artificial media other than that containing live tissue. It is obvious from this fact that the survival of these organisms in nature depends on the accessibility of suitable living hosts, called *reservoirs.* Serving as reservoirs of rickettsiae are rodents, monkeys, dogs, dog ticks and wood ticks. Individuals harboring rickettsiae are likely to exhibit fever and skin eruptions and to be afflicted with disorders of the central nervous system.

Typical of all rickettsial infections is the appearance in the blood serum of a bacterial agglutinin that has the property of agglutinating bacilli of the Proteus OX group. (The reason for this is obscure, for there is no other relationship known between Proteus OX and the rickettsiae.) The phenomenon is the basis for a diagnostic test known as the Weil-Felix test, useful in differentiating this group of diseases, as a whole, from other infectious diseases. Serologic tests using antigens derived from the rickettsiae themselves provide more specific and reliable diagnostic tools. Further differentiation of one rickettsial disease from another is made possible by the use of tissue cultures and protection tests (inoculating suspected material into susceptible animals previously vaccinated with rickettsiae of known identity).

Rocky Mountain Spotted Fever

Rocky Mountain spotted fever typically is characterized by a continuous fever of 3-weeks' duration. It begins abruptly with a chill, severe pains in the bones and muscles, headache and a profuse skin eruption, at first macular and later petechial. In severe

TABLE 37-1. Ricksettsial diseases of man

Group	Principal diseases	Synonyms	Etiologic agent	Reservoir	Usual mode of transmission to man	Known occurrence
Typhus	Epidemic typhus	Classic, historic, European, louse-borne typhus[1]	Rickettsia prowazeki	Man	Human Body louse[2]	Winter and spring in cold climates over most of world
	Brill-Zinsser disease	Brill's disease, recrudescent typhus	Rickettsia prowazeki	Man	Human Body louse[2]	Can be world-wide
	Murine typhus	Endemic typhus, flea-borne typhus	Rickettsia mooseri[3]	Rats	Rat flea[4]	World-wide
Spotted fever	Rocky Mountain spotted fever	Spotted fever, tick fever, tick typhus, etc.	Rickettsia rickettsi	Rabbits and other mammals (possibly dogs) and ticks	Ticks[5]	North and South America
	North-Asian tick-borne rickettsiosis	Siberian tick typhus	Rickettsia siberica	Wild rodents and ticks	Ticks[6]	Asiatic USSR and Mongolia
	African tick typhus	Boutonneuse fever; S. African, Kenya and Indian tick typhus	Rickettsia conori	Dogs, wild rodents and ticks	Ticks[7]	Africa, India and the basins of the Black Sea, Caspian Sea and Mediterranean
	Queensland tick typhus		Rickettsia australis	Marsupials, wild rodents, (? ticks)		Queensland, Australia
	Rickettsialpox	Kew Gardens fever	Rickettsia akari	Mice	Mites[8]	USA, USSR and Korea
Tsutsugamushi disease	Scrub typhus	Mite-borne typhus, Japanese river fever, tropical typhus, Sumatran mite fever, etc.	Rickettsia tsutsugamushi (orientalis)	Rats, other rodents and mites	Mites[9]	South Asia and Western Pacific
Q fever	Q fever	Nine mile fever, Balkan grippe	Coxiella burnetii[10]	Cattle, sheep, goats, marsupials, other mammals and ticks	Principally air-borne; occasionally ticks; possibly milk	World-wide
Trench fever	Trench fever	Wolhynian or five-day fever	Rickettsia quintana	Man	Human body louse[2]	Europe, USSR and Mexico

[1] Jail fever, war fever, camp fever, Fleckfieber (German), typhus exanthematique (French), tifus exantemático (Spanish), dermotypho (Italian).
[2] Pediculus humanus corporis.
[3] Bergey's Manual classification: Rickettsia typhi.
[4] Xenopsylla cheopis.
[5] Dermacentor andersoni; D. variabilis; Amblyomma americanum.
[6] Dermacentor nuttali; D. silvarum; D. marginatus; D. pictus.
[7] Rhipicephalus sanguineus; Amblyomma hebraeum; Haemaphysalis leachi.
[8] Allodermanyssus sanguineus.
[9] Trombicula akamushi; T. deliensis.
[10] Rickettsia diaporica was the name first used for the American variety of Q fever.

(From J. C. Snyder, in Beeson, P. B., and McDermott, W. (eds.): Cecil-Loeb Textbook of Medicine, ed. 12. Philadelphia, W. B. Saunders, 1967)

cases there appear also areas of skin necrosis due to an endarteritis (inflammatory blockage of the arterioles). The disease is prevalent in Montana, Idaho and along the Atlantic seaboard from New York to Georgia (Fig. 37-4).

The organism responsible for Rocky Mountain spotted fever is *Rickettsia rickettsii*. The infection has its reservoirs in rabbits, small wild rodents and in dogs, and its principal or sole vector is the wood tick. Individuals of all ages have been affected. The majority of patients have resided in rural areas and have engaged in removing ticks from dogs.

Clinical Symptoms and Course

The incubation period of this disorder lasts from 2 to 12 days. The skin rash, consisting of rose-colored macules of variable sizes, usually appears on the 3rd day, first on the wrists, the ankles and the back, but it gradually spreads to cover the entire body and sometimes also the mucous membrane of the mouth and the pharynx. After a few days the macules become petechial. Large subcutaneous hemorrhages also may appear. Restlessness, insomnia and hyperesthesias are among the most distressing symptoms of this disease. Delirium is common at the height of the fever, but convulsions rarely occur. The spleen is large and tender. There are a slight leukocytosis and a slight secondary anemia. Pneumonia, not frequent, is the only serious complication reported, but mental confusion, deafness and visual disturbances are common and may last for weeks.

Fatal cases terminate in coma which usually begins between the 6th and the 12th days. In patients who recover, the temperature at the end of the 2nd week falls by lysis and reaches normal by the end of the 3rd week. The rash subsides with the fever, leaving the skin pigmented and somewhat scarred. During the 3rd week necrosis may involve ear lobes, fingers, toes and scrotum, areas at the extreme periphery of the vascular system. The Weil-Felix test and specific complement fixation test become positive.

The prognosis of Rocky Mountain spotted fever differs much in different localities. When specific antibiotics are given the mortality rate is greatly reduced.

Chemotherapy and Nursing Care

Chloramphenicol and tetracyclines have rickettsiostatic properties, and are effective in this disease if administered at an early stage in its course, i.e., concident with the first appearance of the rash. Sedative drugs are indicated for relief of pain, restlessness and exhausting insomnia.

The patient's strength should be maintained early in the disease by a high-protein diet. Liquids should be provided in abundance. Supportive nursing measures are used as needed.

Prevention

Those who are apt to be in an area where ticks abound should be immunized against Rocky Mountain spotted fever. Annual revaccination has been advised. Persons living in tick-infested areas should examine themselves on a twice daily schedule for ticks. Tick repellent should be applied to the clothes. Ticks may be removed from the body by grasping the tick with a pair of forceps and pulling it gently and firmly.

PATIENTS WITH PROTOZOAN INFECTIONS

Protozoa

Protozoa are single-celled animals which, despite their unicellular structure, possess protoplasmic devices adapted for several different functions. They are considerably more complicated structurally than are the bacteria. Most of them possess, to varying degrees, the ability to move about under their own power and are equipped with differential tissue structures that enable them to feed, breathe, eject excreta and attach themselves to other objects.

Varieties of protozoa include the *Sporozoa*, which are without organs of feeding or locomotion; the *Sarcodina*, which move about by means of pseudopodia (temporary projections of their bodies) and the *Mastigophora*, which are protozoa possessing flagella (whiplike appendages) for purposes of locomotion. The Sporozoa of greatest importance to man is the *Plasmodium*, the genus causing malaria. Of the Sarcodina, the most hazardous for humans is of the genus *Endamoeba*, responsible for amebic dysentery. In this country, the most common Mastigophora infestations producing symptoms is that of *Trichomonas vaginalis*, but in Africa and the Orient are to be found diseases of much more serious consequence caused by protozoa of this group, for example, kala-azar, caused by the *Leishmania*, and African sleeping sickness, a *Trypanosoma* infection. The clinical aspects of certain of the more serious protozoan infections are considered in this chapter.

Malaria

Malaria remains one of the most common diseases of the world except for the United States, where it is usually seen in military personnel returning from other countries.

Malaria is an acute, infectious disease caused by protozoa which strongly resemble leukocytes (except that they are much smaller and multiply differently). Their transmission is by way of an intermediate host, the mosquito. There are 4 species of malarial parasites, grouped under the generic name *Plasmodium*, each causing a different type of malaria.

Each malarial parasite lives within a red blood corpuscle, utilizing the hemoglobin as food. When full grown, it divides (segments) into 10 to 20 small, young parasites, called *hyalines* (or segments), which burst the cell; this bursting of cells causes chills in the patient. Free in the plasma, the majority of these hyalines die, but a few find their way into new red cells, and the process described above is repeated.

The tertian parasite (*P. vivax*) is so named because its life cycle requires just 48 hours, hence the chills occur on alternate days (but if two broods of this parasite are present, the patient has a chill each day).

The quartan (*P. malariae*) is so named because its cycle takes just 72 hours: hence, if one brood is present there is a chill each fourth day; if three, one each day. In cases of tertian and quartan malaria the hundreds of millions of parasites of each group are all of the same age, hence their segments are free in the blood at approximately the same time. It is just then that the chill with sharp temperature rise occurs, and it is at that time also that quinine, if present in the blood, will destroy them.

The estivo-autumnal parasite (*P. falciparum*), so named because the malaria that it causes is worse in the summer and the fall, has a cycle which varies between 24 and 72 hours in duration. This is the most virulent of the malarial parasites and is responsible for the most serious form of malaria. The reason for this is that after the first few days parasites of all ages are present in the blood at the same time. Therefore, some of them are segmenting continually (this taking place in the spleen and the bone marrow, not in the peripheral blood as is the case in the other two types). At first there may be a few chills, but as the case goes on they become less and less acute (dumb chills), until the fever is continuous.

We have spoken thus far only of the parasites of each group which cause fever in man. These are the asexual forms. Some hyalines of each group, however, do not segment. These, the sexual forms, remain in the body unchanged, perhaps for months, doing the patient no harm. However, if any are in the blood which a mosquito sucks from the patient, these mature in the body of the insect, producing myriads of young forms, some of which that mosquito will inject into the blood of its next victim, where as asexual forms they will multiply until, in about 2 weeks, they are numerous enough to produce the symptoms of the type of malaria that they cause.

Only one variety of mosquito, the *Anopheles,* can act as the intermediate host of malarial parasite. This mosquito, resting on a wall, can be recognized at a distance, because instead of standing hunchbacked, as does the ordinary mosquito (*Culex*), it stands with body, thorax and bill in a straight line, forming with the wall an angle of about 30°.

Clinical Symptoms and Course

Patients with tertian and quartan malaria feel well on days when they have no chill. The chill, which lasts about 10 minutes, begins suddenly, often with intense headache, nausea and vomiting. During the next 30 minutes to 4 hours the temperature rises rapidly, as high as 41.7° C.,* and the patient becomes intensely hot and flushed. Then, suddenly, with a profuse sweat, the temperature falls rapidly to normal, and in a few minutes the patient feels well. The entire paroxysm lasts from 10 to 14 hours.

Patients with severe malaria of any form may become comatose and die (pernicious malaria); they may develop renal failure (due to the precipitation of free hemoglobin in the kidney tubule); a serious gastrointestinal disturbance or cerebral symptoms (due to an accumulation of the parasites in the blood vessels of the affected organ).

To escape malaria, one must avoid *Anopheles* mosquitoes that have fed on the blood of patients with malaria about 3 weeks previously. This insect usually bites only after sundown, and never a person in motion. Houses should be well screened, especially the room of a patient ill with malaria, lest *Anopheles* mosquitoes become infected from him. Pools of stagnant water (in which mosquitoes breed) should be eliminated. If this is impossible, these accumulations of water should be treated with oil or a preparation of the insecticide DDT.

Diagnosis

The diagnosis of malaria is established by the finding of the plasmodium in the patient's blood. *The most favorable time for the discovery of the parasite is during and to 12 to 18 hours after a chill.*

Chemotherapy

Therapy should be started promptly after the diagnosis is made. The treatment currently recommended for *P. vivax* malaria is chloroquine plus primaquine. A loading dose of 1.0 gm. of chloroquine diphosphate is given by mouth, followed in 6 hours by 0.5 gm., then 0.5 gm. on each of 2 succeeding days. If nausea and vomiting are severe, chloroquine may be given by intramuscular injection, in doses of 0.2 gm. (of the base), the full course then being completed by the oral route.

Primaquine is given in a dose of 10 to 15 mg. (base) daily for 14 days, starting immediately or as soon as the acute phase is controlled by chloroquine.

P. falciparum malaria should be treated with chloroquine alone, 2.5 gm. of the phosphate (or 1.5 gm. of the base) being given in the course of 3 days as outlined above. Cases of chloroquine-resistant *P. falci-*

* 107° F.

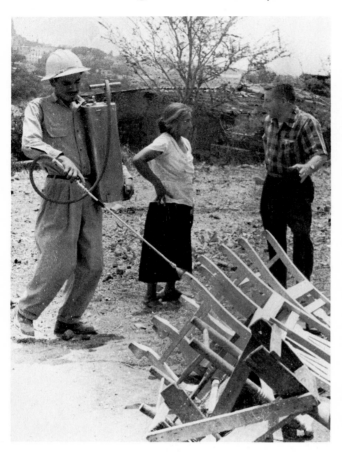

Fig. 37-5. Gentle persuasion is a mighty weapon in malaria campaigns. Here a WHO adviser is explaining to a housewife that spraying is necessary, even if no one of her family is suffering from the disease at the time. (World Health Organization)

Prognosis

The recurrence rate in malaria undoubtedly is destined to be modified to a considerable extent by modern chemotherapy. By using quinine or quinacrine alone, relapses in cases of vivax malaria were regularly anticipated for 3 or 4 years following the initial attack, and in quartan malaria, repeated attacks over a course of 15 to 20 years. Falciparum malaria, on the other hand, rarely relapses after 6 to 9 months. The chief complications attending chronic malaria are anemia, enlargement of the spleen and cachexia. Treatment is carried out as outlined above and is supplemented with iron therapy, blood transfusions and dietary measures as indicated.

Prevention

The essence of malaria control is the eradication of malaria as an endemic disease, which is accomplished if the number of cases in a given area can be reduced and maintained below a certain critical figure for a period of 8 to 10 years. In several areas of the world this goal has been achieved.

Effective control of this disease has relied on two principal measures, employed in combination: (1) the practice of "residual spraying" of dwellings in infested areas with such toxicants as DDT, which has been carried out in systematic, coordinated fashion and on a wide scale for a definitive period of time (e.g., 4 years) so that all, or nearly all, *Anopheles* mosquitoes infected with malarial parasites have been destroyed; and (2) the institution of a "system of surveillance," which has undertaken to investigate every suspected case of malaria occurring in that area following discontinuance of spraying, from the standpoint of its origin, epidemiology and vector, and to initiate and direct whatever corrective measures might be indicated in each case. This program and its rigid timetable are designed to circumvent one important problem which imposes a serious limitation on the use of insecticides, namely, the development of resistance to these agents on the part of insects generally. However, it has been found that eradication of malaria can be accomplished within a period of from 8 to 10 years, including 4 to 6 years of nation-wide spraying, without inducing insect resistance.

The World Health Organization initiated a worldwide eradication of malaria in 1955. This included destruction of not only the malaria-carrying mosquito but also curing all those who are ill with malaria. If two links of the chain exist (a human and a mosquito), and one is infected, the disease may start again and soon reach epidemic proportions. In 1967 an "international achievement unparalleled in the his-

parum are becoming more frequent, especially in Vietnam. Quinine is used in the treatment of such cases, combined with other agents.

Paludrine effectively terminates acute vivax or quartan malaria. Although curing the latter, it is no better than chloroquine as regards a permanent cure of vivax infection. Customarily it is given in a total dosage of 50 to 150 mg., doses as small as 12.5 mg. being effective in some instances. It is highly effective as a prophylactic against falciparum malaria, 0.1 gm. daily completely preventing the infection of individuals who are heavily exposed under natural conditions; it is equally valuable in suppressing vivax infections, only, however, as long as its administration is continued. Due to an almost complete lack of toxicity, Paludrine, chloroquine, Atabrine and quinine are all useful as prophylactic agents.

tory of public health" was announced: 1,304 million people now live where malaria has been eliminated or eradication is under way. However, 362 million people still live in uncontrolled malarious regions. Major problems at this time are the developing resistance of mosquitos to certain insecticides, isolated patients who are unknown reservoirs of disease, and lack of sufficient medical programs in some countries necessary to carry out the unrelenting struggle.

Amebiasis

Amebae are protozoa, larger than leukocytes, which move by ameboid action (they project part of their body at one point as a pseudopod and flow into this). Only a few amebae infect man; the most important of these is *Endamoeba histolytica,* the cause of amebic dysentery. This organism, as seen under the microscope, moves actively, has a small round nucleus and a protoplasm full of leukocytes, red blood cells and bacteria ingested by the parasite. These amebae survive outside the body in resistant encysted forms. From the number of the nuclei of these cysts one may determine the type of ameba.

About 10 per cent of the population harbor *E. histolytica* in their gastrointestinal tracts.

Amebic Dysentery

Amebic dysentery is a disease of the tropics, especially Egypt, India and the Far East, but is common also in our Northern states. It occurs in epidemics spread by water and also by food handled by amebae carriers—persons who may or may not have had amebic dystentery but who harbor this protozoan in their intestinal wall.

The amebae burrow their way into the mucous membranes of the colon and the lower ileum, and in the submucous tissue form pus pockets with only a small orifice opening into the bowel, from which numerous burrows extend for considerable distances in all directions under the mucous membrane. Here the amebae live, probably for years. Later, the protecting mucous membrane roof of this burrowing abscess sloughs, exposing an underlying ulcer. The large bowel may be so covered by such ulcers that very little normal mucous membrane is left. Usually the floor of these ulcers is the muscle wall of the bowel, but they may perforate its entire wall and cause fatal peritonitis.

Clinical Symptoms and Course

The chief symptoms of a case of acute amebic dysentery are slight fever, weight loss and the passage of frequent small stools containing considerable amounts of blood and mucus, the latter swarming with amebae. The two important features of this disease are its chronicity, one attack of acute dysentery following another, separated by periods of constipation which last for months, and the tendency of the infection to cause liver abscesses through its metastases to that organ by way of the portal vein.

Treatment

Drugs especially valuable in the treatment of amebiasis are emetine, chloroquine, diiodohydroxyquin, carbarsone, and humantin.

Amebic Liver Abscess

Amebic liver abscesses differ from those caused by bacteria in that they are more often single than multiple, always are large, have little evidence of real inflammation in their walls and give surprisingly few symptoms. They are merely large holes in the liver, full of necrotic and liquified liver tissue, the walls of which contain hosts of amebae. Such abscesses may heal by perforating and draining through the lung, but the outcome in this event is exceedingly precarious.

Treatment

Chloroquine has been quite effective in causing abscesses to subside. Terramycin also has amebicidal properties. Surgical drainage may have to be resorted to if drug therapy fails. One point to be emphasized is that not infrequently these abscesses are found unexpectedly in patients who have, or have had, few or no symptoms suggesting dysentery.

The treatment is that outlined for amebic dysentery except that emetine is by far the most effective agent for the treatment of liver abscesses.

During the active phase, the patient is supported with fluid, electrolyte and blood replacement. Analgesics with opiates to relieve abdominal pain and tenesmus are given. Monthly follow-up studies of the stools are necessary, because relapses are common.

PATIENTS WITH SYSTEMIC MYCOSES

Introduction

Fungi usually occur in two forms depending on conditions of growth—the unicellular yeast forms and the mycelial or branching forms containing spores. The systemic mycoses (fungal diseases) have become somewhat more frequent in occurrence in recent years with the increased availability and use of potent antibiotics and antimetabolite therapy and chemotherapy of cancer. Many patients who are debilitated, severely ill and whose defenses are reduced become prey to invasion by fungi which they could ordinarily withstand. However, certain drugs have been developed, notably amphoteracin B, which have antifungal properties and lead to favorable therapeutic attacks on mycotic diseases.

The fungi present difficult problems in control because they are so widespread in nature—in soil, decaying vegetation and bird excreta. Infection usually occurs by inhalation, occasionally by traumatic implantation or by the pathologic takeover of a normal inhabitant when resistance of the host is lowered. Transmission is not by person-to-person contact. Lesions are generally granulomatous and antibodies are formed in reaction to them.

Actinomycosis

Actinomycosis is a chronic granulomatous disease caused by fungi of the Actinomyces (ray-fungus) group. The characteristic lesions are local masses of fibrous tissue that suppurate, giving rise to multiple abscesses which discharge through manifold sinuses an exudate containing the characteristic sulfur granules, representing visible masses of the organism. This disease, if untreated, advances indolently but relentlessly for years, destroying all the tissues in its way, frequently, however, disturbing the patient's general health but little.

It is a disease of young adult males in particular and is widely distributed over the United States. The source of this fungus is not known; the mouth probably is its portal of entry, since pathogenic actinomyces often are found in carious teeth and tonsillar crypts of otherwise normal persons. Chewing idly on a piece of straw has allowed entry in some cases.

Clinical Symptoms and Course

Actinomycosis of the head and the neck, the most common locations, starts as a swelling about certain teeth. This, by extension, involves the submaxillary region and the neck, producing a flat, hard, painless tumor mass, with smooth regular surface and uniform dense consistency, which is fixed firmly to the jawbone. From this mass a brawny nodular induration extends into the neck, covered by skin that is wrinkled and dusky red in color. Later this granuloma, breaking down, becomes riddled with abscesses which perforate externally. By extension, this process may involve the cheek, the skull and the brain.

In the abdominal type, any viscera may be affected, including the pelvic organs, especially the ovaries and the tubes, but most commonly the appendix and the cecum. Here in time an uneven tumor mass develops. This resembles carcinoma, and by extension may involve the abdominal wall, discharging externally through open sinuses.

In the pulmonary form, induced by inhaled actinomyces spores, a condition develops usually unilaterally. This simulates tuberculosis with cavity formation, except that usually it involves a lower lobe.

Treatment

Actinomycotic lesions respond to penicillin, which is the drug of choice. Large doses, e.g., 4 to 8 million units, should be given daily, without interruption for 4 to 6 weeks. Tetracyclines, streptomycin and chloramphenicol (Chloromycetin) all have been used with some success and should be tried in the event that penicillin fails to achieve a cure. Surgical drainage and excision of localized lesions occasionally are obligatory.

Histoplasmosis

Histoplasmosis is a chronic systemic fungus infection caused by a spore-bearing mold called *Histoplasma capsulatum*. This disease has been encountered throughout the globe but is especially prevalent in the Eastern Central United States. In its commonest form it presents as a mild, self-limited respiratory illness without distinctive features, manifested solely by low grade fever and cough. In a few instances, however, granulomatous lesions of the proliferative or ulcerative type become disseminated throughout the body, giving rise to all the constitutional symptoms and signs of a severe systemic infection. Such patients face the prospect of a protracted, unpleasant illness, possibly with a fatal outcome.

Histoplasmosis is predominantly a disease of young infants and older adults, especially males over the age of 40 years. The infective fungus is harbored in birds and presumably in animal hosts which as yet are unidentified. One method by which humans acquire the infection is by the inhalation of spore-bearing dust.

Clinical Picture

Some of the clinical features of histoplasmosis resemble closely those of pulmonary tuberculosis, including symptoms of fever, night sweats, anorexia, debility, cough which is productive of purulent sputum, and occasionally hemoptysis. The appearance of parenchymal infiltrates, cavities and calcifications on x-ray examination of the lungs often has led to an erroneous diagnosis of tuberculosis. Other patients present findings that are reminiscent of malignant lymphoma, including anemia, thrombocytopenia, splenomegaly, hepatomegaly and x-ray signs of mediastinal enlargement. Nodules may appear in the skin, and osteolytic bone lesions may be demonstrated by x-ray examination. One group of patients seems prone to develop ulcerations at mucocutaneous junctions, for example, at the lip margins and in the perianal region. Gastrointestinal ulcers may be responsible for massive bleeding, and the syndrome of Addison's disease (see p. 706) may appear as the result of destruction of the adrenal glands by histoplasmosis.

Laboratory Findings

The diagnosis of histoplasmosis is established by culturing *Histoplasma capsulatum* from the sputum or elsewhere, or by identifying this organism morphologically in smears of blood or bone marrow, or in histologic sections of infected tissue obtained by surgical biopsy. Complement fixation tests and histoplasmin skin tests, while not conclusive, are diagnostically helpful. The characteristic radiologic appearance of the lungs, in conjunction with a negative tuberculin skin test, strongly suggest this diagnosis.

Treatment

At present the treatment of choice for histoplasmosis is chemotherapy. Surgical resection of the infected lesions may be required in some instances. The chemotherapeutic agent currently preferred is amphotericin B, administered intravenously.

Amphotericin B has proved to be effective in the treatment of most of the deep mycoses, including histoplasmosis, North American blastomycosis, sporotrichosis, cryptococcosis and aspergillosis. The optimal dose of amphotericin B is 1.0 to 1.5 mg. per Kg. of body weight per day. However, because of the frequency with which severe toxic reactions, including nausea, vomiting, chills and fever, follow the institution of therapy with doses in this range, treatment routinely is started at a much lower level. On day one, for example, 1.0 mg. of the drug dissolved in 250 ml. of 5 per cent dextrose solution is injected intravenously over a 6-hour period; on day 2, the patient receives 5 mg. of amphotericin B in 500 ml., and on day 3, 10 mg. of the drug in 1,000 ml. of dextrose solution. Thereafter, the dose is increased by increments of 5 or 10 mg. each day until the desired level is attained, namely, 1.0 to 1.5 mg. per Kg. injected intravenously in concentrations no greater than 1 mg. per 10 ml. dextrose solution. Should toxic reactions ensue nevertheless, they may be ameliorated (or they may be hopefully prevented) by the administration of a salicylate (e.g., aspirin, 0.6 gm.) and one of the antihistaminic antiemetic drugs (e.g., promethazine hydrochloride, 25 mg.) by mouth 30 minutes prior to each infusion of amphotericin B.

Except in severe disseminated disease, the recovery rate from histoplasmosis is high.

PATIENTS WITH HELMINTHIC INFESTATIONS

Filariasis

Filariasis is due to bodily infestation by the adults and the embryos belonging to roundworms of the filaria group. The most important of these worms is *Wuchereria bancrofti*, a parasite very common in Africa and India. In some regions of India cases of filariasis are as numerous as those of malaria. An occasional case is found in our southern states.

Clinical Course

Its embryos, injected into the skin by the bite of a *Culex* mosquito that previously has bitten a patient with filariasis, locate and reach maturity in the lymph channels and nodes which drain the part bitten (therefore, most often those of the pelvis and the groin). Here the adults, several inches long, block the lymph flow, causing elephantiasis (that is, the legs become huge from a great thickening of the skin), chyluria or hematochyluria (if the lymphatics in the bladder are obstructed) and hydrocele.

The adult worms produce vast numbers of embryos (.033 of a centimeter long) which remain in the bloodstream. These seem to do no harm. The embryos of this parasite appear in the peripheral blood at night, during the day remaining in the capillaries of the lungs and other organs. In the case of night laborers, however, the embryos appear only during the day.

In addition to the above-mentioned local symptoms due to lymphostasis, the patient also suffers certain general symptoms, such as irregular fever, headache, generalized malaise, sweating and pruritus.

Treatment

Diethylcarbamazine (Hetrazan) given orally (2 mg. per Kg. of body weight 3 times daily) for 7 to 14 days kills the microfilariae and kills or sterilizes adult worms. Arsenic and antimony compounds have been used against the adult worms. Antibiotics reduce the secondary infection that may occur. Surgical procedures have been used to remove elephantoid tissue.

Other Types

Other types of filarial worms include *Onchocerca volvulus*, the adults of which locate in colonies in the subcutaneous tissue, giving rise to multiple spongy skin nodules, while the embryos are found in the nearby lymph spaces. They are prevalent in certain parts of Africa and Central America. The adults of *Mansonella ozzardi*, a filarial parasite of the West Indies and South America, locate in the mesenteric lymph vessels, while their embryos appear in the bloodstream. And, finally, the adults of the *Loa loa* (the eye worm) of Africa, travel actively in the subcutaneous and the subconjunctival tissues (whence they are easily removed by operation), while their embryos appear in the bloodstream.

Trichinosis

Trichinosis is infestation by the parasite *Trichinella spiralis*, one of the roundworms.

Clinical Course

This is a disease of pigs, in the muscle fibers of which these tiny embryos lie encysted. These calcified cysts, barely visible to the naked eye, appear in the meat like tiny grains of sand. If such pork is eaten insufficiently cooked, the embryos are set free by the gastric juice and develop in the intestine during the following week to adult worms from 3 to 4 mm. long. These worms make their way into the mucous membrane and there produce myriad embryos. The symptoms of the period of invasion, which last about 1 week, are diarrhea, a fever suggesting typhoid, nausea, vomiting and occasionally abdominal pain.

The embryos, carried by the bloodstream and by their own activity, migrate to all parts of the body. The symptoms during the period of migration, which last about 10 days, are pain and soreness in the muscles, edema of the eyelids, scleral hemorrhages, occasionally cardiac irregularities (due to trichinae in the heart muscle, which may be fatal), redness and swelling of the tongue and a marked eosinophilia (even 50 per cent of a total leukocyte count of 30,000) which continues for months. Very severe cases develop anemia, cachexia, furunculosis and pneumonia. The embryos gradually become encysted, each in a muscle fiber, after which there are no symptoms.

Diagnosis

This is confirmed by the discovery of the embryos themselves in a biopsy specimen of muscle usually removed from the calf of the leg. A skin test using an extract of trichinae as the test antigen becomes positive after 16 to 20 days and may be positive for years afterward. A precipitin test also may yield information useful in diagnosis.

Treatment

Symptomatic treatment, rest, salicylates for pain, adequate fluids and nutrition are important. Steroids, because of their anti-inflammatory properties, give good symptomatic relief but have no effect on the worms or larvae. Thiobendazole, a new antihelminthic drug, has given dramatic relief in a limited number of cases in doses of 25 mg. per Kg. of body weight twice daily for 5 to 7 days. Its side-effects are nausea, vomiting and dizziness.

Mild and moderate infections have a good prognosis. Prognosis has been poor in severe infections, but thiobendazole may prove to change this outlook.

Prevention

The incidence of trichinosis has been estimated between 15 to 20 per cent in the United States. Of these, less than 5 per cent experience symptoms.

A nationwide program for the control and eventual eradication of trichinosis embodies the following proposals:

1. Establishment of state laws forbidding the feeding of hogs with garbage and offal other than that cooked at licensed establishments.
2. Enforcement of interstate quarantine regulations forbidding the shipping across state lines of uncooked garbage that might be used as swine fodder.
3. The forbidding of movement of swine out of any state that does not have or enforce garbage cooking laws.
4. Education of farmers to remove all uncooked pork scraps and offal from the feed given to his own swine.
5. Public education relative to incineration and alternate methods of garbage disposal.
6. Prohibition by state law of the sale of garbage-fed hogs to slaughterhouses that do not operate under Federal inspection or its equivalent.
7. *Public education regarding the importance of cooking thoroughly all pork and pork products.*
8. Support for continued research on methods of destroying *Trichinella* in pork.
9. Improvement of diagnostic procedures for the identification of trichinosis in hogs and man.

Hookworm Disease

Hookworm disease (ancylostomiasis and uncinariasis) is the result of infestation of the upper part of the small intestine by one of two quite similar roundworms about half an inch long: *Uncinaria americana* (the New World hookworm) and *Ancylostoma duodenale* (the Old World form).

Incidence

Hookworm disease is common in rural regions of the tropics, notably of Africa, but also of Europe and of some of our southern states.

Clinical Course

The embryos of this worm, hatched from eggs passed in the stools, live in dirt, sand and clay and easily infest man. They enter by mouth if he eats with dirty hands, or by boring through the skin of bare feet (ground itch). Having gained access to the blood or lymph vessels, they are carried by the bloodstream to the lungs, migrate from the pulmonary capillaries into the air cells, reach the pharynx, are swallowed and mature to adult forms in the bowel. The food of these worms is the patient's blood. To obtain this they wound the mucous membrane at many points and leave bleeding all the wounds they make. The result of these multiple hemorrhages is a severe hypochromic anemia characteristic of chronic blood loss.

The patient, if a child, develops to maturity slowly. He is anemic; his skin has a muddy, pale hue; his eyes are dull and heavy (fish eyes). Later, the skin is edematous, and the patient is weak and short of breath.

The diagnosis of hookworm disease is made easily, because if enough worms are present to cause any symptoms their eggs will be abundant in the stools.

Chemotherapy

Eighty per cent of patients are cured of hookworm disease by a single dose of tetrachlorethylene, the amount given being computed on the basis of 0.12 ml. per Kg. of body weight and not in excess of 5 ml. total at one time. As for the minority of patients whose infestation is not eradicated completely by one dose of the drug, the number of worms that they retain is rarely significant, and this residue can be eliminated completely by repetition of the treatment every 4 or 5 days until the stools are free of eggs. Hexylresorcinol is also useful.

The prevention of hookworm disease depends on sanitary disposal of human excreta and the wearing of shoes.

Roundworm

Ascaris lumbricoides, a roundworm from 4 to 12 inches long, is a common intestinal parasite of children and, as a rule, does no harm. If present in large numbers, however, masses of them may cause intestinal obstruction. This worm may wander up into the stomach, whence it is vomited, or up the esophagus to the pharynx, from which point it may reach the trachea and the bronchi and cause fatal pneumonia. It has been known to enter the nose, or force its way up the eustachian tube, and, having ruptured the drum, appear in the external ear. Also it may enter the common bile duct, causing obstructive jaundice, and occasionally it thrusts its head through a gastric or typhoid ulcer, causing peritonitis.

The diagnosis is made by finding ova in the stools or by the patient passing or occasionally vomiting a worm.

Chemotherapy

Of the many drugs that are available for the treatment of ascaris infection, one of the most effective is piperazine. This drug may be given by mouth or tube, in cases of intestinal obstruction, without preliminary purgation or preparation of any kind, and may be used safely in infants and children as well as adult patients. The recommended dose is 75 mg. per Kg. of body weight per day, not to exceed 3 gm. a day, for each of 2 successive days, the daily dose being divided into 2 or 3 portions. Almost 100 per cent of patients are cured by this treatment. Hexylrescorcinol is also useful.

Prevention depends on the sanitary disposal of human excreta and thorough washing and cooking of vegetables grown with the use of night soil as a fertilizer.

Pinworm

Enterobiasis (oxyuriasis) is the commonest helminthic infection in the United States. The pinworm (*Enterobius vermacularis*) is a small white threadlike worm, about half a centimeter long, commonly found in the rectum of children. The chief symptom it causes is intense itching, especially at night, when the female crawls out of the skin, depositing eggs about the anus. The fingernails should be examined for eggs, and nail-biting children should be encouraged to wear gloves until the infection has been controlled, because this is the common mode of reinfection.

Worms may be seen on freshly passed stool or about the anus. Confirmation of diagnosis can be obtained by preparing the anal impressions on cellophane tape. The percentage of anal impressions that prove to be positive, out of a series made on 7 to 10 successive days, provides a rough index as to the severity of infestation and the likelihood of its recurrence after treatment.

Treatment

Most patients with enterobiasis are relieved completely and conveniently of their infestation by a single oral dose of pyrvinium pamoate suspension (Povan Suspension), ingested by the fasting patient in a dose equivalent to 5 mg. of pyrvinium base per Kg. of body weight (or one 5-ml. teaspoonful of the suspension per 22 lbs.). Patients (or their parents) should be alerted to the fact that their stools will acquire a bright red color following medication, a phenomenon to which no ominous significance is attached. The whole household should be treated.

Tapeworm

Tapeworms are long, flat, segmented worms, with a head, a neck and a chain of thin broad segments, or links. These worms live in the intestines.

Beef Tapeworm

Taenia saginata, the beef tapeworm, the one most common in America, is acquired by eating insufficiently cooked "measled" beef (that is, beef containing this worm in its larval form). In the bowel of man this worm grows to a length of 4.5 to 6 m. (15 to 20 feet). The head, about the size of a common black-headed pin, is provided with suckers only, and the largest links are about a half centimeter broad and one centimeter or more long (quarter inch broad to a half inch or more long). Broken-off chains of links, full of eggs, often are passed in the stools.

Pork Tapeworm

Taenia solium, the pork tapeworm, rare in America, is acquired by eating insufficiently cooked infested pork. It is smaller than the beef tapeworm, being only from 1.8-3.6 m. long, and has somewhat smaller links. Its head, also smaller, is provided with suckers and hooks. This worm is much more difficult than the beef worm to expel.

Cysticercus Disease

If a person swallows an egg instead of the larval form of the pork tapeworm, an embryo will be hatched in the bowel. This penetrates the intestinal mucous membrane and may be carried by the bloodstream to almost any organ of the body. Wherever it settles, it becomes encysted, and in this larval cyst, about a centimeter in diameter, only the head of the tapeworm develops.

The internal organs and the skin of an infested person may contain one or thousands of these cysts. Most of them do no harm; but should one locate in the brain or the eye, its symptoms would be those of any tumor of that size in that location.

No treatment except surgery will remove these cysts.

Fish Tapeworm

Diphyllobothrium latum, a tapeworm common in Europe and the Far East but comparatively rare in America, is acquired by eating uncooked, infested fish. It may grow to a length of 7.6 to 9.1 meters (25 to 30 feet).

Symptoms Caused by Tapeworm

The beef and pork tapeworms cause few if any symptoms, except those suggested by the patient's knowledge that he has the worm. The fish tapeworm, however, occasionally precipitates an anemia which scarcely can be distinguished from pernicious anemia.

Diagnosis. The diagnosis of all large tapeworms is easy, because their links appear in nearly every stool the patient passes, and when seen cannot be mistaken. Ova of the worms may be found on microscopic examination of the stool.

Chemotherapy

All forms of intestinal tapeworm infestation respond to quinacrine (Atabrine) chemotherapy. On the day prior to treatment, the patient's intake is restricted to clear soups, rice, cooked cereal and fruit juices; 60 ml. of saturated solution of magnesium sulfate is ingested during the evening. On the following morning, the patient, still fasting, ingests 3 0.1-gm. tablets of quinacrine as the initial dose. This dose is repeated one half hour later and again in 1 hour following the initial dose, a few ounces of orange juice being given with each dose of tablets. Magnesium sulfate solution (60 ml.) is given 1 or 2 hours following the third and final dose of quinacrine. The liquid stools which are likely to follow soon thereafter are collected in a glass jar to permit observation of the tapeworm, which usually is passed, intact, within a period of a few hours. Failure of the head to emerge with the rest of the worm does not imply, necessarily, that the treatment has failed. Under these circumstances, the patient is advised that, if success has not been achieved, segments again will be passed in the stools within a period of from 6 to 12 weeks, and at that time, but not sooner, retreatment can be carried out. The first treatment is successful in about 70 per cent of cases.

Hydatid Disease (Echinococcosis)

Hydatid disease, the most serious of all tapeworm infestations, is due to *Taenia echinococcus,* a parasite only about one-half centimeter long infesting dogs and sheep. Echinococcus disease is common among sheepherders in Australia, Iceland and the Mediterranean countries.

Clinical Course

If an egg of this worm reaches the stomach, it hatches and the tiny embryo thus set free burrows its way through the intestinal wall and is carried by the bloodstream to some distant organ. Wherever it lodges it forms a little cyst or bladder, the hydatid (drop of water) cyst, which contains the larval head of the worm. Thus far it resembles the cysticercus of the pork tapeworm, but its later development is quite different. This little bladder buds again and again, hundreds of times, each bud producing a new cyst similar to and the same size as the first. These daughter cysts in turn may bud and soon contain many granddaughter cysts.

The one original cyst, now of great size, may contain hundreds of these small cysts.

The symptoms of one of these cysts are those of a tumor of the organ in which it lies. The diagnosis is based upon finding a cystic tumor, for which x-rays are very helpful. The Cason skin test, using hydatid fluid injected intracutaneously, is positive in 90 percent of cases.

Treatment

The treatment is surgical removal of the cysts (always with great care lest it rupture during the operation, setting free one or more tiny embryos, each of which can start a new cyst). Chemotherapy is ineffective.

Fluke Infestations: Distomiasis

Flukes are parasitic, leaf-shaped flatworms; their infestations of man are called *distomiasis*. The life history of flukes is most complicated, since 1, 2 or 3 intermediate hosts are necessary for the life cycle of the worm. These cycles include free-swimming larval stages, hence fluke infestations are most common among people who must work in water, or who eat water plants or raw fish from infested water. Distomiasis, therefore, is endemic only in regions where exactly the right conditions are present; but where it is endemic, it usually affects a large percentage of the population. These infestations must be massive to occasion any symptoms. The diagnosis is always made by finding the fluke eggs (distinctive for each type) in the stools.

Intestinal Flukes

The most important fluke that infests the bowel is *Fasciolopsis buski* (a flatworm about 2.5 cm. long and 1.25 cm. wide), the larvae of which are ingested with aquatic plant foods. If the patient harbors many of these flukes, the symptoms are weakness, chronic diarrhea of blood-free stools and abdominal pain. After months, edema, often marked, appears. It starts as an ascites, then involves the lower extremities and, extending upward, the face or even the lungs. In marked cases the temperature is subnormal, and the skin is yellow, harsh and dry; cardiac insufficiency occasionally arises. Death apparently is from malnutrition and dehydration resulting from the continuous diarrhea.

Treatment. Tetrachlorethylene is effective in treatment as a single dose. Hexylresorcinol is also useful.

Blood Flukes: Bilharziasis

Bilharziasis, or infestation of the blood vessels by one of several types of blood flukes, produces first an initial urticarial and petechial skin rash (due to the invasion of the skin by the larval forms of the fluke) and later hematuria or dysentery, according to the location of the infestation. The liver always is enlarged.

Types. One type of blood fluke, *Schistosoma haematobium* (an elongated fluke about 1.25 cm. long and 0.1 cm. wide, common in some regions of Africa and Asia Minor), resides in the pelvic veins—especially in those of the bladder and the rectum. Some persons harbor these flukes for years, the only evidence of their presence, if in the bladder wall, being the constant or occasional appearance of small clots of blood in the urine. More serious infestations, however, cause thickening and ulceration of the bladder, hence urinary stasis, bladder calculi or ureteral obstruction. Dysentery with severe tenesmus indicates infestation of the rectal veins. The ova, by embolism, may reach the brain, giving rise to symptoms simulating brain tumor. After persisting for variable lengths of time, this parasite often disappears spontaneously.

Another blood fluke, *Schistosoma mansoni*, found in Africa, the West Indies and South America, infests the mesenteric veins, causing emaciation, colic and chronic dysentery. A third blood fluke, *Schistosoma japonicum*, common among the workers of Japan and the Far East, causes a serious disease characterized by diarrhea with or without fever, painful enlargement of the liver and the spleen, edema, anemia and occasionally pulmonary and cerebral symptoms.

All blood flukes seem to develop from their free-swimming larval forms, either those in drinking water or in water in which the person wades, in which circumstance the larvae penetrate the skin.

The diagnosis is based on finding ova in the stools or urine or in the biopsy specimen of affected tissue.

Chemotherapy. The treatment of choice for *S. haematobium* and *S. mansoni* infestations is the intramuscular injection of stibophen (Fuadin), 1 ml. per 13.6 Kg. of body weight, on 20 consecutive days. The maximal dose for any one day should not exceed 5 ml. The rate of administration, but not the total dosage, may be modified in the event of severe vomiting. Dosage schedules entailing the administration of 90 to 100 ml. of the drug are associated with cure rates approximating 100 per cent. *S. japonicum* infestation is treated most effectively by the intravenous injection of tartar emetic on alternate days until a total dose of 2.5 gm., or 500 ml. of the 0.5 per cent solution, has been received, the initial dose being 8 ml., and the maximal dose for a single day being 28 ml. For vesical infection, Miracil D is very useful.

Liver Flukes

Hepatic distomiasis caused by tiny liver flukes (*Clonorchis sinensis*) acquired by eating raw fish infested with larvae, is a disease common in the Far East. If a sufficient number of flukes are present (more than

21,000 were found in the liver of one patient), the infestation causes a bloody diarrhea with subsequent ascites, jaundice, marked anemia and fatal cachexia. The liver at first becomes large, but later, small and cirrhotic; the spleen is enlarged.

Treatment. Currently favored as the treatment of choice in cases of liver fluke infestation is chloroquine diphosphate, given in 250-mg. doses twice daily for 7 or 8 weeks.

Lung Fluke: Pulmonary Distomiasis

Pulmonary distomiasis, or infestation of the lung by the lung fluke *Paragonimus westermani* (which has the shape and size of a coffee bean), is a disease common in the Far East and also in Yucatán and Peru. It is acquired by eating raw crabs or crayfish or by drinking water containing larvae liberated from disintegrating crabs. It is characterized chiefly by thoracic pain, cough and signs of chronic lung infection, with hemoptysis or blood-stained or purulent sputum in which the eggs of this fluke are found easily. This fluke, however, may infest any other organ, with symptoms depending on the organ involved.

Diagnosis. The eggs of the lung fluke may be found in the sputum, the feces and the body fluids obtained by puncture.

Treatment. Chloroquine, 0.75 gm. daily to a total of 40 to 120 gm., has been found of some value. Emetine 0.065 gm. IM daily for 12 days reduces egg productivity. Prevention is by eating only well-cooked crayfish and crabs.

BIBLIOGRAPHY

(The Bibliography also includes less frequently encountered diseases not covered in the text.)

BOOKS

Anderson, G. W., Arnstein, M. G., and Lester, M. R.: Communicable Disease Control. New York, Macmillan, 1962.

Brockington, F.: World Health. London, Churchill, 1967.

Catterall, R. D.: The Venereal Diseases. London, Evans, 1967.

Cockburn, A.: Infectious Diseases. Springfield, Ill., Charles C Thomas, 1967.

Corrigan, M. J., and Corcoran, L. E. (eds.): Workshop on Epidemiology in Nursing. Washington, D. C., Catholic University of America Press, 1961.

Felsenfeld, O.: The Cholera Problem. St. Louis, Warren H. Green, 1967.

Goerke, L. S., and Stebbins, E. L.: Mustard's Introduction to Public Health. New York, Macmillan, 1968.

Gordon, J. E. (ed.): Control of Communicable Diseases in Man. New York, American Public Health Association, 1965.

Greenberg, M.: Studies in Epidemiology. New York, Putnam, 1965.

Hinman, E. H.: World Eradication of Infectious Diseases. Springfield, Ill., Charles C Thomas, 1966.

Horsfall, F. L., and Tamm, I.: Viral and Rickettsial Infections of Man. Philadelphia, J. B. Lippincott, 1965.

Horstmann, D. M.: Virology and Epidemiology. Hamden, Conn., Archon Books, 1962.

Kallins, E. L.: Textbook of Public Health Nursing. St. Louis, C. V. Mosby, 1967.

LeRiche, W. H., Balcom, C. E., and Van Belle, G.: The Control of Infections in Hospitals. Springfield, Ill., Charles C Thomas, 1966.

Minnesota Dept. of Health: Venereal Disease Education—A Teaching Guide. Minneapolis, Minnesota Dept. of Health, 1966.

National Communicable Disease Center: International Epidemiologic Report. Atlanta, National Communicable Disease Center, 1967.

Paul, J. R.: Clinical Epidemiology. Chicago, University of Chicago Press, 1966.

Pulaski, E. J.: Common Bacterial Infections. Philadelphia, W. B. Saunders, 1964.

Rhodes, A. J., and Van Rooyen, C. E.: Textbook of Virology. Baltimore, Williams & Wilkins, 1968.

Schwartz, B.: Clinical Venereology for Nurses and Students. Oxford, Pergamon Press, 1966.

Thompson, L. R.: Microbiology and Epidemiology. Philadelphia, W. B. Saunders, 1962.

Top, F. H.: Communicable and Infectious Diseases. St. Louis, C. V. Mosby, 1968.

U. S. Dept. of H. E. W.: Proceedings of World Forum on Syphilis and Other Treponematoses. Washington, D. C., U. S. Government Printing Office, 1964.

———: Syphilis—A Synopsis. Washington, D. C., U. S. Government Printing Office, 1968.

Bacterial Infections

Ackerman, A. B., et al.: Asymptomatic gonorrhea; the gonococcal carrier state and gonococcemia in men. J.A.M.A., *196*: 101-193, 1966.

An epidemiologist's view of leprosy. WHO Chronicle, *20*:460-461, Dec., 1966.

Artenstein, M. S., et al.: Acute respiratory disease and meningococcal infection in army recruits. J.A.M.A., *201*:1004-1008, 1967.

Bayer, L. M.: Maturation, mores and morals. Postgrad. Med., *44*:176-180, Oct., 1968.

Brubaker, M. L., et al.: Ten-year review of hospital admissions of patients with leprosy. Pub. Health Rep., *83*:155-160, Feb., 1968.

Browne, S. G.: Advances in the treatment of leprosy. Practitioner, *199*:525-531, Oct., 1967.

Catalano, P. M.: Early and latent syphilis. Current management. Arch. Dermat. *92*:433-435, Oct., 1965.

Cholera: Prevention and treatment. WHO Chronicle, *21*:135-139, April, 1967.

Christensen, N. A., and Thurber, D. L.: Current treatment of clinical tetanus. Mod. Treatment, *5*:729-757, July, 1968.

Collins, R. N., et al.: Interstate outbreak of salmonella newbrunswick infection traced to powdered milk. JAMA, *203*: 838-844, 1968.

Corothers, T. E., et al.: An outbreak of diphtheria: a story of investigation and control. Clin. Ped., *5*:29-33, Jan., 1966.

Curtis, A. C.: The reported and actual morbidity of syphilis and gonorrhea. Arch. Environ. Health, *13*:381-384, Sept., 1966.

Fasal, P.: Leprosy occurs everywhere. G.P., *32*:95-102, Oct., 1965.

Feldman, W. H.: Yesterday's triumphs: today's problems. JAMA, *194*:33-37, 1965.

Fleming, W. L.: The problem of syphilis and gonorrhea today. Arch. Environ. Health, *13*:357-366, Sept., 1966.

Gangarosa, E. J.: Cholera pandemic poses threat to world travelers. Hospitals, *41*:64-65, Sept. 16, 1967.

Guckian, J. C.: Treatment of salmonellosis and shigellosis. Mod. Treatment, *3*:1003-1015, Sept., 1966.

Gunn, A. D.: Leprosy—not an exclusively tropical disease. Nurs. Times, *62*:280-281, March, 1966.

Hasselblad, O. W.: End of social dislocation of leprosy patients. Rehab. Record, *8*:6-8, May-June, 1967.

Hornick, R. B., *et al.*: Typhoid fever vaccine—yes or no? Med. Clin. N. Amer., *51*:617-623, May, 1967.

Kampmeier, R. H.: The rise in venereal disease: epidemiology and prevention. Med. Clin. N. Amer., *51*:735-751, May, 1967.

Kaul, P. M.: Trends of cholera. Amer. J. Pub. Health, *56*:1010-1012, July, 1966.

Klein, F., *et al.*: Pathophysiology of anthrax. J. Infect. Dis., *116*:123-138, April, 1966.

Koenig, M. G., *et al.*: Type B botulism in men. Amer. J. Med., *42*:208-219, Feb., 1967.

King, S.: Diphtheria immunization. Practitioner, *195*:289-291, Sept., 1965.

McGarity, W. C., *et al.*: Brucellosis. Indications for splenectomy. Amer. J. Surg., *115*:355-363, March, 1968.

MacKenzie, D. J.: Cholera: whither prevention? Med. Clin. N. Amer., *51*:625-635, May, 1967.

Mechie, A. M., *et al.*: Venereal infection in old age: an autopsy study. Geriatrics, *22*:176-179, Sept., 1967.

Nicholas, L., *et al.*: Late syphilis: a review of some of the recent literature. Amer. J. Med. Sci., *254*:549-569, Oct., 1967.

Olansky, S.: Syphilis—rediscovered. Disease-A-Month, 3-30, May, 1967.

————: Some aspects of the management of venereal disease. Arch. Environ. Health, *13*:376-380, Sept., 1966.

Parry, W. H.: The scourge of cholera. Nurs. Times, *62*:1197-1199, Sept. 9, 1966.

————: Whooping cough. Nurs. Times, *61*:1534-1536, Nov. 12, 1965.

Phillips, R. A.: Twenty years of cholera research. JAMA, *202*:610-614, 1967.

Polk, L. D.: Nursing responsibilities in a salmonella outbreak. Nurs. Outlook, *13*:56-58, Dec., 1965.

Rantz, L. A. (ed.): Symposium on treatment of infectious diseases. Mod. Treatment, *1*, July, 1964.

Schulte, W. J., *et al.*: Surgical implications in salmonellosis. Arch. Surg., *96*:593-598, April, 1968.

Shapiro, L. H., *et al.*: Clinical evaluation of treatment of gonorrhea in the female. Obstet. Gynec., *97*:968-973, April, 1967.

————: Large doses of penicillin for treatment of gonorrhea in women. Obstet. Gynec. *30*:89-92, July, 1967.

Simon, H. J., *et al.*: Ampicillin in the treatment of chronic typhoid carriers. New Eng. J. Med., *274*:807-815, 1966.

Swartz, M. N.: Treatment of opportunistic salmonella infections. Mod. Treatment, *3*:1578-1584, Sept., 1966.

Werrin, M., *et al.*: Salmonella control in hospitals. Amer. J. Nurs., *66*:528-531, March, 1966.

Viral Infections

Baum, S. G., *et al.*: Epidemic nonmeningitic lymphocytic choriomeningitis-virus infection. An outbreak in a population of laboratory personnel. New Eng. J. Med., *274*:934-936, 1966.

Bender, C. E.: The value of corticosteroids in the treatment of infectious mononucleosis. JAMA, *199*:529-531, 1967.

Bond, J. O.: St. Louis encephalitis. Nurs. Outlook, *14*:26-27, 1966.

Brown, G. C.: Coxsackie virus infections and heart disease. Amer. Heart J., *75*:145-146, Feb., 1968.

Burke-Gaffney, H. J.: Yellow fever. Trop. Dis. Bull., *63*:113-115, Feb., 1966.

Calafiore, D. C.: Eradication of measles in the U. S. Amer. J. Nurs., *67*:1871-1874, Sept., 1967.

Cifarelli, P. S., *et al.*: Rubella encephalitis. New York J. Med., *66*:1117-1122, May, 1966.

Constantine, D. G.: Bat rabies in the southwestern United States. Pub. Health Reports, *82*:867-888, Oct., 1967.

Davenport, F. M.: Prospects for the control of influenza, Amer. J. Nurs., *69*:1908-1911, Sept., 1969.

Davidson, W. L., *et al.*: Vaccination of adults with live attenuated mumps virus vaccine. JAMA, *201*:995-998, 1967.

Dooley, J. R., *et al.*: Three faces of dengue. Arch. Int. Med., *117*:170-174, Feb., 1966.

Downs, W. G.: The story of yellow fever since Walter Reed. Bull. New York Acad. Med., *44*:721-727, June, 1968.

Fiumara, N. J.: Use of mumps vaccine. New Eng. J. Med., *278*:681-682, 1968.

Francis, T., Jr.: Epidemic influenza: immunization and control. Med. Clin. N. Amer., *51*:781-790, May, 1967.

Gold, E.: Serologic and virus-isolation studies of patients with varicella or herpes-zoster infections. New Eng. J. Med., *274*:181-185, 1966.

Grant, M.: An epidemiologic investigation of suspected smallpox. G.P., *32*:106-112, Dec., 1965.

Horstmann, D. M.: Enterovirus infections of the central nervous system. The present and future of poliomyelitis. Med. Clin. N. Amer., *51*:681-692, May, 1967.

Jones, R. C.: Rabies: present attitudes. Postgrad. Med., *43*:141-147, March, 1968.

Kempe, C. H., *et al.*: Smallpox immunization in the U. S., JAMA, *194*:161-166, 1965.

Lawrenson, J. A.: Virus encephalitis. Nurs. Times, *61*:1613-1614, Nov. 26, 1965.

Measles immunization: current status. Clin. Pediat., *5*:325-326, May, 1966.

Miller, G. D., *et al.*: Hand-foot-and-mouth disease. JAMA, *203*:827-830, 1968.

Minkowitz, S., *et al.*: Acute glomerulonephritis associated with varicella infection. Amer. J. Med., *44*:489-492, March, 1968.

Oberman, J. W.: Measles vaccination: a review. G.P., *35*:106-107, May, 1967.

Parry, W. H.: Yellow fever, Nurs. Times, *64*:152-153, Feb. 2, 1968.

Quie, P. G., *et al.*: Treatment of smallpox and complications of smallpox vaccination. G.P., *36*:130-136, Oct., 1967.

Rabies 1968 model. JAMA, *203*:420, 1968.

Rabies prophylaxis. Ann. Intern. Med., *67*:159-163, 1967.

Randall, H. B.: Measles eradication. J. Sch. Health, *37*:458-459, Nov., 1967.

Sabin, A. B.: Oral poliovirus vccaine. History of its development and prospects for eradication of poliomyelitis. JAMA, *194*:872-876, 1965.

Seabury, C. J.: A nurse's observations on post-encephalitis patients. Nurs. Outlook, *14*:28-29, Oct., 1966.

Smallpox vaccination. Recommendations of the U. S. Public Health Service Advisory Committee on Immunization Practices. Ann Intern. Med., *66*:358-364, 1967.

Soper, F. L.: Smallpox—world changes and implications for eradication. Amer. J. Pub. Health, *56*:1652-1656, Oct., 1966.

———: *Aedes aegypti* and yellow fever. Bull. WHO, *36*:521-527, 1967.

The vaccinated world. JAMA, *200*:637-638, 1967.

Specific systemic prophylaxis for rabies. G.P., *35*:76-77, April, 1967.

Steele, J. H.: Treatment of persons exposed to rabies. Amer. J. Pub. Health, *56*:338-339, March, 1966.

Weinstein, E. G., *et al.*: Lymphogranuloma venereum. J. Amer. Geriat. Soc., *14*:80-84, Jan., 1968.

Welch, E. M., *et al.*: Variola minor. Nurs. Times, *62*:928-930, July 15, 1966.

Wilkins, R. H., *et al.*: Encephalitis lethargica. Arch. Neurol., *18*:324-328, March, 1968.

Witte, C. L., *et al.*: Pancreatitis due to mumps. JAMA, *203*:1068-1069, 1968.

Witte, J. J., *et al.*: Surveillance of mumps in the U. S. as background for use of vaccine. Pub. Health Reports, *83*:95-100, Feb., 1968.

Protozoal Infections

Amebic infection in the U. S. New Eng. J. Med., *275*:960-961, 1966.

Daroff, R. B., *et al.*: Cerebral malaria. JAMA, *202*:679-682, 1967.

Doxiades, T.: The significance of amoebiasis. Amer. J. Proct., *17*:29-31, Feb., 1966.

Hinman, E. H.: Malaria: the changing outlook. Med. Clin. N. Amer., *51*:729-734, May, 1967.

Juniper, K., Jr.: Treatment of amebiasis. Mod. Treatment, *3*:1016-1031, Sept., 1966.

Neva, F. A.: Malaria—recent progress and problems. New Eng. J. Med., *277*:1241-1252, 1967.

Preventing the re-introduction of malaria. WHO Chronicler, *22*:150-154, April, 1968.

Ruiz-Moreno, F.: Perianal skin amebiases. Dis. Colon and Rectum, *10*:65-69, Jan.-Feb., 1967.

Seaton, D. R.: The malaria situation. Nurs. Times, *62*:215-216, Feb. 18, 1966.

Sheehy, T. W., *et al.*: Complications of falciparum malaria and their treatment. Ann. Intern. Med., *66*:807-809, April, 1967.

Torres, A.: Amebiasis. The hazards of surgical intervention in unsuspected amebic disease. Arch. Surg., *95*:249-252, Aug., 1967.

Wharton, G. K., *et al.*: Clinical evaluation of an intradermal skin test for amebiasis. Amer. J. Gastroent., *48*:233-243, Sept., 1967.

Systemic Mycoses

Briney, R. R.: Primary cutaneous actinomycosis. JAMA, *194*:679-680, 1965.

Coodley, E. L.: Disseminated coccidioidomycosis: diagnosis by liver biopy. Gastroent., *53*:947-952, Dec., 1967.

Goldman, L.: How I treat blastomycosis, actinomycosis and coccidioidomycosis. Postgrad. Med., *42*:A65-A66, July, 1967.

Louria, D. B.: Deep-seated mycotic infections, allergy to fungi and mycotoxins. New Eng. J. Med., *277*:1065-1071, 1967.

———: Treatment of opportunistic fungal infections. Mod. Treatment, *3*:1099-1106, Sept., 1966.

Prolo, J. J., *et al.*: Secondary actinomycotic brain abscess: isolation of a new species and review. Arch. Surg., *96*:58-64, Jan., 1968.

Roberts, P. L.: Primary coccidioidomycosis. Military Med., *132*:625-633, Aug., 1967.

Salkin, D.: Clinical examples of reinfection in coccidioidomycosis. Amer. Rev. Resp. Dis., *95*:603-611, April, 1967.

Shanholtz, M. I.: Histoplasmosis. Virginia Med. Monthly, *94*:123-124, Feb., 1967.

Utz, J. P.: Antimicrobial therapy in systemic fungal infections. Amer. J. Med., *39*:826-830, Nov., 1965.

Utz, J. P., and Benson, M. E.: The systemic mycoses. Amer. J. Nurs., *65*:103-110, Sept., 1965.

Weaver, D. K., *et al.*: Histoplasma endocarditis. Arch. Surg., *96*:158-162, Jan., 1968.

Winn, W. A.: Tuberculosis and coccidioidomycosis. Amer. Rev. Resp. Dis., *96*:229-236, Aug., 1967.

Wright, N. L.: Cervical infections. Amer. J. Surg., *113*:379-386, March, 1967.

Rickettsial Infections

Apted, F. I.: Rickettsial diseases. Trop. Dis. Bull., *63*:825-832, Aug., 1966.

Johnson, J. E., *et al.*: Rocky Mountain spotted fever acquired in a laboratory. New Eng. J. Med., *277*:842-847, 1967.

Wisseman, C. L., Jr.: Rickettsial diseases. Military Med., *132*:449-451, June, 1967.

Parasitic Infections

Higdon, R. S.: Common insect, mite and parasite problems in the United States. G.P. *37*:84-98, May, 1968.

Immunology and parasitic diseases. WHO Chronicle, *20*:87-91, March, 1966.

Iron deficiency anemia due to hookworm infection in man. Nutr. Rev., *26*:47-49, Feb., 1968.

Roche, M., *et al.*: The nature and cause of hookworm anemia. Amer. J. Trop. Med., *15*:1029-1102, Nov., 1966.

PATIENT EDUCATION

Inquiries Branch
Public Health Service
U. S. Department of Health, Education and Welfare
Washington, D. C. 20201

Amebiasis. (HIS-49)
Brucellosis. (HIS-42)
Chickenpox. (HIS-38)
Common Cold. (HIS-29)
Diphtheria. (HIS-37)
Hepatitis. (HIS-82)
Home Food Protection. Cold Facts About. (HIS-121)
You Can Prevent Foodborne Illness. (HIS-1105)
Home Sanitation. (HIS-39)

Insects That Carry Disease. (HIS-90)
Keep Your Drinking Water Safe. (HIS-1511)
Hookworm Disease. (HIS-52)
Immunization Health Benefits for You and Your
    Family. (OM-1781)
Influenza. (HIS-36)
Leptospirosis. (HIS-93)
Louse Infestation. (HIS-26)
Malaria. (HIS-41)
Measles. (HIS-24)
Meningococcal Meningitis. (HIS-26)
Mumps. (HIS-22)
Pinworms. (HIS-51)
Poliomyelitis. (HIS-8)
Rabies. (HIS-30)
Rocky Mountain Spotted Fever. (HIS-20)
Smallpox. (HIS-27)
Syphilis and Gonorrhea. (HIS-84)
Tapeworm. (HIS-48)
Trichinosis. (HIS-47)
Tularemia. (HIS-44)
Typhoid Fever. (HIS-72)
Whooping Cough. (HIS-60)

AGENCIES

Governmental

National Communicable Disease Center
    Atlanta, Georgia 30333

U. S. Department of Health, Education and Welfare
    U. S. Public Health Service
    Washington, D. C. 20201

International

World Health Organization (Regional Office for the Americas)
    525 23rd Street, N. W.
    Washington, D. C. 20037

World Health Organization
    Avenue Appia
    Geneva, Switzerland

Voluntary

The American Public Health Association
    1790 Broadway
    New York, New York 10019

CHAPTER **38**

Nursing in Emergency and Disaster Conditions

- *Orientation*
- *Nursing Responsibilities in Relation to Emergencies*
- *Mobilization of Medical and Nursing Services*
- *Principles of Emergency Management*
- *Psychological Management of Patients in Emergency-Disaster Situations*
- *Improvization and Resourcefulness*
- *Poisoning*

ORIENTATION

Discussions of nursing principles and practices in preceding portions of this text are based on the assumption that adequate facilities for patient care are available. Therapy has been described in ideal terms, according to modern standards, on the assumption that its selection and the method by which it is conducted are dictated by the patient's needs in every case. The fact is, of course, that in certain emergencies it becomes impossible to render ideal medical and nursing care. Circumstances may arise that result in a sudden, unprecedented demand for treatment of a type or on such a scale that the needs cannot possibly be met with the limited facilities and the available personnel.

The Meaning of Disaster

A *disaster* is a catastrophe which is man-made, produced accidentally or by design, such as a hostile enemy act, or which is of natural origin. Disasters caused by war may be thermonuclear, biologic, chemical or psychological. Man-made catastrophes may be train, plane or automobile accidents, or fires, explosions or civil disturbances. Examples of natural disasters are epidemics, floods, hurricanes, blizzards, droughts, earthquakes and tornadoes.

Each kind of disaster takes its toll in its own particular way: property is damaged and destroyed; people are injured and killed. A traffic accident involves an automobile and its occupants, a tornado plays havoc with 1 or 2 city blocks, a thermonuclear attack may strike a large metropolitan center; whatever the cause, the product is casualties. The average hospital is able to cope with minor disasters. The nursing student has valuable learning experiences on the clinical units and in the emergency and the operating rooms to prepare her to function adequately and intelligently.

However, a major disaster, such as might occur during thermonuclear warfare, will present additional problems, even though the principles of care are basically the same. When large numbers of casualties need attention, priority must be given to those having the greatest need who yet, with care, are likely to survive; this is determined in large measure by the availability of medical resources. One major factor distinguishing a thermonuclear attack from all other types of catastrophe would be extensive radioactive contamination of terrain, food, water, clothing and all exposed persons and matériel.

Emergency medical care in the broadest sense of the term refers to the care of patients whose needs are urgent and critical; care administered under cir-

946

cumstances that may or may not be optimal, utilizing whatever facilities are at hand in the most effective manner possible. The proper management of the patient requiring emergency care depends on a broad knowledge of nursing principles and intimate acquaintance with a wide variety of nursing techniques. So equipped, the nurse is in a position to function effectively in the event of an emergency, whether this is the result of an accident involving a few individuals or a catastrophe involving thousands.

NURSING RESPONSIBILITIES IN RELATION TO EMERGENCIES

It is the nurse's responsibility to assume leadership in the planning, the organizing, the directing and the provision of emergency nursing service. Acceptance of this important role assumes a knowledge on her part that must include:

1. An understanding of survival procedures and emergency life-saving measures
2. Familiarity with community plans for emergency action
3. Complete knowledge of warning signals and proper action to be taken in the event of an enemy attack
4. Ability to initiate protective measures against radioactive fallout

The American Nurses Association Committee on Nursing in National Defense has released a publication on *The Role of the Nurse in Disaster.* Our professional organization recognizes that nurses should have additional preparation in applying nursing knowledge and skills "to emergency situations in a disaster environment."

The American Medical Association has developed a list of functions for nurses under mass casualty situations. The functions include:

A. First aid, including but not limited to artificial respiration; emergency treatment of open chest wounds; relief of pain; treatment of shock and the preparation of casualties for movement
B. Control of hemorrhage
C. Attainment and maintenance of patent airway, and intratracheal catheterization, to include emergency tracheotomy
D. Proper and adequate cleansing and treatment of wounds
E. Bandaging and splinting
F. Administration of anesthetics under medical supervision
G. Assisting in surgical procedures
H. Insertion of nasogastric tubes to include lavage and gavage, as directed
I. Administration of whole blood and intravenous solutions, as directed
J. Administration of parenteral medications, as directed

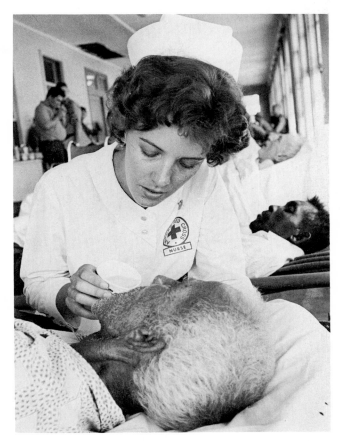

Fig. 38-1. A nurse tends an elderly victim who found a safe haven in a Red Cross shelter during a destructive hurricane. During this disaster over 200,000 persons were housed and fed as well as given necessary nursing and medical care. (American Red Cross Photo)

K. Catheterization of males and females
L. Administration of immunizing agents, as directed
M. Management of the psychologically disturbed
N. Management of normal deliveries
O. Operation of treatment and aid stations in reception areas and in communities where physicians are inadequate in number, to include the diagnosis and the treatment of minor illnesses and injuries, institution of life-saving measures and the referral of more serious cases to physicians*

MOBILIZATION OF MEDICAL AND NURSING SERVICES

Packaged Disaster Hospitals

Under normal conditions, community hospital facilities are usually adequate to meet health needs. However, in the event of a disaster such as a devastat-

* Summary Report on National Emergency Care. American Medical Association, pp. 16-17, Feb., 1962.

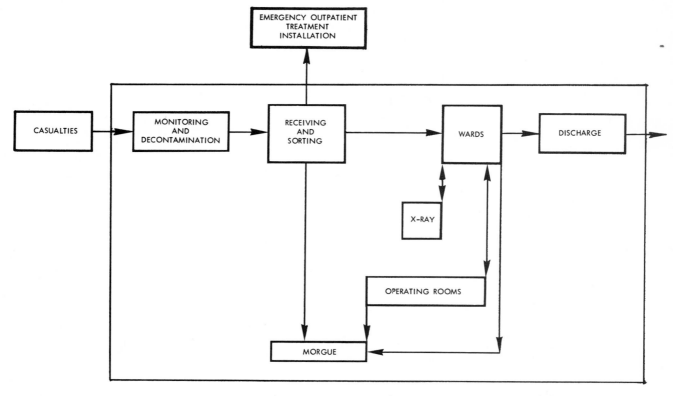

Fɪɢ. 38-2. Patient Flow Chart. (U.S.P.H.S.)

ing flood, a tornado or a nuclear attack, there would be an acute shortage of hospital space and medical supplies. The Federal Government* has stockpiled medical supplies and equipment to help individual communities meet emergency health needs and improve mass casualty care. Stocked hospital units are now placed in strategic positions throughout the country ready to be set up for emergency use. The Packaged Disaster Hospital (PDH) consists of hospital supplies, equipment and pharmaceuticals packaged for long term storage. All hospital sections, including operating room, central sterile supply, pharmacy, laboratory and patient units are included in the Packaged Disaster Hospital components. In case of disaster, the PDH may be used to expand existing hospital facilities or be set up as a separate 200-bed facility in a school or armory and operated as an adjunct to its affiliated hospital. Each PDH contains a 30-day supply of essential medical supplies and equipment. Local community volunteers are trained to perform the setting-up operation in a matter of hours. The PDH is inspected periodically

* United States Public Health Service: The Packaged Disaster Hospital. Washington, D. C., 1967. Health Mobilization Series D-6.

to ensure its constant readiness. Training sessions for professional personnel and lay volunteers are carried out so that the PDH may be activated effectively in an emergency.

The basic plan of operation of medical and nursing services in an emergency is to set up first aid and emergency hospital units and organize professional and auxiliary personnel. Details of such planning should be reviewed as they apply to the local hospital unit, the community and the state. During an emergency, there is an increased demand for many skills usually regulated by law—the nurse may be called to perform tasks usually done by a physician. Upgrading and regrading of functions often are necessary.

Sorting

The *sorting* of casualties (formerly called *triage*) requires clinical judgment of the highest degree. The most responsible and able persons of the medical team should be assigned this difficult operation. Sorting is a continuous process, and it must be borne in mind that trauma can produce profound changes in an individual almost minute by minute.

The initial examination should be done quickly to detect threats to life and evaluate the patient's general condition. Classification for priority in treatment would be based on the casualties' probability of responding to what is immediately available in the way of medical personnel and supplies.

1. *Minimal Treatment:* Patients who can be returned to active duty immediately.

2. *Immediate Treatment:* Patients for whom the available expedient procedures will save life or limb

3. *Delayed Treatment:* Patients who, after emergency treatment, will incur little increased risk by having surgery withheld temporarily

4. *Expectant Treatment:* Critically injured patients who will be given treatment if time and facilities are available

The following is a priority schedule which serves as a guide to establish the flow of casualties from the disaster area through the First Aid Station to Forward Treatment Center and Hospital.

Priorities of Treatment.* *First Priority* (individuals needing immediate attention to save life):

1. Any wound interfering with airway or causing airway obstruction. (This includes sucking chest wounds, tension pneumothorax and maxillofacial wounds in which asphyxia is present or an impending threat.)

2. Any wound requiring immediate pressure

3. Shock due to major hemorrhage, to wounds of any organ system, fractures, etc.

Some of these conditions may be so urgent that immediate life-saving measures are required. The person responsible for sorting would plug a sucking chest wound, clear the airway, etc., before sending the patient for emergency treatment.

Second Priority (individuals needing early surgery):

1. Visceral injuries, including perforations of the gastrointestinal tract; wounds of the biliary and pancreatic system; wounds of the genitourinary tract; and thoracic wounds without asphyxia

2. Vascular injuries requiring repair. All injuries in which the use of a tourniquet is necessary fall into this group

3. Closed cerebral injuries with increasing loss of consciousness

Third Priority (patients who require surgery but can tolerate a delay):

1. Spinal injuries in which decompression is required

2. Soft-tissue wounds in which débridement is necessary, but in which muscle damage is less than major

* Adapted from United States Department of Defense: *Emergency War Surgery.* p. 172. Washington, D. C., United States Government Printing Office, 1959.

3. Lesser fractures and dislocations
4. Injuries of the eyes
5. Maxillofacial injuries without asphyxia

Identification of casualties is done by an emergency medical tag which should be fastened to a part of the body, preferably the wrist (not to clothing, because the tag may be lost). Details of methods used can be obtained in local and state civil defense manuals. Information about special care or handling of casualties can be noted by a simple initial about 7.5 cm. (3 inches) high printed on the tag:

H—severe hemorrhage
L—litter case
T—tourniquet case (add time of application)
X—person who is definitely dead

A clerk accompanies the sorting officer and completes admission records, clinical records and emergency tags. The sorting officer should not take time to write but uses his skill for patient examination and life-saving care.

PRINCIPLES OF EMERGENCY MANAGEMENT

In this discussion the care of the patient as a whole is to be considered first. Then the care of the patient with injury of component body parts is presented. The principles of mass casualty management comprise a broad outline of care that involves the exercise of sound clinical judgment and performance that is based on detailed nursing knowledge.

General Considerations

In caring for a patient in an emergency situation there are many crucial decisions to be made. These require sound judgment based on an understanding of the conditions that produced the emergency and their effect on the injured person. The major objectives of emergency medical treatment are (1) *to preserve life;* (2) to restore the patient to useful living, and (3) to prevent deterioration before more definitive treatment can be done.

Principles of Emergency Management. Certain basic principles are applicable to the emergency management of any patient. These include:

1. Maintaining a patent airway
2. Stopping bleeding
3. Preventing and treating shock
4. Protecting wounds with sterile dressings or dressings as clean as possible
5. Keeping injured persons lying down and covered
6. Allaying anxiety, and keeping patients as comfortable as possible
7. Observing and re-evaluating patients at frequent intervals

Mouth-to-mouth resuscitation
Inspiration **Expiration**

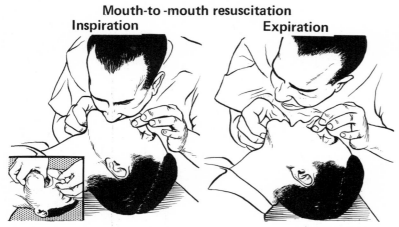

Fig. 38-3. Technics for mouth-to-mouth and mouth-to-nose resuscitation. (Gordon, Archer S., *et al.*: Mouth-to-mouth versus manual artificial respiration for children and adults, J.A.M.A., *167*:326)

Mouth-to-nose resuscitation
Inspiration **Expiration**

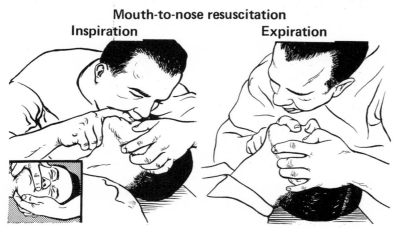

Maintenance of Respiration: Rescue Breathing; Artificial Respiration

The *first requisite* in the treatment of any emergency condition is the maintenance of an open airway. If the airway is obstructed, the ensuing hypoxia will produce permanent brain damage or death in 3 to 5 minutes.

To determine if the patient is breathing, place the palm of the hand over his mouth and nose and feel for air movement. *If the patient is not breathing, some form of pulmonary ventilation should be started immediately.*

Mouth-to-Mouth or Mouth-to-Nose ·Resuscitation. The most practical method of ensuring pulmonary ventilation in an emergency situation (if resuscitation equipment is unavailable) is by the mouth-to-mouth or mouth-to-nose technique. The normal expired air contains approximately 16 per cent oxygen and 4 per cent carbon dioxide. Approximately 1,000 ml. or more of air can be expelled with each expiration, and this is blown into the mouth of the patient at the rate of 12 to 20 times a minute. Adequate oxygenation may be maintained, especially if the rescuer breathes more deeply than normally.

The first requirement is that the airway be open. Most obstructions to the airway occur in the larynx. Therefore, freeing of the larynx by removal of foreign bodies or mucus, etc., with a finger is the first measure to be used. Occasionally, it may be necessary to place the patient on his abdomen and to pat the chest gently to dislodge foreign materials.

The technique of mouth-to-mouth artificial respiration depends on holding the jaw forward so that it "juts out." This pulls the tongue forward and opens the air passage and permits inflation of the lungs. The rescuer's expired air is blown into the mouth or the nose of the patient. In mouth-to-mouth artificial respiration, the nose must be held closed to seal the nasopharynx, so that the air goes into the lungs. When mouth-to-nose artificial respiration is given, the mouth is held closed, and the air is blown through the nose into the nasopharynx and the lungs. With either method, it is important that the jaw be held forward in order to open the airway into the lungs. The expired air is blown with a smooth steady action until the chest is observed to rise. This indicates inflation of the lungs with expired air. When the lungs have been inflated, the mouth of the rescuer is removed, and the lungs are allowed to empty. This cycle should be continued at the rate of about 12 to 20 cycles per minute. The rescuer should take a breath about twice the volume of ordinary respiration, and every 20 cycles he should take one deep breath himself. This type of mouth-to-mouth breathing may be maintained for an hour or more without fatigue in indicated cases. If during the active mouth-to-mouth respiration there appears to be a barrier to the flow of the air into the patient's lungs, this usually indicates an obstruction in the larynx or the pharynx that should be removed before continuing with artificial respiration.

Principles of Mouth-to-Mouth Artificial Respiration.

1. Clear the mouth of mucus and foreign objects
2. Lift up the jaw
   Insert the fingers in the corner of the mouth. Grasp the bony portion of the jaw and lift upward *or* push up on the angle of the jaw.
3. Pinch the nostrils to provide a closed system
4. Open the mouth wide and blow until the patient's chest rises
5. After blowing, turn the head to the side, and *watch* the patient's chest expansion, and *listen* to hear if air is leaving the lungs. (*Blow, watch, listen!*)
6. Repeat at the rate of 12 to 20 times per minute.

Prone-Pressure Method of Artificial Respiration. If there are poisonous gases in the air, mouth-to-mouth resuscitation procedures are not effective. Under these circumstances a prone-pressure method of artificial respiration should be used. Of course, the patient must wear a gas mask.

The prone-pressure method of artificial respiration is based on two principles. The first is compression of the chest against the ground by pressure applied to the back (expiration). The second is expansion of the chest by raising the arms and taking the pressure off the chest (inspiration). This method ensures good expansion of the lungs and helps to oxygenate the blood reaching the heart muscle. Quick oxygenation of the blood is essential in respiratory arrest.

This method of artificial respiration, which is conducted in cycles, is carried out as follows:

1. The patient is placed face down, with the head turned to one side and the arms bent, so as to keep the mouth and nose free from obstruction.
2. The operator kneels at the casualty's head, with one knee near the head and the other foot alongside the casualty's elbow. From time to time the position of the knee and the foot is alternated.
3. The operator's hands are placed over the casualty's shoulder blades, with the thumbs touching in the midline, the fingers spread out, and the arms straight.
4. The operator bends forward, still keeping the arms straight, and applies pressure over the casualty's chest by the weight of the upper part of his own body. As he executes this movement, he counts steadily and regularly, "One-er, two-er, and three-er," over a period of 2½ seconds. This maneuver forces out the air (deflation).
5. The operator then gradually releases the pressure on the casualty's chest by lifting the weight of his own body off it. At the same time he slides his hands to just above the casualty's elbows and counts, "Four-er," over a period of 1 second.
6. The operator then raises the casualty's arms and shoulders by bending backward, with his arms straight, until tension and resistance are felt; the chest is not lifted off the ground. While this maneuver, which draws air into the lungs (inflation) is being carried out, he counts, "Five-er, six-er, and seven-er," over a period of 2½ seconds.
7. The operator then lays the casualty's arms down and replaces his own hands on the casualty's back, thus returning to the original position, while counting, "Eight-er," over a period of 1 second.
8. This cycle is repeated with rhythmic rocking at the rate of about 9 times per minute until breathing is reestablished. Then the arm-raising and the arm-lowering movements (movements 6 and 7) are carried out 12 times to the minute. The operator counts, "One-er, two-er, and three-er," over a 2½-second period during the inspiratory (arm-raising) phase and counts, "Four-er, five-er, and six-er," during the expiratory (arm-lowering) phase.
9. If there are special regional injuries, the procedure must be modified. If the chest is injured, chest pressure is avoided; the patient lies supine, and only the arm-raising and the arm-lowering movements are executed, at the rate of 12 times to the minute. If the arms are injured, they are placed by the side of the body, and the complete procedure is carried out as described except that the operator's hands are placed under the hips, and a back-pressure, hip-lift technic is employed. If both the arms and the chest are injured, limited arm-raising and arm-lowering movements are carried out by inserting the hands only under the shoulders.
10. If necessary, artificial respiration can be continued in the vehicle while the patient is evacuated.*

Control of Hemorrhage

One of the primary causes of shock is the reduction in the circulating blood volume. Only a few conditions, such as obstructed airway or a sucking wound of the chest, take precedence over the immediate control of hemorrhage. "Stop the bleeding" is fundamental to the care and the survival of patients in an emergency or a disaster situation. (Control of hemorrhage is discussed in detail on pp. 149-150).

* United States Department of Defense: Emergency War Surgery. pp. 187-189. Washington, D. C., United States Government Printing Office, 1959.

Principles of Control of Hemorrhage.

1. Apply firm manual pressure over the wound or the artery involved. Unchecked arterial bleeding produces death.
2. Apply a firm pressure bandage. Do not constrict the circulation
3. Immobilize an injured extremity to control the blood loss
4. Elevate the affected part
5. If the patient is hemorrhaging internally, whole blood or plasma expanders, given at the rate of blood loss, are indicated. The patient who is bleeding internally requires surgery
6. Apply a tourniquet only as a *last resort* when the hemorrhage cannot be controlled by any other method.
    A. Apply the tourniquet, just above the wound. Apply it tightly enough to control arterial blood flow
    B. Tag the patient with a notation stating the location of the tourniquet and time applied. (Mark the patient's forehead with a "T")
    C. Once applied, the tourniquet remains in place until it can be released by a trained medical person who is prepared to control hemorrhage and to replace blood volume as necessary
    D. In the event of a traumatic amputation, apply a tourniquet

Control of Shock

Any injured patient should be assessed immediately to determine the presence of shock. If shock is present, it must be treated promptly. (Shock is discussed in detail on pp. 146-149.)

The following signs and symptoms in varying combinations indicate that the patient is in some degree of shock: cold, moist extremities, pallor, colorless lips,

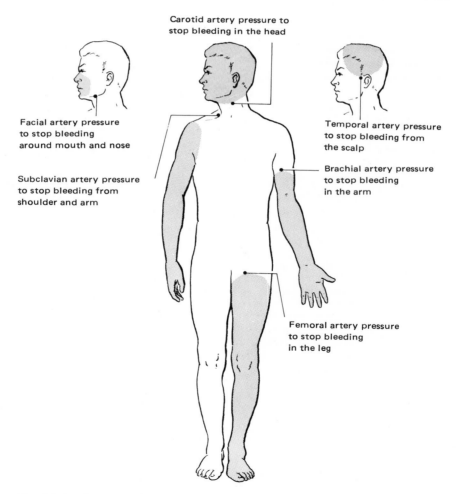

Carotid artery pressure to stop bleeding in the head

Facial artery pressure to stop bleeding around mouth and nose

Subclavian artery pressure to stop bleeding from shoulder and arm

Temporal artery pressure to stop bleeding from the scalp

Brachial artery pressure to stop bleeding in the arm

Femoral artery pressure to stop bleeding in the leg

FIG. 38-4. The six principal pressure points for the control of arterial bleeding.

tachycardia, decreased blood pressure, apathy and thirst. Of these, the most dependable criterion is the level of the arterial pressure.

Principles of Shock Management.

1. Remove the cause of shock
   A. Control hemorrhage
   B. Relieve the pain by splinting, supporting, positioning, and proper bandaging
   C. Treat the wound as soon as possible
   D. Splint the fracture
   E. Institute measures to prevent infection
2. Restore the circulating blood volume
   A. Control hemorrhage
   B. Give whole blood or one of the plasma volume expanders
   C. Give oral fluids to replace volume lost unless contraindicated by abdominal, gastrointestinal injuries or by the patient's condition
3. Support the defense mechanisms of the body
   A. Reassure and comfort the patient
   B. Relieve pain by cautious use of narcotics
   C. Maintain the body temperature. (Do not get the patient too warm, as heat produces vasodilatation, which counteracts the body's compensatory mechanism of vasoconstriction and also increases fluid loss by perspiration)
   D. Protect the patient from cold and dampness
   E. Elevate the feet slightly to improve cerebral circulation. (This position is contraindicated in patients with head injuries)
   F. Give oxygen if indicated

Emergency Use of Blood Derivatives and Substitutes. In the event of mass disaster, whole blood would not be available in the quantities needed. Other materials may be used in its stead for the restoration of deficient blood volume in cases of oligemic shock. Agents that are suitable for this purpose include human plasma, human albumin (plasma Fraction V) and other plasma fractions containing albumin, now under investigation, as well as a variety of products from sources other than human blood that are referred to as "plasma expanders."

Whole plasma, in contrast with certain of its derivatives, cannot be subjected to temperatures that are sufficiently high to achieve sterility, and for that reason its use is attended by the risk of transmitting viral hepatitis. Plasma fractions containing albumin are available, however, that can be pasteurized by exposure to a temperature of 60° C.* for 10 hours, can be used with safety as regards infectivity and are eminently suitable for the treatment of shock from every standpoint but one, namely, their failure to supply red

* 140° F.

CAUSES OF OLIGEMIC SHOCK

HEMATOGENIC OR SECONDARY SHOCK
CAUSED BY LOSS OF FLUID IN ACTIVE CIRCULATION

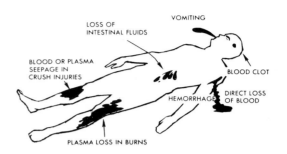

SYMPTOMS

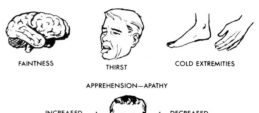

MANAGEMENT

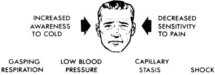

ARREST OF HEMORRHAGE

REMOVE NEUROGENIC CAUSATIVE FACTORS

PREVENTION OF INFECTION AND TOXEMIA

RELIEF OF PAIN

PROTECT PATIENT FROM HEAT, COLD & WET

BALANCE FLUIDS AND ELECTROLYTES

CONSTANT WATCHING OF VITAL SIGNS

PHYSICAL, MENTAL AND NUTRITIONAL COMFORT

Fig. 38-5. Causes, symptoms and management of oligemic shock. (Army War Surgery)

cells, a deficiency of relatively minor importance in the early phases of shock. However, it must be emphasized that in an emergency, whatever is available is used, even if some risk is involved.

Plasma expanders include certain materials that possess in common a molecular size such that they are retained in the circulating blood long enough after injection to cause the blood volume to expand, the prime objective of shock therapy. Such agents include dextran, produced by a bacterium; polyvinyl-pyrrolidone (PVP), a synthetic product; and oxypoly-gelatin. Attached to dextran is the disadvantage of increased cost and potential antigenicity for persons possessing antibodies against certain strains of pneumococci. Gelatin products exhibit gelation when cool, creating difficulties in the mechanics of injection when the latter must be accomplished in unheated quarters or out-of-doors in cold weather.

Wounds

Wounds will vary from minor lacerations to severe crushing injuries. The aims of emergency treatment are to stop bleeding, relieve shock, maintain an adequate airway and control infection. The principles of emergency care of wounds must be shared jointly by the trained personnel available. The nurse may be called on to carry out some of these procedures as instructed by a physician working with her.

Principles of Wound Management.

1. Stop bleeding
   A. Apply sterile pressure dressing
   B. Elevate extremity if this is part involved
   C. Apply tourniquet as low on limb of casualty as possible *if hemorrhage is not controllable any other way.* Apply it tightly and do not loosen it at periodic intervals. A physician should evaluate the situation
2. Relieve shock (see p. 148)
3. Prevent injuries to respiratory tract
   A. Maintain adequate airway. Proper positioning—on side or on back with head turned to side to allow drainage of pharyngeal secretions
   B. Cover gaping chest wounds with an airtight dressing and adhesive
4. Relieve pain: sedation not to exceed 10 mgm. morphine
5. Control infection
   A. Keep wound covered
   B. Give antibiotic therapy
   C. Give Tetanus prophylaxis (see p. 906)
6. Débride wounds
   A. Open wound for inspection
   B. Remove devitalized tissue and foreign bodies
   C. Irrigate gently with saline
   D. Pack loosely with dry gauze and cover with sterile dressings; immobilize part
7. Suture of wounds
   A. *Primary*—face, scalp and hand wounds may be cleaned and sutured primarily. Blood supply is abundant, and these parts are sufficiently resistant to infection
   B. *Secondary*—wounds other than the above mentioned may be closed primarily, or if deep and obviously contaminated, left open
8. Change of dressings: Only for removal of sutures, ischemia, infection or serious hemorrhage

Intra-abdominal Wounds. Intra-abdominal wounds are serious and almost always require surgery. The patient should not be moved until initial assessment has been carried out, because movement may fragment a clot in a large vessel and produce massive hemorrhage. Evidence of rapid concealed hemorrhage may be detected by looking at the patient and by evaluating his vital signs. Hemorrhage is a frequent accompaniment of abdominal injuries, especially if the liver has been injured. The first objective is to control the bleeding and maintain the blood volume until surgery can be performed. If the abdominal contents are protruding, cover them with a sterile saline dressing (warm water will suffice if saline is not available). This prevents drying of the viscera. No attempt should be made to manipulate or replace protruding viscera, because this maneuver enhances the possibility of peritonitis and increases the danger of additional trauma and shock. Flex the knees of the victim —the flexed position prevents further protrusion. Fluids are withheld, because intake of oral fluids increases peristalsis, leading to further contamination by fecal matter. In general, the earlier the patient is taken to the operating room for exploratory laparotomy, the more favorable will be his prognosis.

Mass Management of Wounds. In handling large numbers of injured persons with wounds, it is not possible to carry out ideal wound treatment. However, the objective is to do the best one can for the greatest number of casualties.

It is generally agreed that wounds should be left open until adequate personnel and facilities are available.

Principles of Mass Management of Wounds.

1. Control the hemorrhage
2. Clean the wounds with soap and water
3. Dress the wounds with material as clean as is available
4. Apply a splint if indicated to prevent further tissue damage caused by motion

Many wounds may not be closed for several days. Thus the healing would be by secondary intention. Broad spectrum antibiotics if available, is given to those with the more severe types of contaminated wounds.

Crush Injury. An individual who has been crushed beneath debris, or who has been run over, or whose

Fɪɢ. 38-6. The treatment of the patient with multiple injuries. Priorities of treatment. This is a patient who has a cranial injury (without signs of increased intracranial pressure), a fracture of the mandible with some obstruction of the airway, an open sucking wound of the chest and an open fracture of the femur. The patient has bled considerably and is in shock. Priority treatment would be: (1) Establish adequate airway—endotracheal tube. (2) Close thoracic wound with an occlusive dressing. (3) Start whole blood transfusion as therapy for shock. (4) Sterile dressing to the fracture wound and emergency splinting. (5) Observe for vital and neurologic signs—head injury. (6) Postpone definitive therapy of the fracture of the femur until the life-endangering injuries have been brought under control. (Rhoads, J. E., *et al.*: Surgery, Principles and Practice, Philadelphia, J. B. Lippincott, 1970)

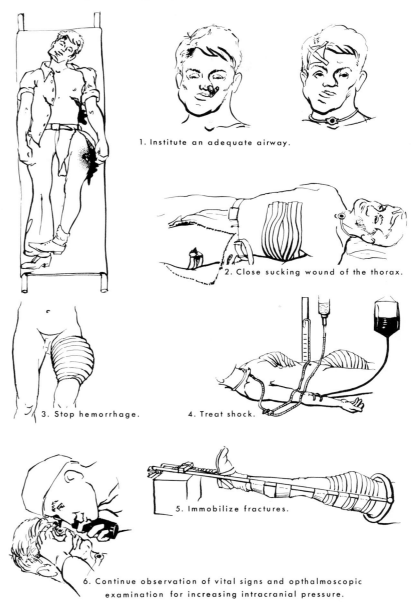

1. Institute an adequate airway.

2. Close sucking wound of the thorax.

3. Stop hemorrhage.

4. Treat shock.

5. Immobilize fractures.

6. Continue observation of vital signs and opthalmoscopic examination for increasing intracranial pressure.

limbs have been compressed in some manner for an hour or more is likely to develop the crush or compression syndrome. Paralysis of the part, erythema, and blistering of the skin may develop as first signs of damage. Shortly after release from compression, swelling due to extravasation of plasma may appear. This initiates oligemic shock, and the patient's condition worsens. The damaged part, usually an extremity, becomes swollen, tense and hard. Later symptoms include anorexia, hiccoughs, tongue dryness, drowsiness or mental disturbances. Renal dysfunction develops.

Principles of Crush Injury Management.

1. Splint early major soft-tissue injuries to control bleeding and pain, and to reduce shock
2. Expose limb to air to reduce tissue metabolism
3. Incise fascia if blood supply is blocked to relieve pressure or extravasated fluid
4. Apply pressure bandages
5. Administer medication for pain and anxiety

Chest Injuries. Injuries of the chest are potentially life-threatening because of danger of disturbances to cardiorespiratory physiology. In penetrating chest injuries, some air escapes into the pleural space (negative intrapleural pressure is replaced by atmospheric pressure). A loss of negative pressure within the pleural cavity may cause collapse of the lung. The changes in pressure interfere with the expansion of the uninvolved lung and there is a shifting back and forth of the collapsed lung and mediastinum. This shifting interferes with filling of the right side of the heart lessening cardiac output and causing cardiopulmonary collapse. *The underlying principle of treatment is to restore normal cardiorespiratory function as quickly as possible.*

Sucking wounds of the chest require immediate treatment. While the patient is exhaling, apply a pressure dressing against the wound and secure it with elastic adhesive or strapping (Fig. 38-6). Assess respiratory status and treat symptomatically until further treatment can be obtained.

Crushing injuries of the chest may produce multiple rib fractures and damage to the sternum. This may cause paradoxical (reverse of normal) respiratory motion, which seriously interferes with ventilatory function and requires immediate treatment. The treatment is to immobilize the flail portion of the chest by stabilizing it with a pressure dressing secured with adhesive strapping. (If necessary, use a sheet, the patient's shirt, etc.) Then place the patient on his *injured* side. In the hospital or treatment center, external traction applied through wires under the ribs or costal cartilages may be employed.

Unless these patients are in shock, they are more comfortable if the head and chest are elevated. Blood replacement should be started as early as possible. Respiratory obstruction is an ever present threat and is treated by nasotracheal catheter suction, bronchoscopic aspiration or tracheostomy.

(The treatment of hemothorax and tension pneumothorax is discussed on p. 270.)

Burns

It is anticipated that burns would be the most serious problem resulting from nuclear warfare. Burns are often associated with other types of injuries that are sometimes more serious than the burn.

Types of burns:

1. Thermal Burns
   A. *Flash burns* are caused by exposure to radiation. They vary in depth and are usually limited to exposed parts of the body. White clothing reflects radiant heat, thereby preventing or lessening the severity of flash burns. Dark colors absorb heat; hence, skin under dark-colored clothing may be burned.
   B. *Contact burns* are caused by heated objects (gases, liquids, solids) coming in contact with the body surface.
2. *Chemical Burns.* These are seen more frequently in industrial accidents. Some chemical agents continue to destroy tissue as long as they remain on the body. It is imperative that a history be elicited from the patient or bystander as to the cause of the burn (identification of chemical).
3. *Electrical Burn.* Electrical burns are usually deep and require prolonged healing time.

Ordinarily the chief dangers from burns are shock and infection (p. 659).

Estimation of Extent and Severity of Burns.
The severity of burns may be determined as follows:
First degree—edema; erythema; pain (epidermis injured but not destroyed)
Second degree—prompt formation of blisters; pain (injury extends into dermis)
Third degree—deep burns with charring of the skin; pain around the edges of the wound

Immediate Treatment. An excellent first aid measure for a burn is to submerge the burned area *immediately* in a cold solution 5° C. (41° F.). Surface cooling has been found to inhibit capillary permeability and resultant edema formation. Cooling is most effective if instituted immediately after the thermal insult and continued at least 30 minutes. Surface cooling may be beneficial up to 3 hours.

In the event of mass casualties, cover the burns with clean dry dressings such as ironed old sheets or towels. This excludes air and lessens pain. Do not apply ointment or other medication as a first-aid measure. Do not disturb blisters. Evaluate extent of burns; make the casualty as comfortable as possible; loosen constricting clothing and treat for shock.

Sorting for Treatment. The most experienced person available should classify patients for treatment. Some suggestions that may be helpful are:

Group 1—patients who can care for themselves
Group 2—patients having moderately severe burns but in no immediate danger
Group 3—patients with severe burns who require vigorous therapy
Group 4—individuals with overwhelming burns.*

Specific Treatment. *Fluid Therapy.* The purpose of fluid therapy in the burn casualty is to replace the water, salt and protein which are lost from the circulation, largely into the burned area, and to restore or to maintain adequate plasma volume and urine output.

---

* It has been estimated that the majority of patients to reach the medical aid center will have second degree burns.

Dressings. Use simple sterile dressings for minor burns. The "universal protective dressing"* may be used as a compression dressing for burns as well as for other types of injuries. As a pressure dressing it can be left on for 10 to 12 days. These dressings are available in an emergency from the State Emergency Medical Service for Civil Defense. For burns of face or the perineum, the trunk or the thorax, the exposure method may be used; obviously, a warm clean environment is essential for this method. Tetanus toxoid is given to all patients. If supplies are available, antibiotics are given to patients having wounds that have a high probability of infection.

Respiratory Tract Burns. Burn victims may suffer respiratory tract burns from inhalation of hot air, noxious gases or hot particles. This can be an extremely serious injury. Symptoms of mild injury are hoarseness, sore throat and coughing. For severe injury, laryngeal edema progresses to complete obstruction, dyspnea and cyanosis. Emergency treatment for laryngeal obstruction is tracheotomy, employing postural drainage, suction, and oxygen therapy.

Mass Casualty Management of Burns. *When there are thousands of casualties, the major emphasis is on supporting the patient systemically.* Fluid replacement is given by the oral route. The following solution is an excellent formula for fluid replacement and oral administration of electrolytes.

1 teaspoon salt
½ teaspoon soda
1 quart of water

Patients who can care for themselves can be given this salt and soda to drink and a supply of antibiotic medications to take. The exposure method of treatment is the treatment of choice. These individuals can be encouraged to return to work or· to help in the care of others.

Patients with moderate burns should be given oral fluids and kept undisturbed in a recumbent position to prevent or to treat shock.

When mass casualties are encountered, local burn therapy may have to be delayed. In patients with moderate or severe burns, the burn is covered with the cleanest available material to protect the area from contamination. The original dressings and the patient's clothing should be left undisturbed, as these offer some protection from infection.

It has been found that even severely burned patients can be evacuated if the evacuation is done within a reasonable length of time after the injury. Patients with severe burns should be evacuated as soon as possible to areas where intravenous therapy and

* This cellulose-pad dry dressing was approved by the National Research Council, Subcommittee on Burns, and has been adopted by the Department of Defense and FCDA.

trained teams can institute the treatment that they require.

Principles of Burn Management.

1. Relieve pain with analgesics and sedation and attempt to make patient as comfortable as possible
2. Assess for shock, pulmonary edema and blood in the urine
3. Estimate carefully or measure intake and output
4. Replace fluids by way of oral route or parenterally, as patient's condition indicates
5. Cleanse flash and flame burns with gentle surface cleaning and apply sterile dressings
6. Check dressings for signs of constriction
7. Give antibiotics and tetanus prophylaxis as indicated
8. Encourage patient to take fluids as ordered
9. Reassure patient and make him as comfortable as possible

Craniocerebral Injuries

Approximately 15 to 20 per cent of patients coming to emergency rooms for treatment have some form of craniocerebral trauma. Craniocerebral injuries are classified as (1) open or (2) closed injuries. The brain is very sensitive to lack of oxygen. Hypoxia of the brain, which leads to increased intracranial pressure, is the most frequent cause of death after head injury. In the initial evaluation of the patient, the treatment of respiratory insufficiency (clearing the airway, endotracheal intubation, tracheostomy) has first priority. Adequacy of brain oxygenation may be determined, in part, by the patient's level of response or consciousness; this is the most important indication of the patient's condition. The level of response, when the patient is first assessed, should be described in exact terms so that it may serve as a basis for comparison as the patient's condition changes. For example, the admission data might read "alert and talking," "confused but states his name when asked," "drowsy and moans when spoken to," etc. A deterioration in the level of consciousness is an indication for surgical intervention, since compression of the brain may be rapidly fatal. Other indications of patient deterioration are slowing of pulse, alterations in vital signs, pupillary changes and loss of motor function and reflexes. Patients with signs of increasing intracranial pressure and with large open head wounds should be taken to surgery immediately. (See pp. 815-821 for a more complete discussion.)

Principles of Craniocerebral Injury Management.

1. Maintain the airway and exchange of air
   A. Keep the patient prone (or semiprone) with head to one side

B. Clear the respiratory passages
C. Insert intraoral airway
D. Perform mouth-to-mouth breathing if required. (In hospital, use appropriate form of assisted ventilation.)
E. Perform tracheostomy if indicated
F. Administer oxygen if available
2. Stop bleeding
3. Evaluate level of response and reassess at frequent intervals
   A. Ascertain the patient's response to commands ("stick out your tongue," etc.)
   B. Pinch Achilles tendon or other body site to assess spinal motor reflexes
   C. Evaluate changes in vital signs

Mass Management of Casualties. In the event of large numbers of craniocerebral injuries, as from a thermonuclear catastrophe, casualties who have critical head injuries could not receive the time-consuming surgical and medical care needed. These patients would be assigned to expectant treatment so that personnel and facilities could be provided for the largest number of individuals possible. Those patients who can tolerate delayed treatment should have head wounds cleansed and dressings applied until more definitive treatment is available.

Eye Injuries*

Wounds. Blunt trauma to the eye is the most common direct ocular injury. It is not always possible to distinguish between a minor and a major injury when the patient is first seen. What may appear minor evidence of external injury may be associated with severe intraocular damage. Therefore, the first principle of treatment is *do no harm*. Suspect a penetrating ocular injury with every eye wound until it is proved otherwise. Tiny penetrating foreign particles may not cause immediate symptoms but can produce blindness later from degenerative changes. Never remove anything actually embedded in the eye. Apply a light dressing to the injured eye and refer the patient at once to an ophthalmologist. If the injury is severe the patient should be transported on a stretcher.

Chemical Burns. Chemical burns may be either alkali or acid in nature; both types cause intense pain and inflammation. The *first action is to irrigate the eye with copious amounts of water* for at least 5 minutes, and repeat every 15 to 20 minutes until the patient is seen by an ophthalmologist. (Holding the patient's head and eye directly under running water is the best way to irrigate the eye when immediate irrigation is required.)

* See also page 727.

Superficial Foreign Bodies and Abrasions of Cornea and Conjunctiva. In these conditions, the patient complains of a "scratchy" feeling that becomes increasingly painful. (As the patient blinks, the corneal irritation increases.) A superficial foreign body should be removed at once by irrigation or lifted out with a moistened sterile applicator. Abrasions of the cornea are painful, and the patient may require a systemic analgesic agent.

Mass Casualty Treatment. The highest priority for evacuation of ophthalmologic patients is given to those with intraocular injuries and perforating wounds of the eyeball.

Principles of Mass Management of Eye Injuries.

1. Prevent infection and shock
2. Prevent further injury to the eyes
3. Apply dressings and bandages gently and *lightly*
4. Occlude both eyes when one is seriously injured
5. Keep the patient at rest when both eyes are seriously injured
6. Evacuate casualties with severe eye injuries on litters

Orthopedic Emergencies (See also pp. 840-863.)

The immediate management of a fracture may determine the patient's outcome and make the difference between recovery or disability. In examining for fracture, handle the part gently and as little as possible. Evaluate for pain over or near a bone, swelling (from tissue infiltration of blood, lymph and exudate), and circulatory disturbance. Keep in mind that the patient may have multiple fractures accompanied by head, chest and other serious injuries.

Principles of Fracture Management

1. Control hemorrhage and prevent and treat shock if present
2. Immobilize the patient when a fracture is suspected
3. Apply the splint before the patient is moved. ("Splint 'em where they lie")
   A. Immobilize the joint above and below the fracture
   B. Extend the splints well beyond the joints adjacent to the fracture
   C. Use the patient's clothing for padding (tie, shirt) if nothing else is available
   D. Use newspapers, magazines, pillows, tree limbs and boards for splints if necessary
   E. Splint joints in functional positions
4. Observe the circulation in the affected part by checking for warmth, color and pulsation
5. Investigate any complaint of pain or pressure
6. Transport the patient carefully and gently

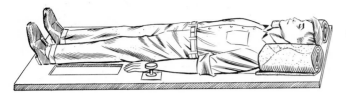

FIG. 38-7. Transporting a patient with a cervical injury of the spine. While transporting patient, assign someone to stabilize the patient's head.

Guidelines to Emergency Splinting and Transporting.

1. Skull—Elevate the head slightly. Transport with head to one side to promote drainage of mucus, blood, vomitus.
2. Jaw—Hold jaw up and in by tying with bandage. Transport in a sitting position with head slightly forward.
3. Cervical spine—Hold the patient's head, keeping it in line with the body. Slide the patient on a rigid surface *flat on his back, face up.* The entire body is moved as a unit. Avoid twisting, turning or pulling of the spine (Fig. 38-7).

   Immobilize the head on each side with padded stones, bricks, sandbags, etc. Assign someone to keep head immobilized while transporting.
4. Lumbar spine—Straighten patient carefully and place him on a rigid surface. If a rigid surface is not available, transport him face down on a blanket using at least 4 persons.
5. Pelvis—Turn the patient carefully on his back. Immobilize the pelvis by binding a folded blanket around the pelvis. Place padding between the legs and splint them together to prevent unnecessary motion. Transport on a stretcher (Fig. 38-8).
6. Shoulder, Arm and Elbow—Place elbow at right angle and apply sling. Bind arm and sling to body with a circular bandage or binder. Allow patient to walk (if able) to evacuation area.
7. Forearm, Wrist, Hand—Immobilize with news-

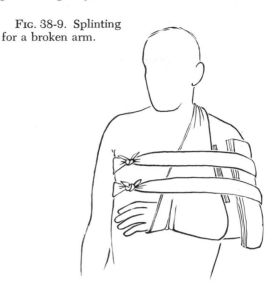

FIG. 38-9. Splinting for a broken arm.

paper splint (or other suitable splinting apparatus) and place in sling. Allow patient to walk to evacuation center if able (Fig. 38-9).
8. Hip—Splint from axilla to ankle with board or bind legs together. Use Thomas splint if available. Transport on a stretcher.

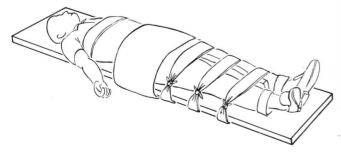

FIG. 38-8. Emergency splinting of a pelvic fracture. Immobilize the pelvis as much as possible.

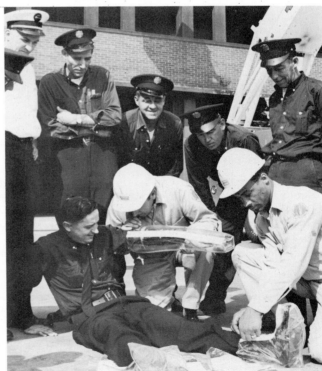

FIG. 38-10. Ambulance crew practicing with application of plastic air splints. (Mine Safety Appliance Company)

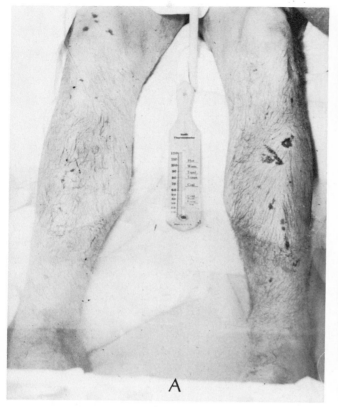
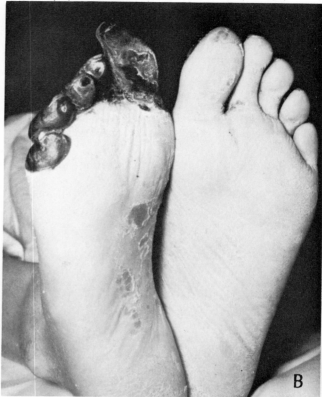

FIG. 38-11. (A) The simple technique used for rapid rewarming. The padding on the tub prevents further injury. The water, which covers the entire frozen area, is maintained between 103° and 107.5° F. by adding warm water. (B) Typical appearance of frostbite. The gangrene, which gives the toes a shriveled and blackened appearance, proved to be superficial. The eschar eventually sloughed and amputation was unnecessary. (Thomas E. Starzl, M.D.: Consultant, January, 1967. Smith Kline & French Laboratories)

9. Lower extremity—Apply steady even traction and splint fracture from hip to ankle. Transport on stretcher.

Mass Management of Fractures. Uncomplicated fractures are low in priority of treatment. Fractures complicated by vascular injury and marked displacement that predisposes to shock and severe injury should have more immediate treatment. With overwhelming numbers of patients, the simple splinting of fractures is done with any material available. Even tying the legs together will serve to splint a broken leg. Hemorrhage has to be controlled, and wounds have to be dressed. The extremity can be elevated to lessen swelling. After 2 or 3 days, sufficient help probably will be available to put more definitive plans of treatment into effect. At this time patients with open fractures are among those selected for early treatment. Tetanus prophylaxis and antibiotic therapy is instituted.

Cold Injury

When a disaster occurs under freezing-weather conditions, the problem may be complicated even further by cold injury. Casualties, whether seriously traumatized or not, may become injured by cold during evacuation if they are immobilized or inadequately clothed. To prevent injury, armored and insulated boots are available.

Hypothermia. In hypothermia there is a progressive deterioration with ataxia, dysarthria, drowsiness and, eventually, coma. Shivering is suppressed below a temperature of 30° C. (86° F.). Below this temperature the body's self-warming mechanisms become ineffective. The heart beat and the blood pressure may be so weak that the peripheral pulsation becomes undetectable. To determine whether the victim is still alive, check his pupillary light reflex and tendon reflexes, all of which remain active until shortly before death.

Rewarming for Hypothermia. The safest and the

best technique for rewarming is still controversial; however, it is generally agreed that artificial ventilation is essential. At temperatures below 30° C.* cardiac irregularities may occur; therefore, it seems advisable to raise the temperature to 30°* to 32° C.† without delay. Thereafter the warming process should be achieved slowly over many hours. Patients who have been severely hypothermic are seriously ill with considerable instability in thermoregulation and vasomotor control; hence they should be observed for 20 or 30 days after restoration to a normothermic state.

Local Cold Injury. This may be of two types: (1) nonfreezing cold injury—"immersion foot" or "trench foot"—and (2) frostbite.

The objectives of therapy are to restore circulation to the part and to relieve vasospasm. *Rapid rewarming* of the affected extremities is now the treatment of choice. The part is immersed in water 40 to 42° C. (104° to 107.5° F.). The temperature of the water is controlled by adding warm water as necessary. After rewarming, the patient is placed on bed rest and given antibiotics and vasodilator drugs. If no bleeding injury is present, heparin may be given.

Follow up study of patients with frostbite reveal that many continue to suffer from cold feet in winter, numbness, pain, sweating of extremities and impairment of joint function. After a patient has been treated for frostbite, he should be warned to avoid subsequent exposure to cold.

Principles of Management of Local Cold Injury.

1. For involvement of lower extremities, do not allow individual to walk but transport otherwise
2. Remove all constrictive clothing
3. Rewarm extremity rapidly by immersing in water (40 to 42° C.; 103 to 107.5° F.)
4. Sterile, dry loose dressings should be applied
5. Keep body warm and encourage patient to sleep and to rest

Radiation Injury

Radiation injury ranges from acute effects to long-term genetic disturbances. Radiation affects the critical tissues of the blood-forming system, the epithelial lining of the gastrointestinal tract and other mucosal areas and the nervous system. In mass casualties caused by thermonuclear warfare, it would be difficult to determine how much radiation a person has absorbed. Under such conditions, incoming patients would be monitored for radioactive contaminants on clothing, on body surfaces, in wounds and in body exudates. This is a measure to protect both the patient

* 86° F.
† 89.6° F.

TABLE 38-1. The patient with a cold injury

Conditions	Factors
Chilblains	Above freezing High humidity
Trench foot	Above freezing Damp environment Immobilization
Immersion foot	Exposure of foot Temperature below 10° C. (50° F.)
Frostbite	Freezing temperature Crystallization of tissue fluids Time: minutes to hours
Space frostbite	High altitude Low temperature May be instantaneous

Clinical manifestations			
1st degree:	Hyperemia Edema Skin peeling Slight swelling Redness Mild cyanosis	3rd degree:	Vesicles Edema Black, hard dry eschar Shrivelling toes
2nd degree:	Redness and slight swelling Vesicles Black eschars	4th degree:	Destruction of entire area involved Gangrene

and personnel caring for him. Standard decontamination procedures exist for disposing of a casualty's clothing, cleaning body surfaces and irrigating open wounds.

Radiation casualties may arrive at the emergency medical center hours or days after radiation exposure, since acute signs and symptoms may not be manifested immediately. If the casualty has been exposed sufficiently to produce symptoms, his symptoms would range from transient weakness to prolonged vomiting, diarrhea and collapse. Table 38-2 shows the relationship between the radiation dose and expected symptomatology.

Treatment. The treatment given is symptomatic. Parenteral fluids and electrolytes are administered to replace fluid losses due to diarrhea, vomiting and profuse sweating. Vomiting may be controlled with antiemetics and intravenous fluids. Antibiotics, in larger than usual doses, are used to control infection. The nutritional status is supported with a high protein and high vitamin diet if tolerated. If not, the patient is fed parenterally. Supportive measures are administered as the various symptoms are encountered.

TABLE 38-2. Summary of clinical symptoms of radiation sickness*

Time after exposure	Survival improbable (700 r or more)	Survival possible (550 r to 300 r)	Survival probable (250 r to 100 r)
1st week	Nausea, vomiting and diarrhea in first few hours No definite symptoms in some cases (latent period)	Nausea, vomiting and diarrhea in first few hours	Possibly nausea, vomiting and diarrhea on first day
2nd week	Diarrhea Hemorrhage Purpura Inflammation of mouth and throat Fever Rapid emaciation Death (mortality probably 100%)	No definite symptoms (latent period) Epilation Loss of appetite and general malaise Fever	No definite symptoms (latent period)
3rd week		Hemorrhage Purpura Petechiae Nosebleeds Pallor Inflammation of mouth and throat Diarrhea Emaciation	Epilation Loss of appetite and malaise Sore throat Hemorrhage Purpura Petechiae Pallor Diarrhea Moderate emaciation
4th week		Death in most serious cases (mortality 50% for 450 r)	Recovery likely in about 3 months unless complicated by poor previous health or superimposed injuries or infections

*Glasstone, S.: The Effects of Nuclear Weapons, p. 477. United States Atomic Energy Commission.

PSYCHOLOGICAL MANAGEMENT OF PATIENTS IN EMERGENCY-DISASTER SITUATIONS

In dealing with patients who are under unusual emotional strain and stress, the nurse must look at her own psychological defenses. Through an understanding of herself the nurse is better able to cope with and to control her own anxieties in an emergency situation.

Certain patterns of individual reactions are common in disaster. By the application of basic principles the nurse is able to administer emergency medical care to injured individuals. By a similar application of psychological principles the nurse is in a better position to understand herself, her colleagues and casualties.

The American Psychiatric Association Committee on Civil Defense has identified 5 types of reactions to disaster and offers 4 basic principles for better understanding of the emotionally disturbed person.

Reactions to Disaster*

1. Normal—Some obvious signs of disturbance are shown, such as trembling, profuse perspiring, feeling weak and even nauseated. Composure is gained fairly soon after the first impact of a trying experience.

2. Individual panic—Judgment seems to disappear and to be supplanted by an unreasoning attempt to flee. This type of reaction occurs in a very few individuals; its danger lies in the fact that it can excite others and may result in mass panic.

3. Depressed reactions—These individuals react as

* Adapted from the American Psychiatric Association, Committee on Civil Defense: Psychological First Aid in Community Disasters. Washington, The Association, 1954.

though they were numbed; they are unable to help themselves without guidance.

4. Overly active responses—These responses are poorly directed, because the individual is easily distracted as he jumps from one task to another. Often he is intolerant of any ideas other than his own and may cause disturbances.

5. Bodily reactions—Severe nausea and vomiting, hysteria.

Four Basic Principles for Better Understanding of the Emotionally Disturbed Person

1. Accept Every Person's Right to Have His Own Feelings. Remember that each person has had certain unique experiences that can strongly affect his feelings in relation to subsequent events in his life. Years of analysis may often fail to explain fully *why* a person feels as he does. Letting a casualty know that you want to understand *how* he feels can be the first step toward helping him. Establish contact with him; do not overwhelm him with pity nor deprive him of *his* world, which appears to have collapsed.

2. Accept a Casualty's Limitations as Real. Then treat him as a potentially valuable member of the disaster team. He cannot be expected to function normally; therefore, there is no place for such remarks as "Pull yourself together," or "Snap out of it." The nurse should guard against being impatient, which may result from fatigue and resentment.

3. Size up a casualty's potentialities as accurately and as quickly as possible. The person caring for the casualty should act immediately while the patient is still suggestible, as anxiety tends to increase unless the situation is dealt with quickly and decisively. A calm, reassuring person will help the emotionally disturbed individual to mobilize his own psychological resources. Direct the casualty away from the area. Provide for a brief rest period of one or several hours. As soon as possible, give him something to do. The axiom "Action absorbs anxiety" has definite application in the management of frightened individuals.

4. Accept Your Own Limitations in a Relief Role. Know your own weaknesses well enough to handle them in a time of crisis. Are you impulsive, easily angered, sensitive to criticism, and so forth? By understanding yourself reasonably well, you may hope justifiably to control and even to divert reactions into some more effective channel.

Psychological first aid can help many emotionally disturbed victims to get back into useful activity more quickly. Sedatives never are administered to psychological casualties except as a last resort, and then the administration is done only on the consultation with a physician. Sedation would only add to

the casualty's confusion and make him even more inaccessible to more effective treatment.

Special Psychological Problems

Fatigue. It is important to recognize fatigue in one's self and coworkers. This is a common product in a disaster situation and may be heralded by evidence of mounting tension.

Shelter Living. This presents many unique problems that can complicate the disaster situation. Material is available to assist the nurse in shelter organization and management. She needs to be able to recognize and to manage psychological disturbances that result from confined living.

IMPROVISATION AND RESOURCEFULNESS

When the principles of medical emergency management are clearly understood, one does not need hospital equipment in order to function effectively. By using imagination and ingenuity, many commonplace items can be used by the first-aider. Resourcefulness is an essential component of emergency and disaster nursing. Sloane* states that in emergency nursing, students are not taught the types of bandages that are seldom used today. Instead, they learn to improvise pressure bandages from bias-cut sheeting, cross-cut T-shirts and old stockings, and they learn to apply triangle, cravat and stocking bandages. A good exercise for the nurse is to take the patient's temperature, pulse and respiration merely by observing him and by touching his skin, then to take the readings in the conventional way and to compare the results. With practice, the nurse can become quite adept in her evaluations.

POISONING

Acute Poisoning

Poisoning from the inhalation and the ingestion of toxic materials, both accidental and by design, constitutes a major health hazard. The problem is one of real magnitude as reflected in the number of cases and the number of deaths at different ages due to specific poisons. More than one million cases of poisoning occur in the U.S. annually. Three thousand of these patients die.

Approximately one half of all poison ingestions involve drugs; other products that are commonly implicated include household preparations, pesticides and petroleum distillates Preschool-age children have accounted for over 80 per cent of all poison cases and

---

* Sloane, A.: Disaster nursing in the curriculum. Nurs. Outlook 5(2):75-77, Feb., 1957.

TABLE 38-3. Examples of improvised equipment

Needs	Improvised equipment
Making holes in rubbers:	Large nails, safety pins, forceps, wire, pen knives, nail files
Cleaning aids:	Pipe cleaners (to clean hollow tubing), soap and water, linen, old clothing and paper, sand, abrasion creams and beauty aids
Sealing bandages:	Cellophane tape, adhesive, putty, wax
Fire:	Wood, paper, waste materials, wood shavings, alcohol lamps, gasoline stoves, glass over paper and sun, fuel oil and kerosene, hair tonics
Refrigeration:	Seal a bottle, place it in cold water, place moistened net over bottle; dig a hole in ground (9 feet); ice wrapped in newspaper
Marking:	Charred material, ink, pencils, lipstick
Picking up hot materials:	Scissors, tweezers, coat hangers
Restraints:	Canvas, raincoats, plastics, clothing
A bed for a casualty:	6 or 8 straight chairs fastened together. They even have built-in side rails. Chairs might be available from hotels, schools, or an undertaking establishment
A crib for a child:	Arm chairs tied together
An occlusive burn dressing:	Soft, absorbent bath towels encased in an old pillow case. Wash clothes in old muslin will do well for smaller burns
A makeshift autoclave:	A household pressure cooker or a pressure canner. Materials will have to be oven-dried after sterilization

Materials	Uses
Cardboard and cardboard boxes:	Mattress, beds, baby cribs, tables Oxygen tents Shade, screening Trays, waste containers, bedpans Props and supports, splints
Rubber tubing:	Tourniquets, holding splints, traction Drinking straws, catheters, rectal and enema tubing, drains, airways, suction, oxygen tubing and infusions
Rubber stoppers:	Tops for infusion bottles, airtight storage, suction apparatus, enema apparatus (bottle, plus top)
Bottles:	Drinking water, storage, water bottle Urinals, enema apparatus, suction equipment, chest drainage bottles, specimens Bottle filled with sand may be used for traction and weights
Paper:	Warmth, padding, protective covers for heat and cold, splints, plaster casts, protection of surfaces Absorption—towels, toilet paper, diapers Wrapping—sterile dressings, waste Containers—food, drinking cups, waste containers Fire starters
Tin cans:	Containers for water, storage, cooking, dishes and drinking Containers for specimens, emesis basins, bedpans, enema cans, waste Shovels Bed blocks
Rope and string:	Ties, traction, holding bandages, splints, restraints, and tagging
Plastic bottles and bags:	Many of the above uses

almost one third of all accidental deaths due to poisoning.

Principles of Poisoning Management.

1. Give immediate supportive treatment, paying particular attention to respiratory and circulatory states (p. 277) and organs of excretion and detoxification

2. Remove the poison from the patient's body
3. Give the appropriate antidote

Emergency Management of Patients With Poisoning. The following instructions are those proposed by the Committee of Toxicology of the American Medical Association.* These refer to emergency measures to

* Committee on Toxicology, *J.A.M.A., 165*:686-688, 1957.

be taken as soon as a poisoning has been discovered, and they specify the precautions that are indicated for the prevention of poisoning accidents.

The steps listed below are to be taken with all possible speed.

Save the poison container and any contents that may remain. If the identity of the poison is not known, save a sample of vomitus.

1. Swallowed Poisons:

In all cases, *except those indicated below*, REMOVE POISON FROM PATIENT'S STOMACH IMMEDIATELY BY INDUCING VOMITING. (See B,2 below.) This cannot be overemphasized, for it is the essence of the treatment and is often a life-saving procedure. Prevent chilling by wrapping patient in blankets if necessary. Do not give alcohol in any form.

A. Do Not Induce Vomiting If:
  1. Patient is in coma or unconscious
  2. Patient is in convulsions
  3. Patient has swallowed petroleum products (i.e., kerosene, gasoline, lighter fluid)
  4. Patient has swallowed a corrosive poison (symptoms: severe pain, burning sensation in mouth and throat, vomiting)
  CALL PHYSICIAN IMMEDIATELY

  (a) Acid and acidlike corrosives: sodium acid sulfate (toilet bowl cleaners), acetic acid (glacial), sulfuric acid, nitric acid, oxalic acid, hydrofluoric acid (rust removers), iodine, silver nitrate (styptic pencil)
  (b) Alkali corrosives: sodium hydroxide—lye (drain cleaners), sodium carbonate (washing soda), ammonia water, sodium hypochlorite (household bleach)
  (c) If the patient can swallow after ingesting a *corrosive poison,* the following substances (and amounts) may be given:
    For acids: milk, water or milk of magnesia (1 tablespoon to 1 cup of water)
    For alkalies: milk, water, any fruit juice or vinegar (1 to 2 cups for patients aged 1 to 5, or up to 1 quart for individuals 5 years old or older)

B. Induce Vomiting When Noncorrosive Substances Have Been Swallowed:
  1. Give milk or water (for patient from 1 to 5 years old—1 to 2 cups; for patient over 5 years—up to 1 quart)
  2. Induce vomiting by placing the blunt end of a spoon or your finger at the back of the patient's throat, or by use of an emetic— such as syrup of ipecac or mustard. When retching and vomiting begin, place patient face down with head lower than hips. This prevents vomitus from entering the lungs and causing further damage. Gastric lavage is a thorough way to evacuate the stomach.

2. Inhaled Poisons:
  A. Carry patient to fresh air immediately
  B. Open all doors and windows
  C. Loosen all tight clothing
  D. Apply artificial respiration if breathing has stopped or is irregular
  E. Prevent chilling (wrap patient in blankets)
  F. Keep patient as quiet as possible
  G. If patient is convulsing, keep him in bed in a semidark room; avoid jarring or noise
  H. Do not give alcohol in any form

3. Skin Contamination:
  A. Drench skin with water (shower, hose, faucet)
  B. Apply stream of water on skin while removing clothing
  C. Cleanse skin thoroughly with water; rapidity in washing is most important in reducing extent of injury

4. Eye Contamination:
  A. Hold eyelids open, wash eyes with gentle stream of running water *immediately.* Delay of a few seconds greatly increases extent of injury
  B. Wash until physician arrives
  C. *Do not use chemicals;* they may increase extent of injury

5. Injected Poisons (scorpion and snake bites):
  The objectives are to remove as much venom as possible and to retard the spread of venom.
  A. Make patient lie down as soon as possible
  B. Do not give alcohol in any form
  C. Apply tourniquet above injection site (e.g., between arm or leg and heart). The pulse in vessels below the tourniquet should not disappear, nor should the tourniquet produce a throbbing sensation. Tourniquet should be loosened for 1 minute every 15 minutes.
  D. Make linear incisions through the fang marks
  E. Apply suction to remove venom
  F. Apply icepack to the site of the bite
  G. Carry patient to physician or hospital; DO NOT LET HIM WALK.

6. Chemical Burns:
  A. Wash with large quantities of running water (except those caused by phosphorus)
  B. Immediately cover with loosely applied clean cloth

C. Avoid use of ointments, greases, powders and other drugs in first-aid treatment of burns

D. Treat shock by keeping patient flat, keeping him warm and reassuring him until arrival of physician

Measures to Prevent Poisoning Accidents

1. Keep all drugs, poisonous substances and household chemicals out of the reach of children.

2. Do not store nonedible products on shelves used for storing food.

3. Keep all poisonous substances in their original containers; do not transfer to unlabeled containers.

4. When medicines are discarded, destroy them. Do not throw them where they might be reached by children or pets.

5. When giving flavored and/or brightly colored medicine to children, *always* refer to it as medicine— *never* as candy.

6. Do not take or give medicine in the dark.

7. *READ LABELS* before using chemical products.

Barbiturate Poisoning. This accounts for approximately 50 per cent of all deaths caused by drug ingestion. It has been estimated that more than 50,000 such cases are hospitalized each year in this country, a large proportion of these being instances of attempted suicide.

The picture is one of stupor, or coma, and respiratory depression; mental response, if obtained at all, is quite adequate, although slow; the face is flushed, the pupils dilated, the reflexes usually depressed. Death can occur, due to cerebral edema, respiratory failure or pneumonia (not an uncommon sequela). Practically all these patients can be saved, despite a huge dose of the drug—even 19.2 Gm (300 grains) and more—if the proper measures are instituted within a few hours of the time of ingestion.

Treatment. The treatment consists of gastric lavage, to remove any drug still remaining in the stomach, and nervous system stimulation. Gastric lavage may be carried out by stomach tube, using water, or by induced vomiting (see B, p. 965).

The most important aspect of treatment is supportive therapy, including measures for the stimulation of the depressed respiration, artificial respiration, if necessary, circulatory stimulants, maintenance of fluid and electrolyte balance, close observation and good nursing care. Supportive care is the major treatment.

The role of analeptic drugs in barbiturate poisoning is still not settled; some centers use them while others do not. Recently, Ritalin has been used with appa-

rent success. Hemodialysis with the artificial kidney clears the bloodstream of barbiturates very rapidly and reduces the duration of coma induced by the long-acting preparations.

Morphine Poisoning

Morphine in overdosage may cause death through respiratory failure. The respiratory rate of a patient receiving morphine therapy must be followed carefully, and the proper measures should be taken if the rate drops below 10 or 12 per minute. Acute morphinism is suspected in all patients in coma with pinpoint pupils and slow respiration.

Treatment. A specific antidote for morphine is available in the form of N-allylnormorphine. Given intravenously in doses of 5 to 20 mg., it counteracts practically every effect of morphine within a period of 1 to 2 minutes. The respiratory rate is restored to normal with great regularity within 10 to 20 seconds after intravenous injection, the respirations thereafter becoming more rapid for a time. Consciousness is restored only partially, if at all, in response to N-allylnormorphine. The circulatory status is improved to a degree commensurate with the respiratory function.

Carbon Monoxide Poisoning

This may occur as an industrial or a household accident, or by design in attempted suicide. The most common source is atmosphere containing an appreciable concentration of automobile exhaust gases, such as might develop, for example, in a closed garage. A concentration of carbon monoxide as low as 0.03 per cent is potentially dangerous. The effect of carbon monoxide is to render the hemoglobin useless as an oxygen-carrying chemical, because it unites so firmly with the pigment in place of oxygen. One liter of the gas is sufficient to combine with all the blood in the body.

The chief signs and symptoms of this poisoning are due to failure of the body tissues to obtain oxygen, from which lack the nervous system suffers first and most severely. These symptoms include headache, lassitude, drowsiness and coma. The skin color usually is pink. Neuritis, tremor, psychoses, spastic paralyses and visual disturbances may persist following resuscitation.

Treatment. This consists in stimulating, as rapidly as possible, the inhalation of atmosphere of high-oxygen concentration, such as with the use of a 95 per cent oxygen—5 per cent carbon dioxide mixture delivered with a closed mask, with the help of artificial respiration (but not a positive-pressure device) if necessary.

Tranquilizer Intoxication

The phenothiazine group (Thorazine, Compazine, Trilafon, Prolixin, Mellaril) may cause cholestatic jaundice, blood dyscrasias, mental depression, extrapyramidal symptoms (Parkinson's syndrome), acute torticollis, oculogyric crisis, tonic spasms of an extremity, extreme restlessness, insomnia, and in large overdoses, coma and hypotension. After gastric lavage, the management is supportive. Levophed and Neosynephrine are the pressor agents of choice.

Reserpine and other rauwolfia compounds may have a cumulative effect leading to mental depression and a coma state in which the patient appears to be sleeping. The patient's pupils are small and he breathes through his mouth because of his nasal congestion. This state may go on several days after stopping the drug. Treatment consists of stopping the drug and giving supportive care.

Large doses of meprobamate may cause coma and vasomotor collapse and on withdrawal after chance addiction, convulsions may occur. Gastric lavage, supportive therapy and if necessary, analeptic agents are given.

Librium and Valium can cause confusion and ataxia and in large overdose, coma and hypotension. Gastric lavage and supportive therapy are used. Pressor agents such as Levophed or Aramine may be needed. Ritalin has been used to help lighten the coma or somnolence.

Sedative Overdosage

Glutethimide (Doriden) is a sedative which, in overdosage, can cause coma and death. The findings are coma, hypothermia followed by fever, tachycardia, hypotension and decreased deep tendon reflexes, dilated and fixed pupils and depressed respirations. Gastric lavage is performed. Supportive therapy consists of pressor agents, assisted respiration (p. 282) and if necessary, hemodialysis (p. 553). In chronic intoxication, withdrawal is accompanied by central nervous system effects, including at times convulsions.

Salicylate Poisoning

Salicylate poisoning, of which aspirin is a common example, is manifested at first by tinnitus and vertigo followed by nausea, vomiting, headache, mental aberration, hyperventilation and coma. Occasionally one sees restlessness and talkativeness—the so-called "salicylate jag." Ketoacidosis develops and hyponatremia appears.

Therapy consists of gastric lavage, supportive treatment with intravenous fluids and combatting acidosis with sodium bicarbonate or sodium lactate parenterally. Peritoneal dialysis (p. 554) or hemodialysis (p. 553) have been successfully used in severe cases.

BIBLIOGRAPHY

Books

American Hospital Association: Readings in Disaster Planning for Hospitals. Chicago, The Association, 1966.
American National Red Cross: Disaster Handbook for Physicians and Nurses. 1966.
American Nurses Association: ANA Guidelines: Nursing in National Defense. New York, ANA, 1962.
———: The Role of the Nurse in National Disaster. Washington, D. C., U. S. Dept. of H.E.W., 1965.
Bailey, H.: Emergency Surgery. Bristol, John Wright Ltd., 1967.
Ballinger, F. F., *et al.*: The Management of Trauma. Philadelphia, W. B. Saunders, 1968.
Cole, W. H., and Puestow, C. B.: First Aid. Diagnosis and Management. New York, Appleton-Century-Crofts, 1965.
Curry, G. J.: Immediate Care and Transport of the Injured. Springfield, Charles C Thomas, 1965.
Eckert, C.: Emergency Room Care. Boston, Little, Brown, 1967.
Garb, S., and Eng, E.: Disaster Handbook. New York, Springer, 1964.
Grosser, G. H., *et al.*: The Threat of Impending Disaster. Cambridge, The M.I.T. Press, 1964.
Henderson, J.: Emergency Medical Guide. New York, McGraw-Hill, 1963.
Flint, T.: Emergency Treatment and Management. Philadelphia, W. B. Saunders, 1965.
Kennedy, R. H. (ed.): Emergency Care. Philadelphia, W. B. Saunders, 1966.
Mahoney, R. F.: Emergency and Disaster Nursing. New York, Macmillan, 1965.
Nahum, A. M. (ed.): Early Management of Acute Trauma. St. Louis, C. V. Mosby, 1966.
Neal, M. (ed.): Disaster Nursing Preparation. New York, National League for Nursing, 1963.
New England Journal of Medicine: The Management of Emergencies. Boston, Mass. Medical Society, 1966.
Shires, G. T.: Care of the Trauma Patient. New York, McGraw-Hill, 1966.
U. S. Department of Defense: Emergency War Surgery. Washington, D. C., U. S. Government Printing Office, 1959.
U. S. Public Health Service:
   Austere Medical Care for Disasters. 1964.
   Disaster Nursing Preparation in a Basic Professional Program. (Publication No. 1071-D-5) 1965.
   Disaster Nursing Preparation in a Hospital Nursing Service. (Publication No. 1071-D-3) 1965.
   Disaster Nursing Preparation in a Practical Nursing Program. (Publication No. 1071-D-4) 1965.
   Hospital Planning for National Disaster. (Health Mobilization Series G-1) 1968.
   The Packaged Disaster Hospital. (Health Mobilization Series D-6) 1968.
Williams, D. W., *et al.*: Review of Combined Trauma: Research, Clinical Management and Planning. Washington, D. C., U. S. Dept. of Health, Education and Welfare, 1966.

Articles

Adler, L., *et al.*: Anaesthesia for mass casualties. Another possible solution for disaster circumstances, Anaesthesia, *22*:29-36, Jan., 1967.

Arena, J. M. (ed.): The treatment of poisoning. Clinical Symposia, *18*:1-31, Jan.-Feb.-March, 1966.

Costello, D., and Elliman, V. B.: I. Emergency Nursing. II. Disaster Nursing. Nurs. Clin. N. Amer., *2*, June, 1967.

Eicherly, E. E.: Civil defense in a nuclear age. Living and nursing in a fallout shelter. Amer. J. Nurs., *65*:123-125, Nov., 1965.

Giorgi, B.: Emergencies and pain. The role of the occupational nurse. Amer. Assoc. Ind. Nurses J., *14*:17-18, April, 1966.

Grested, N.: Emergency services and first aid: The nurse's point of view. Amer. Assoc. Ind. Nurses J., *14*:19-20, April, 1966.

King, T. C., and Zimmerman, J. M.: First aid cooling of the fresh burn. Surg. Gynec. Obstet., *120*:1271-1273, June, 1965.

Kirk, D.: It was 2:00 A.M. Saigon time. Amer. J. Nurs. *65*:77-79, Dec., 1965.

Magruder, D.: Disaster planning. Hosp. Management, *105*:79-80, May, 1968.

Malone, R. H., *et al.*: Handling a large influx of patients in a disaster situation. Hospitals, *42*:67-70, Feb. 16, 1968.

Sullivan, C. M.: Civil defense in a nuclear age. Preparedness may mean survival. Amer. J. Nurs., *65*:121-123, Nov., 1965.

Walt, A. J., *et al.*: The anatomy of a civil disturbance. Its impact on disaster planning. J.A.M.A., *202*:394-397, 1967.

AGENCIES

Voluntary

The American National Red Cross
Washington, D. C. 20006

Federal

U. S. Dept. of Health, Education and Welfare
Public Health Service
Division of Health Mobilization
Chevy Chase, Maryland 20015

U. S. Dept. of the Army
Office of the Secretary of the Army
Office of Civil Defense
Washington, D. C. 20310

Diagnostic Studies and Their Meaning

- *Normal Values—Hematology*
- *Normal Blood or Serum Values—Chemistry*
- *Normal Values—Urine Chemistry*
- *Normal Values—Cerebrospinal Fluid*
- *Miscellaneous Values*

NORMAL VALUES—HEMATOLOGY

DETERMINATION	NORMAL VALUE	CLINICAL SIGNIFICANCE
Bleeding time	30 sec.-6 min.	Prolonged in purpura hemorrhagica, where platelets are reduced, and in chloroform and phosphorus poisoning
Clotting time	5-10 min.	Prolonged in hemorrhagic disease and in various coagulation factor deficiencies
Factor V assay	75-125%	Pro-accelerin factor
Factor VIII assay (antihemophiliac factor)	50-200%	Deficient in classical hemophilia
Factor IX assay (plasma thromboplastin component)	75-125%	Deficient in Christmas disease (pseudohemophilia)
Factor X (Stuart factor)	75-125%	Stuart clotting defect
Fibrinogen	0.2-0.4 gm./100 ml.	Increased in pregnancy, pneumonia, infections accompanied by leukocytosis,' and nephrosis. Decreased in acute yellow atrophy of liver, cirrhosis, typhoid fever, chloroform poisoning, abruptio placentae
Fibrinolysins (whole blood clot lysis time)	No lysis in 24 hrs.	Increased activity associated with massive hemorrhage, extensive surgery, and transfusion reactions
Partial thromboplastin time (cephalin time)	35-45 sec.	Prolonged in factor VIII, IX, and X deficiency

969

NORMAL VALUES—HEMATOLOGY (*Continued*)

DETERMINATION	NORMAL VALUE	CLINICAL SIGNIFICANCE
Prothrombin consumption	Over 25 sec.	Impaired in factor VIII, IX, and X deficiency
Prothrombin time	70-100% of control	Prolonged in factor X deficiency and other hemorrhagic diseases, and in cirrhosis, hepatitis, and acute toxic necrosis of the liver
Erythrocyte count	Male: 4,600,000-6,200,000 per cu mm. Female: 4,200,000-5,400,000 per cu mm.	Increased in severe diarrhea and dehydration, polycythemia rubra vera, secondary polycythemia, acute poisoning, pulmonary fibrosis, and Ayerza disease. Decreased in all anemias, leukemia, and after hemorrhage, when blood volume has been restored
Erythrocyte sedimentation rate	Male: 0-9 mm./hr. Female: 0-20 mm./hr.	Increased in tissue destruction, whether inflammatory or degenerative, and during menstruation, pregnancy, and in acute febrile diseases
Hematocrit	Male: 42-50% Female: 40-48%	Decreased in severe anemias, anemia of pregnancy, acute massive blood loss. Increased in erythrocytosis of any cause, and in dehydration or hemoconcentration associated with shock
Hemoglobin	Male: 13-16 gm./100 ml. Female: 12-14 gm./100 ml.	Decreased in various anemias, pregnancy, severe or prolonged hemorrhage, and with excessive fluid intake. Increased in polycythemia, chronic obstructive pulmonary diseases, failure of oxygenation because of congestive heart failure, and normally, in people living at high altitudes
Leukocyte count	Total: 5,000-10,000 cu. mm.	Elevated in acute infectious diseases—predominately in the neutrophilic fraction with bacterial diseases, and in the lymphocytic and monocytic fractions in viral diseases. Eosinophils elevated in collagen diseases, allergy, intestinal parasitosis. Elevated in acute leukemia, following menstruation, and following surgery or trauma, Depressed in aplastic anemia, agranulocytosis, and by toxic agents, such as chemotherapeutic agents used in treating malignancy
Neutrophils	60-70%	
Eosinophils	1-4%	
Basophils	0-0.5%	
Lymphocytes	20-30%	
Monocytes	2-6%	
Erythrocyte indices		
Mean corpuscular volume (MCV)	80-94 cu. μ	Increased in macrocytic anemias, decreased in microcytic anemia
Mean corpuscular hemoglobin (MCH)	27-32 $\mu\mu$g. per cell	Increased in macrocytic anemias, decreased in microcytic anemia
Mean corpuscular hemoglobin concentration (MCHC)`	33-38%	Decreased in severe hypochromic anemia
Reticulocytes	0.5-1.5% of red cells	Increased with any condition stimulating increase bone marrow activity, i.e., infection, blood loss (acute and chronic), following iron therapy in iron deficiency anemia, polycythemia rubra vera. Decreased with any condition depressing bone marrow activity, acute leukemia, late stage of severe anemias
Leukocyte alkaline phosphatase	Score of 40-100	Decreased in chronic myelocytic leukemia and chronic lymphocytic leukemia. Increased in nonleukemic leukocytosis and myeloproliferative diseases
Osmotic fragility of red cells	Increase if hemolysis occurs in over 0.5% NaCl. Decrease if hemolysis is incomplete in 0.3% NaCl	Increased in congenital spherocytosis, idiopathic acquired hemolytic anemia, isoimmune hemolytic disease, ABO hemolytic disease of newborn. Decreased in sickle-cell anemia, thalassemia
Platelet count	200,000-350,000 per cu. mm.	Increased with chronic granulocytic leukemia, hemoconcentration. Decreased in thrombocytopenic purpura, acute leukemia, aplastic anemia, and during cancer chemotherapy

NORMAL BLOOD OR SERUM VALUES—CHEMISTRY

DETERMINATION	NORMAL ADULT VALUES	CLINICAL SIGNIFICANCE (Increased)	(Decreased)
Acetoacetate and acetone	0.3-2.0 mg./100 ml.	Diabetic acidosis Fasting Toxemia of pregnancy Carbohydrate-free diet High-fat diet	
Aldolase	3-8 units/ml.	Hepatic necrosis Granulocytic leukemia Myocardial infarction Skeletal muscle disease	
Alpha amino nitrogen	3.0-5.5 mg./100 ml.	Phosphorus, arsenic, chloro-form, carbon tetrachloride poisoning Infectious hepatitis Eclampsia	Pneumococcal pneumonia Administration of anterior pituitary extracts Administration of insulin
Ammonia	50-170 μg./100 ml.*	Severe liver disease Hepatic decompensation	
Amylase	80-150 units/ml.	Acute pancreatitis Mumps Duodenal ulcer Carcinoma of head of pancreas Prolonged elevation with pseudocyst of pancreas	Chronic pancreatitis Pancreatic fibrosis and atrophy Cirrhosis of liver Acute alcoholism Toxemias of pregnancy
Ascorbic acid	0.4-1.5 mg./100 ml.		Rheumatic fever Collagen diseases Deficient vitamin C intake Renal and hepatic disease Congestive heart failure
Bilirubin	Total: 0.1-1.0 mg./100 ml. Direct: 0.1-0.2 mg./100 ml. Indirect: 0.1-0.8 mg./100 ml.	Hemolytic anemia (indirect) Biliary obstruction Hepatocellular damage Pernicious anemia Hemolytic disease of newborn Eclampsia	
Bromsulfalein (BSP)	Less than 5% retention in 45 min.	Acute hepatic diseases	
Calcium	9-11 mg./100 ml.	Tumor or hyperplasia of parathyroid Hyperparathyroidism Hypervitaminosis D Multiple myeloma Nephritis with uremia	Hypoparathyroidism Diarrhea Celiac disease Rickets Osteomalacia Malnutrition Nephrosis After parathyroidectomy
CO_2 content	Adults: 24-32 mEq./L. Infants: 20-26 mEq./L.	Tetany Respiratory disease Intestinal obstruction Vomiting	Acidosis Nephritis Eclampsia Diarrhea Anesthesia

* Whole blood

NORMAL BLOOD OR SERUM VALUES (*Continued*)

DETERMINATION	NORMAL ADULT VALUES	CLINICAL SIGNIFICANCE (Increased)	(Decreased)
Carotene, Beta	100-300 µg./100 ml.	Carotenemia Hypothyroidism Diabetes Hyperlipemia	Malabsorption syndromes Hepatic disease Dietary deficiencies
Cephalin flocculation	Negative to 1+	Severe liver disease Atypical viral pneumonia Malaria Lues Infectious mononucleosis Congestive heart failure	
Ceruloplasmin	0.14-0.57 O.D. units	Pregnancy Myocardial infarction Hepatic cirrhosis	Wilson's disease (hepato-lenticular degeneration)
Chloride	95-105 mEq./L.	Nephritis Urinary obstruction Cardiac decompensation Anemia Ether anesthesia	Diabetes Diarrhea Vomiting Pneumonia Heavy metal poisoning Cushing's syndrome Burns Intestinal obstruction Febrile conditions
Cholesterol	150-270 mg./100 ml.	Lipemia Obstructive jaundice Diabetes Hypothyroidism	Pernicious anemia Hemolytic jaundice Hyperthyroidism Severe infection Terminal states of debilitating disease
Cholesterol esters	65-70% of total		The esterified fraction decreases in liver disease
Cholinesterase	Plasma: 1.15-1.65 units Red cells: 0.65-1.0 units	Nephrosis Exercise	Nerve gas intoxication (greater effect on red cell activity) Insecticides, organic phosphates (greater effect on plasma activity)
Congo red	60-100% retained in bloodstream		Deposits of amyloid in tissue absorb congo red. In amyloid disease, less than 40% of the dye will remain in the plasma. In severe cases, less than 10% is retained
Copper	Males: 97-130 µg./100 ml. Females: 105-140 µg. 100 ml.	Cirrhosis of liver Pregnancy	Wilson's disease
Creatine phosphokinase (CPK)	Male: 0-20 I.U./L. Female: 0-14 I.U./L.	Myocardial infarction Skeletal muscle diseases	
Creatine	3-7 mg./100 ml.	Biliary obstruction Pregnancy Nephritis Renal destruction Trauma to muscle Pseudohypertrophic muscular dystrophy	

NORMAL BLOOD OR SERUM VALUES (*Continued*)

DETERMINATION	NORMAL ADULT VALUES	CLINICAL SIGNIFICANCE	
		(Increased)	(Decreased)
Creatinine	1-2 mg./100 ml.	Nephritis Chronic renal disease	
Cryoglobulin	Zero	Multiple myeloma Chronic lymphocytic leukemia Lymphosarcoma Systemic lupus erythematosus Rheumatoid arthritis Subacute bacterial endocarditis Some malignancies	
Fatty acids	Total: 250-390 mg./100 ml.	Diabetes Anemia Nephrosis Hypothyroidism Nephritis	Hyperthyroidism
Fibrinogen**	0.1-0.4 gm./100 ml.	Pneumonia Acute infections Pregnancy Nephrosis Carcinoma	Cirrhosis Acute toxic necrosis of liver Anemia Typhoid fever Chloroform or phosphorus poisoning Abruptio placentae
Glucose	65-110 mg./100 ml.	Diabetes Nephritis Hyperthyroidism Early hyperpituitarism Cerebral lesions Infections Pregnancy Uremia	Hyperinsulinism Hypothyroidism Late hyperpituitarism Pernicious vomiting Addison's disease Extensive hepatic damage
Icterus index	1-6 units	Biliary obstruction Hemolytic anemias	Secondary anemias
Iodine, protein-bound	4.0-8.0 μg./100 ml.	Hyperthyroidism	Hypothyroidism
Iron	65-150 μg./100 ml.	Pernicious anemia Aplastic anemia Hemolytic anemia Hepatitis Hemochromatosis	Iron deficiency anemia
Iron binding capacity	150-225 μg./100 ml.	Iron deficiency anemia	Chronic infectious diseases
Lactic acid*	6-16 mg./100 ml.	Increased muscular activity Congestive heart failure Hemorrhage Shock	
Lactic dehydrogenase (LDH)	60-100 units/ml.	Untreated pernicious anemia Myocardial infarction Pulmonary infarction Liver disease	

* Whole blood

** Plasma

NORMAL BLOOD OR SERUM VALUES (*Continued*)

DETERMINATION	NORMAL VALUE	CLINICAL SIGNIFICANCE (Increased)	(Decreased)
Leucine aminopeptidase	1-3 micromoles/hr./ml.	Liver or biliary tract diseases Pancreatic disease Metastatic carcinoma of liver and pancreas Biliary obstruction	
Lipase	0.2-1.5 units/ml.	Acute and chronic pancreatitis Biliary obstruction Cirrhosis Hepatitis Peptic ulcer	
Total lipids	400-1000 mg./100 ml.	Hypothyroidism Diabetes Nephrosis Glomerulonephritis	Hyperthyroidism
Phospholipids	125-300 mg./100 ml.	Diabetes Nephritis	
Magnesium	1.8-2.2 mEq./L.	Ingestion of epsom salts Parathyroidectomy	Chronic alcoholism Toxemia of pregnancy Severe renal disease
Nonprotein nitrogen	20-35 mg./100 ml.	Acute nephritis Polycystic kidneys Obstructive uropathy Peritonitis Congestive heart failure Pregnancy	
Osmolality	285-295 milliosmoles/L.		Inappropriate secretion of anti- diuretic hormone
Oxygen saturation, arterial*	96-100%	Polycythemia Anhydremia	Anemia Cardiac decompensation Chronic obstructive pulmonary disease
pCO_2*	35-45 mm. Hg.	Respiratory acidosis Metabolic alkalosis	Respiratory alkalosis Metabolic acidosis
pH*	7.35-7.45	Vomiting Hyperpnea Fever Intestinal obstruction	Uremia Diabetic acidosis Hemorrhage Nephritis
pO_2*	75-100 mm. Hg.	Directly related to oxygen saturation	
Pepsinogen	200-425 units/ml.		Conditions which decrease gastric acidity Pernicious anemia Achlorhydria
Phenylalanine	0-2 mg./100 ml.	Phenylketonuria Oasthouse urine disease	
Phosphatase, acid	0-2 units/ml. (Shinowara- Jones-Reinhart units)	Carcinoma of prostate Advanced Paget's disease Hyperparathyroidism	

* Whole blood

NORMAL BLOOD OR SERUM VALUES (*Continued*)

DETERMINATION	NORMAL VALUE	CLINICAL SIGNIFICANCE	
		(Increased)	(Decreased)
Phosphatase, alkaline	4-17 King-Amstrong units/ml.	Conditions reflecting increased osteoblastic activity of bone Rickets Hyperparathyroidism Liver disease	
Phosphorus, inorganic	3.0-4.5 mg./100 ml.	Chronic nephritis Hypoparathyroidism	Hyperparathyroidism
Potassium	3.5-5.0 mEq./L.	Addison's disease Oliguria Anuria Tissue breakdown or hemolysis	Diabetic acidosis Diarrhea Vomiting
Protein, total	6-8 gm./100 ml.	Hemoconcentration Shock	Malnutrition Hemorrhage
Albumin	3.5-5 gm./100 ml.	Multiple myeloma (globulin fraction)	Loss of plasma from burns Proteinuria
Globulin	1.5-3 gm./100 ml.	Chronic infections (globulin)	
Paper electrophoresis	% of total proteins	Liver disease (globulin)	
Albumin	45-60%		
Alpha 1 globulin	2.7-6.1%		
Alpha 2 globulin	7.7-16.2%		
Beta globulin	10-17%		
Gamma globulin	8.7-27%		
Sodium	135-145 mEq./L.	Hemoconcentration Nephritis Pyloric obstruction	Alkali deficit Addison's disease, Myxedema
Sulfate	0.5-1.5 mg./100 ml.	Nephritis Nitrogen retention	
Thymol turbidity	1-4.5 units/ml.	Liver disease Infectious diseases with antibody production	
Transaminase (SGOT)	15-45 units/ml.	Myocardial infarction Skeletal muscle disease Liver disease	
Transaminase (SGPT)	5-36 units/ml.	Same conditions as SGOT, but increase is more marked in liver disease than SGOT	
Urea nitrogen	10-20 mg./100 ml.	Acute glomerulonephritis Obstructive uropathy Mercury poisoning Nephrotic syndrome	Severe hepatic failure Pregnancy
Uric acid	1-6 mg./100 ml.	Gouty arthritis Acute leukemia Lymphomas treated by chemotherapy Toxemia of pregnancy	
Vitamin A	0.5-2.0 units/ml.	Hypervitaminosis A	Vitamin A deficiency
Zinc turbidity	2-12 units/ml.	Same clinical significance as thymol turbidity	

NORMAL VALUES—URINE CHEMISTRY

DETERMINATION	NORMAL VALUE	CLINICAL SIGNIFICANCE (Increased)	(Decreased)
Acetone and acetoacetate	Zero	Uncontrolled diabetes mellitus Starvation	
Alpha amino nitrogen	64-199 mg./24 hrs.	Leukemia Diabetes Phenylketonuria Other metabolic diseases	
Ammonia	20-70 mEq./L. 0.6 gm./L.	Diabetes mellitus Pernicious vomiting Cirrhosis and other destructive diseases of the liver	
Calcium	Less than 150 mg./ 24 hrs.	Hyperparathyroidism	
Catecholamines	Epinephrine: less than 10 μg./24 hrs. Norepinephrine: less than 100 μg./24 hrs.	Pheochromocytoma	
Chorionic gonadotropin	Zero	Pregnancy Chorionepithelioma Hydatidiform mole	
Copper	0-100 μg./24 hrs.	Wilson's disease Cirrhosis of liver	
Coproporphyrin	50-200 μg./24 hrs.	Poliomyelitis Lead poisoning	
Creatine	Less than 100 mg./24 hrs.	Muscular dystrophy Fever Carcinoma of liver Pregnancy	
Creatinine	1-2 gm./24 hrs.	Typhoid fever Salmonella infections Tetanus	Muscular atrophy Anemia Advanced degeneration of kidneys Leukemia
Chlorides	9 gm./L (as NaCl)		
Bile melanin	Zero	Advanced melanoma Ochronosis	
Creatinine clearance	150-180 L./24 hrs./1.73 sq. M. of body surface		Measures glomerular filtration rate Renal diseases
Cystine	Zero	Cystinuria	
Hemoglobin and myoglobin	Zero	Extensive burns Transfusion of incompatible blood Myoglobin increased in severe crushing injuries to muscle	
Homogentisic acid	Zero	Alkaptonuria Ochronosis	
5-Hydroxyindoleacetic acid	Zero	Malignant carcinoid syndrome	
Lead	120 μg. or less/24 hrs.	Lead poisoning	

NORMAL VALUES—URINE CHEMISTRY (*Continued*)

DETERMINATION	NORMAL VALUE	CLINICAL SIGNIFICANCE	
		(Increased)	(Decreased)
Phenolphthalein (PSP)	At least 25% excreted in 15 min., 40% by 30 min., and 60% by 120 min.		Delayed in renal diseases Low in nephritis, cystitis, pyelonephritis, congestive heart failure
Phenylpyruvic acid	Zero	Phenylketonuria	Primarily measures of renal tubular function
Phosphorus, inorganic	Average 1 gm./24 hrs. Varies with intake	Fever Nervous exhaustion Tuberculosis Rickets Chronic lead poisoning	Acute infections Nephritis Chlorosis Pregnancy
Pituitary gonadotropin	Males: 6-24 mouse units/24 hrs. Females: 5-40 mouse units/24 hrs.	Seminoma Teratoma of testis Pregnancy Menopause	
Porphobilinogen	Zero	Acute porphyria Liver disease	
Protein	Zero	Nephritis Cardiac failure Mercury poisoning Bence-Jones protein in multiple myeloma Febrile states Hematuria Amyloidosis	
17-Ketosteroids	Males: 10-22 mg./24 hrs. Females: 6-18 mg./24 hrs.	Masculinizing tumors of testes	Addison's disease,
17-Hydroxycorticoids	2-12 mg./24 hrs.	Cushing's syndrome	Addison's disease Anterior pituitary hypofunction
Glucose	Zero	Diabetes mellitus Pituitary disorders Intracranial pressure Lesion in floor of 4th ventricle	
Titratable acidity	20-40 mEq./24 hrs.	Metabolic acidosis	Metabolic alkalosis
Urea clearance	Over 40 ml. blood cleared of urea/min., or greater than 60%		Renal diseases
Urobilinogen	Up to 4 mg./24 hrs.	Liver and biliary tract disease Hemolytic anemias	Complete or nearly complete biliary obstruction Diarrhea Renal insufficiency
Uroporphyrins	Zero	Porphyria	
Vanilmandelic acid	0.7-6.8 mg./24 hr.	Pheochromocytoma	
D-Xylose absorption	5-hr. excretion of 16-33% of test dose		Malabsorption syndromes
Urea	25-35 gm./24 hrs.	Excessive protein catabolism	Impaired kidney function
Uric acid	0.6-1 gm./24 hrs. as urate	Gout (see blood uric acid)	Nephritis (see blood uric acid)

CEREBROSPINAL FLUID—NORMAL VALUES

DETERMINATION	NORMAL VALUE	CLINICAL SIGNIFICANCE (Increased)	(Decreased)
Cell count	0-5 mononuclear cells/ cu. mm.	Bacterial meningitis Neurosyphilis Anterior poliomyelitis Encephalitis lethargica	
Chloride	100-130 mEq./L.	Uremia	Acute generalized meningitis Tubercular meningitis
Colloidal gold	0000000000	Acute meningitis Neurosyphilis	
Glucose	50-75 mg./100 ml.	Diabetes mellitus Diabetic coma Epidemic encephalitis Uremia	Acute meningitides Tuberculous meningitis Insulin shock

Protein
  Lumbar
  Cisternal
  Ventricular
	
	15-45 mg./100 ml.
	15-25 mg./100 ml.
	5-15 mg./100 ml.
		
		Acute meningitides
		Tubercular meningitis
		Neurosyphilis
		Poliomyelitis
		Guillain-Barré syndrome	

MISCELLANEOUS VALUES

TOXICOLOGY

DETERMINATION	NORMAL VALUE	CLINICAL SIGNIFICANCE
Barbiturate	Zero	Coma level approximately 11 mg./100 ml. for phenobarbital; most other compounds 1.5 mg./100 ml.
Bromide	Zero	Toxic level = 17 mEq./L.
Carbon monoxide	0-2%	Symptoms with over 20% saturation
Dilantin	Zero	Therapeutic level = 1-11 mg./100 ml.
Ethanol	0-0.05%	Maximal level allowable by courts = 0.15% 0.3-0.4% = marked intoxication 0.4-0.5% = alcoholic stupor
Methanol	Zero	May be fatal in concentrations as low as 10 mg./100 ml.
Salicylate	Zero	Therapeutic level = 20-25 mg./100 ml. Toxic level = over 30 mg./100 ml.

Sulfonamide	Zero	Therapeutic levels:
		  Sulfadiazine 8-15 mg./100 ml.
		  Sulfaguanidine 3-5 mg./100 ml.
		  Sulfamerazine 10-15 mg./100 ml.
		  Sulfanilamide 10-15 mg./100 ml.

GASTRIC ANALYSIS

DETERMINATION	NORMAL VALUE	(Increased)	(Decreased)
Free HCl	0-30 mEq./L.	Neuroses	Pernicious anemia
Total acidity	15-45 mEq./L.	Peptic ulcer	Gastric carcinoma
Combined acid	10-15 mEq./L.	Zollinger-Ellison syndrome	Chronic atrophic gastritis Decreases normally with age

Principles of Antisepsis and Asepsis

- *Development of Asepsis*
- *Principles of Sterilization—Definitions*
- *Heat Sterilization*
- *Radiant Energy Sterilization*
- *Gaseous Energy Sterilization*
- *Chemical Methods of Disinfection—Antiseptics*

Surgery as practiced up to the 19th century was a discouraging and distressing branch of medicine. Pus formed in a majority of all open wounds, whether accidental or as a result of operation. Many patients developed more serious complications, such as septicemia (blood poisoning), hemorrhage and gangrene. As a consequence, amputations were frequent, prolonged illness with crippling disability often resulted and, only too often, death occurred.

The first advance toward the present-day practice of surgery was made by a chemist, Louis Pasteur. In 1857, while studying the phenomena of fermentation, he demonstrated the presence and the activity of microorganisms or bacteria. Later, he showed that "putrefaction was a fermentation caused by the growth of microbes." These organisms, he found, were killed by heat, and putrefaction could be avoided by preventing further entrance of the germs, the present-day concept of prophylaxis in surgery.

A short time later, an English surgeon, Joseph Lister, directed his attention to Pasteur's work. He attempted first to prevent putrefaction and pus formation in wounds infected with microbes by destroying the germs with carbolic acid, a solution of which, he had found, would kill bacteria. Later, he developed an elaborate technique for operation on clean wounds, with the carbolization of the patient's skin and wound, the surgeon's hands and all the materials used at the operation. He even attempted to destroy the germs in the surrounding air by the use of a carbolic acid spray.

DEVELOPMENT OF ASEPSIS

Surgery has made great strides since Lister's time. The principles that he laid down are still adhered to, but with fuller knowledge and added experience his methods have been modified. It is known now that the materials used in the treatment of wounds may be freed from living organisms by heat, thus largely replacing chemical disinfection. It has been found unnecessary to attempt to rid the air of bacteria because, when germs are excluded from entrance to the wound by other paths, healing occurs usually without infection. Experience has shown that tissues have a natural power of self-protection against the action of bacteria. The power is lessened markedly by the application of strong antiseptics but, in most cases of clean wounds, is sufficient in itself to kill organisms that gain entrance to the wound during an operation.

For these reasons, surgical procedures have been changed largely from the *antiseptic* (against putrefaction) methods of Lister to the *aseptic* (without infection) technique of today. An effort is made to operate without any initial entrance of bacteria into the wounds. This object is gained by *sterilizing* (killing the bacteria in) all materials used in the operation.

Principles of Aseptic Surgery

The successful practice of aseptic surgery requires a strict observance of preoperative sterilization of the surgical materials, of rigid precautions against infection during the course of the operation, and of guarding the wound from infection afterward until such time as it is healed.

Preoperative Treatment. This comprises sterilizing and keeping sterile (free from microorganisms) all surgical materials that are to come in contact with the wound and exposed tissues or that are to be handled by the surgeon or his assistants. These include all instruments, needles, sutures, dressings, gloves, covers and so forth. In addition, the surgeon and his assistants and nurses must prepare themselves before touching any of these materials. While their hands and arms cannot be rendered absolutely sterile, they must be made as clean as possible by the use of soap, water and chemicals, and then covered with sterile rubber gloves. A cap is used to cover the head and enclose the hair. Masks covering the nose and the mouth are employed to prevent bacteria from the upper respiratory system from entering the wound. A long-sleeved sterile gown must be worn over the clothing. The patient's skin, over an area considerably larger than that requiring exposure during the course of operation, also demands the highest possible degree of cleanliness and the application of some chemical agent. The rest of the patient's body is covered with sterile drapes.

During Operation. During the operation neither the "scrubbed" surgeon nor his nurses or assistants touch anything that has not been rendered and kept sterile. "Nonscrubbed" assistants refrain from touching or contaminating anything that is sterile.

After Operation. After the operation the wound is protected from possible infection by means of sterile dressings and by an occasional disinfection of the surrounding skin with chemical agents. Particular care is taken to prevent contact of anything that is not sterile with the unhealed wound. In most cases not previously infected, this aseptic regimen is all that is necessary to ensure rapid aseptic healing. In recently infected wounds, it is necessary to remove and destroy such microorganisms as are already in the tissues, and also to prevent subsequent infection from without. The first condition is affected by the removal of foreign bodies and devitalized tissues from the wound (*débridement*). The second condition is fulfilled by the use of a rigid aseptic technique during the course of the treatment.

When infection already has developed in the tissues, the chief indication is to help the body to eliminate the organisms by incision and to prevent the entrance of further infection from without.

It must be recognized then that, although the surgical technique of today is said to be aseptic, there are still many uses for chemical disinfection in the treatment of infected, and even of aseptic, wounds.

PRINCIPLES OF STERILIZATION— DEFINITIONS

Sterilization, in surgery, means the destruction of all organisms, including spores.

Disinfection is the act of destroying all nonspore-bearing pathogenic organisms, i.e., those responsible for the communicable diseases. This method would be applicable for the disinfection of clothing, bedding, bedpans, and so forth.

Disinfectants are agents, usually chemical, that destroy disease-producing organisms.

Antiseptics are agents that prevent the growth of microorganisms without necessarily destroying them.

Germicides or **bactericides** are agents that kill microorganisms.

Deodorizers or **deodorants** are agents employed to destroy or prevent offensive odors.

Mechanical Disinfection. When a physician or a nurse "scrubs" or prepares the skin of the operative site, it is an effort to cleanse mechanically the skin surfaces that may be exposed during the operation. This means removal of the surface dirt and fat and the organisms that are found normally on the skin. Usually, this is accomplished by the use of warm water and a soap that produces an abundant lather. Some surgeons prefer soaps containing antiseptics that appear to be more efficient in reducing the bacterial habitants of the skin surface. Others use detergents containing antiseptics for the same purpose (see Technique of Scrubbing, p. 993).

A further method of mechanical disinfection is utilized in recently infected traumatic wounds. Under sterile conditions an effort is made to cut away all the devitalized tissue, so as to remove foreign materials and contaminating bacteria. This procedure is known as *débridement*.

HEAT STERILIZATION

Sterilization by heat ensures the destruction of microorganisms and their spores. It is the method to be chosen for all materials, except those that suffer damage from repeated exposure to heat. Before subjecting a material to sterilization by heat, it is essential that it be clean and free from any dirt, threads, ravelings and so forth that might remain as foreign

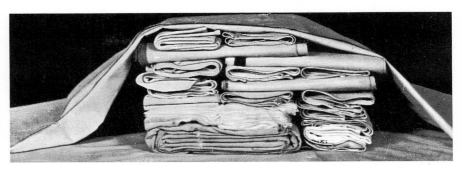

Fig. A-1. A model heavy pack arrangement. None should be larger than 12″x12″x20″, or more densely arranged than illustrated. Note how alternate layers are crossed to promote free circulation of steam through the mass. Note also that gauze sponges are located near the center of the pack to break up close contact between masses of more tightly woven fabrics. (The Surgical Supervisor, American Sterilizer Co., Erie, Pa.)

bodies in the wound. The mode of applying heat varies with the nature of the material to be sterilized and with the circumstances under which the sterilization is to be carried out. The two main forms of heat are moist heat and dry heat.

Moist Heat

Moist heat may be applied as steam or boiling water.

Steam Under Pressure

This is the most desirable method of sterilizing nearly all surgical supplies. The sterilizer or *autoclave* is built in such a manner that steam enters the sterilizing chamber under pressure for the purpose of attaining high temperatures. Materials thus sterilized are subjected to a temperature of 115° to 123° C. (240° to 254° F.). The steam of the autoclave at these temperatures destroys all vegetative bacteria and even the most resistant pathogenic spores in a relatively brief interval of time. Tests have proved that the spores of *Cl. oedematiens, Cl. tetani* and *Cl. welchii* are destroyed in direct contact with steam at 121° C. (250° F.) in 1 minute, at 115° C. (240° F.) in 4 minutes and at 110° C. (230° F.) in 10 minutes. Since these are the absolute minimal requirements, a considerably longer period of time is necessary in order to provide for the steam to permeate the mass, whatever it is. Surrounding the sterilizing chamber is a steam jacket, where from 15 to 17 pounds of pressure is maintained before, during and after the sterilization period. One purpose of the jacket is to prevent condensation of the water vapor, with consequent wetting of the supplies.

The principle of sterilization by the use of steam is the same as in other methods of sterilization—the coagulation of the proteins in the bacterial body, which destroys the bacteria. It has been found by experiment that coagulation occurs at a much lower temperature with moist heat than with dry heat, which is the reason for the use of boiling water and of steam under pressure as sterilizing agents. Steam at atmospheric pressure can transmit a temperature of only 100° C. (212° F.). This temperature is able to kill all living or vegetative forms of bacterial life, but many spores are resistant to this temperature and are not killed.

Removal of Air. In order to reach such high temperatures, it is necessary that the air be removed as completely as possible from the sterilizing chamber. The temperature can be gauged by the pressure indicator only when the pressure represents that of steam and not that of steam plus air in the sterilizing chamber. Therefore, an attempt is made in all types of sterilizers to remove the air from the sterilizing chamber. This is accomplished best by permitting the air to escape through a drain controlled thermostatically from the bottom of the chamber, including an accurate mercury thermometer that indicates consequently the temperature of the coolest medium surrounding the load, since air or steam mixed with air gravitate unfailingly below pure steam in the chamber. The thermostatic valve remains open and permits air and condensate to escape freely. It closes only after the air has been driven out, and relatively pure steam follows. This thermometer thus becomes the one gauge (rather than the pressure indication) under which all sterilization is controlled. Every performance is timed when the thermometer indicates 115° C. (240° F.) in its advance toward the regulated maximum of 123° C. (254° F.).

The importance of withdrawing the air is due to the fact that the presence of air reduces the ultimate temperature of the steam at any given pressure, because steam and air do not blend; therefore, the materials at the top of the sterilizer, heated by pure steam, become sterilized easily and rapidly, and those at the bottom of the sterilizer, where most of the air accumulates, are heated by a mixture of warm air and steam, and the temperature does not rise to the point

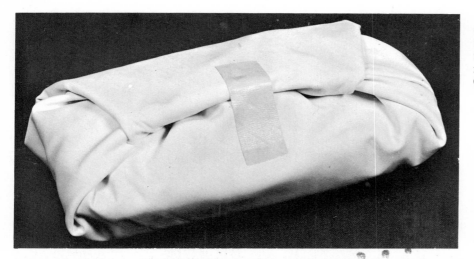

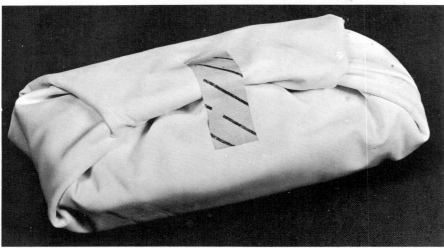

Fɪɢ. A-2. Pressure-sensitive (autoclave) tape before and after sterilization. Dark striped lines appear on the tape when it is autoclaved. (Minnesota Mining and Manufacturing Co.)

that will produce sterilization for a considerable period of time. Furthermore, the presence of air in the sterilizer reduces very materially the power of the steam to penetrate and sterilize large packages of materials, because the penetration of steam into these packages depends upon the displacement of air due to gravity. If the chamber is two-thirds filled with air, there is no displacement by gravity and, therefore, poor penetration of the materials by steam.

In the operation of the sterilizer, no matter what type, the process by which sterilization is accomplished is much the same. In the stage of preparation, steam is admitted to the outer or steam jacket until the pressure of from 15 to 17 pounds is reached. In this way the sterilizing chamber is heated and is prepared for the reception of the materials to be sterilized. After the materials have been introduced into the chamber, air is evacuated from the chamber by

gravity, as explained above. The operator should keep close watch until the thermometer indicates 115° C. (240° F.); then the period of exposure, which is governed by the particular load, is timed.

At the close of the period of sterilization, the operating valve is turned to "exhaust" until chamber pressure has reduced to "zero." Jacket pressure is maintained until drying is complete. When chamber pressure has reduced to zero, the operating valve (for dry loads only) is turned to the "vacuum" or "dry" position, in which a partial vacuum is created in the chamber, rarefying the vapor and hastening drying to some extent. This position is maintained for not more than 3 to 5 minutes, and the operating valve is turned to the "off" position until the chamber gauge again indicates zero pressure. Then the door is unlocked and loosened slightly but opened not more than ½ inch for about 10 minutes, depending upon the size

Fig. A-3. (*Left*) One large pack. (*Right*) Same pack broken down into four small packs, and these are separated slightly from each other in the sterilizer. The single large pack shows why there is oversterilization of the outer portions when exposure has continued long enough to permit steam to penetrate adequately to the interior for sterilization. In the smaller packs, steam permeates the entire mass quickly, and a much shorter period of exposure is needed.

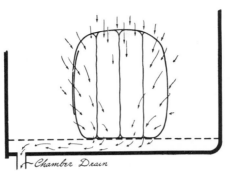 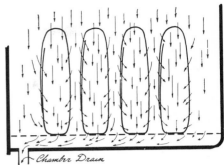

and the density of the load. Vapor will escape into the room from the top of the door, and drying results.

For cooling down solution loads—any aqueous solution in bottles or flasks—exhaust of the chamber steam must be controlled precisely or blown stoppers and undue loss of fluid will result. Steam exhaust can be controlled easily in the following way:

At the close of the period of sterilization, turn the operating valve toward the exhaust position so that the steam from the chamber escapes very slowly. Exhaust to the zero pressure should occur in not less than 6 to 10 minutes, and the door must not be unlocked until all pressure has been exhausted completely. This permits the fluid in the flasks or the bottles to lose its heat without violent ebullition down to the boiling point.

Packaging.

1. All articles must be absolutely clean and freshly laundered (or hydrated) to guard against superheating with resultant injury to the fabric.

2. All linens are checked for holes and tears; these can be mended. Threads and ravelings must be removed.

3. Sheets and covers are folded to facilitate their use, such as fanfolding, etc. Such foresight prevents undue handling and flourishing of sterile drapes. Covers and towels should be folded, so that the edges and not the center part will be handled when opened. Gowns must be folded wrong side out, so that the inner side only is touched by the ungloved hand when they are put on by the surgeon and his assistants. This is accomplished very easily by first folding the gown lengthwise and then, starting at the hem, rolling it into a compact bundle. A 5-inch length of 2-inch stockinet makes a very comfortable cuff for operating gowns and also one that is folded in more readily under the cuff of rubber gloves.

4. The contents of a pack are arranged in such a way that the articles to be used first appear on top.

The arrangement should facilitate steam penetration (Fig. A-1). Basins should not be included with fabrics in one package, since basins interfere with steam permeation and retard drying after sterilization.

5. The size of any pack should not exceed the dimensions of 12″ × 12″ × 20″. A pack arranged as described in Figure A-1 can be sterilized in 30 minutes at 121° C. (250° F.). A properly packaged and arranged kit provides a sterile wrapper for the table, enough supplies for a procedure arranged in the order of use and a wrapper that allows prompt penetration by steam.

6. Two double-thickness muslin wrappers are ideal to wrap supplies.

7. Packages must be wrapped securely and fastened with cord, twill tape or pressure-sensitive tape (Fig. A-2). Pins should not be used, since they cause excessive wear on linen, increase the tendency of tight wrapping, and the holes they produce may permit contamination of the contents.

8. All packages should be marked legibly to identify contents and date of sterilization. When pressure-sensitive tape is used, this information can be written on the tape (Fig. A-2). To facilitate removal of tape, slightly invert one corner.

Loading of Sterilizer.

1. Prepare all packs and arrange the load in the sterilizer so as to present the least possible resistance to the passage of steam through the load, from the top of the chamber toward the bottom (Fig. A-3).

2. All jars, test tubes and other nonporous containers of dry material should be loaded in the sterilizer, with a horizontal path for the escape of air. "Imagine that the container is filled with water. Then place it in the sterilizer in a horizontal position so that the water would drain out freely."*

---

* Perkins, J. J.: Principles and Methods of Sterilization, Springfield, Ill., Charles C Thomas, 1956.

Period of Exposure.

1. Establish a period of exposure that will provide for complete penetration of the load and ensure destruction of microbial life with a liberal margin of safety.

2. Time the sterilizing period from the moment that saturated steam at 121° C. (250° F.) fills the chamber as indicated by the thermometer located in the chamber drain line.

Drying of Load.

1. Provide a minimal drying period of 15 minutes for all bulk loads of supplies.

2. Do not place freshly sterilized packages on cold surfaces, since condensation and wetting will take place, which results in contamination.

Nursing Responsibility. Of all the sterilizers the autoclave is probably the most important. The principles just described apply to any autoclave, be it small, large, round or square. This sterilizing unit is found in the central supply division, the operating and the delivery rooms and even in the utility or treatment rooms on the patient divisions. It is important that such a vital piece of equipment be kept in excellent working order, be kept clean and be checked frequently for its effectiveness in sterilizing. The nurse should learn how to operate the autoclave and to recognize her responsibility for supervising nonprofessional workers as they use it. Sterilization must be timed accurately. No guess work can be sanctioned when a patient's life may depend upon the sterility of a dressing or an instrument. To avoid error some central clock should be used and not an individual's wrist watch, which may allow timing discrepancies to occur.

Boiling Water

The once widely used technique of boiling instruments for surgery is open to question today. The boiling process should be discouraged,* and used only when steam under pressure is not available.

Boiling water (212° F. or 100° C.) destroys all living bacteria in a few seconds, but the spores of some organisms are very resistant and require boiling for a longer time (at least 30 minutes) to ensure their destruction. Some of the most difficult spores to kill, such as tetanus and gas gangrene organisms, resist many hours of boiling. The disadvantage of boiling is that it dulls the edge of cutting instruments— scalpels and so forth; also, the usual tap water leaves

---

* Perkins considers it more appropriate to designate the boiling water process as one of disinfection or sanitization, rather than sterilization.

a deposit of scale (lime) in the joints and on the surfaces of instruments and utensils that can be removed only by vigorous scouring.

The usual technique for sterilization of instruments requires that they boil in plain water for 30 minutes or in water containing 2 per cent of sodium carbonate (from 3 to 4 teaspoonfuls to the quart of water) for not less than 15 minutes. The addition of sodium carbonate brings about the destruction of the more resistant spores in a shorter period of time than is possible in plain water. The following are important points for the nurse to remember when boiling articles: *The article must be clean.* Blood, pus, oils, grease and so forth hinder the sterilizing process. The timing of sterilization is started when the water begins to boil. *All articles must be submerged completely.* The speed at which the water boils does not change the time element; therefore, it is better to have the water boiling quietly.

Specialty Sterilizers

In addition to the autoclave, described in detail on pp. 981-983, there are specialty sterilizers.

Instrument Washer Sterilizer. Instruments can be washed by means of a vigorously agitated detergent bath. Blood, grease and tissue debris is loosened and is drawn off the top of the container and directed to an overflow valve. In the operating process the temperature reaches 132° C. (270° F.) in about 12 minutes. Upon release of water and steam, instruments are thoroughly dried and ready for use or storage.

Instrument Sterilizer. This is similar in construction to the autoclave, but is smaller. In sterilizing instruments a layer of muslin is placed on the bottom of a wire meshed or perforated tray. Instruments are then arranged in the manner in which they will be used later. All jointed instruments must be open or unlocked to allow steam to come in contact with all surfaces. A top muslin cover is added if the tray is eventually to be carried a distance. Sterilizing time is 15 minutes at 121° C. (250° F.) or 7 minutes at 132° C. (270° F.). For emergency use a single instrument or two can be sterilized at 132° C. (270° F.), 27 lb. pressure in 3 minutes.

Water Sterilizer. There is a trend away from using the water sterilizer (in which water is sterilized at 121° C. under pressure every 12 hours) to individual flasks of sterile water or isotonic solutions. The reasons are several: (1) one of the problems is to maintain the sterility of water in the large tank (there is danger of air-borne, insect and contact contamination, especially at the outlet or draw-off point); (2) the pitcher used to transfer sterile water from the tank to the sterile basin is a receptacle difficult to keep sterile because of the human element in handling it over and over again; and (3) surgeons prefer isotonic autoclaved solutions for sponges and irrigation of wounds.

Testing for Sterility

Because of the probability of human error in operating a sterilizer and the possibility of mechanical failure within the equipment itself, sterilization failures may occur. There are several ways of checking proper function and adequate sterilization.

The Recording Thermometer. This instrument contains a clock, mechanically operated, which revolves an 8-inch diameter chart once in 24 hours. The chart records the temperature in the discharge outlet and also the duration of each exposure. It is a valuable means of checking when it is properly installed and used.

Sterilization Indicators. These indicators are of many types, varying from simple paper strips that change color to hermetically sealed glass tubes containing a pellet that melts and changes color when sterilization temperatures are reached. Perkins has observed "that all sterilization indicators possess the same general disadvantage, to a greater or lesser degree, in that a percentage will be found to react to a time-temperature ratio inadequate for sterilization or that the end points are not sufficiently clear so as to permit accurate interpretation of the results. These controls do not indicate the actual build-up of temperature in the test pack nor do they indicate how much over-exposure may have been applied."*

Culture Tests. The best way of determining the sterility of an article is to perform a bacteriologic culture test. Periodic checks on a bimonthly basis is recommended. The spore-bearing organisms used in culture tests are *Bacillus subtilis* and *Bacillus stearothermophilus*.

Perkins describes an effective and simple means by using bacterial spore strips. These are small strips (2″ × ½″) of filter paper upon which a specific number of dry bacterial spores of established heat resistance are placed. They are dried, and then 2 strips are placed side by side in a steam-permeable paper envelope. Then this is placed in the center of the most densely packed package; this in turn is placed in the front bottom portion of the sterilizer. Following the usual sterilizing and drying process, the envelope is sent to the laboratory where, under sterile procedure, the strips are removed and placed in sterile medium to incubate for 7 days.

* Perkins, *op. cit.*, p. 231.

Dry Heat

Cautery

This is used to sterilize cut tissue surfaces—for example, the base of the appendix in an appendectomy.

Hot Air

Some surgical supplies, such as various forms of oil, bone wax and talcum powder in bulk, cannot be sterilized properly by any method other than prolonged exposure to dry heat in the hot-air oven. The moist heat of the autoclave is inadequate because the moisture factor of the steam, essential to autoclave sterilization, does not permeate such masses. Such materials should be sterilized in a dry-heat sterilizer at a temperature of 160° C. (320° F.) for 1 hour or at 121° C. (250° F.) for 4 hours. Usually it is not advisable to attempt sterilization of such materials except in relatively small quantities; that is to say, in small jars or containers.

Another advantage of dry heat is that it does not destroy finely polished cutting edges of instruments, such as scissors, knife blades, osteotomes, etc. It is also a desirable method for syringes, since dry heat does not attack the ground surfaces as moist heat does.

A hot-air oven can be created in the ordinary autoclave. Steam is allowed to enter the jacket but not the chamber; in this way, syringes, needles, sharp-edged instruments, etc., can be adequately sterilized overnight or for a minimum of 4 hours at 121° C. (250° F.).

RADIANT ENERGY STERILIZATION

Ultraviolet Light

There are many limitations to the use of ultraviolet light in the operating room. Since radiation does not penetrate the surface of liquids because the light is reflected, droplets are not sterilized. Every surface must be exposed for sterilization; bacteria are protected in the shadows. Sufficient time must be provided for sterilization, since it is not instantaneous. Prolonged exposure injures skin, tissues and eyes; therefore, the head and the neck of operating room personnel should be protected if ultraviolet light is used.

GASEOUS STERILIZATION

Ethylene Oxide

C_2H_4O is a moderately toxic gas which is able to sterilize effectively many items that are sensitive to heat and moisture, such as telescopic instruments, electric cords, rubber goods and so forth. In an ethylene oxide sterilizer, several conditions must obtain for proper sterilization: (1) air must be evacuated from the chamber; (2) a relative humidity of between 25 and 50 per cent is then created, using vaporized distilled water; (3) temperature between 37.8° and 60° C. is provided; (4) a concentration of 760 mg./L. of ethylene oxide is introduced (at 60° C. the exposure time is 3 hours; for a lower temperature, the time is increased); (5) ethylene oxide is evacuated mechanically; (6) air, sterilized by filtration and exposure to ultraviolet radiation, is admitted.

CHEMICAL METHODS OF DISINFECTION—ANTISEPTICS

Since many chemical agents are not capable of destroying all forms of microbial life, e.g., tubercle bacillus, bacterial spores and the filterable viruses, it is more nearly accurate to refer to the process as "chemical disinfection" rather than "chemical sterilization."

Chemical disinfection is used only when it is not feasible to sterilize an article by heat. Chemical disinfectants tend to congeal proteinaceous material such as blood, and organisms contained within this protein precipitate may well survive. Accordingly, chemical disinfection should not be used for instruments contaminated with blood or tissue fluid.

Factors That Influence Disinfectant Action

1. **Cleanliness.** The presence of blood, pus, oil or grease interferes with the action of all germicides. The effective use of soap and water for cleansing is a necessary preliminary step to ensure optimal effectiveness of a disinfectant.

2. **Concentration.** Usually a weak solution is not as effective as a strong solution of the same disinfectant. An exception is ethyl alcohol; 70 per cent aqueous solution is more germicidal than absolute alcohol.

3. **Time.** This factor varies from seconds to hours, depending on the kind of disinfectant, the strength of the disinfecting agent, and the characteristics of the organisms to be eliminated. Vegetative organisms may be destroyed in 30 minutes by some of the chemical disinfectants, whereas no amount of time (hours or days) by the same agent would result in sporicidal action.

4. **Type of Organism.** Some organisms are killed more readily than others. Examples of the resistant forms are the virus of serum hepatitis, tubercle bacillus and certain bacterial spores.

5. **Temperature.** Usually, room temperature is used; however, most chemical agents are more effective if the temperature is raised.

The Use of Disinfectants

Skin Application

Disinfectants are used to remove as many resident and transient organisms of the skin as is possible. In surgery the preoperative preparation of the skin is necessary to prevent unnecessary contamination of the surgical wound. The hands and the arms of the surgical team likewise must be prepared by scrubbing and the application of appropriate disinfectants.

Application to Tissues

Antiseptics are applied to tissues that are or may be the seat of infection, in order to assist them in destroying germs and their products rapidly and completely. When used in this way "the ideal antiseptic should effect complete sterilization within its sphere of action without causing any damage to tissue cells" (Dakin). However, the disadvantage of most antiseptics is that in killing the bacteria they tend also to destroy tissue cells. For this reason they should be used in wounds in weak solutions, and for only a short period of time. Many antiseptics have been suggested and used in tissues, and their very multiplicity would indicate that the ideal antiseptic has not been found yet. It is being recognized more and more that the body tissues have a natural resistance to infection, and that antiseptics are of value only occasionally in the treatment of certain specific types of infection, especially those on the surface of the body.

Instruments and Materials

Chemicals are used to disinfect certain instruments and materials that cannot be sterilized by heat; for example, cystoscopes, bougies and cataract knives must be immersed in a germicide. Most of the chemicals are used in the form of solutions, being dissolved in water or in alcohol. From time to time new chemical compounds appear on the market, all of them with certain advantages and disadvantages.

Groups of Disinfectants

Disinfectants are classified as follows: (1) alcohols, (2) phenols and cresols, (3) quaternary ammonium compounds, (4) aldehydes and acids, (5) oxidizing agents, (6) halogen compounds, (7) furan derivatives and (8) ointments.

Alcohols

Ethyl Alcohol. This is one of the most useful disinfectants. It has a high degree of antiseptic power and has the advantage of being a fat solvent, dissolving out the fat on the surface and in the follicles of the skin, thus permitting the antiseptic to act on the more deeply situated organisms. In 70 per cent solution by weight (81.5% by volume), it is used frequently in disinfection of the patient's skin and as an evaporating lotion. Because it is a fat solvent, it is used frequently in combination with other antiseptics.

Disadvantages. Alcohol causes considerable pain when applied to raw tissues and produces irritation of mucous surfaces; therefore, it should not be used in fresh, open wounds, for the eye, the urethra and so forth.

As a disinfectant for instruments, it must be remembered that they must be cleansed thoroughly because of the protein-coagulating action of alcohol. Greater effectiveness is brought about when alcohol is combined with other disinfectants.

Isopropyl Alcohol is displacing ethyl alcohol in many instances, since it exhibits slightly greater germicidal action, has a lower surface tension, is a better fat solvent and is less expensive. The dilution need not be as stable as ethyl alcohol.

Phenols and Cresols

Phenol or carbolic acid probably was the first recognized antiseptic. About a 95 per cent solution ("pure phenol" or "pure carbolic acid") is used by many surgeons to sterilize and cauterize the cut edges of intestinal mucosa; for example, the stump of the appendix is often touched with "pure phenol" before it is inverted into the cecal wall.

Disadvantages. Phenol is extremely toxic and highly destructive to tissues. Even in germicidal concentrations, it is an irritant to the skin. It is not effective against spores, and as a practical disinfectant its use is limited.

Cresols are derivatives of phenol, which they have largely replaced. They are much more effective germicides than the phenols; however, they are not effective against spores.

Hexachlorophene (G-11) is a phenol derivative which, when incorporated into soaps, detergent creams, etc., is one of the most effective agents for the preoperative preparation of the skin (see p. 107).

Quaternary Ammonium Compounds

Zephiran, Phemerol, Ceepryn. The chief property is that of lowering the surface tension of solutions. They are stable and nonirritating.

Disadvantages. These compounds are incompatible with soap, and they are not effective against tubercle bacillus and spores. In addition, certain gram-negative bacilli, especially *Pseudomonas aeruginosa,* are not inhibited by the quaternary ammoniums and may even proliferate luxuriantly in such solutions.

Aldehydes and Acids

Formaldehyde is a gas with high disinfecting properties. A 40 per cent solution of the gas in water is known as *formalin.* Since it is too irritating for living tissue, it is mainly used as a preservative of specimens.

A solution of 20 per cent formalin and 70 per cent isopropyl alcohol solution is an effective chemical disinfectant and sporicide (exposure time, 30 minutes immersion) for clean instruments that cannot be exposed to steam under pressure sterilization, and are of a material or property that will not be destroyed by the solution.

Oxidizing Agents

The antiseptic properties of this group are due to their property of liberating oxygen that has a mild germicidal action.

Hydrogen Peroxide. This is a clear, watery solution that decomposes readily in the light or on heating. When applied to wound tissues, there is an immediate effervescence that marks the liberation of gaseous oxygen.

Its chief value lies probably in the mechanical effect of its effervescence, in loosening necrotic tissues and dressings and in breaking up thick adherent masses of pus that float to the surface in a sort of foam. Because of this property and its ability to give off oxygen, it is of special value in the treatment of anaerobic infections, such as those caused by the gas bacillus.

Hydrogen peroxide decomposes rapidly unless protected from light, heat and air.

Potassium Permanganate. This occurs as purple crystals, is soluble easily in water and gives a wine-colored solution.

Special Uses. In solution of 1:1,000 to 1:10,000 in sloughing wounds, as an antiseptic and deodorant.

Disadvantages. The solutions decompose rapidly, losing their antiseptic power on contact with dead organic material, rubber or rusty metal, as in chipped enamel ware. The change is accompanied by a conversion of the purple to a brown color.

Halogen Compound

Iodine. This antiseptic ordinarily is used as a tincture. It is one of the most useful when conditions are such that rapid and complete disinfection may be effected by a single application.

Special Uses. (1) As a 3 to 5 per cent solution in the preparation of the skin of the patient for operation. (2) As a 2 per cent solution for the emergency treatment of contaminated wounds. (3) An iodine solution of 0.5 to 1 per cent in 70 per cent alcohol is the agent of choice for the disinfection of clinical thermometers.

Disadvantages. Iodine solutions often irritate the skin. On wet skin, iodine loses much of its effectiveness as a skin disinfectant and frequently causes blisters or vesicles. For this reason it is used only on dry surfaces, never on the palms of the hands, the soles of the feet, the axillae and the perineum. During the summer months, when profuse sweating occurs, iodine should not be used on the face, the scrotum and any other tender parts of the skin.

The strength of iodine solutions increases on standing. This is due to evaporation of the alcoholic solvent. Therefore, they should be kept tightly corked and renewed frequently.

Ioprep. This preparation utilizes the rapid and complete killing-power of iodine against all species of bacteria in a nonstaining and nonirritating solution. A 3-minute application to the operative site, after a thorough cleansing, is recommended and has been used with good results.

Betadine. This chemical agent has been used successfully in the preoperative preparation of the skin, both as a scrubbing agent for the hands of the operating team, and for the skin disinfection of the patient. It is an aqueous solution of povidone-iodine (N.N.D.), a nonstinging and nonstaining soluble iodine complex. It is not irritating to skin or mucous membranes, and unlike tincture of iodine, it can be safely bandaged with no undesirable effects. It kills on contact fungi, viruses, protozoa and yeasts, and has a more prolonged germicidal action than ordinary iodine solutions.

Iodoform. Its chief use is in the form of "iodoform gauze"—gauze impregnated with a 10 to 20 per cent emulsion of iodoform. Used especially for packing in foul discharging wounds, it is now seldom used.

Furan Derivative

Nitrofurazone, N.N.D. (Furacin). An effective agent against many gram-positive and gram-negative bacteria, Furacin is used in the form of a solution in the local treatment of infections and may be applied in the form of an ointment for surface lesions.

Ointments

These are used in surgery when it is inadvisable to apply watery lotions and when it is desired to protect the surrounding skin from the irritating discharges of a wound. Ointments are used also as mildly antiseptic applications in superficial wounds and ulcers, as stimulating applications to sluggish wound surfaces and as a means of administering medicines.

The bland ointments, such as petrolatum, lanolin and cold cream, are used to soften dry and scaly skin and to prevent dressings from adhering to secreting wounds. Mildly antiseptic ointments, such as the ointments of boric acid or zinc oxide, are used in much the same manner. The zinc oxide ointment is useful especially in the treatment of the irritating excoriation of the skin that surrounds a wound having secretion. Ointments containing scarlet red and balsam of Peru have a reputation for stimulating granulation tissue and epithelial growth. They are applied to wounds that seem to be slow in healing.

Few ointments are used in surgery as a means of administering drugs. However, there are some notable exceptions to this statement. Mercury is given in the form of mercurial ointment (blue ointment). This ointment is useful also in the early treatment of local superficial infections, such as boils, infected sebaceous cysts and so forth. Methylsalicylate ointment is useful in the treatment of joint and muscle affections. It produces a local hyperemia, and its effectiveness may be due more to a local counterirritant than to its absorbed drug.

Antibiotics and certain sulfonamides in the form of ointments also are used as local antiseptics for infected wounds, burns and so forth. The antibiotic ointments may produce local sensitivity. Those which are least apt to give local skin reaction are ointments of neomycin and bacitracin. Ointments particularly effective in the treatment of skin infections such as dermatitis and pruritus are the corticosteroids.

---

* A product of Johnson & Johnson.

Operating Room Nursing*

- *Teamwork in the Operating Room*
- *Maintenance of Surgical Asepsis*
- *Technique of Scrubbing, Putting on Gown and Gloves*
- *Surgical Draping*
- *The Circulating Nurse*
- *Preparation of Tables for the Operation*
- *Ligatures and Sutures*
- *Immediately Before the Operation, During the Operation, Between Operations*
- *At the End of the Operative Schedule*
- *Safety Practices in the Operating Room*
- *Sterilization and Care of Various Articles*

The student of nursing will enjoy her experience in the operating room because she will find the answers to many of the problems she has encountered in her care of surgical patients on the divisions. Only by observing, assisting with and understanding the experiences of the operative patient can the nurse interpret intelligently her own function in relation to each individual surgical patient. For the experience to be a satisfying one, the student must learn the principles involved in surgical asepsis as well as those related to the psychological and physical experiences of the patient.

Alexander† has expressed the significance of patient-centered care in the operating room as follows:

> We would all agree that persons who enter our operating rooms as patients are very important people. We would agree that the people who care for patients are important. We know that good nursing care is given when all personnel carry out their prescribed tasks correctly, completely, and safely. We also know that optimum care requires expert assistance from the personnel in other departments in the hospital—the bacteriologist, the pathologist, the engineer, the nursing teams

stationed in the units, the supply room, and the recovery room, as well as the educational leaders, the medical staff, and the administrators.

> The gowned, masked personnel who hurry down the halls as they pass the worried patients, the many instruments lined row upon row on the numerous draped tables, the odor of disinfectants, the searching lamps, the buzzing saw, the placing of a patient on the operating table as if he were a contortionist—all are necessary in our operating room, but they should not push away the personal, gentle touch in caring for each patient. How the personnel accept their duties and work together influence and often determine how the patients accept their problems.

The nurse consciously uses her voice, her hands and her movements with gentleness because she knows that it is a manifestation of good nursing. She is aware that all activity in the operating room is carried out primarily and solely for the patient. *Whether he is conscious or anesthetized, the patient must be respected, protected and cared for as carefully as we would want those dearest to us to be treated.*

Other important objectives are:

To see and appreciate surgical problems as they affect the patient; to observe the skill necessary to correct these problems.

To understand and apply the principles of surgical

* Revised with the assistance of Jean DeVries, R.N., Operating Room Supervisor, Alexandria Hospital, Alexandria, Virginia.

† Alexander, E.: Patient-centered care, Hospital Topics 33.

asepsis in the clinical area where such technique is practiced in its fullest sense.

To learn to work effectively on a team in which every member is necessary and important, and the element of time is a precious one.

To recognize the value of emotional stability and mental alertness, particularly in a tense or emergency situation.

To appreciate the responsibility of the professional nurse in maintaining a well-organized unit and in practicing satisfactory interpersonal relations.

To appreciate the underlying safety measures which dictate the specific way in which technique is practiced, thus providing the safest possible care for the patient.

TEAMWORK IN THE OPERATING ROOM

When a patient arrives in the operating room, essentially 4 different groups are preparing for their roles in his care. The first group is the anesthesiologist and his assistants who greet the patient, administer the anesthetic agent and place him in the proper position on the operating table. The second team is the nurses who prepare the operating room for the reception of the patient and assist throughout the operation. Such a nurse does not scrub but remains unsterile and often is referred to as the circulating nurse (unsterile nurse). The third group is the nurses who scrub, set up the sterile tables to include all the instruments, sponges, sutures, etc., that will be necessary for the particular operation, and this nurse is referred to as a "scrub" nurse (sterile nurse). The fourth group is the surgeon and his assistants who scrub and perform the operation. Auxiliary personnel, such as surgical technicians and licensed practical nurses are also members of the team.

Regardless of the particular responsibilities of each worker, the concept of teamwork should be practiced. Every member of an operating room group must work together so that the corps of workers may function, not as individuals but as one unit, having one common interest—the welfare of the patient.

The responsibilities of everyone associated with the operating room should be outlined clearly. This avoids many errors and fixes responsibility at all times. If lists enumerating the duties of each person are placed where all may see and read them, endless difficulties will be avoided. More work will be accomplished in a shorter length of time, one person will not wait for another to do some task if she knows it to be part of her own particular duties, and, if something has not been done or has been done improperly, the head nurse will be in a better position to handle the situation.

MAINTENANCE OF SURGICAL ASEPSIS

Principles Regarding Health and Operating Room Attire

Good health is essential for any professional person in the operating room. Colds, sore throats and infected fingers are a distinct menace and must be reported at once to the nurse in charge. A series of wound infections in postoperative patients was traced in one instance to a mild throat infection among operating room nurses. Therefore, it can be understood readily how very important it is for nurses to report any seemingly slight ailment without delay.

Wearing apparel must be clean. All clothing, including the headgear, should be changed daily. A mask requires changing much more frequently, certainly between operations, and oftener if necessary. Operating room dress should be worn on the operating floor only. Shoes used in the operating room should not be worn on the street.

The style of the clothing and the shoes should be plain. This will facilitate cleaning, allow ease in dressing and ensure the comfort of the wearer. For example, a turban or headpiece that requires skill and practice to put on properly may be applied poorly by the novice, and the purpose for which it is intended is lost.

Garments and shoes must be safe.

1. *Headgear* should completely cover the hair so that single strands of hair, bobby-pins, clips, or particles of dandruff or dust do not fall on sterile fields.

2. *Mask.* This is worn to minimize airborne contamination. The mask must do this effectively; in addition, it should leak no air, not interfere with breathing, be compact, comfortable, and not hinder speech or vision. Many effective disposable masks are available. Tests prove their superiority over gauze masks. Forced expiration, such as that produced by talking, laughing, sneezing and coughing, should be avoided, since it deposits organisms on the masks.

3. *Conductive Shoes.* Shoes with rubber soles are nonconducters of electricity, and there is danger of generation of static electricity under such conditions. Static electricity may ignite anesthetic gases to produce explosions in the operating room. Shoes with conductive soles or conductive slip-ons produce a grounding of the wearer that avoids the generation of static electricity and so removes the danger from this source. Soles must be conductive and should be cleaned after each wearing to remove bacteria lodged in blood stains and dirt, which tend to insulate the bottom of the shoe. Shoes can be tested for conductivity by using an insulation tester. In the absence

of conductive shoes, conductive slip-ons or booties may be worn.

4. *Clothing.* Cotton clothing must be worn in the operating room. Wool, nylon, rayon, sharkskin, Orlon, Dacron, celanese and cellulose acetate are potential sources of hazard because the rate of static build-up is so rapid with these materials that sparking is hard to control with certainty. It is acceptable to wear nylon or other synthetic undergarments if the whole garment is in contact with the skin. A nylon slip is not acceptable; the bodice of the slip qualifies, but the free-hanging skirt is dangerous.

Principles of Surgical Asepsis

Ways and means of making an article sterile have been discussed in Appendix II, "Antisepsis and Asepsis." Following the sterilization process, the responsibility of the operating room personnel is to maintain asepsis by practicing a well-defined technique or procedure based on sound principles. Conscientiousness, alertness and honesty are personal qualifications necessary to execute these principles. Table A-1 will serve to emphasize the principle involved, what is implied and how the nurse can apply the principle concerned.

TABLE A-1. Outline of Principles of Asepsis and Applications

Principle	Implication	Guides to action
An article that is sterile remains so until it is contaminated	A package of sterile dressings on a shelf will remain sterile unless organisms are introduced	If commercially prepared sterile goods are cautiously handled and stored in a dry clean area free from vermin, dust and other contaminating sources, they may be considered sterile indefinitely. Items processed by the hospital and not stored in plastic covers are considered sterile for 4 weeks.
A sterile area or field can become contaminated:		
1. By becoming wet if the underlying area is unsterile	A sterile drape on a table can become wet from splashing water or fluid dropped from a container of surgical gut	1. Disposable sterile packs contain a moisture-proof polyvinyl table cover as well as drapes made of soft moisture-resistant fabric. If linen drapes are used, place polyvinyl over the table before opening the pack. If articles (such as ampules, cystoscope) have been soaked in a germicide solution, allow excess solution to drain off and then place in a sterile metal tray lined with a towel to absorb moisture and protect items from damage.
2. By dropping anything unsterile onto a sterile field	Powder falling from surgically clean hands prior to donning sterile gloves. An unsterile arm reaching over a sterile field	2. Avoid powdering hands over or near sterile field. A separate table should be used for gowning and gloving materials. Avoid reaching over a sterile field (1) to drop a sterile object, (2) to pour solutions, (3) to fix suction, cautery or drainage tubes, or (4) to reposition the head light.
3. By infectious or soiled materials from a wound	*E. coli* and other organisms are present in the gastrointestinal tract Pathogenic organisms are present in an abscess	3. Limit the contaminated field to as small an area as is practical. Following the procedure, all linens, dressings, instruments and gloves must be handled with special care.
4. From airborne sources, since air currents are capable of transporting contaminants	Dust, human expirations from the nose and the throat, and thrown soiled sponges are possible sources	4. Anyone with a respiratory infection should not work in an operating room. The nose and mouth must be covered with an effective mask; clearing the throat, coughing or sneezing if necessary should be done with the head turned away from the sterile field. Unnecessary conversation should be kept at a minimum. Excessive traffic should be forbidden. All persons other than the operating room staff must be properly attired before entering the suite, such as members of the x-ray department, consulting physicians, etc. Floors must be damp-mopped with an effective detergent-germicide between each procedure.

TABLE A-1. Outline of Principles of Asepsis and Applications (*Continued*)

Principle	Implication	Guides to action
A sterile area (field) remains sterile even when sterile articles are added to it	A sterile article may be moved to another sterile area by 1. The use of a sterile gloved hand 2. The use of sterile-tipped transfer forceps 3. Being dropped onto it, such as dressings or a knife blade	Sterile gloved hands must remain within constant view of their owner; hence it is desirable to keep hands at or above the waistline.

Over and above these principles, many policies or procedures need to be reviewed to emphasize the many activities that are related to the successful practice of aseptic technique. The most important of these procedures are the following:

PRINCIPLE: Keep sterile areas in view to prevent accidental contamination.

APPLICATION

Sterile Areas	Unsterile Areas
Top of a sterile drape.	Sides and back of a sterile draped table. (A suture or a ligature hanging over the edge of a table is considered unsterile.)
Above the anterior waist and anterior aspect of sleeves of a sterile gown.	Back of sleeves of sterile gown. Below waist of sterile gown. Under arm of sterile gown. Collar area of sterile gown.
Sterile gloved hands resting on a sterile drape or kept within the individual's view, always above the waist.	Sterile gloved hands on the waist at the side or below the waist.
A table, draped from front to back, which permits full view of the sterile area.	Draping a table from back to front is awkward, and all parts of the top side of the drape may not be visible.
Innermost side of a wrapper or cap that encloses a sterile article.	Edge of wrapper on a sterile package or edge of cap on a sterile flask or tube.

PRINCIPLE: "Scrubbed" persons keep away from unsterile areas; circulating personnel keep away from sterile areas.

APPLICATION

"Scrubbed" Persons	Circulating Persons
Stand a safe distance from operating table while patient is being draped. Face sterile areas when passing them. Turn back toward circulating persons or unsterile areas. Keep hand dips and sterile table at a safe distance from operating area so that one's back will not touch them. Never squeeze through a narrow space; rather, ask the "unsterile" person to move, or ask someone to move unsterile equipment.	Face sterile areas or scrubbed persons to prevent accidental contact.

TECHNIQUE OF SCRUBBING, PUTTING ON GOWN AND GLOVES

Scrubbing

Preoperative skin disinfection is done to remove from the hands and the arms as much dirt, fats, transient and resident bacterial flora as is possible. During an operation, should a glove become torn, the possibility of introducing organisms into the wound is lessened provided that a satisfactory preoperative scrub has been done. The normal bacteria on a person's skin vary in different parts of the body. On smooth surfaces, they may be few, whereas, in protected areas, such as creases, there may be many.

Immediately before scrubbing, the headgear can be adjusted and the mask tied so that the nose and the mouth are completely covered. For those who wear glasses, an effective method of preventing foggy glasses ("steaming up") is to rub them with a piece of soap and then wipe them clean. At the scrub sink, the water is adjusted to the proper temperature and flow.

The kind of surgical scrub (which consists of mechanical cleansing of the hands and the arms) depends on the needs of the individual scrubbing. Persons who participate in gardening, painting, mechanics or other activities which bring them in contact with soil need longer periods of scrubbing. Likewise, one who scrubs less frequently, such as once every 3 or 4 days, will need a longer scrub than the person who scrubs daily. Whatever the procedure, and there are several, certain principles must be observed:

1. The nails should be kept short; special attention must be given to the subungual space (beneath nail) with a sterile nail cleaner early in the scrub.

2. Use a soft but firm bristled brush or one of the numerous polyurethane disposable sponges which are impregnated with soap.

3. There are many acceptable antiseptic detergents, such as the hexachlorophenes and the iodophors.

4. Lather well and rinse frequently. No chemical agent can be relied upon as a substitute for conscientious mechanical cleansing of the skin.

5. The duration of the scrub may be determined by a time limit set on the conscientious scrubbing of one part after another in a prescribed manner, or it may be determined by a certain number of strokes per part. A practical, reliable and intelligent procedure should be followed. Scrubbing with circular brush motion is more effective than straight strokes. The long scrub done at the beginning of the day may vary from 7 to 10 minutes, depending upon recent past contamination as described earlier in this section. Because the moisture and warmth present under

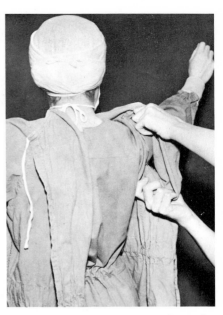

Fig. A-4. Method of putting on sterile gown. The unsterile nurse at the back of the scrub nurse or doctor grasps the axillary seam from within the gown. By pulling on this seam toward the chest wall, the sleeve is drawn easily over the damp hand to its proper position.

surgical gloves provides an ideal growing medium for bacteria, it is essential that a 3-minute scrub be done between cases.

6. Following the scrub, rinse hands and arms thoroughly, discard soap, and turn off water, using the elbow or knee. Hands are held higher than the elbows and away from the body; this allows water to run off at the elbow and prevents contaminated water from above the elbow to run down to the scrubbed hands. Proceed to the operating room.

7. When drying hands, care is taken to prevent the towel from touching the scrub dress or suit. One hand, then the arm, are dried with a towel proceeding from the finger tips to the elbow; the other hand and arm are dried in similar fashion using a dry segment of the towel.

Gowning and Gloving

After scrubbing and disinfecting the hands and the arms, a sterile gown and gloves are put on. These are worn to allow the wearer to participate in the surgical operation while maintaining a state of asepsis in as practical a way as is possible. The sterile gown may be obtained from an open pack, or it may be handed by someone already scrubbed. Since gowns are folded inside out to facilitate donning without touching the outside, the scrubbed person will hold the neckband and gently let the gown unfold from his extended hands. As the gown unfolds, the armholes should face the wearer. Slip the hands into the armholes and hold the hands upward.

The circulating nurse can assist by reaching inside the gown and pulling the sleeves over the hands on the scrubbed person (Fig. A-4). Tapes at the back

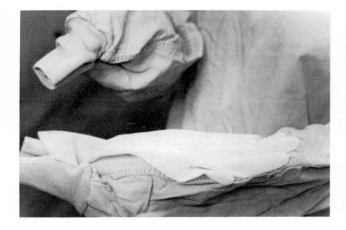
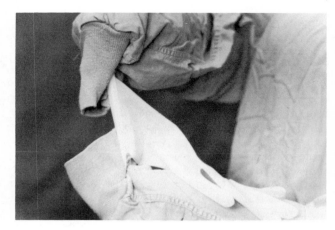
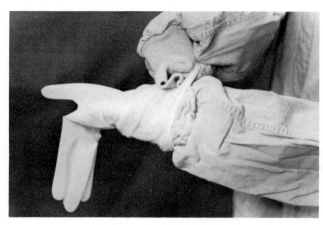
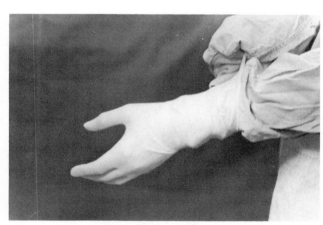

Fig. A-5. Closed method of donning gloves. (From Ginsberg, F., Brunner, L., and Cantlin, V.: A Manual of Operating Room Technology. p. 95. Philadelphia, J. B. Lippincott, 1966)

are tied. If the gown has tapes at the waist, the circulating nurse reaches for the ends of them without touching the gown, draws them back and ties them. Surgeons usually prefer to have their gowns tied loosely, whereas nurses often want the gown tied more snugly.

Note: A gown is sterile only as long as it is dry. If it is wet from perspiration or in any other way, it must be considered contaminated.

In the entire procedure of putting on sterile gloves, one principle must be followed; the surgically clean hand may touch the inside of the glove only; should it touch the outside, the glove is considered contaminated and must be discarded.

Glove lubricant that goes on as cream and dries as a powder minimizes the spread of dust particles. The purpose of powdering the hands is to ease the donning of sterile rubber gloves.

With the acceptance of disposable gloves, manufacturers are using silicone filming, which allows for easy donning. If the hands are dried thoroughly, the necessity of using powder is eliminated.

Steps in Putting on Sterile Gloves. Gloves are packaged with a cuff of at least 2 inches. The objective is to put on the gloves without touching the outside of the glove or the gown with the bare hands.

Open Method. In putting on the right glove, grasp its cuff on the *inside* with the left hand, insert the right hand into the glove and pull it in place with the left hand. Leave the cuff turned and release the grasp. Now the right gloved hand can pick up the left glove by inserting the fingers under its cuff (the outside is the sterile side). Insert the left hand in the left glove and pull into place leaving the cuff turned. By folding the gown wristlet snugly and holding this fold in place, that hand's fingers can safely pull up the rubber glove cuff over the gown wristlet. Repeat for the other glove (Fig. A-5).

Closed Method. Slide hands in sleeves only as far as sleeve-cuff seam. Grasp the inside of sleeve-cuff seam with thumb and index finger. After the gown is tied, (1) pick up a glove with one sleeve-covered hand and place it, thumb down on the palm side of

GUIDE FOR HANDLING OF DRAPES

Activity	Principles
Drapes are folded acording to "use" patterns to eliminate unnecessary handling. Avoid shaking and flourishing of linens.	Air currents carry contaminants.
Making a cuff by turning corners of the drape over the gloved hand will afford protection while placing the drape in position.	Contact with an unsterile surface contaminates a sterile object.
Always drape table or patient in such a way that the side closest to you is covered first.	Contact with an unsterile surface contaminates a sterile object.
The part of the drape that falls below the level of the table is considered contaminated.	When a question exists regarding sterility, the object (or field) is considered unsterile.
Do not use drapes that have holes, tears or worn spots.	A portal of entry that allows contact with an unsterile surface immediately renders an otherwise sterile field contaminated.
Once a drape is in place, it should not be moved.	Contact with an unsterile surface contaminates a sterile object.
If drapes, suction, cautery or drains are secured with towel clips, the portion of the clip that has gone through the drape must be considered unsterile.	
All drapes must be handled carefully. They should be held in such a way as to prevent any contact with areas other than the intended sterile field. Lights, I.V. poles and specialty machines must be watched during this process.	

the other arm with glove fingers pointing toward the shoulder. Glove cuff lies over gown wristlet; (2) grasp the wrist edge of the glove that is against the sleeve with the finger that holds the seam, and grasp the uppermost glove wrist edge with the sleeve-covered fingers of the other hand; (3) pull the glove wrist over the gown cuff, using care not to fold the gown cuff back or to expose the fingers inside it, and (4) as cuff is drawn onto wrist, fingers are directed into cots in glove, adjust the glove to hand. Put the second glove on in the same manner, using the newly gloved hand to hold the glove (Fig. A-5).

Offering the Gown and the Gloves to the Surgeon

The scrub nurse holds the sterile gown and gloves for the surgeon in such a way that he is able to get into them easily. In this procedure, the following steps are taken:

1. The nurse grasps the folded gown at the neck band, holds it out at arm's length and lets it unfold. Care must be taken not to shake the gown.
2. By making a cuff, using the neck area of the gown, the scrub nurse can protect her gloved hands underneath this cuff.
3. She offers the inside of the gown to the surgeon. (The circulating nurse pulls the gown on and ties it.)

4. The lubricant is put on the hands.
5. The scrub nurse places her fingers on each hand beneath the cuff, care being taken to keep the thumbs turned outward and stretching the cuff as the surgeon slips his hand into the glove, exerting a firm downward thrust (Fig. A-6).

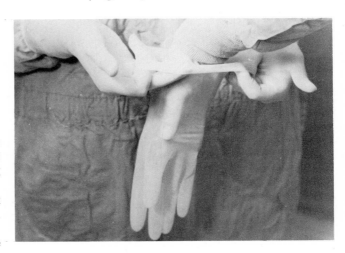

Fig. A-6. The glove cuff is spread wide to allow the donner to slip his hand into the glove without touching the holder of the glove. Note that the thumb is facing toward the person who will wear the glove.

GUIDE FOR HANDLING OF FORCEPS

Activity	Principle

When withdrawing the forceps from the germicide container, do not allow the forceps to touch the side or the top of the container.

A sterile object becomes contaminated when it touches an unsterile area. (The area not covered with germicide solution cannot be considered sterile.)

Keep the forceps blades pointed downward at all times. If this is not done, germicide solution will flow toward the unsterile handle. When the forceps are returned to the correct position, the blades become contaminated.

Gravity pulls liquids downward.

When using the forceps, keep them within view at the level of the waistline or above it.

A sterile object or area remains sterile unless it is contaminated. (A possibility of contamination exists when a sterile object is out of view.)

Drop the sterile article gently on the sterile field; the forceps must not touch the field.

After an operation has begun, the sterile set-up is sterile for that patient alone; should a sterile transfer forceps touch such a field, it is no longer sterile for any other field.

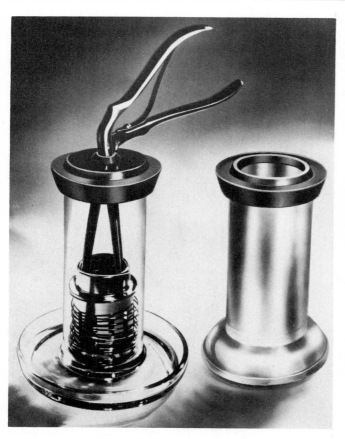

FIG. A-7. Bard-Parker forceps. (From Ginsberg, F., Brunner, L., and Cantlin, V.: Manual of Operating Room Technology. p. 104. Philadelphia, J. B. Lippincott, 1966)

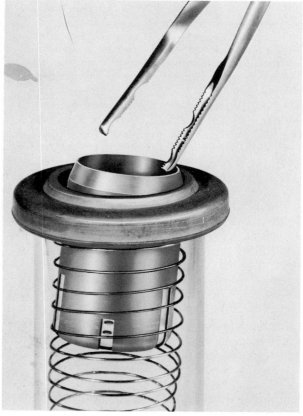

FIG. A-8. Bard-Parker transfer forceps. (From Ginsberg, F., Brunner, L., and Cantlin, V.: Manual of Operating Room Technology. p. 105. Philadelphia, J. B. Lippincott, 1966)

SURGICAL DRAPING

The purpose of draping is to provide a sterile field. Many types of drape materials are available, but the two most popular are (1) linen (broad term to indicate woven cloth) and (2) nonabsorbent synthetic drapes. Disposable drapes are desirable because they are superior bacterial barriers. They are soft, lightweight, lint free, compact, sterile, moisture-resistant and static free. When used in conjunction with the plastic polyvinyl self-adherent drape through which the incision is made, an effective covering is achieved. Regardless of the kind of material used, the principles of handling remain the same.

THE CIRCULATING NURSE

The circulating nurse constantly observes the surgical field and replenishes items used, contaminated or needed for the procedure. Some of her most frequent activities are: (1) using a sterile transfer forcep; (2) opening sterile packages; (3) opening jars; (4) pouring sterile solutions.

Use of Transfer or Pick-Up Forceps

The use of transfer forceps implies that stock materials are used on many cases and are removed from a container as needed. The unit system, in which all items are packaged individually, is by far the best technique. This virtually eliminates potential sources of contamination through faulty handling of transfer forceps (Figs. A-7, A-8). If used, such a forceps and its container are first sterilized (a single forceps for each container); then a germicide is added to the container, and the forceps is placed so that the prongs or the legs are immersed. Thereafter, only that end of the forceps which is in the germicide is considered sterile.

Transfer forceps should be used with the prongs pointed downward. The prongs permit the grasping of circular objects, gloves, drains, sutures as well as fine surgical needles.

Caution: Do not use transfer forceps to pick up anything with an adhering base, such as petroleum gauze. Should this occur, clean and resterilize the forceps; otherwise, anything picked up by the forceps will adhere to it.

Opening a Sterile Package

This may be done by placing the package on a table and undoing the wrapper in such a way that only the outside cover is touched by the circulating nurse. Or she may hold the package in her left hand and unwrap with the right hand (Fig. A-9).

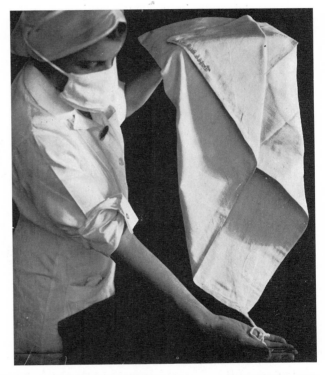

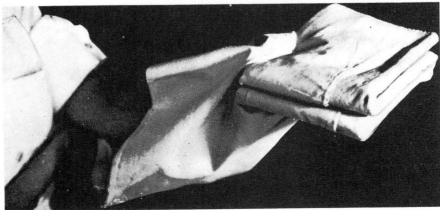

Fig. A-9. (*Top*) The first step is unwrapping the package. (*Bottom*) The package completely unwrapped and ready to hand to a sterile nurse or to place on a sterile table. (The Surgical Supervisor, American Sterilizer Co., Erie, Pa.)

GUIDE FOR HANDLING OF STERILE COVERED CONTAINER

Activity	Principle
Remove the lid only when necessary and replace it as soon as possible.	The possibility of air-borne contamination exists.
In removing the lid, hold it in such a way that the sterile undersurface faces downward.	Because of gravity, dust particles, etc., fall downward.
If it is necessary to set the lid down, the sterile undersurface faces upward.	Contact with an unsterile surface contaminates a sterile object.
The rims of the lids and the container are considered unsterile.	(Proximity to unsterile surfaces makes the rim of the lid and container a doubtful area.) When sterility is doubted, consider the object (or field) as contaminated.
Unused sterile objects are not to be returned to the sterile container.	Air currents carry contaminants.

The scrub nurse may take the offered package, or it may be dropped safely on a sterile field. The loose ends of the wrapper must be drawn back and away from the inner sterile package and the sterile field. The arm and the hand of the circulating nurse must not reach over the sterile field.

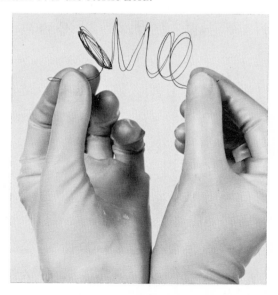

Handling a Sterile Covered Container

The hazards of using sterile covered containers must be understood. Each time the lid is removed there is a possibility of air-borne contamination; hence, unnecessary or prolonged removal of the lid should be avoided. When several persons use a common container, the risk of contamination exists. To minimize these problems, each person using such a container must be thoroughly familiar with the handling of it.

Pouring Sterile Solutions

Sterile flasks or pitchers are covered with a top that fits over the outer edge of the flask or bottle. To remove the cap, touch only the top outer surface and avoid touching the edge. If the flask or the bottle has a pouring lip, such as the "Pour-O-Vac," sterile fluids can be dispensed safely. These flasks and pour bottles may be resealed and opened many times during a procedure, but should only be used for one procedure.

When pouring solutions or medications, the flask or pitcher must be held high enough so that the unsterile outside of the container or the hand of the person pouring do not touch the receiving sterile basin. It should not be held so high that the solution

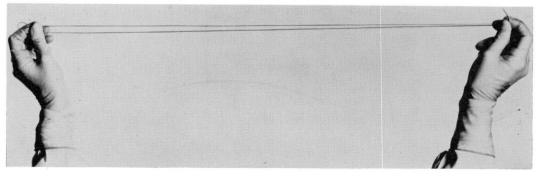

FIG. A-10. Unwinding surgical gut sutures. Strand is gently pulled out straight with an even pull to remove kinks. (Davis & Geck, Division of American Cyanamid Company)

Fig. A-11. Types of sutures commonly used. Types 4, 5 and 8 are utilized on the intestine, Types 3 and 10 on the skin, Type 11 on the fascia and Type 12 on the entire thickness of the abdominal wall (or thoracic wall). The other sutures depicted have more general applications. (Rhoads, J. E., *et al.*: Surgery: Principles and Practice, ed. 4, Philadelphia, J. B. Lippincott, 1970)

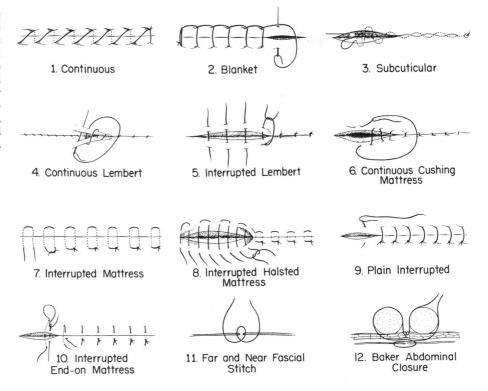

1. Continuous
2. Blanket
3. Subcuticular
4. Continuous Lembert
5. Interrupted Lembert
6. Continuous Cushing Mattress
7. Interrupted Mattress
8. Interrupted Halsted Mattress
9. Plain Interrupted
10. Interrupted End-on Mattress
11. Far and Near Fascial Stitch
12. Baker Abdominal Closure

splashes and wets the sterile field if linen drapes are used. Long cotton flannel gloves are provided as a precaution against burns from hot bottles and solutions.

PREPARATION OF TABLES FOR THE OPERATION

At this point the circulating nurse and the scrub nurse work together to set up the various tables needed for a specific operation.

Laparotomy Pack. The outer cover, when unwrapped, serves as the drape for the table. When the inner wrap is unfolded, it reveals the cover for the Mayo stand, towels, and drapes for the patient, including the fenestrated sheet. Materials included are a matter of preference; however, the significant points of packaging are (1) to keep the size consistent with proper sterilization qualifications, (2) to arrange materials in order of use, and (3) to place the pack where it will be used.

Basin Set. The contents vary according to the procedure. Most basin sets for major surgery contain medicine glasses (for xylocaine, mineral oil, antibiotics, etc.), basins for hand-dip, specimen and sutures.

Gown Pack. The outer wrap also provides the drape for this table. The gowns are arranged on the table and the gloves are added. This unit should be separate and apart from the instrument and prep table.

Surgical Scrub 'Prep' Table. It is necessary to scrub the operative site with soap and germicidal solutions; the person assigned does this with his gloved hand in order to develop the friction necessary for cleansing. Cotton-tipped applicators are essential for cleansing the umbilicus and other hard to reach areas. This set contains towels that are placed on each side of the patient to absorb solutions, sponges, cotton-tipped applicators and basins for soap solution and germicide.

LIGATURES AND SUTURES

After the instruments are placed (according to the prescribed pattern in the local hospital), the "scrubbed" nurse will select and prepare ligatures and sutures according to the needs of the operation and the preference of the surgeon.*

Generally, a *ligature* (a tie) is a free piece of suture material, not threaded on a needle, and of considerable length (10 to 18 in.) or on a spool, for the purpose of tying blood vessels that have previously been clamped with an artery forceps. Spiral-wound suture material is available and is more convenient to use than a suture wound on a reel.

* Types of suture materials are discussed on pages 1007-1008.

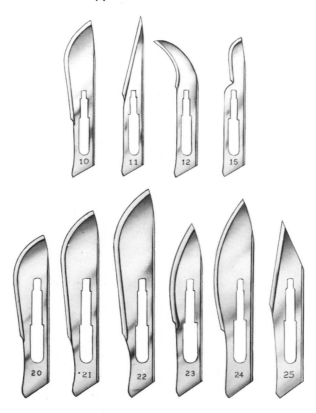

FIG. A-12. The most common kinds of knife blades. (Bard-Parker Co., Danbury, Conn.)

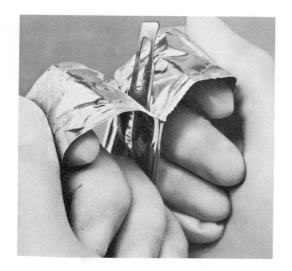

FIG. A-13. Unopened packets of individually wrapped knife blades are put in the instrument pack and autoclaved with them. The scrub nurse opens the packet by pulling two tabs which expose the sterile blade for use. (A-S-R Products Corporation)

A *suture* is either a surgical gut, or a silk, cotton or metal thread, 18 or more inches long, threaded on a needle. It is used for sewing or suturing together the edges and the surfaces of tissue, for checking the flow of blood, fastening drainage tubes in position, etc. Sutures are either *interrupted*, each stitch tied separately, or *continuous*, the thread running in a series of stitches, only the first and last of which are tied. The length of sutures naturally varies considerably. Each depends on the character of the work and the nature of the operation. Deep work, in the pelvis for instance, requires a much longer suture than would be necessary in suturing in an area closer to the surface of a wound. Experience and judgment, along with the desire of the surgeon, must be the determining factors in details of sutures and ligatures.

Testing of suture material is usually unnecessary if it is purchased from reliable firms who gauge and test for tensile strength. However, if testing is undertaken, it must be done carefully. A length of suture material is tested by holding the ends in each hand and exerting a firm, steady pull. Any jerking will weaken it considerably (Fig. A-10). It is injurious to handle suture material any more than is absolutely necessary, such as constantly drawing it through the fingers, etc. If a suture is tightly wound, it may develop a kink, which is easily removed by a brief solution dip and gentle stretching. Do not soak sutures in solution, because this reduces the tensile strength and prematurely hastens the absorption process.

When a suture is being used (Fig. A-11), a duplicate should be kept in reserve. The end of a suture never should be wrapped around a needle holder nor should it be dragged over the instruments or drapings. A needle that has been used should be replaced in the holder as soon as the surgeon lays it down. Constant checking to see that all needles are accounted for is necessary. Suture material cut on the bias facilitates threading. Gloves that are clean and wet make the handling of instruments and sutures much easier than dry, sticky gloves.

IMMEDIATELY BEFORE THE OPERATION

Before the patient is wheeled into the operating room, the circulating nurse checks the patient's chart, identification band and then spends a few moments speaking with her patient. If everything is in order, she assists the anesthesiologist and orderly in moving the patient into the operating room and onto the table. Remembering to consider the patient's modesty, the sheet is turned down or removed to expose the operative site. The knee strap is in place before the anesthesia is started. When the patient is anesthetized, the preparation of the skin is then carried out by a member of the team.

The surgical drapes are positioned and a screen over the head of the patient holds the drapes away from his face and affords visibility and working space for the anesthesiologist. When necessary, plastic or metal clips are used to hold the towels or drapes in place.

Responsibilities of the "Scrub" Nurse:

1. Arrange the instruments on Mayo tray and back table so they are readily accessible.

2. Place knife blades on handles (Figs. A-12, A-13).

3. Count sponges, needles (eye and atraumatic), instruments, and other small items with the circulating nurse.

4. Arrange suture material and prepare the ligatures and sutures that will be used first.

5. Check the performance of all items that will be used during the procedure.

DURING THE OPERATION

Principles of Operative Procedure

Surgery may be done for a variety of reasons: to remove foreign bodies, to remove diseased parts, to repair poorly functioning parts, to diagnose or to explore. Whatever the reason, all precautions are taken to handle tissue gently and carefully. The incision heals best when a clean smooth cut is made; the scalpel blade must not produce a jagged tear. For adequate exposure and a minimum of trauma from retractors, the incision should be adequate.

Hemostasis is the process of controlling hemorrhage and is of importance for these reasons: (1) it prevents blood loss and shock; (2) the likelihood of postoperative hematoma is lessened; (3) the surgeon is able to dissect more accurately in a bloodless field.

Naturally, blood vessels will be severed. In order to make the operative field dry and visible, it is necessary to minimize bleeding by *sponging* as well as using other means of control. A sponge must be used to blot by gentle pressure; rubbing or using force injures delicate tissues. It is much better to conserve the patient's own blood by controlling bleeding areas than to replace lost blood.

Methods of Controlling Blood Loss. Next to the scalpel, the *hemostat* probably is the most common of all surgical instruments. It is of simple design with a screw lock having slender jaws for grasping and compressing a blood vessel. Hemostats may have straight or curved tips, and are of various sized blades according to the needs of the operative procedure and the preference of the surgeon. Sometimes the pressure of the instrument on the vessel is sufficient to con-

strict and seal it; however, the surgeon may slip a *ligature* (a thread or a tie) around the captured vessel. After tying it securely, the hemostat is released, the excess thread is cut, and the vessel is sealed.

In neurosurgery, two common methods of controlling hemorrhage are the use of *bone wax* and *silver clips*. Bone wax, composed mainly of beeswax, is used to seal bleeders in bone. The wax must be broken into small pieces and kneaded between the gloves until it is soft and pliable. It is then rubbed into the bleeding surface of the bone to act as an hemostatic substance. Silver clips are placed in a special holder and used to occlude a bleeding vessel when electrocoagulation or ligature is not used. Many types are available.

Oxidized cellulose (Oxycel, Surgicel) is a hemostatic absorbable substance made of specially treated gauze or cotton, which, when applied directly to a bleeding area, checks capillary oozing. It absorbs fluids, and it swells and becomes sticky, forming a jellylike mass or coagulum. It is available in gauze-type pads, pledgets or strips.

Gelatin sponge (Gelfoam, Gelfoam Powder, Gelfilm) is an absorbable substance made from gelatin that has been beaten to a foamy consistency, dried and heat sterilized. It may be cut to any size or shape; when placed in an area of capillary bleeding, fibrin is deposited within its spaces, the sponge swells, and an effective clot is formed.

Hot Packs. Hot gauze compresses are sometimes used to control superficial bleeding.

Electrocoagulation. The electrocautery is principally used to control bleeding by sealing blood vessels; it is also used to cut with a knife-like tip, to desiccate and cauterize areas such as the cervix. Maximal performance is obtained when the cautery is used in a dry field.

Responsibilities of the Circulating Nurse

The circulating nurse has many functions during an operation. Stated simply, she is responsible for maintaining a neat, quiet, well-organized operating room and must be able to anticipate and meet the needs of the "scrub" nurse, the surgeon, the anesthesiologist and the patient. *Above all, she is responsible for the safety and the comfort of the patient.* Some of her activities include the following:

1. Observe technique at all times to see that it is maintained properly. If there is a break, it must be remedied.

2. Assume responsibility with the other members of the team for the comfort and the safety of the patient.

3. Keep the "scrub" nurse supplied with dressings, suture materials, etc.

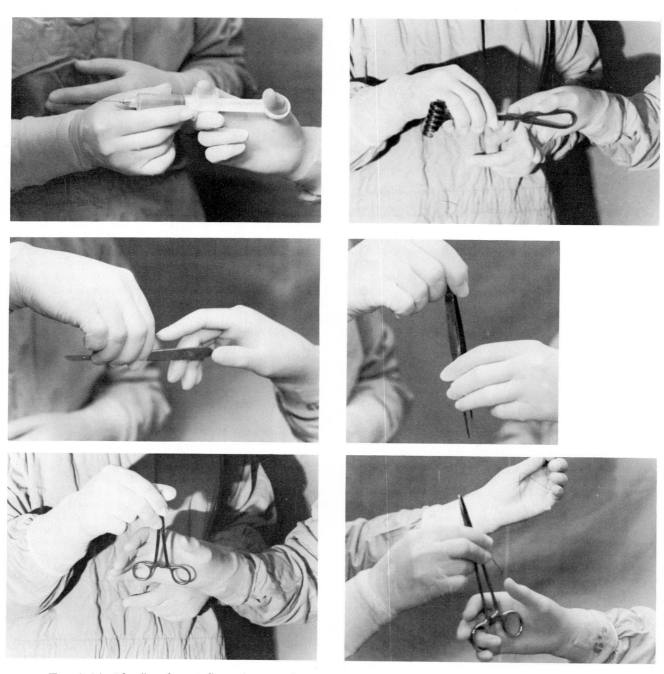

FIG. A-14. The "scrub nurse"—technique of passing sutures and instruments. (*Top left*) Passing the syringe. The ring-type syringe should be passed so that the rings may be grasped easily by the surgeon in the fingers of the right hand. (*Middle left*) Passing the scalpel. The handle is to be directed to the surgeon's hand with the blade pointing downward. (*Bottom left*) Passing an hemostat. The handle is slapped into the receiving hand of the surgeon. (*Top right*) Passing a rake retractor. Handle is slapped into the surgeon's hand with the prongs of the retractor facing downward. (*Middle right*) Forceps to be passed by grasping the end in the fingers, the open part of the forceps down. As most surgeons are right-handed, the forceps usually are passed to the surgeon's left hand. (*Bottom right*) Passing a threaded needle holder. Handle directed to surgeon's hand and the needle in position to be directed downward. Note the scrub nurse's hand guiding the suture material away from the receiving hand of the surgeon.

4. Attach the suction apparatus and check to see that it is functioning properly.

5. Place buckets strategically to receive discarded sponges.

6. Retrieve instruments, etc., that accidentally fall from the table.

7. Replace saline or water in basins as necessary.

8. Regulate temperature of the room as necessary.

9. Count, with the "scrub" nurse, all sponges opened for use, and permit no gauze of any kind to be carried from the operating room during an abdominal operation.

10. Take care of specimens.

11. Prepare dressing materials to be used following wound closure.

12. Direct the cleaning and the preparation of the room for the next patient.

From the responsibilities listed, it is evident that the circulating nurse must be prepared for her position. Essential attributes which she should possess are these: (1) ability to organize activities and direct personnel, with due understanding of interpersonal relations; (2) ability to anticipate needs; (3) ability to differentiate between situations that demand immediate attention and those of lesser import; (4) ability to maintain a quiet, neat and well-equipped unit; (5) understand thoroughly the principles of asepsis and (6) ability to teach actively and by the example she sets.

Responsibilities of the "Scrub" Nurse

Individual surgeons have individual preferences in their effort to standardize operative procedures. The "scrubbed" assistants learn how best to work with each surgeon as a smooth-working team. Some general suggestions are offered to help the "scrub" nurse in her important role.

To begin with, she is guided and directed constantly by what the surgeon is doing. This means almost constant attention to the wound. The scalpel is discarded, after the skin incision is made, and replaced with a fresh one. Since the skin cannot be sterilized, the blade used on the skin is considered contaminated.

The next step is to provide ligatures for tying the vessels that are clamped. If the nurse holds each end of a surgical gut "tie," the surgeon is able to grasp the suture in the middle. When cotton, nylon or silk ligatures are used, the surgeon often ties from a reel or a bobbin of ligature material. In such case the bobbin should be handed to the surgeon, with a 6″ or 8″ length of ligature material hanging free. All ligatures must have excess threads cut after the tie is completed; therefore, an assistant must be provided with scissors.

By knowing these basic steps, a nurse is soon able to anticipate the needs of the surgeon and his assistants without being told. Some surgeons use a sign language, so that the nurse knows by a gesture what he would like next. The simple routine of scalpel, sponges, hemostat, ligature and scissors is fairly consistent. Common sense has to be practiced too. For example, suppose that after a ligature has been passed to the surgeon, he ties the bleeding vessel, and his assistant releases the hemostat. In the usual order, the scissors would be passed next. However, suppose that at that instant, a vessel begins to bleed profusely. The wisdom of passing a scissors or a hemostat can be readily determined.

The "scrub" nurse learns to anticipate intelligently the needs of the surgeon. This can be done only by watching the field of operation carefully. There may be instances in which the view of the nurse is obstructed, but she should make every effort to see and understand the progress of the operation. She is responsible for keeping the field neat and uncluttered —this includes removal of loose ends of suture or ligature material. She should ask quietly for new supplies, work rapidly and efficiently. This implies that her tables should be arranged in such a way (and she should know the arrangement) that she can reach any article without having to turn her head to look for it. Obviously, this can come only with practice. The surgeon should not expect a new nurse to have this skill, nor should a new nurse be placed in a situation for which she is not properly prepared and supervised.

Passing Instruments. In passing an instrument, place it in the surgeon's hand in the position in which he is going to use it. Pass a needle in a needle holder the same way; support the suture so that it does not drag, and have the needle pointing in the direction in which the surgeon will use it (Fig. A-14).

A basin should be provided to receive any specimen. Care must be taken that cultures or other specimens are cared for properly.

Sponge and Item Count. This is necessary in all large wounds and when body cavities (abdominal and chest) are entered during operation. To ensure the patient's safety in the operating room, it is strongly recommended that sponges containing radiopaque materials be used.

The most common and effective procedure is to have the count taken 3 or 4 times for each operation. Since most items in the sponge variety are factory-counted, 3 counts have proven adequate. The following items are counted: sponges, needles (eye and atraumatic), laparotomy packs, instruments and small items such as neurosurgical patties, dissector sponges, "bull dogs" and umbilical tapes.

1. The circulating nurse and scrub nurse or technician count together before the operation begins and records the exact number of each item. As additional items are required, these are also counted together and recorded.

2. The count is taken again when the closure of the wound begins.

3. After the peritoneum has been closed, the final count is taken. The instrument count need not be done for a third time. It is essential that no loose sponges be used during the closure, because they can be masked by blood and lost in the muscle or fascia.

If there is an incorrect count, it must be verified by x-ray that the item is not in the patient. The count should be recorded and kept as a permanent part of the patient's operative record.

After the skin is closed and dressings have been applied, the "scrub" nurse collects all drapes and removes all tables from the operating room. She is personally responsible for taking care of any specimens and seeing that they are labeled properly and transported to the laboratory. She also should remove needles from holders, knife blades from knife handles, etc., so that whoever is responsible for instrument cleaning is not cut accidentally. Dressings and linens that were not used do not have to be discarded. They can be repackaged later and autoclaved

Drainage Materials. Drainage is required to permit easy escape of pus, blood, or such fluids that might collect in wounds and delay their healing; the most common materials used are gauze, rubber tissue, rubber tubes, catheters, plastic tubes and self-contained suction units. The drain selected for use must not clog or adhere to the edges of the wound. All drainage should be recorded and measured when necessary.

BETWEEN OPERATIONS

Every possible precaution should be taken to avoid undue haste; at the same time, as little time as possible should be lost in going from one operation to another. Sufficient time must be allowed for the proper cleaning of the room and the floor. Nothing—instruments, supplies, suture material, etc.—that has been used for one operation should be used for another without resterilization. Gowns, masks and gloves must be changed between patients.

Care of Specimens

A *specimen* is any tissue removed from a patient during an operation. Most specimens are sent to the pathology laboratory for examination, whereas cultures, spinal fluid, urine and smears are sent to the bacteriology laboratory. The nurse's responsibility is twofold: (1) the specimen must be labeled properly, and (2) it must be sent to the proper laboratory.

Each specimen should be handled carefully so as not to destroy any natural landmarks or characteristics that might aid in the diagnosis. Each specimen should be placed in a container of adequate size and covered with the solution recommended by the local laboratory. Allowing a specimen to dry produces autolysis, and the specimen becomes useless for study. There are several exceptions to this general rule, and the nurse should familiarize herself with the policies of the local laboratory. For example, specimens for frozen section are taken to the laboratory immediately after they are obtained. For D and C specimens, some surgeons prefer to have the specimen rinsed of excess blood, with citrate, before placing in formalin. Smears may be placed in equal parts of 95 per cent alcohol and ether. The disposition of the specimen is recorded on the operative record.

Early in the nurse's orientation to the operating room, she should become familiar with the correct procedure to follow in the local hospital. When it is realized that the future of many patients depends on a small specimen of tissue and its laboratory studies, the nurse's responsibility for safeguarding and caring for it is a real and great one.

AT THE END OF THE OPERATIVE SCHEDULE

After the day's operations, the entire operating suite must receive a thorough cleaning, with particular attention to the operating room proper. Soiled linen must be sorted carefully to prevent valuable instruments being sent to the laundry.

Floors should be cleaned and disinfected daily with a detergent germicide; the iodophors and the phenolics combine these actions. All tables, stools, basin racks, etc., must be washed well to remove blood stains and any other foreign material. The operating table and pad should be cleaned thoroughly with a detergent germicide.

All unused sterile supplies, including packages that have been opened, must be resterilized, even though the contents apparently have not been touched. When in doubt, resterilize.

Utensils and special apparatus must be cleansed and sterilized or put away, as the case may demand. Everything that has been used during the course of the day's operations should be returned to its rightful place in condition to be used again at a moment's notice. The operating room must always be in a state of preparedness.

SAFETY PRACTICES IN THE OPERATING ROOM

Throughout the chapter devoted to operating room nursing, safety measures have been emphasized. However, inasmuch as safety practices never can be overemphasized, this section explores further the conditions and the activities that are potentially hazardous and what might be done to eliminate them.

The operating room nurse has a responsibility for the safety of every patient who comes to her department. Emergency equipment always should be available and in usable condition. This includes suction apparatus, airways, drugs, etc. No excuse is acceptable when a patient's life is lost due to negligence.

All solutions that are used in the operating room should be labeled plainly. In order that mistakes may be averted, the policy of tinting solutions is helpful. There is no justification for a patient's receiving an injection of ether when the surgeon assumed that he was using procaine.

Although it is not the direct responsibility of the nurse to check anesthesia equipment, she must be aware of the importance of maintaining proper connections of tubing leading to gas machines, suction outlets, air under pressure, etc. For example, a wrong connection made by a well-intentioned nurse or auxiliary worker may result in a patient's receiving carbon dioxide when his precarious condition demands oxygen.

Occasionally, a needle breaks and is lost in the tissues of the patient. This may be a hollow needle, which can break at the hub during an injection, or it may be a suture needle. It is extremely important that such an accident be reported to the surgeon, who will initiate steps to localize and remove the foreign object.

The recovery of all instruments and sponges used during an operation is imperative. Even though the surgeon assumes the responsibility for a correct count, the nurse is in a unique position to verify such an accounting.

Explosive Hazards and Safety Precautions

Four factors operate simultaneously to produce explosive combustion of anesthetic gases in the operating room: (1) a flammable gas, (2) the presence of oxygen, (3) a source of ignition and (4) carelessness. To control the first 2 factors, a closed technique of administering the gas is recommended. All personnel should keep away from the anesthesia area, at least 2 feet away from anesthesia equipment and the patient securing the anesthetic agent. A source of ignition may be from:

Flammable Anesthesia Drugs	
Ether	Ethylene
Vinethene	Cyclopropane
Ethyl Chloride	Divinyl Ether

Any of these in a gaseous vapor form, mixed with nitrous oxide, air or oxygen, form explosive mixtures.

Nonflammable Anesthesia Drugs	
Nitrogen	Penthrane
Carbon Dioxide	Chloroform
Helium	Nitrous Oxide
Oxygen	Trichlorethylene
	Fluothane

---

1. Flames, such as cigarettes, alcohol lamps;
2. Electrical equipment, such as motors, heaters, hot plates, x-ray equipment, cauteries, switches, lamps, endoscopes;
3. Static electricity, such as friction from rubber goods, clothing, tearing of adhesive, shuffling of feet or personnel moving about the room; and
4. Clicking together of metal parts, such as slip joints, dropping of instruments, or dragging I.V. poles.

All electric equipment should be Underwriters'-approved. Cords of portable lamps and electrical appliances should be flexible, continuous and without connections or switches. They should be equipped with explosion-proof plugs.

Another essential safety factor in the operating room is to maintain conductive pathways so that electrical contact is provided. Conductive parts of tables or equipment that are worn should be replaced. Suture ends, dirt, blood or pus must not be allowed to accumulate on castors of tables that tend to insulate them from the floor. Wax that is nonconductive should not be applied to the floor. A system of checking or testing the safety of equipment is essential to the safety of the surgical patient and should be enforced rigorously.

Wool blankets and plastic sheets should not be used around anesthetic-gas equipment or patients anesthetized with combustible-gas mixtures. Cotton blankets are preferred; however, these blankets must be free of synthetic fibers such as nylon, dacron, etc. It is preferable not to warm cotton blankets, since this removes moisture, which cuts down on the possibility of static sparks. (Physiologically, a superwarmed blanket may be more harmful to the anesthetized patient than one at room temperature.) Conductive rubber mattresses, pads and pillows, breathing tubes, bags and masks should be used. Operating tables should be fitted with conductive straps for connecting the bare skin of the patient with the conductive system. Receptacles and plugs that cannot be pulled apart accidentally should be installed where needed. Unless they are of the explosion-proof type, they should not be placed lower than 5 feet above the floor.

Personnel contribute to the fourth factor mentioned above, namely, carelessness. Proper wearing apparel has been described on page 990. The nurse is in a position to be informed and to pass this information on to others not so informed. This responsibility for teaching, particularly in the operating room, is one major area of difference between professional and nonprofessional personnel. Only by accepting fully her obligations to her patient and to her profession will the nurse justify assuming a key position in the operating room.

STERILIZATION AND CARE OF VARIOUS ARTICLES

Instruments

Instruments have been designed for specific purposes such as cutting, holding, clamping, exposing, etc. They should be used correctly, since misuse will cause deterioration and breakage. Instruments may be cleaned in a washing sterilizer or manually.

Soiled instruments washed manually:

1. Soak in detergent-germicide to prevent drying of soil.
2. Assembled instruments should be disassembled after use and cleaned. All instruments should be opened for cleaning.
3. Place in a deep basin with ordinary cleaners, such as mild soaps or free-rinsing detergents.
4. Instruments with serrations and box-locks must be scrubbed with a brush.
5. Instruments should be thoroughly rinsed with water.
6. Instruments must be completely dry for storage.

To prevent rusting, complete drying can be obtained by placing instruments in a dry heat oven, a sonic energy unit or steam sterilizer that has heat in the jacket only.

For lubrication, only water-soluble lubricants are recommended. These are non-oily, non-sticky liquids that keep the instruments working better longer and do not interfere with steam sterilization.

The following suggestions will prolong the use of an instrument:

1. Do not handle instruments unnecessarily. The habit of idly opening and closing a hemostat merely to feel it click causes more wear than ordinary surgery.
2. Heavy instruments should be placed in the bottom of the tray. Lightweight, delicate and small items should be placed on top.

3. Instruments with movable parts should be taken apart, sterilized and reassembled before use and for storage.
4. Never use the instrument for other than its intended purpose.
5. Do not "soak" instruments in normal saline during the procedure. Salt has an extremely high corrosive action on all steel.

Let the surgeon who uses the instrument be the judge of its performance. If the instrument is not perfect, it should be sent for repair and not returned to the field until its performance is perfect.

Sterilization. Instruments should be unlocked before sterilization; this allows for proper sterilization of all surfaces. The preferred method of sterilizing instruments preoperatively is steam under pressure, 120° C. (250° F.) for 15 minutes, with 15 to 17 lbs. of pressure. Instruments may also be sterilized in a hot oven for 1 hour at 160° C. (320° F.). The disadvantage here is the length of time.

For routine washing and sterilizing of soiled or contaminated instruments, the instrument-washer-sterilizer is recommended. The cleansing process is accomplished chiefly by exposing the instruments to an effective detergent solution in the washer; ultimately, sterilization takes place when the temperature reaches 132.2° C. (270° F.).

For emergency sterilization 132.2° C. (270° F.) at 27 lbs. for 3 minutes is perfectly safe.

Boiling water for 30 minutes may be used; it is recognized that some spores can withstand this method. When an alkali has been added to the water, the time of boiling may be reduced to 15 minutes.

Chemical disinfection is discussed on p. 986.

Cutting Instruments

Knives, scissors, chisels and other sharp instruments depend on the sharpness of their edges for proper performance. Every effort must be exerted to protect the blades from injury. This is accomplished by cleaning them carefully, avoiding abrasives and preventing them from coming in contact with hard surfaces. They must be sterilized in the least injurious and safest way.

Knives may have the blade permanently attached, or it may be detached. One of the safest methods of attaching or removing a detachable blade is by using a special forceps.

Scissors are made in a variety of types for various uses; on the whole, they are delicate and should not be used for purposes other than the use specifically intended. They are easily sprung, and the fine adjustments can be damaged with very little effort.

Sterilization. Cutting-edge instruments and those so delicate that moist heat destroys them should be sterilized by dry heat at 160° C. (320° F.) for 1 hour. Scissors and instruments of stainless steel that are made properly are not injured by heat and can be sterilized safely by autoclaving at 121° C. for 15 minutes. Sharp instruments should not be piled on top of one another, because of the possibility of injuring the cutting edges. Knife blades may be purchased individually wrapped and sterile, and that is the safest method. Blades can be disinfected in a germicide; however, the hazards involved in germicidal disinfection must be recognized. When germicides are used, the blade must be washed carefully before use. The germicide is so powerful that if it comes in contact with tissue, it produces an immediate death of tissues, with consequent complications in wound healing.

Instrument Setups

After the instruments have been sterilized, the nurse arranges them for the next operation. For a simple operation such as a biopsy of lymph node, suturing of a laceration, etc., the instruments, suture materials, drapes and dressings may be conveniently placed on one table. Basic instruments for a simple setup are as follows:

Sponge forceps and towel clips
Scalpel
Scissors (dissecting and nurse's)
Forceps, plain and toothed
Hemostats, straight and curved
Allis forceps
Retractors
Suture needles and needles
Grooved director and/or probe

Modifications of this setup are made in terms of the type of operation and the preference of the surgeon. If the arrangement of this table is standardized, it becomes a simple matter to make minor additions for such operations as hemorrhoidectomy, minor amputations, minor plastic operations, tonsillectomy, etc. For an incision and drainage of an abscess, a culture tube and drainage material should be added.

For a simple abdominal procedure, such as an appendectomy or herniorrhaphy, or a larger dissecting operation such as a mastectomy or radical neck dissection, a Mayo instrument stand plus an instrument table is usually used. The Mayo stand ordinarily contains the basic instruments found in the simple setup described above. The instrument table is convenient for the specialty instruments as well as drains, suture material, dressings, etc. From such a setup as the basic Mayo stand and appendectomy instrument table, the more major procedure setups can be developed.

Fig. A-15. U.S. Pharmacopoeia suture gauges. (Ziegler, P. F.: Text Book of Sutures, Bauer & Black, Chicago, Ill.)

Gauge		mm.
0000000	———	0.038 mm.
000000	———	0.077
00000	———	0.127
0000	———	0.178
000	———	0.229
00	———	0.292
0	———	0.368
1	———	0.445
2	———	0.521
3	———	0.597
4	———	0.671
5	———	0.762
6	———	0.864
7	———	0.965

Suture Materials

Surgical gut (catgut) is made from the submucous layer of sheep's intestine, which is cleaned, dried and twisted into threads of various sizes and prepared for use by special processes, which include innumerable inspections of gauge and tensile strength and scrupulous sterilization. Standard length of gut is between 54 and 60 inches. They range in size from a fine 7-0 to a heavy No. 5. These sutures come in plastic or foil inner envelopes and are opened at the time of use. Some absorbable sutures are collagen tape, surgical gut, cargile membrane, kangaroo tendon and fascia lata. Some nonabsorbable sutures are silk, wire, cotton, linen and dermal. Some synthetics are nylon, polyester fiber, polyethylene and polypropylene.

It may be helpful to remember absorbable as "temporary" and nonabsorbable as "permanent."

Surgical Gut. The length of time for complete absorption of surgical gut in a wound varies according to the action of certain hardening agents. Therefore, "plain surgical gut" has not been treated to alter its digestion rate and is absorbed in 5 to 10 days. Chromic gut that has been treated by tanning with chromic salts may have a prolonged absorption time of 10 to 40 days.

Advantages of surgical gut are: (1) it is absorbed eventually, (2) easily handled, (3) comes in a multitude of sizes, and (4) may be used for all tissue beneath the skin.

Fascia Lata. This muscle connective tissue of beef has been used in reconstructive orthopedic surgery and for the repair of hernias. It is not a true absorbable suture, but becomes a part of the tissue after the wound has healed.

EYED NEEDLES

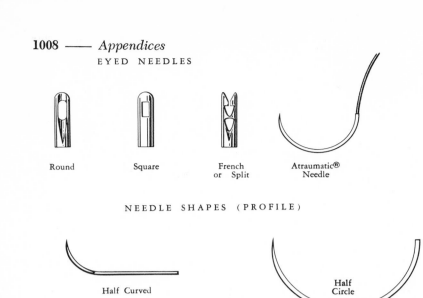

FIG. A-16. Basic needle chart. (American Cyanamid Co., Surgical Products Div., Danbury, Conn.)

Round   Square   French or Split   Atraumatic® Needle

NEEDLE SHAPES (PROFILE)

Half Curved

Half Circle

Straight

Three-eighths Circle

NEEDLE SHAPES (SECTION)

Taper   Cutting   Inverted Cutting   Elliptron*
                                        * Trademark

Nonabsorbable Sutures. Silk. This is prepared from the thread spun by the silkworm larva in making its cocoon. It may be twisted or braided, and it comes in sizes comparable with surgical gut. Its advantages are: (1) high tensile strength, (2) relatively inexpensive, and (3) less tissue reaction than occurs with surgical gut.

Cotton. This is made from cotton fibers. The strands are twisted and used for both internal and external suture. It should always be used wet for maximal strength.

Nylon. Synthetic polyamide available in two forms: monofilament and multifilament (braided). The chief disadvantage is that a triple knot must be tied in the small sizes and a double square knot in the larger sizes.

Wire. This material has maximal flexibility and tensile strength, yet causes little or no local reaction in the tissue in which it is placed.

Dacron. This is a synthetic polyester fiber that has greater tensile strength, minimal tissue reaction, maximal visibility, nonabsorbent and nonfraying qualities.

Linen. This is made of twisted linen thread; it has sufficient tensile strength but is rarely used as suture material.

Silver Wire Clips. Many styles of clips are available for the purpose of holding the edges of tissue in approximation. They tend to produce some scarring when used on the skin, but may be used when the wound is infected.

Silkworm Gut. This is made from the fluid secreted by the silkworm when they are ready to form their cocoons. The disadvantage is that they must be soaked in normal saline for about 10 minutes before use to make them pliable.

Mesh. Stainless steel—used for hernia repairs and large defects. It is rarely used.

Tantalum—a bluish gray metal that is nonirritating to the body tissues. It is used because of its high tensile strength and its inert reaction to tissues.

Teflon and Dacron. These are available in a variety of meshes, fabrics, felts, tapes and sutures. They are used for repair of hernial defects, patch grafts for septal defects, arterial grafts as well as for aortic bifurcated grafts.

Suture Needles

The surgeon's needle must be sharp and made of properly tempered steel so that it is sufficiently malleable not to break easily. Classification of needles may be done in several ways. They may be grouped *according to shape,* such as straight, curved or half-curved (Fig. A-16).

Another classification is *according to the tip* of the needle: cutting-point or taper-point. Cutting needles may be the conventional 3-edged triangular style, reversed cutting edge (an improved design) and trocar (not widely used). These needles may cut into tissue to allow for the easier passage of the suture. This is necessary in suturing dense tissue such as skin, cervix of the uterus and tendon. The taper needle is used for the suturing of such delicate structures as the intestine, brain, mucous membranes and nerves.

A third classification may be *according to the eye* of the needle: ordinary eye, French or split eye and atraumatic or swaged-on needle. The French eye has a slit from the end of the needle to the eye, through which the suture is drawn to thread it. This kind of needle can be threaded more quickly than the ordinary eye needle (Fig. A-17). The atraumatic or swaged-on needle is really an eyeless needle. In the manufacturing process the suture is inserted within the metal of the needle so that the diameter of the suture is not greater than the needle.

Eyeless needles are popular for several reasons: (1) they do not have to be threaded, (2) they produce a minimum of tissue trauma, and (3) there is less damage to the suture strand (Fig. A-17).

Needles also come in various sizes. Different surgeons, with their individual techniques, use different needles. Experience and the wish of the surgeon are the only real guides as to the various uses of needles, although good judgment on the nurse's part is always a valuable asset. Straight needles are generally used without a needle holder, while all curved needles are used with a holder. The jaws of the needle holder should be placed so as to grasp the needle about ⅔ of the distance from the needle tip to the eye end. The clamps of the holder never should come together directly on the eye of the needle. Almost invariably the needle will break if this is done.

Sterilization. Suture needles are arranged in some

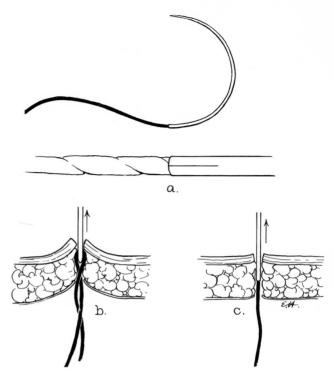

FIG. A-17. Atraumatic needle and suture for intestinal sutures. Needle and suture are of same size, and, when pulled through tissue, suture fills needle hole (c). Ordinary suture and needle (b) for comparison.

definite order on a towel or an anchor-spring needle holder. After use, they are placed in a perforated stainless steel box and washed with the instruments in the instrument-washer-sterilizer. They may be scoured or run through emery powder, washed, rinsed thoroughly and dried.

BIBLIOGRAPHY

Alexander, E. L., Burley, W., Ellison, D., and Valleri, R.: Care of the Patient in Surgery. St. Louis, C. V. Mosby, 1967.

Ginsberg, F., Brunner, L., and Cantlin, V.: A Manual of Operating Room Technology. Philadelphia, J. B. Lippincott, 1966.

Index

Note: **Page numbers in italics refer to figures, tables, graphic and illustrative material.**

1011